Endocrine Surgery Comprehensive Board Exam Guide

Alexander L. Shifrin • Marco Raffaelli
Gregory W. Randolph • Oliver Gimm
Editors

Endocrine Surgery Comprehensive Board Exam Guide

Springer

Editors
Alexander L. Shifrin
Department of Surgery
Jersey Shore University
Medical Center
Neptune, NJ, USA

Gregory W. Randolph
The Claire and John Bertucci
Endowed Chair in Thyroid
Surgical Oncology
Harvard Medical School
Boston, MA, USA

Marco Raffaelli
Division of Endocrine and
Metabolic Surgery, Fondazione
Policlinico Universitario
Agostino Gemelli IRCCS
Università Cattolica del
Sacro Cuore
Rome, Italy

Oliver Gimm
Department of Surgery
Linköping University
Linköping, Sweden

ISBN 978-3-030-84736-4 ISBN 978-3-030-84737-1 (eBook)
https://doi.org/10.1007/978-3-030-84737-1

This Springer imprint is published by the registered company Springer Nature Switzerland AG
The registered company address is: Gewerbestrasse 11, 6330 Cham, Switzerland

To everyone involved in the surgical care of patients with endocrine gland diseases; to all endocrine, head and neck, otolaryngology, oncological, and general surgeons devoting their lives to cure patients with endocrine diseases; to those surgeons who are looking to obtain the highest level of certification in endocrine surgery; to our families, loved ones, and our children, supporting us and patiently waiting for us to complete this book; to our teachers, who taught us the science of medicine and surgery; and to all of our patients that we had the pleasure of taking care, we learned from them and presented some of their cases in this book.

Preface

> To study the phenomena of disease without books is to sail an uncharted sea, while to study books without patients is not to go to sea at all. – William Osler

Every surgical subspecialty has been rapidly developing with the establishment of board certification. The Division of Endocrine Surgery (DES) of the European Board of Surgery has defined the curriculum for endocrine surgery to include thyroid, parathyroid, and adrenal and GEP-NET surgery, and handles accreditation in endocrine surgery. The first examinations in endocrine surgery in Europe were introduced in 2003. The main goal of these exams is to maintain a uniform and high standard of endocrine surgical professionalism across Europe.

This important book project, *Endocrine Surgery Comprehensive Board Exam Guide*, was completed with the expectation that it would benefit all European surgeons looking to be certified in endocrine surgery; additionally, surgeons from the United States and other non-EU countries will also benefit from this book when the Endocrine Surgery Board Exam is introduced in the United States or other non-EU countries.

Collaboratively publishing the first Endocrine Surgery Board Exam preparation manuscript, *Endocrine Surgery Comprehensive Board Exam Guide*, was a detailed process involving collaborative efforts of world leaders in endocrine surgery and the co-editors: Alexander L. Shifrin, MD, Director of Endocrine Oncology at Hackensack Meridian Health of Monmouth and Ocean Counties of New Jersey; Langenbeck's Archives of Surgery Journal, Guest Editor, Endocrine Surgery Section. Marco Raffaelli, MD, the Chairman of the Board of the Division of Endocrine Surgery (DES) of the European Union of Medical Specialists (UEMS); Gregory W. Randolph, MD, President of the American Academy of Otolaryngology Head and Neck Surgery 2016–2017; and Oliver Gimm, MD, the Chairman of the DES.

The book contains knowledge that is expected to be known for the board examination of the DES. In general, chapters start with a patient's case followed by questions. The subsequent comprehensive yet concise main text provides all the information needed and cites important references. The chapters end with the answers to questions. Each chapter is authored by experts in the field of endocrine surgery. Each chapter is written by a DES-certified endocrine surgeon, and some chapters are co-authored with US endocrine or otolaryngology head and neck surgeons.

We hope that this book will be the main source of preparation for the endocrine surgery examination and will bring endocrine surgery to a higher level of expertise by helping to raise the standard of training for future endocrine surgeons.

Alexander L. Shifrin — Neptune, NJ, USA
Marco Raffaelli — Rome, Italy
Gregory W. Randolph — Boston, MA, USA
Oliver Gimm — Linköping, Sweden

Acknowledgments

The creation of this textbook, covering the entire scope of endocrine surgery, was dependent on team effort, which was possible only with the support and enthusiasm of the many individuals who contributed to this book, and our colleagues who trusted us and dedicated their time and effort to make it happen, without whom this book would have never come to life!

Special thanks to the Executive Editor Richard Hruska, who believed in us, and Senior Editor Lee Klein of Springer, for his hard work and dedication.

Finally, we would like to thank the entire staff at Springer, who was very supportive from the first idea of this atlas and maintained their enthusiasm until the end.

Contents

II Parathyroid

III Adrenals

Contributors

Orhan Agcaoglu Department of General Surgery, School of Medicine, Koc University Hospital, Istanbul, Turkey
oagcaoglu@ku.edu.tr

Martin Almquist Lund University, Skåne University Hospital, Department of Clinical Sciences Lund, Departments of Surgery Section of Endocrine and Sarcoma Lund, Lund, Sweden
martin.almquist@med.lu.se

Peter Angelos MacLean Center for Clinical Medical Ethics, University of Chicago, Chicago, IL, USA
pangelos@surgery.bsd.uchicago.edu

Megan K. Applewhite Ethics Education and Research, Albany Medical College, Albany, NY, USA
applewm@amc.edu

Marcin Barczyński Department of Endocrine Surgery, Third Chair of General Surgery, Jagiellonian University – Medical College, Kraków, Poland

Clinical Ward of Surgery and Oncology, Gabriel Narutowicz Memorial Municipal Hospital, Kraków, Poland
marcin.barczynski@uj.edu.pl

Benoît Bédat Division of Thoracic and Endocrine Surgery, University Hospitals of Geneva, Geneva, Switzerland
Benoit.bedat@hcuge.ch

Rocco Bellantone Department Center of Endocrine and Obesity Surgery, Fondazione Policlinico Universitario Agostino Gemelli IRCCS – Università Cattolica del Sacro Cuore, Rome, Italy
rocco.bellantone@unicatt.it

Iuliana D. Bobanga Case Western Reserve University School of Medicine, University Hospitals Portage Medical Center, Ravenna, OH, USA
Iuliana.Bobanga@UHhospitals.org

Robert Bränström Endocrine and Sarcoma Surgery Unit, Department of Molecular Medicine and Surgery, Karolinska Institutet, Karolinska University Hospital, Stockholm, Sweden
robert.branstrom@ki.se

Talia Burneikis Case Western Reserve University, School of Medicine and Lerner College of Medicine, Cleveland Clinic Foundation, Cleveland, OH, USA
burneit@ccf.org

Denise Carneiro-Pla Division of Oncologic and Endocrine Surgery, Medical University of South Carolina, Charleston, SC, USA
Carneiro@musc.edu

Amy Y. Chen Willard and Lillian Hackerman Professor of Otolaryngology Head and Neck Surgery, Emory University School of Medicine, Atlanta, GA, USA
achen@emory.edu

Janet Chiang Division of Endocrinology, Department of Medicine, University of California, San Francisco, CA, USA

Zuckerberg San Francisco General Hospital, San Francisco VA Medical Center, San Francisco, CA, USA
Janet.Chiang@ucsf.edu

Thomas Clerici Head Endocrine Surgery, Kantonsspital St. Gallen, St. Gallen, Switzerland
thomas.clerici@kssg.ch

Louise Davies Otolaryngology – Head & Neck Surgery, Geisel School of Medicine, Hanover, NH, USA
Louise.Davies@Daratmouth.edu

Carmela De Crea Division of Endocrine and Metabolic Surgery, Fondazione Policlinico Universitario Agostino Gemelli IRCCS – Università Cattolica del Sacro Cuore, Rome, Italy
carmela.decrea@unicatt.it

Mechteld C. de Jong Department of Endocrine Surgery, Churchill Cancer Centre, Oxford University Hospitals NHS Foundation Trust, Oxford, UK
Mechteld.dejong@ouh.nhs.uk

Gerard Doherty Surgery, Harvard Medical School, Boston, MA, USA
gmdoherty@bwh.harvard.edu

Cornelia Dotzenrath Helios University Wuppertal, Department of Endocrine Surgery, Wuppertal, Germany
cornelia.dotzenrath@helios-gesundheit.de

Quan-Yang Duh Department of Surgery, University of California, San Francisco, CA, USA

Surgical Service, Veterans Health Administration Medical Center, San Francisco, CA, USA
quan-yang.duh@ucsf.edu

Caitlin Egan Department of Surgery, New York Presbyterian Hospital and Weill Medical College of Cornell University, New York, NY, USA
cee9007@med.cornell.edu

Anton F. Engelsman Department of Surgery, Amsterdam UMC, Amsterdam, The Netherlands

Amsterdam Center for Endocrine and Neuroendocrine Tumors, Amsterdam, The Netherlands
a.f.engelsman@amsterdamumc.nl

Thomas J. Fahey III Department of Surgery, New York Presbyterian Hospital and Weill Medical College of Cornell University, New York, NY, USA
tjfahey@med.cornell.edu

Alexandra Gangi Gastrointestinal Tumor Program, Cedars Sinai Medical Center, Los Angeles, CA, USA
alexandra.gangi@cshs.org

Oliver Gimm Department of Surgery and Department of Biomedical and Clinical Sciences, Linköping University, Linköping, Sweden
oliver.gimm@liu.se

Andrea Goldmann Head Endocrine Surgery, Kantonsspital Winterthur, Winterthur, Switzerland
andrea.goldmann@ksw.ch

Joaquin Gómez-Ramírez Current National Delegate of the Spanish Society of Endocrine Surgeons, Madrid, Spain

Universidad Alcalá de Henares, Madrid, Madrid, Spain

Hospital Ramón y Cajal, Madrid, Madrid, Spain

Jacques Greenberg Department of Surgery, New York Presbyterian Hospital and Weill Medical College of Cornell University, New York, NY, USA
jag9178@med.cornell.edu

Per Hellman Department of Surgery, University Hospital, Uppsala, Sweden
per.hellman@surgsci.uu.se

Miguel F. Herrera National Institute of Medical Science and Nutrition Salvador Zubirán, Mexico City, Mexico

National Autonomous University of Mexico, Mexico City, Mexico

James R. Howe University of Iowa Carver College of Medicine, University of Iowa Hospitals and Clinics, Iowa City, IA, USA
james-howe@uiowa.edu

Johnathan G. Hubbard Endocrine Surgery, Guys and St Thomas' Hospitals London, London, UK
johnathan.hubbard@gstt.nhs.uk

Maurizio Iacobone Endocrine Surgery Unit, Department of Surgery, Oncology and Gastroenterology, University of Padua, Padua, Italy
maurizio.iacobone@unipd.it

A. Micheil Innes Departments of Medical Genetics, Cumming School of Medicine, University of Calgary, Calgary, AB, Canada
Micheil.Innes@albertahealthservices.ca

Reto M. Kaderli Department of Visceral Surgery and Medicine, Inselspital, Bern University Hospital, Bern, Switzerland
Reto.kaderli@insel.ch

Shahab Khan Department of Endocrine Surgery, Churchill Cancer Centre, Oxford University Hospitals NHS Foundation Trust, Oxford, UK
Shahab.Khan@ouh.nhs.uk

Roswitha Koeberle-Wuehrer Division of Endocrine Surgery, Department of Surgery, Kantonsspital Baselland, Liestal, Switzerland
roswitha.koeberle-wuehrer@ksbl.ch

Ioannis Koutelidakis Department of Surgery, "G. Gennimatas" Hospital of Thessaloniki Medical School, Aristoteleio University of Thessaloniki, Thessaloniki, Greece

Alexander A. Leung Departments of Medicine, Sections of Endocrinology and Metabolism, Cumming School of Medicine, University of Calgary, Calgary, AB, Canada
aacleung@ucalgary.ca

Leyre Lorente-Poch Universitat Autònoma de Barcelona, Barcelona, Spain

Hospital del Mar, Barcelona, Barcelona, Spain

Kerstin Lorenz Department of Visceral, Vascular and Endocrine Surgery, Martin-Luther University of Halle-Wittenberg, Halle, Germany
kerstin.lorenz@uk-halle.de

Özer Makay Department of General Surgery, School of Medicine, Ege University Hospital, Izmir, Turkey

Department of Surgery, Ege University, Izmir, Turkey
ozer.makay@ege.edu.tr

Cristina Martínez-Santos Endocrine Surgery Unit, Department of General Surgery, Hospital Costa del Sol, Marbella, Spain

Christopher R. McHenry Case Western Reserve University School of Medicine, Cleveland, OH, USA

Department of Surgery, MetroHealth Medical Center, Cleveland, OH, USA
cmchenry@metrohelth.org

Radu Mihai Department of Endocrine Surgery, Churchill Cancer Centre, Oxford, UK
Radu.Mihai@ouh.nhs.uk

Kelly F. Moyer Department of Otorhinolaryngology, University of Maryland School of Medicine, Baltimore, MD, USA
kmoyer@som.umaryland.edu

Thomas J. Musholt Department of General, Visceral and Transplant Surgery, University Medicine of the Johannes Gutenberg-University, Mainz, Germany
musholt@uni-mainz.de

Bruno Niederle Division of General Surgery, Department of Surgery, Medical University of Vienna, Vienna, Austria
bruno.niederle@meduniwien.ac.at

Martin B. Niederle Division of General Surgery, Department of Surgery, Medical University of Vienna, Vienna, Austria

General Intensive Care and Pain Management Section, Department of General Anesthesia, Medical University of Vienna, Vienna, Austria
martin.niederle@meduniwien.ac.at

Els J. M. Nieveen van Dijkum Department of Surgery, Amsterdam UMC, Amsterdam, The Netherlands

Amsterdam Center for Endocrine and Neuroendocrine Tumors, Amsterdam, The Netherlands
e.j.nieveenvandijkum@amsterdamumc.nl

Inga-Lena Nilsson Department of Molecular Medicine and Surgery, Endocrine Tumors and Sarcoma Unit, Karolinska Institutet, Karolinska University Hospital, Stockholm, Sweden
inga-lena.nilsson@ki.se

Iain Nixon NHS Lothian, Edinburgh, Scotland, UK

Edinburgh University, Edinburgh, Scotland, UK

Vicky Parkins Departments of Medicine, Sections of Endocrinology and Metabolism, Cumming School of Medicine, University of Calgary, Calgary, AB, Canada
Vicky.Parkins@albertahealthservices.ca

Janice L. Pasieka Departments of Medicine, Sections of Endocrinology and Metabolism, Cumming School of Medicine, University of Calgary, Calgary, AB, Canada

Departments of Surgery, General Surgery and Surgical Oncology, Cumming School of Medicine, North Tower Foothills Medical Center, University of Calgary, Calgary, AB, Canada
janice.pasieka@ahs.ca

Natalia S. Pellegata Division Neuroendocrinology, Institute for Diabetes and Cancer, Helmholtz Center Munich, Neuherberg, Germany
natalia.pellegata@helmholtz-muenchen.de

Rafael H. Pérez-Soto National Institute of Medical Science and Nutrition Salvador Zubirán, Mexico City, Mexico

Nancy D. Perrier Section of Surgical Endocrinology, Multidisciplinary Endocrine Center, and Fellowship Program of Surgical Endocrinology, Department of Surgical Oncology, The University of Texas MD Anderson Cancer Center, Houston, TX, USA
nperrier@mdanderson.org

Pietro Princi UOC Chirurgia Endocrina e Metabolica, Fondazione Policlinico Universitario Agostino Gemelli – IRCCS, Rome, Italy
pietro.princi@policlinicogemelli.it

Marco Raffaelli Division of Endocrine and Metabolic Surgery, Fondazione Policlinico Universitario Agostino Gemelli IRCCS, Università Cattolica del Sacro Cuore, Rome, Italy
marco.raffaelli@unicatt.it

Gregory W. Randolph Division of Thyroid and Parathyroid Surgery, Department of Otolaryngology, Massachusetts Eye and Ear, Harvard Medical School, Boston, MA, USA

Division of Surgical Oncology, Endocrine Surgery Service, Department of Surgery, Massachusetts General Hospital, Harvard Medical School, Boston, MA, USA
Gregory_randolph@meei.harvard.edu

Marika D. Russell Head and Neck Surgery, Division of Head and Neck Oncologic and Endocrine Surgery, University of California, San Francisco, San Francisco, CA, USA

Head and Neck Surgery, Zuckerberg San Francisco General Hospital, San Francisco, CA, USA
Marika.Russell@ucsf.edu

Samira Mercedes Sadowski Surgical Oncology Program, Endocrine Surgery Section, National Cancer Institute, NIH, Bethesda, MD, USA
Samira.sadowski@nih.gov

David M. Scott-Coombes University Hospital of Wales, Cardiff, UK
david.scott-coombes@wales.nhs.uk

Frederic Sebag Endocrine, Metabolic and General Surgery, La Conception University Hospital, Aix-Marseille University, Marseilles, France
Frederic.SEBAG@ap-hm.fr

Ashok R. Shaha Memorial Sloan Kettering Cancer Center, New York, NY, USA
shaha@mskcc.org

Wen T. Shen University of California, San Francisco, Endocrine Surgery Section, San Francisco, CA, USA
Wen.shen2@ucsf.edu

Alexander L. Shifrin Department of Surgery, Jersey Shore University Medical Center, Neptune, NJ, USA

Sami Shoucair Department of Surgery, The Johns Hopkins University School of Medicine, Baltimore, MD, USA
sshouca1@jh.edu

Angelica Silva-Figueroa Universidad Finis Terrae Medical School, Santiago, Chile

Department of Head and Neck Surgery at Hospital Barros Luco-Trudeau and Clinic Redsalud Avansalud, Santiago, Chile
angelica.silva@uft.cl

Dietmar Simon Department of General, Visceral and Endocrine Surgery, Specific Genetic Counseling, Fellow of the European Board of Surgery (FEBS) – Endocrine Surgery, Ev. Krankenhaus BETHESDA Duisburg, Academic Teaching Hospital HHU Duesseldorf, Duisburg, Germany
chirurgie@bethesda.de
d.simon@bethesda.de

Catherine F. Sinclair Department of Otolaryngology, Icahn School of Medicine at Mount Sinai, New York, NY, USA

Division of Head and Neck Surgery, Mount Sinai West Hospital, New York, NY, USA
casinclair@chpnet.org

Allan E. Siperstein Case Western Reserve University, School of Medicine and Lerner College of Medicine, Cleveland Clinic Foundation, Cleveland, OH, USA
sipersa@ccf.org

Cristian M. Slough Hawke's Bay Fallen Soldiers Memorial Hospital, Hastings, New Zealand

Carmen C. Solórzano Department of Surgery, Vanderbilt University, Nashville, TN, USA
carmen.solorzano@vumc.org

Julie Ann Sosa University of California, San Francisco, Endocrine Surgery Section, San Francisco, CA, USA
Julie.sosa@ucsf.edu

Michael J. Stechman Department of Endocrine Surgery, University Hospital of Wales, Cardiff, UK
michael.stechman@wales.nhs.uk

Serkan Teksöz Istanbul University-Cerrahpaşa, Cerrahpaşa Medical Faculty, Department of General Surgery, Division of Endocrine Surgery, Fatih/İstanbul, Turkey

David J. Terris Augusta University Thyroid and Parathyroid Center, Augusta University, Augusta, Georgia
dterris@augusta.edu

Francesca Torresan Endocrine Surgery Unit, Department of Surgery, Oncology and Gastroenterology, University of Padua, Padua, Italy
francesca.torresan@unipd.it

Frédéric Triponez Division of Thoracic and Endocrine Surgery, University Hospitals of Geneva, Geneva, Switzerland
Frederic.triponez@hcuge.ch

Alicia M. Trolle-Silva National Institute of Medical Science and Nutrition Salvador Zubirán, Mexico City, Mexico

Kyriakos Vamvakidis Department of Endocrine Surgery, "Henry Dunant" Hospital Center, Athens, Greece
info@drvamvakidis.gr

Klaas Van Den Heede Selwyn Taylor Senior Clinical Fellow Endocrine Surgery, Imperial College Healthcare NHS Trust, Hammersmith Hospital, London, UK
klaas.vandenheede@nhs.net

Paulien van Galen Departments of Medical Genetics, Cumming School of Medicine, University of Calgary, Calgary, AB, Canada
Paulien.VanGalen@albertahealthservices.ca

Sam Van Slycke General and Endocrine Surgery, OLV Clinic Aalst, Aalst, Belgium
sam.van.slycke@olvz-aalst.be

Elisabeth-Ann Vandenwyngaerden Ghent University, Ghent, Belgium
elisabethann.vandenwyngaerden@ugent.be

Jesús M. Villar-del-Moral Department of General, Digestive and Transplant Surgery, Division of Endocrine Surgery, Hospital Universitario Virgen de las Nieves, Granada, Spain
jesusm.villar.sspa@juntadeandalucia.es

Jiping Wang Surgery, Brigham and Women's Hospital, Harvard Medical School, Boston, MA, USA
jwang39@bwh.harvard.edu

Christopher Wolfgang Departments of Surgery, Oncology, and Pathology, The Pancreatic Cancer Precision Medicine Center of Excellence, The Sidney Kimmel Cancer Center at Johns Hopkins, The Johns Hopkins University School of Medicine, Baltimore, MD, USA
cwolfga2@jhmi.edu

Richard J. Wong Head and Neck Service, Memorial Sloan Kettering Cancer Center, New York, NY, USA
wongr@mskcc.org

William F. Young Jr. Division of Endocrinology, Diabetes, Metabolism and Nutrition, Mayo Clinic, Rochester, MN, USA
young.william@mayo.edu

Abbreviations

CCH	C-cell hyperplasia
CLA	Cutaneous lichen amyloidosis
FMTC	Familial medullary thyroid cancer
HD	Hirschsprung's disease
MEN	Multiple endocrine neoplasia
MTC	Medullary thyroid cancer
PCC	Pheochromocytoma
PHPT	Primary hyperparathyroidism
RET	Rearranged during transfection

Thyroid

Contents

Thyroid Gland: Anatomy, Physiology, Pathophysiology, and Ultrasonography

Cristian M. Slough and Gregory W. Randolph

Contents

A. L. Shifrin et al. (eds.), *Endocrine Surgery Comprehensive Board Exam Guide*,
https://doi.org/10.1007/978-3-030-84737-1_1

Case Presentation:

A 57-year-old woman presents to her provider with complaints of fatigue, low mood, weight gain, and constipation. She reports that her weight has gradually increased over the past 18 months despite no change in her activity level or eating habits. She works full time as a lab tech, and finds herself more distracted at work than normal and intermittent dozes off in front of the computer during downtimes. She has found this unsettling.

She feels her mood is down, and she lacks motivation to do anything during the weekend. Upon questioning, the patitent reports the following changes: thinning of her scalp hair and cold intolerance. Physical examination confirms dry skin, and coarse and dry hair. The only medication she takes is a multivitamin daily. She has a positive family history for autoimmune disorders and thyroid cancer.

Questions

1. What are criteria to establish the diagnosis of overt hypothyroidism?
   1. A TSH level above the reference range
   2. A free T4 concentration below the reference range
   3. Elevated antithyroglobulin autoantibodies
   4. Thyroglobulin levels that are undetectable
   5. A total serum T4 below the reference range
      (a) Only (1) and (2) and (5) are correct.
      (b) Only (3) and (5) are correct.
      (c) Only (1) and (2) are correct.
      (d) Only (2) and (4) and (5) are correct.
      (e) All are correct.
2. What are criteria to establish the diagnosis of subclinical hypothyroidism?
   1. A TSH level above the reference range
   2. A total T4 concentration below the reference range
   3. Elevated antithyroglobulin autoantibodies
   4. Thyroglobulin levels that are undetectable
   5. A free T4 concentration within the reference range
      (a) Only (1) and (2) and (5) are correct.
      (b) Only (1) and (5) are correct.
      (c) Only (1) and (2) are correct.
      (d) Only (2) and (4) and (5) are correct.
      (e) All are correct.
3. What are the critical components of thyroid hormone synthesis?
   1. Dietary iodine
   2. The Na/I symporter located on the basolateral membrane
   3. Activation of adenylyl cyclase by TSH
   4. Enzymatic reactions mediated by thyroperoxidase
   5. The presence of thyroid globulin in the colloid
      (a) Only (1) and (2) and (5) are correct.
      (b) Only (1) and (5) are correct.

   (c) Only (1) and (2) are correct.
   (d) Only (2) and (4) and (5) are correct.
   (e) All are correct.

4. Once intravascularly, the vast majority of the thyroid hormones are bound to binding hormones with only 0.03% of total serum T4 and 0.3% of total serum T3 found in unbound forms. What are the most common hormone-binding proteins?
   1. Thyroglobulin
   2. Human serum albumin
   3. Thyroxine-binding hormone
   4. Thyroperoxidase
   5. Transthyretin
      (a) Only (1) and (2) and (5) are correct.
      (b) Only (1) and (5) are correct.
      (c) Only (1) and (2) are correct.
      (d) Only (2) and (3) and (5) are correct.
      (e) All are correct.
5. Several disease states and medications can alter the activity of deiodinase (DIO) enzymes. Which of the following statements are true?
   1. Deiodinase (DIO) enzymes can enhance the signaling and activation of T4 and T3.
   2. Deiodinase (DIO) enzymes can diminish the signaling and activation of T4 and T3.
   3. The signaling and activation of T4 and T3 is regulated by cell-specific iodothyronine (DIO) enzymes.
   4. T4 also exerts its action through ion flux regulation.
   5. T3 binds to thyroid hormone nuclear receptors, modulating gene expression and altering cellular function.
      (a) Only (1) and (2) and (5) are correct.
      (b) Only (1) and (5) are correct.
      (c) Only (1) and (2) are correct.
      (d) Only (2) and (3) and (5) are correct.
      (e) All are correct.
6. The hypothalamic-pituitary-thyroid axis is responsible for thyroid hormone regulation. Which of the following statements are correct?
   1. The major regulator of thyroid hormone production and secretion is synthesized and secreted by the thyrotroph cells of the anterior pituitary.
   2. Exposure to the thyrotrophs by circulating T4 and T3 stimulates the secretion of TSH and TRH.
   3. TSH secretion is pulsatile in nature.
   4. TSH secretion is affected by glucocorticoids, retinoids, somatostatin, and dopamine.
   5. TRH is not affected by glucocorticoids, retinoids, somatostatin, and dopamine.
      (a) Only (1) and (3) and (4) are correct.
      (b) Only (1) and (5) are correct.

(c) Only (1) and (2) are correct.
(d) Only (2) and (3) and (5) are correct.
(e) All are correct.

7. A TSH and free T4 panel is a preferred strategy for diagnosing thyroid dysfunction in ambulatory patients with which of the following conditions?
    1. Patients where central hypothyroidism is suspected
    2. Hashimoto's thyroiditis
    3. TSH-secreting pituitary tumor
    4. As a screening tool for thyroid dysfunction
    5. Patients suspected of having a subclinical hypothyroidism
        (a) Only (1) and (3) and (5) are correct.
        (b) Only (1) and (5) are correct.
        (c) Only (1) and (2) are correct.
        (d) Only (2) and (3) and (5) are correct.
        (e) All are correct.
8. Thyroglobulin assessment is particularly useful in the following scenarios.
    1. Presence of thyroglobulin antibodies
    2. Hashimoto's thyroiditis
    3. Surveillance following treatment for well-differentiated thyroid cancer
    4. Presence of interfering heterophile antibodies
    5. A circumstance of suspected excessive exogenous ingestion
        (a) Only (1) and (3) and (5) are correct.
        (b) Only (3) and (5) are correct.
        (c) Only (2) and (3) are correct.
        (d) Only (1) and (3) and (4) are correct.
        (e) All are correct.
9. The signs and symptoms of hypothyroidism include all of the following?
    1. Weight gain
    2. Impaired concentration
    3. Infertility
    4. Muscle cramps
    5. Cold intolerance
        (a) Only (1) and (3) and (5) are correct.
        (b) Only (3) and (5) are correct.
        (c) Only (2) and (3) are correct.
        (d) Only (1) and (3) and (4) are correct.
        (e) All are correct.
10. Ultrasonography (US) of the thyroid and neck has the following advantages?
    1. Provides great detail of the gland
    2. Allows real-time assessment of tissue mobility
    3. Assessment of cervical lymph node status
    4. Good screening tool for asymptomatic patients.
    5. Works well for the assessment of substernal extension of the thyroid

(a) Only (1) and (2) and (3) are correct.
(b) Only (3) and (5) are correct.
(c) Only (2) and (3) are correct.
(d) Only (1) and (2) and (4) are correct.
(e) All are correct.

11. There are distinctive ultrasonographic characteristics of thyroid malignancy that can be identified on US. Which of the following are these?
    1. Nodular echogenicity
    2. Irregular or blurred margins
    3. Microcalcifications
    4. Taller than wider shape
    5. Intranodular blood flow
       (a) Only (1) and (2) and (3) are correct.
       (b) Only (3) and (5) are correct.
       (c) Only (2) and (3) are correct.
       (d) Only (1) and (2) and (4) are correct.
       (e) All are correct.

1.1 Thyroid Physiology

1.1.1 Thyroid Cellular Physiology

The reason iodine is an essential human nutrient is due to its intrinsic role in the synthesis of two thyroid hormones, namely, triiodothyronine (T3) and tetraiodothyronine (T4 or thyroxine). The crucial first step for thyroid hormone biosynthesis is the active transport of iodine (I-) into the thyroid follicular cells. This is mediated by the Na/I symporter (NIS), an integral plasma membrane glycoprotein located on the basolateral membrane of the thyroid follicular cell [1]. The functional units of the thyroid are follicular structures that are formed by the thyroid epithelial cells orienting in a basal and apical direction. The apical membrane is adjacent to the follicular lumen, which is filled with colloid, and the basolateral membrane is in contact with capillaries and the circulatory system (◘ Fig. 1.1).

The proximity of the basolateral membrane to the circulatory system allows the thyroid-stimulating hormone (TSH) receptor to be activated by TSH, initiating the cascade of thyroid hormone synthesis and secretion. Upon binding of TSH to its receptor, there is activation of adenylyl cyclase with a subsequent increase in cyclic adenosine monophosphate (cAMP) formation, leading to phosphorylation of protein kinase A and to activation of targets in the cytosol and the nucleus of the thyroid cell [2]. Through this cAMP pathway, TSH stimulates the accumulation of iodide in the thyroid [3]. Consequently, the ability of the thyroid to accumulate iodide intracellularly has provided the basis for diagnostic scintigraphic imaging of the thyroid and served as an effective means for therapeutic doses of radioiodide to target and destroy hyperfunctioning

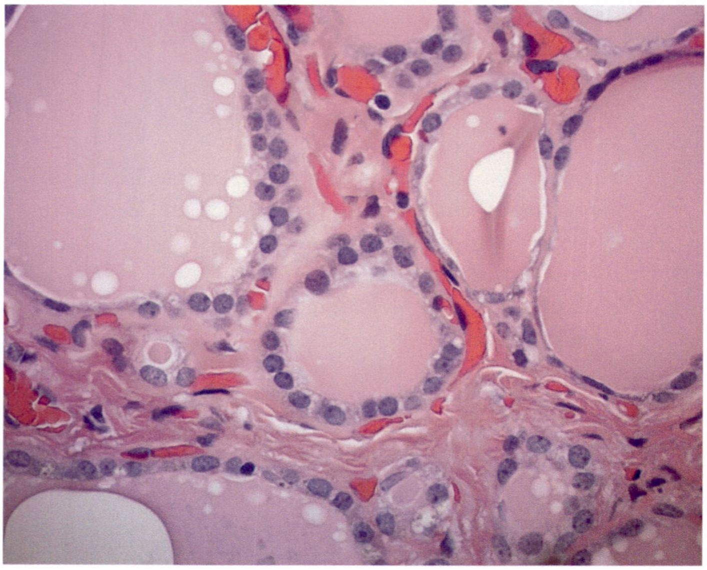

Fig. 1.1 Thyroid Follicles: The functional units of the thyroid are follicular structures that are formed by the thyroid epithelial cells orienting in a basal and apical direction. The apical membrane is adjacent to the follicular lumen, which is filled with colloid, and the basolateral membrane is in contact with capillaries and the circulatory system

thyroid tissue as well as differentiated malignant thyroid cells. The intracellularly accumulated iodide ion is then passively translocated across the apical membrane into the colloid via pendrin proteins and Cl- channels [4]. The effluxed iodide ion then becomes covalently attached to thyroglobulin, at the interface of the apical membrane and the follicular lumen, through an enzymatic reaction mediated by thyroperoxidase (TPO) [5]. Further iodinization (organification) of tyrosine molecules on the thyroglobulin glycoprotein then occurs via TPO facilitating the further incorporation of iodide onto the tyrosine residues. This process forms monoiodotyrosines (MITs) and diiodotyrosines (DITs), which are then coupled to create the bioactive thyroid hormones T4 and T3 again catalyzed via TPO [2]. It should be noted that this process of oxidation of iodide, organification, and coupling is dependent on the presence of hydrogen peroxide present intralumenally and truly occurs simultaneously. The formed thyroid hormones attached to thyroglobulin are then stored in the follicular lumen in the form of colloid. The majority of thyroid hormone stored in the colloid comes in the form of T4 versus T3 [5]. In response to demand for thyroid hormone, which requires further processing intracellularly, stimulation by TSH of its receptor commences the uptake of colloid into the follicular cell by micropinocytosis and subsequent vesicular internalization. These vesicles then fuse with lysosomes intracellularly. Through digestion of this thyroglobulin by lysosomal extracts and a resulting proteolytic breakdown of the thyroglobulin, T4 and T3 are released into

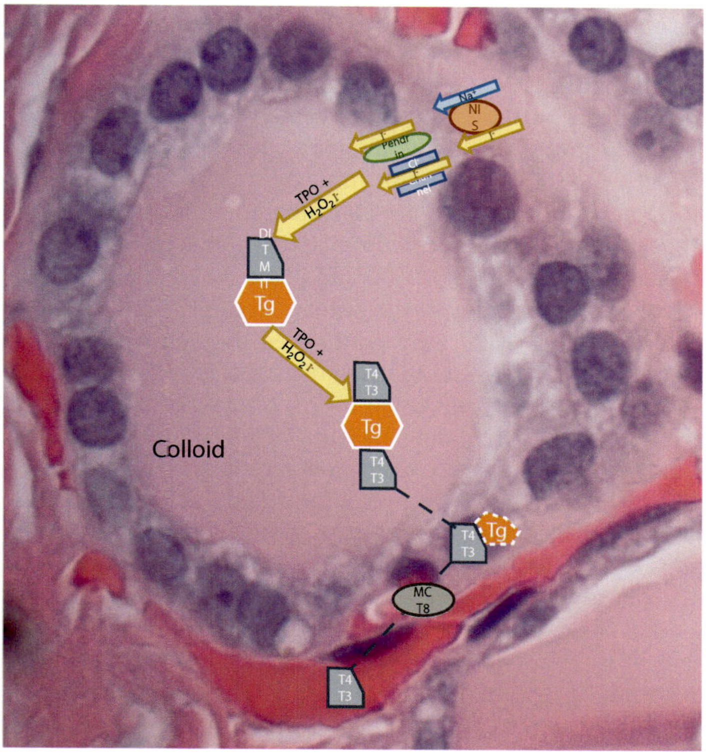

Fig. 1.2 Schematic of Thyroid Hormone Synthesis. Active transport of iodine (I-) into the thyroid follicular cells is mediated by the Na/I symporter (NIS). Intracellular accumulated iodide ion is then passively translocated across the apical membrane into the colloid via pendrin proteins and Cl- channels. The effluxed iodide ion becomes covalently attached to thyroglobulin mediated by thyroperoxidase (TPO). Further iodinization of tyrosine molecules on the thyroglobulin glycoprotein then occurs via TPO forming monoiodotyrosines (MIT) and diiodotyrosines (DIT) which are then coupled to create the bioactive thyroid hormones T4 and T3 again catalyzed via TPO. Colloid is taken up into the follicular cell by micropinocytosis Through digestion of this thyroglobulin by lysosomal extracts and a resulting proteolytic breakdown of the thyroglobulin, T4 and T3 are released into the cytoplasm. Finally T4 and T3 are transported into the circulation by a hormone transporter (monocarboxylate transporter 8 (MCT8))

the cytoplasm [6]. Finally, through a process likely involving the thyroid hormone transporter (monocarboxylate transporter 8 (MCT8)) expressed on the basolateral membrane of the thyroid cell, T4 and T3 are transported into the circulation (Fig. 1.2) [7].

Once intravascularly the vast majority of the thyroid hormones are bound to binding hormones with only 0.03% of total serum T4 and 0.3% of total serum T3 found in unbound forms [8]. The three major binding carriers of thyroid hormone are thyroxine-binding hormone (TBG), transthyretin (TTR), and albumin (HSA), while some minor carriers have also been identified [9]. Of the binding proteins, TBG binds approximately 75% of both T4 and T3 in circulation, while TTR binds approximately 20% of the circulating T4 and <5%

of T3; conversely, HSA binds 5% of the T4 and 20% of the T3 [8]. The physiological significance of this is that bound thyroid hormone is biologically inactive, while "free" T4 and T3 are biologically active and able to enter almost all target cells through transporters in the plasma membrane such as MCT8 [10]. An additional attribute of the extensive binding of thyroid hormone is a resulting long half-life and circulatory concentration [11]. Thyroid hormone receptors on target cells have a higher affinity to T3 than T4, binding for a greater duration and therefore regarded as the primary active thyroid hormone [5]. While T4 is exclusively synthesized by the thyroid gland, only 20% of T3 is produced in the thyroid cell, with the remaining majority being produced at the peripheral tissue level by the deiodination of circulating T4 [10]. Thyroid hormones exert a biological effect at the cellular level via the binding of free T3 to thyroid hormone nuclear receptors, modulating gene expression and altering cellular function. The signaling and activation of T4 and T3 is regulated by cell-specific iodothyronine deiodinase (DIO) enzymes, which can enhance or diminish the thyroid hormone effect once they are intracellular [10]. The clinical significance of this is that several disease states and medications can alter the activity of DIO enzymes [5]. Among the intracellular actions of thyroid hormone at the genomic level, T4 also exerts its action through ion flux regulation, resulting in actions and mechanisms with important effects of the hormone on brain function [12].

1.2 Hypothalamic-Pituitary-Thyroid Axis

A full appreciation of thyroid function and its testing is dependent on a thorough understanding of its axis of regulation. TSH, the major regulator of thyroid hormone production and secretion, is synthesized and secreted by the thyrotroph cells of the anterior pituitary. The main stimulator of TSH production by the anterior pituitary is thyrotropin-releasing hormone (TRH) via the hypothalamic-pituitary portal system [2]. Conversely, exposure to the thyrotrophs by circulating T4 and T3 inhibits the secretion of TSH and TRH via a negative feedback loop, decreasing gene expression of these hormones and therefore its activity. As with other pituitary hormones, TSH secretion is pulsatile in nature, with higher levels seen at night than during the day; however, despite this diurnal variation, serum TSH concentrations generally remain in the reference range when drawn during the day but may be elevated if drawn at night [13]. Among TRH and thyroid hormone itself, TSH secretion is also affected by glucocorticoids, retinoids, somatostatin, and dopamine [2]. Consequently, several disease states and medications can affect TSH levels such as pituitary or hypothalamic dysfunction, recent hyperthyroidism, critical illness, starvation, use of certain medications, interference with serum thyroid autoantibodies, and thyroid hormone resistance syndromes [14]. Given this, thyroid physiology can be affected in nonthyroidal illness (euthyroid sick syndrome) and it is important that the diagnosis of primary thyroid dysfunction not be established during severe illness based solely on an abnormal serum TSH. In these conditions, serum TSH concentrations may be low, normal, or high, due to the TSH-lowering effects of medications or from an acquired central hypothyroidism and therefore, when possible, assessment of thyroid function should be done after recovery from an acute illness [5].

1.3 Thyroid Function Testing

1.3.1 Serum TSH

The main diagnostic strategy for detecting euthyroidism, hypothyroidism, and hyperthyroidism is the measurement of serum TSH. TSH measurement is a more sensitive test than free T4 for identifying these conditions. A TSH-first strategy for diagnosing thyroid dysfunction in ambulatory patients suggests that a TSH within the reference range is evidence of normal thyroid function and requires no additional testing [15]. A TSH and free T4 panel approach more accurately assesses for central hypothyroidism, a TSH-secreting pituitary and allows for evaluations of interferences or detection of unusual conditions characterized by discordance in the ratio of TSH/FT4 [15]. If a TSH first strategy is adopted and an abnormal TSH is encountered, subsequent assessment of additional thyroid hormones levels should be assessed.

1.3.2 Total Thyroid Hormone

Recent increased accuracy of measurements of serum free T4 and free T3 has contributed to the decreased popularity of total thyroid hormone assessments. Total T4 and Total T3 concentrations are an assessment of both bound and free levels of T4 and T3. The clinical utility of this has been particularly impacted by the recognition that many conditions, commonly encountered in clinical practice during the assessment of thyroid function, affect the concentrations of thyroid-hormone-binding proteins and/or compete for binding and therefore do not accurately reflect bioactive free levels of the hormone [5]. Additionally, medications and thyroid hormone autoantibodies can also render total thyroid hormone measurements diagnostically unreliable [2]. The one general exception to this rule is during the assessment of the thyrotoxic patient when the clinician is attempting to differentiate stimulation-induced thyrotoxicosis (Graves' disease) from destruction-induced thyrotoxicosis (painless thyroiditis and subacute thyroiditis). The total T_3/T_4 ratio appears to be relatively useful in the differentiation of these thyrotoxic conditions where Graves' patients usually have a ratio >20, while a ratio of <20 was indicative of a destructive process [16, 17]. This assessment can be further augmented when TSH is considered as serum levels of TSH are generally suppressed in most untreated Graves' patients, whereas they usually were not completely suppressed in patients with painless thyroiditis or subacute thyroiditis [18].

1.3.3 Serum Free T4 and Free T3

The available free hormone fraction in the circulation is believed to be 0.03% for free T4 (FT4) and 0.3% for free T3 (FT3) and is responsible for the biological activity at the cellular level. The concentrations of free thyroid hormones are generally estimated using a variety of indirect (analog, immunometric, and two-step labeled hormone assays) or direct methods (equilibrium dialysis, ultrafiltration), with the concentrations of FT4 having the most clinical relevance [19]. FT3 is usually only measured in a small subset of patient with suspected T3 toxicosis and is not recommended for routine measurement [2].

As previously mentioned, although a TSH-first testing algorithm is sufficient for general screening, both FT4 and TSH assays are needed for diagnosing subclinical thyroid dysfunction, central hypothyroidism, and in the assessment of elderly and hospitalized patients, as well as for accurate assessment of treatment effects [20]. Guidelines from multiple thyroid and endocrine societies have also endorsed a TSH-first strategy in most clinical scenarios with FT4 testing when clinically indicated or TSH is found to be abnormal [15, 21–23]. Work by Henze et al. goes even further suggesting that a TSH-first strategy can be further perfected by widening the TSH reference range from 0.4–4.0 mIU/L to 0.2–6.0 mIU/L with minimal impact on case detection. They found that only 4.2% of TSH values between 0.2 mIU/L and 0.4 mIU/L would not have led to detection of a high FT4 and equally, only 2.5% of TSH values between 4.0 mIU/L and 6.0 mIU/L were associated with low FT4 level [24]. It is likely that this small additional group of patients outside the wider range with abnormal FT4 is clinically unimportant in most cases.

1.3.4 Serum Thyroid Autoantibodies

Autoimmune thyroid disease often accounts for a large proportion of patients with hyperthyroidism and hypothyroidism. Testing for autoantibodies, in particular anti-TSH receptor autoantibodies (TSHRabs), antithyroid peroxidase autoantibodies (TPOabs), and antithyroglobulin autoantibodies (Tgabs), is central to the diagnosis of autoimmune thyroid disease [2]. The evaluation of TSHRab is generally recommended when Graves' disease is suspected and can be done via a measurement of TSH receptor binding or in a functional bioassay of thyroid-stimulating immunoglobulin [5]. The suspected mechanism of action of these autoantibodies is believed to be via direct stimulation of the TSH receptor with increased metabolic activity of the thyroid gland. TSHRab are also believed to be responsible for metabolic changes in TSH receptor positive fibroblast cells in target orbital tissues leading to Graves' orbitopathy [2]. However, in some cases, TSHRabs act as antagonists competing with TSH for receptor binding and prevent the stimulating activity of TSH, resulting in hypothyroidism [25, 26].

The presence of TPOab is commonly associated with patients with hypothyroidism, but can be present in normal individuals who do not display any obvious symptoms of clinical thyroid disease. TPOabs are present in approximately 10% of normal individuals, while it was detected in almost 100% of samples of patients with autoimmune hypothyroidism [27, 28].

Antibodies to thyroglobulin can also be indicative of autoimmune hypothyroidism but are most clinically relevant in testing on patients with differentiated thyroid carcinomas. The presence of Tgab does not correlate with abnormal TSH levels and is not indicated in that assessment of thyroid autoimmunity screening [29]. However, its assessment with the assessment of TPOab may allow prediction of future hypothyroidism in some patients [30]. The most clinically relevant assessment of Tgab is made in conjunction with thyroglobulin, the primary tumor marker used to monitor patients with differentiated thyroid cancer. The presence of Tgab can compromise the accuracy and reliability of thyroglobulin as a tumor marker; however, Tgab trends can be used as a surrogate differentiated thyroid cancer tumor marker in preference to Tg [31].

In general, thyroid autoantibodies should not be measured in the setting of normal thyroid function except in special circumstances.

1.3.5 Serum Thyroglobulin

Thyroglobulin (Tg) represents the primary storage vehicle for precursor for thyroid hormone and serves as the main reservoir of iodine for thyroid hormone production. Tg is regularly released into the circulation as a consequence of thyroid hormone secretion and is present in all subjects with an intact thyroid gland. In view of this, its assessment in patients with intact thyroid glands has limited clinical utility. The caveat to this notion is in the circumstance of suspected excessive exogenous ingestion versus endogenous thyroid hormone release;

in the former scenario, TSH and Tg will be suppressed, while in the latter, only TSH levels will be decreased, while Tg will be increased [32].

The main clinical relevance of Tg testing is in differentiated thyroid carcinoma (DTC) as a tumor marker. Typically, papillary thyroid cancer cells and follicular thyroid cancer cells retain many characteristics of thyroid follicular cells including the expression of thyroid-specific proteins thyroglobulin (Tg). By leveraging this fact, the clinician is able to detect persistent or recurrent disease after treatment with surgery and/or radioactive iodine ablation [33]. Detection of Tg can be further augmented via conventional thyroid hormone withdrawal and subsequent endogenous TSH stimulation of any remaining thyroid cells or via the use of recombinant human thyrotropin stimulation, avoiding thyroid hormone withdrawal [34]. As previously mentioned, Tg serum measurements need to be assessed in conjunction with serum Tg Ab assays as unmeasurable Tg in the backdrop of positive Tg Ab does not eliminate the possibility of recurrent disease [29]. Additionally of note, undetectable Tg levels in the setting of rising Tg Ab are suggestive of recurrent/persistent disease in the setting of DTC [35].

Finally, when Tg levels appear discordant with clinical status or fail to change with TSH stimulation or suppression, the presence of interfering heterophile antibodies (antibodies against the animal-derived antibodies used in the immunometric assay) should be considered [5]. The most common heterophile antibody is human antimouse antibodies and can cause interference in accurate Tg measurements [2]. There is no entirely reliable method to avoid or detect heterophile antibody interference, but clinician awareness is critical and repeating the test using a heterophile-blocking tube (HBT) or measure Tg with an RIA assay should be considered [36, 37].

1.3.6 Hypothyroidism

There is extensive variation of symptoms and signs of hypothyroidism (◘ Table 1.1), and these can often be insidious and nonspecific and if left untreated can lead to serious morbidity and even mortality [38]. The biochemical presence of hypothyroidism is however often easily identified through laboratory testing. Hypothyroidism can be biochemically divided into clinical hypothyroidism and subclinical hypothyroidism. Clinical hypothyroidism can be defined as a TSH level above the reference range associated with a free T4 concentration below the reference range, while subclinical hypothyroidism is considered with a TSH above the reference range but a normal free T4 level.

Primary hypothyroidism, due to thyroid hormone deficiency, represents 99% of the cases while the remaining 1% of cases represent secondary (due to TSH deficiency), tertiary

Table 1.1 Signs and symptoms of hypothyroidism

System	Symptoms	Signs
General	Weight gain, fatigue, cold intolerance	Hyponatremia, hypothermia, increased BMI
Dermatological	Dry coarse skin and hair, hair loss	Pretibial myxedema
Otolaryngological	Hoarseness, tongue enlargement	Periorbital edema, goiter
Musculoskeletal	Myalgia, muscle cramps, muscle weakness	Carpal tunnel syndrome, elevation of serum creatine phosphokinase, Hoffman's syndrome
Neurological	Depression, impaired concentration, memory loss, changes in vision, hearing, and taste	Impaired cognitive function, neuropathy, cochlear dysfunction, decreased olfactory and gustatory sensitivity, delayed relaxation of tendon reflexes
Cardiovascular	Fatigue on exertion, shortness of breath	Dyslipidemia, bradycardia, hypertension, congestive heart failure, diastolic dysfunction, pericardial effusion, hyperhomocysteinemia, electrocardiogram changes, hyperlipidemia
Endocrinological	Infertility and subfertility, menstrual disturbance, galactorrhea, miscarriage	Goiter, glucose metabolism dysregulation, infertility, increased prolactin, pituitary hyperplasia
Hematological	Bleeding, fatigue	Mild anemia, acquired von Willebrand disease, decreased protein C and S, increased red cell distribution width, increased mean platelet volume
Gastrointestinal	Constipation	Reduced esophageal motility, nonalcoholic fatty liver disease

(due to thyrotropin-releasing hormone deficiency), and peripheral (consumptive hypothyroidism) [39, 40]. Environmental iodine deficiency continues to be the most common cause of all thyroid disorders, including hypothyroidism worldwide, but in areas of iodine sufficiency, the most common cause of primary hypothyroidism is chronic autoimmune thyroiditis (Hashimoto's disease) [41]. Hypothyroidism is also caused by various other etiologies listed on ◘ Table 1.2. When considering the diagnosis of hypothyroidism, it is important to differentiate the etiologies responsible for transient hypothyroidism from the clinical conditions presenting with long-term thyroid function failure. Examples of the transient etiologies of hypothyroidism include subacute, silent thyroiditis, postpartum thyroiditis among others, all with varying degrees of duration of biochemical thyroidal derangement. These conditions often follow a triphasic pattern with an initial thyrotoxic phase followed by a hypothyroid phase and an eventual return to a euthyroidism. Their management is generally directed toward controlling patient symptoms associated with the initial thyrotoxic phase with beta-blockers and the hypothyroid phase may or may not require thyroid hormone replacement [42].

1.3.7 Hyperthyroidism

The symptoms and signs of hyperthyroidism are also quite varied as with hypothyroidism but often more characteristic of the condition (◘ Table 1.3). The most common symptoms are palpitations, weakness, heat intolerance, and disturbed sleep with the most frequent physical findings being tachycardia, tremor of the extremities, and weight loss [43]. In clinical practice, the symptoms and signs of hyperthyroidism are often not necessarily correlated with the biochemical severity of the thyroid dysfunction and can be variable and less prevalent in the elderly [44].

As with hypothyroidism, hyperthyroidism can be biochemically defined as clinical (overt) or subclinical: With the former being characterized by low serum TSH with raised serum thyroid hormones while the later showing a low serum TSH associated with normal serum thyroid hormone levels [43]. The most common causes of hyperthyroidism are Graves' disease, followed by toxic multinodular goiter, while rarer causes include an autonomously functioning thyroid adenoma or thyroiditis [45]. Thyrotoxicosis itself can also occur without hyperthyroidism and is caused by extrathyroidal sources of thyroid hormone or by a release of preformed thyroid hormones into the circulation despite a low thyroid radioactive iodine uptake [43]. The underlying etiologies of hyperthyroidism and thyrotoxicosis are complex and varied (◘ Table 1.4). Hyperthyroidism and thyrotoxicosis have an increased risk of all-cause mortality with heart failure being the main cause of cardiovascular events [46]. Given this complexity and higher risk of mortality, identification of the underlying etiology is key prior to treatment. Generally, the diagnosis and management of hyperthyroidism and thyrotoxicosis is best initially deferred to an endocrinologist and, when surgical management is necessary, coordinated via a multidisciplinary team approach.

Table 1.2 Etiologies for hypothyroidism

	Etiology	Example
Primary hypothyroidism	Chronic autoimmune thyroiditis	Hashimoto's thyroiditis
	Dietary	Severe iodine deficiency, mild and severe iodine excess
	Medications	Amiodarone, lithium, tyrosine kinase inhibitors, interferon-alfa, thalidomide, monoclonal antibodies (ipilimumab and nivolumab), antiepileptic drugs (valproate), drugs for second-line treatment of multidrug-resistant tuberculosis
	Iatrogenic	Radioiodine ablation, thyroid surgery, radiotherapy or surgery in the neck or head region
	Transient thyroiditis	Subacute granulomatous (De Quervain's syndrome), postpartum, silent thyroiditis, destructive thyroiditis
	Thyroid gland infiltration	Infectious (mycoplasma), malignant (thyroid malignancy, lymphoma, metastasis), autoimmune (sarcoidosis), inflammatory (Riedel's thyroiditis)
	Genetic	Autoimmunity-related genes general and thyroid-specific genes
Central hypothyroidism	Pituitary tumors	Secreting or nonsecreting
	Pituitary dysfunction	Sheehan's syndrome
	Hypothalamic dysfunction	Posttraumatic
	Resistance to thyroid-stimulating hormone (TSH) or thyrotropin-releasing hormone	
	Medications	Dopamine, somatostatins, glucocorticosteroids, and retinoid X receptor selective ligands
Peripheral hypothyroidism	Consumptive hypothyroidism	
	Tissue-specific hypothyroidism due to decreased sensitivity to thyroid hormone	Mutations in MCT8

Adapted from Chaker et al. [38]

Table 1.3 Signs and Symptoms of hyperthyroidism

System	Symptoms	Signs
General	Weight loss, Increased appetite, heat intolerance, polydipsia	Weight loss
Dermatological	Diaphoresis	Warm skin, Palmer erythema
Ophthalmological	Diplopia; sense of irritation in the eyes; eyelid swelling; retro-orbital pain or discomfort	Proptosis; eyelid retraction and lag; periorbital edema; conjunctival injection and chemosis; ophthalmoplegia
Musculoskeletal	Tremor; muscle weakness; disturbed sleep; poor concentration	Tremor of the extremities; pelvic and girdle muscle weakness, osteoporosis
Neurological	Anxiety, nervousness, anxiety; fatigue, disturbed sleep; poor concentration	Hyperactivity, hyperreflexia, hyperkinesis
Cardiovascular	Palpitations, shortness of breath	Tachycardia; systolic hypertension; irregular heartbeat (atrial fibrillation), tachypnoea
Endocrinological	Irregular menstrual periods/amenorrhea	Irregular menstrual periods/amenorrhea Light menstrual flow Infertility Gynecomastia (males)
Gastrointestinal	Hyperdefecation, nausea, vomiting	Abdominal tenderness

Adapted from De Leo et al. [43]

1.4 Thyroid Anatomy

The foundation of performing safe and effective thyroid surgery is a clear and in-depth understanding of thyroid anatomy, its anatomical relationships, and congenital variations.

The thyroid gland consists of two lobes connected in the midline by a central isthmus. Under normal circumstances, each lobe is approximately 4 cm in length, 2 cm in width, and 2–3 cm in depth, with the majority of glands weighing 15–25 g in adults; however, these dimensions can be drastically different in thyroid disease processes [47].

Table 1.4 Etiologies of hyperthyroidism and thyrotoxicosis

	Etiology	Example
Primary hyperthyroidism	TSH receptor antibodies	Graves' disease
	Dietary	Excess exogenous thyroid hormone (iatrogenic or factitious), iodine-induced hyperthyroidism
	Medications	Amiodarone, lithium, interferon-alfa
	Autonomous thyroid function	Solitary hyperfunctioning adenoma, toxic multinodular goiter
	Transient thyroiditis	Subacute granulomatous (De Quervain's syndrome), postpartum, silent thyroiditis, destructive thyroiditis
	Thyroid gland infiltration	Bacterial or fungal infection with acute suppurative thyroiditis
	Genetic	Familial nonautoimmune hyperthyroidism
	Iatrogenic	Radiation-induced thyroiditis
Central hyperthyroidism	Pituitary tumors	TSH-secreting adenoma
	Pituitary dysfunction	Pituitary resistance to thyroid hormone
	Hypothalamic dysfunction	Posttraumatic
Peripheral hyperthyroidism	Excess hCG secretion	Trophoblastic tumors, hyperemesis gravidarum
	Ectopic thyroid hormone production	Struma ovarii, functional thyroid cancer metastasis

The anatomical boundaries of the normal thyroid gland lobes are the larynx and trachea medially, sternocleidomastoid muscle laterally and carotid sheath posterolaterally, the sternothyroid and sternohyoid muscles anteriorly, and the condensation of the deep cervical fascia forming the suspensory ligament of Berry affixing to the cornu of the cricoid cartilage extending inferiomedially onto the tracheal wall [47]. The isthmus of the thyroid glands is generally related anteriorly to the level of the second, third, and fourth tracheal rings. The superior pole of the thyroid lies lateral to the inferior constrictor muscle, and posterior to the sternothyroid muscle with the inferior pole extending to the level of the fifth or sixth tracheal ring [48]. The thyroid is enveloped by the layers of the deep cervical fascia, and the true thyroid capsule is tightly adherent to the gland and continues into the parenchyma to form fibrous septae often separating the gland into lobules. When a pyramidal lobe is present, it will be directed superiorly and may arise from the isthmus, or either lobe, occurring in 50% of cases.

1.4.1 Blood Supply and Lymphatics

The blood supply of the superior pole of the thyroid is derived from the superior thyroid artery, the first branch off the external carotid artery and less commonly the common carotid, and lies anterior to the external branch of the superior laryngeal nerve as it courses to supply the cricothyroid muscle [48]. Inferiorly, the thyroid is supplied by the inferior thyroid artery by way of the thyrocervical trunk from the subclavian artery. Furthermore, a thyroid ima artery may be additionally present or replace the inferior thyroid artery supplying the thyroid in the midline. The venous drainage is similar to the arterial supply with two or three pairs of veins traveling in association with their arterial pedicle along with a separate middle thyroid vein that drains directly into the internal jugular vein [49]. The lymphatic drainage of the thyroid gland is predominantly via the accompanying venous drainage with the superior and middle thyroid lymphatics draining into the upper and middle deep cervical chain and the inferior thyroid lymphatics draining into lower deep cervical chain nodes, the pretracheal, paratracheal, and supraclavicular nodes.

1.5 Surgical Thyroid Anatomy

1.5.1 External Branch of the Superior Laryngeal Nerve

The superior laryngeal nerve consists of two branches: the internal branch, which supplies sensory fibers to the pharynx, and the external laryngeal nerve (EBSLN), which innervates the cricothyroid muscle. The function of the cricothyroid muscle is to lengthen, stiffen, and thin the true vocal cord and therefore tense the vocal cords when they are approximated, providing timbre to the voice. There is also some evidence that the EBSLN may also be involved in reflex glottic closure, which prevents aspiration during deglutition [50]. The EBSLN is most commonly deep to the superior thyroid artery, but it can cross anterior, or between branches of the artery in 14–18% of cases

[51]. The external branch of the superior laryngeal nerve has highly variable anatomical patterns epitomized by the multiple classification schemes for its anatomy and consequently a thorough preoperative knowledge of its anatomy can be crucial in minimizing iatrogenic injury [52–55].

1.5.2 Recurrent Laryngeal Nerve

The recurrent laryngeal nerve (RLN) via its motor and sensory fibers supplies all of the intrinsic muscles of the larynx other than the cricothyroid while receiving sensory and secretomotor fibers from the glottis, subglottis, and trachea.

The left RLN arises off the vagus nerve at the level of the aortic arch, while the right RLN arises anterior to the right subclavian artery prior to their ascent into the neck. The right RLN generally courses more obliquely in the sagittal plane as it ascends the neck, while the left RLN ascends more vertically just anterior to the tracheal esophageal groove [56]. The terminal part of the RLN enters the larynx, underneath the thyroid gland, deep to the inferior border of the inferior pharyngeal constrictor, posterior to the cricothyroid joint making this a consistent surgical landmark. There have been multiple variations described as to the relationship of the RLN to inferior thyroid with three basic configurations including anterior to the artery, nerve between branches of the artery, and posterior to the artery [48].

The clinician must also be familiar with the occurrence of a nonrecurrent laryngeal nerve (NRLN). The NRLN is an anatomic variant and has been reported in 0.52% of cases on the right and 0.04% on the left by Henry et al. [57]. Almost invariably, this anatomic variant is also associated with the presence of an aberrant right subclavian artery when on the right and a situs inversus or right aortic arch when on the left [58, 59].

1.5.3 Parathyroid Glands

Typically, the inferior parathyroid glands are often found ventral to the plane of the RLN but deep to the thyroid gland [5]. However, 17% are found on or within the capsule of the thyroid gland, 26% are found within the cervical part of the thymus, and 2.8% found superior to the intersection of the recurrent nerve and the inferior thyroid artery [48] The superior parathyroid glands are typically found dorsal to the plane of the RLN. Due to its shorter embryological descent compared to the inferior parathyroid glands, its location is less variable. The superior parathyroid can often be found at the posterior aspect of the thyroid lobe in a 2-cm diameter area centered 1 cm above the junction of the inferior thyroid artery and the RLN [5].

1.6 Ultrasonography of the Thyroid Gland

Ultrasonography (US) is the modality of choice in the evaluation of the thyroid gland and its surrounding associated structures [33]. Given the gland's location, its distinct sonographic features, and signature echogenicity (◘ Fig. 1.3), ultrasound is a powerful tool in the assessment of the thyroid and its pathology, often providing greater detail of the gland than CT, MRI, or radionuclide studies [60]. The majority of thyroid ultrasounds are performed for thyroid nodules, many of which are discovered incidentally on other imaging studies. The current indications for US of the thyroid include evaluation of a palpable nodule, workup of incidentally found nodules, or assessment of suspected thyroid enlargement. Caution should be exercised in using thyroid US as a screening tool for the detection of nodules given the high prevalence rate (50%) [61]. US of the thyroid achieves multiple goals when imaging a nodule as it is also able to characterize its size, location, presence of benign or suspicious features, and evaluate for cervical lymphadenopathy [62]. It also permits greater accuracy when performing an ultrasound-guided fine-needle aspiration (USgFNA), if so indicated.

There are distinctive characteristics of thyroid malignancy that can be identified on US that not only offer high sensitivity, but when several of these characteristics are present, they increase sensitivity. The specific US features that have been recognized as suggestive of malignancy comprise namely hypoechogenicity, irregular or blurred margins, microcalcifications, taller than wider shape, and abnormal vascular signals (◘ Fig. 1.4) [63]. A hypoechoic nodule has a higher propensity for malignancy compared to an iso-/hyperechoic nodule

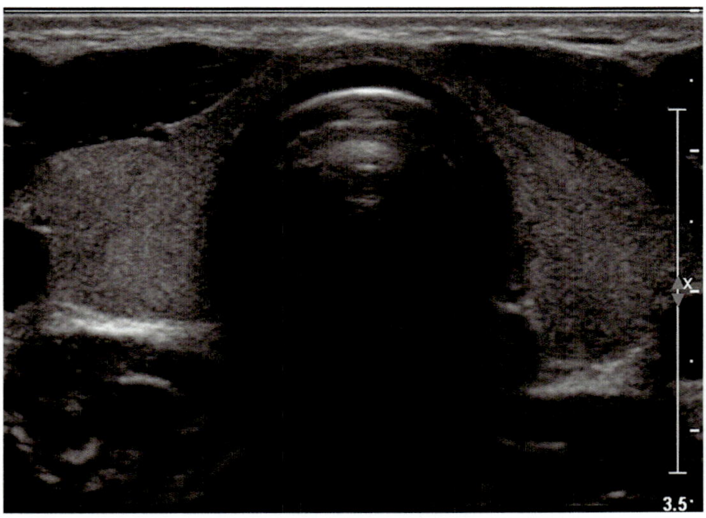

◘ **Fig. 1.3** Normal thyroid ultrasound image with signature thyroid echogenicity

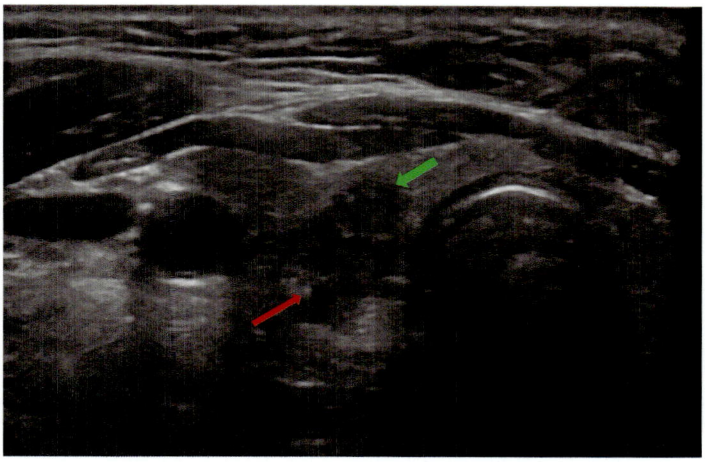

■ **Fig. 1.4** Papillary thyroid cancer within the thyroid illustrating microcalcifications (red arrow), irregular boarders (green arrow), hypoechogenicity

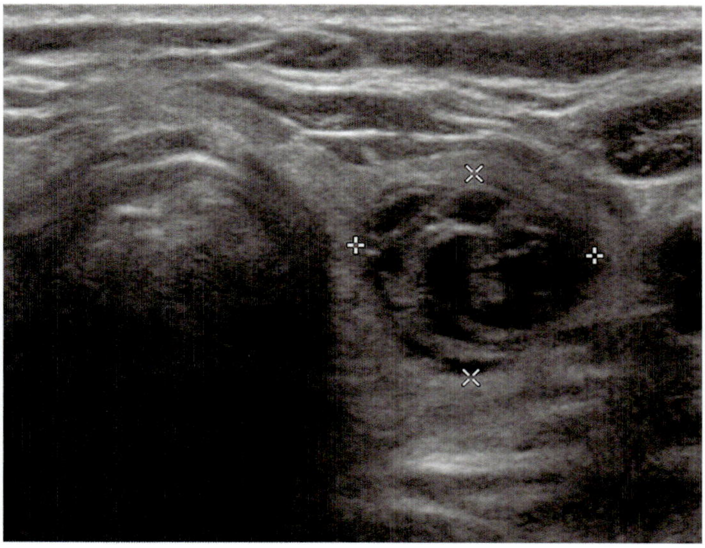

■ **Fig. 1.5** Spongioform thyroid nodule

[63, 64]. A solid composition of a nodule is more suggestive of malignancy when compared to a spongiform one (■ Fig. 1.5), and an increasingly cystic structure is more likely benign, with a completely cystic nodule being certainly benign [65]. Irregular or blurred margins are suggestive of malignancy via malignant extension of the carcinoma [64]. When concern for malignant extension is seen, an assessment of mobility of the nodule with respect to surrounding structures can be made, fixation suggests invasion of surrounding tissue [60]. Microcalcifications within the nodule have been shown to increase the risk of malignancy and have been corroborated by several studies (■ Fig. 1.6) [63, 64, 66]. These microcalcifications are thought to represent psammoma bodies, which are a histopathologic

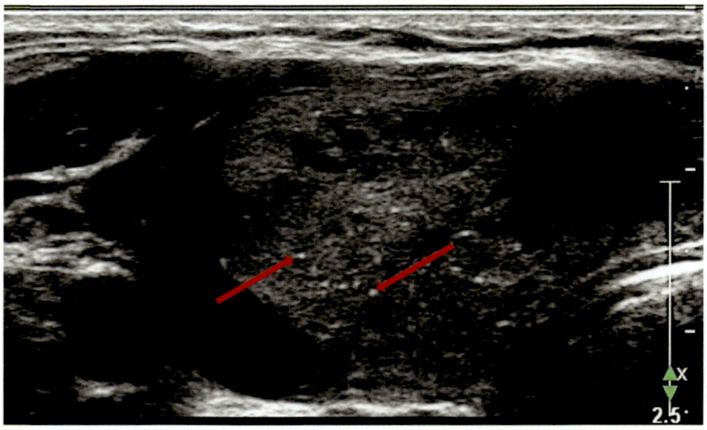

Fig. 1.6 Thyroid ultrasound image illustrating microcalcifications (red arrows)

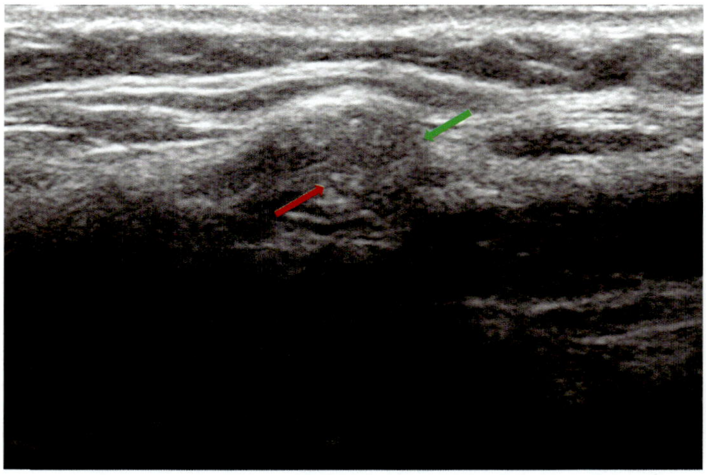

Fig. 1.7 Level V metastatic papillary carcinoma in a cervical lymph node. Illustrative of microcalcifications (red arrow) and ill-defined margins (green arrow)

feature considered pathognomonic of papillary thyroid cancer. The predictive value of the "taller than wider" nodular shape has been questioned by some authors with studies suggesting spherical nodules having a higher incidence of malignancy [60]. Finally, an intranodular blood flow pattern that becomes more dominant has been correlated with an increased risk of malignancy [67].

Ultrasound-guided fine-needle aspiration (USgFNA) is an integral part of ultrasonography of the thyroid in the assessment of suspicious lesions within the thyroid and in the neck (Fig. 1.7). USgFNA allows a greater sensitivity (83.3%), specificity (98.8%), positive predictive value (97.0%), and negative predictive value (92.5%) when compared to conventional FNA of thyroid nodules [62]. When considering the need for proceeding to FNA, it is useful to use one of the recognized guidelines for thyroid nodule classification. There are three main published and validated US classification criteria for stratifying risk of malignancy and determining the need for FNA. The American Thyroid Association (ATA) guidelines propose five levels of risk stratification ranging from benign, to very low, low, intermediate, and high suspicion for malignancy [33]. The American Association of Clinical Endocrinologists (AACE), American College of Endocrinology (ACE), and Associazione Medici Endocrinologi (AME) propose three risk categories: low (class 1), intermediate (class 2), and high (class 3) [61]. The American College of Radiology (ACR) Thyroid Imaging Reporting and Data System (TI-RADS) classification categorizes nodules as benign, minimally suspicious, moderately suspicious, or highly suspicious for malignancy depending on their US features [68]. All guidelines for the management of thyroid nodules couple the characteristics delineated above with nodule size thresholds to decide whether an FNA is warranted. The use of these classification systems improves communication among clinicians and helps in standardizing clinical practice [62]. It is also important not only to be knowledgeable of the various validated ultrasound classification systems but to be to be familiar with the Bethesda System for Reporting Thyroid Cytopathology. This is a well-established standardized, category-based cytological reporting system for thyroid fine-needle aspiration (FNA) specimens. The Bethesda system is broken down into six diagnostic categories: (I) nondiagnostic or unsatisfactory; (II) benign; (III) atypia of undetermined significance (AUS) or follicular lesion of undetermined significance (FLUS); (IV) follicular neoplasm or suspicious for a follicular neoplasm; (V) suspicious for malignancy; and (VI) malignant. Each category has an implied risk of malignancy, ranging from 0% to 3% to virtually 100% with a corollary recommended clinical management strategy including observation, repeat biopsy, molecular testing, or surgical removal (◘ Table 1.5) [69].

Thyroid ultrasound can also be used to detect thyroid disease beyond nodularity including Graves' disease, thyroiditis, and subacute or de Quervain's thyroiditis. Graves' disease is characterized by heterogeneous thyroid tissue with diffuse hypoechogenicity and hypervascularity, while Hashimoto's thyroiditis includes ill-defined hypoechoic areas separated by echogenic septa, with increased (early) or decreased (late) vascularity [60]. Subacute or de Quervain's thyroiditis, though more often a clinical diagnosis, has US findings of an ill-defined hypoechoic area, without round or ovoid mass formation on the multiple planes of US, and no vascular flow on color doppler [70].

Finally, US is recommended for surveillance of thyroid nodules. Though malignant transformation of benign thyroid nodules is rare, the 3% or greater false-negative rate of FNA makes US surveillance advocated. The ATA and the AACE/

1

Table 1.5 The 2017 Bethesda System for Reporting Thyroid Cytopathology with corollary risk of malignancy and usual management strategy

	Bethesda category	Cytological findings	Risk of malignancy (%)	Usual management
I	Nondiagnostic or unsatisfactory	Cystic fluid Virtually acellular specimen Other (obscuring blood, clotting artifact, etc.)	5–10	Repeat FNA with ultrasound guidance
II	Benign	Benign follicular nodule Lymphocytic (Hashimoto) thyroiditis Granulomatous (subacute) thyroiditis	0–3	Clinical and sonographic follow-up
III	Atypia of undetermined significance or follicular lesion of undetermined significance		6–18	Repeat FNA, molecular testing or lobectomy
IV	Follicular neoplasm or suspicious for a follicular neoplasm		10–40	Molecular testing or lobectomy
V	Suspicious for malignancy	Suspicious for papillary carcinoma Suspicious for medullary carcinoma Suspicious for metastatic carcinoma Suspicious for lymphoma	45–60	Near-total thyroidectomy or lobectomy (dependent on the type of suspicious malignancy)
VI	Malignant	Papillary thyroid carcinoma Poorly differentiated carcinoma Medullary thyroid carcinoma Undifferentiated (anaplastic) carcinoma Squamous cell carcinoma Metastatic carcinoma Lymphoma	94–96	Near-total thyroidectomy or lobectomy (dependent on the type of suspicious malignancy)

Adapted from Cibas and Ali [69]

AME both recommend that cytologically benign thyroid nodules be followed every 6–18 months with palpation or with US if not easily palpable [33, 61]. Nodules should undergo repeat FNA if there is evidence of nodule growth, defined as more than 50% change in volume or >20% increase or greater than 2 mm in at least two nodule dimensions in solid nodules or in the solid portion of a mixed cystic solid nodule. If there is evidence of nodule growth either by palpation or sonographically, then an FNA should be repeated [33, 61].

Answers to the Questions

1. (c); 2. (b); 3. (e); 4. (d); 5. (e); 6. (a); 7. (a); 8. (b); 9. (e); 10. (a); 11. (e)

References

1. Dohán O, la Vieja DA, Paroder V, Riedel C, Artani M, Reed M, et al. The sodium/iodide symporter (NIS): characterization, regulation, and medical significance. Endocr Rev. 2003;24(1):48–77.
2. Braverman LE. Werner & Ingbar's the thyroid. LWW; 2020. 1 p
3. Weiss SJ, Philp NJ, Ambesi-Impiombato FS, Grollman EF. Thyrotropin-stimulated iodide transport mediated by adenosine 3",5-"mono-phosphate and dependent on protein synthesis. Endocrinology. 1984; 114(4):1099–107.
4. Scott DA, Wang R, Kreman TM, Sheffield VC, Karniski LP. The Pendred syndrome gene encodes a chloride-iodide transport protein. Nat Genet. 1999;21(4):440–3.
5. Randolph GW. Surgery of the thyroid and parathyroid glands e-book. Elsevier Health Sciences; 2020. 1 p
6. Tokuyama T, Yoshinari M, Rawitch AB, Taurog A. Digestion of thyroglobulin with purified thyroid lysosomes: preferential release of iodoamino acids. Endocrinology. 1987;121(2):714–21.
7. Visser WE, Friesema ECH, Visser TJ. Minireview: thyroid hormone transporters: the knowns and the unknowns. Mol Endocrinol. 2011;25(1):1–14.
8. Pappa T, Ferrara AM, Refetoff S. Inherited defects of thyroxine-binding proteins. Best Pract Res Clin Endocrinol Metab. 2015;29(5):735–47.
9. Benvenga S, Lapa D, Trimarchi F. Thyroxine binding to members and non-members of the serine protease inhibitor family. J Endocrinol Investig. 2002;25(1):32–8.
10. Gereben B, McAninch EA, Ribeiro MO, Bianco AC. Scope and limitations of iodothyronine deiodinases in hypothyroidism. Nat Rev Endocrinol. 2015;11(11):642–52.
11. Oppenheimer JH. Role of plasma proteins in the binding, distribution and metabolism of the thyroid hormones. N Engl J Med. 1968;278(21):1153–62.
12. Davis PJ, Zhou M, Davis FB, Lansing L, Mousa SA, Lin H-Y. Mini-review: cell surface receptor for thyroid hormone and nongenomic regulation of ion fluxes in excitable cells. Physiol Behav. 2010;99(2):237–9.
13. Ehrenkranz J, Bach PR, Snow GL, Schneider A, Lee JL, Ilstrup S, et al. Circadian and Circannual rhythms in thyroid hormones: determining the TSH and free T4 reference intervals based upon time of day, age, and sex. Thyroid. 2015;25(8):954–61.
14. Ross DS. Serum thyroid-stimulating hormone measurement for assessment of thyroid function and disease. Endocrinol Metab Clin N Am. 2001;30(2):245–64–vii.
15. Baloch Z, Carayon P, Conte-Devolx B, Demers LM, Feldt-Rasmussen U, Henry J-F, et al. Laboratory medicine practice guidelines. Laboratory support for the diagnosis and monitoring of thyroid disease. Thyroid. 2003;13:3–126.
16. Amino N, Yabu Y, Miki T, Morimoto S, Kumahara Y, Mori H, et al. Serum ratio of triiodothyronine to thyroxine, and thyroxine-binding globulin and calcitonin concentrations in Graves' disease

and destruction-induced thyrotoxicosis. J Clin Endocrinol Metab. 1981;53(1):113–6.
17. Yoshimura Noh J, Momotani N, Fukada S, Ito K, Miyauchi A, Amino N. Ratio of serum free triiodothyronine to free thyroxine in Graves' hyperthyroidism and thyrotoxicosis caused by painless thyroiditis. Endocr J. 2005;52(5):537–42.
18. Yanagisawa T, Sato K, Kato Y, Shimizu S, Takano K. Rapid differential diagnosis of Graves' disease and painless thyroiditis using total T3/T4 ratio, TSH, and total alkaline phosphatase activity. Endocr J. 2005;52(1):29–36.
19. Thienpont LM, Van Uytfanghe K, Poppe K, Velkeniers B. Determination of free thyroid hormones. Best Pract Res Clin Endocrinol Metab. 2013;27(5):689–700.
20. Soh SB, Aw TC. Laboratory testing in thyroid conditions - pitfalls and clinical utility. Ann Lab Med. 2019;39(1):3–14.
21. Baskin HJ, Cobin RH, Duick DS, Gharib H, Guttler RB, Kaplan MM, et al. American Association of Clinical Endocrinologists medical guidelines for clinical practice for the evaluation and treatment of hyperthyroidism and hypothyroidism. Endocr Pract. 2002;8(6): 457–69.
22. Garber JR, Cobin RH, Gharib H, Hennessey JV, Klein I, Mechanick JI, et al. Clinical practice guidelines for hypothyroidism in adults: cosponsored by the American Association of Clinical Endocrinologists and the American Thyroid Association. Thyroid. 2012;22: 1200–35.
23. Ross DS, Burch HB, Cooper DS, Greenlee MC, Laurberg P, Maia AL, et al. 2016 American Thyroid Association guidelines for diagnosis and management of hyperthyroidism and other causes of thyrotoxicosis. Thyroid. 2016;26:1343–421.
24. Henze M, Brown SJ, Hadlow NC, Walsh JP. Rationalizing thyroid function testing: which TSH cutoffs are optimal for testing free T4? J Clin Endocrinol Metab. 2017;102(11):4235–41.
25. Gupta MK. Thyrotropin-receptor antibodies in thyroid diseases: advances in detection techniques and clinical applications. Clin Chim Acta. 2000;293(1–2):1–29.
26. Sanders J, Miguel RN, Furmaniak J, Smith BR. TSH receptor monoclonal antibodies with agonist, antagonist, and inverse agonist activities. Methods Enzymol. 2010;485:393–420.
27. Feldt-Rasmussen U, Høier-Madsen M, Bech K, Blichert-Toft M, Bliddal H, Date J, et al. Anti-thyroid peroxidase antibodies in thyroid disorders and non-thyroid autoimmune diseases. Autoimmunity. 1991;9(3):245–54.
28. Hollowell JG, Staehling NW, Flanders WD, Hannon WH, Gunter EW, Spencer CA, et al. Serum TSH, T(4), and thyroid antibodies in the United States population (1988 to 1994): National Health and Nutrition Examination Survey (NHANES III). J Clin Endocrinol Metab. 2002;87(2):489–99.
29. Spencer C, Petrovic I, Fatemi S. Current thyroglobulin autoantibody (TgAb) assays often fail to detect interfering TgAb that can result in the reporting of falsely low/undetectable serum Tg IMA values for patients with differentiated thyroid cancer. J Clin Endocrinol Metab. 2011;96(5):1283–91.
30. Walsh JP, Bremner AP, Feddema P, Leedman PJ, Brown SJ, O'Leary P. Thyrotropin and thyroid antibodies as predictors of hypothyroidism: a 13-year, longitudinal study of a community-based cohort using current immunoassay techniques. J Clin Endocrinol Metab. 2010;95(3):1095–104.

31. Spencer CA. Clinical review: clinical utility of thyroglobulin antibody (TgAb) measurements for patients with differentiated thyroid cancers (DTC). J Clin Endocrinol Metab. 2011;96(12):3615–27.
32. Mariotti S, Martino E, Cupini C, Lari R, Giani C, Baschieri L, et al. Low serum thyroglobulin as a clue to the diagnosis of thyrotoxicosis factitia. N Engl J Med. 1982;307(7):410–2.
33. Haugen BR, Alexander EK, Bible KC, Doherty GM, Mandel SJ, Nikiforov YE, et al. 2015 American Thyroid Association management guidelines for adult patients with thyroid nodules and differentiated thyroid cancer: the American Thyroid Association guidelines task force on thyroid nodules and differentiated thyroid cancer. Thyroid. 2016;26:1–133.
34. Weiss R, Magner J. Serial measurements of serum thyroglobulin in response to recombinant human thyrotropin stimulation. Thyroid. 2015;25(6):708–10.
35. Kim WG, Yoon JH, Kim WB, Kim TY, Kim EY, Kim JM, et al. Change of serum antithyroglobulin antibody levels is useful for prediction of clinical recurrence in thyroglobulin-negative patients with differentiated thyroid carcinoma. J Clin Endocrinol Metab. 2008;93(12):4683–9.
36. Boscato LM, Stuart MC. Incidence and specificity of interference in two-site immunoassays. Clin Chem. 1986;32(8):1491–5.
37. Algeciras-Schimnich A. Thyroglobulin measurement in the management of patients with differentiated thyroid cancer. Crit Rev Clin Lab Sci. 2018;55(3):205–18.
38. Chaker L, Bianco AC, Jonklaas J, Peeters RP. Hypothyroidism. Lancet. 2017;390(10101):1550–62.
39. Persani L. Clinical review: central hypothyroidism: pathogenic, diagnostic, and therapeutic challenges. 10 ed. J Clin Endocrinol Metab. 2012;97(9):3068–78.
40. Beck-Peccoz P, Rodari G, Giavoli C, Lania A. Central hypothyroidism - a neglected thyroid disorder. Nat Rev Endocrinol. 2017;13(10):588–98.
41. Chiovato L, Magri F, Carlé A. Hypothyroidism in context: where we"ve been and where we"re going. Adv Ther. 2019;36(Suppl 2):47–58.
42. Samuels MH. Subacute, silent, and postpartum thyroiditis. Med Clin North Am. 2012;96(2):223–33.
43. De Leo S, Lee SY, Braverman LE. Hyperthyroidism. Lancet. 2016;388(10047):906–18.
44. Slough CM, Randolph GW. Workup of well-differentiated thyroid carcinoma. Cancer Control. 2006;13(2):99–105.
45. Vanderpump MPJ. The epidemiology of thyroid disease. Br Med Bull. 2011;99:39–51.
46. Selmer C, Olesen JB, Hansen ML, von Kappelgaard LM, Madsen JC, Hansen PR, et al. Subclinical and overt thyroid dysfunction and risk of all-cause mortality and cardiovascular events: a large population study. J Clin Endocrinol Metab. 2014;99(7):2372–82.
47. Mohebati A, Shaha AR. Anatomy of thyroid and parathyroid glands and neurovascular relations. Richards a, editor. Clin Anat. 2012;25(1):19–31.
48. Fancy T, Gallagher D, Hornig JD. Surgical anatomy of the thyroid and parathyroid glands. Otolaryngol Clin N Am. 2010;43(2):221–7–vii.
49. Miller FR. Surgical anatomy of the thyroid and parathyroid glands. Otolaryngol Clin N Am. 2003;36(1):1–7–vii.
50. Folk D, Wahba B, Sasaki CT. Is the external branch of the superior laryngeal nerve dispensable in thyroid surgery? Thyroid. 2016;26(1):169–73.

51. Lennquist S, Cahlin C, Smeds S. The superior laryngeal nerve in thyroid surgery. Surgery. 1987;102(6):999–1008.
52. Cernea CR, Ferraz AR, Furlani J, Monteiro S, Nishio S, Hojaij FC, et al. Identification of the external branch of the superior laryngeal nerve during thyroidectomy. Am J Surg. 1992;164(6):634–9.
53. Kierner AC, Aigner M, Burian M. The external branch of the superior laryngeal nerve: its topographical anatomy as related to surgery of the neck. Arch Otolaryngol Head Neck Surg. 1998;124(3):301–3.
54. Friedman M, LoSavio P, Ibrahim H. Superior laryngeal nerve identification and preservation in thyroidectomy. Arch Otolaryngol Head Neck Surg. 2002;128(3):296–303.
55. Selvan B, Babu S, Paul MJ, Abraham D, Samuel P, Nair A. Mapping the compound muscle action potentials of cricothyroid muscle using electromyography in thyroid operations: a novel method to clinically type the external branch of the superior laryngeal nerve. Ann Surg. 2009;250(2):293–300.
56. Haller JM, Iwanik M, Shen FH. Clinically relevant anatomy of recurrent laryngeal nerve. Spine. 2012;37(2):97–100.
57. Henry JF, Audiffret J, Denizot A, Plan M. The nonrecurrent inferior laryngeal nerve: review of 33 cases, including two on the left side. Surgery. 1988;104(6):977–84.
58. Watanabe A, Kawabori S, Osanai H, Taniguchi M, Hosokawa M. Preoperative computed tomography diagnosis of non-recurrent inferior laryngeal nerve. Laryngoscope. 2001;111(10):1756–9.
59. Bakalinis E, Makris I, Demesticha T, Tsakotos G, Skandalakis P, Filippou D. Non-recurrent laryngeal nerve and concurrent vascular variants: a review. Acta Med Acad. 2018;47(2):186–92.
60. Randolph G. Surgery of the thyroid and parathyroid glands. Elsevier Health Sciences; 2012. 1 p
61. Gharib H, Papini E, Garber JR, Duick DS, Harrell RM, Hegedüs L, et al. American Association of Clinical Endocrinologists, American College of Endocrinology, and Associazione Medici Endocrinologi medical guidelines for clinical practice for the diagnosis and management of thyroid nodules – 2016 update. Endocr Pract. 2016;22:622–39.
62. Slough CM, Kamani D, Randolph GW. In-office ultrasonographic evaluation of neck masses/thyroid nodules. Otolaryngol Clin N Am. 2019;52(3):559–75.
63. Kim E-K, Park CS, Chung WY, Oh KK, Kim DI, Lee JT, et al. New sonographic criteria for recommending fine-needle aspiration biopsy of nonpalpable solid nodules of the thyroid. AJR Am J Roentgenol. 2002;178(3):687–91.
64. Cappelli C, Castellano M, Pirola I, Cumetti D, Agosti B, Gandossi E, et al. The predictive value of ultrasound findings in the management of thyroid nodules. QJM. 2007;100(1):29–35.
65. Frates MC, Benson CB, Doubilet PM, Kunreuther E, Contreras M, Cibas ES, et al. Prevalence and distribution of carcinoma in patients with solitary and multiple thyroid nodules on sonography. J Clin Endocrinol Metab. 2006;91(9):3411–7.
66. Seiberling KA, Dutra JC, Grant T, Bajramovic S. Role of intrathyroidal calcifications detected on ultrasound as a marker of malignancy. Laryngoscope. 2004;114(10):1753–7.
67. Chammas MC, Gerhard R, De Oliveira IRS, Widman A, De Barros N, Durazzo M, et al. Thyroid nodules: evaluation with power Doppler and duplex Doppler ultrasound. Otolaryngol Head Neck Surg (SAGE Publications, Sage CA: Los Angeles, CA). 2016;132(6):874–82.

68. Tessler FN, Middleton WD, Grant EG, Hoang JK, Berland LL, Teefey SA, et al. ACR thyroid imaging, reporting and data system (TI-RADS): white paper of the ACR TI-RADS Committee. J Am Coll Radiol. 2017;14(5):587–95.
69. Cibas ES, Ali SZ. The 2017 Bethesda system for reporting thyroid cytopathology. Thyroid. 2017;27:1341–6.
70. Park SY, Kim E-K, Kim MJ, Kim BM, Oh KK, Hong SW, et al. Ultrasonographic characteristics of subacute granulomatous thyroiditis. Korean J Radiol. 2006;7(4):229.

Non-toxic Thyroid Nodules and Multinodular Goitre

David M. Scott-Coombes and Catherine F. Sinclair

Contents

A. L. Shifrin et al. (eds.), *Endocrine Surgery Comprehensive Board Exam Guide*,
https://doi.org/10.1007/978-3-030-84737-1_2

Case Presentation

A 60-year-old lady presents with a 12-week history of dyspnoea, worse on exercise and when she lies down in bed. She has no hoarseness or dysphagia. There is no family history of goitre. She is previously fit and well aside from controlled essential hypertension (furosemide). She has had a known goitre for many years.

On examination, she has a ruddy complexion and stridor at rest. Palpation reveals a large diffuse nodular goitre, and it is not possible to palpate a lower limit on either side. The images below show a lateral profile of her neck and two representative scans from her CT neck and thorax.

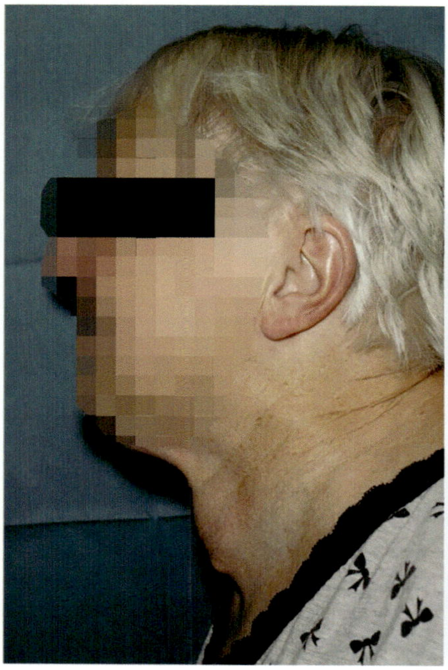

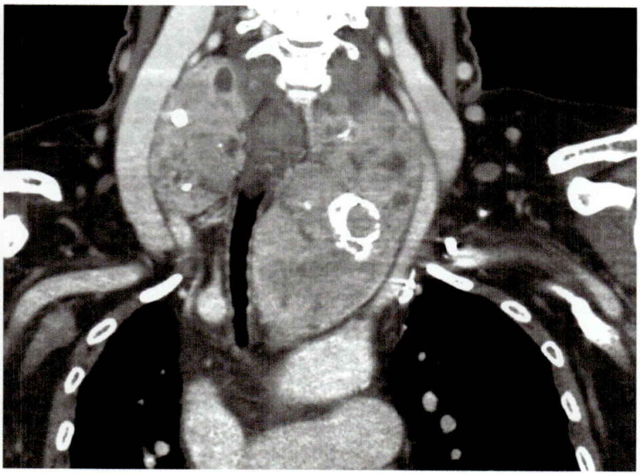

2

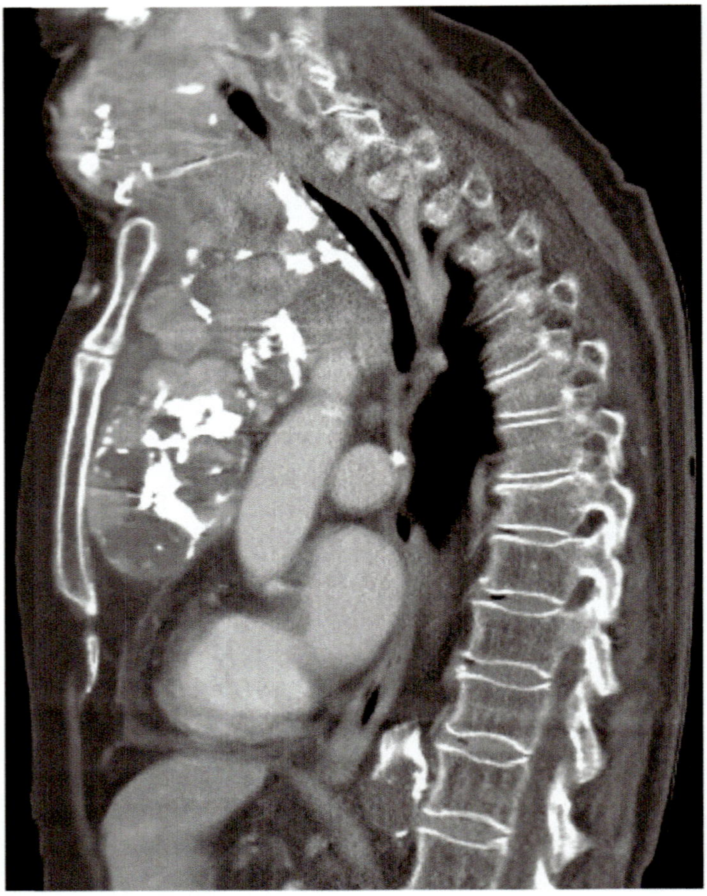

Questions

1. Which of the following statements are true?
    1. Goitre is more common in women.
    2. Goitre is more common in the elderly.
    3. Diffuse goitre is more common than nodular in iodine-sufficient areas of the world.
    4. Smoking is a risk factor for the development of goitre.
    5. Multiple genes are responsible for the pathogenesis of goitre.
        (a) All are correct.
        (b) 1, 2 and 3 only are correct.
        (c) 2, 3, 4, 5 only are correct.
        (d) 1, 2, 4 and 5 only are correct.
        (e) 1, 2 and 4 only are correct.
2. Regarding blood tests
    1. Thyroid function tests are likely to be normal.
    2. A high TSH is associated with malignancy.
    3. A raised thyroglobulin is diagnostic of malignancy.
    4. An elevated anti-TPO titre predicts myxoedema.
    5. Thyrotoxicosis must be excluded.

(a) All are correct.
(b) 1 and 3 only are correct.
(c) 1 and 5 only are correct.
(d) 1, 2 and 5 only are correct.
(e) 2 and 4 only are correct.

3. The following ultrasonographic features are suggestive of malignancy:
   1. The presence of a halo
   2. Microcalcifications
   3. A low elasticity measure
   4. Cervical lymphadenopathy
   5. A nodule greater than 4 cm in maximum diameter
      (a) 1, 2 and 4 only
      (b) 2, 3 and 4 only
      (c) 2, 3, 4 and 5 only
      (d) 2 and 4 only
      (e) 2, 4 and 5 only
4. Regarding biopsy
   1. Ultrasound determines whether to perform an FNAB.
   2. Core biopsy can be used to diagnose thyroid lymphoma.
   3. FNAB of the dominant clinical nodule is the next best step.
   4. Biopsy should not be undertaken for anaplastic cancer.
   5. Biopsy is not necessary for long-standing goitres.
      (a) All are correct.
      (b) All are incorrect.
      (c) 3 and 5 are correct.
      (d) 2 and 5 only are correct.
      (e) 1, 2 and 3 are correct.
5. Regarding dysphagia
   1. It is more likely with retrosternal goitres.
   2. It is more likely with bilaterally enlarged goitres.
   3. It can be secondary to gastro-oesophageal reflux.
   4. It is suggestive of a malignant process.
   5. Upper intestinal endoscopy must be undertaken.
      (a) All are correct.
      (b) 1 only is correct.
      (c) 1 and 2 only are correct.
      (d) 1, 2 and 3 only are correct.
      (e) 1, 2, 3 and 4 only are correct.
6. Which of the following statements are true regarding the goitre in the clinical images above?
   1. This goitre could be treated with 131 iodine ablation.
   2. This goitre could be treated with thermal ablation.
   3. A median sternotomy may be required to excise this goitre.
   4. Preoperative vocal cord inspection is mandatory.
   5. This goitre might be extracted using the cervical approach alone.

   (a) All are correct.
   (b) 4 and 5 only are correct.
   (c) 3 and 4 only are correct.
   (d) 1 and 5 only are correct.
   (e) 3, 4 and 5 only are correct.

7. Which of the following statements are true?
   1. Unilateral nodular disease is best treated by hemithyroidectomy.
   2. A hemithyroidectomy carries a 50% risk of permanent hypothyroidism.
   3. A Dunhill operation has fewer complications compared with total thyroidectomy.
   4. Prescribing levothyroxine after hemithyroidectomy may reduce the risk of contralateral 'recurrence' in a subgroup of patients.
   5. Hemithyroidectomy avoids the risk of hypoparathyroidism.
      (a) 1, 2, 4 and 5 only are correct.
      (b) All are correct.
      (c) 1, 3 and 4 only are correct.
      (d) 1, 4 and 5 only are correct.
      (e) 1, 2, 3 and 4 only are correct.
8. Indications for a median sternotomy for retrosternal goitre include
   1. Pre-existing recurrent laryngeal nerve palsy
   2. Previous median sternotomy
   3. Working in a hospital with thoracic surgeons
   4. A preoperative diagnosis of papillary thyroid carcinoma
   5. Severe stridor
      (a) All are correct.
      (b) 1, 3 and 5 are correct.
      (c) 5 only is correct.
      (d) 3 only is correct.
      (e) None are correct.
9. For retrosternal goitre, the following complications are more common:
   1. Hypoparathyroidism
   2. Recurrent laryngeal nerve injury
   3. Postoperative haemorrhage
   4. Tracheomalacia
   5. Venous thromboembolic disease
      (a) All are correct.
      (b) 1, 2 and 3 only are correct.
      (c) 1, 2, 3, and 4 only are correct.
      (d) 1 and 2 only are correct.
      (e) 2 and 3 only are correct.
10. For a euthyroid benign solitary nodule, indications for surgical management include
    1. A nodule with a maximum diameter >4 cm
    2. The presence of dysphagia

3. In the case of significant cosmetic concerns
4. Tracheal deviation
5. A positive family history of thyroid cancer
   (a) All answers correct.
   (b) None of the answers are correct.
   (c) 2 and 3 only are correct.
   (d) 1 and 4 only are correct.
   (e) 1, 2 and 4 only are correct.

2.1 Introduction

The normal thyroid cannot be seen by inspection nor palpated. A visible or palpable thyroid gland is called a goitre (latin *guttur* = *throat*). A goitre may be large or small, hyper-, eu- or hypothyroid and can either be benign or malignant. So the term *goitre* tells us nothing about the aetiology; it is simply a short-hand term for an enlarged thyroid. Goitres can be *nodular* (solid or fluid-filled) or *diffuse*. A single thyroid nodule can also be called *solitary*. This chapter deals with euthyroid goitre.

2.2 Clinical Presentation

Patients present with a painless lump and are often unsure as to its duration. The increased size of the goitre can lead to symptoms related to pressure effects on adjacent structures such as dysphagia (from pharyngeal and/or oesophageal compression), globus sensation, hoarseness (from laryngeal or recurrent laryngeal nerve compression) or shortness of breath (from tracheal deviation and compression).

An incidental thyroid nodule (ITN) is one of the most common incidental findings on imaging studies that include the neck. Guidelines have been developed to assist the medical provider in deciding when and how to investigate ITN [1].

2.3 Natural History

The presence of goitre was originally determined from autopsy studies that weighed the thyroid gland, but this was superseded by the use of ultrasound by which a goitre is diagnosed if the size of the thyroid gland is greater than three standard deviations of the median (volume 18 ml for women and 25 ml for men). Goitre is more common in iodine-deficient regions of the world, where endemic goitre affects 10% of the population [1, 2]. In Framingham, clinically apparent nodules (palpation) were present in 6.4% of women and 1.5% of men [3]. The presence of single thyroid nodules was 3%, and multinodular goitre was 1%. In an autopsy study in 1955, 50% of people had thyroid nodules and the majority were multiple [4, 5]. Like autopsy, imaging frequently reveals subclinical thyroid nodules and, when ultrasound is used in epidemiological studies, the estimate of goitre prevalence is 19–67% [4]. Incidental thyroid nodules are seen in up to 25% of contrast-enhanced chest CT scans [6]; 16–18% of CT and MR scans of the neck [7, 8] and 1–2% PET scans [9]. In patients under 40 years, the goitre is typically a solitary nodule, whereas diffuse goitre is more common over the age of 65 years. The female to male ratio is 4:1 [10].

2.4 Aetiology

It is generally believed that the development of goitre depends on complex interactions amongst genetic, environmental and endogenous factors. Studies on monozygotic and dizygotic twins provide evidence to suggest that there is a genetic component to the aetiology of goitre [11]. Whilst various candidate genes have been associated with familial goitre, it appears that there is a considerable heterogeneity in familial goitre [11, 12]. The genetic contribution to goitre formation is more pronounced in areas of borderline iodine deficiency compared with areas of endemic goitre. Moreover, goitre with multiple nodules (multinodular goitre, MNG) is clearly influenced by genetic markers, whereas goitre with a solitary nodule most likely develops as a result of environmental exposures [13]. The most important risk factors associated with the genesis of goitre are smoking and iodine deficiency. In iodine-deficient areas of the world, people suffer from nodular goitre, whereas in iodine-abundant areas, diffuse goitre is more common [14]. Tobacco smoking increases the risk of goitre formation probably via iodine-mediated mechanisms. Thiocyanate from the metabolism of cyanide in tobacco smoke is a likely candidate [13].

2.5 Pathogenesis

The genetic development of goitre appears to be polygenic with no single gene being either necessary or sufficient for goitre development. A number of loci (MNG-1, and 3) have been identified on various chromosomes including 14, 19 and the X chromosome [13]. Iodine deficiency triggers hyperplasia and hypertrophy probably via the mutagenic effects of free oxygen radicals generated in the iodine-deficient thyroid and this process is independent of TSH [15]. Both diffuse and nodular goitre may occur secondary to subtle arrangements in thyroid hormonogenesis and TSH overproduction [15]. In smoking, thiocyanate from the metabolism of cyanide in tobacco smoke is a likely mediator for goitre formation [13].

2.6 Diagnosis

The goals from the history, clinical examination and special investigations are as follows:

- To confirm that the patient has a goitre
- To identify patients with thyroid cancer
- To identify patients with benign disease and compressive effects that would benefit from thyroid surgery

When present, growth of the lump is slow unless there has been haemorrhage into a cyst, in which case there is a very sudden onset/expansion. There will be an absence of symptoms of thyroid dysfunction and symptoms to suggest malignancy (rapid growth and hoarseness). A positive family history is common. It is important to enquire about the geographical background – does the patient come from a geographical area with endemic goitre?

2.7 Clinical Examination

Whilst taking the history it will become apparent if the patient has any audible hoarseness of the voice, stridor or breathlessness at rest. Inspection will allow you to form an impression about the patient's thyroid endocrine status. In the neck, any obvious mass is seen and the patient is asked to swallow a cup of water to determine if the mass rises. The examiner should look for dilated veins coursing over the anterior chest wall which would raise the suspicion of mediastinal venous hypertension (◘ Fig. 2.1).

Palpation can be performed standing behind the patient. The mass is confirmed as a goitre by palpation as the patient swallows water (as seen on inspection). The goitre is palpated and the size (cm), extent (solitary or diffuse), surface (smooth or nodular) and consistency (hard, rubbery or soft) are determined. You should examine for the lowest extent of the goitre on swallowing to determine if there is retrosternal extension. The trachea should be palpated (is it palpable and central?) and the lateral neck must be palpated for the presence or absence of lymph nodes. The sternum may be percussed to determine retrosternal dullness (an unreliable physical sign). In the presence of retrosternal extension, ask the patient to elevate their upper limbs to narrow the thoracic inlet and elicit Pemberton's sign (inducing facial plethora). With the arms elevated listen again for the presence of stridor.

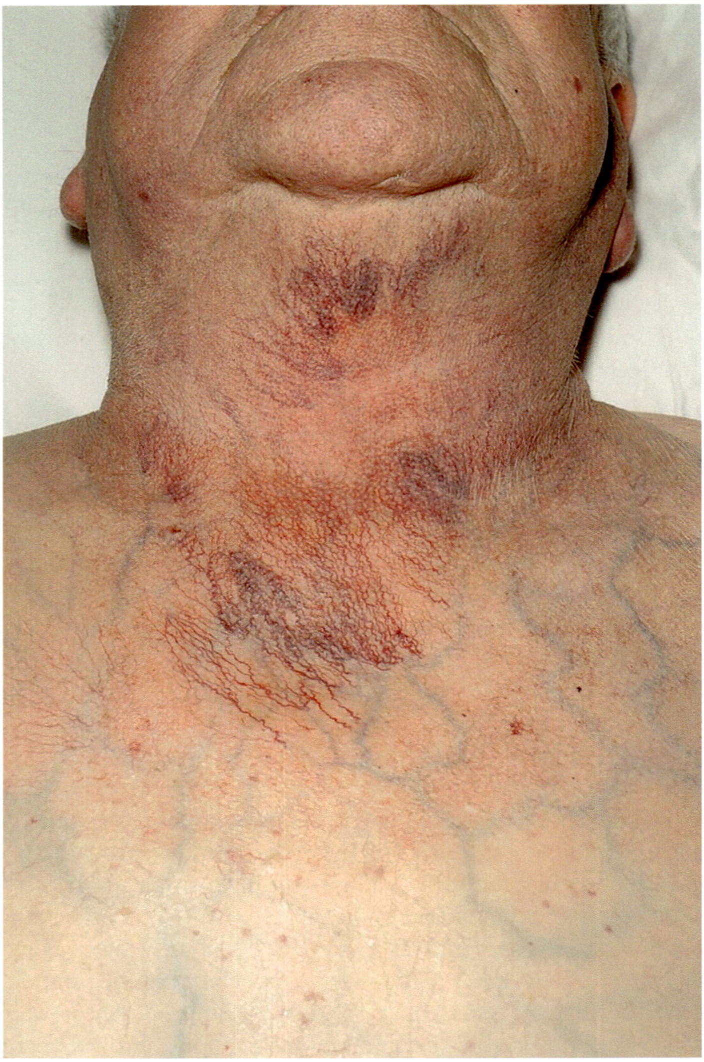

Fig. 2.1 Dilated veins over the chest wall in the presence of significant retrosternal extension

2.8 Thyroid Function Tests

All patients presenting with a goitre should undergo thyroid function tests. If abnormal, auto-antibody titres are measured. An elevated TSH is associated with a higher chance of malignancy [16].

2.8.1 Thyroid Ultrasound

Thyroid ultrasound can

- Confirm the patient has a thyroid lump
- Accurately measure its dimensions

- Provide information about the ultrasound characteristics of the goitre
- Determine the presence of suspicious cervical lymphadenopathy

The pattern of sonographic features confers a risk of malignancy and guides decision making about which nodules should undergo FNAB [17]. For example a hypoechoic solid nodule with calcifications and irregular margins requires a biopsy, whereas a purely cystic or spongiform lesion is less likely to need cytologic evaluation [17, 18]. Elastosonography is a relatively newer technique and nodules with high elasticity have a low probability of malignancy. This can further guide which nodules require FNAB [19].

2.8.2 Fine-Needle Aspiration Biopsy (FNAB)

Most thyroid nodules are benign (95%). The main goal in assessing a patient with a goitre is to identify those patients who require thyroid surgery. FNAB is the most useful preoperative tool to diagnose malignancy. The nodules that should undergo biopsy include the following:

- Nodules >10 mm with high-risk sonographic features (hypoechoic solid nodule with microcalcification, irregularity, taller than wide shape, evidence of extrathyroid extension (ETE))
- Nodules >10 mm with intermediate sonographic suspicion (hypoechoic, solid nodule with smooth margins without microcalcifications, irregularity, ETE, wider than tall shape)
- Nodules >15 mm with low sonographic suspicion (isoechoic or hyperechoic solid nodules, partially cystic nodules with eccentric solid area) [17]

The biopsy result is classified according to the Bethesda (USA) or Thy (UK) classification system.

2.8.3 Precision Medicine

Precision medicine is defined as 'the right treatment for the right patient at the right time'. For the indeterminate thyroid nodule this translates to the 'right clinical decision for the right cytology, with the right test'. A vast amount of effort has been invested in trying to identify cancers in the population of patients with indeterminate cytology. The approach can either be to try and identify cancers by searching for the presence of somatic mutations (rule-in approach) or to try and identify patients with benign nodules (rule-out).

Rule-in tests are designed to drive the clinician to recommend surgery in the case of a positive result. Rule-in searches for a number of mutations simultaneously (*BRAF, NRAS, HRAS* and *KRAS* mutations and *PAX8/PPARG*- and *RET/PTC* rearrangements) and to be successful a high positive predictive value is required. Rule-out tests are designed to identify patients who have benign disease and do not require follow-up. To be successful, it requires a high negative predictive value. The drawback to the test is the lack of long-term outcome data on patients excluded from surgery.

Currently, no test is wholly reliable and the greatest barrier to their use is cost [20, 21].

2.8.4 Cross-Sectional Scans

CT scanning is indicated for retrosternal goitre and can provide information on the following:

- Confirmation of the presence and determination of extent of retrosternal extension
- A 'road map' for the anaesthetist (tracheal deviation and compression)
- Oesophageal compression
- At-risk anatomical structures in the impending surgical field
- An assessment of malignancy (not accessible by ultrasound)
- Anterior versus posterior mediastinal extension
- The likelihood that the goitre can be extracted without the need for a sternotomy (the 'shape' of the goitre)

2.8.5 Laryngeal Examination

Despite a thorough patient history, subtle voice changes are not easily volunteered by patients and may be difficult for clinicians to detect. Also, there is a significant divergence between voice symptoms and objective vocal cord function. Indeed, the sensitivity of voice change in predicting VCP can range from 33% to 68% [22, 23]. Thus, vocal cord paralysis may be present without significant vocal symptoms (and vice versa). Goitres can directly compress the recurrent laryngeal nerve which provides a rationale for the inclusion of a preoperative glottic examination in these patients to facilitate surgical planning, aid intraoperative decision making and optimize patient counselling.

2.9 Management

Indications for treatment include the following:
- Suspicion of malignancy
- Compression of trachea
- Compression of oesophagus
- Quality of life

The patients at particular risk for these symptoms are those with a retrosternal component. When the goitre is confined to the neck, the overlying skin and subcutaneous tissues are stretched and the patient may only notice a visible lump in the neck. However, when the goitre plunges behind the bones (clavicular head and manubrium), the confined space causes adjacent soft tissue structures to become compressed, principally the trachea and oesophagus (◘ Fig. 2.2). Tracheal involvement can either result in deviation or narrowing. Tracheal deviation is typically asymptomatic and does not require surgery (◘ Fig. 2.3). Tracheal compression results in upper airway obstruction (UAO) with suppression of the inspiratory capacity which can be detected on flow loop volume analysis. The patients may have stridor and/or complain of exertional dyspnoea.

Oesophageal compression is less common than tracheal and more difficult to quantify. Contrast swallowing radiologi-

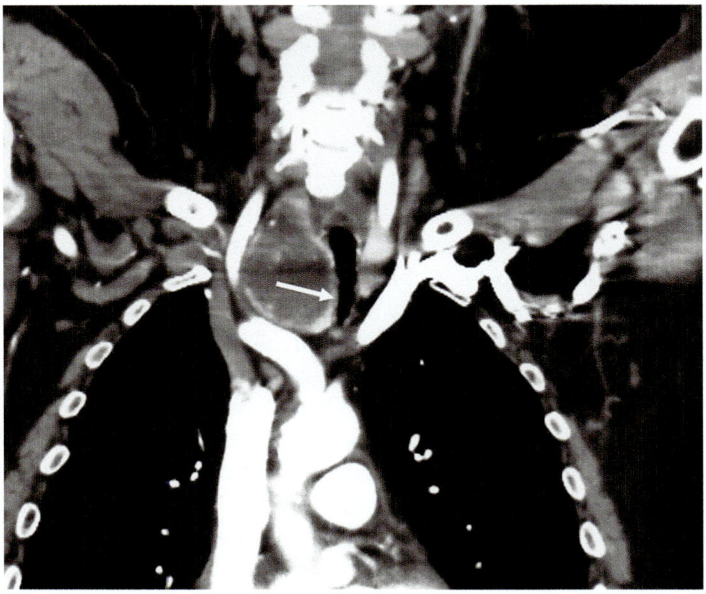

◘ **Fig. 2.2** Coronal plane of CT scan showing retrosternal right goitre with deviation and compression of the trachea (arrow)

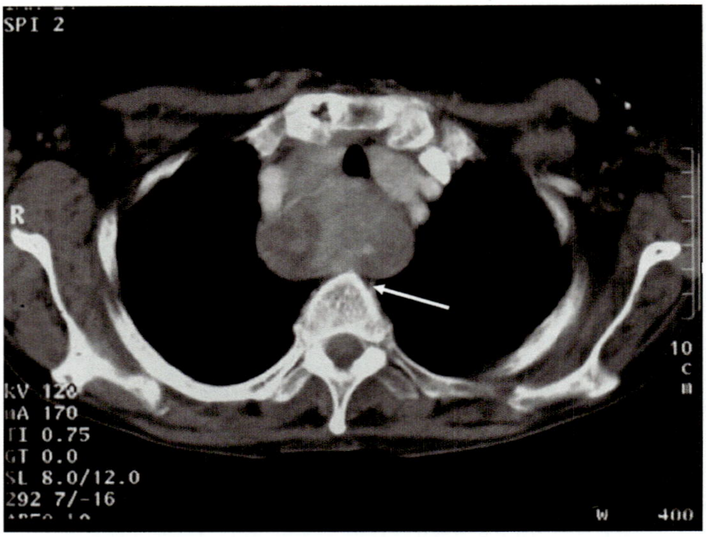

Fig. 2.3 Cross-sectional CT scan of the neck at the level of the manubrium in a patient with dysphagia to solid food. A goitre can be seen to be sited between the trachea and the oesophagus (arrow)

cal studies are often unhelpful and the surgeon should rely on the history and cross-sectional imaging to determine whether surgery is likely to be of benefit (Fig. 2.3). In severe cases, large vessel venous compression may manifest as superior vena cava syndrome.

There are three options for management.

2.9.1 Conservative

Many patients with goitre have no or only a few symptoms. In the absence of any concern about malignancy (either by ultrasound and/or biopsy) or compressive symptoms, it is very reasonable to manage patients with goitre conservatively. Treat the patient, not the X-ray. Be aware that some apparent retrosternal goitres on CT scan may be exaggerated by a patient's flexed neck at the time of the scan. When looking at the CT scan, take note of where the chin is, in relation to the thyroid. Some 'retrosternal goitres' can be cured by neck extension! Most goitres (90%) do not progress in size and those that do, do so slowly [24]. It is reasonable to offer to review the patient after a 6–12-month period and if there has been no progression and the patient is happy to avoid surgery, then the patient can be discharged. Note that there is a poor correlation between goitre size and symptoms. Be aware that some symptoms may be unrelated to the goitre. This is especially so for patients with neck discomfort. Care must be taken in attributing symptoms to a goitre when the patient has an underlying lung condition (e.g. COPD) or gastro-oesophageal reflux disease.

2.10 Non-surgical (Means to Debulk the Thyroid)

2.10.1 Radio-iodine Therapy

Surgery has the uncontested advantage that it provides a rapid and comprehensive removal of the goitre. However, there are certain situations when a non-surgical approach might be considered:

- Previous thyroid surgery
- Severe co-morbidity
- Intrathoracic location

131I therapy reduces the volume of non-toxic nodular goitres by 35–50% within 1 year [25]. A prerequisite is sufficient radio-iodine uptake in the target tissue which can be evaluated qualitatively by thyroid scintigraphy.

Complications can be classified as early and late. A radiation-induced thyroiditis is occasionally seen in the early days after treatment. Adjuvant glucocorticoids might be considered in patients with significant tracheal compression. Patients may also experience a transient hyperthyroid state, but this is usually subclinical. In the longer term, about 20% of patients may develop hypothyroidism. The risk of malignancy remains unproven [25, 26]. For patients requiring a rapid debulking and for those with a larger goitre (>100 ml), surgery remains the preferred option.

2.10.2 Thermal Ablation

There are a number of 'minimally invasive techniques' performed under local anaesthesia. They all induce thermonecrosis via a local circumscribed damage of tissue when temperatures rise to between 65 and 100 degrees Celsius. The cells are irreversibly destroyed and degraded by the body, resulting in a reduction in volume of thyroid tissue over subsequent months. The variety of techniques include the following:

- Laser ablation
- Microwave ablation
- High intensity focused ultrasound
- Mono- and bi-polar radiofrequency ablation

Prerequisites to these forms of treatment include exclusion of malignancy (FNAB), vocal cord assessment and informed consent [27]. These techniques are relatively new, and long-term data is not available. However, the published outcomes suggest that these techniques offer an alternative to surgery especially for the smaller benign nodules. Relative contraindications include diffuse enlargement, larger nodules (>30 ml) and nodules with far caudal extension [28].

2.11 Surgical

2.11.1 Thyroid Surgery

The details of thyroid surgery are covered in ▶ Chap. 11. However, there are different approaches to the treatment of the euthyroid nodular goitre that deserve special consideration.

2.11.2 Hemithyroidectomy

Multinodular goitre is often asymmetric and only one half of the thyroid is affected in about one half of all patients [29]. In this scenario, a hemithyroidectomy is a reasonable option as it avoids the possibility of hypoparathyroidism, halves the risk of recurrent laryngeal nerve injury and reduces the risk of hypothyroidism (22%) [30]. The disadvantage of this approach is the potential for contralateral progression of the goitre and the later need for a second completion operation. This can be mitigated with the prescription of levothyroxine which reduces the risk of progression from 16.7% to 1.4% [31]. All of these issues must be discussed with the patient before a management plan is agreed.

2.11.3 Subtotal Thyroidectomy or Total Thyroidectomy

Historically, the approach for diffuse multinodular goitre was a unilateral total lobectomy and contralateral subtotal lobectomy (Dunhill operation). A total thyroidectomy was proposed in order to abolish the risk of recurrent goitre and the need for re-operative surgery with its much higher morbidity [32]. The concern about shifting to a total thyroidectomy is the higher risks of permanent recurrent laryngeal nerve injury and hypoparathyroidism. However, more recent data suggests that these risks are not greater when the surgery is undertaken by higher volume surgeons [17]. In a randomised study comparing Dunhill with total thyroidectomy, the recurrent goitre rate was 8.6% versus 0.6% with a subsequent re-operative rate of 2.8% versus 0.6% [33]. For bilateral multinodular goitre, total thyroidectomy is the operation of choice.

2.11.4 Retrosternal Goitre

It is desirable to avoid a median sternotomy with its associated morbidity whenever possible. The majority of retrosternal goitres (90%) can be extracted via a cervical excision [34]. Risk factors for a non-cervical approach include involvement of multiple mediastinal compartments, iceberg morphology,

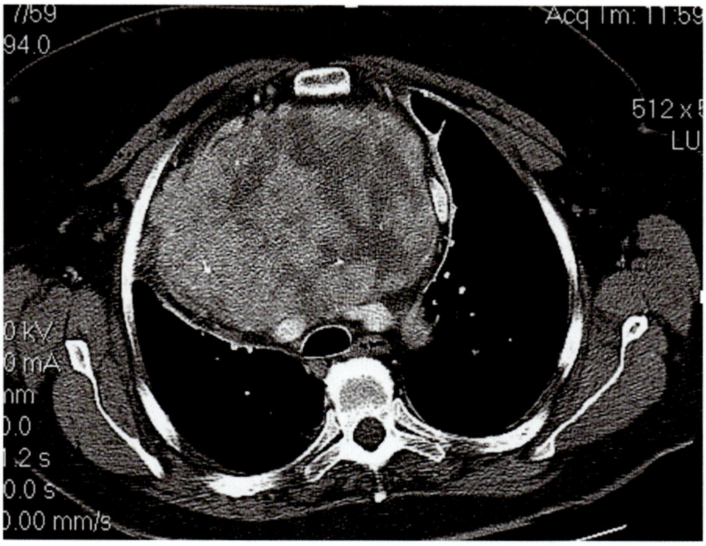

Fig. 2.4 Cross-sectional CT scan demonstrating a huge anterior mediastinal goitre for which a cervical extraction is not possible

extension to the posterior pleura and goitre with separate components (Fig. 2.4) [35]. All of these can be determined by cross-sectional imaging of the neck and thorax. Where there is a risk for an extracervical access, a thoracic surgeon should be engaged early in the planning stage. It is equally important that an anaesthetist with experience in the 'difficult airway' is a member of the multidisciplinary team. There is an increased risk of injury to the recurrent laryngeal nerve due to a combination of distorted anatomy, a longer length of nerve dissection and at times a suboptimal view of the nerve [36]. Intermittent intraoperative nerve monitoring can assist in nerve localisation and continuous monitoring may help prevent traction related nerve injuries. Equally, identification of the inferior parathyroid glands may be more demanding and so, the surgeon must be obsessive in identifying the superior glands to minimise the risk of hypoparathyroidism. Retrosternal goitre is an independent risk factor for postoperative haemorrhage [37]. Whilst tracheomalacia is a justifiable concern in patients with tracheal compression, this complication is very rarely observed in the Western World. Owing to the large dead space at the end of the resection, drains are often deployed.

2.11.5 Video-Assisted Thoracoscopic Thyroidectomy

This minimally invasive approach has been adopted by some thoracic surgeons with less morbidity compared to median sternotomy. Several ports are placed into the chest between the ribs. The conversion rate to open surgery is less than 10% [38].

2

2.11.6 Transoral Thyroidectomy

The minimally invasive approach to thyroidectomy via the oral vestibular route has been developed and is currently under evaluation. It adheres to the principles of minimally invasive surgery using an endoscopic approach anterior to the mandible between the mentalis muscles. Contraindications to this approach are thyroid volume: >45 ml or a dominant nodule size >50 mm [39]. The sole benefit of this novel approach is cosmetic. The technique is very demanding and is yet to be adopted as a mainstream approach by thyroid surgeons.

Answers to the Questions

1. (a); 2. (d); 3. (b); 4. (e); 5. (d); 6. (e); 7. (d); 8. (e); 9. (b); 10. (c)

References

1. Hoang JK, Langer JE, Middleton WD, Wu CC, Hammers LW, Cronan JJ, Tessler FN, Grant EG, Berland LL. Managing incidental thyroid nodules detected on imaging: white paper of the ACR incidental thyroid findings committee. J Am Coll Radiol. 2015;12:143–50.
2. Wang C, Crapo LM. The epidemiology of thyroid disease and implications for screening. Endocrinol Metab Clin N Am. 1997;26:189–218.
3. Vander JB, Gaston EA, Dawber TR. The significance of nontoxic thyroid nodules. Final report of a 15-year study of the incidence of thyroid malignancy. Ann Intern Med. 1968;69:537–40.
4. Tan GH, Gharib H. Thyroid incidentalomas: management approaches to nonpalpable nodules discovered incidentally on thyroid imaging. Ann Intern Med. 1997;126:226–31.
5. Mortensen JD, Woolner LB, Bennett WA. Gross and microscopic findings in clinically normal thyroid glands. J Clin Endocrinol Metab. 1955;15:1270–80.
6. Ahmed S, Horton KM, Jeffrey RB Jr, Sheth S, Fishman EK. Incidental thyroid nodules on chest CT: review of the literature and management suggestions. AJR Am J Roentgenol. 2010;195:1066–71.
7. Youserm DM, Huang T, Loevner LA, Langlotz CP. Clinical and economic impact of incidental thyroid lesions found with CT and MR. AJNR Am J Neuroradiol. 1997;18:1423–8.
8. Nguyen XV, Choudhury KR, Eastwood JD, Lyman GH, Esclamado RM, Werner JD, Hoang JK. Incidental thyroid nodules on CT: evaluation of 2 risk-categorization methods for work-up of nodules. AJNR Am J Neuroradiol. 2013;34:1812–7.
9. Soelberg KK, Bonnema SJ, Brix TH, Hegedüs L. Risk of malignancy in thyroid incidentalomas detected by 18F-fluorodeoxyglucose positron emission tomography: a systematic review. Thyroid. 2012;22:918–25.
10. Tunbridge WM, Evered DC, Hall R, Appleton D, Brewis M, Clark F, Evans JG, Young E, Bird T, Smith PA. Lipid profiles and cardiovascular disease in the Whickham area with particular reference to thyroid failure. Clin Endocrinol. 1977;7:495–508.
11. Hawkes CH. Twin studies in medicine – what do they tell us? QJM. 1997;90:311–21.
12. Brix TH, Hegedüs L. Genetic and environmental factors in the aetiology of simple goitre. Ann Med. 2000;32:153–6.
13. Knudsen N, Brix TH. Genetic and non-iodine-related factors in the aetiology of nodular goitre. Best Pract Res Clin Endocrinol Metab. 2014;28:495–506.

14. Carlé A, Krejbjerg A, Laurberg P. Epidemiology of nodular goitre. Influence of iodine intake. Best Pract Res Clin Endocrinol Metab. 2014;28:465–79.
15. Krohn K, Führer D, Bayer Y, Eszlinger M, Brauer V, Neumann S, Paschke R. Molecular pathogenesis of euthyroid and toxic multinodular goiter. Endocr Rev. 2005;26:504–24.
16. Boelaert K, Horacek J, Holder RL, Watkinson JC, Sheppard MC, Franklyn JA. Serum thyrotropin concentration as a novel predictor of malignancy in thyroid nodules investigated by fine-needle aspiration. J Clin Endocrinol Metab. 2006;91:4295–301.
17. Haugen BR, Alexander EK, Bible KC, et al. 2015 American Thyroid Association management guidelines for adult patients with thyroid nodules and differentiated thyroid cancer: the American Thyroid Association guidelines task force on thyroid nodules and differentiated thyroid cancer. Thyroid. 2016;26:1–133.
18. Gharib H, Papini E, Garber JR, Duick DS, Harrell RM, Hegedüs L, Paschke R, Valcavi R, Vitti P, AACE/ACE/AME Task Force on Thyroid Nodules. American Association of Clinical Endocrinologists, American College of Endocrinology, and Associazione Medici Endocrinologi medical guidelines for clinical practice for the diagnosis and management of thyroid nodules – 2016 update. Endocr Pract. 2016;22:622–39.
19. Rago T, Scutari M, Loiacono V, et al. Low elasticity of thyroid nodules on ultrasound elastography is correlated with malignancy, degree of fibrosis, and high expression of Galectin-3 and Fibronectin-1. Thyroid. 2017;27:103–10.
20. Vargas-Salas S, Martínez JR, Urra S, Domínguez JM, Mena N, Uslar T, Lagos M, Henríquez M, González HE. Genetic testing for indeterminate thyroid cytology: review and meta-analysis. Endocr Relat Cancer. 2018;25:R163–77.
21. González HE, Martínez JR, Vargas-Salas S, et al. A 10-gene classifier for indeterminate thyroid nodules: development and multicenter accuracy study. Thyroid. 2017;27:1058–67.
22. Randolph GW, Kamani D. The importance of preoperative laryngoscopy in patients undergoing thyroidectomy: voice, vocal cord function, and the preoperative detection of invasive thyroid malignancy. Surgery. 2006;139:357–62.
23. Farrag TY, Samlan RA, Lin FR, Tufano RP. The utility of evaluating true vocal fold motion before thyroid surgery. Laryngoscope. 2006;116:235–8.
24. Durante C, Costante G, Lucisano G, et al. The natural history of benign thyroid nodules. JAMA. 2015;313:926–35.
25. Nygaard B, Hegedüs L, Ulriksen P, Nielsen KG, Hansen JM. Radioiodine therapy for multinodular toxic goiter. Arch Intern Med. 1999;159:1364–8.
26. Bonnema SJ, Fast S, Hegedüs L. The role of radioiodine therapy in benign nodular goitre. Best Pract Res Clin Endocrinol Metab. 2014;28:619–31.
27. Dobnig H, Zechmann W, Hermann M, et al. Radiofrequency ablation of thyroid nodules: "Good Clinical Practice Recommendations" for Austria : an interdisciplinary statement from the following professional associations: Austrian Thyroid Association (ÖSDG), Austrian Society for Nuclear Medicine and Molecular Imaging (OGNMB), Austrian Society for Endocrinology and Metabolism (ÖGES), Surgical Endocrinology Working Group (ACE) of the Austrian Surgical Society (OEGCH). Wien Med Wochenschr. 2020;170:6–14.
28. Dobnig H, Amrein K. Value of monopolar and bipolar radiofrequency ablation for the treatment of benign thyroid nodules. Best Pract Res Clin Endocrinol Metab. 2019;33:101283.
29. Gharib H, Papini E, Paschke R, Duick DS, Valcavi R, Hegedüs L, Vitti P, AACE/AME/ETA Task Force on Thyroid Nodules. American Association of Clinical Endocrinologists, Associazione Medici

Endocrinologi, and European Thyroid Association medical guidelines for clinical practice for the diagnosis and management of thyroid nodules: executive summary of recommendations. J Endocrinol Investig. 2010;33:51–6.
30. Louwerens M, Appelhof BC, Verloop H, Medici M, Peeters RP, Visser TJ, Boelen A, Fliers E, Smit JWA, Dekkers OM. Fatigue and fatigue-related symptoms in patients treated for different causes of hypothyroidism. Eur J Endocrinol. 2012;167:809–15.
31. Barczyński M, Konturek A, Hubalewska-Dydejczyk A, Gołkowski F, Cichoń S, Nowak W. Five-year follow-up of a randomized clinical trial of total thyroidectomy versus Dunhill operation versus bilateral subtotal thyroidectomy for multinodular nontoxic goiter. World J Surg. 2010;34:1203–13.
32. Delbridge L, Guinea AI, Reeve TS. Total thyroidectomy for bilateral benign multinodular goiter: effect of changing practice. Arch Surg. 1999;134:1389–93.
33. Barczyński M, Konturek A, Hubalewska-Dydejczyk A, Gołkowski F, Nowak W. Ten-year follow-up of a randomized clinical trial of total thyroidectomy versus Dunhill operation versus bilateral subtotal thyroidectomy for multinodular non-toxic goiter. World J Surg. 2018;42:384–92.
34. Shaha AR, Alfonso AE, Jaffe BM. Operative treatment of substernal goiters. Head Neck. 1989;11:325–30.
35. Simó R, Nixon IJ, Poorten VV, Quer M, Shaha AR, Sanabria A, Alvarez FL, Angelos P, Rinaldo A, Ferlito A. Surgical management of intrathoracic goitres. Eur Arch Otorhinolaryngol. 2019;276:305–14.
36. Testini M, Gurrado A, Bellantone R, et al. Recurrent laryngeal nerve palsy and substernal goiter. An Italian multicenter study. J Visc Surg. 2014;151:183–9.
37. Hanson MA, Shaha AR, Wu JX. Surgical approach to the substernal goiter. Best Pract Res Clin Endocrinol Metab. 2019;33:101312.
38. Gupta P, Lau KKW, Rizvi I, Rathinam S, Waller DA. Video assisted thoracoscopic thyroidectomy for retrosternal goitre. Ann R Coll Surg Engl. 2014;96:606–8.
39. Zhang D, Park D, Sun H, Anuwong A, Tufano R, Kim HY, Dionigi G. Indications, benefits and risks of transoral thyroidectomy. Best Pract Res Clin Endocrinol Metab. 2019;33:101280.

Graves' Disease and Toxic Nodular Goiter (Plummer's Disease)

Marcin Barczyński

Contents

A. L. Shifrin et al. (eds.), *Endocrine Surgery Comprehensive Board Exam Guide*,
https://doi.org/10.1007/978-3-030-84737-1_3

3

Case Presentation

A 48-year-old female, with a past medical history of Graves' disease and 2 years status post–radioiodine ablation, presented to a clinic, after a 2-year lapse in healthcare. She had increasing anxiety over the past several months regarding her perceived worsening state of health, particularly the recent weight gain and facial edema. Upon further questioning, the patient also reported hair loss, dry skin, hoarse voice, constipation, difficulty sleeping, fatigue, depression, anxiety, arthralgias, and myalgias. Her past medical history was significant only for Graves' disease treated with radioiodine ablation. She denied ever taking thyroid replacement medication after her thyroid ablation due to a lack of such a recommendation.

On initial presentation, her body mass index (BMI) was 28.7 kg/m^2, temperature 36.0 °C, blood pressure 100/70 mmHg, and pulse 54 beats per minute. Physical exam was remarkable for hoarse voice, bradycardia, dry skin on her hands and legs bilaterally, tender scalp, and facial edema. Electrocardiogram (ECG) revealed marked sinus bradycardia (heart rate (HR) 44), low voltage, and nonspecific T wave changes.

Although the patient's longstanding untreated hypothyroidism was quickly identified and confirmed with TSH serum level of 102.4 mIU/L (reference range: 0.27–4.5 mIU/L), a comprehensive evaluation was completed to rule out other contributing factors. Lipid panel, comprehensive metabolic panel, and complete blood count revealed hypercholesterolemia, elevated liver enzymes, and mild normocytic anemia, respectively.

The patient was started on levothyroxine 50 mcg/day, and the dose was slowly adjusted according to serial TSH levels. On week 8, from the onset of levothyroxine replacement therapy, the dose was 112 mcg/day and serum TSH level was 2.4 mIU/L. Once she became euthyroid, her cholesterol, low-density lipoprotein (LDL), and triglycerides improved, while her hemoglobin, creatinine, and aspartate aminotransferase (AST) levels normalized. The patient reported improved balance and stability, facial edema disappeared, increased body hair growth, softer skin, more regular bowel movements, uninterrupted sleep, increased energy, and improved mood. She continued to have myalgias and arthralgias, which were treated conservatively with nonsteroidal anti-inflammatory medication with clinical improvement. On exam, her voice was less hoarse, heart rate increased, skin appeared normal, face was normal, and she was more relaxed. Follow-up ECG showed improved sinus bradycardia and nonspecific T wave changes. After treatment, the patient stated that she felt better than she had in many months. She continues to come to the clinic every 6 months for TSH monitoring.

Questions

1. The symptoms of hyperthyroidism include
   1. Nervousness, anxiety, irritability, emotional liability
   2. Weight gain and facial edema
   3. Hair loss, thinning of the hair
   4. More frequent bowel movements/diarrhea
   5. Increased sweating
      - (a) Only (1) and (2) and (3) are correct.
      - (b) Only (1) and (2) and (4) are correct.
      - (c) Only (1) and (3) and (4) are correct.
      - (d) Only (1) and (3) and (4) and (5) are correct.
      - (e) All are correct.

2. Signs of hyperthyroidism include
   1. Menstrual disorders
   2. Tachycardia
   3. Systolic hypertension
   4. Proximal muscle weakness
   5. Diarrhea
      (a) Only (1) and (2) and (3) are correct.
      (b) Only (1) and (2) and (4) are correct.
      (c) Only (1) and (3) and (4) are correct.
      (d) Only (2) and (3) and (4) are correct.
      (e) All are correct.
3. Low serum TSH and normal serum FT4 and FT3 correspond to
   1. Overt hyperthyroidism
   2. Subclinical hyperthyroidism
   3. Overt hypothyroidism;
   4. Subclinical hypothyroidism
      (a) Only (1) and (2) and (3) are correct.
      (b) Only (1) and (2) and (4) are correct.
      (c) Only (2) is correct.
      (d) Only (1) and (2) are correct.
      (e) All are correct.
4. The diagnosis of Graves' disease is very likely in the following situations:
   1. Overt or subclinical hyperthyroidism and an increased anti-TSHR serum level
   2. Hyperthyroidism accompanied by thyroid orbitopathy with clear involvement of the soft tissues of the orbits or thyroid dermopathy
   3. Hyperthyroidism with goiter confirmed by ultrasound (diffuse parenchymal hypoechogenicity) – if anti-TSHR antibodies cannot be determined
   4. Isolated thyroid orbitopathy and increased anti-TSHR serum level
      (a) Only (1) and (2) and (3) are correct.
      (b) Only (1) and (2) and (4) are correct.
      (c) Only (2) and (4) are correct
      (d) Only (2) is correct.
      (e) All are correct.
5. The diagnosis of Graves' disease is likely if
   1. There are relapses of hyperthyroidism, separated by periods of euthyroidism lasting >6 months without the use of antithyroid drugs.
   2. There are cases of Graves' disease or Hashimoto's disease in the family of a patient with hyperthyroidism, or another autoimmune disease.
   3. There is limited but diffuse ^{123}I thyroid uptake on scintigraphy.
   4. There is limited but diffuse ^{99m}Tc thyroid uptake on scintigraphy.

(a) Only (1) and (2) and (3) are correct.
(b) Only (1) and (2) and (4) are correct.
(c) Only (3) and (4) are correct.
(d) Only (1) and (2) are correct.
(e) All are correct.

6. What statements regarding differential diagnosis of hyperthyroidism are correct?
   1. The diagnosis of Graves' disease should be based on signs of thyrotoxicosis, elevation in serum fT4 and fT3 levels, suppression of TSH, and elevated level of anti-TSHR antibody.
   2. Thyroid scintigraphy, which demonstrates diffuse and remarkably elevated uptake of ^{123}I, suggests a diagnosis of Graves' disease.
   3. Patients with Plummer's disease have thyrotoxicosis but are negative for anti-TSHR antibody and show scintigraphic patterns of multifocal uptake of ^{123}I.
   4. Increased thyroid blood flow in whole thyroids on ultrasound in patients with hyperthyroidism suggests the existence of Graves' disease, whereas nodules showing increased thyroid blood flow in anti-TSHR-negative patients with hyperthyroidism are suggestive for Plummer's disease.

   (a) Only (1) and (2) and (3) are correct.
   (b) Only (1) and (2) and (4) are correct.
   (c) Only (3) and (4) are correct.
   (d) Only (1) and (2) are correct.
   (e) All are correct.
7. What statements regarding Graves' disease are correct?
   1. There is no effective causative treatment of Graves' disease, only the symptoms are treated like hyperthyroidism and orbitopathy.
   2. The first goal of treatment is to achieve euthyroidism as soon as possible and to make a decision together with the patient on a further treatment strategy.
   3. There are three therapeutic alternatives for GD: antithyroid drugs, radioactive iodine, and thyroidectomy.
   4. Each modality has its own advantages and disadvantages.

   (a) Only (1) and (4) are correct.
   (b) Only (1) and (3) are correct.
   (c) Only (2) and (4) are correct.
   (d) Only (2) and (3) are correct.
   (e) All are correct.
8. Which statements regarding toxic multinodular goiter are correct?
   1. The etiologic factors involved in the formation of a toxic multinodular goiter include an inherent functional heterogeneity of thyroid follicles.

2. The etiologic factors involved in the formation of a toxic multinodular goiter include the effect of growth factors and goitrogens.
3. The etiologic factors involved in the formation of a toxic multinodular goiter include iodine deficiency.
4. The etiologic factors involved in the formation of a toxic multinodular goiter include genetic abnormalities that include somatic activating mutations of genes that regulate thyroid growth and hormone synthesis.
   (a) Only (1) and (2) and (3) are correct.
   (b) Only (1) and (2) and (4) are correct.
   (c) Only (1) and (3) and (4) are correct.
   (d) Only (2) and (3) and (4) are correct.
   (e) All are correct.

9. Which statement regarding toxic multinodular goiter are correct?
   1. There are two main goals for treatment in patients with TMNG: to eliminate an autonomously functioning thyroid tissue and to alleviate compressive symptom.
   2. Pharmacological treatment with antithyroid drugs (methimazole) allows for controlling the symptoms of hyperthyroidism, but its withdrawal always leads to the relapse of the hyperthyroidism (after a few days to several weeks).
   3. The beta-blocker is used similarly to other types of hyperthyroidism, but in TMNG, it is needed more often and in higher doses than in Graves' disease due to the greater severity of cardiac symptoms.
   4. Definitive treatment options for TMNG are either surgical (subtotal or total thyroidectomy) or radioiodine ablation, and the choice of method is not individualized for each patient.
      (a) Only (1) and (2) and (3) are correct.
      (b) Only (2) and (3) and (4) are correct.
      (c) Only (3) and (4) are correct.
      (d) Only (4) is correct.
      (e) All are correct.

10. Which statements regarding toxic multinodular goiter are correct?
    1. Surgical resection is the preferred treatment option in patients with a nodule with cytological or clinical features of malignancy and also in patients with a large goiter giving compression symptoms, especially in the presence of inactive thyroid nodules, unless there are contraindications for surgery.
    2. The operation is possible only after euthyroid state is achieved.
    3. Treatment with methimazole should be stopped on the day of surgery, and the dose of beta-blocker should be gradually reduced to discontinue it within a few days after surgery.

4. Potassium iodide should be given 5–10 days before surgery.
   (a) Only (1) and (2) are correct.
   (b) Only (1) and (2) and (3) are correct.
   (c) Only (2) and (3) are correct.
   (d) Only (4) is correct.
   (e) All are correct.

11. Which statements regarding toxic multinodular goiter are correct?
    1. The presence of substernal thyroid extension or airway obstruction is a relative contraindication for RAI because of the potential for transient increase in size of the goiter and worsening of airway compromise through RAI-induced transient radiation thyroiditis.
    2. The extent of surgery should be total or near-total thyroidectomy.
    3. Subtotal thyroidectomy (Dunhill operation) may be considered in patient who experienced intraoperative loss of signal of neuromonitoring after removal of the first-attempted lobe, and usually dominant thyroid lobe (a staged thyroidectomy).
    4. The risk of permanent surgical morbidity is low (<1–2%) if surgery is performed by a high-volume thyroid surgeon.
    5. In untreated TMNG, the risk of arrhythmias and other cardiovascular complications as well as thyroid crisis is not increased.
    6. The risk of cancer is far lower than in other forms of nodular goiter.
       (a) Only (1) and (2) and (3) and (4) are correct.
       (b) Only (2) and (3) and (5) and (6) are correct.
       (c) Only (1) and (3) and (4) and (6) are correct.
       (d) Only (2) and (3) and (4) and (6) are correct.
       (e) All are correct.

3.1 Introduction

Primary hyperthyroidism is a set of disorders in which the thyroid gland synthesizes and secretes too much thyroid hormones for the body's needs, which leads to the hypermetabolic condition of thyrotoxicosis. The thyroid gland is a small organ located at the base of the neck. It is responsible for the production and release of two hormones: triiodothyronine (T3) and thyroxine (T4), which regulate the function of most tissues of the body, influence the metabolism of our body and thermogenesis (heat production). The thyroid gland is controlled by the pituitary gland, which releases thyroid-stimulating hormone (TSH), which stimulates the thyroid gland to produce the hormones T3 and T4.

The activities of the thyroid gland and pituitary gland are closely related (known as negative feedback), in which the increased concentration of thyroid hormones reduces the release of TSH by the pituitary gland, and the deficiency of these hormones increases the production of TSH, which in turn stimulates the thyroid to produce more T3 and T4.

The term hyperthyroidism is distinct from thyrotoxicosis, a clinical state in which there is an inappropriately high thyroid hormone action in tissues. Thyrotoxicosis can result from hyperthyroidism as well as from other etiologies like subacute, painless, or radiation-induced thyroiditis, excessive intake of thyroid hormone, struma ovarii, and functional metastatic thyroid cancer.

The most common causes of hyperthyroidism include: Graves' disease (an autoimmune disease in which your own antibodies stimulate the thyroid gland to produce hormones), thyroid nodules (hyperactive [toxic] multinodular goiter [Plummer's disease], or a solitary thyroid autonomic tumor). The less common causes of hyperthyroidism include subacute thyroiditis (a disease associated with a previous viral infection), postpartum thyroiditis, and amiodarone-induced thyrotoxicosis.

The overall prevalence of hyperthyroidism, which is approximately 1.3% (it occurs in 2% of women and 0.5% in men), increases to 4–5% in older women. Hyperthyroidism is also more common in smokers. Graves' disease is seen most often in younger women, while toxic nodular goiter is more common in older women [1].

3.1.1 Clinical Presentation of Hyperthyroidism

The main symptoms and manifestations that suggest thyrotoxicosis are presented in ◘ Box 3.1, while signs of hyperthyroidism are listed in ◘ Box 3.2.

The extent of symptoms may differ from patient to patient. In the elderly, the symptoms of hyperthyroidism may be less pronounced and subtle. Weakness, asthenia, fatigue, and problems with the circulatory system may predominate – heart rhythm disturbances (atrial fibrillation), ischemic heart disease, and symptoms of congestive heart failure.

Box 3.1 Symptoms and Manifestations of Hyperthyroidism

Feeling hot, heat intolerance
- Increased sweating
- Nervousness, anxiety, irritability, emotional liability
- Shaking hands
- Losing weight, despite increased appetite

More frequent bowel movements/diarrhea
Increase in heart rate, feeling your heart racing, palpitations
Muscle weakness
Insomnia
Hair loss, thinning of the hair
Brittle nails
Eye symptoms – exophthalmia, double vision, swelling and redness of the eyelids or conjunctiva (typical for Graves' disease)
Menstrual disorders, infertility
Osteoporosis and increased fracture risk
Atrial fibrillation or other supraventricular arrhythmias
Congestive heart failure
Male gynecomastia and erectile dysfunction

Box 3.2 Signs of Hyperthyroidism

Stare
Lid lag
Tachycardia
Irregular or rapid pulse
Systolic hypertension
Proximal muscle weakness
Hyperreflexia
Resting tremor
Warm, moist skin
Thin, fine hair
Onycholysis

3.1.2 Natural History of Hyperthyroidism

Hyperthyroidism should not be taken lightly, and if left untreated, it can lead to dangerous complications, for example, arrhythmias, heart failure, osteoporosis, or thyroid crisis (with a life-threatening increase in T3 and T4 levels). In pregnant women, hyperthyroidism is detrimental to both the mother and the fetus. Treatment of hyperthyroidism requires compliance with medical recommendations, regular medication, and regular medical check-ups.

3.1.3 Diagnosis of Hyperthyroidism

A person who finds symptoms suggesting the presence of hyperthyroidism should see a general practitioner who, after a medical examination (after taking an anamnesis and after the physical examination), will decide on the need to measure the serum TSH level. The test is performed with a blood sample that does not have to be taken on an empty stomach. In the case of very severe hyperthyroidism, it is necessary to urgently refer the patient to a hospital.

To confirm hyperthyroidism, hormonal tests are performed. The best initial screening test to assess thyroid function is a serum TSH level, and it may be ordered by the general practitioner. If the result is incorrect, it is necessary to measure thyroid hormone tests: free T4 (FT4) and/or free T3 (FT3). Hyperthyroidism is diagnosed if a decreased TSH concentration is accompanied by an increased FT4 and/or FT3 concentration in the serum (the higher FT4 and FT3 serum levels, the more severe is hyperthyroidism).

Patients with a low serum TSH level and normal FT4 and FT3 levels are defined as having subclinical hyperthyroidism. A FT3 serum level is important to make a diagnosis of "T3 thyrotoxicosis" in a patient with a suppressed serum TSH level and a normal FT4 level. In most cases, T3 thyrotoxicosis is an early manifestation of Graves' disease.

If hyperthyroidism is diagnosed, its cause and etiology should be determined, which is important when deciding on the treatment method. The following studies are helpful for this: thyroid ultrasound, serum antithyroid antibodies (especially anti-TSH receptor [anti-TSHR] antibodies, and antithyroid peroxidase [anti-TPO] antibodies), fine-needle aspiration biopsy (if there are focal lesions of the thyroid), and thyroid scintigraphy performed in selected cases. Sometimes clinical examination may readily reveal the etiology of the disease like in case of orbitopathy associated with Graves' disease (◘ Fig. 3.1).

Thyroid uptake scintigraphy with iodine-123 (^{123}I) or technetium-99m (^{99m}Tc) can be helpful in determining the cause of hyperthyroidism. Thyroid uptake is elevated in patients with Graves' disease and may be elevated or normal in patients with toxic multinodular goiter or a solitary toxic nodule [2]. It is low or undetectable in patients with thyrotoxicosis from thyroiditis. Thyroid scintigraphy typically demonstrates diffuse symmetrical uptake in patients with Graves' disease, heteroge-

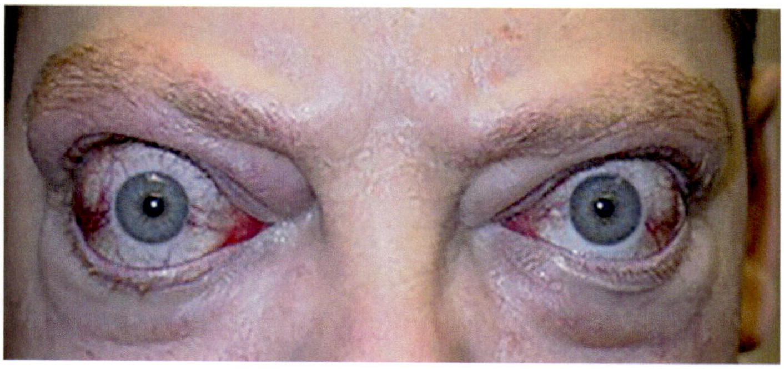

◘ **Fig. 3.1** Orbitopathy associated with Graves' disease

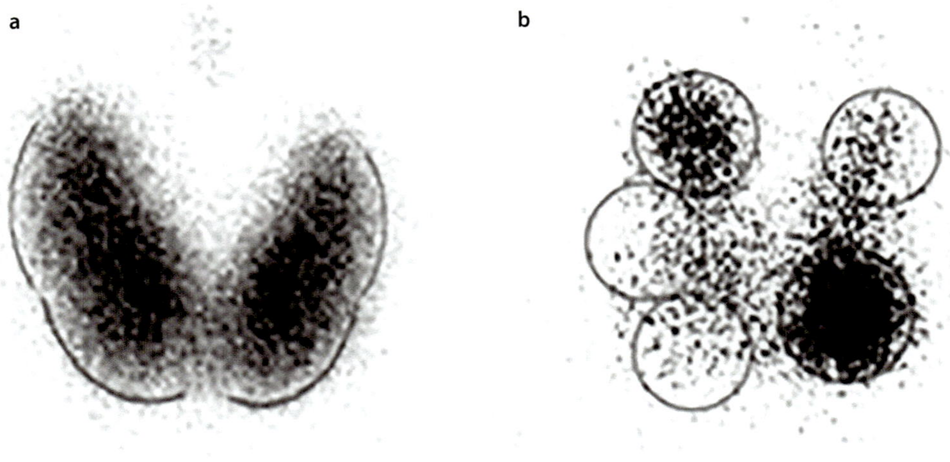

Fig. 3.2 Thyroid scintigraphy typically demonstrates diffuse symmetrical uptake in patients with Graves' disease **a**, and heterogeneous uptake in patients with toxic multinodular goiter **b**

neous uptake in patients with toxic multinodular goiter, and a single area of hyperfunctioning with a variable degree of suppression of the remaining thyroid gland in patients with a solitary toxic nodule (Fig. 3.2).

The diagnosis of Graves' disease should be based on signs of thyrotoxicosis, elevation in serum fT4 and fT3 levels, suppression of TSH and elevated level of anti-TSHR antibody. In addition, thyroid scintigraphy demonstrates diffuse and remarkably elevated uptake of ^{123}I, suggesting a diagnosis of Graves' disease. Contrary to these findings, patients with Plummer's disease have thyrotoxicosis but are negative for anti-TSHR antibody and show scintigraphic patterns of multifocal uptake of ^{123}I. When we consider hyperthyroidism based on thyroid ultrasound, increased thyroid blood flow in whole thyroids in patients with hyperthyroidism suggests the existence of Graves' disease. When we find nodules showing increased thyroid blood flow in anti-TSHR-negative patients with hyperthyroidism, we consider such patients likely having Plummer's disease.

3.1.4 Treatment of Hyperthyroidism

There are many ways to treat hyperthyroidism. There is no single best treatment as each method has advantages and disadvantages that can be discussed with a healthcare professional. In addition, the treatment of hyperthyroidism depends on its cause, severity, age of the patient, and coexisting diseases. Hence, the best method of treatment is tailored individually for each patient. Most often, it begins with the use of drugs that reduce the production of thyroid hormones, usually also when treatment is planned by another method (surgery or radioiodine ^{131}I).

In the treatment of hyperthyroidism, the following are used: drug treatment with antithyroid drugs (thyreostatic drugs), radioiodine treatment (^{131}I), and surgical treatment (strumectomy, thyroidectomy).

3.1.4.1 Antithyroid Drugs

Antithyroid drugs include methimazole (thiamazole) and propylthiouracil. Thyreostatics inhibit the production of hormones in the thyroid gland, and their effect becomes apparent after about 2–4 weeks of use. Each time the physician determines the starting dose of the drug individually. Adjuvant therapy with ß-blockers, for example, propranolol, is also often used, as they do not lower thyroid hormone levels by themselves, but help to control some symptoms, such as trembling hands and the feeling of a rapid heartbeat. During the treatment, the physician controls the effectiveness of the therapy through clinical evaluation (interview and examination of the patient) and determination of the concentration of thyroid hormones, and adjusts the dose accordingly. Undesirable effects may occur during treatment with thyreostatic drugs.

In the event of any side effects that may be related to the commencement of treatment, the patient should report it to the physician as soon as possible. In minor complications (e.g., itching of the skin, joint pain), it is enough to change the drug or its dose. In some, very rare cases, it may be necessary to discontinue thyreostatic treatment.

A particularly dangerous, but fortunately extremely rare complication can be agranulocytosis, a significant decrease in the number of neutrophils (a type of white blood cell) in the serum due to reversible toxic bone marrow damage that resolves after drug discontinuation, but requires close medical supervision. This is a very dangerous condition, because the body's resistance to infection is greatly impaired. Therefore, in the event of fever, weakness, or sore throat, the patient should immediately stop taking the drug and urgently visit the clinic or hospital for complete blood count control with a smear. If the neutrophil count is not decreased, the earlier treatment should be continued immediately. If agranulocytosis is confirmed, this group of drugs must never be used again in the future.

3.1.4.2 Radioactive Iodine (RAI)

A single oral administration of radioiodine is intended to slow irreversible damage to the thyroid cells that actively take up iodine from the blood. The radioiodine effect develops within a few months after therapy. The development of permanent hypothyroidism (requiring treatment with thyroxine tablets) cannot be treated as a complication, but as an effect of effective treatment. This form of therapy must not be used in pregnant women and during breastfeeding. Additionally, the treated person should not contact young children and pregnant women for a period of about a week. Finally, women should not plan a pregnancy for at least 6–12 months after treatment.

3.1.5 Indications for Surgery in Hyperthyroidism

This form of therapy is absolutely indicated in the case of suspected or diagnosed thyroid cancer, including coexisting hyperthyroidism. Moreover, surgical treatment is considered in patients with high volume goiter compressing the trachea (◘ Fig. 3.3). After surgical removal of the thyroid gland, hypothyroidism occurs, which requires constant treatment with levothyroxine. Unfortunately, during the operation, one must take into account the possibility of complications that should be discussed with the consulting surgeon. Serious postoperative complications include paresis/paralysis of one or both vocal cords as a result of intraoperative injury to the recurrent laryngeal nerve(s), damage to the external branch of the superior laryngeal nerve(s), and transient or permanent hypoparathyroidism.

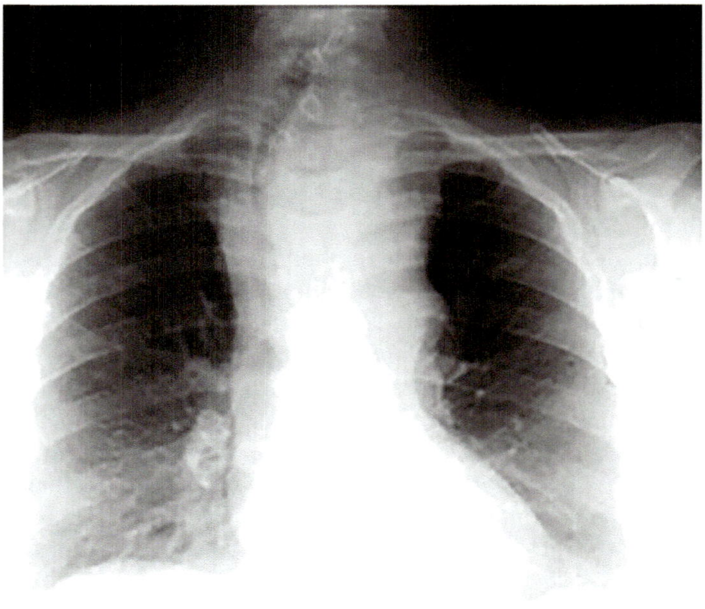

◘ **Fig. 3.3** A large toxic multinodular goiter with retrosternal extension causing trachea deviation and narrowing to the right side can be seen on plain chest X-ray

3.1.6 Prognosis in Hyperthyroidism

The possibility of a complete recovery (the patient does not require any thyroid medication) depends mainly on the cause of the hyperthyroidism. Hypothyroidism is common after radioiodine therapy or thyroidectomy, requiring continued treatment with thyroxine preparations for life.

After the treatment of hyperthyroidism is finished, the patient requires further constant medical care. Periodic hormonal control (serum TSH level) and ultrasound (ultrasound of the thyroid) are recommended. In some cases, there is a possibility of relapse of hyperthyroidism, recurrence of nodular goiter, or development of hypothyroidism after the treatment, even many months after its completion. If the patient, after completing the therapy, requires treatment with oral thyroid hormones due to hypothyroidism, it is necessary to take them regularly and periodically check the effectiveness of this treatment.

This chapter focuses on the clinical presentation, diagnosis, and surgical management of hyperthyroidism caused by Graves' disease and multinodular toxic goiter (Plummer's disease).

3.2 Graves' Disease

3.2.1 Pathogenesis

Graves' disease (GD) is an autoimmune disease in which the autoantigen is the TSH receptor (TSHR). Its activation by anti-TSHR antibodies causes increased secretion of thyroid hormones and leads to symptoms of hyperthyroidism, stimulates the growth of the thyroid gland, and the development of its vascularization [3]. Activation of the cellular response mechanisms against the same antigen, which is present in orbital and skin fibroblasts, leads to increased secretion of proinflammatory cytokines and the development of nonthyroid symptoms of the disease. Thyroid orbitopathy is a set of eye symptoms caused by immunological inflammation of the soft tissues of the orbit in the course of GD, leading to temporary or permanent damage to the organ of vision.

3.2.2 Epidemiology

Graves' disease is the most common cause of hyperthyroidism in developed countries. An annual incidence of Graves' disease is estimated to be 30–38 per 100,000 population [4, 5]. It is more common between 30 and 60 years; 5–10 times more frequent in women [6]. The genetic predisposition accounts for

79% of the risk for GD, while environmental factors for 21%. About 70% of genes associated with autoimmune thyroid disorders are implicated in T-cell function. Among GD environmental risk factors, smoking, iodine excess, selenium or vitamin D deficiency, and interferon- α (IFN-α) treatment in history for chronic HCV hepatitis are well recognized.

It can be also associated with other autoimmune diseases such as rheumatoid arthritis, systemic lupus erythematosus, chronic lymphocytic thyroiditis, Sjögren's syndrome, vitiligo, pernicious anemia, type 1 diabetes mellitus, Addison's disease, myasthenia gravis, and idiopathic thrombocytopenic purpura [7].

3.2.3 Clinical Presentation

The clinical manifestations of GD include typical presentation of symptoms and signs of overt hyperthyroidism (◘ Boxes 3.1 and 3.2) in a patient with diffuse goiter (◘ Fig. 3.4). However, in the elderly, only cardiac symptoms may be present. Typically, GD is characterized by periods of exacerbation and remission, there is a diffuse symmetrical and well-vascularized goiter with a characteristic vascular murmur, there may be exophthalmos (overt orbitopathy is not a necessary condition for the diagnosis of GD), less often symptoms of autoimmune dermatitis – pretibial edema (thyroid dermopathy – a pathognomonic symptom, but rare), and thyroid acropachy (thickened and rounded end phalanges of the hands; symptom very rare).

Orbitopathy manifests itself simultaneously with hyperthyroidism or later within 18 months, may precede other symptoms of hyperthyroidism, and is rarely the only symptom of GD; exceptionally, it may accompany hypothyroidism. Patients complain of pain in the eyeballs, burning sensation, lacrimation, decreased visual acuity, a feeling of sand under the eyelids, photophobia and double vision; physical examination

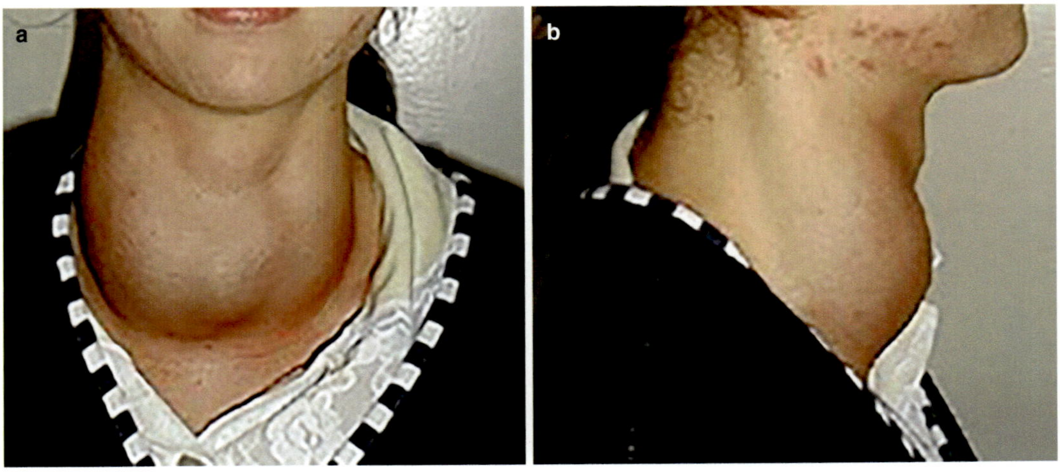

◘ **Fig. 3.4** Visible and palpable diffuse goiter, characteristic for Graves' disease (**a** – front view; **b** – lateral view)

reveals exophthalmos, swelling of the eyelids and periorbital tissues, conjunctival redness, and limited eye movement. The risk of blindness occurs when there is ulceration of the cornea due to regurgitation of the eyelids and when there is pressure on the optic nerve (initially impaired color vision).

Clinically relevant orbitopathy occurs in 20–30% of patients with GD and is vision-threatening in 3–5% of patients [8]. Malignant exophthalmos is a rare but severe form of progressive edematous infiltrative orbitopathy with a particularly high risk of permanent complications [9].

3.2.4 Diagnosis

Graves' disease may present as overt or subclinical primary hyperthyroidism, accompanied by features of autoimmune inflammation, clinically evident or detected in additional tests.

In laboratory tests, decreased serum TSH level and increased (less frequently normal) FT4 and FT3 levels (usually FT4 determination is sufficient; if correct – FT3 determination is needed) is found. In overt hyperthyroidism, the significant advantage of the FT3 increase over the FT4 increase is a prognostic signal – the response to antithyroid therapy is worse. In the remission phase, the results of hormonal tests are normal.

Increased serum level of anti-TSHR antibodies confirms the diagnosis (determine before or during the first 3 months of antithyroid treatment), whereas normalization indicates immune remission of the disease.

Characteristic for GD on ultrasound of the thyroid gland is the hypoechoic parenchyma (◘ Fig. 3.5), enlarged thyroid with increased vascular flow; the presence of thyroid nodules

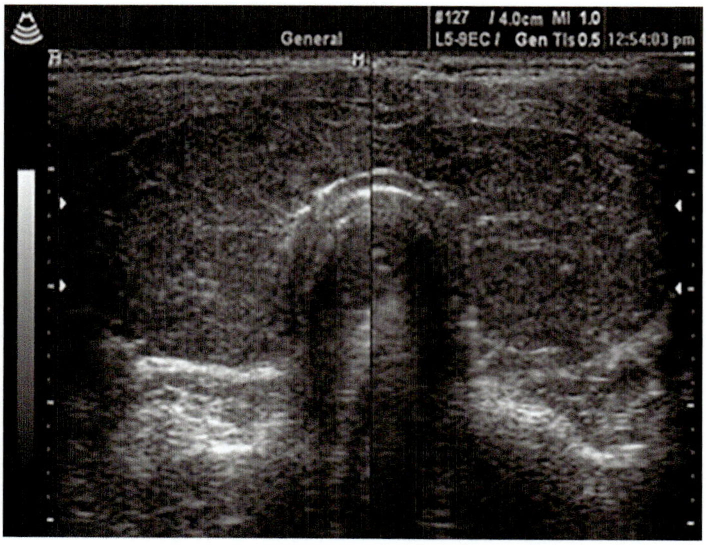

◘ **Fig. 3.5** Diffuse and hypoechoic goiter on thyroid ultrasound is typical for Graves' disease

does not exclude GD. Thyroid scintigraphy is especially helpful in the presence of nodules and qualification for radioiodine treatment.

Computed tomography (CT) of the eye sockets without contrast allows for assessment of the soft tissues of the orbit, its bones (important in planning decompression surgery), and external thickening of the eyeball muscles.

Magnetic resonance imaging (MRI) of the eye sockets allows for assessment of the swelling or fibrosis of the eyeball muscles.

The diagnosis of GD may be certain or probable depending on the set of available data (◘ Table 3.1). An isolated increase in the serum level of anti-TSHR antibodies is not sufficient for the diagnosis of GD (it may occur in relatives of patients with GD who do not develop symptoms of the disease).

It is also important not only to diagnose inflammation of the orbital tissues and to diagnose thyroid orbitopathy (GO), but above all to assess whether the severity of symptoms warrants treatment (requires full ophthalmological examination and often CT of the orbits). Classification of thyroid orbitopathy taking into account the activity of immune inflammation (according to EUGOGO, 2016) distinguishes the following: mild GO with a limited influence on daily functioning, moderate to severe GO without risk of vision loss, and very severe GO with a risk of blindness [10]. In addition, Clinical Activity Score (CAS) serves to assess of the activity of the thyroid orbitopathy based on the presence of inflammatory features including (sign present 1, sign absent 0): spontaneous retro-orbital pain, pain when looking up or down, redness of the eyelids,

◘ **Table 3.1** The diagnosis of GD may be certain or probable depending on the set of available data

The diagnosis of GD is certain in the following situations:	The diagnosis of GD is likely if
1. Overt or subclinical hyperthyroidism and an increased anti-TSHR serum level 2. Hyperthyroidism accompanied by thyroid orbitopathy with clear involvement of the soft tissues of the orbits or thyroid dermopathy 3. Hyperthyroidism with goiter confirmed by ultrasound (diffuse parenchymal hypoechogenicity) – if anti-TSHR antibodies cannot be determined 4. Isolated thyroid orbitopathy and increased anti-TSHR serum level	1. There are relapses of hyperthyroidism, separated by periods of euthyroidism lasting >6 months without the use of antithyroid drugs 2. There are cases of GD or Hashimoto's disease in the family of a patient with hyperthyroidism, or another autoimmune disease

conjunctival redness, inflammation of the lacrimal muscle and/or conjunctival crescent fold, swelling of the eyelids, swelling of the conjunctiva (chemosis). An active GO is indicated by a CAS value of 3 out of 7 or more. Inactive GO is diagnosed at CAS below 3.

3.2.5 Treatment

An ideal treatment of GD would include the following: prompt control of the disease manifestations, return to and maintenance of the euthyroid state, minimal morbidity, no mortality risk, and a reasonable cost.

Unfortunately, there is no effective causative treatment of GD, only the symptoms are treated like hyperthyroidism and orbitopathy.

The first goal of treatment is to achieve euthyroidism as soon as possible and to make a decision together with the patient on a further treatment strategy.

There are three therapeutic alternatives for GD: antithyroid drugs, radioactive iodine, and thyroidectomy. Each modality has its own advantages and disadvantages. Patient, physician, institutional, and geographical preferences often influence the choice of therapy. In the United States, radioactive ablation has traditionally been the primary treatment used. However, a 2011 survey indicates that there has been a trend toward increasing the long-term use of antithyroid drugs in lieu of radioactive iodine [11]. In Europe, Japan, and South America, prolonged antithyroid drugs therapy still remain a preferred option [12–14].

3.2.5.1 Antithyroid Drugs

If the main method of treatment is antithyroid drugs, efforts should be made to achieve and maintain immune remission. The prognosis of anti-TSHR normalization is favorable, as well as a decrease in the volume of the goiter and the disappearance of the vascular features (the stimulating effect of anti-TSHR antibodies decreases and lymphocytic infiltration subsides), which represent indirect features of immune remission. In the event of recurrence of hyperthyroidism, radical treatment – radioiodine treatment or surgery – is preferable, but chronic treatment with a low dose of antithyroid drug is acceptable, if radical treatment cannot be performed or if it is contraindicated or if this is the patient's preferences.

The optimal duration of pharmacological treatment is 18 months, or at least 12 months, if the goal is to achieve permanent immune remission [15]. The risk of relapse increases with the disease severity, and it was reported to be as high as 48% [16].

The classic antithyroid treatment regimen is methimazole (thiamazole) to achieve euthyroidism (which takes 3–6 weeks), usually at a dose of 20–30 mg per day, then gradually reduce the dose to the maintenance dose (continued for 18 months); only if allergic to methimazole, if treatment is necessary, propylthiouracil can be used (as time to achieve euthyroidism is usually longer).

Manifestation of the ineffectiveness of pharmacotherapy in GD is summarized in ◘ Box 3.3.

Propylthiouracil is preferred for the management of GD during pregnancy, because methimazole has been associated with birth defects [17, 18].

Initial pharmacological preparation before radical treatment should last 4–6 weeks (at least 2 weeks) before surgery, and methimazole is preferred due to the shorter time to achieve euthyroid state. On the other hand, methimazole is recommended to be used 1–3 months prior to treatment with radioactive iodine because of the lesser inhibition of thyroid sensitivity to ionizing radiation [2, 13].

Box 3.3 Manifestation of the Ineffectiveness of Pharmacotherapy in GD

1. No hormonal remission – despite the use of antithyroid drugs, thyroid hormones serum levels do not normalize or increase when trying to reduce the dose of the drug.
2. No initial immune remission – the concentration of anti-TSHR antibodies remains above 10 IU/l after 6 months of pharmacotherapy (Resolution of symptoms of hyperthyroidism does not guarantee immunological remission.).
3. No permanent immune remission – an increased concentration of anti-TSHR antibodies after 12 months of treatment indicates a high risk of recurrence (75–90%) despite euthyroidism.
4. Recurrence of hyperthyroidism after hormonal and immune remission; true relapse when posttreatment remission was at 1 year or longer.

3.2.5.2 Radioactive Iodine (RAI)

Radioactive iodine was introduced for treatment of hyperthyroidism in the 1940s (subtotal thyroidectomy was in use before that era) [19]. Radioactive iodine is nowadays the method of choice in the radical treatment of hyperthyroidism in the course of GD (at a dose of 10–15 mCi). ^{131}I emits beta particles, which destroy the follicular cells of the thyroid. In approximately 3/4 of cases, a single administration of ^{131}I is sufficient; in the remaining cases, it is necessary to administer the second dose, usually after 6 months [20]. Treatment with ^{131}I is contraindicated in active severe or moderate orbitopathy [2, 13]. In mild active orbitopathy, treatment with ^{131}I should be performed in a corticosteroid shield (due to the risk of temporary exacerbation) – prednisone 0.3–0.5 mg/kg/d from 1–3 days after ^{131}I administration for 1 month, then gradually reduce the dose to stop treatment within 3 months. The majority of patients with GD gradually enter remission of TSH-receptor autoimmunity during medical or after surgical therapy, with no difference between the types of therapy. Remission of TSH-receptor autoimmunity after radioiodine therapy is less common [21, 22]. Side effects of RAI ablation include neck pain and tenderness from radiation-induced thyroiditis, transient increase in thyroid hormone levels, and worsening of Graves' orbitopathy [2, 13].

3.2.6 Indications for Surgery and Surgical Details

A clear indication for surgery in GD is a coexisting nodule with cytological proven or clinical risk of malignancy (the risk of thyroid cancer in GD is similar to that in other forms of nodular goiter and accounts for 2–7%). Surgical approach is also preferred in the case of coexisting severe orbitopathy and in the case of large goiter (>80 ml) with compressive symptoms, especially in the case of large radioiodine non-avid foci (area of the nodule refractory to RAI).

It can be also considered based on patient preference, and in pregnant women requiring high doses of antithyroid drugs, or who are intolerant to the drugs. Patient preference is often related to desire for the most rapid amelioration of symptoms (RAI take several months to render a patient hypothyroid), a reluctance to receive RAI because of having young children, a planned pregnancy, and a fear of exposure to radiation [2, 13].

The advantages of surgical therapy are the following: euthyroid state is achieved rapidly and consistently, long-term risks of RAI and antithyroid medications are avoided, tissues for histology are provided (concomitant thyroid nodules and carcinoma are removed), childbearing renders immediately possible, with total thyroidectomy risk of recurrent hyperthyroidism is practically abolished, and absolute titration of thyroid hormone is allowed. In addition, total thyroidectomy has been associated with improvement in eye manifestation attributable to excess adrenergic activity [23].

The disadvantage of surgical treatment of Graves' disease is the risk of surgical morbidity, which includes laryngeal nerve(s) injury, hypoparathyroidism, bleeding, hematoma, and thyroid storm. When total thyroidectomy is performed by a high-volume endocrine surgeon, the risk of permanent complication is approximately 1–2%, and neck hematoma is 1% or less. Advancements such as preoperative preparation, intraoperative neural monitoring of the laryngeal nerves, and intraoperative parathyroid hormone monitoring together with novel technologies based on autofluorescence phenomenon and currently available for intraoperative parathyroid glands identification and viability assessment have decreased risks greatly and improved outcomes at hands of high-volume endocrine surgeons [24].

Patients should be rendered euthyroid before operation to decrease thyroid vascularity, to improve surgical planes, and to prevent life-threatening thyroid storm. The latter complication is characterized by severe manifestation of hyperthyroidism along with fever, nausea, vomiting, diarrhea, tachyarrhythmias, congestive heart failure, agitation, and delirium. The risk of thyroid storm can be eliminated by adequate preoperative preparation [25–27]. Antithyroid drugs are used to normalize FT4 and FT3 serum levels before the planned operation. A beta-blocker is used for symptomatic treatment of adrenergic symptoms and tachycardia. Once the patient's FT4 and FT3 are normalized, a saturated solution of potassium iodide (SSKI) or Lugol's solution is administered 5–10 days before surgery. This treatment has also been shown to reduce the thyroid blood flow and vascularity, which allows for surgical dissection in a dry operative field and improves identification and preservation of vital perithyroidal structures like laryngeal nerves and parathyroid glands. Despite convincing data in the literature on utility of preoperative preparation with iodide among patient with GD and the American Thyroid Association (ATA) and European Thyroid Association (ETA) recommendations to use iodide in the presurgical management [2, 13], the need for this treatment approach has recently been challenged [28].

In addition, the vitamin D serum level should be checked and corrected preoperatively to reduce the risk of symptomatic hypocalcemia.

The extent of thyroidectomy for the treatment of GD has been controversial in the past. This controversy regarding the extent of surgical resection in Graves' disease presumably arose because of the previously reported higher prevalence of permanent complications following total thyroidectomy. More recent data support the safety of total thyroidectomy for benign thyroid disease including GD if surgery is performed in a high-volume unit [24]. Subtotal thyroidectomy (leaving unilateral or bilateral thyroid remnants) is associated with a high rate of hypothyroidism (40–60% within 20 years of operation), and large remnants (more than 4 g; volume of the residual thyroid fragments strongly correlates with the risk of GD recurrence) have a potential for recurrence [29, 30].

Total thyroidectomy or near-total thyroidectomy obviates these disadvantages and can be performed without increased complication rates, and hence, it is the preferred surgical option for treatment of GD when thyroid hormone replacement therapy is readily available (However, bilateral subtotal thyroidectomy still remains an option in the treatment of GD, particularly in the low-income countries with limited access to thyroid hormones medication or in case of no patient compliance.). In addition, total thyroidectomy eliminates the antigen that is the source for the TSH receptor antibodies and other antibodies that cross-react with antigens in the extraocular muscles, the retro-orbital connective tissue, and the optic nerve [31–34].

Postoperatively, patients must be monitored carefully for hypocalcemia, a potentially serious complication. Patients will require lifelong thyroid hormone replacement with levothyroxine. Radioactive iodine ablation should be considered for disease recurrence after surgery.

3.2.7 Prognosis

If hyperthyroidism is untreated, sometimes, it comes to spontaneous remission, but sooner life-threatening complications may occur. Pharmacological treatment eliminates the symptoms of thyroid hormones excess and accelerates remission, but relapse occurs in approximately 50% of patients [16]. The concentration of anti-TSHR antibodies is normalized in most patients after approximately 6 months of treatment, but this does not ensure that the achieved remission will be long-lasting. The risk of relapse is increased in men and in those below 20 years of age, as well as in patients with high volume goiter and a high initial FT3/FT4 ratio. Hypothyroidism always occurs after radical surgery (total thyroidectomy) and very often after successful radioiodine treatment; it can also develop in GD treated with pharmacological treatment for a long time.

Untreated Graves' orbitopathy may resolve without permanent sequelae, especially if it is mild, but in the active severe form, the risk of permanent damage to the orbital tissues (impaired eye mobility and visual acuity, and even blindness) is high, especially in malignant exophthalmia. Early treatment (in the active phase of the disease) often avoids serious consequences. If the advancement of exophthalmos and the involvement of the soft tissues and muscles of the eyeball are significant, or if the cornea is affected or the optic nerve is compressed, the risk of permanent damage to the organ of vision and permanent changes in the patient's appearance is high. Strabismus and exophthalmia are surgically corrected after disappearance of the active phase of the disease [10].

3.3 Toxic Multinodular Goiter (Plummer's Disease)

Toxic nodular (hyperactive) goiter (TMNG), also known as Plummer's disease, is a disease in which hyperthyroidism develops on the basis of nodular hyperplasia of the thyroid gland and there is no autoimmune background. A characteristic feature is the presence of a nodule or nodules that secrete thyroid hormones in an autonomous manner independent of TSH regulation.

3.3.1 Pathogenesis

A toxic multinodular goiter contains multiple autonomously functioning nodules, resulting in hyperthyroidism. These nodules function independently of TSH regulation and are almost always benign. However, nonfunctioning thyroid nodules in the same goiter may be malignant.

The etiologic factors involved in the formation of a multinodular goiter include an inherent functional heterogeneity of thyroid follicles, the effect of growth factors and goitrogens, iodine deficiency, and genetic abnormalities that include somatic activating mutations of genes that regulate thyroid growth and hormone synthesis [35–37]. It is postulated that in iodine-deficient areas, chronic TSH stimulation increases the replication of the follicular cells and results in the appearance of expression of mutations in the TSH receptor gene [38, 39]. Nodular growth results from hyperplasia of clusters of follicular cells with abnormal growth potential at scattered sites in the thyroid gland. The final phase in the evolution of goiter is when nodules become autonomous, progress form a nontoxic to a toxic state with loss of TSH regulation and nonsuppressability with thyroxine administration. A nontoxic multinodular goiter is present for 10–25 years before becoming toxic. During this evolution, patients with nontoxic multinodular goiter have a high prevalence of subclinical hyperthyroidism [40–42].

3.3.2 Epidemiology

Autonomous nodules are the second most common overall cause of thyrotoxicosis, accounting for 5–15% of all causes of hyperthyroidism [43]. The prevalence of TMNG increases with age, making it the most common cause of thyrotoxicosis in the elderly, whereas solitary toxic adenomas are more often found in young individuals [35, 36, 44, 45].

3.3.3 Clinical Presentation

Hyperthyroidism usually develops very slowly (the onset of an overt disease is preceded by subclinical hyperthyroidism in nodular goiter), but it can also occur suddenly, under the influence of a large dose of iodine (iodine-induced thyrotoxicosis, or the Jod-Basedow phenomenon), administered, for example, in the form of a radiological contrast agent or contained in drugs (amiodarone or some disinfectants) [46]. The growth of a goiter or the appearance of a lump(s) often goes unnoticed by the patient. If the goiter is large, there may be a feeling of pressure in the neck (compressive symptoms attributable to mass effect, particularly in case of substernal extension), difficulty in breathing (due to trachea deviation or narrowing), or, more rarely, dysphagia and coughing. The hyperthyroidism is usually less severe than in GD. Over manifestations of thyrotoxicosis are often masked in older patients, whereas cardiac manifestations, such as atrial fibrillation, tachycardia, congestive heart failure, and accelerated angina pectoris, are predominant. Unexplained weight loss, anxiety, insomnia, and muscle wasting are also more likely to occur in the elderly hyperthyroid patients [47].

3.3.4 Diagnosis

Visible or palpable nodular goiter of various sizes (the primary importance is the finding of 2 or more nodules or ultrasound), with laboratory findings of hyperthyroidism: marked suppression of TSH secretion and markedly increased concentrations of FT4 and FT3 or only FT3 in the serum, are sufficient findings to make a diagnosis of TMNG.

As TMNG is often asymmetrical, and substernal extension may make it less apparent on physical examination (◘ Fig. 3.6),

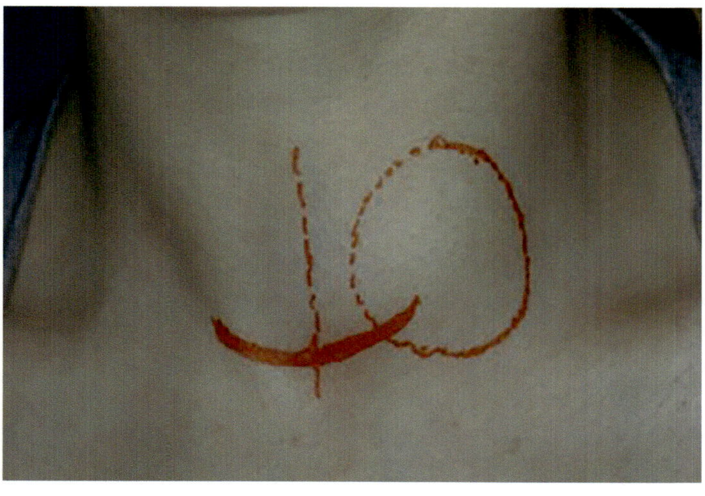

◘ **Fig. 3.6** Toxic multinodular goiter is often asymmetrical, and substernal extension may make it less apparent on physical examination

thyroid imaging tests are helpful. Ultrasound of the thyroid gland allows to measure the size of the goiter and accurately assess the nodules. Thyroid scintigraphy enables an accurate assessment of tracer uptake and distribution and the diagnosis of autonomic nodules, which is the basis for the decision to treat with ^{131}I [47].

An autonomic nodule (hot in scintigraphy), in diameter <3 cm on ultrasound, usually does not require fine-needle aspiration biopsy (FNAB) due to a very low risk of cancer; in other focal lesions, indications for FNAB are the same as in nontoxic nodular goiter.

A CT scan may be necessary to assess for substernal extension, and trachea narrowing, but iodine contrast should only be administered with caution (◘ Fig. 3.7).

3.3.5 Treatment

There are two main goals for treatment in patients with TMNG: to eliminate an autonomously functioning thyroid tissue and to alleviate compressive symptoms.

Pharmacological treatment with antithyroid drugs (methimazole) allows for controlling the symptoms of hyperthyroidism, but its withdrawal always leads to the relapse of the hyperthyroidism (after a few days to several weeks) [48]. The beta-blocker is used similarly to other types of hyperthyroidism, but in TMNG, it is needed more often and in higher doses than in GD due to the greater severity of cardiac symptoms.

Hence, radical treatment is necessary and definitive treatment options are surgical (subtotal or total thyroidectomy) or radioiodine ablation. The choice of method is individual for each patient [2, 37, 43, 47]. Nevertheless, most recent data indicate on safety of long-term, low-dose methimazole treatment for TMNG for 60–100 months, which is not inferior to RAI treatment [49].

3.3.5.1 Radioactive Iodine (RAI)

The radiosensitivity of autonomic nodules is lower than in Graves' disease (this is taken into account when planning RAI treatment). Inactive nodules do not respond to treatment, and most active nodules do not disappear, but only shrink, but the hyperthyroidism subsides (although sometimes ^{131}I must be readministered after 6 months). Small goiter with no signs of malignancy risk is more inclined to treatment with ^{131}I, as are contraindications for surgery (most elderly patients with comorbidities that increase their risk for surgery). Because TMNG contains nonfunctioning nodules and areas of fibrosis and calcifications, RAI treatment is only variably effective in reducing goiter size and relieving compressive symptoms. However, a reduction in thyroid volume and an increase in the

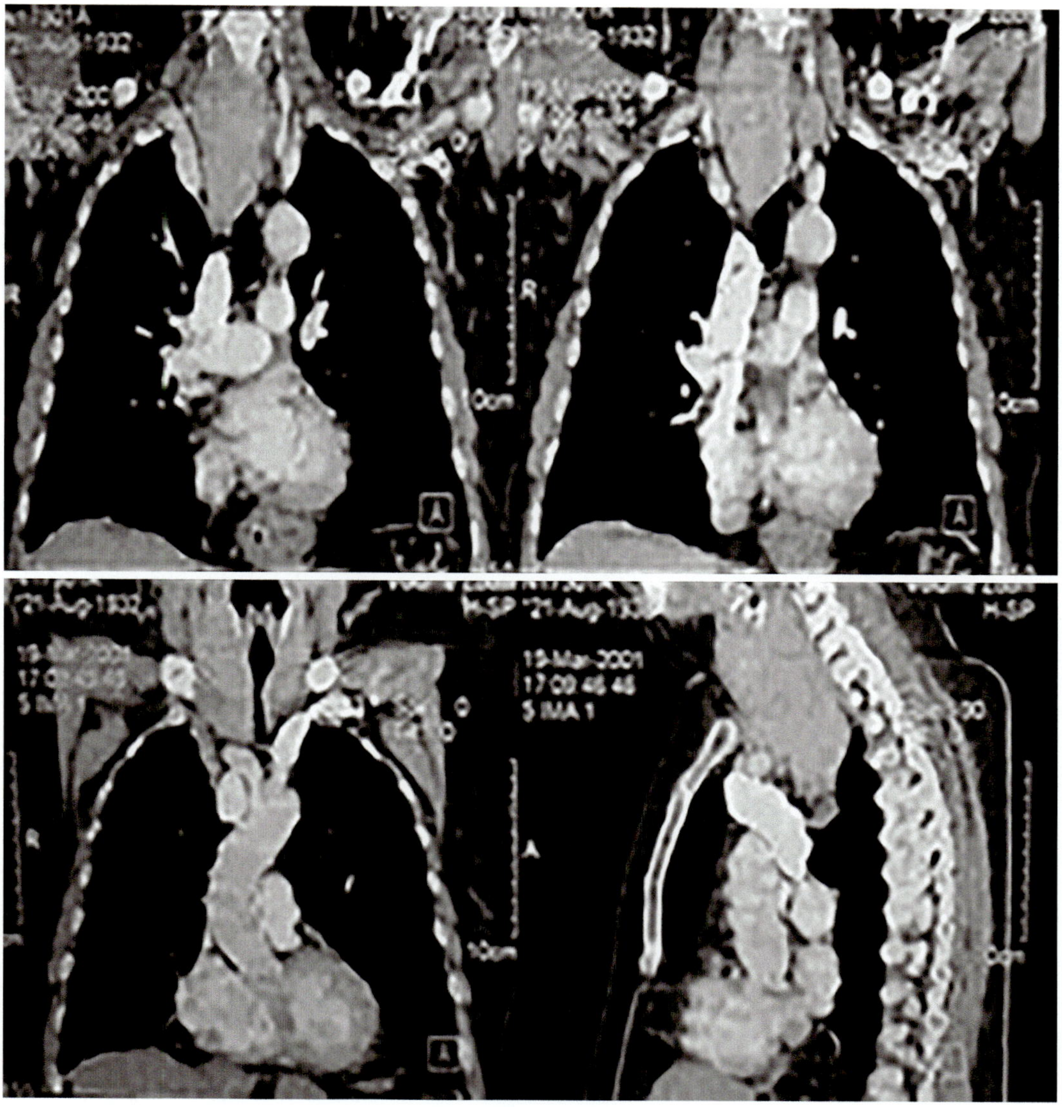

Fig. 3.7 Toxic multinodular goiter is often asymmetrical, and substernal extension may make it less apparent on physical examination, but cross-sectioning imaging reveals real dimensions of the goiter (view in axial and coronal modes on neck CT)

cross-sectional area of the tracheal lumen have been demonstrated by MRI imaging after RAI treatment [50–52].

3.3.6 Indications for Surgery and Surgical Details

Surgical resection is the preferred treatment option in patients with a nodule with cytological or clinical features of malignancy and also in patients with a large goiter giving compression symptoms, especially in the presence of inactive thyroid nodules, unless there are contraindications for surgery [2, 48, 53]. The operation is possible only after euthyroid state is achieved. Treatment with methimazole should be stopped on the day of surgery, and the dose of beta-blocker should be gradually reduced to discontinue it within a few days after surgery. Potassium iodide should not be given before surgery.

The presence of substernal thyroid extension or airway obstruction is a relative contraindication for RAI because of the potential for transient increase in size of the goiter and worsening of airway compromise through RAI-induced transient radiation thyroiditis. The extent of surgery should be total (◘ Fig. 3.8) or near-total thyroidectomy. Subtotal thyroidectomy (Dunhill operation) may be considered in patient who experienced intraoperative loss of signal of neuromonitoring after removal of the first-attempted, and usually, dominant thyroid lobe (a staged thyroidectomy) [54]. The risk of permanent surgical morbidity is low (<1–2%) if surgery is performed by a high-volume thyroid surgeon [55–60]. Surgery was also demonstrated to be more cost-effective than treatment with RAI for TMNG in patients aged 62 years or less [59]. Surgery also allows for curing incidental concomitant thyroid cancer, which was reported in 3–9% of patients with TMNG [61, 62]. In general, age older than 50 years, cold nodule(s), and ultrasound characteristics of nodule(s) may preselect patients with higher risk of malignancy for surgical treatment of TMNG [63, 64].

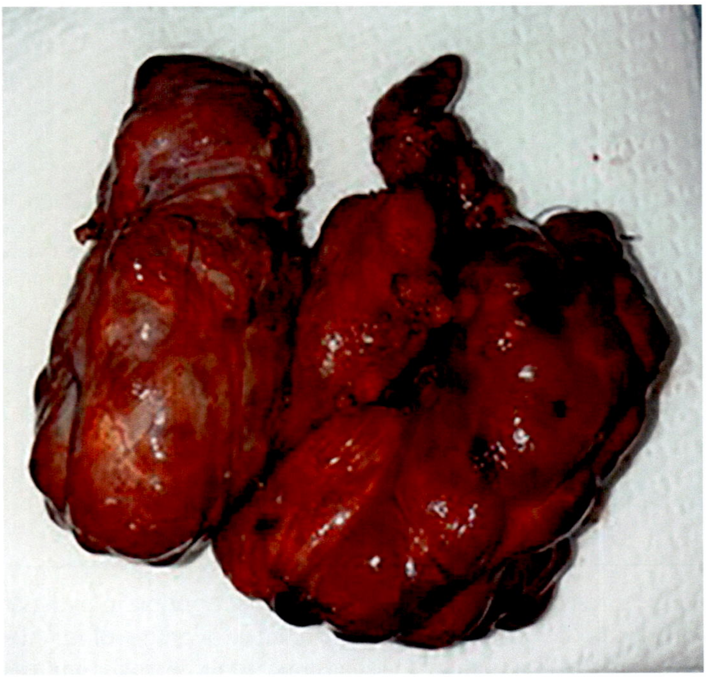

◘ **Fig. 3.8** Total thyroidectomy specimen for asymmetric toxic multinodular goiter

3.3.7 Prognosis

In untreated TMNG, the risk of arrhythmias and other cardiovascular complications as well as thyroid crisis is increased. The risk of cancer is the same as with other forms of nodular goiter. Recurrence of thyrotoxicosis after incomplete surgery for TMNG was reported to be as high as 50–78%. Hence, total or near-total thyroidectomy is the preferred surgical approach in patients not eligible for RAI treatment [55–60].

Answers to the Questions

1. (d); 2. (e); 3. (c); 4. (e); 5. (d); 6. (e); 7. (e); 8. (e); 9. (a); 10. (e); 11. (a)

References

1. Hollowell JG, Staehling NW, Flanders WD, et al. Serum TSH, T-4 and thyroid antibodies in the United States population (1988 to 1994): National Health and Nutrition Examination Survey (NHANES III). J Clin Endocrinol Metab. 2002;87(2):489–99.
2. Ross DS, Burch HB, Cooper DS, et al. 2016 American Thyroid Association guidelines for diagnosis and management of hyperthyroidism and other causes of thyrotoxicosis. Thyroid. 2016;26(10):1343–421.
3. Morshed SA, Latif R, Davies TF. Delineating the autoimmune mechanisms in Graves' disease. Immunol Res. 2012;54(1–3):191–203.
4. Smith TJ, Hegedüs L. Graves' disease. N Engl J Med. 2016;375(16):1552–65.
5. McLeod DS, Cooper DS. The incidence and prevalence of thyroid autoimmunity. Endocrine. 2012;42(2):252–65.
6. McLeod DS, Caturegli P, Cooper DS, Matos PG, Hutfless S. Variation in rates of autoimmune thyroid disease by race/ethnicity in US military personnel. JAMA. 2014;311(15):1563–5.
7. Antonelli A, Ferrari SM, Ragusa F, et al. Graves' disease: epidemiology, genetic and environmental risk factors and viruses. Best Pract Res Clin Endocrinol Metab. 2020;34(1):101387.
8. Bartalena L, Pinchera A, Marcocci C. Management of Graves' ophthalmopathy: reality and perspectives. Endocr Rev. 2000;21(2):168–99.
9. Kubota S, Gunji K, Stolarski C, Kennerdell JS, Wall J. Reevaluation of the prevalences of serum autoantibodies reactive with "64-kd eye muscle proteins" in patients with thyroid-associated ophthalmopathy. Thyroid. 1998;8(2):175–9.
10. Bartalena L, Baldeschi L, Boboridis K, et al. The 2016 European Thyroid Association/European Group on Graves' Orbitopathy guidelines for the management of Graves' orbitopathy. Eur Thyroid J. 2016;5(1):9–26.
11. Burch HB, Burman KD, Cooper DS. A 2011 survey of clinical practice patterns in the management of Graves' disease. J Clin Endocrinol Metab. 2012;97(12):4549–58.
12. Wartofsky L, Glinoer D, Solomon B, et al. Differences and similarities in the diagnosis and treatment of Graves' disease in Europe, Japan, and the United States. Thyroid. 1991;1(2):129–35.
13. Kahaly GJ, Bartalena L, Hegedüs L, Leenhardt L, Poppe K, Pearce SH. 2018 European thyroid association guideline for the management of Graves' hyperthyroidism. Eur Thyroid J. 2018;7(4):167–86.

14. Moon JH, Yi KH. The diagnosis and management of hyperthyroidism in Korea: consensus report of the Korean Thyroid Association. Endocrinol Metab (Seoul). 2013;28(4):275–9.
15. In H, Pearce EN, Wong AK, Burgess JF, McAneny DB, Rosen JE. Treatment options for Graves' disease: a cost-effectiveness analysis. J Am Coll Surg. 2009;209(2):170–9.
16. Masiello E, Veronesi G, Gallo D, et al. Antithyroid drug treatment for Graves' disease: baseline predictive models of relapse after treatment for a patient-tailored management. J Endocrinol Investig. 2018;41(12):1425–32.
17. Yoshihara A, Noh J, Yamaguchi T, et al. Treatment of Graves' disease with antithyroid drugs in the first trimester of pregnancy and the prevalence of congenital malformation. J Clin Endocrinol Metab. 2012;97(7):2396–403.
18. Andersen SL, Olsen J, Wu CS, Laurberg P. Birth defects after early pregnancy use of antithyroid drugs: a Danish nationwide study. J Clin Endocrinol Metab. 2013;98(11):4373–81.
19. Hertz S, Roberts A. Radioactive iodine in the study of thyroid physiology. The use of radioactive iodine therapy in hyperthyroidism. J Am Med Assoc. 1946;131:81–6.
20. Bogazzi F, Giovannetti C, Fessehatsion R, et al. Impact of lithium on efficacy of radioactive iodine therapy for Graves' disease: a cohort study on cure rate, time to cure, and frequency of increased serum thyroxine after antithyroid drug withdrawal. J Clin Endocrinol Metab. 2012;95(1):201–8.
21. Laurberg P, Wallin G, Tallstedt L, et al. TSH-receptor autoimmunity in Graves' disease after therapy with anti-thyroid drugs, surgery, or radioiodine: a 5-year prospective randomized study. Eur J Endocrinol. 2008;158(1):69–75.
22. Ponto KA, Zang S, Kahaly GJ. The tale of radioiodine and Graves' orbitopathy. Thyroid. 2010;20(7):785–93.
23. Bhargav PRK, Sabaretnam M, Kumar SC, Zwalitha S, Devi NV. Regression of ophthalmopathic exophthalmos in Graves' disease after total thyroidectomy: a prospective study of a surgical series. Indian J Surg. 2017;79(6):521–6.
24. Lorenz K, Raffaeli M, Barczyński M, Lorente-Poch L, Sancho J. Volume, outcomes, and quality standards in thyroid surgery: an evidence-based analysis-European Society of Endocrine Surgeons (ESES) positional statement. Langenbeck's Arch Surg. 2020;405(4):401–25.
25. Yilmaz Y, Kamer KE, Ureyen O, Sari E, Acar T, Karahalli O. The effect of preoperative Lugol's iodine on intraoperative bleeding in patients with hyperthyroidism. Ann Med Surg (Lond). 2016;9:53–7.
26. Whalen G, Sullivan M, Maranda L, Quinlan R, Larkin A. Randomized trial of a short course of preoperative potassium iodide in patients undergoing thyroidectomy for Graves' disease. Am J Surg. 2017;213(4):805–9.
27. Erbil Y, Ozluk Y, Giriş M, et al. Effect of Lugol's solution on thyroid gland blood flow and microvessel density in the patients with Graves' disease. J Clin Endocrinol Metab. 2007;92(6):2182–9.
28. Mercier F, Bonal M, Fanget F, et al. Does surgery without Lugol's solution pretreatment for graves' disease increase surgical morbidity? World J Surg. 2018;42(7):2123–6.
29. Jörtsö E, Lennquist S, Lundström B, Norrby K, Smeds S. The influence of remnant size, antithyroid antibodies, thyroid morphology, and lymphocytic infiltration on thyroid function after subtotal resection for hyperthyroidism. World J Surg. 1987;11(3):365–71.
30. Alsnea O, Clark OH. Treatment of Graves' disease: the advantages of surgery. Endocrinol Metab Clin N Am. 2000;29(2):321–37.
31. Barczyński M, Konturek A, Hubalewska-Dydejczyk A, Gołkowski F, Nowak W. Randomized clinical trial of bilateral subtotal thyroid-

ectomy versus total thyroidectomy for Graves' disease with a 5-year follow-up. Br J Surg. 2012;99(4):515–22.
32. Maurer E, Maschuw K, Reuss A, et al. Total versus near-total thyroidectomy in Graves' disease: results of the randomized controlled multicenter TONIG-trial. Ann Surg. 2019;270(5):755–61.
33. Liu ZW, Masterson L, Fish B, Jani P, Chatterjee K. Thyroid surgery for Graves' disease and Graves' ophthalmopathy. Cochrane Database Syst Rev. 2015;(11):CD010576.
34. Bobanga ID, McHenry CR. Treatment of patients with Graves' disease and the appropriate extent of thyroidectomy. Best Pract Res Clin Endocrinol Metab. 2019;33(4):101319.
35. Berghout A, Wiersinga WM, Smits NJ, Touber JL. Interrelationships between age, thyroid volume, thyroid nodularity, and thyroid function in patients with sporadic nontoxic goiter. Am J Med. 1990;89(5):602–8.
36. Gozu HI, Lublinghoff J, Bircan R, Paschke R. Genetics and phenomics of inherited and sporadic non-autoimmune hyperthyroidism. Mol Cell Endocrinol. 2010;322(1–2):125–34.
37. Siegel RD, Lee SL. Toxic nodular goiter: toxic adenoma and toxic multinodular goiter. Endocrinol Metab Clin N Am. 1998;27(1):151–68.
38. Krohn K, Führer D, Bayer Y, et al. Molecular pathogenesis of euthyroid and toxic multinodular goiter. Endocr Rev. 2005;26(4):504–24.
39. Vitti P, Rago T, Tonacchera M, Pinchera A. Toxic multinodular goiter in the elderly. J Endocrinol Invest. 2002;25(10 suppl):16–18.
40. Vadiveloo T, Donnan PT, Cochrane L, Leese GP. The Thyroid Epidemiology, Audit, and Research Study (TEARS): the natural history of endogenous subclinical hyperthyroidism. J Clin Endocrinol Metab. 2011;96(1):E1–8.
41. Rosario PW. Natural history of subclinical hyperthyroidism in elderly patients with TSH between 0.1 and 0.4 mIU/l: a prospective study. Clin Endocrinol (Oxf). 2010;72(5):685–8.
42. Das G, Ojewuyi TA, Baglioni P, Geen J, Premawardhana LD, Okosieme OE. Serum thyrotrophin at baseline predicts the natural course of subclinical hyperthyroidism. Clin Endocrinol. 2011;77(1):146–51.
43. Pearce EN Diagnosis and management of thyrotoxicosis. BMJ. 2006;332(7554):1369–73.
44. Laurberg P, Pedersen KM, Vestergaard H, Sigurdsson G. High incidence of multinodular toxic goitre in the elderly population in a low iodine intake area vs. high incidence of Graves' disease in the young in a high iodine intake area: comparative surveys of thyrotoxicosis epidemiology in East-Jutland Denmark and Iceland. J Intern Med. 1991;229(5):415–20.
45. Abraham-Nordling M, Byström K, Törring O, et al. Incidence of hyperthyroidism in Sweden. Eur J Endocrinol. 2011;165(6):899–905.
46. Fradkin JE, Wolff J. Iodide-induced thyrotoxicosis. Medicine (Baltimore). 1983;62(1):1–20.
47. Nayak B, Hodak SP. Hyperthyroidism. Endocrinol Metab Clin N Am. 2007;36(3):617–56.
48. van Soestbergen MJ, van der Vijver JC, Graafland AD. Recurrence of hyperthyroidism in multinodular goiter after long-term drug therapy: a comparison with Graves' disease. J Endocrinol Investig. 1992;15(11):797–800.
49. Azizi F, Takyar M, Madreseh E, Amouzegar A. Treatment of toxic multinodular goiter: comparison of radioiodine and long-term methimazole treatment. Thyroid. 2019;29(5):625–30. https://doi.org/10.1089/thy.2018.0397.
50. Huysmans DA, Hermus AR, Corstens FH, Barentsz JO, Kloppenborg PW. Large, compressive goiters treated with radioiodine. Ann Intern Med. 1994;121(10):757–62.
51. Nygaard B, Hegedüs L, Ulriksen P, Nielsen KG, Hansen JM. Radioiodine therapy for multinodular toxic goiter. Arch Intern Med. 1999;159(12):1364–8.

3

52. Schiavo M, Bagnara MC, Camerieri L, et al. Clinical efficacy of radioiodine therapy in multinodular toxic goiter, applying an implemented dose calculation algorithm. Endocrine. 2015;48(3):902–8.
53. Ríos A, Rodríguez JM, Balsalobre MD, Torregrosa NM, Tebar FJ, Parrilla P. Results of surgery for toxic multinodular goiter. Surg Today. 2005;35(11):901–6.
54. Schneider R, Randolph GW, Dionigi G, et al. International neural monitoring study group guideline 2018 part I: staging bilateral thyroid surgery with monitoring loss of signal. Laryngoscope. 2018;128(Suppl 3):S1–S17.
55. Miccoli P, Antonelli A, Iacconi P, Alberti B, Gambuzza C, Baschieri L. Prospective, randomized, double-blind study about effectiveness of levothyroxine suppressive therapy in prevention of recurrence after operation: result at the third year of follow up. Surgery. 1993;114(6):1097–101.
56. Agarwal G, Aggarwal V. Is total thyroidectomy the surgical procedure of choice for benign multinodular goiter? An evidence-based review. World J Surg. 2008;32(7):1313–24.
57. Ríos A, Rodríguez JM, Galindo PJ, Montoya MJ, Canteras M, Parrilla P. Surgical treatment of multinodular goiter in young patients. Endocrine. 2005;27(3):245–52.
58. Moalem J, Suh I, Duh QY. Treatment and prevention of recurrence of multinodular goiter: an evidence-based review of the literature. World J Surg. 2008;32(7):1301–12.
59. Vidal-Trecan GM, Stahl JE, Eckman MH. Radioiodine or surgery for toxic thyroid adenoma: dissecting in important decision. A cost-effectiveness analysis. Thyroid. 2004;14(11):933–45.
60. Barczyński M, Konturek A, Hubalewska-Dydejczyk A, Gołkowski F, Nowak W. Ten-year follow-up of a randomized clinical trial of total thyroidectomy versus Dunhill operation versus bilateral subtotal thyroidectomy for multinodular non-toxic goiter. World J Surg. 2018;42(2):384–92.
61. Cerci C, Cerci SS, Eroglu E, et al. Thyroid cancer in toxic and non-toxic multinodular goiter. J Postgrad Med. 2007;53(3):157–60.
62. Alexopoulou O, Beguin C, Buysschaert M, et al. Predictive factors of thyroid carcinoma in non-toxic multinodular goiter. Acta Clin Belg. 2004;59(2):84–9.
63. Senyurek Giles Y, Tunca F, Boztepe H, Kapran Y, Terzioglu T, Tezelman S. The risk factors for malignancy in surgically treated patients for Graves's disease, toxic multinodular goiter, and toxic adenoma. Surgery. 2008;144(6):1028–36.
64. Haugen BR, Alexander EK, Bible KC, et al. 2015 American Thyroid Association management guidelines for adult patients with thyroid nodules and differentiated thyroid cancer: the American Thyroid Association Guidelines Task Force on Thyroid Nodules and Differentiated Thyroid Cancer. Thyroid. 2016;26(1):1–133.

Diagnosis and Management of Thyroiditis: Hashimoto, de Quervain, Riedel

Marika D. Russell and Janet Chiang

Contents

A. L. Shifrin et al. (eds.), *Endocrine Surgery Comprehensive Board Exam Guide*,
https://doi.org/10.1007/978-3-030-84737-1_4

Case Presentation

A 47-year-old woman presented with progressively enlarging thyroid goiter, which had developed over the previous 6-month period. She reported dysphagia to liquids and solids and dyspnea when lying flat. Physical examination revealed firm enlargement of the thyroid. Ultrasound demonstrated symmetric enlargement (approximately 5 × 9 × 4 cm for each lobe) with heterogenous hypoechogenicity and no distinct nodules or increased vascularity (◘ Fig. 4.1). TSH was elevated at 5.74 mIU/mL (normal range 0.37–4.42 mIU/mL) and TPO-Abs were elevated at >1300 U/mL. A diagnosis of Hashimoto's thyroiditis (HT) was rendered, and she was started on LT_4 with a plan to monitor her thyroid enlargement. She was lost to follow-up and returned 1 year later with complaints of persistent compressive symptoms. TSH was found to be elevated to 24.22 mIU/mL, and she acknowledged poor compliance with LT_4 therapy. A repeat US was performed, which showed enlargement of the heterogeneous and hypoechoic thyroid gland compared to 1 year prior (now approximately 7 × 9 × 5 cm for each lobe). The goiter also had a deep retrosternal component. Although the ultrasound did not reveal discrete nodules, an FNA was obtained due to the size and firmness of the thyroid as well as increase in size over 1 year. Pathology showed lymphocytes and bland follicular epithelial cells, felt be consistent with a diagnosis of chronic lymphocytic thyroiditis. However, given the firm and relatively rapid enlargement of the thyroid, Riedel's thyroiditis (RT) and primary thyroid lymphoma (PTL) remained under consideration. To further characterize the thyroid, an MRI was obtained, which showed a markedly enlarged thyroid with T1- and T2-hypointensity and moderate contrast enhancement, displacing but not encasing the great vessels (◘ Fig. 4.2). She was subsequently recommended to undergo thyroid isthmusectomy for histologic characterization. Intraoperatively, the isthmus was noted to be markedly fibrotic and firm but not adherent to surrounding tissues. Pathology showed chronic inflammatory cells, germinal centers, and dense fibrosis, which did not appear to extend outside the thyroid capsule (◘ Fig. 4.3). Abundant IgG4+ plasma cells were noted, up to 30 per high power field. Together these findings suggested IgG4-related variant of HT. Serum IgG4 levels were normal. She was started on high-dose prednisone, which was continued for 4 months. During this time, she reported improvement in dysphagia symptoms, though no change in size of the thyroid was appreciated on physical examination. She was weaned off steroid treatment over the ensuing year. A follow-up US obtained 2 years after treatment showed no change in size or characteristics of the thyroid. At the present time, she has remained on LT_4 therapy for 3 years with stable thyromegaly and no progression of symptoms.

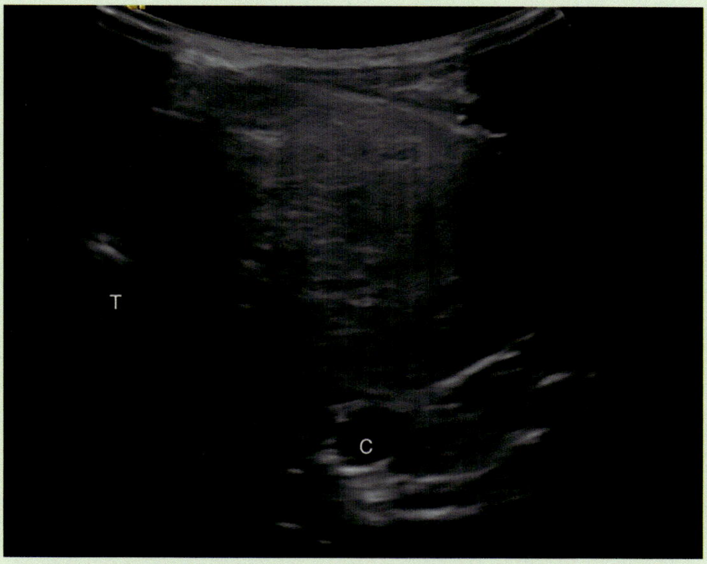

■ **Fig. 4.1** Ultrasound image in axial view demonstrating an enlarged and heterogenous left thyroid lobe without distinct nodules (C = carotid artery, T = trachea)

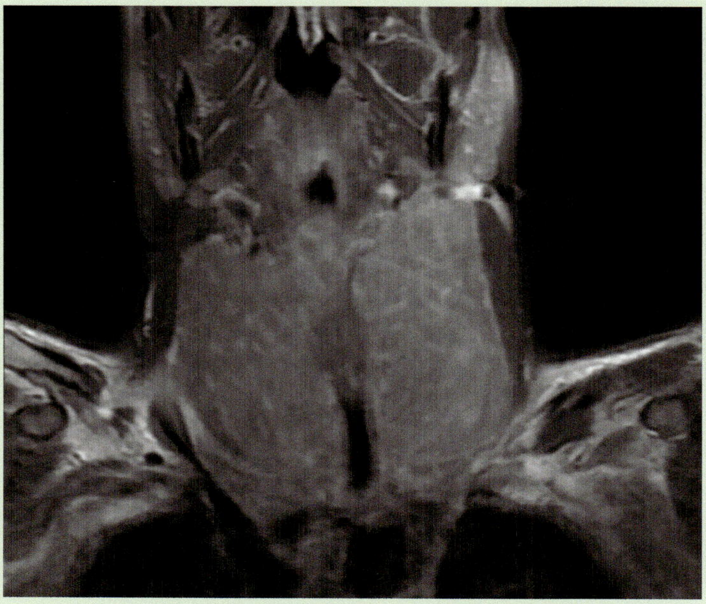

■ **Fig. 4.2** Contrast-enhanced MRI in coronal view demonstrating marked diffuse enlargement of the thyroid

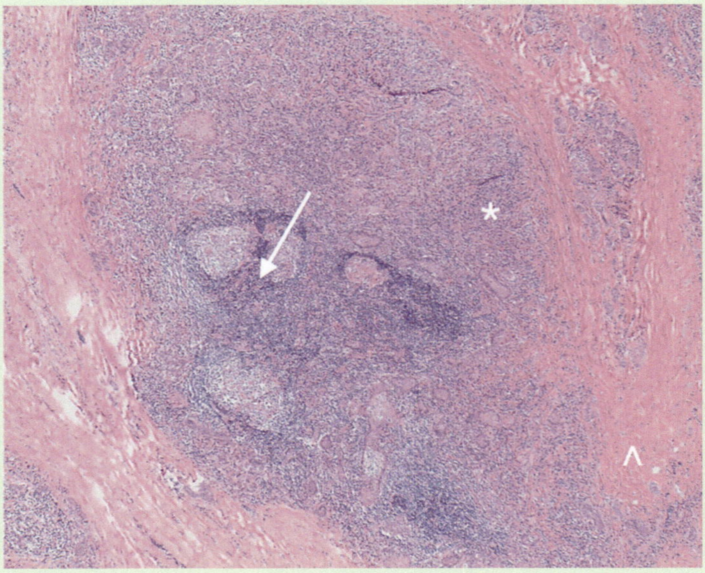

Fig. 4.3 Histologic appearance of IgG4-related Hashimoto's thyroiditis, including chronic inflammatory cells (*) and germinal centers (arrow) in a background of fibrosis (^)

Questions

1. Which of the following can be presenting features of Hashimoto's thyroiditis?
   1. Painless enlargement of the thyroid
   2. Atrophic thyroid gland
   3. Thyroid toxicosis
   4. Hypothyroidism with elevated thyroperoxidase levels
      (a) Only (1) and (2) and (3) are correct.
      (b) Only (1) and (2) and (4) are correct.
      (c) Only (1) and (3) and (4) are correct.
      (d) Only (2) and (3) and (4) are correct.
      (e) All are correct.
2. During the thyrotoxic phase of subacute thyroiditis, what pattern of radioactive iodine uptake would be expected?
   1. Diffuse increased uptake
   2. Focal increased uptake
   3. Focal decreased uptake
   4. Diffuse decreased uptake
      (a) Only (1) is correct.
      (b) Only (4) is correct.
      (c) Only (1) and (2) are correct.
      (d) Only (3) and (4) are correct.
      (e) All are correct.

3. Which of these treatment or supportive options are reasonable for patients presenting with de Quervain's thyroiditis?
   1. Beta-blocker
   2. Levothyroxine
   3. Corticosteroids
   4. Nonsteroidal anti-inflammatory drugs
   5. Methimazole or other antithyroid medications
      (a) Only (1) and (2) and (3) are correct.
      (b) Only (1) and (3) and (5) are correct.
      (c) Only (1) and (3) and (4) are correct.
      (d) Only (2) and (3) and (4) are correct.
      (e) All are correct.
4. Which of the following are features that can be found on ultrasound in patients with Hashimoto's thyroiditis?
   1. Pseudonodules
   2. Heterogeneity with ill-defined areas of hypoechogenicity
   3. Atrophied gland with "honeycomb" appearance
   4. Prominent central neck adenopathy
      (a) Only (1) is correct.
      (b) Only (4) is correct.
      (c) Only (1) and (2) are correct.
      (d) Only (3) and (4) are correct.
      (e) All are correct.
5. Which of these antibodies are often found to be positive in patients with Hashimoto's thyroiditis?
   1. Thyroperoxidase antibodies (TPO)
   2. Thyroglobulin antibodies (Tg)
   3. Thyrotropin receptor antibodies (TRAB)
   4. Thyroid-stimulating immunoglobulin (TSI)
      (a) Only (1) is correct.
      (b) Only (4) is correct.
      (c) Only (1) and (2) are correct.
      (d) Only (3) and (4) are correct.
      (e) All are correct.
6. Which of these statements are true regarding interpretation of ultrasonographic findings in patients with coexistent Hashimoto's thyroiditis (HT) and differentiated thyroid cancer?
   1. Benign central neck nodes are frequently encountered in patients with HT and one must not reflexively characterize prominent neck nodes as metastatic disease.
   2. Sensitivity of ultrasound for detecting central compartment lymphadenopathy is higher when thyroid is present.
   3. Atrophy of the thyroid gland in later HT limits detection of central neck lymphadenopathy.

4. Metastatic central neck lymph nodes are frequently encountered in patients with HT and prominent central nodes should be biopsied.
   (a) Only (1) is correct.
   (b) Only (4) is correct.
   (c) Only (1) and (2) are correct.
   (d) Only (3) and (4) are correct.
   (e) All are correct.

7. Which of the following statements are true regarding the association between Hashimoto's thyroiditis (HT) and papillary thyroid cancer (PTC)?
   1. Chronic inflammation in HT may facilitate malignant transformation.
   2. HT is associated with aggressive PTC including increased rates of metastasis and recurrence.
   3. HT may be an immune response to the tumor.
   4. Patients with HT have lower TSH levels from levothyroxine treatment, which contributes to thyroid epithelial cell proliferation.
   5. Increased expression of the (PI3K)/Akt pathway has been shown in thyroid tissue of those with HT.
   (a) Only (1) and (2) and (3) are correct.
   (b) Only (1) and (3) and (5) are correct.
   (c) Only (1) and (3) and (4) are correct.
   (d) Only (2) and (3) and (4) are correct.
   (e) All are correct.

8. Which of these statements are true regarding postpartum thyroiditis?
   1. Onset of postpartum thyroiditis typically occurs within 2–6 months after delivery.
   2. Postpartum thyroiditis is often transient with return to normal thyroid function within a year.
   3. Postpartum thyroiditis may manifest as mild hyperthyroidism.
   4. Postpartum thyroiditis results in development of permanent hypothyroidism.
   (a) Only (1) and (2) and (3) are correct.
   (b) Only (3) and (4) are correct.
   (c) Only (1) and (3) and (4) are correct.
   (d) Only (2) and (3) and (4) are correct.
   (e) All are correct.

9. In which of the following scenarios are FNAs likely to have pitfalls, either with nondiagnostic samples, low sensitivity, or low positive predictive value?
   1. A patient with thyroid tenderness following an upper respiratory illness
   2. A patient with a rapidly enlarging hypoechoic thyroid mass with variable edge characteristics, homogeneous echotexture without calcifications, and absence of necrosis

3. A patient with firm enlargement of the thyroid associated with compressive symptoms, with sclerotic thyroid, which is hypointense on MRI T1- and T2- weight images
4. A patient with Hashimoto's thyroiditis and a thyroid nodule rich in Hürthle cells
   (a) Only (1) and (2) and (3) are correct.
   (b) Only (3) and (4) are correct.
   (c) Only (1) and (3) and (4) are correct.
   (d) Only (2) and (3) and (4) are correct.
   (e) All are correct.

10. What are some pitfalls of cytologic evaluation of nodules in setting of Hashimoto's thyroiditis (HT)?
    1. Structural or nuclear features of papillary thyroid cancer, including papillary or microfollicular pattern and nuclear groves, can be present in HT without malignancy.
    2. Nondiagnostic samples are commonly encountered in HT due to atrophic thyroid tissue.
    3. Aspirates interpreted as "suspicious for follicular neoplasm, Hürthle cell type" may have low positive predictive value (PPV) for malignancy in those with HT.
    4. Molecular testing platforms such as the Afirma™ gene sequencing classifier (GSC) demonstrate poor performance for samples rich in Hürthle cells.
       (a) Only (1) and (2) and (3) are correct.
       (b) Only (3) and (4) are correct.
       (c) Only (1) and (3) are correct.
       (d) Only (2) and (3) and (4) are correct.
       (e) All are correct.

11. Which of these statements are correct regarding surgical treatment for Riedel thyroiditis?
    1. Complete surgical excision has higher likelihood of success compared to partial thyroid surgery.
    2. Isthmusectomy alone could be considered as treatment to relieve pressure symptoms.
    3. Thyroidectomy is challenging due to obliteration of normal tissue planes.
    4. Significant risk of complications such as temporary and permanent vocal cord paralysis and rates of temporary and permanent hypoparathyroidism may be associated with thyroidectomy.
       (a) Only (1) and (2) and (3) are correct.
       (b) Only (3) and (4) are correct.
       (c) Only (1) and (3) and (4) are correct.
       (d) Only (2) and (3) and (4) are correct.
       (e) All are correct.

12. Which of these are possible medical treatment options for Riedel's thyroiditis?
    1. Corticosteroids
    2. Tamoxifen

3. Mycophenolate mofetil
4. Levothyroxine
5. Methimazole
    (a) Only (1) and (2) and (3) and (4) are correct.
    (b) Only (3) and (4) are correct.
    (c) Only (1) and (3) and (4) are correct.
    (d) Only (2) and (3) and (4) are correct.
    (e) All are correct.

4.1 Introduction

The term "thyroiditis' encompasses a broad spectrum of clinical conditions characterized by inflammation of the thyroid gland with varying causation and clinical manifestations. Both autoimmune and infectious etiologies have been implicated in thyroiditis. These clinical entities may present as isolated disease states or may be coexistent with thyroid nodules or malignancy. Indeed, Hashimoto's thyroiditis (HT) is associated with an increased risk of developing thyroid lymphoma, and a linkage between HT and papillary thyroid carcinoma (PTC) has been proposed [1, 2].

Several thyroiditis syndromes have been described, many sharing overlap in their clinical features [2]. This chapter will address the diagnosis and management of three thyroiditis types: Hashimoto, de Quervain, and Riedel. A summary of clinical characteristics and treatment recommendations discussed in this chapter is presented in ◘ Table 4.1.

While medical management of thyroiditis is paramount, surgical treatment for compressive symptoms or coexistent nodules or malignancy is often indicated. To this end, the surgeon should be familiar with surgical considerations specific to these conditions. It also is important to understand the impact of thyroid inflammation on the assessment of thyroid nodules and malignancy in order to make sound clinical decisions regarding surgical management.

4.2 Clinical Presentation and Diagnosis

4.2.1 Hashimoto's Thyroiditis

Hashimoto's thyroiditis (HT), also called chronic lymphocytic thyroiditis or autoimmune thyroiditis, is the most common autoimmune condition [3] and the leading cause of hypothyroidism in iodine-replete areas of the world [4]. The worldwide incidence is estimated to be 0.3 to 1.5 per 1000 [1]. Women are 8–10 times more likely to suffer from HT than men, with a peak age of onset between 30 and 50 years of age [2, 4]. There is increasing evidence to suggest that genetic susceptibility and

Table 4.1 Characteristics and treatment of thyroiditis syndromes

Syndrome	Hashimoto	de Quervain	Riedel
Etiology	Autoimmune	Infectious	Unknown
Clinical presentation	Symmetric thyroid enlargement; later stages with thyroid atrophy	Thyroid pain/tenderness preceded by viral prodrome or upper respiratory illness	Firm enlargement of thyroid, may include compressive symptoms, hypoparathyroidism, or hoarseness
Thyroid hormone status	Initial hyperthyroidism ("hashitoxicosis") or euthyroid status, progressing to subclinical and overt hypothyroidism	Initial thyrotoxicosis followed by euthyroidism or hypothyroidism; majority return to euthyroid state	Initially may be euthyroid, progressing to hypothyroidism
Thyroid antibodies	High titers of anti-TPO (>90%), anti-Tg (~50%)	Absent, low titers or transient anti-TPO	+/– anti-TPO, +/– anti-Tg
US features	Diffuse heterogeneity with ill-defined areas of hypoechogenicity and "pseudonodules"; atrophied with "honeycomb" appearance in later stages	Patchy, poorly defined areas of hypoechogenicity with decreased vascularity	Heterogeneous hypoechogenicity with decreased vascularity
Histology	Interstitial lymphocytic infiltrate with plasma cells, macrophages; lymphoid follicles with or without germinal centers; hyperplastic or atrophied thyroid follicles with Hürthle cell change; fibrosis	Noncaseating granulomas; disrupted follicles; interstitial inflammatory infiltrate containing lymphocytes and multinucleated giant cells; fibrosis	Diffuse fibrosis extending outside thyroid capsule
Medical treatment	Thyroid hormone replacement	NSAIDs, corticosteroids	Corticosteroids, tamoxifen, mycophenolate mofetil
Surgical indications (excluding coexistent thyroid pathology)	Compressive symptoms, persistent systemic symptoms	Recurrent thyroiditis	Compressive symptoms (isthmusectomy recommended)

environmental triggers contribute to the loss of immune tolerance [5]; nutritional factors, including high iodine intake and dietary deficiencies of selenium and iron, have been implicated in its development [6, 7]. For reasons that are not clear, smoking appears to have a protective effect against levels of autoantibodies and development of hypothyroidism in HT [8, 9].

Hashimoto first described this condition in 1912 as "struma lymphomatosa," based on histopathologic examination of 4 goitrous thyroidectomy specimens from middle-aged women showing diffuse lymphocytic infiltration with formation of lymphoid follicles and degeneration of thyroid follicles [10]. Several variants of thyroiditis along the same clinical and histopathologic spectrum have since been described, including fibrous variant, IgG4-related variant, juvenile form, and painless/postpartum thyroiditis. The defining feature in each of these entities is profound lymphocytic infiltration of the thyroid gland [11].

Classically, HT presents with painless, gradual enlargement of the thyroid, though morphology of the thyroid gland may vary, depending on the timing and circumstances of clinical detection. Patients who present later in the disease process may demonstrate thyroid atrophy resulting from destruction and fibrosis of thyroid parenchyma [5, 12]. Elevated levels of antibodies to thyroperoxidase (TPO) are present in nearly all patients, and antibodies to thyroglobulin (Tg) are present in up to half of patients with HT [11, 13]. Mild hyperthyroidism or so-called Hashitoxicosis, resulting from destruction of follicular cells and release of hormone, has been described as a presenting feature [11, 14], though thyroid function is frequently normal at presentation. While subclinical hypothyroidism may persist for a period of time, most eventually develop overt hypothyroidism [11].

In patients in whom the diagnosis of HT is considered, the presence of anti-TPO and Tg antibodies can be helpful. Notably, ultrasound findings suggestive of HT may precede evidence of elevated antithyroid antibodies in a subset of cases [15]. The characteristic ultrasonographic appearance of HT is of diffuse heterogeneity with ill-defined areas of hypoechogenicity resulting from accumulation of lymphoid tissue. Parenchymal destruction and fibrosis distort thyroid architecture and give the appearance of "pseudonodules." The term "pseudonodule" refers to an area within the thyroid that appears to represent a nodule in one imaging plane but loses its demarcation as such in another plane; this finding is especially marked in the fibrosing variant of Hashimoto's, where dense fibrous bands appear as hyperechoic septations, generating the false appearance of distinct nodules. Vascularity may be increased early in the disease course and decreased as disease progresses. In later stages, the atrophied gland appears shrunken and imparts a "honeycomb" appearance. Central neck adenopathy may be prominent, reflective of increased local immune activity [11, 16, 17].

Histologically, HT shows interstitial lymphocytic infiltrates containing plasma cells and macrophages; lymphoid follicles containing occasional germinal centers are seen. Thyroid follicles range from hyperplastic to atrophic with minimal colloid. Hürthle cell change is often observed, and variable degrees of fibrosis are present. The fibrosing variant of HT, which clinically presents with a large, firm, and nodular thyroid, is characterized by a predominance of fibrosis replacing thyroid parenchyma. This entity must be distinguished from Riedel's thyroiditis (discussed below), which shows a similar extent of fibrosis, but which progresses outside of the thyroid capsule. The IgG4 variant of HT also shows dense stromal fibrosis but with the hallmark finding of increased number of IgG4-

producing plasma cells. This latter disease is clinically characterized by earlier age of onset, decrease in the ratio of women to men, higher levels of circulating antithyroid antibodies, and a more rapid and progressive clinical course [11, 18].

Painless sporadic (silent) thyroiditis and postpartum thyroiditis are autoimmune conditions, which demonstrate similar histologic findings of lymphocytic infiltration and may be considered variants of HT. Contrasting findings include an absence of germinal centers, less extensive fibrosis, minimal Hürthle cell metaplasia, and lack of follicular atrophy [2, 11, 19]. Clinically, silent thyroiditis and postpartum thyroiditis are felt to represent the same disease process, distinguished only by the association of postpartum thyroiditis with pregnancy [2, 11]. The onset of postpartum thyroiditis occurs typically within 2 to 6 months after delivery. Both conditions initially manifest as mild hyperthyroidism caused by destruction of follicular cells and release of thyroid hormone. In some, a brief period of euthyroidism follows before development of hypothyroidism. In about 80% of cases, the disease is transient and normal thyroid function returns within a year [20].

The increased utilization of immunotherapy in oncologic diseases has led to the recognition of checkpoint inhibitor–mediated thyroiditis as another variant of autoimmune thyroiditis. The prevalence of thyroiditis with checkpoint inhibitor treatment (such as nivolumab, ipilimumab, and pembrolizumab) ranges from 6% to 20%. Thyroiditis can present with a thyrotoxic phase lasting an average of 6 weeks, followed by development of hypothyroidism [21]. Histological findings include lymphocytic inflammation and nonnecrotizing colloid granulomas [22].

4.2.2 de Quervain's Thyroiditis

Also known as subacute thyroiditis (SAT) or granulomatous thyroiditis, de Quervain's thyroiditis is a self-limited inflammatory disorder thought to be a sequela of viral infection. The incidence varies geographically but is noted to be higher in women in the fifth and sixth decades of life [23, 24]. Clinical presentation is characterized by a viral prodrome or upper respiratory illness preceding development of fever and thyroid pain or tenderness. Thyrocyte destruction results in thyrotoxicosis, which resolves over a period of several weeks. Hypothyroidism sometimes follows and resolves spontaneously over several months. Approximately 5% experience persistent hypothyroidism; recurrence of subacute thyroiditis has been reported in 2–9% [23–26].

The diagnosis of SAT is primarily clinical. In most patients, the findings of thyroid tenderness, a viral prodrome, and a self-limiting course are enough to establish the diagnosis. If the diagnosis is uncertain, an elevated erythrocyte sedimentation rate (ESR) or C-reactive protein (CRP) may help establish the diagnosis. Antithyroid antibodies are typically absent but may be present transiently or in low levels and may predict development of future hypothyroidism [2]. Extreme tenderness of the thyroid with palpation is characteristic. During the thyrotoxic phase, thyroid-stimulating hormone (TSH) is suppressed and uptake of radioactive iodine on nuclear imaging is low; uptake may be increased during the recovery phase when TSH is elevated [24, 27]. Ultrasonographic findings include patchy, poorly defined areas of hypoechogenicity with decreased vascularity; diffuse heterogeneity may also be seen [28]. Tissue sampling is not required for diagnosis, though cytologic findings reveal noncaseating granulomatous inflammation with disrupted follicles, interstitial inflammatory infiltrate with lymphocytes and multinucleated giant cells, and interfollicular fibrosis [29].

4.2.3 Riedel's Thyroiditis

Riedel's thyroiditis (RT) is a rare form of chronic thyroiditis characterized by dense progressive fibrosis extending outside the thyroid capsule to surrounding tissues. The true incidence is not known but is estimated to be 1.06 per 100,000 based on a large population study [30]. The etiology of RT is unclear, though it has been linked to a generalized fibroinflammatory disorder based on concurrent presentation with other inflammatory conditions, including idiopathic retroperitoneal fibrosis, sclerosing cholangitis, fibrosing mediastinitis, inflammatory pseudotumor, and Tolosa-Hunt syndrome [31–34]. This constellation of findings shares overlapping features with IgG4-related systemic disease, a systemic sclerosing process characterized by infiltration of IgG-4-bearing plasma cells, leading some to suggest they are the same clinical entity [35, 36]. The IgG4 variant of HT also shares similar clinicopathologic characteristics [37–39].

The clinical presentation of RT includes firm enlargement of the thyroid, often associated with compressive symptoms, which worsen as extrathyroidal involvement progresses. Hypoparathyroidism may be a presenting symptom, resulting from extension of fibrosis to the parathyroid glands [40, 41]. Vocal cord paralysis related to involvement of the recurrent laryngeal nerve was reported in 29% in one series [32]. Thyroid function may be normal at presentation though hypothyroidism is frequent, occurring up to 80% [42]. On ultrasonographic examination, the thyroid appears heterogeneously hypoechoic with decreased vascularity; tracheal narrowing or encasement of the carotid artery or jugular vein may be seen. Computed tomography (CT) shows hypodense enlargement of the thyroid with relative lack of contrast enhancement; evidence of extrathyroidal extension can be readily appreciated, along with carotid artery or jugular vein encasement [32, 42]. On magnetic resonance imaging (MRI), the sclerotic thyroid appears hypointense on T1- and T2-weighted images with modest enhancement following administration of gadolinium contrast [43]. Elevated levels of circulating thyroid autoantibodies (anti-Tg, anti-TPO) are commonly encountered in RT, though it is not clear whether this represents a causative element or a reaction to thyroid degeneration [42]. The clinical course of RT is often progressive but may be stabilize over time [32].

The presence of a firm, fixed mass along with clinical and radiographic evidence of extrathyroidal involvement may raise concern for malignancy. Fine-needle aspiration (FNA) biopsy is often nondiagnostic owing to a pauci-cellular sample obtained from densely fibrous tissue [32, 42, 44]. A diagnosis of Riedel's thyroiditis is confirmed by open biopsy with histopathology showing a fibroinflammatory process extending outside the thyroid. Inflammatory infiltrate without the presence of giant cells, lymphoid follicles, oncocytic cells, or granulomas differentiates this condition from other inflammatory disorders, including the fibrous variant of HT and de Quervain's thyroiditis [38, 44, 45].

4.3 Treatment

4.3.1 Hashimoto's Thyroiditis

HT is primarily a medical disease, with thyroidectomy uncommonly indicated as treatment (discussed below). Medical therapy involves levothyroxine (LT_4) administration for patients with thyroid hypofunction. Patients initially require low doses of LT_4, but with gradual loss of thyroid function, full thyroid hormone replacement with LT_4 (1.6 to 1.8 μg per kg of body weight) may ultimately be required [11]. Thyroid hormone replacement may also be effective in reducing thyroid enlargement associated with HT [46, 47]. Selenium (Se) supplementation has been studied as an adjunctive treatment to LT_4. A systematic review and meta-analysis showed reduction in TPO-Ab titers and improvement in mood-related symptoms associated with 3 months of Se supplementation [48], though benefit has not been consistently demonstrated [49]. Corticosteroid treatment may be beneficial in the IgG-4 variant of HT, as IgG-4-related disease is shown to be steroid-responsive [11, 36].

4.3.2 de Quervain's Thyroiditis

Treatment of de Quervain's thyroiditis is supportive and directed at pain relief with administration of nonsteroidal anti-inflammatory drugs (NSAIDS). Caution is advised with use of salicylates, which may increase levels of free thyroid hormone [27, 50]. Corticosteroids may be offered for more severe cases. Dosing of prednisone is 20–40 mg daily, tapered over several weeks to avoid relapse of symptoms [27, 32]. Treatment of hyperthyroidism with antithyroid medications is ineffective, as increased thyroid hormone results from destruction of thyrocytes and release of stored thyroid hormone and not increased production; as such, beta-blockade should be used for treatment of systemic effects. LT_4 therapy is indicated for prolonged or symptomatic hypothyroidism.

4.3.3 Riedel's Thyroiditis

Thyroid isthmusectomy allows for diagnosis of RT and may provide relief of compressive symptoms, but thyroidectomy is associated with increased risk, especially in later stages where invasion may be extensive. As such, medical management is generally advocated, with treatment directed at inhibiting the fibroinflammatory process. Treatment with corticosteroids may reduce thyroid size and improve compressive symptoms. Hypothyroidism in IgG4-related disease has been shown to respond to corticosteroid therapy [36]. Tamoxifen, believed to inhibit fibroblast proliferation through stimulation of transforming growth factor (TGF)-β1, has been used with reports of success in some patients [32, 43, 51–53]. Recommended dosing of tamoxifen is 10–20 mg per day, with or without prednisone therapy [27]. Mycophenolate mofetil, an immune modulator shown to be beneficial in the treatment of fibrotic disorders, has been reported to be effective in treatment of steroid- and tamoxifen-resistant RT [31, 37], and treatment with Rituximab has also been described [54].

4.4 Surgical Indications and Outcomes

4.4.1 Hashimoto's Thyroiditis

Surgical treatment in HT is most commonly recommended for management of coexistent thyroid nodules or malignancy. Thyroidectomy as a treatment for HT alone is not frequently undertaken, but may be indicated in patients with goiters to treat local compressive symptoms or address cosmesis [55]. Several case series have shown thyroid surgery to be effective for relieving compressive symptoms such as dysphagia, dyspnea, and neck discomfort or tightness [55–58]. Heggie et al. [59] compared the resected gland weight for thyroidectomies performed to treat compressive symptoms in HT versus goiter and found lighter gland weights in the HT group, suggesting that thyroid stiffening in HT contributes to pressure symptoms, even without significant gland enlargement.

Thyroidectomy has been explored for some patients who experience systemic symptoms of HT, including fatigue and joint or muscle tenderness, despite normalization of thyroid hormone status. A study of HT patients randomized to total thyroidectomy and hormone replacement versus hormone replacement alone found improved health survey and fatigue scores in the thyroidectomy group at 18 months follow-up, with no significant changes in the medical management group. The authors hypothesize that the improvements were related to normalization of TPO-Ab levels, which declined sharply in the thyroidectomy group but decreased only modestly in the hormone replacement group [60]. This remains a controversial area as the trial was nonblinded and concerns remain regarding whether the findings were placebo-driven.

Potential benefits from thyroid surgery should be considered in the context of surgical risk. Increased risk of recurrent laryngeal nerve or parathyroid injury related to inflammatory changes and adherence of the thyroid to surrounding structures have been raised by many as a concern. A large prospective multicenter study published by Thomusch et al. [61] examined complication rates in 18,955 patients undergoing surgery for autoimmune thyroid disease or multinodular goiter (MNG) without known malignancy. Preoperative and postoperative laryngoscopy was performed for all patients. Among the 1266 patients who underwent thyroid surgery for HT, 67% received total thyroidectomy. No difference was seen in rates of transient and permanent vocal cord paralysis (VCP) between surgery for HT and surgery for MNG. However, rates of transient and permanent hypoparathyroidism were slightly increased for HT compared with MNG (15.3 vs. 12.9% for temporary, 1.1 vs. 0.9% for permanent, $p < 0.001$).

4.4.2 de Quervain's Thyroiditis

Thyroidectomy for SAT is rarely indicated, as the disease is typically self-limiting. However, for the rare cases in which there is repeated recurrence, thyroidectomy may be considered. Despite this uncommon indication, 69 cases of thyroid surgery for SAT were included in the Thomusch et al. study [61], with over half receiving total thyroidectomy. Rates of temporary and permanent VCP were not different than for MNG, though rates of temporary and permanent hypoparathyroidism were higher than for MNG, at 14% and 7%, respectively.

4.4.3 Riedel's Thyroiditis

Thyroidectomy for RT is regarded as challenging due to obliteration of normal tissue planes and may be associated with significant risk of complications. Fatourechi et al. [32] reported a series of 21 patients with RT treated over a 30-year period at the Mayo Clinic, including 18 patients who underwent at least partial thyroid surgery (isthmusectomy, lobectomy, or subtotal thyroidectomy). Complete surgical excision was deemed impossible in all cases. Seven patients (39%) experienced surgical complications involving the recurrent laryngeal nerve or parathyroid glands. Isthmusectomy alone was recommended as treatment to relieve pressure symptoms. By contrast, 10 cases of RT were reported in the large multicenter study described above [61], with 5 receiving total thyroidectomy. Rates of temporary and permanent VCP were 6.7% and 0%, respectively, and rates of temporary and permanent hypoparathyroidism were 16.7% and 0%, respectively. It is not clear whether these disparate findings are the result of selection bias, with patients in the latter study receiving surgery at an earlier stage of disease when fibrosis is less extensive.

4.5 Association with Malignancy

A link between HT and the development of thyroid malignancy has been long surmised [1]. Patients with HT have a 67–80-fold higher risk of developing primary thyroid lymphoma (PTL) [62, 63], though overall, the rate of occurrence in this population is just 0.5% [64]. The pathogenic mechanism underlying this epidemiologic association is not clear; however, the high prevalence of thyroid autoantibodies in cases of PTL suggests autoimmune stimulation plays a role [63, 65, 66]. The most common type of lymphoma occurring in the thyroid is large diffuse B-cell lymphoma, which can present with rapid thyroid enlargement, hoarseness, and dysphagia, and must be differentiated from anaplastic thyroid carcinoma [65]. The ultrasonographic appearance of thyroid lymphoma is a solid hypoechoic mass with variable edge characteristics (well defined to poorly defined) and increased vascularity [67]. Homogenous echotexture without calcifications and absence of necrosis or cystic degeneration can help distinguish its appearance from anaplastic carcinoma [68]. Core needle biopsy has better sensitivity and accuracy than fine-needle aspiration (FNA) in the diagnosis of thyroid lymphoma [67, 69] and should be employed when PTL is suspected.

An association between HT and PTC has also been observed, though the linkage appears inconsistent and a causal relationship has not been established [1]. Whether co-occurrence of HT and PTC is simply coincidental, HT triggers the development of PTC, or HT represents an immune response to tumor remains controversial. A systematic review conducted by Jankovic et al. [70] examined the coexistence of PTC with HT and noted a statistically positive correlation in studies of thyroidectomy specimens (27.2% prevalence of PTC in specimens with HT), but no association in studies of FNA specimens (1.2% prevalence of PTC in FNAs of subjects with HT). Notably, thyroidectomy studies are subject to selection bias; population studies of FNA are more representative of patients with HT but are limited by absence of histologic examination [1, 70]. Despite these challenges, several hypotheses have been proposed to explain a linkage, including chronic inflammation facilitating malignant transformation and elevated TSH levels in hypothyroid patients stimulating thyroid epithelial proliferation [1, 71]. Various molecular mechanisms supporting a linkage have been explored. Larson et al. [72] examined expression of the phosphatidylinositol 3-kinase (PI3K)/Akt pathway in thyroidectomy specimens of patients with HT and PTC and found increased expression in regions of HT and PTC compared with normal thyroid tissue. RET/PTC rearrangement has been implicated as an early oncogenic event in patients with lymphocytic thyroiditis [73, 74], and differential expression of various genes, including CD98 and p63, appears to support a linkage [75, 76]. Several studies have found that PTC coexisting with HT exhibits less aggressive clinicopathologic features and is associated with more favorable outcomes, including decreased rate of metastases, lower recurrence rates, and improved overall and disease-specific survival [77–80].

The diagnostic performance of FNA in the evaluation of thyroid nodules coexisting with HT has been examined in several studies. Overall, the positive predictive value (PPV) of FNA for malignancy is high at 97–99%, with sensitivity of 65–99% and specificity of 72–100% [81]. However, various pitfalls have been described for cytologic evaluation of nodules in the setting of HT, with risk of both false-negatives and false-positives [82, 83]. Structural and nuclear features of PTC, including a papillary or microfollicular pattern and nuclear grooves, can be present in HT without malignancy [82–84]. Furthermore, the frequent presence of Hürthle cells in HT can complicate interpretation of FNA, with aspirates rich in Hürthle cells being interpreted as "suspicious for follicular neoplasm, Hürthle cell type" (Bethesda IV category) [85]. One study found this cytologic designation had a PPV for malignancy of just 9.5% when HT was coexistent, versus 25.2% without HT, though this difference did not meet statistical significance [86]. The presence of Hürthle cells was also found to impact the diagnostic accuracy of early molecular testing platforms, with the Afirma™ gene expression classifier (GEC) disproportionately assigning "suspicious" results to samples rich with Hürthle cells [87–90]. The more recently developed Afirma™ gene sequencing classifier (GSC) addressed this problem by incorporating new classifier algorithms with improved performance for Hürthle cell samples [91, 92].

HT coexistent with PTC should inform the interpretation of ultrasonographic findings, especially as it relates to the presence of lymph nodes in the central compartment. Overall, the sensitivity of ultrasound for detecting central compartment lymphadenopathy is limited when the thyroid is present [93]. However, atrophy of the gland, as occurs in later stages of HT, may allow for improved detection of central neck lymphadenopathy. Benign central neck nodes are frequently encountered in HT, with one study demonstrating a sensitivity of 93.4% in the diagnosis of autoimmune thyroiditis [94]. As such, when evaluating thyroid malignancy coexistent with HT, the clinician must be careful to not reflexively characterize prominent central neck nodes as metastatic disease. Indeed, it has been suggested that an explanation for the finding of decreased central neck metastases in PTC coexistent with HT is increased sampling of benign nodes brought to clinical attention as a result of HT [77].

Answers

1. (e); 2. (b); 3. (c); 4. (e); 5. (c); 6. (a); 7. (b); 8. (a); 9. (d); 10. (c); 11. (d); 12. (a)

References

1. Noureldine S, Tufano R. Association of Hashimoto's thyroiditis and thyroid cancer. Curr Opin Oncol. 2015;27(1):21–5.
2. Pearce EN, Farwell AP, Braverman LE. Thyroiditis. N Engl J Med. 2003;348(26):2646–55.
3. McLeod DSA, Cooper DS. The incidence and prevalence of thyroid autoimmunity. Endocrine. 2012;42(2):252–65.
4. Vanderpump MPJ. The epidemiology of thyroid disease. Br Med Bull. 2011;99(1):39–51.
5. Ragusa F, Fallahi P, Elia G, Gonnella D, Paparo SR, Giusti C, et al. Hashimotos' thyroiditis: epidemiology, pathogenesis, clinic and therapy. Best Pract Res Clin Endocrinol Metab. 2019;33(6):101367.
6. Hu S, Rayman MP. Multiple nutritional factors and the risk of Hashimoto's thyroiditis. Thyroid. 2017;27(5):597–610.
7. Wichman J, Winther KH, Bonnema SJ, Hegedüs L. Selenium supplementation significantly reduces thyroid autoantibody levels in patients with chronic autoimmune thyroiditis: a systematic review and meta-analysis. Thyroid. 2016;26(12):1681–92.
8. Belin RM, Astor BC, Powe NR, Ladenson PW. Smoke exposure is associated with a lower prevalence of serum thyroid autoantibodies and thyrotropin concentration elevation and a higher prevalence of mild thyrotropin concentration suppression in the Third National Health and Nutrition Examination Survey (NHANES III). J Clin Endocrinol Metab. 2004;89(12):6077–86.
9. Effraimidis G, Tijssen JGP, Wiersinga WM. Discontinuation of smoking increases the risk for developing thyroid peroxidase antibodies and/or thyroglobulin antibodies: a prospective study. J Clin Endocrinol Metab. 2009;94(4):1324–8.
10. Takami HE, Miyabe R, Kameyama K. Hashimoto's thyroiditis. World J Surg. 2008;32(5):688–92.
11. Caturegli P, De Remigis A, Rose NR. Hashimoto thyroiditis: clinical and diagnostic criteria. Autoimmun Rev. 2014;13(4):391–7.
12. Caleo A, Vigliar E, Vitale M, Di Crescenzo V, Cinelli M, Carlomagno C, et al. Cytological diagnosis of thyroid nodules in Hashimoto thyroiditis in elderly patients. BMC Surg. 2013;13(Suppl 2):S41.

13. Singer PA. Thyroiditis. Acute, subacute, and chronic. Med Clin North Am. 1991;75(1):61–77.
14. Nabhan ZM, Kreher NC, Eugster EA. Hashitoxicosis in children: clinical features and natural history. J Pediatr. 2005;146(4):533–6.
15. Biondi B, Cooper DS. The clinical significance of subclinical thyroid dysfunction. Endocr Rev. 2008;29(1):76–131.
16. Orloff LA. Head and neck ultrasonography: essential and extended applications. 2nd: Plural Publishing; 2017. 545 p.
17. Kangelaris GT, Kim TB, Orloff LA. Role of ultrasound in thyroid disorders. Otolaryngol Clin N Am. 2010;43(6):1209–27.
18. Li Y, Zhou G, Ozaki T, Nishihara E, Matsuzuka F, Bai Y, et al. Distinct histopatholcgical features of Hashimoto's thyroiditis with respect to IgG4-relatec disease. Mod Pathol. 2012;25(8):1086–97.
19. Samuels MH. Subacute, silent, and postpartum thyroiditis. Med Clin North Am. 2012;96(2):223–33.
20. Bindra A, Braunstein GD. Thyroiditis. Am Fam Physician. 2006;73(10):1769–76.
21. Iyer PC, Cabanillas ME, Waguespack SG, Hu MI, Thosani S, Lavis VR, et al. Immune-related thyroiditis with immune checkpoint inhibitors. Thyroid. 2018;28(10):1243–51.
22. Neppl C, Kaderli RM, Trepp R, Schmitt AM, Berger MD, Wehrli M, et al. Histology of nivolumab-induced thyroiditis. Thyroid. 2018;28(12):1727–8.
23. Benbassat CA, Olchovsky D, Tsvetov G, Shimon I. Subacute thyroiditis: clinical characteristics and treatment outcome in fifty-six consecutive patients diagnosed between 1999 and 2005. J Endocrinol Investig. 2007;30(8):631–5.
24. Fatourechi V, Aniszewski JP, Fatourechi GZE, Atkinson EJ, Jacobsen SJ. Clinical features and outcome of subacute thyroiditis in an incidence cohort: Olmsted County, Minnesota, study. J Clin Endocrinol Metab. 2003;88(5):2100–5.
25. Lio S, Pontecorvi A, Caruso M, Monaco F, D'Armiento M. Transitory subclinical and permanent hypothyroidism in the course of subacute thyroiditis (de Quervain). Acta Endocrinol. 1984;106(1):67–70.
26. Kitchener MI, Chapman IM. Subacute thyroiditis: a review of 105 cases. Clin Nucl Med. 1989;14(6):439–42.
27. Randolph GW, editor. Surgery of the thyroid and parathyroid glands. 3rd ed. Philadelphia: Elsevier Health Sciences; 2020. 1010 p.
28. Frates MC, Marqusee E, Benson CB, Alexander EK. Subacute granulomatous (de Quervain) thyroiditis: grayscale and color Doppler sonographic characteristics. J Ultrasound Med. 2013;32(3):505–11.
29. Ranganath R, Shaha MA, Xu B, Migliacci J, Ghossein R, Shaha AR. de Quervain's thyroiditis: a review of experience with surgery. Am J Otolaryngol. 2016;37(6):534–7.
30. Hay ID. Thyroiditis: a clinical update. Mayo Clin Proc. 1985;60(12):836–43.
31. Levy JM, Hasney CP, Friedlander PL, Kandil E, Occhipinti EA, Kahn MJ. Combined mycophenolate mofetil and prednisone therapy in tamoxifen- and prednisone-resistant Reidel's thyroiditis. Thyroid. 2010;20(1):105–7.
32. Fatourechi MM, Hay ID, McIver B, Sebo TJ, Fatourechi V. Invasive fibrous thyroiditis (Riedel thyroiditis): the Mayo Clinic experience, 1976–2008. Thyroid. 2011;21(7):765–72.
33. Baloch ZW, Saberi M, Livolsi VA. Simultaneous involvement of thyroid by Riedel's [correction of Reidel's] disease and fibrosing Hashimoto's thyroiditis: a case report. Thyroid. 1998;8(4):337–41.
34. Khan MAE, Hashmi SMH, Prinsley PR, Premachandra DJ. Reidel's thyroiditis and Tolosa-Hunt syndrome, a rare association. J Laryngol Otol. 2004;118(2):159–61.

35. Dahlgren M, Khosroshahi A, Nielsen GP, Deshpande V, Stone JH. Riedel's thyroiditis and multifocal fibrosclerosis are part of the IgG4-related systemic disease spectrum. Arthritis Care Res. 2010;62(9):1312–8.
36. Watanabe T, Maruyama M, Ito T, Fujinaga Y, Ozaki Y, Maruyama M, et al. Clinical features of a new disease concept, IgG4-related thyroiditis. Scand J Rheumatol. 2013;42(4):325–30.
37. Falhammar H, Juhlin CC, Barner C, Catrina S-B, Karefylakis C, Calissendorff J. Riedel's thyroiditis: clinical presentation, treatment and outcomes. Endocrine. 2018;60(1):185–92.
38. Kumar N, Gupta R, Sayed S, Moloo Z, Vinayak S, Ahmed M. Difficulties in diagnosis of Riedel's thyroiditis on aspiration cytology: a case report and brief review of the literature. Diagn Cytopathol. 2019;47(5):512–6.
39. Li Y, Nishihara E, Kakudo K. Hashimoto's thyroiditis: old concepts and new insights. Curr Opin Rheumatol. 2011;23(1):102–7.
40. Yasmeen T, Khan S, Patel SG, Reeves WA, Gonsch FA, de Bustros A, et al. Clinical case seminar: Riedel's thyroiditis: report of a case complicated by spontaneous hypoparathyroidism, recurrent laryngeal nerve injury, and Horner's syndrome. J Clin Endocrinol Metab. 2002;87(8):3543–7.
41. Stan MN, Haglind EG, Drake MT. Early hypoparathyroidism reversibility with treatment of Riedel's thyroiditis. Thyroid. 2015;25(9):1055–9.
42. Hennessey JV. Riedel's thyroiditis: a clinical review. J Clin Endocrinol Metab. 2011;96(10):3031–41.
43. Pritchyk K, Newkirk K, Garlich P, Deeb Z. Tamoxifen therapy for Riedel's thyroiditis. Laryngoscope. 2004;114(10):1758–60.
44. Papi G, LiVolsi VA. Current concepts on Riedel thyroiditis. Pathol Patterns Rev. 2004;121(suppl_1):S50–63.
45. Schwaegerle SM, Bauer TW, Esselstyn CB. Riedel's thyroiditis. Am J Clin Pathol. 1988;90(6):715–22.
46. Hayashi Y, Tamai H, Fukata S, Hirota Y, Katayama S, Kuma K, et al. A long term clinical, immunological, and histological follow-up study of patients with goitrous chronic lymphocytic thyroiditis. J Clin Endocrinol Metab. 1985;61(6):1172–8.
47. Hegedüs L, Hansen JM, Feldt-Rasmussen U, Hansen BM, Høier-Madsen M. Influence of thyroxine treatment on thyroid size and anti-thyroid peroxidase antibodies in Hashimoto's thyroiditis. Clin Endocrinol. 1991;35(3):235–8.
48. Toulis KA, Anastasilakis AD, Tzellos TG, Goulis DG, Kouvelas D. Selenium supplementation in the treatment of Hashimoto's thyroiditis: a systematic review and a meta-analysis. Thyroid. 2010;20(10):1163–73.
49. Eskes SA, Endert E, Fliers E, Birnie E, Hollenbach B, Schomburg L, et al. Selenite supplementation in euthyroid subjects with thyroid peroxidase antibodies. Clin Endocrinol. 2014;80(3):444–51.
50. Larsen PR. Salicylate-induced increases in free triiodothyronine in human serum. Evidence of inhibition of triiodothyronine binding to thyroxine-binding globulin and thyroxine-binding prealbumin. J Clin Invest. 1972;51(5):1125–34.
51. Few J, Thompson NW, Angelos P, Simeone D, Giordano T, Reeve T. Riedel's thyroiditis: treatment with tamoxifen. Surgery. 1996;120(6):993–8; discussion 998-999.
52. Jung YJ, Schaub CR, Rhodes R, Rich FA, Muehlenbein SJ. A case of Riedel's thyroiditis treated with tamoxifen: another successful outcome. Endocr Pract. 2004;10(6):483–6.
53. Dabelic N, Jukic T, Labar Z, Novosel SA, Matesa N, Kusic Z. Riedel's thyroiditis treated with tamoxifen. Croat Med J. 2003;44(2):239–41.
54. Soh S-B, Pham A, O'Hehir RE, Cherk M, Topliss DJ. Novel use of rituximab in a case of Riedel's thyroiditis refractory to glucocorticoids and tamoxifen. J Clin Endocrinol Metab. 2013;98(9):3543–9.

55. Shih M-L, Lee JA, Hsieh C-B, Yu J-C, Liu H-D, Kebebew E, et al. Thyroidectomy for Hashimoto's thyroiditis: complications and associated cancers. Thyroid. 2008;18(7):729–34.
56. Wormer BA, McHenry CR. Hashimoto's thyroiditis: outcome of surgical resection for patients with thyromegaly and compressive symptoms. Am J Surg. 2011;201(3):416–9; discussion 419.
57. Shimizu K, Nakajima Y, Kitagawa W, Akasu H, Takatsu K, Ishii R, et al. Surgical therapy in Hashimoto's thyroiditis. J Nippon Med Sch. 2003;70(1):34–9.
58. Promberger R, Hermann M, Pallikunnel SJ, Seemann R, Meusel M, Ott J. Quality of life after thyroid surgery in women with benign euthyroid goiter: influencing factors including Hashimoto's thyroiditis. Am J Surg. 2014;207(6):974–9.
59. Heggie K, Yeung M, Grodski S, Lee J, Serpell J. Total thyroidectomy for pressure symptoms in patients with Hashimoto's thyroiditis. ANZ J Surg. 2018;88(4):359–62.
60. Guldvog I, Reitsma LC, Johnsen L, Lauzike A, Gibbs C, Carlsen E, et al. Thyroidectomy versus medical management for euthyroid patients with Hashimoto disease and persisting symptoms: a randomized trial. Ann Intern Med. 2019;170(7):453–64.
61. Thomusch O, Sekulla C, Billmann F, Seifert G, Dralle H, Lorenz K, et al. Risk profile analysis and complications after surgery for autoimmune thyroid disease. Br J Surg. 2018;105(6):677–85.
62. Holm L-E, Blomgren H, Löwhagen T. Cancer risks in patients with chronic lymphocytic thyroiditis. N Engl J Med. 1985;312(10):601–4.
63. Kato I, Tajima K, SucHI T, Aozasa K, Matsuzuka F. Chronic thyroiditis as a risk factor of B-cell lymphoma in the thyroid gland. Jpn J Cancer Res. 1985;76:1085.
64. Pavlidis ET, Pavlidis TE. A review of primary thyroid lymphoma: molecular factors, diagnosis and management. J Investig Surg. 2019;32(2): 137–42.
65. Kossev P, Livolsi V. Lymphoid lesions of the thyroid: review in light of the revised European-American lymphoma classification and upcoming World Health Organization classification. Thyroid. 1999;9(12):1273–80.
66. Derringer GA, Thompson LD, Frommelt RA, Bijwaard KE, Heffess CS, Abbondanzo SL. Malignant lymphoma of the thyroid gland: a clinicopathologic study of 108 cases. Am J Surg Pathol. 2000;24(5):623–39.
67. Sharma A, Jasim S, Reading CC, Ristow KM, Villasboas Bisneto JC, Habermann TM, et al. Clinical presentation and diagnostic challenges of thyroid lymphoma: a cohort study. Thyroid. 2016;26(8):1061–7.
68. Aiken AH. Imaging of thyroid cancer. Semin Ultrasound CT MR. 2012;33(2):138–49.
69. Ravinsky E, Morales C. Diagnosis of lymphoma by image-guided needle biopsies: fine needle aspiration biopsy, core biopsy or both? Acta Cytol. 2005;49(1):51–7.
70. Jankovic B, Le KT, Hershman JM. Clinical review: Hashimoto's thyroiditis and papillary thyroid carcinoma: is there a correlation? J Clin Endocrinol Metab. 2013;98(2):474–82.
71. McLeod DSA, Watters KF, Carpenter AD, Ladenson PW, Cooper DS, Ding EL. Thyrotropin and thyroid cancer diagnosis: a systematic review and dose-response meta-analysis. J Clin Endocrinol Metab. 2012;97(8):2682–92.
72. Larson SD, Jackson LN, Riall TS, Uchida T, Thomas RP, Qiu S, et al. Increased incidence of well-differentiated thyroid cancer associated with Hashimoto thyroiditis and the role of the PI3k/Akt pathway. J Am Coll Surg. 2007;204(5):764–73; discussion 773–775.
73. Mechler C, Bounacer A, Suarez H, Saint Frison M, Magois C, Aillet G, et al. Papillary thyroid carcinoma: 6 cases from 2 families with associated lymphocytic thyroiditis harbouring RET/PTC rearrangements. Br J Cancer. 2001;85(12):1831–7.

74. Muzza M, Degl'Innocenti D, Colombo C, Perrino M, Ravasi E, Rossi S, et al. The tight relationship between papillary thyroid cancer, autoimmunity and inflammation: clinical and molecular studies. Clin Endocrinol. 2010;72(5):702–8.
75. Unger P, Ewart M, Wang BY, Gan L, Kohtz DS, Burstein DE. Expression of p63 in papillary thyroid carcinoma and in Hashimoto's thyroiditis: a pathobiologic link? Hum Pathol. 2003;34(8):764–9.
76. Anderson CE, Graham C, Herriot MM, Kamel HM, Salter DM. CD98 expression is decreased in papillary carcinoma of the thyroid and Hashimoto's thyroiditis. Histopathology. 2009;55(6):683–6.
77. Jara SM, Carson KA, Pai SI, Agrawal N, Richmon JD, Prescott JD, et al. The relationship between chronic lymphocytic thyroiditis and central neck lymph node metastasis in North American patients with papillary thyroid carcinoma. Surgery. 2013;154(6):1272–80; discussion 1280–1282.
78. Liang J, Zeng W, Fang F, Yu T, Zhao Y, Fan X, et al. Clinical analysis of Hashimoto thyroiditis coexistent with papillary thyroid cancer in 1392 patients. Acta Otorhinolaryngol Ital. 2017;37(5):393–400.
79. Kim EY, Kim WG, Kim WB, Kim TY, Kim JM, Ryu J-S, et al. Coexistence of chronic lymphocytic thyroiditis is associated with lower recurrence rates in patients with papillary thyroid carcinoma. Clin Endocrinol. 2009;71(4):581–6.
80. Kashima K, Yokoyama S, Noguchi S, Murakami N, Yamashita H, Watanabe S, et al. Chronic thyroiditis as a favorable prognostic factor in papillary thyroid carcinoma. Thyroid. 1998;8(3):197–202.
81. Rossi ED, Adeniran AJ, Faquin WC. Pitfalls in thyroid cytopathology. Surg Pathol Clin. 2019;12(4):865–81.
82. Harvey AM, Truong LD, Mody DR. Diagnostic pitfalls of Hashimoto's/Lymphocytic thyroiditis on fine-needle aspirations and strategies to avoid overdiagnosis. Acta Cytol. 2012;56(4):352–60.
83. Haberal AN, Toru S, Ozen O, Arat Z, Bilezikçi B. Diagnostic pitfalls in the evaluation of fine needle aspiration cytology of the thyroid: correlation with histopathology in 260 cases. Cytopathology. 2009;20(2):103–8.
84. Berho M, Suster S. Clear nuclear changes in Hashimoto's thyroiditis. A clinicopathologic study of 12 cases. Ann Clin Lab Sci. 1995;25(6):513–21.
85. Ren Y, Kyriazidis N, Faquin WC, Soylu S, Kamani D, Saade R, et al. The presence of Hürthle cells does not increase the risk of malignancy in Most Bethesda categories in thyroid fine-needle aspirates. Thyroid. 2020;30(3):425–31.
86. Roh MH, Jo VY, Stelow EB, Faquin WC, Zou KH, Alexander EK, et al. The predictive value of the fine-needle aspiration diagnosis "suspicious for a follicular neoplasm, hurthle cell type" in patients with Hashimoto thyroiditis. Am J Clin Pathol. 2011;135(1):139–45.
87. Alexander EK, Kennedy GC, Baloch ZW, Cibas ES, Chudova D, Diggans J, et al. Preoperative diagnosis of benign thyroid nodules with indeterminate cytology. N Engl J Med. 2012;367(8):705–15.
88. McIver B, Castro MR, Morris JC, Bernet V, Smallridge R, Henry M, et al. An independent study of a gene expression classifier (Afirma) in the evaluation of cytologically indeterminate thyroid nodules. J Clin Endocrinol Metab. 2014;99(11):4069–77.
89. Lastra RR, Pramick MR, Crammer CJ, LiVolsi VA, Baloch ZW. Implications of a suspicious afirma test result in thyroid fine-needle aspiration cytology: an institutional experience. Cancer Cytopathol. 2014;122(10):737–44.
90. Harrell RM, Bimston DN. Surgical utility of Afirma: effects of high cancer prevalence and oncocytic cell types in patients with indeterminate thyroid cytology. Endocr Pract. 2014;20(4):364–9.
91. Angell TE, Heller HT, Cibas ES, Barletta JA, Kim MI, Krane JF, et al. Independent comparison of the Afirma genomic sequencing classifier

and gene expression classifier for cytologically indeterminate thyroid nodules. Thyroid. 2019;29(5):650–6.
92. Endo M, Nabhan F, Porter K, Roll K, Shirley LA, Azaryan I, et al. Afirma gene sequencing classifier compared with gene expression classifier in indeterminate thyroid nodules. Thyroid. 2019;29(8):1115–24.
93. Hwang HS, Orloff LA. Efficacy of preoperative neck ultrasound in the detection of cervical lymph node metastasis from thyroid cancer. Laryngoscope. 2011;121(3):487–91.
94. Serres-Créixams X, Castells-Fusté I, Pruna-Comella X, Yetano-Laguna V, Garriga-Farriol V, Gallardo-Agromayor E. Paratracheal lymph nodes: a new sonographic finding in autoimmune thyroiditis. J Clin Ultrasound. 2008;36(7):418–21.

Papillary Thyroid Carcinoma

Iain Nixon and Louise Davies

Contents

A. L. Shifrin et al. (eds.), *Endocrine Surgery Comprehensive Board Exam Guide*,
https://doi.org/10.1007/978-3-030-84737-1_5

Case Presentation

Patient is a 47-year-old woman who presents with a 9 mm right thyroid nodule found after she requested a thyroid ultrasound because her sister was diagnosed with papillary thyroid cancer last year. She has no symptoms referable to the nodule, although she notes some issues with intermittent hoarseness. Her past medical history is significant for treatment of Hodgkin lymphoma as a child with external beam radiation to her chest and low neck. Her family history is significant for a goiter in her maternal grandmother but no other first-degree relatives with thyroid cancer. She takes levothyroxine for hypothyroidism, 100 micrograms daily. She has had no surgery or prior trauma in the head or neck region. Physical examination reveals vital signs in the normal range and a healthy appearing woman who appears her stated age. The neck has no masses or swelling on observation and on palpation, the thyroid gland has a normal thyroid texture and is not fixed. There is no palpable lymphadenopathy Papillary thyroid carcinoma (PTC) patient history in the lateral neck on the left or right.

Questions

1. The most likely type of thyroid cancer in this patient is.
   (a) Follicular thyroid cancer
   (b) Papillary thyroid cancer
   (c) Medullary thyroid cancer
   (d) Anaplastic thyroid cancer
2. The presence of thyroid cancer in her sister as the only first-degree relative with a history of thyroid cancer suggests she has familial thyroid cancer syndrome.
   (a) True
   (b) False
3. Her history of radiation to the thyroid region is meaningful. She should be counseled that "It is more likely that this biopsy will show you have a cancer, but it does not mean that cancer will be more aggressive than if you had not received radiation."
   (a) True
   (b) False
4. The next step in workup of her thyroid nodule is
   (a) Check serum TSH
   (b) Needle biopsy of the thyroid gland
   (c) Nuclear medicine evaluation of the thyroid nodule
   (d) Neck CT scan with and without contrast
5. Her full workup is completed and reveals 9-mm hypoechoic nodule with microcalcifications and regular, smooth borders located in the central aspect of the right thyroid gland. There is no contact of the nodule with the thyroid capsule. The left hemithyroid and isthmus are without nodules or lesions. The lateral necks show no abnormal appearing lymph nodes. Needle biopsy result was Bethesda V – suspicious for papillary carcinoma.

   (a) Nuclear medicine evaluation of the thyroid is not indicated.
   (b) Neck CT scan with and without contrast must be performed.
   (c) No further workup is required.
6. Because the patient reports intermittent hoarseness, you decide to obtain a complete laryngeal exam. It is normal. Her options at this point include
   (a) Total thyroidectomy.
   (b) Hemithyroidectomy.
   (c) Active surveillance.
   (d) All are within the range of current guidelines.
7. Imagine now that her laryngeal exam instead shows a compensated left vocal cord paresis: the left vocal cord rests in a slightly paramedian position and does not move through its full range, but the right vocal cord moves over just past midline to meet it nearly fully. This finding suggests which treatment(s) might best be discussed with her as first-line management?
   (a) Total thyroidectomy
   (b) Hemithyroidectomy
   (c) Active surveillance
   (d) Either (a) or (b)
8. She asks for information about her prognosis. Her 9-mm papillary thyroid cancer confined to the thyroid gland suggests her prognosis is
   (a) Excellent. She is very unlikely to die from her thyroid cancer. However, there is always a small chance that her cancer may recur if removed, or grow and eventually need surgery if she does active surveillance.
   (b) Good. She is at higher risk than others of having recurrence after surgery/cancer growth or spread on active surveillance because of her sister's cancer and her childhood radiation.
   (c) Fair. It would be better if she had not had childhood radiation.
9. As you discuss the prognosis of her 9-mm papillary thyroid cancer confined to the thyroid gland with her, you remember that her cancer was found on a thyroid ultrasound she requested, because her sister had recently been diagnosed with cancer. You explain what may have happened:
   (a) Ultrasound can detect subclinical thyroid cancers.
   (b) Not all ultrasound detected thyroid cancers go on to become clinically evident during the patient's life.
   (c) Thyroid cancer is commonly found at autopsy in people who died of other causes.

(d) Though it is possible her cancer will grow or spread, the data suggest that for the large majority of people, it will not.
(e) All of the above.

10. Imagine now instead that this patient presented with a 2-cm thyroid nodule abutting the trachea by ultrasound. Her vocal cord function is normal. Your physical exam suggests fullness in the right neck. The next imaging step to consider is
(a) Cross-sectional imaging of the neck and chest, without contrast
(b) Cross-sectional imaging of the neck and chest, with contrast
(c) Lateral neck ultrasound and further ultrasound exam of the trachea
11. The imaging shows several rounded lymph nodes in right neck levels III and IV, but they are just 1 cm. The imaging of the trachea suggests the disease might be in the wall of the trachea on the right. The next steps are
(a) Needle biopsy of the lymph nodes
(b) Bronchoscopy and esophagoscopy to fully evaluate the vital central neck structures
(c) Both (a) and (b)
12. Imagine the workup for the lateral neck adenopathy and the tracheal involvement is negative, she has only a 2-cm papillary thyroid cancer. There is no spread to the lymph nodes, and the trachea is not involved. Her thyroid gland treatment options are
(a) Active surveillance
(b) Hemithyroidectomy
(c) Total thyroidectomy
(d) (b) or (c)
13. Imagine the workup is positive and the patient undergoes total thyroidectomy and right central and lateral neck dissection. The trachea is not involved. The patient has classical variant of papillary thyroid cancer and four positive lymph nodes, all with microscopic disease. The initial step in follow-up is
(a) Radioactive iodine.
(b) Check thyroglobulin and do an ultrasound about 6 months after surgery.
(c) Do a neck ultrasound about 6 months after surgery.
14. After initial follow-up, the patient is followed regularly. She is likely to be followed with
(a) Periodic Neck CT scan
(b) Periodic serum thyroglobulin
(c) Periodic neck ultrasound
(d) (a) and (b)
(e) (b) and (c)

15. After several years, she develops metastases to the lungs. They are not avid on PET scan. Commonly used first-line option(s) for management are
    (a) Radioactive iodine
    (b) External beam radiation
    (c) Tyrosine kinase inhibitors
    (d) (b) or (c)

5.1 Introduction

A familiarity with papillary thyroid carcinoma (PTC) is essential for any endocrine surgeon. PTC is by far the most common endocrine malignancy, and the incidence of this disease is rapidly increasing across the world [1, 2]. While the reasons for this are debated, there is little doubt that the increased sensitivity and application of medical imaging is largely responsible for the rise [3–8]. It is now apparent that there is a large reservoir of occult PTC in the otherwise well population. Series of benign thyroidectomy surgery report an unexpected malignancy rate of around 5–10% and autopsy series of people who died of other causes never knowing they had a thyroid cancer have found rates of up to 30% [9]. The autopsy prevalence has remained stable over time, and meta-analysis has shown that autopsy prevalence is higher when glands are more closely sectioned or examined [10]. Therefore, the modern endocrine surgeon will spend much of their time managing patients with suspected, proven, or treated PTC.

Over recent decades, a significant change in our understanding of the biology of PTC has resulted in a revolution in management approach. An appreciation of the background to this contemporary approach to the management of PTC will allow the modern endocrine surgeon to best serve their patients and provide a treatment approach that balances risk of recurrence against functional outcomes and treatment side effects for the individual.

5.2 Clinical Presentation

The most common presentation of PTC is a female patient with a small thyroid nodule, with no symptoms. In developed countries, most patients present with cancers that are too small to feel (2 cm or less). If palpable, the majority will move up and down with the larynx on swallowing. In modern population-based data sets, the most common age range of patients is 45–54 years, and about 80% are female. A significant minority will present with regional spread to the lymph nodes of the central or lateral neck. Fewer than 5% of cases present with locally invasive disease [11]. Local invasion may be a sign of de-differentiation of PTC toward a more aggressive disease type. When local invasion progresses, involvement of the critical structures of the central neck may result in important symptoms including dysphonia, dysphagia, hemorrhage, and even asphyxia.

During clinical assessment, the patient should be queried for symptoms that might suggest invasive local or regional disease – change in voice, and change in swallowing or breathing. The only known risk factors for papillary thyroid cancer are childhood or adolescent exposure to ionizing radiation and family history. In particular, if exposed to ionizing radiation prior to age 19, rates of papillary thyroid malignancy are higher [12]. Those exposed at younger ages (i.e., less than age 5) have the highest risk, and the risk increases with increasing dose. The increased risk of thyroid cancer persists for up to 60 years or more, but the cancer is no more aggressive than nonradiation-induced thyroid cancer [13–15]. Although rare, familial nonmedullary thyroid cancer (most commonly PTC) has also been described and is diagnosed when three *additional* first-degree relatives are also affected by thyroid cancer [16, 17].

In areas where high-resolution cross-sectional imaging is not readily available or not widely used, patients more commonly present with symptoms of their disease. However, in routine clinical practice, in areas with access to a wide array of imaging and health care services, an increasing number of patients will be referred with incidentally discovered disease that is small, and asymptomatic, as described above. Such patients will have undergone examination or imaging for a nonthyroid-directed reason, which identifies a thyroid finding [5]. In turn, this leads to more investigations and the diagnosis of PTC. This group tends to be older, as older adults tend to undergo imaging and receive more healthcare than younger people [18]. The most dramatic example occurred in South Korea, where thyroid ultrasound was offered as a retail add-on by individual health care providers during sanctioned cancer screenings for breast, stomach, and liver cancer, and this resulted in the largest increased incidence of PTC globally, without impacting mortality [19].

Evaluation of the patient with thyroid cancer should include asking about daily activities and voice usage needs. Patients should be educated about the disease and decisions about extent of treatment should be approached jointly. Most patients with PTC will require surgery to remove all or part of the thyroid gland, and that carries the risk of voice change and permanent hypoparathyroidism if the entire gland is removed. Damage to the recurrent nerve or superior laryngeal nerve will adversely affect vocal range, stamina, volume, and quality – making it difficult to talk for long periods or in noisy environments. If these changes in voice occur, it may have a significant impact on their ability to continue in their role. Chronic hypocalcemia requires ongoing treatment and can affect clarity of thinking and muscle function. At the point of presentation, as with any cancer diagnosis, patients with PTC are likely to be highly anxious and fear for themselves as well as their family and others who depend on them.

5.3 Natural History

The natural history of PTC is excellent. The 10-year survival of papillary thyroid cancer of any size localized to the thyroid gland and treated with either hemithyroidectomy or total thyroidectomy is 99% [20]. Though a small proportion of cases are aggressive, the increasing incidence of papillary thyroid cancer across the world has primarily resulted from the detection of subclinical disease, meaning small cancers localized to the thyroid gland that had they not been found would have been unlikely to go on to become clinically apparent [6]. Cohorts of patients followed over time with cancers measuring up to 1.5 cm in size have shown that rates of growth are low and vary by age. Those diagnosed in their 20s will show advancement in their cancer up to 24% of the time, but those in the age 60 or over will have growth less than 3% of the time [21, 22].

In contrast to the hematogenous spread pattern for follicular thyroid cancer, PTC spreads primarily through the lymphatic route. It is now understood that PTC has a slow growth pattern, but paradoxically, a high rate of regional metastasis. This finding runs counter to many of the classical "rules" of oncology. For example, it is widely taught that if a head and neck squamous cell carcinoma negative for human papilloma virus metastasizes to the regional nodes, the chance of survival drops by half. In contrast, although only 20–30% of patients with PTC present with overt nodal disease (cN1), if elective dissection of the regional lymph nodes is performed, occult disease can be detected in over a third of cases who were thought to be cN0 [23]. Although this has long been used as a justification for elective lymph node surgery in the central neck compartment, the outcome of patients who received prophylactic central neck lymph nodes dissection was compared to those who did not, and showed no or minimal clinical difference [24, 25]. This is consistent with autopsy data suggesting that 16–18% of patients who die of other causes never knowing they had thyroid cancer have evidence of metastatic thyroid cancer at the time of their death [26, 27].

Fewer than 5% of patients with papillary thyroid cancer have distant metastases at the time of diagnosis: the most common site of spread is the lung. Although in the distant past, the majority of patients with PTC died of uncontrolled central neck disease, with improvements in management, death is now more commonly associated with progressive distant than uncontrolled locoregional disease [28].

5.4 Diagnosis

Diagnosing and staging PTC requires a history and examination followed by imaging and biopsy. In the clinical history, features associated with involvement of central neck structures should be sought, as outlined above. In addition, past medical and surgical history, family history, comorbidities, and daily activities and life roles should be discussed to gain a full appreciation of the patient's situation.

Physical examination includes observation and palpation of the neck, both the thyroid and the regional lymphatics. Examination of the larynx is also an important part of the initial assessment, particularly if there is any concern related to voice change, or if the patient has had prior thyroid (or parathyroid) surgery. Although pre-existing vocal cord dysfunction is not typical in the absence of a pertinent history or voice finding, results should be available to clinicians involved in the management of thyroid malignancy so that any postoperative changes can be understood, and prognostic estimations of future vocal cord function can be offered.

Biochemical assessment of thyroid function (TSH, and in some locales, calcitonin) should be completed prior to nodule biopsy to guide interpretation of needle biopsy results.

First-line imaging for identified thyroid nodules is ultrasound. Not only is this relatively cheap and avoids ionizing radiation, but in trained hands, it is the most accurate method for assessing the thyroid and facilitates image-guided biopsy. A number of different risk stratification systems are available to guide the need for biopsy [29, 30].

Fine-needle aspiration (FNA) biopsy is the most common method of achieving a tissue diagnosis. This can be taken from the suspicious thyroid nodule or a pathological lymph node. Core biopsy is an alternative, which provides additional tissue and is favored by some groups. Standardized reporting schema now exist to facilitate communication between cytopathologists and other members of the disease management team [31], as discussed in ► Chap. 1.

For many patients, further investigation will not be required. Thyroid function testing, ultrasound, and needle biopsy results will provide adequate information to plan treatment. However, there are some notable exceptions to this. Patients with overt nodal disease may warrant cross-sectional imaging in the form of contrast-enhanced CT scan of neck and chest. Not only does this provide information regarding the presence or absence of metastatic disease in the lung, but it allows accurate characterization of the mediastinal lymph nodes behind the manubrium, which are not visualized on ultrasound. The other setting where cross-sectional imaging is critical is in the setting of invasive primary disease. The relationship of disease to the critical structures of the central and lateral neck allows accurate presurgical planning. This is often combined with formal esophagoscopy and tracheoscopy to fully assess the extent of visceral involvement prior to surgery, which informs the process of presurgical consent. It is worth mentioning at this point that there has historically been concern about the use of iodinated contrast during CT scans and the potential impact that may have on subsequent use of radioactive iodine (RAI). However, these concerns are theoretical and have never been proven clinically. In addition, the need for accurate presurgical information to maximize the chance of a complete surgical excision far outweighs any such concerns. As such, when indicated, the surgeon should have no hesitation in ordering adequate imaging to fully stage all aspects of such advanced disease.

Fluorodeoxyglucose positron emission tomography (FDG-PET) scanning seldom has a role in the investigation of primary PTC. The disease tends not to be FDG avid. It may have a role in detection of de-differentiated disease: FDG avidity tends to increase as RAI avidity decreases.

5.5 Risk Stratification and Treatment

Treatment for PTC is highly controversial and has been for decades: most patients have extremely good outcomes, which translates to very low "event-rates" for clinical outcomes research. This makes planning and execution of prospective randomized controlled trials difficult, as large numbers and prolonged follow-up would be required for some of the important questions [32]. In the absence of prospective randomized evidence, opinions are based on detailed retrospective studies from single institutions or population-based databases that can provide representative results, but with fewer details. The inherent limits can result in conflicting results and interpretations.

Up until the first decade of the 2000s, most patients with PTC were recommended to undergo total thyroidectomy and RAI. Elective central neck dissection, including prophylactic dissection, was supported [33]. However, this chapter is written at a time where international opinion on the optimal management of PTC is slowly moving toward a more conservative approach [34]. Despite this, there remains significant disagreement between experts across the world and we hope to reflect this in a balanced summary below.

The surgeon dealing with PTC must have an appreciation of the impact that initial surgical therapy can have on the case overall. To effectively treat patients with adjuvant RAI, all thyroid tissues must be removed, which is clearly the job of the surgeon. However, variation in surgical practice can also alter subsequent decision-making. For example, those surgeons who perform elective neck surgery identify nodal disease in a significant number of patients [23]. This potentially upstages the disease and may influence clinical decision-making in the postoperative period. Having an understanding of the interplay among surgery, staging, adjuvant therapy, complications, and outcomes is critical for all surgeons involved in the management of PTC.

No discussion about treatment for PTC can start without reviewing the concept of risk stratification. This approach was first suggested in the mid-twentieth century and has been more fully developed since. Initially, there was a recognition that prediction of survival in all thyroid cancers could be based on variables, the most important of which was histology [35]. However, refinements within differentiated thyroid cancers recognized advancing age, tumor size, presence of gross extrathyroidal extension, and distant metastases as predictive of survival.

A number of risk stratification systems were developed, which would allow young patients with small volume disease to be categorized as low risk, whereas older patients with advanced disease were recognized as high risk of cause-specific mortality [36–39]. These staging systems were eventually incorporated into the AJCC staging systems [40].

Despite advances in risk stratification, therapy for the majority of patients with PTC remained total thyroidectomy, consideration of elective central neck dissection, and postoperative adjuvant radioactive iodine (RAI) based on early data suggesting a recurrence and survival advantage [41].

Over the past three decades, a significant body of work from groups around the world has helped to refine that approach based upon the original risk stratification systems. For example, it is now accepted that in low-risk patients, there is little to gain from RAI, reducing the need for total thyroidectomy to facilitate this adjuvant therapy. In addition, although microscopic occult nodal disease is common, elective dissection of regional nodes has failed to demonstrate long-term advantage, and again in low-risk patients, there is a move away from this practice [24].

One of the issues with original risk stratification systems was their lack of translatability to clinical practice. The overwhelming majority of patients with PTC will not die. Therefore, systems designed to predict survival lacked clinical utility. Hence, in recent years, there has been a focus on predictors of recurrence rather than survival. In addition to the originally recognized factors, features including multicentricity, the presence of lymphatic and vascular invasion, microscopic extrathyroidal extension, and small volume nodal disease have been combined into a recurrence risk continuum promoted by the American Thyroid Association [34].

Unfortunately, many of these additional features can only be described on postoperative pathology, so they cannot be used at the point of initial diagnosis. As a result, it is critical that the surgeon managing patients with PTC considers the whole case at the outset in order to plan effective treatment. If a patient is to receive RAI, a total thyroidectomy is required. Therefore, this should be considered when making initial treatment recommendations. If a hemithyroidectomy is undertaken and the pathology suggests RAI may provide recurrence benefit, completion thyroidectomy may be required.

The spectrum of risk, both for recurrence and survival, is shown in Table 5.1.

Many patients with PTC present with low-risk disease. In such cases, without evidence of nodal disease, there is no proven advantage of RAI. Therefore, such patients can normally be considered candidates for a thyroid lobectomy. This procedure removes the disease, protects the parathyroids and recurrent laryngeal nerve on the contralateral side, reduces the risk of requiring lifelong thyroxine, and is associated with excellent long-term outcomes.

In contrast, for those patients who present with gross extrathyroidal extension, advanced nodal or even distant disease, there is a well-proven role for RAI. In such patients, treatment should be aimed at eradicating macroscopic disease in the neck and facilitating adjuvant RAI. This requires a total thyroidectomy and compartment-oriented neck dissection.

For patients with nodal disease limited to the central neck, dissection of the central compartment is sufficient. For those

Table 5.1 Spectrum of risk of recurrence and survival in papillary thyroid cancer

	Predictors of survival	Predictors of recurrence
Lower-risk features	Younger age (<55y) Smaller tumor (<4 cm) No gross extrathyroidal extension M0	Unicentric N0 disease Classical histology Microscopic extrathyroid extension
Higher-risk features	Older age (>55y in advanced disease) Larger tumor (>4 cm) Gross extrathyroidal extension M1	Large volume N1 disease Vascular invasion pN1 with extranodal extension

with lateral neck disease, a compartment-oriented level II-V neck dissection is recommended to minimize the chance of recurrent disease [42]. In addition, for patients with advanced primary disease invading structures in the central neck, elective central neck dissection is recommended [43]. Not only does this provide optimal access to the disease, but in aggressive primary disease, rates of occult nodal disease are high. Outside this setting, elective neck dissection is not generally recommended.

In these two examples, the approach to management is fairly clear-cut. However, a great number of patients fall between these two extremes. Many patients present with PTC on the background of multinodular disease. In such patients, a decision is required about the likelihood of those additional nodules harboring disease and a balance must be struck between the need for surveillance of these nodules versus an upfront total thyroidectomy.

Analysis of the postoperative specimen may identify higher-risk features, such as more aggressive variants of PTC (tall cell, insular, solid, etc.), multicentric disease, small associated nodes in the perithyroid tissues, or microscopic extrathyroidal extension. Although treatment intensification (completion thyroidectomy to facilitate RAI) has never been shown to improve either recurrence or survival outcomes based on these individual features, given that total thyroidectomy and RAI was the standard of care for the majority of cases until relatively recently, many disease management teams may still recommend this approach for such intermediate-risk cases.

The surgeon is in a critical position to advise in such cases where definitive oncological evidence is lacking. Other highly pertinent information can be used to aid in decision-making. First is the complication rate of the surgeon themselves. As with many surgeries, association exists between volume and complications in thyroid surgery, with recent data suggesting that an annual volume of thyroidectomies in the low to mid-20s is required to minimize complication rates [44–46]. It is also understood that even high-volume surgeons have higher complication rates in total thyroidectomy versus thyroid lobectomy [44]. Often quoted rates of a 1% RLN injury and similarly low long-term hypocalcemia rates likely represent an underestimate for the average surgeon, based on population-based estimates, registry data, and careful institutional reports, which show short-term hypocalcemia following total thyroidectomy is around 20%, with long-term risk 1.8–5%, and vocal cord paralysis rates around 8% [47–49]. Overall complication rates of unilateral thyroid surgery are around 10% versus 20% for bilateral surgery [44]. Although complication rates are lower for high-volume surgeons, a higher rate is observed following bilateral versus unilateral surgery, even in expert hands.

Although an appreciation of the literature is useful, only the surgeon themselves can understand their individual complication rate through self-audit. This can then be balanced against the potential for oncological benefit. This is particularly evident when the patient has been diagnosed following thyroid lobectomy and the disease management team is considering the need for completion thyroidectomy [50]. In this setting, if the patient suffered an RLN injury during the initial surgery, or one is detected during an initial procedure, which was planned as a total thyroidectomy, there is seldom a justification for completion surgery as this carries the risk of tracheotomy.

Another factor, which is central to the decision, is the opinion of the patient, who should be included explicitly in discussions about not just oncological outcomes but side effects of therapy. In particular, patients may be wary of the potential for additional surgical impact on laryngeal function. The long-term impact of hypocalcemia is also not to be underestimated. Lifelong calcium supplementation is highly inconvenient for patients and difficult to manage. These factors should be discussed with patients as possible side effects of total thyroidectomy in comparison with thyroid lobectomy. Additional surgical details on the indications and extent of both primary thyroid and nodal surgery are covered in ► Chaps. 11 and 12, respectively.

It should also be remembered that RAI is not without side effects. Although less in comparison with external beam radiotherapy (EBRT), RAI is associated with dry mouth, dry eyes, and swallowing dysfunction, which can compromise quality of life. Some groups have studied the use of EBRT in advanced local disease with some success [51]. In patients with unresected local disease, or in the setting of disease, which is excised with minimal margin (R1), radiotherapy may be considered in addition to RAI. However, such treatment is not without significant side effects, and management teams must consider the risk–benefit ratio carefully when recommending such an approach. PTC is ot generally considered sensitive to chemotherapy, and in large part, traditional chemotherapy has been superseded by advances in targeted treatments such as tyrosine kinase inhibitors, which are covered in ► Chap. 10.

Within a section dedicated to treatment of PTC, it is now critical to include consideration of "active observation" as a potential method of treatment. This approach was pioneered in Japan for small volume (1 cm or smaller) PTC [52, 53]. Such cases were diagnosed using US-guided FNA, and following counselling were offered surveillance, with surgery performed if the cancers grew or spread. When followed in this manner, only a small proportion of patients, predictable by age at diagnosis, demonstrate progression on ultrasound and go on to require surgery [22]. No patient who followed this strategy has succumbed to thyroid cancer and all patients with cancer growth or spread have been successfully rescued. In this manner, many patients can avoid surgery in the medium to long term without any negative oncological impact on the group as a whole. The ideal patient has a rim of normal thyroid tissue around the cancer, can present for regular follow-up, has access to a medical team with the ability to follow with ultrasound, and the patient is interested in active surveillance [54]. This approach is being adopted now internationally with success in selected patients [21, 55–62]. Although currently 1 cm is generally considered the upper size limit to recommend a surveillance approach, groups are now investigating with success a similar approach in larger tumors (<2 cm) [58]. It seems likely that the option of treating patients with active surveillance will play a larger part in PTC management in the future.

In summary, when recommending treatment for PTC, a number of patient- and tumor-related factors must be considered. A select group of the smallest, lowest-risk PTC may be suitable for observation. For high-risk patients, aggressive treatment with total thyroidectomy and adjuvant RAI is justifiable. In contrast, for low-risk patients, a conservative approach with thyroid lobectomy achieves excellent oncological outcomes while minimizing the chance of surgical complications. For patients who lie between these extremes, additional factors relating to both the patient, their tumor, and the chance of surgical (and RAI) complications should be balanced to optimize oncological and functional outcomes in the long term (▣ Fig. 5.1).

5.6 Follow-Up

The aims of follow-up include detection of recurrent disease, management of thyroid function (and calcium if required), detection of the complications of treatment, and provision of cancer survivorship support. Initial treatment ends either at the point of surgery or following RAI. Some patients are treated for benign disease, and PTC is diagnosed incidentally. Such cases often fall under low-risk category: in practice, the chance of recurrent disease is so low that this patient group can be discharged without any follow-up [43].

For the majority of patients, the end of treatment represents the start of long-term follow-up. The cornerstones of follow-up for most patients are clinical assessment, periodic ultrasound, and serum thyroglobulin monitoring if the patient has undergone total thyroidectomy.

Recently, risk stratification has been extended beyond the pre- and peritreatment period to follow up with the concept of dynamic risk stratification. This approach uses the 12-month ultrasound and thyroglobulin assessment to stratify patients into excellent response, indeterminate response, biochemically incomplete response, and structurally incomplete response groups [63]. Patients who fall into the lowest-risk category have <5% chance of recurrence in the long term. Patients who have a detectable thyroglobulin (biochemically incomplete

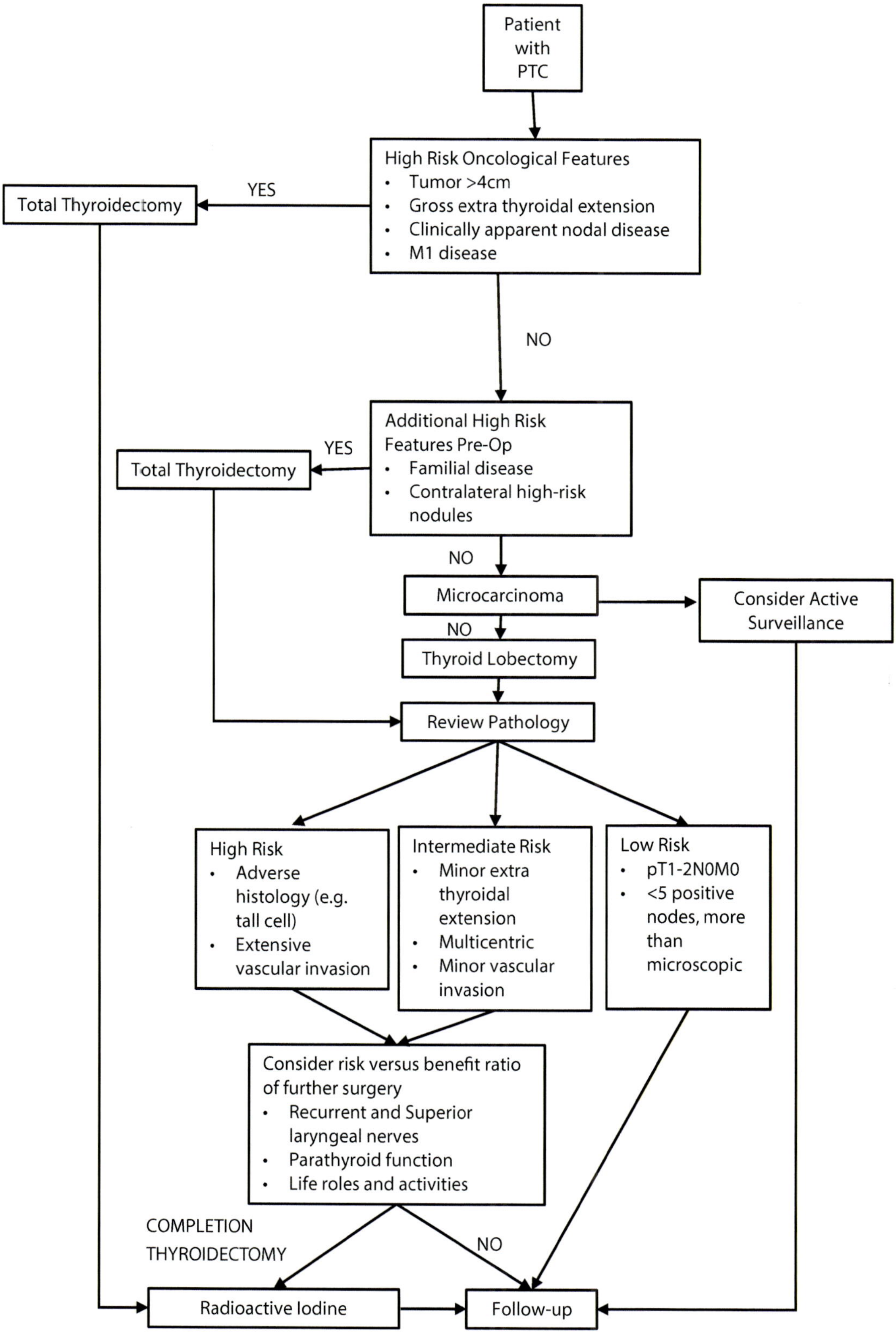

Fig. 5.1 Therapeutic approach to a patient with papillary thyroid carcinoma (PTC)

response) or indeterminate features on ultrasound (indeterminate response group) have around a 20% chance of recurrence. Those who have a structurally incomplete response to therapy have imaging findings consistent with persistent disease and, as such, rates of "recurrence" in this group are high [64]. These definitions were first provided for patients who had undergone total thyroidectomy and RAI. However, in recent years, modifications to this system have been provided for patients who underwent thyroid lobectomy alone [65].

Follow-up protocols can be tailored to the expected level of risk, with those low-risk patients who show an excellent response to initial treatment being reviewed less frequently than higher-risk patients, particularly if there is a less convincing response to treatment.

Patients will tend to be reviewed at 6–12 monthly intervals with ultrasound and thyroglobulin assessments. Any sustained rise in thyroglobulin will lead to a thorough search for evidence of structural disease, if not evident on ultrasound assessment.

Historically, patients were advised to keep their thyroid-stimulating hormone (TSH) suppressed, with a T4 level at the upper end of the normal range and the TSH below 0.1 mU/L. Although this TSH suppression has been shown to have a beneficial effect in patients with high-risk disease, this is not the case with patients at lower risk and may present problems in the elderly. The majority of patients do not require lifelong TSH suppression, and particularly during later stages of follow-up, a more normalized level of thyroid function is desirable. Avoidance of long-term TSH suppression minimizes the risks from cardiovascular disease and osteoporosis. Therefore, for initially high-risk patients and those patients considered to have a structurally incomplete response to initial therapy, suppression of TSH to <0.1 mU/L is reasonable. For patients with an indeterminate response, TSH levels 0.1–0.5 mU/L are acceptable. For low-risk patients, a TSH level 0.5–2 mU/L is acceptable [34].

The duration of follow-up required for patients with PTC is unclear. Although most recurrences occur in the early stages of follow-up, some can occur decades after initial therapy. It is reasonable to consider all patients for at least 5 years of surveillance. After that, if an excellent response to therapy has been achieved, there is little to gain from routine surveillance. In higher-risk patients, and in particular in those who have already recurred, longer-term surveillance is likely to be justified.

5.7 Outcomes

The vast majority of patients will not die from PTC and will have a long survivorship period following diagnosis. Indeed, despite the significant increase in the incidence of PTC, there has not been a proportional increase in the number of deaths, suggesting that detection of subclinical disease has been the main cause of the increased incidence [6]. This well-recognized epidemiologic phenomenon is called "overdiagnosis", the detection of the disease on pre-clinical stage, when the patient is asymptomatic and the disease is very unlikely will become clinically evident [66–69].

As described above, risk stratification can be applied to cohorts presenting with PTC. Around 85% of adults presenting with PTC will be considered low risk, and 15% high risk; 30-year outcomes have now been reported by some groups and <5% of adults with PTC will die from disease. When risk stratified, less than 1% of low-risk adults will die from disease during this time versus up to 30% of high-risk cases [70]. It should be noted, therefore, that for the vast majority of patients, long-term survival is the rule.

Another outcome of interest is recurrence. In contrast to survival, recurrence is relatively common. It can be categorized as development of disease in sites, which are treatment naïve and recurrence in areas of previous treatment. By far the most common recurrence is in regional lymph nodes. The development of overt disease within previously untreated regional nodes is detected during follow-up in up to 20% of cases [71]. However, detection of disease does not mandate treatment. This is because we now appreciate that a significant number of patients who are cN0 do indeed harbor occult nodal disease at presentation, which can slowly progress and present on ultrasound or TG monitoring [23]. Although such patients do indeed have "recurrent" or perhaps more accurately "persistent" nodal disease, slow progression is the rule and serial monitoring has been shown to be clinically safe in the low volume (<1 cm) setting. Clearly, if such disease progresses, treatment will be required in the form of compartment-oriented neck dissection, and cure rates are high [72].

Distant recurrence is rare (<5%) in most series and is often first detected using serial measurements of thyroglobulin. Treatment usually involves RAI treatment, unless disease is considered RAI refractory, in which case, treatment options are more limited. Even in patients who develop distant disease, long-term survival with disease is the rule with generally slow progression of metastatic deposits over time.

Local recurrence can be defined as development of recurrent disease in the operated bed of the thyroid gland. This should be differentiated from contralateral lobar recurrence in a nonoperated thyroid lobe following contralateral lobectomy. True local recurrence is extremely rare (<2%) in contemporary practice following an extracapsular thyroid lobectomy [73]. However, when it occurs, structures including the RLN, airway, and esophagus are at high risk from both disease and from its treatment. Identification of the RLN, for example, in a previously operated thyroid bed is challenging and rates of injury in this setting are far higher than those reported in the primary setting. In contrast, when disease manifests in a contralateral lobe following initial thyroid lobectomy, completion thyroidectomy is required. This procedure is associated with a risk profile similar to initial thyroid lobectomy, although there remains the potential for hypocalcemia (particularly if the contralateral lobectomy resulted in inadvertent parathyroid gland excision) and injury to the RLN. Clearly, if the initial procedure resulted in RLN injury, there is a risk of bilateral injury in this setting, which can be weighed against the oncological benefit of completion surgery.

The details of surgical management for patients with recurrent disease are beyond the scope of this chapter. In brief, for regional recurrence, which occurs in the nonoperated field, a compartment-oriented salvage neck dissection is recommended [42]. If recurrent nodes are detected within the previously operated neck, a more limited and targeted nodal resection is preferred. In the setting of local recurrence, careful staging including cross-sectional imaging and endoscopy is required. Salvage surgery may require resection of critical structures including the larynx or trachea. A careful balance should be struck among the morbidity of resection, the trajectory of disease, and the expected outcome of continued observation or nonsurgical treatments. These cases should be referred to units experienced in the management of recurrent PTC to optimize the chance of favorable outcome.

Alongside oncological outcomes, the surgeon must also consider the impact that treatment has on a patient's life. As shown above, most patients will love long lives following treatment and will therefore have to live with the after-effects of their therapy. Patients who present with invasive or metastatic disease are a small high-risk group who require aggressive primary treatment with neck dissection and adjuvant therapy. Clearly, this approach to treatment carries risks, but they are balanced against a meaningful risk of death. Such patients are in the minority. The vast majority of patients present with localized disease, are at low risk of recurrence, and almost no risk of death. For these patients, definitive evidence regarding the benefits of different approaches to treatment is lacking and a balanced approach, which includes explicit discussion with the patient, must be taken. Overall, the therapeutic choice is among total thyroidectomy, thyroid lobectomy, or active surveillance for the lowest-risk cancers.

The risks of unilateral thyroid lobectomy include damage to the recurrent laryngeal nerve, the external branch of the superior laryngeal nerve, and injury to the parathyroid glands. However, bilateral thyroidectomy not only doubles these risks but introduces the risk of long-term hypocalcemia and tracheotomy.

Given the generally indolent nature of PTC, the ability to accurately risk-stratify patients according to easily available preoperative variables and our understanding about the risks of thyroid surgery, one can appreciate why some groups have now demonstrated that the risk of treatment may outweigh the risk or the disease in the lower-risk group [74].

Overall then, outcomes can be predicted based on the patient and the tumor. Low-risk patients have excellent oncological outcomes, irrespective of treatment approach. For this group, surgeons should balance the chance of surgical complications against the potential that more aggressive therapy has to provide an outcome advantage. In contrast, high-risk patients (although relatively rare) have a significant rate recurrence and are at risk of death. Therefore, a more aggressive approach to such patients is warranted.

Answers to the Questions

1. (b); 2. (b); 3. (a); 4. (a); 5. (c); 6. (d); 7. (c); 8. (a); 9. (e); 10. (b); 11. (c); 12. (d); 13. (b); 14. (e); 15. (a)

References

1. Kim J, Gosnell JE, Roman SA. Geographic influences in the global rise of thyroid cancer. Nat Rev Endocrinol. 2020;16(1):17–29.
2. Li M, Dal Maso L, Vaccarella S. Global trends in thyroid cancer incidence and the impact of overdiagnosis. Lancet Diabetes Endocrinol. 2020;8(6):468–70.
3. Sanabria A, Kowalski LP, Shah JP, Nixon IJ, Angelos P, Williams MD, et al. Growing incidence of thyroid carcinoma in recent years: factors underlying overdiagnosis. Head Neck. 2018;40(4):855–66.
4. Davies L, Morris LG, Haymart M, Chen AY, Goldenberg D, Morris J, et al. American Association of Clinical Endocrinologists and American College of Endocrinology Disease State Clinical Review: the increasing incidence of thyroid cancer. Endocr Pract. 2015;21(6):686–96.
5. Davies L, Ouellette M, Hunter M, Welch HG. The increasing incidence of small thyroid cancers: where are the cases coming from? Laryngoscope. 2010;120(12):2446–51.
6. Davies L, Welch HG. Increasing incidence of thyroid cancer in the United States, 1973-2002. JAMA. 2006;295(18):2164–7.
7. Chen AY, Jemal A, Ward EM. Increasing incidence of differentiated thyroid cancer in the United States, 1988-2005. Cancer. 2009;115(16):3801–7.
8. Malone MK, Zagzag J, Ogilvie JB, Patel KN, Heller KS. Thyroid cancers detected by imaging are not necessarily small or early stage. Thyroid. 2014;24(2):314–8.
9. Harach HR, Franssila KO, Wasenius VM. Occult papillary carcinoma of the thyroid. A "normal" finding in Finland. A systematic autopsy study. Cancer. 1985;56(3):531–8.
10. Furuya-Kanamori L, Bell KJ, Clark J, Glasziou P, Doi SA. Prevalence of differentiated thyroid cancer in autopsy studies over six decades: a meta-analysis. J Clin Oncol. 2016;34(30):3672–9.
11. Wang LY, Nixon IJ, Patel SG, Palmer FL, Tuttle RM, Shaha A, et al. Operative management of locally advanced, differentiated thyroid cancer. Surgery. 2016;160(3):738–46.
12. Efanov AA, Brenner AV, Bogdanova TI, Kelly LM, Liu P, Little MP, et al. Investigation of the relationship between radiation dose and gene

mutations and fusions in post-Chernobyl thyroid cancer. J Natl Cancer Inst. 2018;110(4):371–8.
13. Reiners C, Biko J, Haenscheid H, Hebestreit H, Kirinjuk S, Baranowski O, et al. Twenty-five years after Chernobyl: outcome of radioiodine treatment in children and adolescents with very high-risk radiation-induced differentiated thyroid carcinoma. J Clin Endocrinol Metab. 2013;98(7):3039–48.
14. Furukawa K, Preston D, Funamoto S, Yonehara S, Ito M, Tokuoka S, et al. Long-term trend of thyroid cancer risk among Japanese atomic-bomb survivors: 60 years after exposure. Int J Cancer. 2013;132(5):1222–6.
15. Shaha MA, Wang LY, Migliacci JC, Palmer FL, Nixon IJ, Tuttle RM, et al. Previous external beam radiation treatment exposure does not confer worse outcome for patients with differentiated thyroid cancer. Thyroid. 2017;27(3):412–7.
16. Nixon IJ, Suarez C, Simo R, Sanabria A, Angelos P, Rinaldo A, et al. The impact of family history on non-medullary thyroid cancer. Eur J Surg Oncol. 2016;42(10):1455–63.
17. Nose V. Familial thyroid cancer: a review. Mod Pathol. 2011;24(Suppl 2):S19–33.
18. Hughes DT, Haymart MR, Miller BS, Gauger PG, Doherty GM. The most commonly occurring papillary thyroid cancer in the United States is now a microcarcinoma in a patient older than 45 years. Thyroid. 2011;21(3):231–6.
19. Ahn HS, Kim HJ, Kim KH, Lee YS, Han SJ, Kim Y, et al. Thyroid cancer screening in South Korea increases detection of papillary cancers with no impact on other subtypes or thyroid cancer mortality. Thyroid. 2016;26(11):1535–40.
20. Davies L, Welch HG. Thyroid cancer survival in the United States: observational data from 1973 to 2005. Arch Otolaryngol Head Neck Surg. 2010;136(5):440–4.
21. Tuttle RM, Fagin JA, Minkowitz G, Wong RJ, Roman B, Patel S, et al. Natural history and tumor volume kinetics of papillary thyroid cancers during active surveillance. JAMA Otolaryngol Head Neck Surg. 2017;143(10):1015–20.
22. Miyauchi A, Kudo T, Ito Y, Oda H, Sasai H, Higashiyama T, et al. Estimation of the lifetime probability of disease progression of papillary microcarcinoma of the thyroid during active surveillance. Surgery. 2018;163(1):48–52.
23. Hartl DM, Leboulleux S, Al Ghuzlan A, Baudin E, Chami L, Schlumberger M, et al. Optimization of staging of the neck with prophylactic central and lateral neck dissection for papillary thyroid carcinoma. Ann Surg. 2012;255(4):777–83.
24. Nixon IJ, Wang LY, Ganly I, Patel SG, Morris LG, Migliacci JC, et al. Outcomes for patients with papillary thyroid cancer who do not undergo prophylactic central neck dissection. Br J Surg. 2016;103(3):218–25.
25. Wada N, Duh QY, Sugino K, Iwasaki H, Kameyama K, Mimura T, et al. Lymph node metastasis from 259 papillary thyroid microcarcinomas: frequency, pattern of occurrence and recurrence, and optimal strategy for neck dissection. Ann Surg. 2003;237(3):399–407.
26. Sampson RJ, Oka H, Key CR, Buncher CR, Iijima S. Metastases from occult thyroid carcinoma. An autopsy study from Hiroshima and Nagasaki, Japan. Cancer. 1970;25(4):803–11.
27. Ottino A, Pianzola HM, Castelletto RH. Occult papillary thyroid carcinoma at autopsy in La Plata, Argentina. Cancer. 1989;64(2):547–51.
28. Nixon IJ, Ganly I, Palmer FL, Whitcher MM, Patel SG, Tuttle RM, et al. Disease-related death in patients who were considered free of macroscopic disease after initial treatment of well-differentiated thyroid carcinoma. Thyroid. 2011;21(5):501–4.

29. Tessler FN, Middleton WD, Grant EG, Hoang JK, Berland LL, Teefey SA, et al. ACR thyroid imaging, reporting and data system (TI-RADS): white paper of the ACR TI-RADS Committee. J Am Coll Radiol. 2017;14(5):587–95.
30. Middleton WD, Teefey SA, Reading CC, Langer JE, Beland MD, Szabunio MM, et al. Comparison of performance characteristics of American College of Radiology TI-RADS, Korean Society of Thyroid Radiology TIRADS, and American Thyroid Association guidelines. AJR Am J Roentgenol. 2018;210(5):1148–54.
31. Cibas ES, Ali SZ. The Bethesda system for reporting thyroid cytopathology. Thyroid. 2009;19(11):1159–65.
32. Carling T, Carty SE, Ciarleglio MM, Cooper DS, Doherty G, Kim LT, et al. American Thyroid Association (ATA) - design and feasibility of a prospective randomized controlled trial of prophylactic central lymph node dissection for papillary thyroid carcinoma. Thyroid. 2012;22(3):237–44.
33. Cooper DS, Doherty GM, Haugen BR, Kloos RT, Lee SL, Mandel SJ, et al. Revised American Thyroid Association management guidelines for patients with thyroid nodules and differentiated thyroid cancer. Thyroid. 2009;19(11):1167–214.
34. Haugen BRM, Alexander EK, Bible KC, Doherty G, Mandel SJ, Nikiforov YE, et al. 2015 American Thyroid Association management guidelines for adult patients with thyroid nodules and differentiated thyroid cancer. Thyroid. 2016;26(1):1–133.
35. Byar DP, Green SB, Dor P, Williams ED, Colon J, van Gilse HA, et al. A prognostic index for thyroid carcinoma. A study of the E.O.R.T.C. Thyroid Cancer Cooperative Group. Eur J Cancer. 1979;15(8):1033–41.
36. Hay ID, Bergstralh EJ, Goellner JR, Ebersold JR, Grant CS. Predicting outcome in papillary thyroid carcinoma: development of a reliable prognostic scoring system in a cohort of 1779 patients surgically treated at one institution during 1940 through 1989. Surgery. 1993;114(6):1050–7; discussion 7–8.
37. Hay ID, Grant CS, Taylor WF, McConahey WM. Ipsilateral lobectomy versus bilateral lobar resection in papillary thyroid carcinoma: a retrospective analysis of surgical outcome using a novel prognostic scoring system. Surgery. 1987;102(6):1088–95.
38. Cady B, Rossi R. An expanded view of risk-group definition in differentiated thyroid carcinoma. Surgery. 1988;104(6):947–53.
39. Shah JP, Loree TR, Dharker D, Strong EW, Begg C, Vlamis V. Prognostic factors in differentiated carcinoma of the thyroid gland. Am J Surg. 1992;164(6):658–61.
40. Amin MB, Edge SB, Greene FL, Byrd DR, Brookland RK, Washington MK, et al. AJCC staging manual. Springer; 2017. 1024 p
41. Mazzaferri EL, Jhiang SM. Long-term impact of initial surgical and medical therapy on papillary and follicular thyroid cancer. Am J Med. 1994;97(5):418–28.
42. Scharpf J, Tuttle M, Wong R, Ridge D, Smith R, Hartl D, et al. Comprehensive management of recurrent thyroid cancer: an American Head and Neck Society consensus statement: AHNS consensus statement. Head Neck. 2016;38(12):1862–9.
43. Perros P, Boelaert K, Colley S, Evans C, Evans RM, Gerrard Ba G, et al. Guidelines for the management of thyroid cancer. Clin Endocrinol. 2014;81(Suppl 1):1–122.
44. Hauch A, Al-Qurayshi Z, Randolph G, Kandil E. Total thyroidectomy is associated with increased risk of complications for low- and high-volume surgeons. Ann Surg Oncol. 2014;21(12):3844–52.
45. Meltzer C, Hull M, Sundang A, Adams JL. Association between annual surgeon total thyroidectomy volume and transient and permanent complications. JAMA Otolaryngol Head Neck Surg. 2019;145(9):830.

46. Adam MA, Thomas S, Youngwirth L, Hyslop T, Reed SD, Scheri RP, et al. Is there a minimum number of thyroidectomies a surgeon should perform to optimize patient outcomes? Ann Surg. 2017;265(2):402–7.
47. Chadwick D, Kinsman R, Walton P. The British Association of Endocrine and Thyroid Surgeons: fifth national audit report. Dendrite Clinical Systems Ltd; 2017. 196 p
48. Francis DO, Pearce EC, Ni S, Garrett CG, Penson DF. Epidemiology of vocal fold paralyses after total thyroidectomy for well-differentiated thyroid cancer in a Medicare population. Otolaryngol Head Neck Surg. 2014;150(4):548–57.
49. Oda H, Miauchi A, Ito Y, Yoshioka K, Nakayama A, Sasai H, Masuoka H, Yabuta T, Fukushima M, Higashiyama T, Kihara M, Kobayashi K, Miya A. Incidences of unfavorable events in the management of low-risk papillary microcarcinoma of the thyroid by active surveillance versus immediate surgery. Thyroid. 2016;26(1):150–5.
50. Sawant R, Hulse K, Sohrabi S, Yeo JCL, Pal K, Gibb FW, et al. The impact of completion thyroidectomy. Eur J Surg Oncol. 2019;45(7):1171–4.
51. Kiess AP, Agrawal N, Brierley JD, Duvvuri U, Ferris RL, Genden E, et al. External-beam radiotherapy for differentiated thyroid cancer locoregional control: a statement of the American Head and Neck Society. Head Neck. 2016;38(4):493–8.
52. Ito Y, Miyauchi A, Inoue H, Fukushima M, Kihara M, Higashiyama T, et al. An observational trial for papillary thyroid microcarcinoma in Japanese patients. World J Surg. 2010;34(1):28–35.
53. Ito Y, Uruno T, Nakano K, Takamura Y, Miya A, Kobayashi K, et al. An observation trial without surgical treatment in patients with papillary microcarcinoma of the thyroid. Thyroid. 2003;13(4):381–7.
54. Brito JP, Ito Y, Miyauchi A, Tuttle RM. A clinical framework to facilitate risk stratification when considering an active surveillance alternative to immediate biopsy and surgery in papillary microcarcinoma. Thyroid. 2016;26(1):144–9.
55. Sugitani I, Fujimoto Y, Yamada K. Association between serum thyrotropin concentration and growth of asymptomatic papillary thyroid microcarcinoma. World J Surg. 2014;38(3):673–8.
56. Smulever A, Pitoia F. Active surveillance in papillary thyroid carcinoma: not easily accepted but possible in Latin America. Arch Endocrinol Metab. 2019;63(5):462–9.
57. Sanabria A. Experience with active surveillance of thyroid low-risk carcinoma in a developing country. Thyroid. 2020;30(7):985–91.
58. Sakai T, Sugitani I, Ebina A, Fukuoka O, Toda K, Mitani H, et al. Active surveillance for T1bN0M0 papillary thyroid carcinoma. Thyroid. 2019;29(1):59–63.
59. Ohtsuru A, Midorikawa S, Ohira T, Suzuki S, Takahashi H, Murakami M, Shimura H, Matsuzuka T, Yasumura S, Suzuki S, Yokoya S, Hashimoto Y, Sakai A, Ohto H, Yamashita S, Tanigawa K, Kamiya K. Incidence of Thyroid Cancer among children and young adults in Fukushima, Japan, screened with 2 rounds of ultrasonography within 5 years of the 2011 Fukushima Daiichi nuclear power station accident. JAMA Otolaryngol Head Neck Surg. 2019;145(1):4–11.
60. Oh HS, Ha J, Kim HI, Kim TH, Kim WG, Lim DJ, et al. Active surveillance of low-risk papillary thyroid microcarcinoma: a multi-center cohort study in Korea. Thyroid. 2018;28(12):1587–94.
61. Molinaro E, Campopiano MC, Pieruzzi L, Matrone A, Agate L, Bottici V, et al. Active surveillance in papillary thyroid microcarcinomas is feasible and safe: experience at a Single Italian Center. J Clin Endocrinol Metab. 2020;105(3):e172.
62. Kwon H, Oh HS, Kim M, Park S, Jeon MJ, Kim WG, et al. Active surveillance for patients with papillary thyroid microcarcinoma: a single center's experience in Korea. J Clin Endocrinol Metab. 2017;102(6):1917–25.

63. Tuttle RM, Alzahrani AS. Risk stratification in differentiated thyroid cancer: from detection to final follow-up. J Clin Endocrinol Metab. 2019;104(9):4087–100.
64. Pitoia F, Jerkovich F. Dynamic risk assessment in patients with differentiated thyroid cancer. Endocr Relat Cancer. 2019;26(10):R553–R66.
65. Momesso DP, Vaisman F, Yang SP, Bulzico DA, Corbo R, Vaisman M, et al. Dynamic risk stratification in differentiated thyroid cancer patients treated without radioactive iodine. J Clin Endocrinol Metab. 2016;101(7):2692–700.
66. Welch HG, Black WC. Overdiagnosis in cancer. J Natl Cancer Inst. 2010;102(9):605–13.
67. Feinstein AR, Sosin DM, Wells CK. The Will Rogers phenomenon. Stage migration and new diagnostic techniques as a source of misleading statistics for survival in cancer. N Engl J Med. 1985;312(25):1604–8.
68. Black WC, Welch HG. Advances in diagnostic imaging and overestimations of disease prevalence and the benefits of therapy. N Engl J Med. 1993;328(17):1237–43.
69. Black WC, Ling A. Is earlier diagnosis really better? The misleading effects of lead time and length biases. AJR Am J Roentgenol. 1990;155(3):625–30.
70. Hay ID, Johnson TR, Kaggal S, Reinalda MS, Iniguez-Ariza NM, Grant CS, et al. Papillary thyroid carcinoma (PTC) in children and adults: comparison of initial presentation and long-term postoperative outcome in 4432 patients consecutively treated at the Mayo Clinic during eight decades (1936-2015). World J Surg. 2018;42(2):329–42.
71. Chereau N, Buffet C, Tresallet C, Tissier F, Leenhardt L, Menegaux F. Recurrence of papillary thyroid carcinoma with lateral cervical node metastases: predictive factors and operative management. Surgery. 2016;159(3):755–62.
72. Tufano RP, Clayman G, Heller KS, Inabnet WB, Kebebew E, Shaha A, et al. Management of recurrent/persistent nodal disease in patients with differentiated thyroid cancer: a critical review of the risks and benefits of surgical intervention versus active surveillance. Thyroid. 2015;25(1):15–27.
73. Sanabria A, Rojas A, Arevalo J, Kowalski LP, Nixon I. Microscopically positive surgical margins and local recurrence in thyroid cancer. A meta-analysis. Eur J Surg Oncol. 2019;45(8):1310–6.
74. Oda H, Miyauchi A, Ito Y, Yoshioka K, Nakayama A, Sasai H, et al. Incidences of unfavorable events in the management of low-risk papillary microcarcinoma of the thyroid by active surveillance versus immediate surgery. Thyroid. 2016;26(1):150–5.

Follicular Thyroid Cancer

Wen T. Shen and Julie Ann Sosa

Contents

A. L. Shifrin et al. (eds.), *Endocrine Surgery Comprehensive Board Exam Guide*,
https://doi.org/10.1007/978-3-030-84737-1_6

Case

A 45-year-old woman is detected to have a right thyroid nodule on annual physical examination. Past medical and surgical histories are unremarkable. She reports no local compressive symptoms and no signs or symptoms of hyper- or hypothyroidism. Her family history is notable for Hashimoto's thyroiditis and hypothyroidism in a sister, but no known thyroid cancers or other endocrine diseases. She has no history of exposure to therapeutic or ionizing radiation. She is euthyroid and has no evidence of autoimmune thyroiditis on antibody testing.

Further evaluation with ultrasound demonstrates a 2 cm right thyroid nodule that is solid and hypoechoic (TIRADS 4a). No additional thyroid nodules are identified. She undergoes ultrasound-guided FNA interpreted as Bethesda IV (follicular neoplasm). She is offered the opportunity for repeat biopsy with molecular testing but elects to proceed with diagnostic right thyroid lobectomy.

Diagnostic right thyroid lobectomy is performed, and the final pathology demonstrates a 2.1 cm follicular thyroid cancer, unifocal, well-differentiated, negative margins, with a single area of capsular invasion (minimally invasive) and no evidence of vascular invasion.

Questions (Select the Best Single Answer)

1. What are the defining histopathologic characteristics of FTC?
   (a) Lymphatic invasion
   (b) Poorly differentiated features
   (c) Full-thickness invasion of surrounding capsule, or vascular invasion
   (d) Absence of mitoses and/or nuclear atypia
2. Which of the following statements is true regarding the incidence of FTC?
   (a) It is more likely in men than women.
   (b) It is increasing in incidence, but at a slower rate compared with papillary thyroid cancer.
   (c) The peak age of diagnosis is 30.
   (d) Incidence is inversely correlated with iodine deficiency.
3. Possible histopathologic diagnoses from a patient with Bethesda IV (follicular neoplasm) cytology include all of the following *except*:
   (a) Medullary thyroid cancer
   (b) Noninvasive follicular tumor with papillary-like nuclear features (NIFTP)
   (c) Follicular variant of papillary thyroid cancer
   (d) Follicular adenoma
4. Which of the following is the appropriate initial operation for a patient with solitary 1.5 cm follicular neoplasm?
   (a) Total thyroidectomy
   (b) Total thyroidectomy with bilateral central neck dissection
   (c) Nodulectomy
   (d) Thyroid lobectomy

5. Genetic mutations associated with pathogenesis of FTC include all of the following *except*:
    - (a) PTEN
    - (b) RAS
    - (c) RET
    - (d) PAX8-PPAR-gamma
6. Choose the correct statement regarding metastatic FTC:
    - (a) FTC metastasizes to the lymph nodes in 50% of cases.
    - (b) The lungs and bones are the least common sites of FTC metastasis.
    - (c) FTCs are equally likely to metastasize via lymphatic and hematogenous spread.
    - (d) Presence of angioinvasion correlates with risk of distant metastases of FTC.
7. Intraoperative frozen section analysis:
    - (a) Reliably distinguishes follicular adenoma from follicular carcinoma
    - (b) Has limited utility during diagnostic thyroid lobectomy for follicular neoplasm
    - (c) May be used to determine whether a follicular thyroid tumor is NIFTP
    - (d) Should only be used in patients with a family history of thyroid cancer
8. Which of the following statements is false regarding the utility of radioactive iodine therapy for FTC?
    - (a) Radioactive iodine therapy may be useful in patients with intermediate- and high-risk FTC.
    - (b) One of the primary indications for completion thyroidectomy after initial diagnostic lobectomy for FTC is the anticipated need for radioactive iodine.
    - (c) Radioactive iodine therapy is ineffective for FTCs, because the cells are not typically iodine-avid.
    - (d) Distant metastases of FTC may be treated with radioactive iodine.
9. The most widely utilized staging system for follicular thyroid cancer is
    - (a) MACIS
    - (b) AGES
    - (c) ATA
    - (d) AJCC/TNM
10. FDG-PET scan:
    - (a) Is the first-line imaging modality in patients with known or suspected FTC
    - (b) May be useful in postoperative FTC patients with elevated serum thyroglobulin levels but negative radioactive iodine scan
    - (c) Is more accurate than ultrasound for detecting lymph node metastases of FTC
    - (d) Has limited utility for dedifferentiated FTC

6.1 Introduction

Follicular thyroid cancer (FTC) is the second most common type of differentiated thyroid cancer, representing 10–15% of all thyroid cancers. In this chapter, we discuss the clinical, histopathologic, and molecular features of FTC and review treatment options.

6.2 Definition

According to the WHO, the definition of follicular thyroid cancer is a *malignant epithelial thyroid tumor showing follicular cell differentiation, without the nuclear features of papillary thyroid cancer (psammoma bodies, nuclear inclusions, ground-glass appearance, longitudinal grooves, nuclear overlapping)* [1]. Distinction between FTC and follicular thyroid adenoma is based upon capsular and/or vascular invasion identified on histopathologic analysis.

6.3 Epidemiology

The peak incidence of FTC is in patients between 40 and 60 years old [2]. FTC occurs in women three times more often than in men [3]. Iodine deficiency is believed to play a role in the development of FTC; iodine-deficient regions exhibit a higher prevalence of FTC compared to iodine-sufficient regions, and declining rates of FTC observed in certain geographic areas have been attributed to implementation of iodine supplementation [4, 5]. While exposure to ionizing radiation is considered a risk factor for the development of all types of differentiated thyroid cancers, papillary thyroid cancer (PTC) is by far the most common radiation-induced thyroid cancer. Obesity has been implicated as a risk factor for developing differentiated thyroid cancers; a 2015 meta-analysis revealed that obese patients have a 61% increased risk of developing follicular thyroid cancer compared to matched patients of normal weight [6].

PTC is the most common type of thyroid cancer, (~85%), while FTC represents approximately 11% of thyroid cancers [7]. A 2013 review of the SEER database collected during the period 1980–2009 reported an incidence rate of FTC of 0.88 per 100,000 person-years, as compared with an incidence rate for PTC of 6.21 per 100,000 person-years over the same time interval [8]. The worldwide increase in thyroid cancer diagnoses observed over the past few decades has been largely due to increases in PTC diagnoses; FTC incidence has also increased, but at a significantly lower rate [9].

6.4 Clinical Presentation

Patients with FTC typically present with a thyroid nodule, detected either on physical examination or radiographic imaging. These nodules are usually painless, but may cause local compressive symptoms of dysphagia, dyspnea, or dysphonia if they abut the aerodigestive tract or recurrent laryngeal nerve. Most patients will be euthyroid, although some may have coexistent autoimmune thyroiditis and hypothyroidism, and there are rare cases of hyperfunctioning FTCs causing thyrotoxicosis (usually from metastatic disease) [10, 11].

There are no distinct radiologic features that reliably distinguish between follicular adenoma and FTC. Follicular thyroid tumors are typically solitary, solid, hypervascular, and homogeneous, with varying echogenicity. Ultrasound findings that may suggest increased risk of malignancy include irregular borders, calcifications, hypoechogenicity, and taller-than-wide shape. Numerous classification systems for ultrasound examination of thyroid nodules have been studied in patients with cytologically indeterminate nodules. The ATA and TI-RADS systems have both demonstrated reasonable utility for risk stratification in patients with indeterminate nodules, and can help guide clinical decision-making in conjunction with cytology and molecular testing [12–14]. PET-FDG scan does not reliably diagnose malignancy in patients with cytologically indeterminate thyroid nodules [15].

Unlike PTCs, FTCs typically metastasize hematogenously. Lymph node metastases of FTC are therefore rare (~5% of patients) [16]. The most common distant metastatic sites of FTC are the lungs and bones; less commonly, FTC may metastasize to the liver, brain, and other solid organs, as well as the skin; 15–25% of patients with FTC will have distant metastases upon presentation [17, 18].

6.5 Molecular Pathogenesis

Multiple oncogenes and pathways have been identified in the molecular pathogenesis of FTCs. The two most commonly involved genetic alterations identified in FTCs are RAS mutations and PAX-8-PPAR-gamma rearrangements.

The RAS proto-oncogene activates the MAP-kinase pathway, and RAS point mutations are commonly identified in both follicular adenomas (20–40%) and follicular carcinomas (30–50%) [19, 20]. The presence of RAS mutations is not a reliable indicator of FTC, but may be suggestive of increased malignant potential. RAS activation is believed to be an important early step in the development of follicular adenoma and the progression of follicular adenoma to FTC [19, 21, 22].

PAX-8-PPAR-gamma is a fusion protein of PAX-8 (a thyroid-specific transcription factor) and PPAR-gamma (a regulator of lipid metabolism and insulin sensitivity), and rearrangements of this fusion protein are found in 5–20% of follicular adenomas and 20–50% of FTCs [23–25]. PAX-PPAR-gamma translocation has been implicated as another critical step in FTC tumorigenesis.

Other oncogenes and genetic alterations have been identified in FTCs. These include deletions of the tumor suppressor gene PTEN, seen in Cowden's Syndrome; TERT promoter mutations; TSH-receptor mutations; and presence of proto-oncogenes p53, c-myc, and c-fos [26].

FTCs are not associated with the mutations of BRAF or RET/PTC, which are commonly identified in PTCs.

6.6 Diagnosis

FTCs and follicular adenomas cannot be distinguished from each other based upon cytology alone; the diagnosis of FTC is determined by the presence of capsular or vascular invasion identified on histopathologic analysis. The most common FNA diagnoses for FTCs are atypia of undetermined significance/follicular lesion of undetermined significance (AUS/FLUS, Bethesda 3) and follicular neoplasm (Bethesda 4) [27]. The diagnosis of AUS/FLUS (Bethesda class 3) is designated for thyroid nodule biopsies with mild nuclear or architectural atypia. The cytologic diagnosis of follicular neoplasm (Bethesda class 4) is made in thyroid nodule samples with high cellularity, microfollicular architecture, and scant or absent colloid. The possible histologic diagnoses from Bethesda 3 or Bethesda 4 cytology include follicular adenoma, FTC, follicular variant of papillary thyroid carcinoma, and noninvasive follicular thyroid neoplasm with papillary-like nuclear features (NIFTP). Molecular profiling is a useful adjunct for risk stratification and improved characterization of indeterminate thyroid nodules in selected patients; the details of molecular testing for thyroid nodules are covered in a separate chapter of this text.

FTCs are further subclassified as minimally invasive, encapsulated angioinvasive, and widely invasive. Minimally invasive FTC is defined by microscopic foci of capsular invasion. Encapsulated angioinvasive FTC exhibits an intact capsule with adjacent vascular invasion. Angioinvasive FTC is associated with higher risk for metastases and recurrence; invasion of greater than 4 blood vessels has a negative impact on overall survival [28, 29]. Widely invasive FTC is defined by extensive invasion of the thyroid capsule, often with concurrent invasion of surrounding blood vessels, with possible involvement of adjacent tissues and structures.

Follicular variant of papillary thyroid carcinoma (FVPTC) is a distinct subtype of thyroid cancer that should be distinguished from other types of papillary or follicular thyroid cancers [30]. FVPTCs are follicular tumors with other histologic features of papillary thyroid cancer such as psammoma bodies and clear nuclei (Orphan Annie eyes).

A recent change in thyroid tumor nomenclature involved the reclassification of encapsulated follicular variant of papillary thyroid cancer without capsular or vascular invasion as noninvasive follicular thyroid neoplasm with papillary-like nuclear features (NIFTP). This reclassification was based upon multiple studies demonstrating indolent clinical behavior of these encapsulated tumors, with negligible risk of metastasis, recurrence, or other adverse outcomes [31–33]. It should be noted, however, that NIFTP is a postsurgical diagnosis requiring complete excision and histopathologic analysis, and cannot be reliably diagnosed based upon cytology or molecular profiling. Patients diagnosed with NIFTP are likely adequately treated with lobectomy alone and do not require radioactive iodine therapy.

6.7 Staging and Prognostic Features

The most widely used staging system for well-differentiated thyroid cancers is the American Joint Committee on Cancer/Union for International Cancer Control (AJCC/UICC) TNM (tumor/node/metastasis) classification scheme (most recent update 2016, 8th edition) [34]. This classification scheme utilizes the standard metrics of tumor size, nodal involvement, and distant metastases for risk stratification, but also includes patient age at diagnosis as a significant determining factor: patients younger than 55 years at diagnosis are limited to stages I and II, even if they have distant metastases or locally advanced disease.

Other prognostic clinical and pathologic variables include patient age, tumor size, angioinvasion, extrathyroidal extension, margin status, lymphovascular invasion, and distant metastases.

While many clinical guidelines and practice algorithms consider the various subtypes of differentiated thyroid cancer to be interchangeable and similar in behavior, each has its own distinct biology, clinical profile, and prognosis. The overall prognosis of FTC is worse than that of papillary thyroid cancer [10]. Patients with FTC are more likely to present with distant metastases and at a higher stage than patients with papillary thyroid cancers [35]. Extent of invasion plays a significant role in the prognosis of FTCs. A 2013 analysis of the SEER database demonstrated that patients with minimally invasive FTC rarely develop distant metastases or recurrent disease, and have a long-term survival similar to that of the general US population [36]. In contrast, patients with angioinvasion (especially ≥4 vessels involved) and/or widely invasive FTC are more likely to develop distant metastases and disease recurrence, and have decreased overall survival [28, 29].

6.8 Treatment

Most patients with cytologically indeterminate thyroid nodules, with or without adjunctive molecular profiling, will be recommended for diagnostic thyroid lobectomy. Thyroid lobectomy is sufficient treatment for the majority of low-risk FTCs. Total thyroidectomy may be considered for first-line operation in patients with tumors >4 cm, bilateral nodular disease, high-risk clinical features such as family history of thyroid cancer or a history of radiation exposure, worrisome radiologic findings such as local invasion or distant metastases, and patient preference.

Intraoperative frozen section does not reliably diagnose follicular thyroid cancer in patients with indeterminate nodules undergoing thyroid lobectomy. Numerous retrospective studies have demonstrated minimal clinical utility for frozen section in distinguishing between follicular adenomas and carcinomas [37–39]. The only randomized prospective trial of frozen section analysis for patients with follicular neoplasm reported that frozen section showed no benefit in >96% of patients [40].

When follicular thyroid cancer is diagnosed on final pathology following initial diagnostic thyroid lobectomy for indeterminate cytology, completion thyroidectomy should be considered for patients with intermediate- to high-risk features who are candidates for radioactive iodine therapy. Until recently, completion thyroidectomy was routinely performed in patients with a final pathology diagnosis of follicular thyroid cancer after diagnostic lobectomy. However, data from multiple studies demonstrating similar oncologic outcomes for lobectomy versus total thyroidectomy for low-risk differentiated thyroid cancers have resulted in a more selective approach to surgical decision-making for follicular thyroid cancer [41]. Findings that may warrant consideration for completion thyroidectomy include tumor size >4 cm, wide capsular invasion, angioinvasion (especially if ≥4 vessels are involved), positive margin, poorly differentiated or undifferentiated tumor, and patient preference.

Radioactive iodine therapy should be reserved for patients with intermediate- to high-risk FTC. The ATA definition for intermediate-risk disease includes tumor size >4 cm, microscopic extrathyroidal extension, and nodal metastases; high-risk is defined by gross extrathyroidal extension and distant metastases [42]. Patients with low-risk FTC do not benefit from radioactive iodine therapy.

6.9 Recurrence

Reported recurrence rates for follicular thyroid cancers vary widely in the literature (3–44%) [10]. Recurrent follicular thyroid cancer may occur locally in the thyroid bed or at distant sites such as bone, lungs, liver, brain, or other organs. Lymph node metastases are rare (<5% of FTC cases). Recurrent disease is more commonly seen in patients with angioinvasive and widely invasive FTC.

Follow-up protocols for FTC include thyroglobulin measurement and serial ultrasound, in conjunction with TSH suppression in the majority of patients. Other imaging modalities such as radioiodine scan, CT, and FDG-PET also may be utilized, depending on clinical suspicion and institutional availability.

6.10 Summary and Conclusion

FTC is the second most common differentiated thyroid cancer, representing ~11% of all thyroid cancers. It is defined by capsular or vascular invasion identified on histopathologic analysis and cannot be reliably diagnosed by fine-needle aspiration cytology or molecular testing. The most common genetic mutations identified in FTCs are RAS mutations and PAX8-PPAR-gamma rearrangements. Clinical and pathologic features influencing prognosis of FTC include AJCC stage, angioinvasion, extent of capsular invasion, and distant metastases. Low-risk FTC is almost always adequately treated with thyroid lobectomy alone; patients with intermediate- and high-risk FTC should be considered for total thyroidectomy and radioactive iodine therapy.

Answers

1. (c); 2. (b); 3. (a); 4. (d); 5. (c); 6. (d); 7. (b); 8. (c); 9. (d); 10. (b)

References

1. Lloyd RV, Osamura RY, Klöppel G, Rosai J. WHO classification of tumours of endocrine organs. 4th ed. Geneva: World Health Organization; 2017.
2. Milano AF. Thyroid cancer: 20-year comparative mortality and survival analysis of six thyroid cancer histologic subtypes by age, sex, race, stage, cohort entry time-period and disease duration (SEER*Stat 8.3.2) a systematic review of 145,457 cases for diagnosis years 1993-2013. J Insur Med. 2018;47(3):143–58.

3. Aschebrook-Kilfoy B, Ward MH, Sabra MM, Devesa SS. Thyroid cancer incidence patterns in the United States by histologic type, 1992-2006. Thyroid. 2011;21(2):125–34.
4. Nettore IC, Colao A, Macchia PE. Nutritional and environmental factors in thyroid carcinogenesis. Int J Environ Res Public Health. 2018;15(8):1735.
5. Vuong HG, Kondo T, Oishi N, Nakazawa T, Mochizuki K, Inoue T, Tahara I, Kasai K, Hirokawa M, Tran TM, Katoh R. Genetic alterations of differentiated thyroid carcinoma in iodine-rich and iodine-deficient countries. Cancer Med. 2016;5(8):1883–9.
6. Schmid D, Ricci C, Behrens G, Leitzmann MF. Adiposity and risk of thyroid cancer: a systematic review and meta-analysis. Obes Rev. 2015;16(12):1042–54.
7. Lim H, Devesa SS, Sosa JA, Check D, Kitahara CM. Trends in thyroid cancer incidence and mortality in the United States, 1974-2013. JAMA. 2017;317(13):1338–48.
8. Aschebrook-Kilfoy B, Grogan RH, Ward MH, Kaplan E, Devesa SS. Follicular thyroid cancer incidence patterns in the United States, 1980-2009. Thyroid. 2013;23(8):1015–21.
9. Kitahara CM, Sosa JA. The changing incidence of thyroid cancer. Nat Rev Endocrinol. 2016;12(11):646–53.
10. Grani G, Lamartina L, Durante C, Filetti S, Cooper DS. Follicular thyroid cancer and Hürthle cell carcinoma: challenges in diagnosis, treatment, and clinical management. Lancet Diabetes Endocrinol. 2018;6(6):500–14.
11. Nishihara E, Amino N, Miyauchi A. Fractionated radioiodine therapy for hyperthyroidism caused by widespread metastatic follicular thyroid carcinoma. Thyroid. 2010;20(5):569–70.
12. Chng CL, Kurzawinski TR, Beale T. Value of sonographic features in predicting malignancy in thyroid nodules diagnosed as follicular neoplasm on cytology. Clin Endocrinol. 2015;83(5):711–6.
13. Ha SM, Ahn HS, Baek JH, Ahn HY, Chung YJ, Cho BY, Park SB. Validation of three scoring risk-stratification models for thyroid nodules. Thyroid. 2017;27(12):1550–7.
14. Ahmadi S, Herbst R, Oyekunle T, Jiang X, Strickland K, Roman S, Sosa JA. Using the ATA and ACR TI-RADS sonographic classifications as adjunctive predictors of malignancy for indeterminate thyroid nodules. Endocr Pract. 2019;25(9):908–17.
15. Deandreis D, Al Ghuzlan A, Auperin A, Vielh P, Caillou B, Chami L, Lumbroso J, Travagli JP, Hartl D, Baudin E, Schlumberger M, Leboulleux S. Is (18)F-fluorodeoxyglucose-PET/CT useful for the presurgical characterization of thyroid nodules with indeterminate fine needle aspiration cytology? Thyroid. 2012;22(2):165–72.
16. Alfalah H, Cranshaw I, Jany T, Arnalsteen L, Leteurtre E, Cardot C, Pattou F, Carnaille B. Risk factors for lateral cervical lymph node involvement in follicular thyroid carcinoma. World J Surg. 2008;32(12):2623–6.
17. Sugino K, Ito K, Nagahama M, Kitagawa W, Shibuya H, Ohkuwa K, Yano Y, Uruno T, Akaishi J, Kameyama K, Ito K. Prognosis and prognostic factors for distant metastases and tumor mortality in follicular thyroid carcinoma. Thyroid. 2011;21(7):751–7.
18. Parameswaran R, Shulin Hu J, Min En N, Tan WB, Yuan NK. Patterns of metastasis in follicular thyroid carcinoma and the difference between early and delayed presentation. Ann R Coll Surg Engl. 2017;99(2):151–4.
19. Howell GM, Hodak SP, Yip L. RAS mutations in thyroid cancer. Oncologist. 2013;18(8):926–32.
20. Esapa CT, Johnson SJ, Kendall-Taylor P, Lennard TW, Harris PE. Prevalence of Ras mutations in thyroid neoplasia. Clin Endocrinol. 1999;50(4):529–35.

21. Garcia-Rostan G, Zhao H, Camp RL, Pollan M, Herrero A, Pardo J, Wu R, Carcangiu ML, Costa J, Tallini G. Ras mutations are associated with aggressive tumor phenotypes and poor prognosis in thyroid cancer. J Clin Oncol. 2003;21(17):3226–35.
22. Namba H, Rubin SA, Fagin JA. Point mutations of ras oncogenes are an early event in thyroid tumorigenesis. Mol Endocrinol. 1990;4(10): 1474–9.
23. Marques AR, Espadinha C, Catarino AL, Moniz S, Pereira T, Sobrinho LG, Leite V. Expression of PAX8-PPAR gamma 1 rearrangements in both follicular thyroid carcinomas and adenomas. J Clin Endocrinol Metab. 2002;87(8):3947–52.
24. Dwight T, Thoppe SR, Foukakis T, Lui WO, Wallin G, Höög A, Frisk T, Larsson C, Zedenius J. Involvement of the PAX8/peroxisome proliferator-activated receptor gamma rearrangement in follicular thyroid tumors. J Clin Endocrinol Metab. 2003;88(9):4440–5.
25. Nikiforova MN, Biddinger PW, Caudill CM, Kroll TG, Nikiforov YE. PAX8-PPARgamma rearrangement in thyroid tumors: RT-PCR and immunohistochemical analyses. Am J Surg Pathol. 2002;26(8): 1016–23.
26. Yip L. Molecular markers for thyroid cancer diagnosis, prognosis, and targeted therapy. J Surg Oncol. 2015;111(1):43–50.
27. Cibas ES, Ali SZ. The 2017 Bethesda system for reporting thyroid cytopathology. Thyroid. 2017;27(11):1341–6.
28. Ito Y, Hirokawa M, Masuoka H, Yabuta T, Kihara M, Higashiyama T, Takamura Y, Kobayashi K, Miya A, Miyauchi A. Prognostic factors of minimally invasive follicular thyroid carcinoma: extensive vascular invasion significantly affects patient prognosis. Endocr J. 2013;60(5):637–42.
29. Lee YM, Song DE, Kim TY, Sung TY, Yoon JH, Chung KW, Hong SJ. Risk factors for distant metastasis in patients with minimally invasive follicular thyroid carcinoma. PLoS One. 2016;11(5):e0155489.
30. Tallini G, Tuttle RM, Ghossein RA. The history of the follicular variant of papillary thyroid carcinoma. J Clin Endocrinol Metab. 2017;102(1) 15–22.
31. Nikiforov YE, Seethala RR, Tallini G, Baloch ZW, Basolo F, Thompson LD, Barletta JA, Wenig BM, Al Ghuzlan A, Kakudo K, Giordano TJ, Alves VA, Khanafshar E, Asa SL, El-Naggar AK, Gooding WE, Hodak SP, Lloyd RV, Maytal G, Mete O, Nikiforova MN, Nosé V, Papotti M, Poller DN, Sadow PM, Tischler AS, Tuttle RM, Wall KB, LiVolsi VA, Randolph GW, Ghossein RA. Nomenclature revision for encapsulated follicular variant of papillary thyroid carcinoma: a paradigm shift to reduce overtreatment of indolent tumors. JAMA Oncol. 2016;2(8):1023–9.
32. Haugen BR, Sawka AM, Alexander EK, Bible KC, Caturegli P, Doherty GM, Mandel SJ, Morris JC, Nassar A, Pacini F, Schlumberger M, Schuff K, Sherman SI, Somerset H, Sosa JA, Steward DL, Wartofsky L, Williams MD. American Thyroid Association guidelines on the management of thyroid nodules and differentiated thyroid cancer task force review and recommendation on the proposed renaming of encapsulated follicular variant papillary thyroid carcinoma without invasion to noninvasive follicular thyroid neoplasm with papillary-like nuclear features. Thyroid. 2017;27(4):481–3.
33. Thompson LD. Ninety-four cases of encapsulated follicular variant of papillary thyroid carcinoma: a name change to noninvasive follicular thyroid neoplasm with papillary-like nuclear features would help prevent overtreatment. Mod Pathol. 2016;29(7):698–707.
34. American Joint Committee on Cancer. Thyroid – differentiated and anaplastic. In: AJCC cancer staging manual. 8th ed. New York: Springer; 2017.

35. Goffredo P, Sosa JA, Roman SA. Differentiated thyroid cancer presenting with distant metastases: a population analysis over two decades. World J Surg. 2013;37(7):1599–605.
36. Goffredo P, Jillard C, Thomas S, Scheri RP, Sosa JA, Roman S. Minimally invasive follicular carcinoma: predictors of vascular invasion and impact on patterns of care. Endocrine. 2016;51(1):123–30.
37. Kennedy JM, Robinson RA. Thyroid frozen sections in patients with preoperative FNAs: review of Surgeons' preoperative rationale, intraoperative decisions, and final outcome. Am J Clin Pathol. 2016;145(5):660–5.
38. Huber GF, Dziegielewski P, Matthews TW, Warshawski SJ, Kmet LM, Faris P, Khalil M, Dort JC. Intraoperative frozen-section analysis for thyroid nodules: a step toward clarity or confusion? Arch Otolaryngol Head Neck Surg. 2007;133(9):874–81.
39. Cohen MA, Patel KR, Gromis J, Kutler DI, Kuhel WI, Stater BJ, Schulman A, Hoda RS, Scognamiglio T. Retrospective evaluation of frozen section use for thyroid nodules with a prior fine needle aspiration diagnosis of Bethesda II-VI: the Weill Cornell Medical College experience. World J Otorhinolaryngol Head Neck Surg. 2015;1(1):5–10.
40. Udelsman R, Westra WH, Donovan PI, Sohn TA, Cameron JL. Randomized prospective evaluation of frozen-section analysis for follicular neoplasms of the thyroid. Ann Surg. 2001;233(5):716–22.
41. Adam MA, Pura J, Gu L, Dinan MA, Tyler DS, Reed SD, Scheri R, Roman SA, Sosa JA. Extent of surgery for papillary thyroid cancer is not associated with survival: an analysis of 61,775 patients. Ann Surg. 2014;260(4):601–5; discussion 605–7.
42. Haugen BR, Alexander EK, Bible KC, Doherty GM, Mandel SJ, Nikiforov YE, Pacini F, Randolph GW, Sawka AM, Schlumberger M, Schuff KG, Sherman SI, Sosa JA, Steward DL, Tuttle RM, Wartofsky L. 2015 American Thyroid Association management guidelines for adult patients with thyroid nodules and differentiated thyroid cancer: the American Thyroid Association guidelines task force on thyroid nodules and differentiated thyroid cancer. Thyroid. 2016;26(1):1–133.

Hürthle Cell Carcinoma

Inga-Lena Nilsson

Contents

A. L. Shifrin et al. (eds.), *Endocrine Surgery Comprehensive Board Exam Guide*,
https://doi.org/10.1007/978-3-030-84737-1_7

Case Presentation

A 74-year-old man was referred to the endocrine surgeon in February 2020 because of an incidental finding of a lesion in the left thyroid lobe that was visualized on a magnetic resonance (MR) scanning of the spine. The indication for MR was pain in the neck and shoulder, and there was suspicion of a spinal hernia. The thyroid lesion was observed to bulge into, deviate, and partially compress the trachea.

The patient presented with a palpable lump, about 5 cm in diameter. Interestingly, the patient had not noticed the lump himself nor noted any local symptoms of dysphagia or airway obstruction. The patient was a non-smoker with no history of malignancy; he had a history of past surgical procedures due to inguinal hernia and meniscectomy, yet had no medicinal treatment other than painkillers and antihypertensives. Ultrasound examination visualized an almost solid hypoechoic lesion where the shape was wider-than-tall, measuring 2.9 cm in anterioposterior, 3.4 cm in transverse, and 5.1 cm in longitudinal diameter. The lesion was surrounded by a halo, contained some microcalcifications, and the margin was well defined. According to the EU-TIRADS, the lesion would be categorized as having an intermediate risk of malignancy or, according to ACR-TIRADS, as moderately suspicious for malignancy. The right thyroid lobe was normal with the exception of a cyst 4 mm in size.

Fine-needle aspiration cytology showed increased cellularity with predominance (about 90%) of Hürthle cells, absence of background colloid or chronic inflammation, and classified as Bethesda IV. The proliferation rate was low (Ki-67 <1%).

The patient underwent a left-sided hemithyroidectomy. No lymph nodes were removed.

The histopathological examination verified a radically removed Hürthle cell carcinoma with multifocal invasion of the tumor capsule, yet without lymphovascular invasion or extrathyroidal extension. The pTNM was classified as pT3aNx (◘ Figs. 7.1, 7.2, 7.3, and 7.4). The cells were characterized by large, bulky, and eosinophilic cytoplasm and carried a low nuclei-cytoplasmic ratio. The nuclei were relatively monomorphic with compact chromatin, and puncta formed nucleoli without nuclear changes characteristic for papillary thyroid cancer. The growth pattern was mixed: solid, trabecular, and microfollicular. Less than 1 mitosis per 10 high-power fields was observed and no obvious tumor necrosis was seen. Immunohistochemical analyses showed immuno reactivity against TTF-1, PAX8 and thyroglobulin, with the latter positive in 75–100% of cells. The Ki-67-index was 2.1%. According to the local routine, molecular genetic examination of tumor DNA

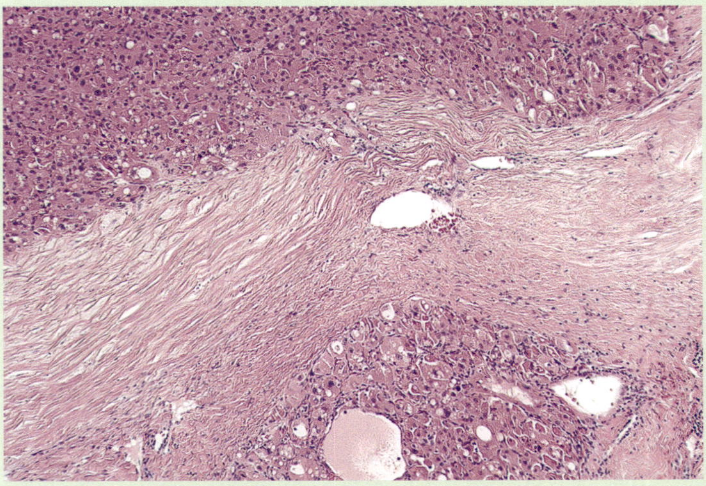

◘ **Fig. 7.1** Hürthle cell carcinoma; capsular invasion, original magnification ×100; hematoxylin and eosin (H&E) stain. (All histology images provided by C. Christofer Juhlin, Associate Professor, Department of Pathology and Cytology, Karolinska University Hospital, Stockholm, Sweden)

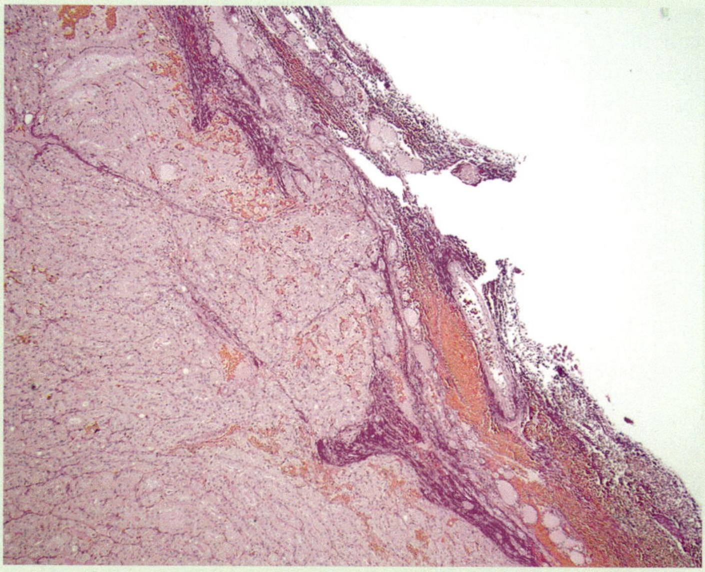

Fig. 7.2 Hürthle cell carcinoma; capsular invasion, original magnification ×20; Van Gieson stain

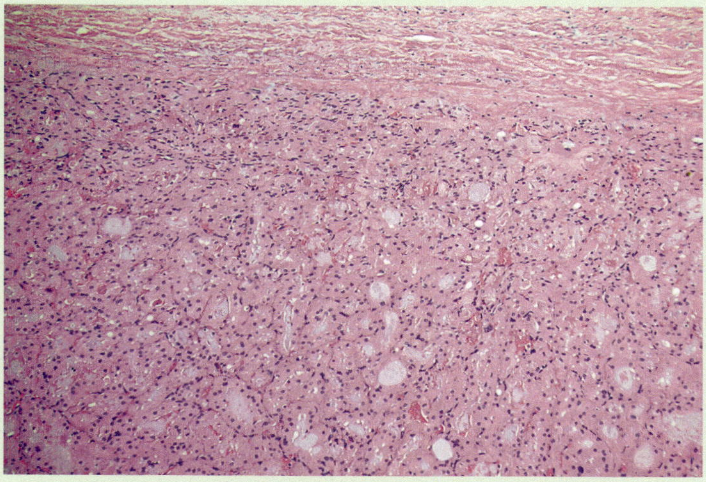

Fig. 7.3 Hürthle cell carcinoma; cellular attributes, original magnification ×100; H&E stain

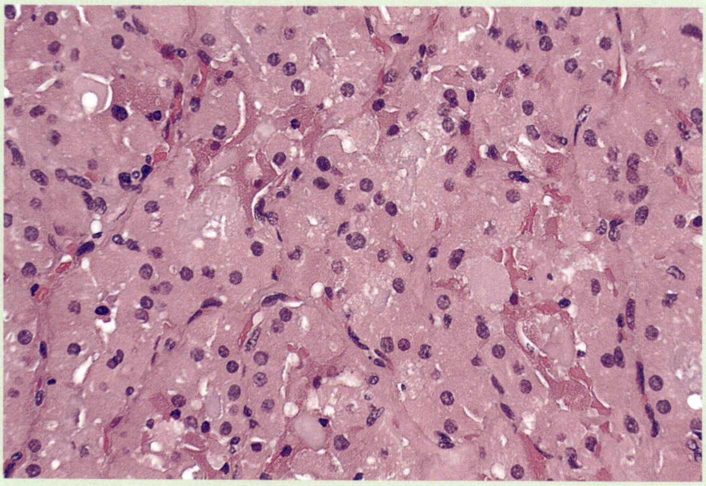

Fig. 7.4 Hürthle cell carcinoma; cellular attributes, original magnification ×400 H&E stain

with *TERT* promoter sequencing was performed and verified a *TERT* promoter mutation, C228T.

The patient underwent completion thyroidectomy. The subsequent histopathological examination revealed a colloid nodule but no sign of tumor. Thyroxine treatment followed and included a daily dose of 125 micrograms in order to maintain a circulating thyroid-stimulating hormone concentration below 0.01 mIU/L. Based upon a multidisciplinary board decision, the patient received radioiodine treatment in the dose of 3.7 gigabecquerel (GBq) (100 Millicurie (mCi)). A full-body scan after the procedure showed local uptake of radioactivity in the thyroid bed.

Questions

1. In which of the following would you establish the diagnosis of Hürthle cell carcinoma?
   1. Cytology specimen from a solid thyroid nodule showing greater than 70% of Hürthle cells
   2. Cytology specimen from a solid thyroid nodule showing greater than 70% of Hürthle cells, classified as Bethesda V
   3. Intraoperative frozen section of intrathyroidal lesion containing greater than 70% of Hürthle cells
   4. Histopathological verification of intrathyroidal lesion with full-thickness capsular invasion containing greater than 70% of Hürthle cells
      (a) All are correct.
      (b) Only 2, 3, and 4 are correct.
      (c) Only 2 and 4 are correct.
      (d) Only 4 is correct.
      (e) None are correct.
2. What is true about Hürthle cells?
   1. Presence of Hürthle cells, per se, increases the risk of malignancy.
   2. Hürthle cells are also called oncocytes.
   3. Hürthle cells can be present in benign goiter.
   4. Hürthle cells are characterized by a high content of mitochondria.
      (a) All are correct.
      (b) Only 3 and 4 are correct.
      (c) Only 2, 3, and 4 are correct.
      (d) Only 4 is correct.
3. How would you classify a Hürthle cell carcinoma?
   1. A variant of follicular thyroid cancer
   2. A variant of papillary thyroid cancer
   3. A variant of differentiated thyroid cancer
   4. A separate entity
      (a) All are correct.
      (b) Only 1, 2, and 3 are correct.
      (c) Only 3 and 4 are correct
      (d) Only 4 is correct.
      (e) None are correct.

4. Which of the following preoperative preparative examinations are advisable for patients with Hürthle cell neoplasia, presenting with hoarseness?
   1. Ultrasound
   2. Laryngoscopy
   3. MR scanning to detect extrathyroidal extension
   4. Contrast-enhanced CT scanning to detect extrathyroidal extension
      (a) All are correct.
      (b) Only 1 and 2 are correct.
      (c) Only 1, 2, and 4 are correct
      (d) All but 4 are correct
5. Which of the following statements are correct about ultrasound?
   1. Thyroid Imaging Reporting and Database Systems are developed to provide a structured ultrasound reporting template.
   2. Ultrasound is effective for detection of lymph node metastases in region VI.
   3. Ultrasound is effective for differentiation between Hürthle cell carcinoma and adenoma.
   4. Protrusion into adjacent structures and disruption of the capsular margin indicate extrathyroidal extension.
      (a) All are correct.
      (b) Only 1 is correct.
      (c) Only 1 and 2 are correct.
      (d) Only 1 and 4 are correct.
6. Which of the following statements are correct for Bethesda classification?
   1. Introduced to standardize the terminology for reporting of thyroid cytopathology.
   2. Grouped into six categories based on the risk of malignancy.
   3. Hürthle cell carcinoma are often classified as follicular lesion of undetermined significance.
   4. Cytology may be diagnostic for Hürthle cell carcinoma in patients with metastatic disease.
      (a) Only 1 and 2 is correct.
      (b) Only 1, 2, and 3 are correct.
      (c) Only 1, 2, and 4 are correct.
      (d) All are correct.
7. Which are the goals of radioiodine therapy?
   1. Remnant ablation meant to facilitate detection of recurrent disease
   2. Adjuvant therapy intended to destroy suspected residual disease
   3. Therapy intended to treat persistent disease
   4. Therapy intended to improve disease-specific and disease-free survival
      (a) All are correct.
      (b) Only 1 is correct.

(c) Only 1 and 2 are correct.
(d) Only 1, 3, and 4 are correct.
(e) Only 2 and 3 are correct.

8. Why treat patients with recombinant TSH?
   1. To suppress TSH
   2. To avoid negative effects on Quality of Life from thyroxin withdrawal
   3. To achieve a TSH greater than 30 mIU/L
   4. To increase the effect of radioiodine treatment
      (a) All are correct.
      (b) Only 4 is correct.
      (c) Only 2 and 3 are correct.
      (d) Only 2, 3 and 4 are correct.
9. Which of the following risk factors have been found to be negative prognostic signs in Hürthle cell carcinoma?
   1. Age over 45 years
   2. Female gender
   3. Tumor size and extension at diagnosis
   4. Hot nodule with hyperfunction
      (a) All are correct.
      (b) Only 3 is correct.
      (c) Only 1 and 3 are correct.
      (d) Only 1, 3, and 4 are correct.
10. Which of the following statements are true for Hürthle cell carcinoma?
   1. Accounts for about 3% of all thyroid malignancies.
   2. 10-year survival of 92.6% has been reported.
   3. The majority presents with local disease.
   4. $_{18}$FDG-PET/CT can be useful for detection of recurrent disease.
      (a) All are correct.
      (b) Only 3 is correct.
      (c) Only 1 and 3 are correct.
      (d) Only 1, 3, and 4 are correct.

7

7.1 Introduction

Hürthle cell carcinoma is defined as a malignant thyroid tumor that is predominantly (at least 75%) composed of metaplastic thyroid follicular cells with abundant granular eosinophilic cytoplasm. These cells, also called oncocytes, may also be present in nontumor tissue such as nodular goiter, lymphocytic thyroiditis, and other variants of thyroid neoplasia [1, 2]. The granular eosinophilic cytoplasm results from excessive accumulation of mitochondria. The name is actually a misnomer; the cells, as described by Hürthle in 1894, were actually parafollicular C cells [3]. Hürthle cell carcinoma accounts for about 3% of thyroid malignancies [4]. Traditionally, Hürthle cell carcinoma has been considered a histopathological variant of follicular carcinoma, yet is now defined as a separate entity based upon its unique biological behavior, genetic alterations, and differences in prognosis as compared to follicular carcinoma [5, 6]. Hürthle cell carcinoma has historically been found to be more aggressive, carrying a higher risk for distant metastases and poor prognosis when compared to other differentiated thyroid cancers; however, the survival rate has improved dramatically over time [7–9]. The majority of patients with Hürthle cell carcinoma can today be effectively treated.

7.2 Clinical Presentation

Most Hürthle cell cancer patients present with a single, painless thyroid nodule. In a recent analysis of 2101 patients with Hürthle cell carcinoma identified in the database from the Surveillance, Epidemiology and End Results (SEER) and who were diagnosed between 2004 and 2016 with an average age of 55, +/− 15 years, it was found that 29% were men and 83% had local disease at the time of diagnosis. Patients with distant disease were older, more often males, and more often exhibited extensive and multifocal tumors [10].

Compared to follicular thyroid carcinoma, Hürthle cell carcinoma seems to be diagnosed in older patients and in more advanced stages where lymph node metastases are more frequent; however, T1 tumors do occasionally exhibit metastatic disease [1, 11–14]. Symptoms such as hoarseness, airway obstruction, dysphagia, and hyperthyroidism can exist in advanced cases [12, 15]. Hürthle cell carcinoma is sometimes detected as an incidental finding of other imaging for nonthyroidal disorders, especially in an $_{18}$FDG-PET [16]. Both malignant and benign forms of Hürthle cell neoplasia have high FDG avidity. The increased utilization of $_{18}$FDG-PET during the diagnostic workup of several malignant and nonmalignant disorders leads to the detection of an increasing number of focal thyroid lesions requiring workup [17].

Hürthle cell carcinoma is divided into two types based on the pathological presentation: minimally invasive Hürthle cell carcinoma and widely invasive Hürthle cell carcinoma. Generally, minimally invasive Hürthle cell carcinoma demonstrates much less aggressive behavior compared to widely invasive Hürthle cell carcinoma, which is associated with a higher rate of distant metastases [18].

7.3 Natural History

The natural history of Hürthle cell carcinomas has not been systematically studied. The biological behavior varies. Often, Hürthle cell carcinomas have been included as a part of follicular thyroid carcinomas. Some are slow-growing lesions, while others grow aggressively and spread hematogenously. Also, Hürthle cell carcinomas may be diagnosed as incidental findings of microcarcinoma, while others exhibit extrathyroidal spread [1, 10, 13, 19]. A history of childhood head and neck radiation has been associated with risk of more extensive and bilateral thyroid lobe involvement [20]. Hürthle cell carcinomas have been reported to differ from follicular carcinomas by having a higher prevalence of lymph node metastases and more frequent locoregional recurrence as soft tissue implants [21, 22]. Recent independent categorization of Hürthle cell carcinoma as a separate entity from follicular carcinoma, together with advances in molecular pathology, will facilitate future studies and in time our understanding [5].

7.4 Diagnosis

Patients with Hürthle cell carcinoma often exhibit a solitary thyroid nodule, either as a palpable nodule or as an incidental finding on an imaging modality for reasons not related to clinical suspicion of a thyroid disorder. Some may be autonomously hyperfunctioning [14, 15]. The recommendation for evaluation of clinically or incidentally detected thyroid lesions follows the guidelines for thyroid nodules and differentiated thyroid cancer [23, 24].

Generally, only nodules larger than 1 cm in size need to be evaluated, with the exception of those associated with clinical symptoms or associated lymphadenopathy, which require the need for further evaluation [19, 25]. A diagnostic ultrasonography of the thyroid and the cervical lymph nodes should be performed in order to evaluate size, location, sonographic characteristics of thyroid lesions, and the presence or absence of any suspicious cervical lymph nodes in the central or lateral compartments [23, 24]. Based upon the sonographic appearance, ultrasound-based risk stratification systems are developed and modified to identify lesions that warrant fine-needle biopsy or sonographic follow-up [26–28]. Follow-up should be considered for nodules that do not meet criteria for fine-needle aspiration at the initial ultrasound examination. For optimal planning of all procedures related to thyroid nodules, such as fine-needle cytology and surgical procedures, access to a high-resolution system, a high-frequency linear probe, and, last but not least, an experienced ultrasound operator are all essential [24]. The main limitations of thyroid ultrasound are the operator dependency and the difficulty of analyzing lymph nodes in the central compartment [16, 29]. The Thyroid Imaging Reporting and Database System (TIRADS) has been introduced to allow for systematic reporting of sonographic characteristics of thyroid nodules and to simplify communication. Different variants, including web-based versions, have been introduced and found to provide high sensitivity, negative predictive value, and interobserver reproducibility for stratification of malignancy [26, 30]. Generally, only lesions classified as intermediate or high risk for malignancy are referred for surgery [26].

At this time, neither ultrasound nor any other imaging has provided the ability to distinguish between Hürthle cell carcinoma and adenoma, except for when extrathyroidal extension or lymph node metastases are confirmed. The differentiation between benign and malignant is dependent on histopathological verification of full-thickness capsular and/or vascular invasion. Hürthle cells are typically large, polygonal follicular cells with a prominent nucleolus and display eosinophilic cytoplasm on hematoxylin and eosin stains (H&E) [3]. The eosinophilic granularity of the cytoplasm is due to accumulation of mitochondria [31, 32]. Hürthle cell lesions are defined as lesions with a predominating expression of Hürthle cells (>75% of the cellular population). Based on the latest WHO classification, Hürthle cell carcinoma is defined as a separate entity without subclassification [5]. Expression of Hürthle cells, per se, does not increase the risk of malignancy. It is often possible to differentiate between neoplasia and nontumor tissue, such as nodular goiter and lymphocytic thyroiditis but not between cancer and adenoma. The Bethesda System for reporting thyroid cytopathology was introduced in 2007 to help standardize the terminology for reporting of thyroid cytopathology and has been shown to be reliable and valid [33]. The results are grouped into six Bethesda categories based on risk of malignancy: nondiagnostic (I); benign (II); atypia of undetermined significance/follicular lesion of undetermined significance (III), follicular neoplasm/ suspicious for follicular neoplasm (IV), suspicious for malignancy (V) and malignant (VI). An increased risk of malignancy of specimens defined as benign (Bethesda II) has been reported [34–36]. Fine-needle cytology from Hürthle cell carcinoma is often classified into category IV with the expected risk of cancer as 20–30%. In the context of multiple thyroid noduli, fine-needle specimens showing predominant expression of Hürthle cells are often classified as follicular lesion of undetermined significance (Bethesda III) rather than suspicious for Hürthle cell neoplasm (Bethesda IV). It was recently shown that the risk of malignancy did not differ between cases with or without multiple nodules or the presence of lymphocytic thyroiditis [37]. In the latest WHO classification, Hürthle cell carcinoma was defined as a specific entity without subclassification [5]. However, in practice, the tumors are often further categorized, based on their extent of invasion, into minimally and widely invasive. Encapsulated Hürthle cell carcinoma with microscopically identifiable foci of capsular and/or a few foci(<4) of vascular invasion are often defined as minimally invasive, in contradistinction to tumors with extrathyroidal and/or extensive vascular invasion, categorized as widely invasive [23]. However, controversy still remains concerning the prognostic importance of the degree of angioinvasion and, if encapsulated, tumors with angioinvasion should be defined as a separate group [24].

Recent advances in cancer genomics and molecular testing have enabled evolvement of tests that have progressed from single gene to broad genomic panels. Identification of distinct genomic alterations in Hürthle cell carcinoma with widespread losses of heterozygosity/chromosomes and prominent mitochondrial DNA mutations has formed the basis for recently available, modified next-generation sequencing tests [6, 31, 38]. At the present time, genomic panels have shown accuracy in correctly classifying hyperplastic nodules as likely to be benign, yet are not adequate for differentiating malignant Hürthle neoplasia from benign. The amount of nucleic acids needed is very low. An input as low as 2.5 nanograms is sufficient as long as the concentration of tumor cells is at least 12% [31]. Prospective clinical studies with long-term ultrasound follow-ups are needed in order to determine when molecular rule-in tests for cytology samples with potential malignancy can guide surgical decision-making [24, 31, 39]. Testing for prognostic markers such as *TERT*- and *TP53*-mutations that are interpreted in the context of the *BRAF*-mutation status may be helpful in the planning of treatment and accurate follow-up [24, 31, 40, 41].

For patients with advanced disease or with clinically evident extensive lymph node involvement, cross-sectional imaging, such as magnetic resonance imaging (MRI) or computer tomography without contrast, may be necessary for effective surgical planning. After contrast administration, radioiodine treatment needs to be withheld for at least 3 months [24].

7.5 Treatment

The basic goals of treatment are to improve survival, reduce risk of persistent or recurrent disease, and to permit accurate risk stratification while minimizing unnecessary therapy and morbidity related to therapy. Adequate surgery is the primary and most important treatment, while treatment with radioactive iodine, TSH suppression, as well as other treatments play adjunctive roles [23, 24]. Before surgery, accurate staging including clinical examination, ultrasound, and fine-needle cytology is mandatory. For patients with clinical suspicion of advanced disease, cross-sectional images are recommended as is discussed in the previous section.

In the majority of cases, it is not possible to distinguish between Hürthle cell adenoma and carcinoma preoperatively. The first step is usually ipsilateral hemithyroidectomy/isthmusectomy. Partial thyroidectomy can be sufficient for single tumors without extrathyroidal invasion, yet the acceptable size limit for partial thyroidectomy is controversial. For patients with indeterminate nodules that are cytologically or sonographically suspicious for malignancy, large (>4 cm), positive for known mutations associated with a higher cancer risk, familial disease, or history of radiation exposure, an initial total thyroidectomy may be performed [23, 24]. Still, there is no evidence for benefit of total compared to partial thyroidectomy [10]. For patients planning to receive radioactive iodine treatment postoperatively, near-total or total thyroidectomy is necessary in order to enable efficient radioiodine therapy [23, 24]. Hürthle cell carcinoma has been reported to more likely be associated with lymph node metastases than follicular thyroid cancer [21]. The risk of lymph node metastases is related to size of lesion, age, and male gender. Prophylactic ipsilateral central neck dissection at the time of initial operation has been suggested for older male patients with HCC greater than 5 cm [21]. The current guidelines do not address Hürthle cell carcinoma specifically [23, 24]. Prophylactic central-compartment dissection is only recommended for patients with papillary thyroid cancer and an advanced primary tumor or clinically involved lateral neck nodes [23, 24].

Due to the less aggressive behavior of a minimally invasive Hürthle cell carcinoma as compared to the more aggressive behavior of a widely invasive Hürthle cell carcinoma, a lesion that is less than 4 cm in size can be treated with thyroid lobectomy alone, because it does not require adjuvant treatment with radioactive iodine. This approach is applied to the tumor that has been removed during a thyroid lobectomy for "follicular neoplasm" or "follicular lesion of undetermined significance" and diagnosed as a minimally invasive Hürthle cell carcinoma on final pathological evaluation [18].

According to guidelines, the decision of adjuvant treatment and surveillance after radical surgical removal of a differentiated thyroid cancer is based on stratification of risk for recurrence into three groups: low, intermediate, and high risk. Hürthle cell carcinoma is not specifically addressed in the guidelines. In the WHO classification from 2017, Hürthle cell carcinoma is defined as a specific entity without subclassification. In everyday practice, the stratification of Hürthle cell carcinoma often follows that for follicular thyroid carcinoma.

Initial TSH suppression treatment is recommended for patients with follicular-derived thyroid cancers of high and intermediate risk and is based on the reported effect on overall survival and the documented stimulating effects of TSH on growth and proliferation of follicular thyroid cells [23, 24, 42]. Data regarding the optimal intensity and duration of TSH suppression therapy are weak. For patients with persistent disease, treatment is life-long; however, for patients with high risk of adverse effects on heart and bone, the benefits should be weighed against the potential risks [23].

Data concerning the benefits on outcome of radioiodine treatment are conflicting. Generally, the European experts prefer a wider use of radioactive treatment as compared to the ATA. In the ATA guidelines, radioiodine treatment is considered for patients with aggressive histology, vascular invasion, and tumor size larger than 4 cm or having extrathyroidal extension [23]. In the European revised version, radioiodine administration is classified by goal as remnant ablation meant to facilitate staging and detection of recurrent disease by measurement of thyroglobulin or scintigraphy; also adjuvant therapy intended to improve disease-free survival by destroying suspected but unproven residual disease and as therapy intended to treat persistent disease and improve disease-specific and disease-free survival [24]. Based on observational research, the goal is to elevate TSH to greater than 30mIU/L in preparation for radioiodine treatment. Treatment with recombinant human thyrotropin should be considered before thyroid hormone withdrawal due to the aspects for quality of life [23, 24]. In terms of radioiodine treatment used as therapy, higher versus lower initial activities and fewer high-activity administrations versus more numerous low-activity administrations are preferred [24]. The use of remnant ablation solely for facilitating follow-up is questioned. Survival benefits with or without postoperative radioiodine will be analyzed in two on-going European randomized, multicenter studies [24].

Generally, Hürthle cell carcinoma is less sensitive to radioactive radioiodine therapy than other differentiated thyroid cancers, yet survival benefits from adjuvant radioiodine treatment have been exhibited. In a study including 2799 patients with Hürthle cells from the SEER database, an increase of overall survival was observed for patients (n = 1529) receiving adjuvant radioiodine treatment [43]. It has also been verified that some but not all distant metastases of Hürthle cells can concentrate radioiodine [44, 45]. In one study where Hürthle cells and follicular thyroid cancer were analyzed together, two-thirds of 394 patients with lung and/or bone metastases had verified radioactive iodine uptake, but only 46% achieved complete response and the age of the patient seemed to affect the uptake. Uptake with response was coupled to a 15-year survival rate of 89% as compared to 8% for patients who did not achieve response [46].

Surveillance is guided by dynamic risk stratification. Patients that have undergone treatment with thyroidectomy and radioiodine ablation are usually examined with full-body scintigraphy within 6–9 months in order to evaluate the effect of ablation. After 9–12 months, a risk re-evaluation is performed based on clinical examination, measurement of thyroglobulin, and neck ultrasound, after which the TSH suppression therapy may be substituted with TSH supplementation. Patients with persistent disease continue with lifelong TSH suppression therapy.

For advanced or metastatic Hürthle cell carcinoma refractory to radioactive iodine therapy, several different anticancer agents outside or inside clinical trials are available. The challenge remains to correctly identify which patients will benefit from these treatments and when to start and when to end treatment. For patients who are asymptomatic, stable, or minimally progressive, TSH-suppressive thyroid hormone therapy and close monitoring may be preferable. Conventional cytotoxic chemotherapy is not recommended. Treatment with kinase inhibitors has been shown to improve progression-free survival in prospective trials and should therefore be considered; preliminary data also indicate the option of resensitization to radioiodine treatment [23, 24]. Focal palliative approaches such as bronchial stenting or bronchial laser therapy may be considered [24]. For patients with pathological fractures and spinal cord compression, external radiation and antiresorptive agents such as bisphosphonates should be considered [47].

7.6 Surgical Details

Surgical resection is the primary and curative treatment of Hürthle cell carcinoma. Substantial controversy still surrounds the selection of initial partial or near-total/total thyroidectomy and or lymph node clearance [23, 24]. Since it is generally not possible to distinguish between Hürthle cell adenoma and carcinoma preoperatively, ipsilateral lobectomy and isthmusectomy are frequently the initial routine procedures for patients with a single dominant nodule. The surgical risks of two-stage thyroidectomy (lobectomy followed by completion thyroidectomy) are similar to those of one-stage total thyroidectomy. Initial thyroidectomy is recommended for patients with obvious malignant disease when the strategy includes radioactive iodine treatment postoperatively. Findings elicited during the preoperative workup may indicate the need for more extensive procedures including the need for sternotomy and/or tracheal or laryngeal resection and reconstruction. Total thyroidectomy is also preferred for patients with a history of cervical head and neck radiation in childhood, which has shown to be associated with an increased incidence of multifocal disease and concomitant papillary cancer [23]. The pros and cons of choice of the surgical procedure must be carefully considered in each case, and the surgeon should communicate the surgical risks to the patient. Contralateral nodular disease/goiter or a high risk for a second surgical procedure could advocate for a one-stage total thyroidectomy [23]. For minimally invasive Hürthle cell carcinoma, the risk of recurrence is very low and lobectomy may be sufficient [1]. For widely invasive Hürthle cell carcinoma, completion thyroidectomy and subsequent radioiodine ablation are often advocated to facilitate follow-up and earlier detection of recurrence; however, controversies regarding indication for thyroidectomy still remain [8].

A preoperative laryngoscopy should be routinely performed. The correlation between vocal symptoms and actual vocal status is poor. Vocal cord paralysis is indicative of invasive disease. The surgical procedure should include a careful exploration to detect tumor invasion into adjacent structures, contralateral nodular disease, and metastatic nodal and soft tissue disease in the central neck [23, 24]. Frozen section is neither diagnostic nor informative in the differentiation between Hürthle cell carcinoma and Hürthle cell adenoma [48]. Care should be taken to preserve the parathyroid glands and their blood supply. Visual identification of the recurrent laryngeal nerve is required in all cases, and during dissection of the superior pole, care should be taken to preserve the external branch of the superior laryngeal nerve. Intraoperative neuromonitoring is favored in order to help prevent bilateral paresis by avoiding contralateral resection when nerve paralysis is detected on the initial side [24]. Neuromonitoring may also facilitate nerve identification and protection. If completion thyroidectomy is recommended based upon the histopathological examination, the surgeon should check a laryngeal exam prior to the completion surgery.

7.7 Outcomes or Prognosis

The majority of patients with HCC can be treated effectively. From the SEER's database, 5-year and 10-year survival rates of 95.4% and 92.6%, respectively, have been reported [10].

Compared to other differentiated thyroid cancers, Hürthle cell carcinoma has been found to be more aggressive, carrying a higher risk of distant metastases and poor prognosis, yet the rate of survival has improved dramatically over time [7, 8]. Size and extension of the tumor at diagnosis, presence of vascular invasion and/or of residual tumor after surgery, patients age over 45 years, and male gender have all been identified as negative prognostic factors [1, 10, 13, 49–51]. Patients with Hurthle cell microcarcinomas more oftenly present with distant metastases and have compromised survival as compared to patients with papillary thyroid microcarcinoma and carry less than a 10-year overall survival rate of 89.3% versus 94.3% for the latter [19, 25].

For dynamic risk stratification, one may take advantage of the postoperative doubling-time for thyroglobulin levels and assess imaging with an 18FDG-PET/CT in order to optimize staging and plans for follow-ups and eventual treatment therapy [24, 52, 53]. The value of 18FDG-PET/CT in the initial diagnostic workup is limited due to the fact that even benign adenoma may present with high FDG avidity [17].

Answers to the Questions

1. (d); 2. (c); 3. (c); 4. (d); 5. (d); 6. (b); 7. (a); 8. (d); 9. (c); 10. (a)

References

1. Chindris AM, Casler JD, Bernet VJ, Rivera M, Thomas C, Kachergus JM, et al. Clinical and molecular features of Hurthle cell carcinoma of the thyroid. J Clin Endocrinol Metab. 2015;100(1):55–62.
2. DeLellis RA. Pathology and genetics of thyroid carcinoma. J Surg Oncol. 2006;94(8):662–9.
3. Martin JD, Elkin DC. Hurthle cell tumors of the thyroid. Ann Surg. 1939;110(2):169–76.
4. Hundahl SA, Fleming ID, Fremgen AM, Menck HR. A National Cancer Data Base report on 53,856 cases of thyroid carcinoma treated in the U.S., 1985-1995 [see comments]. Cancer. 1998;83(12):2638–48.
5. WHO. WHO classification of tumours of endocrine organs. 4th ed. Geneva: World Health Organization; 2017.
6. Ganly I, Makarov V, Deraje S, Dong Y, Reznik E, Seshan V, et al. Integrated genomic analysis of Hurthle cell cancer reveals oncogenic drivers, recurrent mitochondrial mutations, and unique chromosomal landscapes. Cancer Cell. 2018;34(2):256–70 e5.
7. Nagar S, Aschebrook-Kilfoy B, Kaplan EL, Angelos P, Grogan RH. Hurthle cell carcinoma: an update on survival over the last 35 years. Surgery. 2013;154(6):1263–71; discussion 71.
8. Goffredo P, Roman SA, Sosa JA. Hurthle cell carcinoma: a population-level analysis of 3311 patients. Cancer. 2013;119(3):504–11.
9. Sugino K, Kameyama K, Ito K, Nagahama M, Kitagawa W, Shibuya H, et al. Does Hurthle cell carcinoma of the thyroid have a poorer prognosis than ordinary follicular thyroid carcinoma? Ann Surg Oncol. 2013;20(9):2944–50.
10. Zhou X, Zheng Z, Chen C, Zhao B, Cao H, Li T, et al. Clinical characteristics and prognostic factors of Hurthle cell carcinoma: a population based study. BMC Cancer. 2020;20(1):407.

11. Ernaga Lorea A, Migueliz Bermejo I, Anda Apinaniz E, Pineda Arribas J, Toni Garcia M, Martinez de Esteban JP, et al. Comparison of clinical characteristics of patients with follicular thyroid carcinoma and Hurthle cell carcinoma. Endocrinol Diabetes Nutr (Engl Ed). 2018;65(3):136–42.
12. Grani G, Lamartina L, Durante C, Filetti S, Cooper DS. Follicular thyroid cancer and Hurthle cell carcinoma: challenges in diagnosis, treatment, and clinical management. Lancet Diabetes Endocrinol. 2018;6(6):500–14.
13. Stojadinovic A, Hoos A, Ghossein RA, Urist MJ, Leung DH, Spiro RH, et al. Hurthle cell carcinoma: a 60-year experience. Ann Surg Oncol. 2002;9(2):197–203.
14. Wong CP, AuYong TK, Tong CM. Thyrotoxicosis: a rare presenting symptom of Hurthle cell carcinoma of the thyroid. Clin Nucl Med. 2003;28(10):803–6.
15. Russo D, Wong MG, Costante G, Chiefari E, Treseler PA, Arturi F, et al. A Val 677 activating mutation of the thyrotropin receptor in a Hurthle cell thyroid carcinoma associated with thyrotoxicosis. Thyroid. 1999;9(1):13–7.
16. Yu R, Auerbach MS. FDG-avid Hurthle cell thyroid adenoma. Clin Nucl Med. 2019;44(9):752–3.
17. Nilsson IL, Arnberg F, Zedenius J, Sundin A. Thyroid incidentaloma detected by fluorodeoxyglucose positron emission tomography/computed tomography: practical management algorithm. World J Surg. 2011;35(12):2691–7.
18. Ahmadi S, Stang M, Jiang X, Sosa J. Hürthle cell carcinoma: current perspectives. Onco Targets Ther. 2016;9:6873–84.
19. Khokar AM, Holoubek SA, Kuchta KM, Winchester DJ, Prinz RA, Moo-Young TA. Survival with follicular and Hurthle cell microcarcinoma compared to papillary thyroid microcarcinoma: a population study of 84,532 patients. World J Surg. 2020;44(2):469–78.
20. Samaan NA, Schultz PN, Ordonez NG, Hickey RC, Johnston DA. A comparison of thyroid carcinoma in those who have and have not had head and neck irradiation in childhood. J Clin Endocrinol Metab. 1987;64(2):219–23.
21. Guerrero MA, Suh I, Vriens MR, Shen WT, Gosnell J, Kebebew E, et al. Age and tumor size predicts lymph node involvement in Hurthle cell carcinoma. J Cancer. 2010;1:23–6.
22. Bishop JA, Wu G, Tufano RP, Westra WH. Histological patterns of locoregional recurrence in Hurthle cell carcinoma of the thyroid gland. Thyroid. 2012;22(7):690–4.
23. Haugen BR, Alexander EK, Bible KC, Doherty GM, Mandel SJ, Nikiforov YE, et al. 2015 American Thyroid Association management guidelines for adult patients with thyroid nodules and differentiated thyroid cancer: the American Thyroid Association guidelines task force on thyroid nodules and differentiated thyroid cancer. Thyroid. 2016;26(1):1–133.
24. Luster M, Aktolun C, Amendoeira I, Barczynski M, Bible KC, Duntas LH, et al. European perspective on 2015 American Thyroid Association management guidelines for adult patients with thyroid nodules and differentiated thyroid cancer: proceedings of an interactive international symposium. Thyroid. 2019;29(1):7–26.
25. Kuo EJ, Roman SA, Sosa JA. Patients with follicular and Hurthle cell microcarcinomas have compromised survival: a population level study of 22,738 patients. Surgery. 2013;154(6):1246–53; discussion 53-4.
26. Russ G, Bonnema SJ, Erdogan MF, Durante C, Ngu R, Leenhardt L. European thyroid association guidelines for ultrasound malignancy risk stratification of thyroid nodules in adults: the EU-TIRADS. Eur Thyroid J. 2017;6(5):225–37.

27. Kim PH, Suh CH, Baek JH, Chung SR, Choi YJ, Lee JH. Diagnostic performance of four ultrasound risk stratification systems: a systematic review and meta-analysis. Thyroid. 2020;30(8):1159–68.
28. Bahl M, Sosa JA, Eastwood JD, Hobbs HA, Nelson RC, Hoang JK. Using the 3-tiered system for categorizing workup of incidental thyroid nodules detected on CT, MRI, or PET/CT: how many cancers would be missed? Thyroid. 2014;24(12):1772–8.
29. Santana NO, Freitas RMC, Marcos VN, Chammas MC, Camargo RYA, Schmerling CK, et al. Diagnostic performance of thyroid ultrasound in Hurthle cell carcinomas. Arch Endocrinol Metab. 2019;63(3):300–5.
30. Noto B, Eveslage M, Pixberg M, Gonzalez Carvalho JM, Schafers M, Riemann B, et al. Prevalence of hyperfunctioning thyroid nodules among those in need of fine needle aspiration cytology according to ATA 2015, EU-TIRADS, and ACR-TIRADS. Eur J Nucl Med Mol Imaging. 2020;47(6):1518–26.
31. Nikiforova MN, Mercurio S, Wald AI, Barbi de Moura M, Callenberg K, Santana-Santos L, et al. Analytical performance of the ThyroSeq v3 genomic classifier for cancer diagnosis in thyroid nodules. Cancer. 2018;124(8):1682–90.
32. Straccia P, Rossi ED, Bizzarro T, Brunelli C, Cianfrini F, Damiani D, et al. A meta-analytic review of the Bethesda system for reporting thyroid cytopathology: has the rate of malignancy in indeterminate lesions been underestimated? Cancer Cytopathol. 2015;123(12):713–22.
33. Bongiovanni M, Spitale A, Faquin WC, Mazzucchelli L, Baloch ZW. The Bethesda system for reporting thyroid cytopathology: a meta-analysis. Acta Cytol. 2012;56(4):333–9.
34. Ren Y, Kyriazidis N, Faquin WC, Soylu S, Kamani D, Saade R, et al. The presence of Hurthle cells does not increase the risk of malignancy in most Bethesda categories in thyroid fine-needle aspirates. Thyroid. 2020;30(3):425–31.
35. Slowinska-Klencka D, Wysocka-Konieczna K, Wozniak-Osela E, Sporny S, Popowicz B, Sopinski J, et al. Thyroid nodules with Hurthle cells: the malignancy risk in relation to the FNA outcome category. J Endocrinol Investig. 2019;42(11):1319–27.
36. Anila KR, Nayak N, George PS, Jayasree K. Cytomorphologic Spectrum of Hurthle cell lesions of thyroid: a study of 54 cases. Gulf J Oncolog. 2018;1(26):6–10.
37. Wong KS, Jo VY, Lowe AC, Faquin WC, Renshaw AA, Shah AA, et al. Malignancy risk for solitary and multiple nodules in Hurthle cell-predominant thyroid fine-needle aspirations: a multi-institutional study. Cancer Cytopathol. 2020;128(1):68–75.
38. Gopal RK, Kubler K, Calvo SE, Polak P, Livitz D, Rosebrock D, et al. Widespread chromosomal losses and mitochondrial DNA alterations as genetic drivers in Hurthle cell carcinoma. Cancer Cell. 2018;34(2):242–55 e5.
39. Endo M, Nabhan F, Angell TE, Harrell RM, Nasr C, Wei S, et al. Use of molecular diagnostic tests in thyroid nodules with Hurthle cell-dominant cytology. Thyroid. 2020;30(9):1390–2.
40. Melo M, da Rocha AG, Vinagre J, Batista R, Peixoto J, Tavares C, et al. TERT promoter mutations are a major indicator of poor outcome in differentiated thyroid carcinomas. J Clin Endocrinol Metab. 2014;99(5):E754–65.
41. Melo M, Gaspar da Rocha A, Batista R, Vinagre J, Martins MJ, Costa G, et al. TERT, BRAF, and NRAS in primary thyroid cancer and metastatic disease. J Clin Endocrinol Metab. 2017;102(6):1898–907.

42. Jonklaas J, Sarlis NJ, Litofsky D, Ain KB, Bigos ST, Brierley JD, et al. Outcomes of patients with differentiated thyroid carcinoma following initial therapy. Thyroid. 2006;16(12):1229–42.
43. Yang Q, Zhao Z, Zhong G, Jin A, Yu K. Effect of adjuvant radioactive iodine therapy on survival in rare oxyphilic subtype of thyroid cancer (Hurthle cell carcinoma). PeerJ. 2019;7:e7458.
44. Chen H, Nicol TL, Zeiger MA, Dooley WC, Ladenson PW, Cooper DS, et al. Hurthle cell neoplasms of the thyroid: are there factors predictive of malignancy? Ann Surg. 1998;227(4):542–6.
45. Samaan NA, Schultz PN, Haynie TP, Ordonez NG. Pulmonary metastasis of differentiated thyroid carcinoma: treatment results in 101 patients. J Clin Endocrinol Metab. 1985;60(2):376–80.
46. Schlumberger M, Challeton C, De Vathaire F, Travagli JP, Gardet P, Lumbroso JD, et al. Radioactive iodine treatment and external radiotherapy for lung and bone metastases from thyroid carcinoma. J Nucl Med. 1996;37(4):598–605.
47. Farooki A, Leung V, Tala H, Tuttle RM. Skeletal-related events due to bone metastases from differentiated thyroid cancer. J Clin Endocrinol Metab. 2012;97(7):2433–9.
48. Udelsman R, Westra WH, Donovan PI, Sohn TA, Cameron JL. Randomized prospective evaluation of frozen-section analysis for follicular neoplasms of the thyroid. Ann Surg. 2001;233(5):716–22.
49. Mai KT, Khanna P, Yazdi HM, Perkins DG, Veinot JP, Thomas J, et al. Differentiated thyroid carcinomas with vascular invasion: a comparative study of follicular, Hurthle cell and papillary thyroid carcinoma. Pathology. 2002;34(3):239–44.
50. Lopez-Penabad L, Chiu AC, Hoff AO, Schultz P, Gaztambide S, Ordonez NG, et al. Prognostic factors in patients with Hurthle cell neoplasms of the thyroid. Cancer. 2003;97(5):1186–94.
51. Petric R, Gazic B, Besic N. Prognostic factors for disease-specific survival in 108 patients with Hurthle cell thyroid carcinoma: a single-institution experience. BMC Cancer. 2014;14:777.
52. Kelders A, Kennes LN, Krohn T, Behrendt FF, Mottaghy FM, Verburg FA. Relationship between positive thyroglobulin doubling time and 18F-FDG PET/CT-positive, 131I-negative lesions. Nucl Med Commun. 2014;35(2):176–81.
53. Robbins RJ, Wan Q, Grewal RK, Reibke R, Gonen M, Strauss HW, et al. Real-time prognosis for metastatic thyroid carcinoma based on 2-[18F]fluoro-2-deoxy-D-glucose-positron emission tomography scanning. J Clin Endocrinol Metab. 2006;91(2):498–505.

Medullary Thyroid Carcinoma: Diagnosis and Treatment of Sporadic and Hereditary Tumors

Bruno Niederle and Martin B. Niederle

Contents

A. L. Shifrin et al. (eds.), *Endocrine Surgery Comprehensive Board Exam Guide*,
https://doi.org/10.1007/978-3-030-84737-1_8

Cases

Case 1

62-year-old female

Palpable nodule, left thyroid lobe

US: solitary nodule in the left thyroid lobe, size – 30 mm; ovoid, hypoechogenic, regular sharp margins, no macro–/microcalcification

Scintigraphy: "non-functioning" nodule on right side

Thyroid-stimulating hormone (TSH): 0.9 (0.4–4.0 u/L); free triiodothyronine (FT3), free thyroxine (FT4) normal – normal thyroid metabolism

Ca: 2.3; parathyroid hormone (PTH): 29, calcifediol (25(OH)D3) n.d.

Ct: 4 pg/mL (Immulite 2000; Diagnostic Products Corporation [ICMA] reference range: F: –6.4 pg/mL)

Creatinine (Cr): 0.9 mg/dL

FNAB: follicular neoplasm/suspicious for follicular neoplasm (Bethesda 4)

Surgery: left hemithyroidectomy, left CND

Frozen section: no signs of malignancy

Histology: microfollicular adenoma; medullary thyroid microcarinoma (near the upper left pole: multifocal [three lesions], each measuring 1 mm), pN0 (0/5)

(1) Follow-up only
(2) Completion of thyroidectomy en principe? With/without CND/LND?
(3) Completion of thyroidectomy after specific "testing"? With/without CND/LND?

If (1) Follow-up
(1a) US, every 6 months
(1b) Biochemistry (Ct), every 6 months
(1c) 1a + 1b
If (2) Right lobectomy en principe
(2a) Without CND
(2b) With CND
If 3
(3a) Biochemistry (Ct) with Ca stimulation
(3b) Biochemistry (Ct), plasma metanephrine, plasma normetanephrine, genetic testing (RET proto-oncogene)

Case 2

66-year-old female

Palpable nodule, right thyroid lobe

US: solitary nodule in the right thyroid lobe, 39 mm – mild hypoechogenic, regular sharp margin, no macro–/microcalcification

Scintigraphy: "non-functioning" nodule on the right side

TSH: 1.2 (0.4–4.0 u/L); FT3, FT4 normal

Ca: 2.4 PTH 26, 25(OH)D3 42

Ct: 1549 pg/mL (Immulite 2000; Diagnostic Products Corporation [ICMA] reference range: F: –6.4 pg/mL)

Cr: 1.0 mg/dL

CEA: 1690 ng/mL (Elecsys System 2010 (Roche-Diagnostics, Germany) (reference range – 3.8 μg/L)

plasma metanephrines/plasma normetanephrines: normal catecholamines/metanephrines and normetanephrines (24-h urine): normal

(1) Follow-up
(2) Surgery

(2a) Thyroidectomy
(2b) Thyroidectomy with unilateral CND
(2c) Thyroidectomy with bilateral CND, bilateral LND
(2d) Thyroidectomy with bilateral CND, frozen section

Case 3

60-year-old male

No palpable nodules in both thyroid lobes

US: small thyroid gland, inhomogeneous echogenicity, nodules less than 3 mm

Appearance as in autoimmune thyroiditis

Scintigraphy: not performed

TSH: 85 (0.4–4.0 u/L); FT3 1.2 (1.8–4.2 ng/mL), FT4 0.7 (0.8–1.9 ng/mL) – hypothyroidism.

Microsomal antibodies: 1403 (normal range <80 U/mL)

Ca: 2.34 PTH 31, 25(OH)D3 n.d.

Ct: 685 pg/mL (Immulite 2000; Diagnostic Products Corporation [ICMA] reference range: M: – 9.5 pg/mL)

Cr: 0.7 mg/dL

Plasma metanephrines/plasma normetanephrines: normal catecholamines/metanephrines and normetanephrines (24-h urine): normal

(1) Follow-up
(2) Further diagnostic tests (stimulation tests)
(3) Surgery – MTC suspected: thyroidectomy, bilateral CND, if tumor DSR-negative: bilateral LND

Case 4

63-year-old male

Palpable nodule in the right thyroid lobe

US: right thyroid lobe nodule – 49 mm, ovoid, hypoechogenic, regular sharp margins; left lobe is inhomogeneous

TSH: 0.03 (0.4–4.0 u/L); FT3, FT4 – normal

Scintigraphy: "non-functioning" nodule on the right side – multifocal thyroid autonomy in both thyroid lobes

Ca: 2.23 PTH 40, 25(OH)D3–24, reduced vitamin D uptake

Ct < 2 pg/mL (Immulite 2000; Diagnostic Products Corporation [ICMA] reference range: M: –9.5 pg/mL)

Cr: 0.9 mg/dL

FNAB: follicular neoplasm/suspicious for follicular neoplasm (Bethesda 4)

Surgery: thyroidectomy, frozen section: inconclusive – follicular neoplasia

Histology: encapsulated follicular variant of papillary thyroid carcinoma, pT2–36 mm, pNx

medullary thyroid microcarcinoma with DSR, left lobe – pT1a – <1 mm pNx

(1) Ct
(2) Completion surgery with left CND
(3) Molecular genetic analysis
(4) Ct, molecular genetic analysis

Case 5

42-year-old male

No palpable thyroid nodule

Prophylactic health examination

Carotid US: incidentally – left lobe: solitary nodule, 9 mm – mild hypoechogenic, regular shape, no macro-/microcalcification

TSH: 1.67 (0.4–4.0 u/L); FT3, FT4 – normal

Scintigraphy: not performed

Ca: 2.54 PTH 43, 25(OH)D3: 40

Ct: 10 pg/mL, follow-up 13 pg/mL (Immulite 2000; Diagnostic Products Corporation [ICMA] reference range: M: –9.5 pg/mL)

Cr: 0.85 mg/dL

(1) Ct follow-up in 1 year
(2) Stimulation test to select patient for surgery
(3) Hemithyroidectomy with left CND
(4) Molecular genetic analysis

8.1 Introduction

Medullary thyroid cancer (MTC) is a rare ("orphan") disease. MTC accounts for approximately 3% of all thyroid cancers in unselected American and European series (USA: 177/5583; Germany: 79/2537) [1, 2]. The overall prevalence of occult MTC was 0.14% among 7897 autopsies from 24 published series [3], increasing to 0.85% in North American and European clinical series routinely applying calcitonin (Ct) measurements in the biochemical workup of thyroid nodules (0.13–0.85%; 238 [0.34%] of 70,286 patients; 13 authors) [4].

In contrast to well-differentiated, follicular-cell-derived thyroid cancer, MTC originates from the parafollicular (neuroendocrine) C cells (CCs) of the thyroid. CCs comprise a minor population of the thyroid, representing approximately 2–4% of the organ's cells, and secrete Ct in the low normal range. The CC belongs to the group of neuroendocrine cells. Therefore, it may to a lesser degree secrete smaller quantities of several other neuroendocrine peptides, such as somatostatin, Ct gene–related peptide, and serotonin.

8.2 Clinical Presentation

In former clinical studies, patients with MTC (sporadic or hereditary index patients) presented clinically in 45–94% with a palpable thyroid mass [5, 6]. Less symptomatic patients are dominant in current surveys [7].

Neck masses may provoke symptoms reported in up to 30%, such as dysphagia, shortness of breath, hoarseness, or diarrhea. In patients with a palpable primary, MTC has already metastasized clinically to the cervical lymph nodes (LN; 42–52%). Spread is most frequent to the central compartment (Robbins level VI [8]); Dralle central neck = C1a/C1b [9]), followed by the ipsilateral jugular chain of nodes and the contralateral cervical nodes (levels II–V; C2 and C3), but it is also seen to the upper and anterior mediastinum (level VII; C4) [9–11] – ◘ Table 8.1.

Distant metastasis may occur in the lungs, liver, bones, brain, and soft tissues (documented in 12–28%). Metastatic spread may be difficult to assess by cross-sectional imaging because of the fine, miliary pattern of these lesions. Laparoscopy with direct imaging of the liver may identify small metastatic deposits not visible by conventional imaging in 25% of patients with elevated Ct levels following therapeutic surgery [12].

Computed tomography (CT) or magnetic resonance imaging (MRI) studies for distant disease are done preoperatively if Ct levels are higher than 500 pg/mL. Neither fluorodeoxyglucose- (FDG-) positron emission tomography (PET)/CT nor fluorodopa- (F-DOPA-) PET/CT is used routinely for preoperative staging but may contribute information in doubtful individual cases.

◘ **Table 8.1** Correlation between Robbins LN levels [8] and Dralle compartments [9]

Robbins (level)	Dralle (compartment)		Neck dissection
VI	C1	1a – central right 1b – central left	Central
(I), II–V	C2/3	C2 – right lateral C3 – left lateral	Lateral
VII	C4	Upper/lower mediastinal	Mediastinal

8.3 Ultrasonography

Ultrasound (US) examination is a valuable diagnostic tool to diagnose MTC. Typical MTC appears as a solid, (often markedly) hypoechogenic lesion without a halo and quite commonly containing micro- or macrocalcifications. However, the first three features are known to be very unspecific and the other two are less sensitive.

The presence of a lesion with the appearance described above should lead to suspicion of MTC and be considered as an argument for further diagnostic steps such as Ct measurements [13]. However, most MTCs do not present all of the mentioned features, and some of them can have a relatively benign US appearance [14].

Neck US revealed an overall sensitivity of only 90% in detecting MTC with a mean tumor size of 20 mm and larger. In the subgroup of patients with tumors ≤10 mm, the sensitivity was even lower (71%) [15].

The sensitivity of US to diagnose LN metastasis was overall only 6% and 56% in the central and lateral neck, respectively [15].

8.4 FNAB

A meta-analysis demonstrated that fine-needle aspiration biopsy (FNAB) is able to detect approximately one half of MTC lesions [16]. These low diagnostic rates suggest that other techniques are needed in combination with FNAB to improve the diagnosis of MTC and to avoid false-negative results. The majority of small nodules are difficult or are even impossible to examine by FNAB. Small MTC size (≤10 mm) and a smooth margin may be factors predicting false-negative FNAB results [17].

Routine basal Ct (bCt) measurements have been documented to show a higher sensitivity to diagnose MTC compared with FNAB cytology, especially in diagnosing small (≤10 mm) MTCs [18].

Desmoplastic stromal reaction (DSR) appears to be an excellent (intraoperative) marker to predict LN involvement with a high specificity. Initial lateral neck dissection (LND) may be avoided in MTC patients without DSR, because these tumors never metastasize, independent of tumor size and bCt levels [19–21].

Therefore, FNAB should be avoided as a first-step diagnostic procedure, as traumatizing the tumor capsule may trigger the development of scar tissue in the tumor, leading to be misinterpreted as DSR positivity [22].

8.5 FNAB and Evaluation of Ct in the Fine-Needle Aspirate

Boi et al. [23] were the first to recommend Ct measurements in wash-out fluids from fine-needle aspiration to improve the diagnosis in primary (and metastatic) MTC in the workup of thyroid nodules to avoid false-negative or inconclusive results from cytology [24].

Almost all MTC lesions >10 mm were correctly diagnosed. However, even this modification of FNAB may be inconclusive or hardly possible in small (≤10 mm) tumors [25].

8.6 Carcinoembryonic Antigen

Besides Ct, carcinoembryonic antigen (CEA) is a widely used tumor marker for the diagnosis and postoperative follow-up of patients with MTC. However, not all patients with MTC are characterized by elevated CEA levels.

8.7 Procalcitonin

It was suggested that procalcitonin (PCT) may be an accurate biomarker in the diagnosis and follow-up of MTC. In the first systematic review to analyze the value of PCT, a total of 15 out of 184 articles were retrieved and analyzed [26]. Of these 15 studies, 3 were case reports. In these studies, the values of Ct and PCT were assessed in a group of patients with MTC versus another consisting of healthy volunteers and patients with benign/malignant thyroid nodular disease or bacterial infection. *The authors suggested that PCT would seem to be a useful biomarker for the diagnosis and follow-up of MTC when used in conjunction with Ct, particularly in a small proportion of tumors that are Ct-negative or secrete low levels of Ct.* So far, the data have not been sufficient to suggest a specific threshold for normal PCT. However, most studies indicate a value of 0.1 μg/mL as an acceptable cut-off in everyday clinical practice. The authors concluded that Ct should continue to be the primary biomarker in MTC, with the addition of PCT in some patient groups (e.g., Ct-negative MTC). Nevertheless, larger patient series were suggested in order to provide safer and more accurate results.

In a prospective study [27] among 2705 patients, 9 with positive serum PCT (i.e., above 0.1 μg/L) and 370 with negative PCT underwent thyroid surgery. MTC was histologically confirmed in all patients with positive PCT but not found in patients with negative PCT. The serum PCT levels were significantly higher in patients with MTC (median 0.64 μg/L, range 0.16–12.9 μg/L) than in those without (median 0.075 μg/L, range 0.075–0.16 µg/L; $P < 0.0001$). ROC curves were plotted to calculate the optimal PCT value separating patients with MTC from those without. The best cut-off was 0.155 µg/L with sensitivity, specificity, positive, and negative predictive values as well as accuracy of 100%, 99.7%, 91.7%, 100%, and 99.7%, respectively. Positive and negative likelihood ratios were 329 and 0, respectively. *It was concluded that the measurement of PCT may be a sensitive and accurate method for detecting MTC in patients with thyroid nodules and thus could be a reliable alternative to, but not completely replace, Ct measurement.*

8.8 Ct

Ct is a polypeptide hormone consisting of 32 amino acids with a disulfide bridge between position 1 and 7 and is involved in calcium (Ca)-phosphorus metabolism.

Elevations in serum Ca trigger release of Ct from CCs. Ct release from CCs in response to elevated serum Ca provides the basis for the Ca stimulation test. Other hormones such as gastrin have been reported to stimulate Ct release as well. The sensitivity of CC to gastrin led to the application of pentagastrin (Pg) to increase the Ct secretion in CC disease. However, widely used previously, Pg is no longer available [28].

CCs become clinically relevant when they change their normal "morphology." Oncogenic transformation of the thyroid CC is thought to progress through a hyperplastic process prior to malignancy with increasing levels of serum Ct serving as a biomarker for tumor burden [29]. Repeatable elevated bCt levels may indicate CC disease [30].

Ct is the established gold-standard biomarker for the diagnosis and follow-up of MTC. Reliable and sensitive Ct assays applied to screen sporadic and hereditary MTC are important for health and economic reasons, as they facilitate early diagnosis [31, 32]. However, the normal ranges and cut-offs of bCt levels differ in the literature because Ct is measured by different assays, resulting in difficulties in interpreting and comparing the results.

Over the past decade, commercial assays for measuring Ct have progressed to the newest immunochemiluminometric assays (ICMAs) that are highly sensitive and specific for monomeric Ct. With ICMAs, cross-reactivity with other Ct-related peptides is largely eliminated. Ultrasensitive Ct assays have mostly eliminated false-negative rates of bCt measurements when diagnosing CC disease [33].

The growth of MTC is relatively slow, but if metastasized to the LNs or distant organs, or if it persists or recurs after surgery, it may become very aggressive, causing more than 13% of all thyroid-cancer-related deaths.

Lacking alternative treatment (e.g., radioiodine, chemo-/radiotherapy), stage-adapted (= adequate) surgery is the only curative therapeutic modality with a high chance for cure if surgery is performed as long as MTC is limited to the thyroid. Since surgical treatment for even small MTCs must be more radical compared to other types of thyroid cancer, the preoperatively definitive (early) diagnosis of MTC significantly influences management. Delayed diagnosis and inadequate initial treatment deteriorate the prognosis. In two retrospective North American cohort studies of patients with MTC, 15–41% of patients did not receive appropriate surgical therapy because the malignant disease was unknown preoperatively [34, 35]. Adherence rates to the American Thyroid Association (ATA) recommendations for the treatment of MTC increased modestly following the publication of guidelines in 2009. However, only 66.8% of patients treated between 2009 and 2013 received care in accordance with the recommendations, compared to 61.4% of patients treated between 2004 and 2008 [36]. In another report, only half of the MTC patients in California underwent central LN dissection (CLND) at the time of thyroidectomy, which may suggest a lack of appropriate care across a range of healthcare systems [37].

Overall, poor prognosis is linked with late diagnosis. It is well documented that early diagnosis based on preoperatively established Ct levels followed by adequate surgery improves prognosis [38, 39].

Although Cheung et al. [40] concluded that routine Ct screening in patients undergoing evaluation for thyroid nodules appears to be cost-effective in the United States, comparable to the measurement of thyroid-stimulating hormone, colonoscopy, and mammography screening, there is still an ongoing discussion concerning the benefits of early diagnosis [41].

Proponents of Ct evaluation during the diagnostic workup of thyroid nodule(s), regardless of their sizes and function, clearly state the benefits of early diagnosis of MTC, which facilitate one-step (adequate) surgery and therefore a greater potential for cure.

While European guidelines recommend this procedure [42], Anglo-American guidelines are more restricted [13, 33, 43].

Because expert opinions vary regarding the usefulness of routinely measuring serum Ct levels in patients with nodular thyroid disease, the members of the ATA Guidelines Task Force suggested that covering physicians should decide whether Ct determinations are useful in establishing a management strategy in any particular situation [33].

8

8.9 Interpretation of bCt Levels

Adequate interpretation of Ct results during the diagnostic workup of thyroid nodules allows the supervising team of specialists to appropriately select patients for surgery.

Tumor volume correlates with bCt levels [44–46]. Therefore, it is very important to correlate bCt and the results of ultrasonography, documenting the size of the lesion(s) in the thyroid gland and LN status. A careful interrelation of these findings guides subsequent diagnostic procedures such as the application of further diagnostic tests (e.g., stimulation test) and finally the indication to surgery and surgical decision-making [47, 48]. Elevated bCt levels must always be questioned and reasons for non-CC-derived Ct elevations or the rare cases of false-positive results due to heterophilic antibodies have to be considered [49].

Especially in the absence of thyroid nodules in US (no indication per se to determine Ct), or *if there is a discrepancy between the size of a thyroid nodule and bCt level (a small nodule and an inadequately high bCt level), stimulation tests may help to differentiate thyroid from non-thyroid sources of Ct production* [50–52]. Ectopic Ct production by neuroendocrine tumors has to be taken into account, characterized by no or a less than twofold increase in Ct levels after stimulation. *When stimulation exceeds bCt by more than twofold, MTC is found exclusively* [50].

Up to now, there are no generally accepted Ct cut-off levels to predict MTC, as different Ct assays are used in different laboratories.

In a recently published paper, four different assays based on three assay types were used for Ct measurements [53]. Each assay has its specific gender-dependent cut-off value for positivity. In this chapter, the most precise bCt thresholds for the identification of MTC were ≥46 pg/mL for males and ≥35 pg/mL for females. Using these cut-offs, only 6% of the male patients were not identified as having MTC, whereas 5% were false-positive, having CC hyperplasia (CCH) instead. In females, the discrepancy was higher, since 13% of the female MTC patients were false-negative by using the cut-off of ≥35 pg/mL missing MTC, and 13% had false-positive results (suffering from CCH), which retrospectively led to "unnecessary" surgery. Therefore, "cut-off levels" recommended for decision-making should be applied with caution. Based on various publications and respecting conversion factors [31, 32, 54], ◘ Table 8.2 shows the three most frequently used assay variants in the literature and their gender-specific cut-off values, which definitively predict MTC.

Table 8.2 bCt "cut-off levels" for the most commonly used Ct assays – predicting MTC in 100%

Gender	CIS (Cisbio)	Immulite DPC (Siemens)	DiaSorin (Liaison)	Cobas (Roche)	Mean
	IRMA bCt pg/mL	ICMA bCt pg/mL	ICMA bCt pg/mL	ECLIA bCt pg/mL	bCt pg/mL
Female	>28	>23	>33	>29	>28
Male	>53	>43	>58	>52	>51

IRMA immunoradiometric assay, *ICMA* immunochemiluminescent assay, *ECLIA* electrochemiluminescence immunoassay, *DPC* Diagnostic Products Corporation, *bCt* basal calcitonin
Conversion formula [31, 32, 54]
Immulite 2000 DPC (Siemens) = 0.8 × DiaSorin(Liaison) – 3.4
DiaSorin (Liaison) = 1.24 × (Immulite 2000 DPC /Siemens) + 4.24
Cobas (Roche) = Immulite 2000 DPC × 1.17 + 1,2
Immulite 2000 DPC (Siemens) = (Cobas –1.2)/1.17
Immulite 2000 DPC (Siemens) = CIS × 0.8
Cis (Cisbio) = Immulite 2000 DPC (Siemens): 0.8

The gender-specific mean upper limits for bCt concentrations that led to a recommendation to operate a suspected thyroid nodule as MTC were around 30 pg/mL in women and 50 pg/mL in men.

As a rule, males have higher bCt values than females. Without specifying the characteristics of the Ct assay and without respecting gender differences, concentrations between 60 and 100 pg/mL have been assessed as highly suggestive/pathognomonic of MTC in recently published guidelines [43]. After excluding non-CC-derived Ct elevations [49] and considering the assay and gender, patients may be subdivided into those with "mildly" elevated and others with "highly" elevated bCt levels.

8.10 Surgery

Surgery is the most effective option for curative therapy, reduction in tumor burden, or effective palliation in sporadic and hereditary (index) patients and also for prophylactic and early surgery for those with hereditary MTC.

Surgical decision-making is based on bCt values in sporadic and hereditary patients [47, 55, 56].

8.11 Clinically Occult MTC – "Mildly" Elevated bCt Levels

By definition, in patients with "mildly" elevated bCt levels (= gray zone), the Ct values are documented below assay and gender-specific cut-off Ct values for MTC. In these patients, there is an indistinct overlap between CCH and micro-MTC (mMTC).

If treated surgically, mMTC (≤10 mm; pT1, pN0 or exceptionally pN1a) is expected. mMTC is clinically "silent" and predominantly found beside a clinically dominant benign or a follicular-cell-derived malignant tumor [57].

As shown recently, the bCt levels were documented in the "gray zone" in 41/70 (58.6%) females and 58/79 (73.4%) males [48]. The final histological examination of the thyroid glands and the central LNs revealed MTC in more males (19/58 [32.8%]) than in females (7/41 [17.1%]). All MTCs in the male and female patients in this group were classified as pT1. While all tumors in the 19 males were staged pN0, central LN metastases (pN1a) were documented in 1/7 females. Independent of gender, unilateral or bilateral multifocality was documented in hereditary (89%) but also in sporadic mMTCs (23%) [48].

The goal of surgical treatment is to perform thyroidectomy as long as the malignancy is still confined to the thyroid gland and, if the tumors have early spread locally, to remove micrometastasis in the central LNs. While a more liberal indication for surgery may be considered in men, a restricted indication for surgery may theoretically exist in women, as MTC was found in fewer females than males. However, CLND should be an integral strategy in females. Because bCt levels did not sufficiently specify the possible causes of mildly elevated Ct values, stimulation tests have been recommended in the literature [13, 58, 59].

Ct stimulations either with Ca or Pg have failed to improve diagnostic quality. Neither bCt nor stimulated Ct (sCt) levels (or the combination of both) were able to discriminate between CCH and MTC in either gender within the "gray zone" [28].

The Ca stimulation test may be helpful to theoretically subclassify patients with "mildly" elevated bCt, who are definitively not candidates for surgery. In a previous investigation (cited by many following studies), surgery was recommended in all subjects with an abnormal Ct response to stimulation above 100 pg/mL. This was because peak Ct levels exceeding 100 pg/mL were considered to be indicative of MTC, and MTC was definitively documented in many patients [60].

Costante et al. [61] reported that sCt values after Pg infusion of above 100 pg/mL predicted MTC in at least 40%. However, CCH was revealed in the majority of females (83%) and less frequently in males (66%) [48].

Frank-Raue et al. [62] recommended to re-evaluate patients with "mildly" elevated bCt values in intervals of 3 to 6 months and advise surgery in patients only with rising Ct levels, which may indicate MTC. However, the clinical experience with this concept is marginal. There is only one series of 171 patients who were followed for 2 to 4 years and in 170 of those basal levels remained stable. Only one man experienced an increase after 2 years of follow-up. He underwent a stimulation test (with Pg) with positive results and a peak level above 100 pg/mL. Surgery demonstrated the presence of CCH only [61].

Many patients are aware that Ct is a sensitive tumor marker for MTC. Reproducible "mildly" elevated bCt levels may be the first sign of MTC in those presenting with thyroid nodules ≤10 mm. With regard to the psychological burden accompanying such awareness, keeping some patients in persistent anxiety and uncertainty, many call for surgery even after having been informed about the minor long-term consequences of "mildly" elevated bCt. Potential morbidity must be carefully discussed with the patients and be balanced against unnecessary thyroid surgery and continuous follow-up.

In experienced surgical teams, patients with "mildly" elevated Ct values who decide for surgery may be treated early by (total) thyroidectomy and bilateral CLND, which seems mandatory, because LN micrometastasis may also be present in patients with "mildly" elevated bCt levels (at least in females). "First-step CLND" is recommended to keep permanent morbidity low [63].

Initial (total) thyroidectomy and bilateral CLND is recommended if patients and their supervising physicians decide upon surgical treatment in the presence of "mildly" elevated Ct levels and suspected clinically occult MTC.

In all patients with documented sporadic hypercalcitoninemia, rearranged during transfection (*RET*) proto-oncogene mutation analysis by screening exons 8, 10, 11, 13, 14, 15, and 16 to establish the possible genetic basis for the disease within an individual is mandatory, even in the absence of a positive family history.

In a prospective study in approximately 13% of patients with presumed sporadic CCH or MTC, a germline *RET* mutation was verified. Consequently, pheochromocytoma and primary hyperparathyroidism as part of multiple endocrine neoplasia (MEN) type 2A have to be excluded [56].

If pheochromocytoma is diagnosed biochemically and confirmed by imaging, it is to be treated surgically before treating MTC.

8.12 Biochemically and Clinically Apparent MTC – "Highly" Elevated bCt Levels

By definition, patients with bCt values above the assay and gender-specific cut-off levels suffer from MTC (no false-positive patients!) and therefore are definitive candidates for surgery [48]. "Biochemically apparent MTCs" (= T1a, ≤10 mm, (N0) N1, M0) and "clinically apparent (=palpable) tumors," staged as pT1b-4 (>10 mm, N0 or N1; M0 or M1), are included in this patient group.

In a recently published series of patients with various thyroid nodules prospectively screened for MTC, fulfilling the criteria of biochemically or clinically apparent MTC, overall LN metastases were revealed in 12/21 (57.1%) males and in 8/29 (27.6%) females. Radiologically distant metastasis were found in 3/21 (14.3%) males and in 1/29 (3.5%) females, respectively [48].

In a subanalysis, "biochemically apparent pT1a tumors" were documented in 7/21 (33.3%) males and 15/29 (51.7%) females, with positive LNs in 2/7 (28.6%) males and 2/15 (13.3%) females, respectively [48].

The aim of initial surgery is to control locoregional disease with the prevention of locoregional persistence/recurrence and long-term disease-free survival with biochemical as well as clinical cure [47, 64]. The special biology of MTC is to be respected in selecting the adequate surgical strategy to reach this aim.

8.13 Surgical Strategy – Central Neck

Independent of the genetic background, up to 15% of sporadic MTCs are multifocal and 5% bilateral, with higher rates in patients with germline *RET* mutations because of widespread CCH resulting in multiple foci of MTC [65].

LN metastases occur early in the course of MTC. The pattern of LN metastatic distribution in the neck areas varies between patients and is not related to tumor size [66].

Accidental horizontal (central to lateral) and vertical (central to paratracheal [prelaryngeal/pretracheal] to mediastinal or contralateral central/lateral) lymphatic flows are the cause of formation of LN metastasis. Reviewing the literature, LN involvement was identified in 10–30% of tumors ≤10 mm [11, 57, 67]. Overall, at the time of initial surgery, the involvement of central LNs has been documented in 50–100% in the literature [10, 11, 66].

In terms of diagnosing central LN metastasis, neck US demonstrated a sensitivity of only 6%. In particular, micrometastasis may be hidden by the thyroid gland and may therefore be missed on US [15].

Therefore, (total) thyroidectomy and bilateral CLND (level VI) is recommended initially in all patients with biochemically and clinically apparent tumors [33, 43].

For completeness of CLND, Perros et al. [43] recommended to extend dissection down to the innominate artery (Robbins levels VI and VII).

8.14 Surgical Strategy – Lateral Neck

Independent of size, the occurrence of malignant ipsilateral nodes ranges from 48% to 81% [10, 11, 66]. Furthermore, contralateral LN metastases were found on histology in 44% of patients with palpable unilateral and in 49% with bilateral MTC [10, 11, 66].

Skip metastasis (= negative central but positive lateral or mediastinal LNs) may occur in 21.3% [68]. Mediastinal LN metastases were revealed in 32% [10].

The presence [7, 69] and the higher numbers of removed and affected LNs [70] predict a lower chance of biochemical cure and negatively influence disease-free survival.

The biochemical cure rate was 33% in node-positive patients; the latter was improved to 45% after four compartment lymphadenectomies [71].

Quantitative LN analysis of MTC improves prediction of Ct normalization. When more than two compartments are involved, normalization of serum Ct cannot be attained. Surgery should then be less extensive and directed rather at preventing local complications [50].

Individually, the extent of neck dissection did not alter disease-specific survival. But patients who underwent both central neck dissection (CND) and LND at the time of initial surgery were less likely to require reoperation for locoregional recurrence [70].

There is a general consensus to dissect central and lateral compartments with clinical or radiological evidence of involved LNs to prevent local recurrence and, if possible, persistence [33, 43].

However, as shown recently [15], the sensitivity of US to correctly document lateral LN metastasis was only 56% with a specificity of 97% (overall accuracy: 84%).

The prophylactic dissection of ipsilateral or bilateral lateral LNs in node-negative patients is part of an ongoing discussion. The oncological benefit of more extended (lateral) LN dissection is to be weighed against higher rates of surgical complications compared with total thyroidectomy and CLND alone.

Patients with tumor multiplicity based on preoperative imaging evaluations more frequently showed lateral node positivity based on pathological examination than those without tumor multiplicity. However, 28% of solitary MTCs based on preoperative findings were histopathologically positive for lateral LN metastasis. Twenty-nine percent of the MTCs measuring 2 cm or less were lateral-node-positive [72].

Machens et al. [73] investigated the rates of occult lateral compartment metastases in patients with central compartment nodal disease, and identified a risk of ipsilateral lateral compartment metastasis of 77% if one to three central compartment nodes were involved, and the same risk of contralateral lateral compartment involvement if more than 10 central compartment nodes were involved.

Bilateral LND for thyroid cancers confers a significant amount of morbidity. Knowledge of the complications of this procedure, especially in the setting of questionable survival benefit, may assist in preoperative decision-making and patient counseling [74].

The morphology of the primary tumor (DSR – yes/no) and the involvement of central LNs (yes/no) influence the indication for a more extended lateral LN dissection (LLND).

8

An observational study [19] confirmed that the extent of LN surgery may be individualized based on intraoperative frozen sections documenting DSR negativity. DSR is defined as the presence of a newly formed fibrotic (collagenous) stroma surrounding the invasive epithelial tumor cells, which is not found in the non-neoplastic thyroid parenchyma. Patients with DSR-negative tumors are always LN-negative (pN0: negative predictive value 100%) and have an excellent long-term prognosis without persisting or recurrent disease, even without lateral LN surgery, regardless of tumor size, thus reducing the surgical trauma and possible complications [20]. FNAB should be avoided during the diagnostic workup of a thyroid nodule because a DSR may be triggered by inserting a needle into the nodule [22].

Perros et al. [43] recommended ipsilateral prophylactic LLND only after documenting histologically proven central compartment node metastasis because of the higher risk of lateral LN involvement [75]. However, this recommendation does not consider the phenomenon of skip lesions.

CLND and ipsilateral (or contralateral) LN dissection may be performed as a one-stage or a two-stage procedure (= delayed LLND in a second operation) [76].

Two-stage LLND has the advantage of providing the pathological nodal status of the central compartment, as well as postoperative Ct levels, both of which may influence the decision to follow a supplementary approach. If there is no histopathologic evidence of central LN metastasis and postoperative Ct is normal, then delayed LN dissection is unlikely to confer any benefit. The disadvantage of two-stage LN dissection is the requirement for a second hospital stay and general anesthesia.

While the classification of LN levels by Robbins [8] is used in the Anglo-American literature, the classification of LN compartments by Dralle [9] is applied in Central Europe. ■ Table 8.1 shows the correlation of both nomenclatures.

There is a close correlation among Ct levels, tumor size, and tumor stage. Higher biomarker levels reflect larger primary tumors and/or more severely involved LNs and/or distant metastasis.

Therefore, Ct levels allow for a "tailored" surgical strategy [77].

Preoperative Ct levels may guide the extent of LN dissection. Disregarding gender-specific cut-off bCt levels, LN metastases were present in the ipsilateral central and lateral neck, contralateral central neck, contralateral lateral neck, and upper mediastinum, respectively, beyond bCt thresholds of 20, 50, 200, and 500 pg/mL applying an Immulite 2000 automated Ct assay (Diagnostic Products Corp., Los Angeles, CA) [47].

In most newly diagnosed MTC patients, that is, those with pretherapeutic bCt levels greater than 200 pg/mL, bilateral compartment-oriented neck surgery is recommended to reduce the number of reoperations [47].

Applying the same Ct assay and respecting gender [48], all male patients with LN metastases were diagnosed with bCt levels ≥100 pg/mL (sensitivity: 100%). The specificity for the diagnosis of any LN metastases (pN1a or pN1b) was 82% and 74% for the presence of lateral LN metastases (pN1b only).

Among the female patients, one woman was diagnosed with a single LN metastasis in the central compartment (N1a) with a bCt level of 23 pg/mL. Therefore, the cut-off of ≥23 pg/mL was used to diagnose any LN metastases (pN1a or pN1b) and specificity was only 22% with a sensitivity of 100%. However, all other women with LN metastases had bCt levels ≥85 pg/mL and metastases in the lateral compartment (specificity: 57%).

8.15 Locally Advanced MTC and Distant Metastasis

In patients with suspected locally advanced MTC, invasion of the aerodigestive tract or involvement of the mediastinum has to be ruled out using CT or MRI. These techniques clarify the technical resectability of the tumor from the neck or mediastinum.

Functional imaging with F-DOPA-PET (CT or MRT) may confirm LN metastases in the mediastinum, which are revealed in 32% [10]. When there is strong suspicion or evidence of mediastinal node involvement below the brachiocephalic vein, and no evidence of distant metastases, the patient should be considered for mediastinal dissection, which will require sternotomy [71, 78].

Functional imaging with F-DOPA-PET (CT or MRT) is able to ensure the diagnosis of distant metastasis [15]. Patients with distant metastases at presentation often have prolonged survival. Even in the presence of disseminated disease, less aggressive surgery in the central and lateral neck may be appropriate to preserve speech, swallowing, parathyroid function, and shoulder mobility. External beam radiotherapy, systemic medical therapy, and other non-surgical therapies should be considered to achieve local tumor control [33, 43].

8.16 Special Situations

As shown previously [57] in systematically performed determinations of Ct levels during the diagnostic workup of unselected thyroid nodules, 153/159 (96.2%; pT1a: 91/159 [57.2%], pT1b-pT4: 62/159 [39%]) were screened positive and 6/159 (3.8%; pT1a: 6/159 [3.8%]) screened negative for MTC.

In these rare cases, incidentally discovered mMTCs with preoperatively normal bCt levels are revealed in final histological/immunohistochemical examinations. These tumors are predominantly ≤5 mm in diameter and show no LN metastasis.

Analysis of germline RET proto-oncogene mutations (hereditary or de novo) should be undertaken to identify hereditary cases. Completion thyroidectomy should be performed in genetically positive patients because of the high risk of a contralateral focus of MTC.

In sporadic patients, the necessity for reoperation (completion thyroidectomy, uni-/bilateral CND) depends on the results of bCt. Surgery is recommended if postoperative levels are elevated 3 months postoperatively or if there is radiological evidence of residual disease [57].

8.17 TNM Classification and Staging

The Union for International Cancer Control system is recommended for staging all MTC patients [79].

The eighth edition introduced important changes in the criteria used for staging MTC. In the absence of gross extracapsular extension, the primary will be staged solely on the basis of its size (pT1, pT2, or pT3a). Tumors of any size with gross extrathyroidal extension invading the strap muscles (sternohyoid, sternothyroid, or omohyoid muscles) are classified as pT3b (◘ Table 8.3a, b).

Table 8.3 **a** TNM classification and staging of hereditary and sporadic MTC [79]. **b** TNM staging of hereditary and sporadic MTC [79]

Table 3a			
T – primary tumor			
Tx	Primary tumor cannot be assessed		
T0	No evidence of primary tumor		
T1	Tumor 2 cm or less in greatest dimension, limited to the thyroid T1a		
T1b	Tumor >1 cm but ≤2 cm in greatest dimension, limited to the thyroid		
T2	Tumor >2 cm but ≤4 cm in greatest dimension, limited to the thyroid		
T3	Tumor >4 cm in greatest dimension, limited to the thyroid or with gross extrathyroidal extension invading only strap muscles (sternohyoid, sternothyroid, or omohyoid muscles)		
T3a	Tumor >4 cm in greatest dimension, limited to the thyroid		
T3b	Tumor of any size with gross extrathyroidal extension invading strap muscles (sternohyoid, sternothyroid, or omohyoid muscles)		
T4a	Tumor extends beyond the thyroid capsule and invades any of the following: subcutaneous soft tissues, larynx, trachea, esophagus, recurrent laryngeal nerve		
T4b	Tumor invades prevertebral fascia or encasing the carotid artery or mediastinal vessels from a tumor of any size		
N – Regional lymph nodes			
N0	No evidence of locoregional lymph node metastasis N		
N1a	Metastasis to level VI (pretracheal, paratracheal, and prelaryngeal/Delphian lymph nodes) or upper/superior mediastinum		
N1b	Metastasis in other unilateral, bilateral, or contralateral cervical compartments (levels I, II, III, IV or V) or retropharyngeal		
M – Distant metastasis			
M0	No distant metastasis		
M	Distant metastasis		
Table 3b			
Stage	**T**	**N**	**M**
I	1a, 1b	0	0
II	2, 3	0	0
III	1–3	1a	0

(continued)

Table 8.3 (continued)

IVA	1–3	1b	0
	4a	Any N	0
IVB	4b	Any N	0
IVC	Any T	Any N	1

The pT and pN categories correspond to the T and N categories
pN0 histological examination of a selective neck dissection specimen will ordinarily include 6 or more lymph nodes. If the lymph nodes are negative, but the number ordinarily examined is not met, classify as pN0
The eighth edition of the UICC TNM staging system introduced several changes compared with the seventh edition. The main changes are noted with superscript numbers and are described in detail as following:
Minor extrathyroidal extension was removed from the definition of T3 disease
Two new categories, T3a and T3b, were introduced
N1a was expanded to include the upper mediastinum (previously included in the N1b category)

8.18 Hereditary MTC

Approximately 3–7% of patients with presumed sporadic MTC actually have hereditary MTC, including about 2–9% with de novo germline mutations [80–85].

Approximately 98% of "index patients" with hereditary CC disease have identifiable mutations that are caused by several missense gain-of-function mutations of the RET proto-oncogene, which encodes the receptor tyrosine kinase on chromosome 10. RET encodes a receptor tyrosine kinase, which is expressed in neural-crest-deriving cells and involved in cell proliferation control.

In a prospective investigation [56], germline mutations in the RET proto-oncogene were documented in 22 (8.5%) of 260 patients with apparently sporadic CC diseases, in 4 (3.2%) of 126 patients with various types of CCH, and in 18 (13.4%) of 134 patients with MTC.

It is important to test for germline RET mutations in any patient with MTC, regardless of their family history [86].

The mutations can be distributed in several codons (including non-hot-spot). Codons are located in different exons of the RET gene. It is recommended that RET genetic screening should cover not only exons 10, 11, and 16 but also 5, 8, 13, 14, and 15 [33].

Hereditary MTC represents a progression from normal histopathology to preneoplastic CCH and to MTC [87]. Hereditary and sporadic MTCs do not differ morphologically. In pathological reports, however, the presence of CCH should always be mentioned. Still, its usefulness alone for indicating familial risk is limited.

Hereditary CC disease (CCH and/or MTC) may be part of one of the three autosomal-dominant hereditary cancer syndromes (Table 8.4). Familial MTC "only" is documented in

Table 8.4 Current classification of hereditary MTC tumor syndromes [33]

Classification	Definition
MEN 2A	Classic: MTC, PHEO, PHPT
	MEN 2A with lichen amyloidosis
	MEN 2A with Hirschsprung's disease
	FMTC
MEN 2B	MTC, PHEO

MEN multiple endocrine neoplasia, *MTC* medullary thyroid cancer, *PHEO* pheochromocytoma, *PHPT* primary hyperparathyroidism, *FMTC* familial medullary thyroid cancer "only"

approximately 15%, MEN 2A in 80%, and MEN 2B in 5% of affected patients [88].

Multifocal tumors are more often found in a genetic background.

Hereditary MTC is a potentially lethal disease. MTC remains confirmed to the thyroid gland for a distinct period of time. Once spread beyond the thyroid gland, it is incurable in the majority of patients, spreading on to the regional LNs and subsequently to the liver, lung, bone, and brain.

Thyroidectomy (without CLND) should be offered to mutation carriers before the development of MTC ("prophylactic surgery"; CCH is expected) or while the malignancy is still confirmed to the thyroid gland ("early surgery," surgery in a "preclinical stage"; mMTC without expected LN metastasis).

Ultrasonography is insufficient to identify MTC of any size or micrometastasis in LNs in hereditary CC disease [89].

Applying direct DNA analysis, mutation carriers (patients at risk to develop MTC) can be specified within a family. A given patient's genotype (specific *RET* mutation) predicts per se the aggressiveness of the clinical course.

Patients carrying the same mutation may show a heterogenic progression of disease. Even within the same family, the natural course of disease may vary. Neoplastic CCH is the precursor lesion of hereditary MTC. MTC develops over time. There is a well-documented age-related progression from neoplastic CCH to asymptomatic micro- and to clinically apparent macrocarcinoma (including LN and distant metastasis).

The current ATA risk levels stratify very well all known RET mutations into one of three risk levels (highest risk, high risk, moderate risk; Table 8.5).

Thyroid surgery is generally recommended based on the ATA risk levels (Table 8.6) [33].

There is also a positive correlation among bCt and sCt levels, tumor size, and stage of hereditary MTC.

Table 8.5 The current American Thyroid Association (ATA) risk levels: risk classification in correlation to (common) RET proto-oncogene mutations [33]

Risk classification	RET mutation
Moderate (ATA-MOD)	790, 791, 804, 609, 611, 618, 620
High (ATA-H)	634, 883
Highest (ATA-HST)	918

ATA American Thyroid Association, *MOD* moderate risk, *H* high risk, *HST* highest risk

Table 8.6 Risk classification of (common) RET proto-oncogene mutations – timing of surgery following the **G** (enetic) **A** (ge) **C** (alcitonin) concept [33]

Risk classification	RET mutation	Timing of surgery
Moderate (ATA-MOD)	790, 791, 804, 609, 611, 618, 620	Based on serum calcitonin levels
High (ATA-H)	634, 883	≤5 years (or earlier based on the elevated serum calcitonin levels)
Highest (ATA-HST)	918	<1 year (3 months)

ATA American Thyroid Association, *MOD* moderate, *H* high, *HST* highest

The moment of transition from CCH to MTC seems to occur when Ct levels rise upon stimulation. In patients with normal bCt but increased sCt levels, the chance of mMTC increases significantly (Table 8.7). In this situation, "early thyroidectomy" should definitively be performed (minimum total thyroidectomy). Elevated bCt and sCt levels may indicate MTC with LN metastasis. Therefore, CND (level VI) is mandatory for staging and to remove micrometastasis in patients with elevated bCt levels [90] (Table 8.8).

Postponing surgery and avoiding CND (level VI) in patients with moderate-risk levels are only justified in families with a less aggressive MTC history and in combination with the results of normal bCt and (Ca-) stimulated serum Ct levels.

Table 8.7 Pretherapeutic calcitonin levels and histology [90]

Calcitonin		*n* (%)	Normal CCH	MTC pN0	MTC pN1	Cured
Basal	**Stimulated**		**92**	**76**	**46**	
Normal	Normal	34 (16)	32	2	0	34 (100)
Normal	Increased	40 (19)	26	14	0	33 (100)
Increased	Increased	140 (65)	34	60	46	87 (69)
Cured		154 (79)	79 (100)	69 (100)	7 (15)	

MTC medullary thyroid cancer, *N* lymph node

Table 8.8 Indication for prophylactic and early thyroidectomy and central neck dissection [33]; see also Table 8.7

Calcitonin		Thyroidectomy		Central neck dissection
Basal	**Stimulated**			
Normal	Normal	Prophylactic	Yes	No
Normal	Increased	Early	Yes	No/Yes[a]
Increased	Increased		Yes	Yes

[a]If bCt is less than 40 pg/mL, a total thyroidectomy without central (level VI) neck dissection is adequate therapy

Thyroidectomy can be delayed in some children with MEN 2A if the serum Ct and neck ultrasonography results are normal [33].

bCt (and sCt) levels, determined in periodical intervals, may help to individually schedule timely surgery and to minimize the extent of the surgical procedure. This may satisfy parents who wish to postpone surgery in their children.

Although no data are as yet available, Ct measurements are recommended based on the ATA risk levels: every 6 months in the high and annually in the moderate levels [33].

Considering genotype, age, and bCt (and sCt) levels, the time of surgery may be postponed individually and the extent of the surgical intervention (CND [level VI]: yes/no) may be modified (▣ Table 8.6).

If bCt is less than 40 pg/mL, total thyroidectomy without CND (level VI) may be an adequate therapy ([33]–▣ Table 8.8).

The timing of surgery in asymptomatic disease requires a balance between the prevention of thyroid malignancy and the risks of the operation (permanent hypoparathyroidism, permanent paralysis of the recurrent laryngeal nerve) [91].

"Prophylactic" and "early" thyroidectomy (with and without neck dissection) should be performed by high-volume endocrine neck surgeons to reduce morbidity to the lowest possible extent [92].

The surgical strategy to treat "hereditary, clinically apparent MTC" (index patients) follows the same guidelines as for sporadic disease.

8.19 MEN 2A

Besides premalignant or malignant thyroid lesions, tumors in the adrenal glands (pheochromocytoma) and/or the parathyroid glands may develop with variable penetrance and must be ruled out, first, by measuring 24-h urinary catecholamine or, preferably, metanephrine concentrations to exclude pheochromocytoma and, second, by determining serum Ca concentrations and the serum parathyroid hormone to exclude primary hyperparathyroidism before planning thyroid surgery [93].

Table 8.9 summarizes the recommendations when screening for pheochromocytoma, and primary hyperparathyroidism should start depending on the given RET proto-oncogene mutation.

8

8.20 MEN 2B

In the clinical setting of MEN 2B, MTC is highly aggressive and associated with a very early onset of metastasis (ATA risk level "D"). LN metastases are documented within the first year of life. Most frequently, MEN 2B arises as a result of a de novo mutation, with the child having unaffected parents. In the past, the diagnosis has often been delayed because

Table 8.9 Hereditary MTC – Recommendation: age of screening considering the (common) RET proto-oncogene mutation for screening pheochromocytoma and primary hyperparathyroidism [33]

Risk classification	Start for screening for Pheo/PHPT (a)
Moderate (ATA-MOD)	16
High (ATA-H)	11
Highest (ATA-HST)[a]	

Pheo pheochromocytoma, *PHPT* primary hyperparathyroidism, *a* age, *ATA* American Thyroid Association, *MOD* moderate, *H* high, *HST* highest
[a]No PHPT screening necessary

the typical phenotype is often not apparent in early childhood or the typical symptoms were not appreciated on time. Awareness of non-endocrine components (tearless crying, constipation) may help to diagnose this syndrome earlier. In the presence of genetically verified MEN 2B, children should undergo thyroidectomy as soon as possible within the first year of life (preferably within the first 6 months of life). CND (level VI) should be considered particularly when bCt (and more importantly, stimulated Ct) is elevated, and in children older than 6 months [94].

8.21 Prognosis and Postoperative Follow-Up

Early detection and adequate surgical treatment is followed by cure and disease-free survival (defined by normal or undetectable Ct values) in over 98% of patients.

At clinical presentation, about 50% of patients with MTC show LN metastasis. Distant metastases are detected in 10% of newly diagnosed patients, and more than 20% of patients will die from progressive metastatic disease.

The 10-year survival rates for all patients with MTC range from approximately 61–76% [7, 95–97].

The 5-year and 10-year survival rates for all patients with MTC in a Ct screening program were 96 +/− 2% (patients at risk: 43) and 93 +/− 3% (patients at risk: 6), respectively [56].

Patients with distant metastases at diagnosis have a poor prognosis, with a 10-year survival rate of merely 40% [97].

Prognosis is directly related to postoperative staging considering tumor size (in former studies, extrathyroidal invasion – however, not respected in the current TNM classification), nodal and distant metastasis. The quantities of involved LNs and compartments are also prognostically relevant.

Postoperative measurements of bCt (and CEA) are widely used as tumor markers also for postoperative follow-up. The bCt levels indicate cure and persisting or recurring disease [98].

Ct levels typically normalize within 1 week and within a fortnight in patients with node-positive MTC and preoperative Ct levels of 500–1000 pg/mL. Ct normalization takes longer with node-positive MTC and preoperative Ct levels exceeding 1000 pg/mL, and with more than ten nodal metastases [99]. In cases with very high preoperative bCt levels, a decrease in bCt might be delayed for 24 h to 12 weeks after surgery [100]. Therefore, 3 months following surgery appears to be the optimal time point for determining Ct levels [100, 101].

Postoperative, undetectable bCt levels (optimal documentation together with a negative provocative test) are strong predictors of complete remission [98].

Serum bCt determinations should be repeated every 3 to 6 months for the first 2 to 3 years. When bCt stays unmeasurable, it should be determined annually thereafter. Patients with biochemical remission after an initial treatment have a 3% chance of recurrence during long-term follow-up [102].

Patients with biochemically and clinically apparent MTC have tumors very frequently metastasized to regional LNs and to distant organs. This condition cannot be cured biochemically, despite aggressive surgery, including bilateral LLND [47, 103].

Despite meticulous surgical techniques, Ct levels remain detectable in 40–66% of patients after initial surgery, and the optimal surgical management for persistent or recurrent disease remains controversial.

Localized and limited locoregional disease can be treated with resections, with the intention to cure. However, in more advanced localized or in residual/recurrent disease, a multimodal approach is generally recommended to control local disease and to reduce tumor progression. The extent of surgery will depend on the types of surgical procedures performed previously and on the nature of the relapse and bCt level.

When the extent of initial surgery was incomplete, the preferred surgery protocol is always resection. Patients with residual LN metastases after initial thyroidectomy are likely to benefit from reoperation [103].

In 59 (44.4%) of 133 patients who had no LN metastases removed at the initial operation, systematic CLND, and LLND attained biochemical cure. Conversely, biochemical cure was reached in only 12 (18.5%) of 65 patients in whom 1 to 5 LN metastases had been previously cleared. If more than five LN metastases were dissected at prior surgery, the biochemical cure rate fell to 4.7% (2 of 43 patients). When preoperative serum Ct levels exceeded 1000 pg/mL, biochemical cure was exceptional (1 of 76 patients). Based on these data, systematic LN dissection in patients who had inadequate neck surgery is worthwhile as long as the preoperative serum Ct level is <1000 pg/mL and no more than five LN metastases were removed. Beyond these thresholds, the focus of surgical treatment shifts to the maintenance of local control in the neck [103].

The rate of Ct normalization after reoperation for MTC is enhanced by applying meticulous compartment-oriented LN dissection. Compartment-oriented LN dissection results in Ct normalization in 18.6% of reoperated MTC patients [104].

When patients have bCt levels less than 150 pg/mL following thyroidectomy, any persistent or recurrent disease is nearly always confined to LNs in the neck. When the postoperative Ct level exceeds 150 pg/mL, patients should be evaluated with imaging procedures, including CT of the neck and chest, contrast-enhanced MRI and US of the liver and bone, and PET-CT to exclude distant metastasis [47].

One can estimate the growth rate of MTC metastases by quantifying increases in tumor size over time from sequential imaging studies analyzed with the response evaluation criteria in solid tumors (RECIST).

The tumor burden and proliferation characteristics can be estimated from imaging studies and measurements of tumor marker doubling times.

In patients with elevated serum Ct and CEA, the tumor dynamics can be described by calculating the time to double the serum concentration (tumor doubling time).

bCt and CEA doubling times of less than 2 years are negative prognostic factors for MTC progression-free and total survival in patients with persistent or recurrent disease [105].

When the doubling time of bCt was less than 6 months, the 5- and 10-year survival rates were 25% and 8%, respectively; when the doubling time was longer than 2 years, all patients were alive at the end of follow-up [106].

Once metastases appear, clinicians must decide which patients require therapy. They must balance the often slow rate of tumor progression, which is associated with good quality of life, against the limited efficacy and potential toxicities of local and systemic therapies [33].

Only patients with significant tumor burden and those with symptomatic or progressive, measurable disease are candidates for systemic therapy.

Progression is defined as a ≥20% increase in the sum of the longest lesion diameters or the appearance of one or more new lesions within a given time interval (e.g., 12 months) [33].

8.22 Unresectable, Progressive, and Symptomatic Sporadic and Hereditary MTC

Unresectable and progressive MTC affects both patients' health-related quality of life and survival. A systematic review [107] identified two placebo-controlled trials. Schlumberger et al. [108] evaluated the efficacy and safety of cabozantinib, while the Zactima Efficacy in Thyroid Cancer Assessment (ZETA) trial evaluated the efficacy and safety of vandetanib [109, 110].

Both drugs significantly improved progression-free survival compared to placebo ($P < 0.001$). Within the symptomatic and progressive MTC population, the effects on progressive-free survival were similar (vandetanib vs. cabozantinib: hazard ratio 1.14, 95% credible interval 0.41–3.09). Neither trial demonstrated a significant overall survival benefit for cabozantinib or vandetanib versus placebo, although data from ZETA were subject to potential confounding.

Answers to the Questions

Case 1: (3)

Completion thyroidectomy, CND only if: bCt [and/or sCt] elevated – genetic background

Specific "testing" – Ca stimulation 2 (0 min) – 21 (3 min) pg/mL; plasma metanephrine, plasma normetanephrine normal range; exon 14 – codon V804L – [GTG > TTG: val – leu];

Right lobectomy with right CND – MTC 1 mm, pN0 (0/6) – hereditary MTC, pT1mpN0 (0/11) – no CCH.

Case 2: (2d)

Adequately high bCt level in correlation with the size of the nodule: thyroidectomy, bilateral CND – frozen section DSR: yes/no

MTC – pT2–39 mm; pN0 (0/8), DSR negative – no bilateral neck dissection – follow-up: 164 months, bCt <1 pg/mL; CEA: 1.0 μg/L.

Case 3: (2)

Inadequately high bCt level in correlation with the size of the nodules – other than thyroid CC disease

Ca stimulation test: 704 pg/mL (0 min) – 1219 pg/mL – sCt less than twofold bCt – lung X-ray: 36 mm lesion right intermediate lobe, enlarged paratracheal and infracarinal lymph nodes – paraneoplastic Ct secretion by a neuroendocrine neoplasia of the lungs.

Case 4: (3)

Incidentally discovered mMTCs with preoperatively normal bCt levels

Except for molecular genetic analysis (in this particular patient: no RET proto-oncogene mutation), no further treatment.

Case 5: (2)

Clinically asymptomatic/mildly elevated bCt – reproducible – anxious patient – to select patients for surgery – stimulation test: 21 pg/mL (0 min) – 1664 pg/mL (3 min) – MTC suspected - plasma metanephrines/plasma normetanephrines: normal catecholamines/metanephrines and normetanephrines (24-h urine): normal – RET proto-oncogene mutation (exon 10, codon C611Y – GTG>TTG; cys – tyr)

Thyroidectomy, bilateral CND (early thyroidectomy) – multifocal, bilateral mMTC (pT1am; L: 5 mm; R: 1 mm with DSR; neoplastic CCH – N: pN0 (0/15); M: M0

References

1. Holzer S, Reiners C, Mann K, Bamberg M, Rothmund M, Dudeck J, et al. Patterns of care for patients with primary differentiated carcinoma of the thyroid gland treated in Germany during 1996. U.S. and German Thyroid Cancer Group. Cancer. 2000;89(1):192–201. https://doi.org/10.1002/1097-0142(20000701)89:1<192::aid-cncr26>3.0.co;2-7.
2. Hundahl SA, Cady B, Cunningham MP, Mazzaferri E, McKee RF, Rosai J, et al. Initial results from a prospective cohort study of 5583 cases of thyroid carcinoma treated in the United States during 1996.

U.S. and German Thyroid Cancer Study Group. An American College of Surgeons Commission on cancer patient care evaluation study. Cancer. 2000;89(1):202–17. https://doi.org/10.1002/1097-0142(20000701)89:1<202::aid-cncr27>3.0.co;2-a.

3. Valle LA, Kloos RT. The prevalence of occult medullary thyroid carcinoma at autopsy. J Clin Endocrinol Metab. 2011;96(1):E109–13. https://doi.org/10.1210/jc.2010-0959.
4. Daniels GH. Screening for medullary thyroid carcinoma with serum calcitonin measurements in patients with thyroid nodules in the United States and Canada. Thyroid. 2011;21(11):1199–207. https://doi.org/10.1089/thy.2010.0297.
5. Bergholm U, Adami HO, Bergstrom R, Johansson H, Lundell G, Telenius-Berg M, et al. Clinical characteristics in sporadic and familial medullary thyroid carcinoma. A nationwide study of 249 patients in Sweden from 1959 through 1981. Cancer. 1989;63(6):1196–204. https://doi.org/10.1002/1097-0142(19890315)63:6<1196::aid-cncr2820630626>3.0.co;2-o.
6. Kebebew E, Ituarte PH, Siperstein AE, Duh QY, Clark OH. Medullary thyroid carcinoma: clinical characteristics, treatment, prognostic factors, and a comparison of staging systems. Cancer. 2000;88(5):1139–48. https://doi.org/10.1002/(sici)1097-0142(20000301)88:5<1139::aid-cncr26>3.0.co;2-z.
7. Torresan F, Cavedon E, Mian C, Iacobone M. Long-term outcome after surgery for medullary thyroid carcinoma: a single-center experience. World J Surg. 2018;42(2):367–75. https://doi.org/10.1007/s00268-017-4321-z.
8. Robbins KT, Clayman G, Levine PA, Medina J, Sessions R, Shaha A, et al. Neck dissection classification update: revisions proposed by the American Head and Neck Society and the American Academy of Otolaryngology-Head and Neck Surgery. Arch Otolaryngol Head Neck Surg. 2002;128(7):751–8. https://doi.org/10.1001/archotol.128.7.751.
9. Dralle H. Lymph node dissection and medullary thyroid carcinoma. Br J Surg. 2002;89(9):1073–5. https://doi.org/10.1046/j.1365-2168.2002.02160.x.
10. Machens A, Hinze R, Thomusch O, Dralle H. Pattern of nodal metastasis for primary and reoperative thyroid cancer. World J Surg. 2002;26(1):22–8. https://doi.org/10.1007/s00268-001-0176-3.
11. Moley JF, DeBenedetti MK. Patterns of nodal metastases in palpable medullary thyroid carcinoma: recommendations for extent of node dissection. Ann Surg. 1999;229(6):880–7; discussion 7-8. https://doi.org/10.1097/00000658-199906000-00016.
12. Tung WS, Vesely TM, Moley JF. Laparoscopic detection of hepatic metastases in patients with residual or recurrent medullary thyroid cancer. Surgery. 1995;118(6):1024–9; discussion 9-30. https://doi.org/10.1016/s0039-6060(05)80109-6.
13. Gharib H, Papini E, Garber JR, Duick DS, Harrell RM, Hegedus L, et al. American Association of Clinical Endocrinologists, American College of Endocrinology, and Associazione Medici Endocrinologi medical guidelines for clinical practice for the diagnosis and management of thyroid nodules--2016 update. Endocr Pract. 2016;22(5):622–39. https://doi.org/10.4158/EP161208.GL.
14. Wolinski K, Rewaj-Losyk M, Ruchala M. Sonographic features of medullary thyroid carcinomas--a systematic review and meta-analysis. Endokrynol Pol. 2014;65(4):314–8. https://doi.org/10.5603/EP.2014.0043.
15. Brammen L, Niederle MB, Riss P, Scheuba C, Selberherr A, Karanikas G, et al. Medullary thyroid carcinoma: do ultrasonography and F-DOPA-PET-CT influence the initial surgical strategy? Ann Surg Oncol. 2018;25(13):3919–27. https://doi.org/10.1245/s10434-018-6829-3.

16. Trimboli P, Treglia G, Guidobaldi L, Romanelli F, Nigri G, Valabrega S, et al. Detection rate of FNA cytology in medullary thyroid carcinoma: a meta-analysis. Clin Endocrinol. 2015;82(2):280–5. https://doi.org/10.1111/cen.12563.
17. Choi N, Moon WJ, Lee JH, Baek JH, Kim DW, Park SW. Ultrasonographic findings of medullary thyroid cancer: differences according to tumor size and correlation with fine needle aspiration results. Acta Radiol. 2011;52(3):312–6. https://doi.org/10.1258/ar.2010.100247.
18. Essig GF Jr, Porter K, Schneider D, Debora A, Lindsey SC, Busonero G, et al. Fine needle aspiration and medullary thyroid carcinoma: the risk of inadequate preoperative evaluation and initial surgery when relying upon FNAB cytology alone. Endocr Pract. 2013;19(6):920–7. https://doi.org/10.4158/EP13143.OR.
19. Scheuba C, Kaserer K, Kaczirek K, Asari R, Niederle B. Desmoplastic stromal reaction in medullary thyroid cancer-an intraoperative "marker" for lymph node metastases. World J Surg. 2006;30(5):853–9. https://doi.org/10.1007/s00268-005-0391-4.
20. Niederle MB, Riss P, Selberherr A, Koperek O, Kaserer K, Niederle B et al. Omission of lateral lymph node dissection in medullary thyroid cancer without a desmoplastic stromal reaction. Br J Surg. 2021;108 (2):174–181. https://doi.org/10.1093/bjs/znaa047.
21. Andreas, Machens Peter, Kaatzsch Kerstin, Lorenz Lars-Christian, Horn Claudia, Wickenhauser Kurt Werner, Schmid Henning, Dralle Udo, Siebolts. Abandoning node dissection for desmoplasia-negative encapsulated unifocal sporadic medullary thyroid cancer. Surgery. 2021 https://doi.org/10.1016/j.surg.2021.07.035.
22. Aubert S, Berdelou A, Gnemmi V, Behal H, Caiazzo R, D'Herbomez M, et al. Large sporadic thyroid medullary carcinomas: predictive factors for lymph node involvement. Virchows Arch. 2018;472(3):461–8. https://doi.org/10.1007/s00428-018-2303-7.
23. Boi F, Maurelli I, Pinna G, Atzeni F, Piga M, Lai ML, et al. Calcitonin measurement in wash-out fluid from fine needle aspiration of neck masses in patients with primary and metastatic medullary thyroid carcinoma. J Clin Endocrinol Metab. 2007;92(6):2115–8. https://doi.org/10.1210/jc.2007-0326.
24. Trimboli P, Guidobaldi L, Bongiovanni M, Crescenzi A, Alevizaki M, Giovanella L. Use of fine-needle aspirate calcitonin to detect medullary thyroid carcinoma: a systematic review. Diagn Cytopathol. 2016;44(1):45–51. https://doi.org/10.1002/dc.23375.
25. Diazzi C, Madeo B, Taliani E, Zirilli L, Romano S, Granata AR, et al. The diagnostic value of calcitonin measurement in wash-out fluid from fine-needle aspiration of thyroid nodules in the diagnosis of medullary thyroid cancer. Endocr Pract. 2013;19(5):769–79. https://doi.org/10.4158/EP12420.OR.
26. Karagiannis AK, Girio-Fragkoulakis C, Nakouti T. Procalcitonin: a new biomarker for medullary thyroid cancer? A systematic review. Anticancer Res. 2016;36(8):3803–10.
27. Giovanella L, Imperiali M, Piccardo A, Taborelli M, Verburg FA, Daurizio F, et al. Procalcitonin measurement to screen medullary thyroid carcinoma: a prospective evaluation in a series of 2705 patients with thyroid nodules. Eur J Clin Investig. 2018;48(6):e12934. https://doi.org/10.1111/eci.12934.
28. Niederle MB, Scheuba C, Gessl A, Li S, Koperek O, Bieglmayer C, et al. Calcium-stimulated calcitonin - The "new standard" in the diagnosis of thyroid C-cell disease - clinically relevant gender-specific cut-off levels for an "old test". Biochem Med (Zagreb). 2018;28(3):030710. https://doi.org/10.11613/BM.2018.030710.
29. Cote GJ, Grubbs EG, Hofmann MC. Thyroid C-cell biology and oncogenic transformation. Recent Results Cancer Res. 2015;204:1–39. https://doi.org/10.1007/978-3-319-22542-5_1.

30. Costante G, Meringolo D. Calcitonin as a biomarker of C cell disease: recent achievements and current challenges. Endocrine. 2020;67(2):273–80. https://doi.org/10.1007/s12020-019-02183-6.
31. Bieglmayer C, Vierhapper H, Dudczak R, Niederle B. Measurement of calcitonin by immunoassay analyzers. Clin Chem Lab Med. 2007;45(5):662–6. https://doi.org/10.1515/CCLM.2007.124.
32. Bieglmayer C, Scheuba C, Niederle B, Flores J, Vierhapper H. Screening for medullary thyroid carcinoma: experience with different immunoassays for human calcitonin. Wien Klin Wochenschr. 2002;114(7):267–73.
33. Wells SA Jr, Asa SL, Dralle H, Elisei R, Evans DB, Gagel RF, et al. Revised American Thyroid Association guidelines for the management of medullary thyroid carcinoma. Thyroid. 2015;25(6):567–610. https://doi.org/10.1089/thy.2014.0335.
34. Kebebew E, Greenspan FS, Clark OH, Woeber KA, Grunwell J. Extent of disease and practice patterns for medullary thyroid cancer. J Am Coll Surg. 2005;200(6):890–6. https://doi.org/10.1016/j.jamcollsurg.2004.12.011.
35. Panigrahi B, Roman SA, Sosa JA. Medullary thyroid cancer: are practice patterns in the United States discordant from American Thyroid Association guidelines? Ann Surg Oncol. 2010;17(6):1490–8. https://doi.org/10.1245/s10434-010-1017-0.
36. Chang EHE, Lutfi W, Feinglass J, Reiher AE, Moo-Young T, Bhayani MK. National trends in the surgical treatment of non-advanced medullary thyroid cancer (MTC): an evaluation of adherence with the 2009 American Thyroid Association guidelines. World J Surg. 2016;40(12):2930–40. https://doi.org/10.1007/s00268-016-3643-6.
37. Cox C, Chen Y, Cress R, Semrad AM, Semrad T, Gosnell JE, et al. Are there disparities in the presentation, treatment and outcomes of patients diagnosed with medullary thyroid cancer?-An analysis of 634 patients from the California Cancer Registry. Gland Surg. 2016;5(4):398–404. https://doi.org/10.21037/gs.2016.04.02.
38. Karga H, Giagourta I, Papaioannou G, Doumouchtsis K, Polymeris A, Thanou S, et al. Changes in risk factors and tumor node metastasis stage of sporadic medullary thyroid carcinoma over 41 years, before and after the routine measurements of serum calcitonin. Metabolism. 2011;60(5):604–8. https://doi.org/10.1016/j.metabol.2010.06.004.
39. Machens A, Dralle H. Surgical cure rates of sporadic medullary thyroid cancer in the era of calcitonin screening. Eur J Endocrinol. 2016;175(3):219–28. https://doi.org/10.1530/EJE-16-0325.
40. Cheung K, Roman SA, Wang TS, Walker HD, Sosa JA. Calcitonin measurement in the evaluation of thyroid nodules in the United States: a cost-effectiveness and decision analysis. J Clin Endocrinol Metab. 2008;93(6):2173–80. https://doi.org/10.1210/jc.2007-2496.
41. Verbeek HH, de Groot JWB, Sluiter WJ, Muller Kobold AC, van den Heuvel ER, Plukker JT, et al. Calcitonin testing for detection of medullary thyroid cancer in people with thyroid nodules. Cochrane Database Syst Rev. 2020;3:CD010159. https://doi.org/10.1002/14651858.CD010159.pub2.
42. Pacini F, Castagna MG, Brilli L, Pentheroudakis G, Group EGW. Thyroid cancer: ESMO clinical practice guidelines for diagnosis, treatment and follow-up. Ann Oncol. 2012;23(Suppl 7):110–9. https://doi.org/10.1093/annonc/mds230.
43. Perros P, Boelaert K, Colley S, Evans C, Evans RM, Gerrard Ba G, et al. Guidelines for the management of thyroid cancer. Clin Endocrinol. 2014;81(Suppl 1):1–122. https://doi.org/10.1111/cen.12515.
44. Cohen R, Campos JM, Salaun C, Heshmati HM, Kraimps JL, Proye C, et al. Preoperative calcitonin levels are predictive of tumor size and postoperative calcitonin normalization in medullary thyroid carcinoma. Groupe d'Etudes des Tumeurs a Calcitonine (GETC). J Clin

Endocrinol Metab. 2000;85(2):919–22. https://doi.org/10.1210/jcem.85.2.6556.
45. Pomares FJ, Rodriguez JM, Nicolas F, Sola J, Canteras M, Balsalobre M, et al. Presurgical assessment of the tumor burden of familial medullary thyroid carcinoma by calcitonin testing. J Am Coll Surg. 2002;195(5):630–4. https://doi.org/10.1016/s1072-7515(02)01499-0.
46. Yip DT, Hassan M, Pazaitou-Panayiotou K, Ruan DT, Gawande AA, Gaz RD, et al. Preoperative basal calcitonin and tumor stage correlate with postoperative calcitonin normalization in patients undergoing initial surgical management of medullary thyroid carcinoma. Surgery. 2011;150(6):1168–77. https://doi.org/10.1016/j.surg.2011.09.043.
47. Machens A, Dralle H. Biomarker-based risk stratification for previously untreated medullary thyroid cancer. J Clin Endocrinol Metab. 2010;95(6):2655–63. https://doi.org/10.1210/jc.2009-2368.
48. Niederle MB, Scheuba C, Riss P, Selberherr A, Koperek O, Niederle B. Early diagnosis of medullary thyroid cancer: are calcitonin stimulation tests still indicated in the era of highly sensitive calcitonin immunoassays? Thyroid. 2020;30(7):974–84. https://doi.org/10.1089/thy.2019.0785.
49. Toledo SP, Lourenco DM Jr, Santos MA, Tavares MR, Toledo RA, Correia-Deur JE. Hypercalcitoninemia is not pathognomonic of medullary thyroid carcinoma. Clinics. 2009;64(7):699–706. https://doi.org/10.1590/S1807-59322009000700015.
50. Machens A, Haedecke J, Holzhausen HJ, Thomusch O, Schneyer U, Dralle H. Differential diagnosis of calcitonin-secreting neuroendocrine carcinoma of the foregut by pentagastrin stimulation. Langenbeck's Arch Surg. 2000;385(6):398–401. https://doi.org/10.1007/s004230000169.
51. Schneider R, Waldmann J, Swaid Z, Ramaswamy A, Fendrich V, Bartsch DK, et al. Calcitonin-secreting pancreatic endocrine tumors: systematic analysis of a rare tumor entity. Pancreas. 2011;40(2):213–21. https://doi.org/10.1097/MPA.0b013e3182015f5d.
52. Vahidi S, Stewart J, Amin K, Racila E, Li F. Metastatic medullary thyroid carcinoma or calcitonin-secreting carcinoid tumor of lung? A diagnostic dilemma in a patient with lung mass and thyroid nodule. Diagn Cytopathol. 2018;46(4):345–8. https://doi.org/10.1002/dc.23852.
53. Allelein S, Ehlers M, Morneau C, Schwartz K, Goretzki PE, Seppel T, et al. Measurement of basal serum calcitonin for the diagnosis of medullary thyroid cancer. Horm Metab Res. 2018;50(1):23–8. https://doi.org/10.1055/s-0043-122237.
54. Kahaly GJ, Algeciras-Schimnich A, Davis TE, Diana T, Feldkamp J, Karger S, et al. United States and European multicenter prospective study for the analytical performance and clinical validation of a novel sensitive fully automated immunoassay for calcitonin. Clin Chem. 2017;63(9):1489–96. https://doi.org/10.1373/clinchem.2016.270009.
55. Niederle B, Sebag F, Brauckhoff M. Timing and extent of thyroid surgery for gene carriers of hereditary C cell disease – a consensus statement of the European Society of Endocrine Surgeons (ESES). Langenbeck's Arch Surg. 2014;399(2):185–97. https://doi.org/10.1007/s00423-013-1139-5.
56. Scheuba C, Kaserer K, Moritz A, Drosten R, Vierhapper H, Bieglmayer C, et al. Sporadic hypercalcitoninemia: clinical and therapeutic consequences. Endocr Relat Cancer. 2009;16(1):243–53. https://doi.org/10.1677/ERC-08-0059.
57. Scheuba C, Kaserer K, Bieglmayer C, Asari R, Riss P, Drosten R, et al. Medullary thyroid microcarcinoma recommendations for treatment - a single-center experience. Surgery. 2007;142(6):1003–10. https://doi.org/10.1016/j.surg.2007.09.016.
58. Daumerie C, Maiter D, Gruson D. Serum calcitonin estimation in medullary thyroid cancer: basal or stimulated levels? Thyroid Res. 2013;6(Suppl 1):S4. https://doi.org/10.1186/1756-6614-6-S1-S4.

59. Fugazzola L, Di Stefano M, Censi S, Repaci A, Colombo C, Grimaldi F, et al. Basal and stimulated calcitonin for the diagnosis of medullary thyroid cancer: updated thresholds and safety assessment. J Endocrinol Investig. 2021;44(3):587–97. https://doi.org/10.1007/s40618-020-01356-9.
60. Barbot N, Calmettes C, Schuffenecker I, Saint-Andre JP, Franc B, Rohmer V, et al. Pentagastrin stimulation test and early diagnosis of medullary thyroid carcinoma using an immunoradiometric assay of calcitonin: comparison with genetic screening in hereditary medullary thyroid carcinoma. J Clin Endocrinol Metab. 1994;78(1):114–20. https://doi.org/10.1210/jcem.78.1.7904611.
61. Costante G, Meringolo D, Durante C, Bianchi D, Nocera M, Tumino S, et al. Predictive value of serum calcitonin levels for preoperative diagnosis of medullary thyroid carcinoma in a cohort of 5817 consecutive patients with thyroid nodules. J Clin Endocrinol Metab. 2007;92(2):450–5. https://doi.org/10.1210/jc.2006-1590.
62. Frank-Raue K, Schott M, Raue F. Im Namen der Sektion Schilddruse der DGE. [recommendation for calcitonin screening in nodular goiter]. Dtsch Med Wochenschr. 2018;143(15):1065–9. https://doi.org/10.1055/a-0585-8097.
63. Selberherr A, Riss P, Scheuba C, Niederle B. Prophylactic "first-step" central neck dissection (level 6) does not increase morbidity after (total) thyroidectomy. Ann Surg Oncol. 2016;23(12):4016–22. https://doi.org/10.1245/s10434-016-5338-5.
64. Moley JF. Medullary thyroid carcinoma: management of lymph node metastases. J Natl Compr Cancer Netw. 2010;8(5):549–56. https://doi.org/10.6004/jnccn.2010.0042.
65. Essig GF Jr, Porter K, Schneider D, Arpaia D, Lindsey SC, Busonero G, et al. Multifocality in sporadic medullary thyroid carcinoma: an international multicenter study. Thyroid. 2016;26(11):1563–72. https://doi.org/10.1089/thy.2016.0255.
66. Scollo C, Baudin E, Travagli JP, Caillou B, Bellon N, Leboulleux S, et al. Rationale for central and bilateral lymph node dissection in sporadic and hereditary medullary thyroid cancer. J Clin Endocrinol Metab. 2003;88(5):2070–5. https://doi.org/10.1210/jc.2002-021713.
67. Kim JH, Pyo JS, Cho WJ. Clinicopathological significance and prognosis of medullary thyroid microcarcinoma: a meta-analysis. World J Surg. 2017;41(10):2551–8. https://doi.org/10.1007/s00268-017-4031-6.
68. Machens A, Holzhausen HJ, Dralle H. Skip metastases in thyroid cancer leaping the central lymph node compartment. Arch Surg. 2004;139(1):43–5. https://doi.org/10.1001/archsurg.139.1.43.
69. Mathiesen JS, Kroustrup JP, Vestergaard P, Stochholm K, Poulsen PL, Rasmussen AK, et al. Survival and long-term biochemical cure in medullary thyroid carcinoma in Denmark 1997-2014: a Nationwide study. Thyroid. 2019;29(3):368–77. https://doi.org/10.1089/thy.2018.0564.
70. Momin S, Chute D, Burkey B, Scharpf J. Prognostic variables affecting primary treatment outcome for medullary thyroid cancer. Endocr Pract. 2017;23(9):1053–8. https://doi.org/10.4158/EP161684.OR.
71. Gimm O, Ukkat J, Dralle H. Determinative factors of biochemical cure after primary and reoperative surgery for sporadic medullary thyroid carcinoma. World J Surg. 1998;22(6):562–7; discussion 7-8. https://doi.org/10.1007/s002689900435.
72. Ito Y, Miyauchi A, Kihara M, Higashiiyama T, Fukushima M, Miya A. Static prognostic factors and appropriate surgical designs for patients with medullary thyroid carcinoma: the second report from a single-institution study in Japan. World J Surg. 2018;42(12):3954–66. https://doi.org/10.1007/s00268-018-4738-z.
73. Machens A, Hauptmann S, Dralle H. Prediction of lateral lymph node metastases in medullary thyroid cancer. Br J Surg. 2008;95(5):586–91. https://doi.org/10.1002/bjs.6075.

74. McMullen C, Rocke D, Freeman J. Complications of bilateral neck dissection in thyroid cancer from a single high-volume center. JAMA Otolaryngol Head Neck Surg. 2017;143(4):376–81. https://doi.org/10.1001/jamaoto.2016.3670.
75. Machens A, Gimm O, Ukkat J, Hinze R, Schneyer U, Dralle H. Improved prediction of calcitonin normalization in medullary thyroid carcinoma patients by quantitative lymph node analysis. Cancer. 2000;88(8):1909–15.
76. Polistena A, Sanguinetti A, Lucchini R, Galasse S, Monacelli M, Avenia S, et al. Timing and extension of lymphadenectomy in medullary thyroid carcinoma: a case series from a single institution. Int J Surg. 2017;41(Suppl 1):S70–S4. https://doi.org/10.1016/j.ijsu.2017.04.026.
77. Scheuba C, Kaserer K, Weinhausl A, Pandev R, Kaider A, Passler C, et al. Is medullary thyroid cancer predictable? A prospective study of 86 patients with abnormal pentagastrin tests. Surgery. 1999;126(6):1089–95; discussion 96.
78. Machens A, Holzhausen HJ, Dralle H. Prediction of mediastinal lymph node metastasis in medullary thyroid carcinoma. Br J Surg. 2004;91(6):709–12. https://doi.org/10.1002/bjs.4525.
79. Brierley J, Gospodarowicz MK, Wittekind C. TNM classification of malignant tumours. 8th ed. Chichester, West Sussex/Hoboken: John Wiley & Sons, Inc.; 2017.
80. Bugalho MJ, Domingues R, Santos JR, Catarino AL, Sobrinho L. Mutation analysis of the RET proto-oncogene and early thyroidectomy: results of a Portuguese cancer centre. Surgery. 2007;141(1):90–5. https://doi.org/10.1016/j.surg.2006.03.025.
81. Elisei R, Romei C, Cosci B, Agate L, Bottici V, Molinaro E, et al. RET genetic screening in patients with medullary thyroid cancer and their relatives: experience with 807 individuals at one center. J Clin Endocrinol Metab. 2007;92(12):4725–9. https://doi.org/10.1210/jc.2007-1005.
82. Eng C, Smith DP, Mulligan LM, Healey CS, Zvelebil MJ, Stonehouse TJ, et al. A novel point mutation in the tyrosine kinase domain of the RET proto-oncogene in sporadic medullary thyroid carcinoma and in a family with FMTC. Oncogene. 1995;10(3):509–13.
83. Romei C, Cosci B, Renzini G, Bottici V, Molinaro E, Agate L, et al. RET genetic screening of sporadic medullary thyroid cancer (MTC) allows the preclinical diagnosis of unsuspected gene carriers and the identification of a relevant percentage of hidden familial MTC (FMTC). Clin Endocrinol. 2011;74(2):241–7. https://doi.org/10.1111/j.1365-2265.2010.03900.x.
84. Schuffenecker I, Ginet N, Goldgar D, Eng C, Chambe B, Boneu A, et al. Prevalence and parental origin of de novo RET mutations in multiple endocrine neoplasia type 2A and familial medullary thyroid carcinoma. Le Groupe d'Etude des Tumeurs a Calcitonine. Am J Hum Genet. 1997;60(1):233–7.
85. Wiench M, Wygoda Z, Gubala E, Wloch J, Lisowska K, Krassowski J, et al. Estimation of risk of inherited medullary thyroid carcinoma in apparent sporadic patients. J Clin Oncol. 2001;19(5):1374–80. https://doi.org/10.1200/JCO.2001.19.5.1374.
86. Elisei R, Alevizaki M, Conte-Devolx B, Frank-Raue K, Leite V, Williams GR. 2012 European thyroid association guidelines for genetic testing and its clinical consequences in medullary thyroid cancer. Eur Thyroid J. 2013;1(4):216–31. https://doi.org/10.1159/000346174.
87. Hubert J, Wolfe Kenneth EW., Melvin Sergio J, Cervi-Skinner Abdul A, AL Saadi Joseph F, Juliar Charles E, Jackson Armen H, Tashjian. C-Cell Hyperplasia Preceding Medullary Thyroid Carcinoma. New England Journal of Medicine 1973;289(9):437–41 https://doi.org/10.1056/NEJM197308302890901.
88. Samuel A., Wells Furio, Pacini Bruce G., Robinson Massimo, Santoro. Multiple Endocrine Neoplasia Type 2 and Familial Medullary Thyroid

Carcinoma: An Update. The Journal of Clinical Endocrinology & Metabolism 2013;98(8):3149–64. https://doi.org/10.1210/jc.2013-1204.
89. Morris LF, Waguespack SG, Edeiken-Monroe BS, Lee JE, Rich TA, Ying AK, et al. Ultrasonography should not guide the timing of thyroidectomy in pediatric patients diagnosed with multiple endocrine neoplasia syndrome 2A through genetic screening. Ann Surg Oncol. 2013;20(1):53–9. https://doi.org/10.1245/s10434-012-2589-7.
90. Machens A, Lorenz K, Dralle H. Individualization of lymph node dissection in RET (rearranged during transfection) carriers at risk for medullary thyroid cancer: value of pretherapeutic calcitonin levels. Ann Surg. 2009;250(2):305–10. https://doi.org/10.1097/SLA.0b013e3181ae333f.
91. Machens A, Elwerr M, Thanh PN, Lorenz K, Schneider R, Dralle H. Impact of central node dissection on postoperative morbidity in pediatric patients with suspected or proven thyroid cancer. Surgery. 2016;160(2):484–92. https://doi.org/10.1016/j.surg.2016.03.007.
92. Kluijfhout WP, van Beek DJ, Verrijn Stuart AA, Lodewijk L, Valk GD, van der Zee DC, et al. Postoperative complications after prophylactic thyroidectomy for very young patients with multiple endocrine Neoplasia type 2: retrospective cohort analysis. Medicine (Baltimore). 2015;94(29):e1108. https://doi.org/10.1097/MD.0000000000001108.
93. R., Elisei M., Alevizaki B., Conte-Devolx K., Frank-Raue V., Leite G.R., Williams. 2012 European Thyroid Association Guidelines for Genetic Testing and Its Clinical Consequences in Medullary Thyroid Cancer. European Thyroid Journal 2012;1(4)216–31 https://doi.org/10.1159/000346174.
94. Brauckhoff M, Machens A, Lorenz K, Bjoro T, Varhaug JE, Dralle H. Surgical curability of medullary thyroid cancer in multiple endocrine neoplasia 2B: a changing perspective. Ann Surg. 2014;259(4):800–6. https://doi.org/10.1097/SLA.0b013e3182a6f43a.
95. Cupisti K, Wolf A, Raffel A, Schott M, Miersch D, Yang Q, et al. Long-term clinical and biochemical follow-up in medullary thyroid carcinoma: a single institution's experience over 20 years. Ann Surg. 2007;246(5):815–21. https://doi.org/10.1097/SLA.0b013e31813e66b9.
96. Kebebew E, Kikuchi S, Duh QY, Clark OH. Long-term results of reoperation and localizing studies in patients with persistent or recurrent medullary thyroid cancer. Arch Surg. 2000;135(8):895–901. https://doi.org/10.1001/archsurg.135.8.895.
97. Roman S, Lin R, Sosa JA. Prognosis of medullary thyroid carcinoma: demographic, clinical, and pathologic predictors of survival in 1252 cases. Cancer. 2006;107(9):2134–42. https://doi.org/10.1002/cncr.22244.
98. Engelbach M, Görges R, Forst T, Pfützner A, Dawood R, Heerdt S, et al. Improved diagnostic methods in the follow-up of medullary thyroid carcinoma by highly specific calcitonin measurements. J Clin Endocrinol Metab. 2000;85(5):1890–4. https://doi.org/10.1210/jcem.85.5.6601.
99. Machens A, Lorenz K, Dralle H. Time to calcitonin normalization after surgery for node-negative and node-positive medullary thyroid cancer. Br J Surg. 2019;106(4):412–8. https://doi.org/10.1002/bjs.11071.
100. Ismailov SI, Piulatova NR. Postoperative calcitonin study in medullary thyroid carcinoma. Endocr Relat Cancer. 2004;11(2):357–63. https://doi.org/10.1677/erc.0.0110357.
101. Elisei R, Pinchera A. Advances in the follow-up of differentiated or medullary thyroid cancer. Nat Rev Endocrinol. 2012;8(8):466–75. https://doi.org/10.1038/nrendo.2012.38.
102. Franc S, Niccoli-Sire P, Cohen R, Bardet S, Maes B, Murat A, et al. Complete surgical lymph node resection does not prevent authentic recurrences of medullary thyroid carcinoma. Clin Endocrinol. 2001;55(3):403–9. https://doi.org/10.1046/j.1365-2265.2001.01339.x.

103. Machens A, Dralle H. Prognostic impact of N staging in 715 medullary thyroid cancer patients: proposal for a revised staging system. Ann Surg. 2013;257(2):323–9. https://doi.org/10.1097/SLA.0b013e318268301d.
104. Rowland KJ, Jin LX, Moley JF. Biochemical cure after reoperations for medullary thyroid carcinoma: a meta-analysis. Ann Surg Oncol. 2015;22(1):96–102. https://doi.org/10.1245/s10434-014-4102-y.
105. Gawlik T, d'Amico A, Szpak-Ulczok S, Skoczylas A, Gubala E, Chorazy A, et al. The prognostic value of tumor markers doubling times in medullary thyroid carcinoma - preliminary report. Thyroid Res. 2010;3(1):10. https://doi.org/10.1186/1756-6614-3-10.
106. Barbet J, Campion L, Kraeber-Bodere F, Chatal JF, Group GTES. Prognostic impact of serum calcitonin and carcinoembryonic antigen doubling-times in patients with medullary thyroid carcinoma. J Clin Endocrinol Metab. 2005;90(11):6077–84. https://doi.org/10.1210/jc.2005-0044.
107. Tappenden P, Carroll C, Hamilton J, Kaltenthaler E, Wong R, Wadsley J, et al. Cabozantinib and vandetanib for unresectable locally advanced or metastatic medullary thyroid cancer: a systematic review and economic model. Health Technol Assess. 2019;23(8):1–144. https://doi.org/10.3310/hta23080.
108. Schlumberger M, Elisei R, Muller S, Schoffski P, Brose M, Shah M, et al. Overall survival analysis of EXAM, a phase III trial of cabozantinib in patients with radiographically progressive medullary thyroid carcinoma. Ann Oncol. 2017;28(11):2813–9. https://doi.org/10.1093/annonc/mdx479.
109. Wells SA Jr, Gosnell JE, Gagel RF, Moley J, Pfister D, Sosa JA, et al. Vandetanib for the treatment of patients with locally advanced or metastatic hereditary medullary thyroid cancer. J Clin Oncol. 2010;28(5):767–72. https://doi.org/10.1200/JCO.2009.23.6604.
110. Wells SA Jr, Robinson BG, Gagel RF, Dralle H, Fagin JA, Santoro M, et al. Vandetanib in patients with locally advanced or metastatic medullary thyroid cancer: a randomized, double-blind phase III trial. J Clin Oncol. 2012;30(2):134–41. https://doi.org/10.1200/JCO.2011.35.5040.

Anaplastic Thyroid Carcinoma, Thyroid Lymphoma, and Metastases

Kelly F. Moyer, Richard J. Wong, and Ashok R. Shaha

Contents

A. L. Shifrin et al. (eds.), *Endocrine Surgery Comprehensive Board Exam Guide*,
https://doi.org/10.1007/978-3-030-84737-1_9

Case Presentation

Patient is an 80-year-old man who first noted a lump in his neck about 2 years ago. It was initially thought to be infectious and no workup was pursued, but over time became concerning because it began to grow rapidly over the last month prior to presentation. A thyroid ultrasound demonstrated a large right thyroid lobe nodule measuring 7.8 x 5.4 x 5.1 cm. Two weeks following ultrasound, the patient was admitted to the emergency room with hemoptysis. He also complained of cough, fatigue, headaches, and shortness of breath. He reported tolerating a regular diet, but had recent weight loss. A CT scan with contrast of the neck then revealed a large, right thyroid mass measuring 10.3 x 8.9 x 9.3 centimeters with signs of metastatic adenopathy in the neck, including a node in the right carotid sheath measuring 2.4 x 2.6 cm. The mass was shown to be invading the right sternocleidomastoid muscle and abutting the larynx, with infiltration of the thyroid lamina on the right side and into the paraglottic space. There is mass effect noted on the trachea.

Physical examination reveals vital signs within normal range, a well-nourished man in no acute distress. There is an extremely large, fixed mass filling the entire right neck and extending across the midline. It is fixed to the larynx. There is no obvious palpable lymphadenopathy. His voice is hoarse, but he has no dyspnea or stridor. Endoscopic laryngoscopy shows an immobile right vocal cord, edematous pyriform sinus, and right hemilarynx.

Labs are remarkable for calcium 9.2, albumin 3.8, thyroglobulin antibody 1.5, calcitonin <0.5, T3 73, Free T4 1.05, TSH 4.46, Thyroglobulin 50. CBC with WBC 13, platelets 400, neutrophils 80, ANC 10.3.

9

Questions

1. What diagnoses are most likely in a patient with a rapidly growing thyroid mass?
    1. Anaplastic thyroid carcinoma
    2. Renal cell carcinoma metastasis
    3. Papillary thyroid cancer
    4. Primary thyroid lymphoma
    5. Medullary thyroid cancer
        (a) Only (1) and (2) and (3) are correct.
        (b) Only (1) and (2) and (4) are correct.
        (c) Only (1) and (4) are correct.
        (d) Only (3) and (4) and (5) are correct.
        (e) All are correct.
2. FNA of a rapidly growing thyroid mass is nondiagnostic. What is the next best step?
    1. Core needle biopsy
    2. Repeat FNA
    3. Open surgical biopsy
    4. Total thyroidectomy
    5. Thyroid lobectomy
        (a) (1)
        (b) (2)
        (c) (3)
        (d) (4)
        (e) (5)

3. Biopsy of a thyroid mass reveals high mitotic activity, bizarre cells, and extensive necrosis. ATC is diagnosed, and early molecular markers are sent for targetable treatment options. Which molecular markers should be studied?
   1. NTRK
   2. RET
   3. BRAF
   4. RAS
   5. Overall high mutational load
      (a) Only (1) and (2) and (3) are correct.
      (b) Only (1) and (2) and (4) are correct.
      (c) Only (1) and (2) and (3) and (4) are correct.
      (d) Only (1) and (2) and (5) are correct.
      (e) All are correct.
4. What is the most common primary malignancy with metastases to the thyroid gland?
   1. Renal cell carcinoma (RCC)
   2. Prostate cancer
   3. Rhabdomyosarcoma
   4. Colorectal cancer
   5. Breast cancer
      (a) Only (1) is correct.
      (b) Only (2) is correct.
      (c) Only (3) is correct.
      (d) Only (4) is correct.
      (e) Only (5) is correct.
5. Airway management in rapidly enlarging thyroid mass should include the following:
   1. Physical examination
   2. Fiber-optic laryngoscopy
   3. Bronchoscopy
   4. Pulmonary function tests
   5. CT neck with contrast
      (a) Only (1) and (2) are correct.
      (b) Only (1) and (2) and (3) are correct.
      (c) Only (1) and (2) and (3) are correct.
      (d) Only (1) and (2) and (3) and (5) are correct.
      (e) All are correct.
6. Surgical management is most often indicated for the following thyroid pathologies:
   1. Stage IVA + B anaplastic thyroid cancer
   2. Renal cell carcinoma metastasis to the thyroid
   3. Stage IE thyroid lymphoma
   4. Stage IIE thyroid lymphoma
   5. Colorectal cancer metastasis to the thyroid
      (a) Only (1) and (2) are correct.
      (b) Only (1) and (2) and (3) are correct.
      (c) Only (1) and (2) and (5) are correct.
      (d) Only (1) and (2) and (3) and (5) are correct.
      (e) All are correct.

7. Promising targeted therapies for treatment of anaplastic thyroid cancer include the following molecular targets:
   1. BRAF
   2. NTRK
   3. RET fusion
   4. TP53
   5. VEGF
      (a) (1) and (2) and (3) only
      (b) (1) and (2) and (5) only
      (c) (1) and (2) and (4) only
      (d) (1) and (2) only
      (e) (1) and (3) only
8. The preferred chemotherapy regimen for advanced stage thyroid lymphoma is
   1. EPOCH (etoposide, prednisone, vincristine, cyclophosphamide, doxorubicin)
   2. RCHOP (rituximab, cyclophosphamide, doxorubicin, vincristine, prednisolone)
   3. FOLFOX (5-FU, leucovorin, oxaliplatin)
   4. TPF (docetaxel, cisplatin, 5-FU)
   5. GVD (gemcitabine, vinorelbine, doxorubicin)
      (a) (1)
      (b) (2)
      (c) (3)
      (d) (4)
      (e) (5)

9. Mortality in anaplastic thyroid cancer can be related to the following:
   1. Airway obstruction
   2. Catastrophic hemorrhage
   3. Distant metastasis
   4. Circulatory failure due to compression of mediastinal vasculature
   5. Local invasion
      (a) Only (1) and (2) are correct.
      (b) Only (1) and (2) and (4) are correct.
      (c) Only (1) and (2) and (4) and (5) are correct.
      (d) Only (1) and (4) and (5) are correct.
      (e) All are correct.
10. Surgical management of metastases to the thyroid gland most commonly includes
    1. Metastectomy
    2. Thyroid lobectomy
    3. Total thyroidectomy
    4. Total thyroidectomy with central neck dissection
    5. Tracheal resection
       (a) Only (1) and (2) are correct.
       (b) Only (1) and (2) and (3) are correct.
       (c) Only (1) and (2) and (4) are correct.
       (d) Only (1) and (2) and (3) and (4) are correct.
       (e) All are correct.

9.1 Introduction

Thyroid cancer is typically classified based on cell of origin, with the more common cancers being of follicular cell origin, including papillary, follicular, and Hurthle cell cancers. Less common cancers of neuroendocrine origin include medullary thyroid cancer [1]. When presented with a thyroid mass, clinicians must also consider the rarer tumors of the thyroid gland including anaplastic thyroid carcinoma, lymphoma, and metastatic tumors to the thyroid gland.

Anaplastic thyroid carcinoma (ATC) is an aggressive, undifferentiated tumor originating from the follicular epithelium of the thyroid gland [1]. It is postulated this tumor may develop from the dedifferentiation of existing well-differentiated thyroid cancers, but there is evidence that quite often may develop de novo [2]. ATC is quite rare, with approximately one to two cases per one million persons [3]. It is more prevalent in the elderly, with the mean age at diagnosis of 65 years. It is more common in women than men [4, 5]. Although it comprises only 1% of all thyroid cancers, ATC has significant mortality and accounts for up to 35% of all deaths from thyroid cancer in some series [6, 7].

Lymphoma of the thyroid gland is almost always non-Hodgkin's lymphoma; it is very rare to have a Hodgkin's lymphoma arise in the thyroid gland [8]. When considering all extranodal lymphomas, only about 2% occur in the thyroid gland [9]. By subtype, there are two distinct groups of thyroid lymphoma. The more common type, comprising approximately 70% of cases, is diffuse large B-cell lymphoma (DLBCL). This subtype has a more aggressive clinical course with the majority of patients diagnosed with already disseminated disease. Another subtype includes mucosa-associated lymphoid tissue (MALT) lymphoma, only up to 25% of thyroid lymphomas. These have relatively indolent course [10]. Similar to anaplastic disease, the mean age of thyroid lymphoma at diagnosis is 65 years and several series indicate a female predominance [11–14]. Hashimoto's thyroiditis is a known risk factor for thyroid lymphoma, seen in about 50% of patients [15–17].

Metastases of nonthyroid malignancies to the thyroid gland are very uncommon, however, must remain on the differential. It is important to consider metastases in patients who present with a thyroid mass and any history, however remote, of prior malignancy. Nonthyroid malignancies have been reported in 1–3% of all patients who have surgery for suspected cancer in the thyroid gland [18]. The most commonly reported malignancies with metastases to the thyroid are renal cell carcinoma (RCC) and lung, colorectal, and breast carcinoma [19–22]. Metastatic melanoma is also relatively common in this group. The literature reports isolated cases of numerous carcinomas metastasizing to the thyroid gland, including urothelial sarcomatoid, bladder, endometrial, neuroendocrine, gastrointestinal stromal tumor (GIST), intraductal papillary-mucinous carcinoma of the pancreas, ovarian, testicular seminoma, and uterine [19–25].

Although these rare tumors of the thyroid gland will be seen infrequently, the presentation, diagnosis, and management are clinically significant. Because of clinical parallels in their presentation and the rarity of occurrence, they are addressed together as a group.

9.2 Clinical Presentation

As a classic teaching, patients with anaplastic thyroid carcinoma first present with a rapidly expanding neck mass [26]. Physical examination typically reveals a diffuse, enlarged thyroid. The mass is firm, immobile, and may be tender. There can be multifocal nodules in the gland or one large index nodule, but often ill-defined in nature. At the time of presentation, the diameter of the tumor can be quite large and exceed 5 cm [27]. A rapidly enlarging thyroid mass should also prompt consideration for thyroid lymphoma. Thyroid lymphoma is similarly firm to palpation and possibly tender, and may be fixed to adjacent structures. Substernal extension is common [28].

With both anaplastic thyroid carcinoma and thyroid lymphoma, because of the rapid progression and large size, local invasion is frequently seen at presentation of disease. Nearby structures, including muscles, lymph nodes, esophagus, larynx, and trachea, can be involved and cause clinical symptoms. The most frequent symptoms are hoarseness, dysphagia, dyspnea, and stridor [6, 11–13, 15, 29–32]. When hoarseness is present in either disease, flexible laryngoscopy is indicated and will commonly reveal vocal cord immobility [28].

Some differentiating features between anaplastic thyroid carcinoma and lymphoma may be accompanying symptoms, as well as thyroid function. Classic systemic "B" symptoms associated with lymphomas, such as fever, night sweats, and weight loss, should be elicited in the history of a patient with an enlarging thyroid mass. These "B" symptoms can be seen in about 10% of patients with thyroid lymphoma [33].

Thyroid function tests are usually normal in anaplastic thyroid carcinoma; however, laboratory tests should include electrolytes, serum urea nitrogen, creatinine, glucose, and liver function tests. Thyroid function tests should be obtained because large masses may have compromised thyroid function, and some cases of ATC are associated with significant thyrotoxicosis [34, 35]. In approximately 10% of patients with thyroid lymphoma, thyroid dysfunction can be seen. It is usually related to underlying Hashimoto's, but occasionally secondary to infiltration of the thyroid gland with lymphoma [33]. Hyperthyroidism has also been described secondary to tumor-induced inflammation or pre-existing Graves' disease [36].

About 50% of thyroid non-Hodgkin's lymphomas have a clinical history of chronic lymphocytic thyroiditis and two-thirds show histology consistent with chronic lymphocytic thyroiditis [37]. It is thought that lymphomas originating in a wide variety of primary sites represent a malignant transformation of lymphocytic tissue during a chronic inflammatory or an autoimmune process [38].

Metastases to the thyroid gland are typically found in routine workup of a new thyroid nodule. The majority of symptoms described in large retrospective studies include new or enlarging thyroid nodule, neck swelling, dysphagia, dysphonia, or cough. It has been described that metastatic disease can also present with a rapidly enlarging mass, however, much less commonly [39, 40]. Up to 25% of cases of metastases to the thyroid gland are incidentally found. The literature describes numerous cases of patients undergoing thyroidectomy for other indications and only after histological examination of the specimen is metastatic disease identified. Routine imaging studies for other indications are commonly the first indicator of metastatic disease [41].

9.3 Diagnosis

In a patient who presents with a new thyroid mass, particularly a rapidly enlarging one, it is critical to obtain a complete history, paying special attention to any known risk factors. For anaplastic thyroid carcinoma, the history may include a patient of older age, history of radiation, established goiter, or family history of thyroid disease [5, 42]. A comprehensive review of symptoms will elicit possible systemic "B" symptoms for patients with lymphoma, as previously described.

Any history of other cancers should be discussed with the patient and, when present, timely consideration to the possibility of metastases. Metastases can be synchronous or metachronous. Thyroid metastases can present many years after initial diagnosis and treatment for another malignancy [43]. In some series, the mean interval of metachronous thyroid metastases is approximately 6 years [20, 24]. The most common synchronous thyroid metastasis is renal cell carcinoma [21].

A full diagnostic physical examination should be performed. Anaplastic carcinoma and lymphoma may reveal a fixed mass indicating local invasion. With large thyroid masses, respiratory symptoms, or hoarseness, careful attention to airway management is warranted. To evaluate the airway and mobility of vocal cords, all patients should undergo fiber-optic laryngoscopy. Local invasion of the larynx may result in an immobile vocal cord through direct extension to the paraglottic space or paratracheal involvement, damaging the recurrent laryngeal nerve [6].

A bronchoscopy should be planned to evaluate the trachea if the laryngoscopy shows evidence of airway invasion. Bronchoscopy is useful for determining extent of disease, evaluation of the tracheal lumen, luminal obstruction, and resectability of the tumor, if indicated. Similarly, an esophagoscopy should be performed if there is suspected esophageal invasion, particularly when there is dysphagia or odynophagia [44]. A clinical neck exam will often reveal metastatic disease in anaplastic thyroid carcinoma with locoregional spread to lymph nodes noted in over 50% of cases [6].

As with any new clinically evident thyroid nodule, initial workup should include imaging with ultrasound. Thyroid and neck ultrasounds should be performed to evaluate the primary tumor and assess cervical lymph nodes for metastatic disease. The basins of interest include the central and lateral compartments of the neck [44]. On ultrasound, lymphoma will appear hypoechoic and pseudocystic. A series of 46 patients with thyroid lymphoma described the vast majority with a characteristic asymmetrical pseudocystic pattern [45].

The National Comprehensive Cancer Network (NCCN) guidelines recommend fine-needle aspiration biopsy or core biopsy for preoperative diagnosis of ATC and lymphoma. If the FNA results are limited or nondiagnostic, open biopsy should be performed in order to confirm the diagnosis [46]. However, core biopsy with appropriate immunohistochemistry and flow cytometry will help to confirm the diagnosis.

Anaplastic thyroid carcinomas exhibit wide variations of morphology and cytologic patterns, with many tumors manifesting mixed morphology [47, 48]. Cytology from ATC nodules typically reveals multinucleated cells with large, bizarre nuclei and atypical mitotic features, without features of thyroid differentiation [1]. Commonly, the biphasic spindle and giant cell tumor are seen [49]. There is usually extensive necrosis, often so diffuse that that the only viable tumor is preserved around blood vessels. Inflammatory infiltrates are frequently seen with necrosis. Osteoclast-like giant cells may be identified and have been shown by immunohistochemical studies to be of the monocytic or histiocytic lineage [50, 51].

Well-differentiated papillary carcinoma, often the tall cell variant, is the most common coexistent carcinoma with anaplastic thyroid carcinoma, followed by conventional follicular carcinoma or Hürthle cell type [52]. Molecular profiling in anaplastic thyroid carcinoma is fast becoming the most important step in the initial workup. New data on actionable mutations including *BRAF* V600E, *NTRK* gene fusion and *RET* fusion are revolutionizing treatment for ATC. Genomic testing and mutational tumor burden are now imperative recommended initial diagnostic studies in treating this disease [46]. Exciting new treatments based on molecular profiling will be discussed in the treatment section.

When FNA is obtained in lymphoma, it will likely show a highly cellular sample comprised predominantly of a monomorphic population of lymphoid cells with high nuclear: cytoplasmic (N:C) ratio and scant cytoplasm. Nuclei are typically round to oval with fine chromatin. Centrocytes, mature lymphocytes, macrophages, plasma cells, and occasionally mast cells may be seen in the background [53]. Immunohistochemical staining and flow cytometry are usually necessary to confirm monoclonal populations in lymphoma and characterize surface markers. FNA can suggest lymphoma, but typically is nondiagnostic [45].

Generally, for all lymphomas, including thyroid lymphomas, the addition of flow cytometry yields a sensitivity of 97% and specificity of 87% for the detection of B-cell lymphoma. Inadequate sampling is a limiting factor for performing flow cytometry [54, 55]. A small retrospective study demonstrates that core biopsy can improve the diagnostic accuracy when compared with FNA and flow cytometry alone [56]. Open surgical biopsy is recommended only when less invasive techniques cannot achieve a definitive diagnosis or when identification of the exact subtype is required for specific treatment [32].

In metastases to the thyroid gland, FNA may be inaccurate. In a series of 167 patients with thyroid metastases, FNA was correct in approximately 75% of the cases. However, in the other 25%, the FNA diagnosed primary thyroid malignancy instead of metastatic disease. When there is a history of previous cancer, a high suspicion for metastases must always be maintained [18]. A review and comparison of the previous index tumor pathology will help the pathologist to suspect metastatic tumor.

With large, rapidly enlarging thyroid masses, cross-sectional imaging is appropriate to adequately evaluate the airway at the time of diagnosis. High-resolution cross-sectional imaging is critical for surgical planning, when indicated. Computed tomography (CT) with contrast of the neck and mediastinum provides high-resolution assessment of locoregional involvement and invasion of critical aerodigestive structures. On CT, anaplastic masses appear isodense or slightly hyperdense relative to muscle [57, 58]. These masses are frequently heterogeneous with areas of necrosis and calcifications. Careful attention must be paid to the imaging in cases of surgical resection, as local structures must be clearly delineated from the heterogeneous, poorly defined nature of the mass.

Staging of anaplastic thyroid carcinoma, based on the American Joint Committee on Cancer (AJCC) 8th edition (October 2016), helps to provide stratification of management. As all anaplastic thyroid carcinomas are stage IV tumors, they are subclassified as Stage IVA (intrathyroidal tumor), IVB [gross extrathyroidal extension (ETE) or cervical lymph node metastasis] or IVC (distant metastasis). The T stage is dependent on tumor size and ETE. T1 disease is less than or equal to 2 centimeters, T2 is 2–4 centimeters, and T3 tumors are greater than 4 centimeters. T3a is disease limited to the thyroid and T3b has gross ETE into strap muscles. T4 disease occurs when there is gross ETE into major neck structures [59, 60]. The staging system can be used to ensure that patients receive the appropriate treatment in order to maximize survival.

The Lugano staging system is used for staging primary thyroid lymphoma [61]. PET/CT can be used for FDG-avid lymphoma staging and CT alone can be used for small lymphocytic lymphomas. Approximately 50% of patients presenting with thyroid lymphoma will have Stage IE disease, defined as being limited to the thyroid gland. Another 45% of patients will have Stage IIE disease with the presence of locoregional nodes. Only the remaining 5% will have distant disease or diffuse organ involvement (Stage IIIE or IV). Almost 80% of patients have limited disease on presentation [15, 28].

9.4 Treatment

Treatment of anaplastic thyroid cancer is largely multimodal, with the most recent NCCN Guidelines recommending surgery, external beam radiation, and chemotherapy/radiosensitizing agents. Different combinations are recommended depending on the characteristics of each particular case [46]. The multidisciplinary approach maximizes survival and provides for a well-balanced treatment plan to optimize quality of life. It is also important in the management of anaplastic thyroid carcinoma to achieve the best balance between quality of life and longevity in a generally fatal disease.

Unlike differentiated thyroid carcinomas, poorly differentiated or undifferentiated tumors cannot concentrate iodine, express TSH receptor, or produce thyroglobulin (Tg). Therefore, 131I imaging and thyroglobulin measurement are not used in anaplastic thyroid carcinoma and radioactive iodine treatment is not effective [44, 62].

Cytogenetics of anaplastic thyroid carcinoma is complex and often shows progressive accumulation of chromosomal alterations (numerical and structural aberrations). The most common mutations are in TP53 (nuclear expression), but BRAF V600E, RAS, PIK3CA, and PTEN are also present in about 10–20% of cases [63, 64]. TP53 gene inactivation plays a role in the progression from differentiated to undifferentiated carcinoma [65].

Groundbreaking data published by Subbiah et al. in 2018 in the *Journal of Clinical Oncology* reported efficacy and safety of dabrafenib (BRAF inhibitor) and trametinib (MEK inhibitor) combination therapy in *BRAF* V600E–mutated anaplastic thyroid cancer. This series cites up to 50% of anaplastic thyroid carcinoma cases possessing the *BRAF* V600E mutation. Animal models cited suggest the combined inhibition of BRAF and MEK improves treatment response and can prevent MAPK pathway reactivation, a known resistance mechanism. This combination has previously shown efficacy in melanoma and lung cancer. The overall response rate of dabrafenib and trametinb in ATC was 69% in this series with a 12-month estimate of duration of response of 90%. The Kaplan-Meier 12-month estimate of overall survival was remarkable at 80% [66]. This data led to the FDA approval of this combination for *BRAF* V600E-mutant anaplastic thyroid carcinoma without locoregional treatment options, making it the first newly approved therapy for ATC in approximately 50 years.

Important other new data also emphasizes the utilization of next-generation sequencing (NGS) in thyroid cancer. Neurotrophic receptor tyrosine kinase genes *NTRK1, NTRK2*, and *NTRK3* encode TRK proteins. Fusion events involving these genes have been identified across diverse cancers that occur in children and adults. Animal models suggest TRK fusions may be implicated in up to 1% of all solid tumors [67–70]. Larotrectinib and entrectanib are highly selective small-molecule inhibitors of TRK proteins and have significant and durable therapeutic effects in TRK fusion–positive cancers. This new data underscores the need to routinely test mutations to increase the therapeutic options available for patients who previously suffered from untreatable diseases like anaplastic thyroid carcinoma [71, 72].

RET gene fusions were previously identified in more well-differentiated thyroid cancers, but were absent from anaplastic thyroid carcinoma. However, in newer data, patients with metastatic ATC have identifiable RET fusions that have been treated with lenvatinib and selpercatinib with acceptable partial response [73, 74] New data even suggests that tumors with high mutational burden (≥10 mut/Mb) will be sensitive to pembrolizumab and is recommended as an additional possible treatment [46, 75].

Histological subtype and staging of thyroid lymphoma will guide treatment. Combined chemotherapy and radiation therapy for limited lymphoma is associated with a higher survival rate versus chemotherapy alone [76]. Advanced stage disease is treated with chemotherapy alone. The preferred regimen is R-CHOP (rituximab, cyclophosphamide, doxorubicin, vincristine, prednisolone). Distant disease is the most commonly seen treatment failure. Surgery is generally not recommended with additional benefit compared to chemoradiation therapy [32].

Obstructive symptoms associated with thyroid lymphomas usually improve within hours of initiating R-CHOP because of steroid action. With rapid diagnosis and initiation of treatment, tracheostomy and thyroidectomy can be avoided even in severe cases. Thyroid hormone replacement is the management strategy for hypothyroidism due to Hashimoto thyroiditis, diffuse thyroid gland infiltration, or radiation-associated dysfunction [32].

Because of possible inaccuracy of FNA in metastatic disease, some authors recommend thyroidectomy as treatment in patients with nodular goiters with a history of malignancy [21, 77]. As an abnormal thyroid gland may increase the likelihood of metastatic deposits, patients with abnormal thyroid lesions should be followed carefully with regular clinical exam and serial ultrasounds. This follow-up is especially important in those patients with nondiagnostic or equivocal FNA who do not undergo thyroidectomy [18].

9.5 Indications for Surgery and Surgical Details

Surgery is a critical component of treatment for anaplastic thyroid carcinoma. Primary surgical resection can be considered for patients with stage IVA or IVB disease, specifically, patients without aerodigestive tract involvement. Primary surgical treatment should be planned when gross resection (R1) is anticipated [44, 78]. There are several studies that have demonstrated survival benefit in patients with ATC if complete resection can be achieved [26, 42]. The ATA guidelines recommended a lobectomy or near-total thyroidectomy with lymph node dissection for patients with intrathyroidal disease (Stage IVA). En-bloc resection is advocated if grossly negative margins (R1) can be achieved for patients with extrathyroidal invasion (Stage IVB) [44].

It is important to note, however, that although most studies do show a survival benefit with R0 or R1 resection, because of the rapidly progressive nature of ATC, very few patients present with fully resectable disease. Ultimately, the surgeon must decide whether a resection can be attempted with acceptable risk and morbidity. Many patients with initially unresectable disease may benefit from external beam radiation (full or partial course) or neoadjuvant chemotherapy to shrink the tumor before undergoing surgical resection [44].

Exciting new data using targeted therapies describes successful outcomes in six patients with a BRAF-V600E mutated ATC using neoadjuvant dabrafenib and trametinib followed by complete surgical resection [79]. By using the combination targeted therapy, this important new data demonstrated that it is possible to achieve complete resection, decrease need for tracheostomy, and provide symptom relief and locoregional control. This type of targeted treatment is changing the paradigm for treating ATC. The 2020 NCCN Guidelines provide a significant focus on multimodal treatment, including this new systemic treatment option for ATC.

Additionally, data published in Thyroid in 2018 by Cabanillas et al. describe another surgical strategy with the use dabrafenib, trametinib, and pembrolizumab ("DTP") in an unresectable, end-stage, *BRAF*-mutated case of anaplastic thyroid carcinoma. Complete surgical resection was only possible after a meaningful clinical response to these agents. Using BRAF- and immune-directed drugs combined with surgical treatment is another approach that is changing the overall landscape of treatment for anaplastic thyroid carcinoma. Survival is significantly improved, patients can avoid tracheostomy, and overall quality of life is greatly enhanced [80]. The new 2020 NCCN Guidelines for thyroid cancer reflect these exciting new developments and recommend targeted and immune-directed therapies in conjunction with surgery in the treatment of anaplastic thyroid carcinoma.

Thyroid lobectomy or total thyroidectomy is usually considered in the cases of thyroid metastases either with the aim of long-term cure or achieving local control [23]. Careful consideration must be given to the balance between the course of systemic disease versus the morbidities associated with uncontrolled local disease. The data regarding those patients with thyroid metastases who should undergo surgery is unclear. Local invasion causing aerodigestive symptoms typically is an indication for surgical intervention to prevent airway compromise. If the metastasis is confined to the thyroid gland without significant extrathyroidal extension, thyroidectomy may be performed with minimal morbidity [18, 81, 82]. When considering thyroid surgery for palliative intent, the burden of disease, overall risk-benefit analysis, and individual patient characteristics should be thoughtfully deliberated [83].

Mean survival after surgical intervention for thyroid metastases is approximately 2 years, with 5-year overall survival of 42%. However, in the majority of those patients who are selected for surgical removal of metastases, long-term control of the central neck can be achieved [84, 85]. A recent meta-analysis suggests that those patients managed with surgery have better outcomes than those managed expectantly. This benefit was most significant for renal cell carcinoma (RCC), where median survival for expectant management was 6 months versus 27 months for surgical treatment [86]. However, this retrospective analysis and inherent biases must be interpreted carefully.

For any patient considered to be candidate for thyroid surgery, regardless of the pathology, the aim should be to ensure removal of all gross disease with an adequate margin. This resectability will dictate the extent of surgery. For any of the pathology discussed, in unilateral disease, most authors favor thyroid lobectomy, when possible, to minimize risk to the contralateral recurrent laryngeal nerve and parathyroid glands. The advantages to total thyroidectomy are improved oncologic margins [83].

Traditionally, in thyroid lymphoma, surgery is indicated for diagnostic biopsy only and debulking surgery has been thought to add no benefit to treatment and may contribute to risk [32]. However, there are always selected cases where there may be a role for surgery depending on the response to treatment and clinical indication. Surgery should be reserved for those situations and at the discretion of the treating surgeon and medical oncology management team.

9.6 Prognosis

Anaplastic thyroid carcinoma historically has a poor prognosis, with high metastatic rate and often rapidly fatal course [87]. Although distant metastases are found in at least 50% of patients at presentation, the immediate cause of mortality in most patients is secondary to local complications, such as airway obstruction. Disease-specific mortality has historically been reported as exceedingly high, often documented as approaching 100% [88]. Older data reports the median survival after diagnosis is between 3 and 7 months and classic publications describe 5-year survival is as low as 5% [87]. Favorable prognostic factors for anaplastic thyroid carcinoma are young age, absence of metastatic disease, small tumors (considered 5–7 centimeters), unilateral tumors, absence of local invasion, and an incidental finding on pathology [89].

With new, promising treatment regimens on the horizon, the survival estimates of anaplastic thyroid carcinoma are greatly changing. As previously mentioned, data shows the combination of dabrafenib and trametinb in ATC has a nearly 70% response rate and 12-month overall survival of 80%. These are dramatically improved outcomes compared to expectations in the past with ATC [66]. Targeted therapies, immune-directed treatments, and radiosensitizing agents are promising new treatments for this previously universally fatal disease. The 2020 NCCN Guidelines for anaplastic thyroid carcinoma reflect these changes and recommend early molecular testing and directed therapy.

Thyroid lymphoma has a variable prognosis depending on the histology, tumor burden, stage, age, performance status, and treatment type. A series of 51 patients with limited (Stage I or II) disease demonstrates a 5-year survival rate of 91% in those who received combined chemotherapy and radiation. The same series has 76% survival for radiation alone and 50% survival for chemotherapy alone. Thyroid lymphoma, in general, has an excellent prognosis [76].

With thyroid lymphoma, the relative prognosis depends on the histological classification of the tumor and the stage. MALT lymphomas, due to a more indolent behavior and more favorable response to therapy, have a better prognosis compared to

DLBCL. The 5-year-survival rate in patients with intrathyroidal disease is 90% and decreases to 35% in patients with extrathyroidal disease. Clinical factors that may predict a worse prognosis include large tumor (>10 cm), advanced stage (greater than stage IE), presence of obstructive local symptoms, rapid growth, mediastinal involvement, elderly patients (>60 years), and elevated LDH and b2microglobulin levels [28].

Although distant metastases are widely considered as a poor prognostic factor, thyroid metastases may be an exception. While metastases to the thyroid show better outcomes than other sites, studies show 35–80% of patients with thyroid involvement present with multiorgan metastases concurrently. The overall prognosis can be most closely linked to the inherent features of the primary tumor [18].

Answers to the Questions

1. (c); 2. (a); 3. (e); 4. (a); 5. (d); 6. (c); 7. (a); 8. (b); 9. (e); 10. (d)

References

1. O'Neill JP, Shaha AR. Anaplastic thyroid cancer. Oral Oncol. 2013;49:702–6.
2. Molinaro E, Romei C, Biagini A, et al. Anaplastic thyroid carcinoma: from clinicopathology to genetics and advanced therapies. Nat Rev Endocrinol. 2017;13:644–60.
3. Davies L, Welch HG. Increasing incidence of thyroid cancer in the United States. JAMA. 2006;295:2164–7.
4. Kebebew E, Greenspan FS, Clark OH, et al. Anaplastic thyroid carcinoma. Treatment outcome and prognostic factors. Cancer. 2005;103:1330–5.
5. Hundahl SA, Cady B, Cunningham MP, et al. Initial results from a prospective cohort study of 5583 cases of thyroid carcinoma treated in the united states during. U.S. and German Thyroid Cancer Study Group. An American College of Surgeons Commission on Cancer Patient Care Evaluation study. Cancer. 2000;89:202–17.
6. Hundahl SA, Fleming ID, Fremgen AM, Menck HR. A National Cancer Database report on 53,856 cases of thyroid carcinoma treated in the US. Cancer. 1998;83:2638–48.
7. Besic N, Auersperg M, Us-Krasovec M, et al. Effect of primary treatment on survival in anaplastic thyroid carcinoma. Eur J Surg Oncol. 2001;27:260–4.
8. Wang SA, Rahemtullah A, Faquin WC, et al. Hodgkin's lymphoma of the thyroid: a clinicopathologic study of five cases and review of the literature. Mod Pathol. 2005;18:1577.
9. Freeman C, Berg JW, Cutler SJ. Occurrence and prognosis of extranodal lymphomas. Cancer. 1972;29:252.
10. Gupta N, Nijhawan R, Srinivasan R, Rajwanshi A, Dutta P, Bhansaliy A, et al. Fine needle aspiration cytology of primary thyroid lymphoma: a report of ten cases. Cytojournal. 2005;2:21.
11. Skarsgard ED, Connors JM, Robins RE. A current analysis of primary lymphoma of the thyroid. Arch Surg. 1991;126:1199.
12. Junor EJ, Paul J, Reed NS. Primary non-Hodgkin's lymphoma of the thyroid. Eur J Surg Oncol. 1992;18:313.

13. Logue JP, Hale RJ, Stewart AL, et al. Primary malignant lymphoma of the thyroid: a clinicopathological analysis. Int J Radiat Oncol Biol Phys. 1992;22:929.
14. Wolf BC, Sheahan K, DeCoste D, et al. Immunohistochemical analysis of small cell tumors of the thyroid gland: an Eastern Cooperative Oncology Group study. Hum Pathol. 1992;23:1252.
15. Pedersen RK, Pedersen NT. Primary non-Hodgkin's lymphoma of the thyroid gland: a population based study. Histopathology. 1996;28:25.
16. Holm LE, Blomgren H, Löwhagen T. Cancer risks in patients with chronic lymphocytic thyroiditis. N Engl J Med. 1985;312:601.
17. Hyjek E, Isaacson PG. Primary B cell lymphoma of the thyroid and its relationship to Hashimoto's thyroiditis. Hum Pathol. 1988;19:1315.
18. Chung AY, Tran TB, Brumund KT, Weisman RA, Bouvet M. Metastases to the thyroid: a review of the literature from the last decade. Thyroid. 2012;22(3):258–68.
19. Calzolari F, Sartori PV, Talarico C, Parmeggiani D, Beretta E, Pezzullo L, Bovo G, Sperlongano P, Monacelli M, Lucchini R, Misso C, Gurrado A, D'Ajello M, Uggeri F, Puxeddu E, Nasi P, Testini M, Rosato L, Barbarisio A, Avenia N. Surgical treatment of intrathyroid metastases: preliminary results of a multicentric study. Anticancer Res. 2008;28:2885–8.
20. Papi G, Fadda G, Corsello SM, Corrado S, Rossi ED, Radighieri E, Miraglia A, Carani C, Pontecorvi A. Metastases to the thyroid gland: prevalence, clinicopathological aspects and prognosis: a 10-year experience. Clin Endocrinol. 2007;66:565–71.
21. Wood K, Vini L, Harmer C. Metastases to the thyroid gland: the Royal Marsden experience. Eur J Surg Oncol. 2004;30:583–8.
22. Kumamoto K, Utsumi Y, Sugano K, Hoshino M, Suzuki S, Takenoshita S. Colon carcinoma metastasis to the thyroid gland: report of a case with a review of the literature. Tumor. 2006;92:252–6.
23. Cichon S, Anielski R, Konturek A, Barczynski M, Cichon W. Metastases to the thyroid gland: seventeen cases operated on in a single clinical center. Langenbeck's Arch Surg. 2006;391:581–7.
24. Mirallie E, Rigaud J, Mathonnet M, Gibelin H, Regenet N, Hamy A, Bretagnol F, de Calan L, Le Neel JC, Kraimps JL. Management and prognosis of metastases to the thyroid gland. J Am Coll Surg. 2005;200:203–7.
25. Peteiro A, Duarte AM, Honavar M. Breast carcinoma metastatic to follicular adenoma of the thyroid gland. Histopathology. 2005;46:587–8.
26. McIver B, Hay ID, Giuffrida DF, et al. Anaplastic thyroid carcinoma: a 50-year experience at a single institution. Surgery. 2001;130:1028–34.
27. Aldinger KA, Samaan NA, Ibanez M, Hill CS. Anaplastic carcinoma of the thyroid: a review of 84 cases of spindle and giant cell carcinoma of the thyroid. Cancer. 1978;41:2267–75.
28. Tupchong L, Hughes F, Harmer CL. Primary lymphoma of the thyroid: clinical features, prognostic factors, and results of treatment. Int J Radiat Oncol Biol Phys. 1986;12:1813.
29. Faulkner A, Maguire P. Teaching ward nurses to monitor cancer patients. Clin Oncol. 1984;10:383.
30. Herrmann R, Panahon AM, Barcos MP, et al. Gastrointestinal involvement in non-Hodgkin's lymphoma. Cancer. 1980;46:215.
31. Anscombe AM, Wright DH. Primary malignant lymphoma of the thyroid--a tumour of mucosa-associated lymphoid tissue: review of seventy-six cases. Histopathology. 1985;9:81.
32. Walsh S, Lowery AJ, Evoy D, et al. Thyroid lymphoma: recent advances in diagnosis and optimal management strategies. Oncologist. 2013;18:994.

33. Mazzaferri EL, Oertel YC. Primary malignant thyroid lymphoma and related lymphoproliferative disorders. In: Mazzaferri EL, Samaan NA, editors. Endocrine tumors. Boston: Blackwell Scientific; 1993. p. 348.
34. Alagol F, Tanakol R, Boztepe H, Kapran Y, Terzioglu T, Dizdaroglu F. Anaplastic thyroid cancer with transient thyrotoxicosis: case report and literature review. Thyroid. 1999;9(10):1029–32.
35. Heymann RS, Brent GA, Hershman JM. Anaplastic thyroid carcinoma with thyrotoxicosis and hypoparathyroidism. Endocr Pract. 2005;11:281–4.
36. Zeki K, Eto S, Fujihira T, et al. Primary malignant lymphoma of the thyroid in a patient with long-standing Graves' disease. Endocrinol Jpn. 1985;32:435.
37. Foppiani L, Secondo V, Arlandini A, Quilici P, Cabria M, Del Monte P. Thyroid lymphoma: a rare tumor requiring combined management. Hormones (Athens). 2009;8:214–8.
38. Thieblemont C, Bastion Y, Berger F, Rieux C, Salles G, Dumontet C, et al. Mucosa-associated lymphoid tissue gastrointestinal and nongastrointestinal lymphoma behavior: analysis of 108 patients. J Clin Oncol. 1997;15:1624–30.
39. Cheung AY, Donner L, Capen C. Metastatic adenocarcinoma of the uterine cervix to the thyroid gland. Clin Oncol (R Coll Radiol). 2000;12:60–1.
40. Poon D, Toh HC, Sim CS. Two case reports of metastases from colon carcinoma to the thyroid. Ann Acad Med Singap. 2004;33:100–2.
41. Filosso PL, Arslanian A, Palestini N, Farnetti A, Papotti M, Bongiovanni M, Giobbe R, Ruffini E. Thyroid metastasis after resection of atypical bronchial carcinoid. J Thorac Cardiovasc Surg. 2004;127:1840–3.
42. Kihara M, Miyauchi A, Yamauchi A, Yokomise H. Prognostic factors of anaplastic thyroid carcinoma. Surg Today. 2004;34:394–8.
43. Brandwein-Gensler M, Urken M, Wang B. Collision tumor of the thyroid: a case report of metastatic liposarcoma plus papillary thyroid carcinoma. Head Neck. 2004;26:637–41.
44. Smallridge RC, Ain KB, Asa SL, et al. American Thyroid Association guidelines for management of patients with anaplastic thyroid cancer. Thyroid. 2012;22:1104–39.
45. Matsuzuka F, Miyauchi A, Katayama S, et al. Clinical aspects of primary thyroid lymphoma: diagnosis and treatment based on our experience of 119 cases. Thyroid. 1993;3:93.
46. National Comprehensive Cancer Network. Thyroid Cancer (Version 1.2020). https://www.nccn.org/professionals/physician_gls/pdf/thyroid.pdf. Accessed July 15, 2020.
47. Carcangiu ML, Steeper T, Zampi G, Rosai J. Anaplastic thyroid carcinoma. A study of 70 cases. Am J Clin Pathol. 1985;83:135–58.
48. Venkatesh YS, Ordonez NG, Schultz PN, Hickey RC, Goepfert H, Samaan NA. Anaplastic carcinoma of the thyroid. A clinicopathologic study of 121 cases. Cancer. 1990;66:321–30.
49. Bronner MP, LiVolsi VA. Spindle cell squamous carcinoma of the thyroid: an unusual anaplastic tumor associated with tall cell papillary cancer. Mod Pathol. 1991;4:637–43.
50. Ordonez NG, El-Naggar AK, Hickey RC, Samaan NA. Anaplastic thyroid carcinoma. Immunocytochemical study of 32 cases. Am J Clin Pathol. 1991;96:15–24.
51. Gaffey MJ, Lack EE, Christ ML, Weiss LM. Anaplastic thyroid carcinoma with osteoclast-like giant cells. A clinicopathologic, immunohistochemical, and ultrastructural study. Am J Surg Pathol. 1991;15:160–8.

52. Seethala RR, Nikiforov YE. Anaplastic (undifferentiated) carcinoma. In: Nikiforov YE, Biddinger PW, Thompson LDR, editors. Diagnostic pathology and molecular genetics of the thyroid: a comprehensive guide for practicing thyroid pathology. Philadelphia: Lippincott Williams & Wilkins; 2009. p. 228–48.
53. Verma D, Puri V, Agarwal S, Bhaskar A. Primary thyroid lymphoma: a rare disease. J Cytol. 2014;31(4):218–20.
54. Swart GJ, Wright C, Brundyn K, et al. Fine needle aspiration biopsy and flow cytometry in the diagnosis of lymphoma. Transfus Apher Sci. 2007;37:71–9.
55. Swart GJ, Wright CA. The utilization of fine needle aspiration biopsy (FNAB) and flow cytometry (FC) in the diagnosis and classification of non-Hodgkin B-cell and T-cell lymphomas. Transfus Apher Sci. 2010;42:199–207.
56. Ravinsky E, Morales C. Diagnosis of lymphoma by image-guided needle biopsies: fine needle aspiration biopsy, core biopsy or both? Acta Cytol. 2005;49(1):51–7.
57. Miyakoshi A, Dalley R, Anzai Y. Magnetic resonance imaging of thyroid cancer. Top Magn Reson Imaging. 2007;18:293–302.
58. Chiacchio S, Lorenzoni A, Boni G, et al. Anaplastic thyroid cancer: prevalence, diagnosis and treatment. Minerva Endocrinol. 2008;33:341–57.
59. Perrier ND, Brierley JD, Tuttle RM. Differentiated and anaplastic thyroid carcinoma: major changes in the American Joint Committee on cancer eighth edition cancer staging manual. CA Cancer J Clin. 2018;68:55–63.
60. Tuttle RM, Haugen B, Perrier ND. Updated American Joint Committee on cancer/tumor-node-metastasis staging system for differentiated and anaplastic thyroid cancer (eighth edition): what changed and why? Thyroid. 2017;27:751–6.
61. Cheson BD, Fisher RI, Barrington SF, Cavalli F, Schwartz LH, Zucca E, Lister TA. Recommendations for initial evaluation, staging, and response assessment of Hodgkin and non-Hodgkin lymphoma: the Lugano classification. J Clin Oncol. 2014;32(27):3059–68.
62. Sugino K, Ito K, Mimura T, et al. The important role of operations in the management of anaplastic thyroid carcinoma. Surgery. 2002;131:245–8.
63. Smallridge RC, Marlow LA, Copland JA. Anaplastic thyroid cancer: molecular pathogenesis and emerging therapies. Endocr Relat Cancer. 2009;16(1):17–44.
64. Smallridge RC, Copland JA. Anaplastic thyroid carcinoma: pathogenesis and emerging therapies. Clin Oncol (R Coll Radiol). 2010;22(6):486–97.
65. Soares P, Lima J, Preto A, Castro P, Vinagre J, Celestino R, Couto JP, Prazeres H, Eloy C, Máximo V, Sobrinho-Simões M. Genetic alterations in poorly differentiated and undifferentiated thyroid carcinomas. Curr Genomics. 2011;12(8):609–17.
66. Subbiah V, Kreitman RJ, Wainberg ZA, et al. Dabrafenib and Trametinib treatment in patients with locally advanced or metastatic BRAF V600-mutant anaplastic thyroid cancer. J Clin Oncol. 2018;36(1):7–13.
67. Landa I, Ibrahimpasic T, Boucai L, Sinha R, Knauf JA, Shah RH, Dogan S, Ricarte-Filho JC, Krishnamoorthy GP, Xu B, Schultz N, Berger MF, Sander C, Taylor BS, Ghossein R, Ganly I, Fagin JA. Genomic and transcriptomic hallmarks of poorly differentiated and anaplastic thyroid cancers. J Clin Invest. 2016;126:1052–66.
68. Pozdeyev N, Gay LM, Sokol ES, Hartmaier R, Deaver KE, Davis S, French JD, Borre PV, LaBarbera DV, Tan AC, Schweppe RE, Fishbein

L, Ross JS, Haugen BR, Bowles DW. Genetic analysis of 779 advanced differentiated and anaplastic thyroid cancers. Clin Cancer Res. 2018;24:3059–68.
69. Chen H, Luthra R, Routbort MJ, Patel KP, Cabanillas ME, Broaddus RR, Williams MD. Molecular profile of advanced thyroid carcinomas by next-generation sequencing: characterizing tumors beyond diagnosis for targeted therapy. Mol Cancer Ther. 2018;17:1575–84.
70. Begum S, Rosenbaum E, Henrique R, Cohen Y, Sidransky D, Westra WH. BRAF mutations in anaplastic thyroid carcinoma: implications for tumor origin, diagnosis and treatment. Mod Pathol. 2004;17:1359–63.
71. Drilon A, Laetsch TW, Kummar S, et al. Efficacy of Larotrectinib in TRK fusion-positive cancers in adults and children. N Engl J Med. 2018;378(8):731–9.
72. Doebele RC, Drilon A, Paz-Ares L, et al. Entrectinib in patients with advanced or metastatic NTRK fusion-positive solid tumours: integrated analysis of three phase 1-2 trials. Lancet Oncol. 2020;21(2):271–82.
73. Dias-Santagata D, Lennerz JK, Sadow PM, et al. Response to RET-specific therapy in *RET*Fusion-positive anaplastic thyroid carcinoma [published online ahead of print, 2020 May 19]. Thyroid. 2020;30(9):1384–9.
74. Tahara M, et al. Lenvatinib for anaplastic thyroid cancer. Front Oncol. 2017;7:25.
75. Marabelle A, et al. Association of tumor mutational burden with outcomes in patients with select advanced solid tumors treated with pembrolizumab in KEYNOTE-158. Presented at the Annual Meeting of ESMO in Barcelona, Spain, September 30, 2019.
76. Ha CS, Shadle KM, Medeiros LJ, et al. Localized non-Hodgkin lymphoma involving the thyroid gland. Cancer. 2001;91:629.
77. El Fakih RO, Delgado FA, Harstine LR. Marked thyroid enlargement secondary to renal cell carcinoma metastasis with acute respiratory failure. Thyroid. 2009;19:917–8.
78. Yau T, Lo CY, Epstein RJ, Lam AK, Wan KY, Lang BH. Treatment outcomes in anaplastic thyroid carcinoma: survival improvement in young patients with localized disease treated by combination of surgery and radiotherapy. Ann Surg Oncol. 2008;15(9):2500–5.
79. Wang JR, Zafereo ME, Dadu R, et al. Complete surgical resection following neoadjuvant dabrafenib plus trametinib in BRAFV600E-mutated anaplastic thyroid carcinoma. Thyroid. 2019;29:1036–43.
80. Cabanillas ME, Ferrarotto R, Garden AS, et al. Neoadjuvant BRAF- and immune-directed therapy for anaplastic thyroid carcinoma. Thyroid. 2018;28:945–51.
81. Czech JM, Lichtor TR, Carney JA, van Heerden JA. Neoplasms metastatic to the thyroid gland. Surg Gynecol Obstet. 1982;155:503–5.
82. Ericsson M, Biorklund A, Cederquist E, Ingemansson S, Aker-man M. Surgical treatment of metastatic disease in the thyroid gland. J Surg Oncol. 1981;17:15–23.
83. Ishikawa M, Hirano S, Tsuji T, Ito J. Management of metastasis to the thyroid gland. Auris Nasus Larynx. 2011;38:426–30.
84. Nixon IJ, Whitcher M, Glick J, et al. Surgical management of metastases to the thyroid gland. Ann Surg Oncol. 2011;18:800–4.
85. Iesalnieks I, Winter H, Bareck E, et al. Thyroid metastases of renal cell carcinoma: clinical course in 45 patients undergoing surgery. Assessment of factors affecting patients' survival. Thyroid. 2008;18:615–24.

86. Russell JO, Yan K, Burkey B, Scharpf J. Nonthyroid metastasis to the thyroid gland: case series and review with observations by primary pathology. Otolaryngol Head Neck Surg. 2016;155(6):961–8.
87. Patel KN, Shaha AR. Poorly differentiated thyroid cancer. Curr Opin Otolaryngol Head Neck Surg. 2014;22:121–6.
88. Neff R, Farrar W, Kloos R, Burman K. Anaplastic thyroid cancer. Endocrinol Metab Clin N Am. 2008;37:525–38.
89. Besic N, Hocevar M, Zgajnar J, Pogacnik A, Grazio-Frkovic S, Auersperg M. Prognostic factors in anaplastic carcinoma of the thyroid-a multivariate survival analysis of 188 patients. Langenbeck's Arch Surg. 2005;390(3):203–8.

Surgical Procedures. Thyroidectomy: Indications, Flexible Laryngoscopy, Operative Techniques, Recurrent Laryngeal Nerve Monitoring, and Management of Complications

Iuliana D. Bobanga and Christopher R. McHenry

Contents

A. L. Shifrin et al. (eds.), *Endocrine Surgery Comprehensive Board Exam Guide*,
https://doi.org/10.1007/978-3-030-84737-1_10

Questions

1. A 45-year-old woman is referred for evaluation of a thyroid nodule. She is asymptomatic, and her serum TSH level is normal. She had an ultrasound exam demonstrating a 2.5 cm hyperechoic nodule with ill-defined margins in the right lobe of the thyroid gland. The remainder of the thyroid gland is normal, and there are no abnormal lymph nodes in the central or lateral neck. What is the next most appropriate step in management?
   (a) Follow-up ultrasound in 6–12 months
   (b) I-123 thyroid scintigraphy
   (c) FDG PET imaging
   (d) Fine-needle aspiration biopsy
   (e) Thyroid lobectomy
2. A 54-year-old woman has multiple, bilateral thyroid nodules. She has a 2 cm nodule in the right lobe and a 5 cm nodule in the left lobe extending substernally with displacement and compression of her trachea. Fine-needle aspiration biopsy of the nodule in the right lobe reveals atypia of undetermined significance, and fine-needle aspiration biopsy of the nodule in the left lobe is benign. What is the most appropriate management?
   (a) Molecular testing for the right thyroid nodule
   (b) Repeat fine-needle aspiration biopsy of both nodules in 3 months
   (c) Diagnostic right thyroid lobectomy
   (d) Total thyroidectomy
   (e) Total thyroidectomy and central compartment neck dissection
3. A 40-year-old woman has a 2.5 cm firm nodule palpable in the left lobe of the thyroid gland. She reports hoarseness and difficulty in swallowing pills. Her serum TSH level is normal. Ultrasound exam reveals a 2.5 cm solid hypoechoic nodule with microcalcifications and a 1.3 cm left, level III cervical lymph node without an obvious normal fatty hilum. Fine-needle aspiration biopsy of the thyroid nodule reveals papillary thyroid cancer. What is the most appropriate initial recommendation for this patient?
   (a) Fine-needle aspiration biopsy of the level III lymph node for cytology and thyroglobulin rinsing
   (b) Total thyroidectomy and excisional biopsy of the level III lymph node
   (c) Total thyroidectomy with left lateral neck dissection
   (d) Total thyroidectomy with central and left lateral neck dissection

4. Prior to surgical intervention in this patient, what preoperative evaluation is necessary?
   (a) Serum thyroglobulin and antithyroglobulin antibody titer
   (b) Laryngoscopy
   (c) Molecular testing for B-Raf
   (d) Computed tomography of the chest
   (e) FDG PET imaging
5. In general when performing thyroidectomy, the technique should include
   (a) A curvilinear skin incision above the cricoid cartilage
   (b) Division of the superior pole vessels well away from thyroid parenchyma
   (c) Routine demonstration of all parathyroid glands
   (d) Division of the inferior pole vessels prior to demonstration of the recurrent laryngeal nerve
   (e) Division of the branches of the inferior thyroid artery close to the thyroid gland
6. Neuromonitoring is used intraoperatively, and there is an absent signal in the posterior branch of the left recurrent laryngeal nerve. An electrode check on the neuromonitor reveals that all electrodes are functional. What is the most likely explanation for this finding?
   (a) A normal electrophysiologic response
   (b) Change in position of the endotracheal tube
   (c) Traction injury to the recurrent laryngeal nerve
   (d) Thermal injury to the recurrent laryngeal nerve
   (e) Transection of the recurrent laryngeal nerve
7. At operation, there is extrathyroidal tumor spread of the cancer in the left lobe of the thyroid gland with adherence of the cancer to a functioning left recurrent laryngeal nerve. What is the most appropriate management?
   (a) Preservation of the recurrent laryngeal nerve
   (b) An en bloc resection of the cancer and the recurrent laryngeal nerve
   (c) An en bloc resection with neurorrhaphy
   (d) An en bloc resection with a free ansa cervicalis nerve graft
8. Six hours after operation, the patient develops significant swelling in the neck and complains of difficulty breathing. She is on the hospital ward and appears extremely anxious and is tachycardic. She is on 4 liters nasal cannula oxygen, and her oxygen saturation is 92%. What is the next most appropriate step in her management?
   (a) Ultrasound of the neck and ultrasound-guided drainage, if necessary
   (b) Increase her supplemental oxygen
   (c) Call anesthesia for endotracheal intubation
   (d) Schedule the patient for an operating room emergently
   (e) Open the incision at the bedside

9. On postoperative day #1, the patient's calcium is 7.2 mg/dl (8.4–10.4 mg/dl) and her intact PTH level is 4 pg/ml (12–68 pg/ml). She is complaining of perioral and acral numbness and tingling. How should her hypocalcemia be managed?
   (a) Intravenous calcium gluconate alone
   (b) Oral calcium alone
   (c) Oral calcium and vitamin D
   (d) Intravenous calcium gluconate, oral calcium, and vitamin D
10. At her first follow-up visit, the patient is audibly hoarse and laryngoscopy reveals an immobile left vocal cord and a normal functioning right vocal cord. What is the best recommendation for further evaluation or management?
   (a) Follow-up assessment in 3 months for resolution of symptoms
   (b) Transcutaneous laryngeal ultrasound exam
   (c) Injection laryngoplasty
   (d) Laryngeal reinnervation
   (e) Referral to a voice specialist

10.1 Introduction

Thyroidectomy is one of the most commonly performed operations, with over 130,000 performed annually in the United States [1]. Thyroidectomy is indicated for treatment of thyroid cancer, symptomatic goiter, indeterminate thyroid nodules, and thyrotoxicosis. In general, the rate of complications after thyroidectomy is low; however, recurrent laryngeal nerve (RLN) injury, neck hematoma, and permanent hypoparathyroidism can be life altering for patients. Surgeon experience, meticulous operative technique, and strict attention to detail using a series of well-defined steps when performing thyroidectomy are important to minimize complications.

10.2 Indications for Thyroidectomy

Thyroidectomy is indicated for treatment of benign and malignant thyroid conditions. Three broad categories summarize the most common indications for thyroidectomy: thyroid cancer or an indeterminate thyroid nodule with concern for thyroid cancer, compressive symptoms caused by simple goiter, nodular goiter, or Hashimoto's thyroiditis, and thyrotoxicosis due to a toxic nodule, toxic multinodular goiter, or Graves' disease.

Thyroidectomy is indicated for a thyroid nodule with a fine-needle aspiration biopsy (FNAB) result that is categorized as malignant (Bethesda VI) based on the Bethesda System for

Reporting Thyroid Cytopathology [2]. It is also indicated for a thyroid nodule when thyroid cancer cannot be excluded; this includes an indeterminate FNAB result categorized as persistent atypia/follicular lesion of undetermined significance (Bethesda III); follicular or Hurthle cell neoplasm (Bethesda IV) or suspicious for malignancy (Bethesda V) because of the potential for thyroid cancer. Indeterminate thyroid nodules can also be evaluated with commercially available molecular tests that refine the risk of malignancy. When molecular test results indicate a high risk of malignancy in Bethesda III and IV nodules, thyroidectomy is indicated. Completion thyroidectomy is indicated for patients with a cancer determined to be high risk for recurrence or mortality or for treatment of recurrent thyroid cancer following a diagnostic thyroid lobectomy. Prophylactic thyroidectomy is indicated for patients with known genetic mutations associated with familial medullary thyroid cancer [2].

Compressive symptoms due to an enlarged thyroid gland with or without nodules can manifest as dysphagia, globus sensation, coughing or choking spells, dyspnea, and hoarseness. A very large goiter with substernal extension can impinge on structures in the neck and mediastinum. Mass effect can be seen on chest X-ray or computed tomography of the neck and chest, including deviation or compression of the trachea, esophagus, or superior vena cava and displacement of the great vessels.

Patients with Graves' disease, toxic multinodular goiter, or a single toxic adenoma typically present with signs and symptoms of hyperthyroidism. They may also have compressive symptoms [3]. They are initially treated with antithyroid medications to achieve a euthyroid state and minimize the risk of thyroid storm, a life-threatening condition. Surgery can be performed once their free T3 and free T4 levels normalized. Beta-blockers are often added to control tachycardia and adrenergic symptoms. In addition, patients with Graves' disease are often treated with potassium iodide in the immediate preoperative period to decrease thyroid vascularity and intraoperative blood loss [4].

10.3 Flexible Laryngoscopy

The quality of a patient's voice should be assessed during the initial evaluation for thyroidectomy, and it should be determined if they have had prior neck surgery. While some clinicians advocate preoperative examination of the vocal cords for all patients prior to thyroidectomy, the American Head and Neck Consensus Statement recommends preoperative laryngeal examination in patients undergoing thyroid surgery who have hoarseness of the voice, prior cervical or upper chest surgery where the recurrent laryngeal or vagus nerves were at risk, thyroid cancer with known posterior extension, or extensive cervical node metastases [2, 5].

Preoperative laryngeal examination allows for the visual assessment of vocal cord function prior to surgery. Flexible laryngoscopy can be performed in the outpatient clinic after topical anesthesia to the nasal passage and nasopharynx is administered. Alternatively, the vocal cords may be evaluated with indirect mirror laryngoscopy, rigid transoral laryngoscopy, transcutaneous laryngeal ultrasound, or videolaryngostroboscopy [6]. If there is known or suspected recurrent laryngeal nerve injury after thyroidectomy, patients can be referred to a voice specialist and should be evaluated for vocal cord paresis postoperatively with flexible laryngoscopy.

10.4 Operative Description and Technique

In our practice, thyroidectomy is performed using a series of well-defined steps and maneuvers [7]. In general, routine adherence to these steps helps maintain the flow of the operation. It is also helpful for teaching others how to perform the operation and foremost to minimize complications and enhance patient outcomes.

10.4.1 Airway and Anesthesia

The patient is positioned supine on the operating table and a pneumatic compression device is applied to the lower extremities for deep vein thrombosis prophylaxis. Thyroidectomy is preferably performed under general anesthesia. Intraoperative neuromonitoring to confirm the functional integrity of the recurrent laryngeal nerves throughout the operation is used routinely for all thyroidectomies by one of the authors (CRM), and used selectively for reoperative cases by the other author (IB). As a result, a short-acting neuromuscular blocking agent is utilized for placement of an electrode-embedded endotracheal tube. A number 7-sized electrode embedded endotracheal tube provides for adequate electrode contact with the vocal cords in most adults (◘ Fig. 10.1). A videolaryngoscope is used to properly position the electrodes adjacent to the vocal cords. An esophageal stethoscope is placed for continuous monitoring of core temperature and breath sounds.

After the endotracheal tube has been secured, a grounding electrode for the endotracheal tube recording electrodes and a stimulator probe electrode are placed in the skin of the anterior chest wall over the sternum. The grounding electrode for the endotracheal tube recording electrodes is placed just superior to the grounding electrode for the stimulator probe

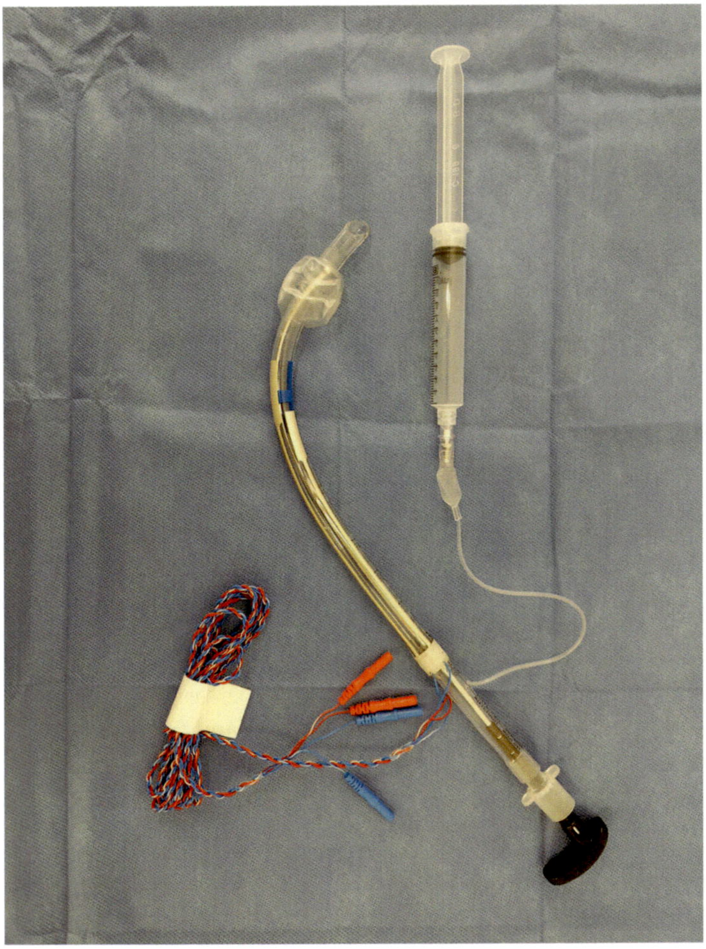

Fig. 10.1 Electrode-imbedded endotracheal tube. The blue area of the endotracheal tube just proximal to the cuff represents the site of the electrodes. The blue and red wires attached to the endotracheal tube are the recording wires, which are plugged into an interface connector box

(Fig. 10.2). The grounding wire, the stimulus return wire, the recording wires from the endotracheal tube, and a stimulator probe, that is used to stimulate the recurrent laryngeal nerve, are all plugged into an interface-connector box, which is connected to a nerve integrity monitor (Fig. 10.3).

10.4.2 Positioning (Fig. 10.4)

A soft roll is placed lengthwise beneath the patient's shoulders to extend the neck, and a foam headrest is placed beneath the occiput. The patient's arms are tucked at their side, and all pressure points are padded. The endotracheal tube and ventilator tubing is directed off the top of the operating table to optimize the surgeon's working space. The head of the bed is

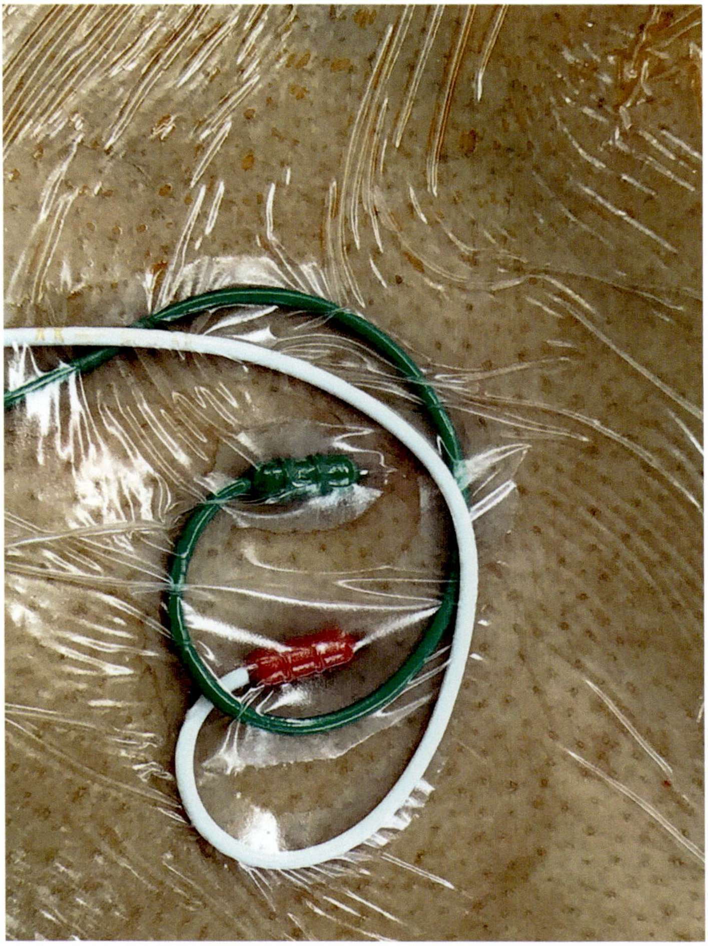

Fig. 10.2 The grounding electrode (green) for the endotracheal tube recording electrodes is placed just superior to the grounding electrode for the stimulator probe (white)

elevated to reduce venous pressure. The patient is then prepped and draped, and a timeout is completed to confirm the correct patient, procedure, and site.

10.4.3 Incision (Fig. 10.5)

Important anatomic landmarks are identified to help determine the optimal site for the skin incision and development of skin flaps; these include the prominence of the thyroid cartilage, the cricoid cartilage, the sternal notch, and the sternocleidomastoid muscles. The site of the low collar skin incision is marked with a 0 silk suture or skin marker. The sternal notch is used to determine the midline of the incision, and a ruler is used to measure the length of the incision.

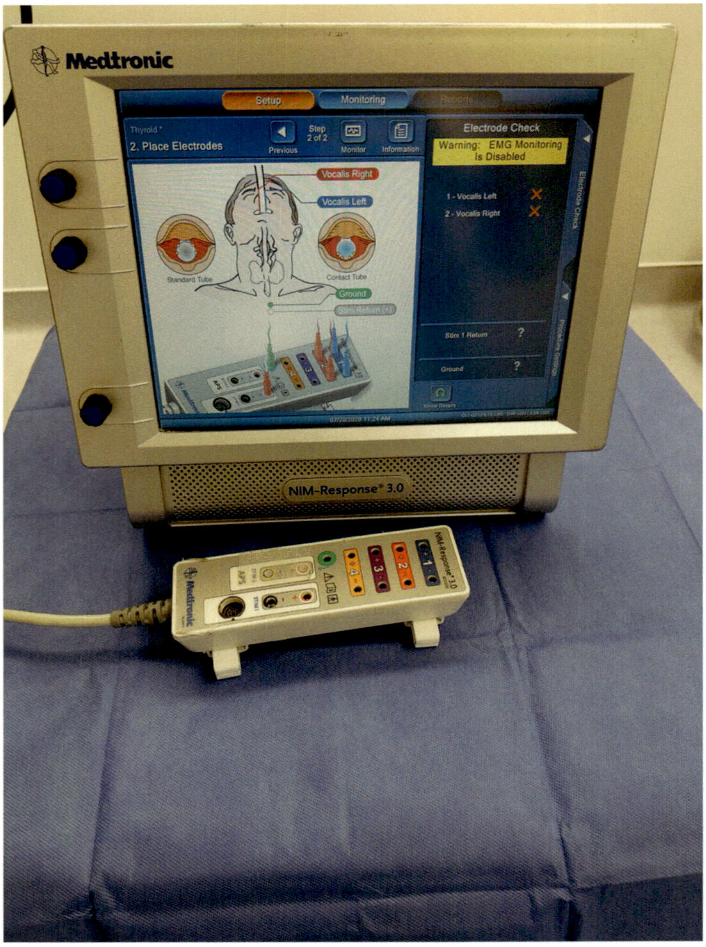

Fig. 10.3 The interface connector box and nerve integrity monitor

Marcaine 0.5% is used to anesthetize the site of the skin incision prior to making the incision to establish preemptive analgesia. A transverse curvilinear incision is made preferably in a normal skin crease approximately two fingerbreadths above the sternal notch with a 15-blade scalpel. The length of the incision is dependent on the size of the thyroid gland. For most thyroid nodules, a 6-cm incision is adequate, recognizing that the incision can always be lengthened if additional exposure is required.

10.4.4 Creation of a Working Space to Remove the Thyroid Gland (Fig. 10.6)

The subcutaneous tissue and platysma muscle are divided with the electrocautery. The anterior jugular veins are identified and preserved. Superior and inferior skin flaps are developed in a plane below the platysma muscle and anterior to the anterior

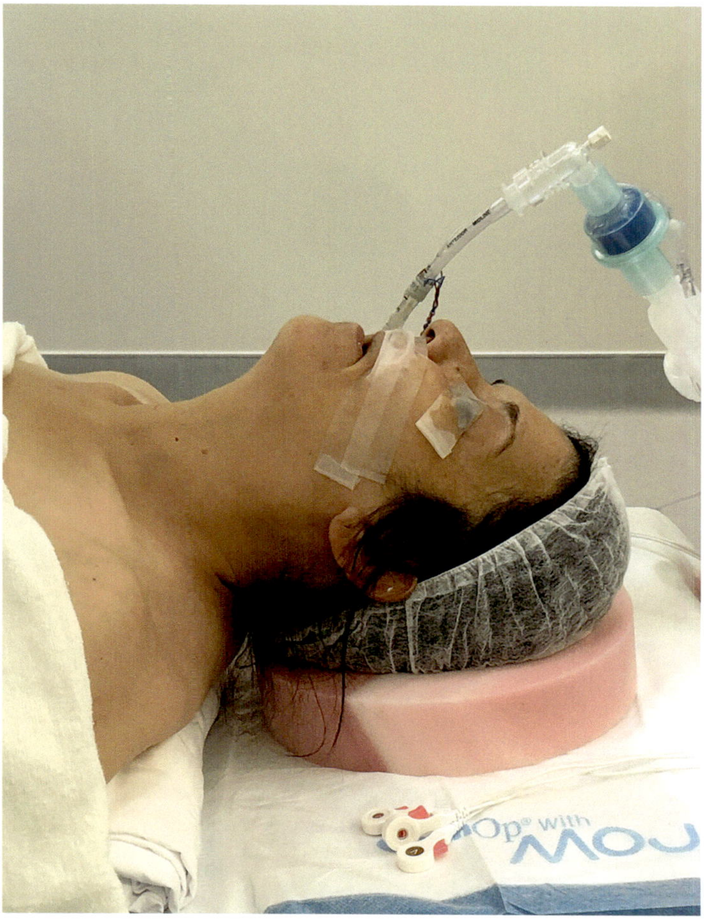

Fig. 10.4 Positioning of the patient for thyroidectomy. A roll is placed beneath the shoulders to extend the neck. The head is positioned on a soft foam headrest. The arms are tucked at the patient's side, and all pressure points are padded. The bed is positioned in slight reverse Trendelenburg to reduce venous pressure. The endotracheal tube and ventilator tubing is directed off the top of the operating table to optimize the space for the surgeon and the assistants

jugular veins using the electrocautery. When developing the skin flaps, traction is applied to the skin using double-armed skin hooks or small Richardson retractors. Alternatively, the surgeon can use his or her hand to elevate the skin. Skin flaps are raised to the prominence of the thyroid cartilage superiorly, the sternal notch inferiorly, and the sternocleidomastoid muscles laterally.

10.4.5 Exposure of the Thyroid Lobe

The median raphe is incised and the sternohyoid muscles are separated in the midline from the thyroid cartilage to the sternal notch. This provides exposure to the prelaryngeal and pre-

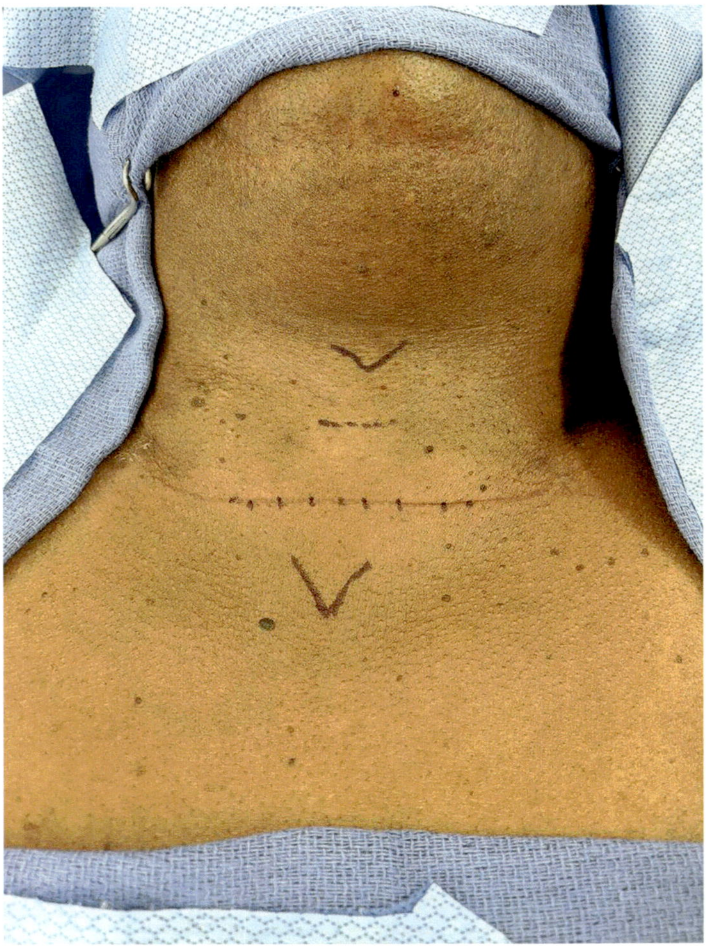

Fig. 10.5 The important anatomic landmarks that are identified when deciding where to make the skin incision include the prominence of the thyroid cartilage, the cricoid cartilage, and the sternal notch. The site of the skin incision is depicted here approximately two fingerbreadths above the sternal notch and inferior to the cricoid cartilage

tracheal fibrofatty and nodal tissue, the isthmus of the thyroid gland, and a pyramidal lobe, which is present in 40–50% of patients. The pyramidal lobe extends inferiorly from above the thyroid cartilage most commonly to the left half of the isthmus. When present, the pyramidal lobe is resected by mobilizing it from above the thyroid cartilage to its attachment to the isthmus.

The sternothyroid muscle on one side of the neck is exposed and is separated from the underlying thyroid lobe by separating and dividing the intervening loose areolar tissue using a combination of blunt dissection and the electrocautery. The strap muscles can be divided when additional exposure is required, especially for patients with massive thyroid enlargement. Alternatively, some surgeons choose not to develop skin flaps and routinely divide the strap muscles.

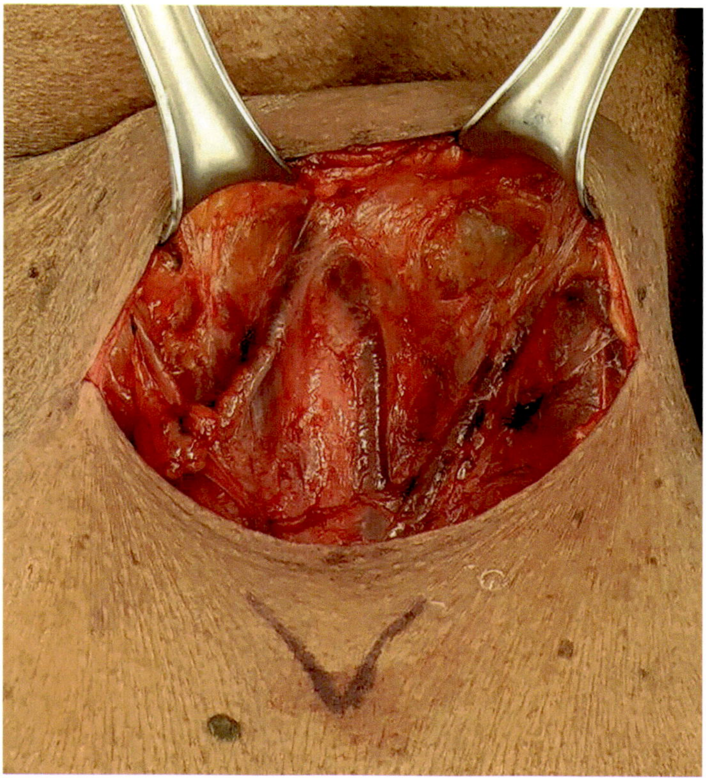

Fig. 10.6 Demonstrating the superior skin flap that has been raised in a subplatysmal plane anterior to the anterior jugular veins that are visualized. The superior skin flap is being elevated with Richardson retractors. This is the working space that is created to remove the thyroid gland

The lobe of the thyroid gland is elevated anteriorly and medially. The common carotid artery is visualized. The middle thyroid vein is exposed and then ligated and divided. Our preference is to ligate the vessel with a suture, and then, divide it using an energy device on the specimen side.

10.4.6 Exposure, Ligation, and Division of the Superior Pole Vessels

The plane between the superior pole vessels and the thyroid parenchyma is exposed. This is facilitated by retracting the strap muscles superiorly and laterally using an appendiceal retractor and applying downward traction on the superior pole of the thyroid lobe using an Allis clamp. The cricothyroid space between the superior vascular pedicle and the cricothyroid muscle is delineated.

A right-angled clamp is then passed beneath the superior pole vessels close to the thyroid gland to avoid injury to the external branch of superior laryngeal nerve. We do not rou-

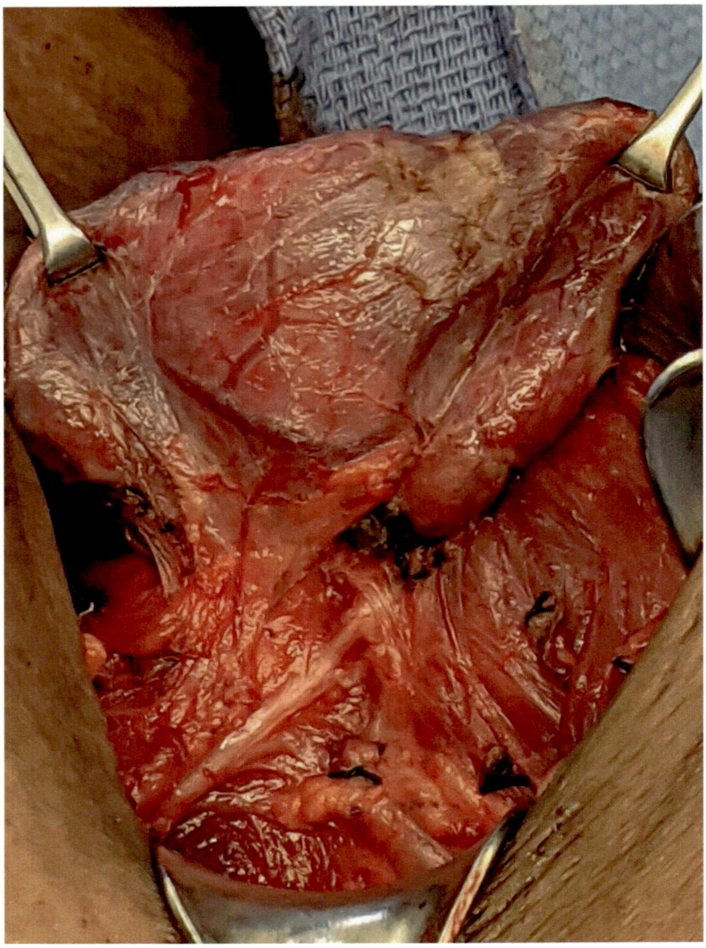

Fig. 10.7 The left lobe of the thyroid gland is being elevated with Allis clamps anteriorly and medially. The left recurrent laryngeal nerve has been exposed

tinely search for and expose the external branch of superior laryngeal nerve. The superior pole vessels are ligated with suture and divided on the specimen side with an energy device.

10.4.7 Identification and Preservation of the Recurrent Laryngeal Nerve (Fig. 10.7)

With the lobe of the thyroid gland retracted anteriorly and medially and the common carotid artery retracted laterally, the inferior thyroid artery is identified. The inferior thyroid artery is an important anatomic landmark to help identify the recurrent laryngeal nerve. The recurrent laryngeal nerve is preferably exposed just inferior to the inferior thyroid artery as it ascends from the chest in the tracheoesophageal groove.

The recurrent laryngeal nerve can pass anterior or posterior to the inferior thyroid artery. In approximately 50% of patients, there is extralaryngeal branching of the recurrent laryngeal nerve and the branches may be anterior and posterior to the inferior thyroid artery. The anterior branch of the recurrent laryngeal nerve is a motor branch, and the posterior branches are sensory.

After the recurrent laryngeal nerve has been identified, intraoperative neuromonitoring is used to confirm the functional integrity of the nerve and then used again intermittently throughout the remainder of the nerve dissection. The recurrent laryngeal nerve is then exposed superiorly using a mosquito clamp to dissect the overlying tissue parallel to the nerve, being careful to minimize contact with the nerve. The recurrent laryngeal nerve is traced through its entire course and is preserved.

10.4.8 Division of the Inferior Pole Vessels

In general, we do not divide the inferior pole vessels until the recurrent laryngeal nerve has been identified to avoid injury to the nerve. The vessels are ligated with suture and are divided on the side of the specimen with an energy device. This exposes the anterior surface of the trachea and allows for division of the ligament of Berry inferiorly. The ligament of Berry is divided sharply with Metzenbaum scissors, which helps enhance the exposure of the recurrent laryngeal nerve superiorly.

10.4.9 Preservation of the Parathyroid Glands

The key to in situ preservation of the parathyroid glands is to delineate the branches of the inferior thyroid artery close to the thyroid gland to preserve the blood supply to the parathyroid glands. The branches of the inferior thyroid artery are ligated with suture and divided on the specimen side with a scalpel rather than an energy device to avoid potential thermal injury to the recurrent laryngeal nerve.

We do not routinely search for and expose the parathyroid glands as this may potentially lead to their devascularization. However, we routinely examine the surface of the thyroid lobe for parathyroid glands that may be within the capsule to avoid removal with the specimen. If a parathyroid gland is found and it cannot be preserved in situ, the parathyroid gland is excised in its entirety.

A small fragment of the excised parathyroid gland is submitted for frozen section exam. If frozen section examination confirms that it is parathyroid tissue, the remainder of the gland is minced and is autotransplanted into a pocket of the sternocleidomastoid muscle. When creating the pocket in the sternocleidomastoid muscle, it is important to avoid causing a hematoma, because this may reduce the viability of the parathyroid gland. The pocket is closed with a single suture ligature.

10.4.10 Separation of the Thyroid Lobe from the Recurrent Laryngeal Nerve

Dissection of the recurrent laryngeal nerve is completed superiorly, separating it from the ligament of Berry. There are small vessels that are a source for troublesome bleeding that need to be ligating preferably with suture rather than an energy device to avoid thermal injury to the nerve. The vessels are divided on the specimen side with a 15-blade scalpel. This allows the recurrent laryngeal nerve to fall away from the thyroid lobe. The remainder of the ligament of Berry can be divided sharply with Metzenbaum scissors.

10.4.11 Removal of the Thyroid Lobe and Isthmus

The lobe and isthmus are mobilized to the contralateral side of the trachea. For a thyroid lobectomy, a Kelley clamp is placed on the medial aspect of the contralateral lobe and the thyroid is divided above the clamp with a 10-blade scalpel. The cut edge of the contralateral lobe is oversewn with a running horizontal mattress technique using 2-0 Vicryl suture. For a total thyroidectomy, the contralateral lobe is removed in a similar fashion.

10.4.12 Closure

The wound is examined for hemostasis. Bleeding adjacent to the recurrent laryngeal nerve can be controlled with precise suture ligation or a small square of gelfoam left adjacent to the trachea. A drain is not used.

The sternohyoid muscles are reapproximated in the midline with a 2-0 Vicryl suture leaving a 3 cm opening inferiorly. This opening is important in the event of postoperative bleeding to prevent blood from accumulating in an enclosed space that may cause tracheal compression or impair venous drainage from the larynx and cause laryngeal edema. The opening allows blood to egress into the subcutaneous space, delaying the onset of airway compromise.

The subcutaneous tissue and platysma muscle are reapproximated with 3-0 Vicryl suture. A subcuticular skin closure is completed with a 4-0 Monocryl suture. Dermabond or Mastisol, steristrips, and a gauze dressing can be applied to the incision.

10.5 Intraoperative Neuromonitoring (IONM)

Prior studies examining the use of IONM for prevention of recurrent laryngeal nerve injury during thyroidectomy have found mixed results. A randomized controlled trial by Barczynski and colleagues found a reduction in transient recurrent laryngeal nerve injury from 5.0% to 2.7% with IONM during bilateral thyroidectomy without reduction in permanent recurrent laryngeal nerve injury [8]. A systematic review and meta-analysis by Yang and colleagues also showed a reduction in transient recurrent laryngeal nerve injury without reduction in permanent recurrent laryngeal nerve injury [9]. In a large multicenter prospective study, Dralle and colleagues reported no significant difference in recurrent laryngeal nerve injury in 16,448 consecutive thyroidectomies with or without the use of IONM [10]. In a meta-analysis performed by Lombardi and colleagues, it was found that there was no benefit of IONM over visualization alone in reducing the rate of permanent recurrent laryngeal nerve injury [11].

Given the low incidence of recurrent laryngeal nerve injury, most studies have been underpowered to demonstrate a statistically significant difference in recurrent laryngeal nerve injury. Additionally, results are hard to interpret when: different definitions for recurrent laryngeal nerve injury are used, studies combine intermittent and continuous monitoring techniques, data is obtained from multiple surgeons with varying degrees of experience and operative volumes, and thyroidectomies are performed on different patient populations. Despite the lack of consensus regarding the potential for reduction in recurrent laryngeal nerve injury, IONM is widely used in thyroid surgery.

In our practice, IONM is utilized as an adjunct to confirm the functional integrity of the recurrent laryngeal nerve after it has been visually identified [12]. Intermittent neuroevaluation is performed throughout the dissection of the recurrent laryngeal nerve.

IONM has been helpful for assessment of anatomic variations in the nerve, particularly for confirming a nonrecurrent laryngeal nerve and for distinguishing motor and sensory branches of the nerve in patients with extralaryngeal branching. It has been helpful to ensure that the anterior motor branch of the recurrent laryngeal nerve is properly exposed. It has also been useful for identifying loss of signal in the nerve with traction, most notably in patients with very firm thyroid glands that make it difficult to retract anteriorly and medially, such as patients with Hashimoto's thyroiditis. Anecdotally, we have documented loss of signal with traction on the nerve that returns with elimination of the traction.

Surgeons who use IONM should familiarize themselves with guidelines for standards of equipment setup, endotracheal tube placement, and intraoperative problem solving, which are intended to improve the quality of neuromonitoring [13]. While there are multiple commercially available systems for IONM, the Medtronic NIM-Response 3.0 system is used and available at our institution, and is described in this chapter. IONM requires placement of a specialized electrode-embedded endotracheal tube (◘ Fig. 10.1). The electrodes are positioned directly adjacent to the vocal cords using a videolaryngoscope, and the endotracheal tube is secured to maintain the proper positioning of the electrodes. This is ensured by maintaining the red recording wires to the patient's right, the blue recording wires to the patient's left, and the numbering on the endotracheal tube anteriorly and in the center (◘ Fig. 10.8).

If the position of the endotracheal tube changes during the operation, the electrodes may no longer be correctly positioned adjacent to the vocal cords and they will not receive the electri-

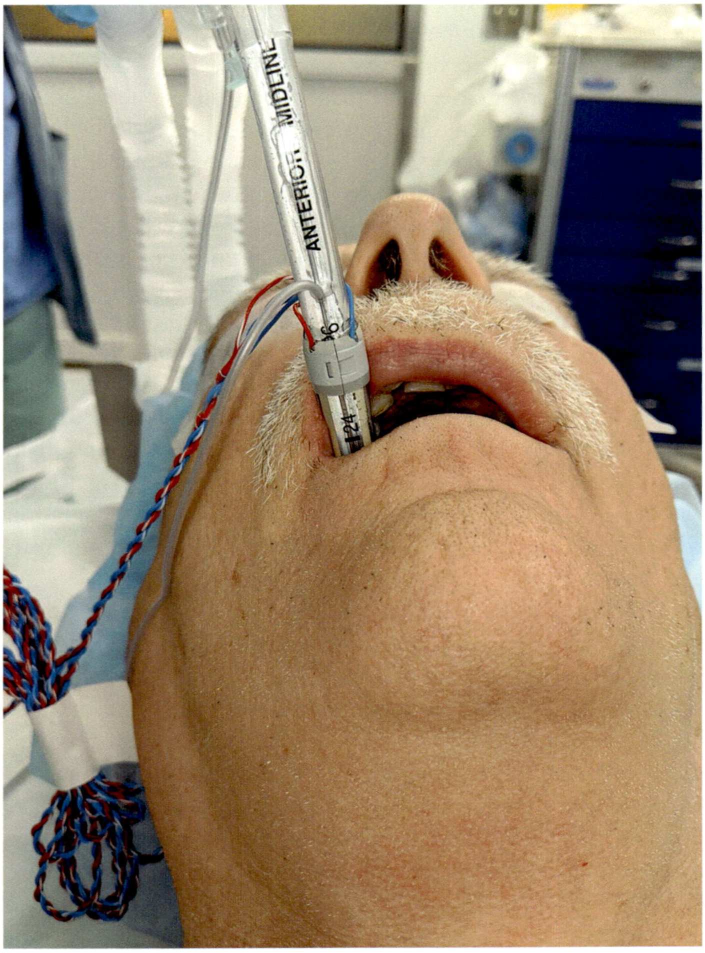

◘ **Fig. 10.8** The endotracheal tube is secured to maintain the proper positioning of the electrodes adjacent to the vocal cords. This is ensured by the correct orientation of the tube with the red recording wires to the patient's right, the blue recording wires to the patient's left, and the numbering on the endotracheal tube anterior and in the center

cal stimulus applied to the recurrent laryngeal nerve. The four wires from the endotracheal tube are plugged into an interface-connector box connected to a nerve integrity monitor (◘ Fig. 10.3) for electromyographic recording of vocal cord contractions. After the endotracheal tube has been placed, neuromuscular blockade is no longer used for the remainder of the case. Incorrect positioning of the endotracheal tube relative to the vocal cords may result from inadequate or excessive depth or rotation of the endotracheal tube. Malpositioning of the endotracheal tube is a common cause for malfunction of IONM.

Grounding electrodes for the endotracheal tube recording electrodes and the stimulator probe electrode are placed in the skin of the anterior chest wall over the sternum. The grounding electrode for the stimulator probe electrode is placed inferior to the grounding probe for the endotracheal tube recording electrodes to help minimize stimulus artifact (◘ Fig. 10.2). The grounding electrodes are plugged into the interface-connector box connected to the nerve integrity monitor. An electrode check on the nerve integrity monitor is used to confirm proper function of the electrodes (◘ Fig. 10.9).

A hand-held probe (◘ Fig. 10.10), used to apply an electrical stimulus to the recurrent laryngeal nerve, is plugged into the interface-connector box. The probe is used to intermittently stimulate the recurrent laryngeal nerve with 1 mA of pulsed current, and the response of the laryngeal muscles is confirmed by hearing a characteristic acoustic tone and is assessed using the laryngeal electromyographic wave forms depicted on the monitor.

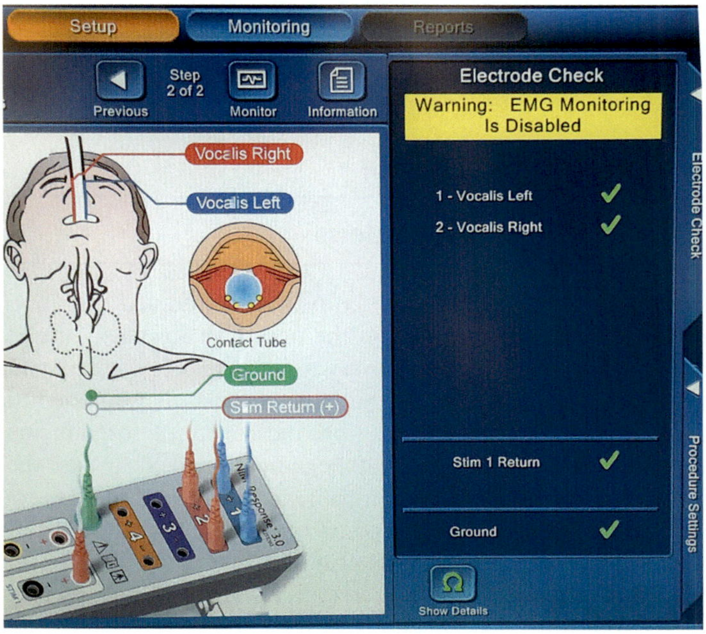

◘ **Fig. 10.9** An electrode check on the nerve integrity monitor is used to confirm proper function of the electrodes

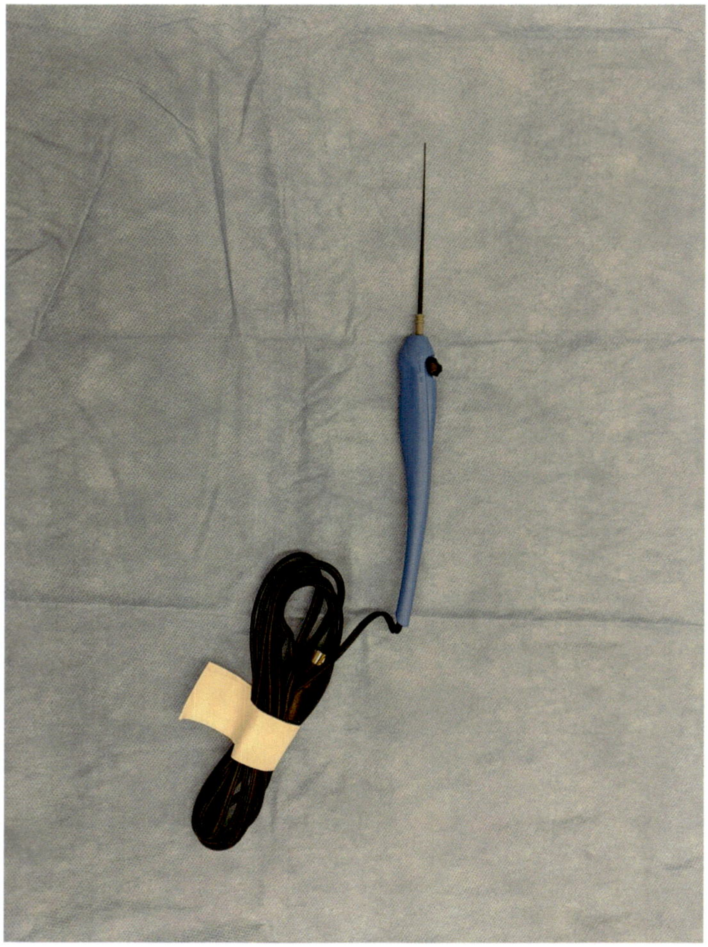

Fig. 10.10 Nerve probe used to apply an electrical stimulus to the recurrent laryngeal nerve

10.6 Postoperative Care

10.6.1 General Instructions

Postoperatively, the head of the bed is maintained at 30° to decrease venous congestion in the neck. An ice pack can be applied to the neck in the recovery room to reduce swelling and help with analgesia [14]. The patient is frequently examined to monitor for hematoma formation and a tray of instruments that includes a scalpel is kept at the patient's bedside in case the incision needs to be opened and a hematoma needs to be evacuated emergently. Dicyclomine or benzocaine/menthol throat lozenges and analgesic throat spray can be used for sore throat related to endotracheal tube irritation. There are no dietary restrictions after thyroidectomy. A regular diet is ordered, and patients self-regulate and start their diet with liquids and softer foods if they choose to. Nausea should be treated with antinausea medications and patients who have vomiting should be made nil per os (NPO), as vomiting and retching can increase the risk of a neck hematoma.

10.6.2 Duration of Observation

The duration of observation after uncomplicated thyroid lobectomy and total thyroidectomy varies widely among surgeons. The main reasons for observation are to monitor for hypocalcemia and for neck hematoma, a potentially lethal complication. Numerous studies have been published on the safety of outpatient thyroidectomy [15–17]. A thyroidectomy followed by observation in the hospital for up to 23 h constitutes same day or outpatient thyroidectomy as defined by the insurance industry [18]. In most studies, the incidence of postoperative neck hematoma is $\leq 1\%$ and the majority occur within the first 24 h, with a range of 10 min to 15 days postoperatively [17]. Two to ten percent of hematomas occur after 24 h [17]. A study by Rosenbaum et al. found that 6 out of 1050 patients developed a neck hematoma (0.6%), 5 after total thyroidectomy and 1 after thyroid lobectomy, with a range of 10 min to 7 days postoperatively. Four of the six hematomas occurred within 4 h of surgery [16].

Due to the occurrence of most hematomas within 4–6 h of surgery, and over 90% of hematomas within the first 23 h, many thyroid surgeons have adapted a routine of outpatient thyroidectomy, with 4-, 6-, or 23-h observation postoperatively. One of the authors routinely admits all thyroidectomy patients for 23-h observation (IDB), while the other author observes patients for 4 h postoperatively after thyroid lobectomy and 23 h after total thyroidectomy (CRM).

10.6.3 Pain Management

Postoperative pain after thyroidectomy has traditionally been managed with narcotic-based analgesia. However, recently, more institutions and surgeons have found narcotic-free regimens in combination with local anesthesia to be adequate for postoperative pain control after thyroidectomy. A recent randomized prospective study comparing a narcotic to a nonnarcotic regimen demonstrated equivalent postoperative pain scores in patients receiving either a narcotic or nonnarcotic medication regimen [19]. This has resulted in the elimination of the routine use of narcotics for postoperative analgesia following thyroidectomy in our practices. A multimodality analgesic regimen consisting of ice, throat lozenges, and 1000 mg acetaminophen alternating with 800 mg ibuprofen every 4 h postoperatively in combination with intraoperative bupivacaine injection into the incision will provide effective pain control in the majority of patients. Patients with pain that is not controlled with this regimen benefit from a median of 2 oxycodone pills and may be discharged with no more than 5 oxycodone pills.

10.6.4 Calcium Monitoring and Supplementation

At minimum, a serum calcium level is obtained on the morning after surgery in patients following total thyroidectomy or completion thyroidectomy. Serum calcium measurement is unnecessary following thyroid lobectomy. Some authors also routinely obtain an intact-parathyroid hormone (PTH) level, which they use to help decide on recommendations for administration of calcium and calcitriol [17]. Various protocols are used to manage hypocalcemia and hypoparathyroidism and supplement calcium in the postoperative period after thyroidectomy. In 2018, the American Thyroid Association published a consensus statement summarizing some of these protocols [20]. Some groups routinely discharge all patients on supplemental oral calcium with or without calcitriol. Others take a more selective approach based on postoperative PTH) and/or calcium levels [17, 20].

Patients with Graves' disease have a higher incidence of profound postoperative hypocalcemia. It is recommended that calcium and vitamin D therapy be started preoperatively in patients with Graves' disease to help reduce the length of hospital stay for treatment of hypocalcemia [4, 21]. All patients should receive instruction preoperatively and postoperatively regarding the symptoms of hypocalcemia and the potential need for calcium and vitamin D replacement to alleviate those symptoms.

10.6.5 Thyroid Hormone Replacement

10.6.5.1 After Total Thyroidectomy

Patients who undergo total thyroidectomy require lifelong thyroid hormone therapy, and dosing is most commonly based on body weight. It has previously been demonstrated that in patients with spontaneous hypothyroidism, a levothyroxine dose of 1.6 mcg/kg/day is required to maintain serum TSH levels in the normal range [22]. Jin and colleagues found that a 1.5 ug/kg/day was the best formula for estimation of an initial replacement dose of levothyroxine following total thyroidectomy [23]. Patients older than 55 years and patients with a body mass index >30 have a lower levothyroxine dosage requirement. As a result, when the dosage calculation is in between two prescription strengths of levothyroxine, the lower of the two is chosen for older and obese patients. A serum TSH level is checked at 6 weeks postoperatively and dosage adjustments are made to ensure that serum TSH is in the normal range. Other protocols exist that are based on BMI in an attempt to achieve a euthyroid state more rapidly [24].

Patients with thyroid cancer require higher doses of levothyroxine to suppress TSH, which has been shown to stimulate tumor growth, invasion, angiogenesis, and dedifferentiation. The degree of TSH suppression is dependent on the stage of the cancer and the risk of recurrence and mortality. Serum TSH levels should be <0.1 uIU/L in patients with metastatic disease, 0.1–0.5 for patients with high-risk cancer who are free of disease, and 0.3–2.0 uIU/L for patients with low-risk cancer [25].

10.6.5.2 After Thyroid Lobectomy

A serum TSH level is obtained 6 weeks after thyroid lobectomy to see if thyroid hormone replacement is warranted. Hypothyroidism occurs in approximately one-third of patients following thyroid lobectomy [26]. Factors predictive of postoperative hypothyroidism after thyroid lobectomy include higher preoperative serum TSH levels and Hashimoto's thyroiditis [26–28]. In patients with a functioning residual lobe of the thyroid gland, the mean levothyroxine dosage to maintain the serum TSH level in a normal range is lower than following total thyroidectomy and has previously been demonstrated to be 1.3 ug/kg/day [26]. After initiating replacement therapy, a serum TSH level is rechecked in 6 weeks.

10.7 Management of Complications

Complications specific to thyroid surgery include neck hematoma, temporary and permanent recurrent laryngeal nerve injury, hypocalcemia, and permanent hypoparathyroidism. The reported rates of complications are highly variable, particularly when outcome studies from national databases are compared to single-institution studies from high-volume thyroid surgeons. The American Association of Endocrine Surgeons guidelines for definitive management of thyroid disease documents an incidence of 0.7–1.3% for neck hematoma, an average incidence of 9.8% for temporary RLN injury and 2.3% for permanent RLN injury, a median incidence of 27% for transient hypocalcemia and 1% for permanent hypoparathyroidism [6, 29–31].

10.7.1 Neck Hematoma

Patients with life-threatening neck hematoma present with respiratory distress manifested by dyspnea, voice change, stridor, neck pain, and dysphagia. On exam, patients appear anxious, struggling to breathe with tachypnea, and visible neck swelling. Respiratory distress is caused by laryngeal edema as a consequence of decreased venous return from the larynx and tracheal compression due to the hematoma [16].

There have been multiple reported risk factors for postthyroidectomy neck hematoma requiring reoperation including age >65, Graves' disease, hypertension, male gender, antithrombotic drug use, prior thyroid surgery, bilateral thyroidectomy, and neck dissection [6, 32]. Additional contributing factors may be excessive coughing, retching, or vomiting.

Patients should be evaluated immediately at the bedside when there is concern for a neck hematoma. If the patient is showing signs of respiratory distress, the incision should be opened at the bedside to rapidly evacuate the hematoma. The sutures in the skin, the subcutaneous tissue and platysma muscle, and the strap muscles are removed and the superficial and deep spaces of the neck are opened to evacuate the hematoma and relieve the pressure on the airway. The wound is then loosely packed and covered, and the patient is taken to the operating room for neck exploration and control of the bleeding [16, 33]. For patients who are clinically stable, consideration may be given to transporting the patient to the operating room for management.

10.7.2 Recurrent Laryngeal Nerve Injury

Patients with unilateral RLN injury may experience hoarseness or dysphonia, loss of strength of the voice, and, less commonly, dysphagia or aspiration. Patients with bilateral RLN injury present with stridor. The most common mechanism for injury of the RLN is traction. Other mechanisms include transection, thermal injury, suture impingement, and crush injury [6, 34]. Vocal fold dysfunction (VFD) may also result from direct injury due to endotracheal intubation. Routine identification and delineation of the course of the RLN in the neck during thyroidectomy is the gold standard to help prevent injury. Excessive traction injury or thermal injury is mechanism of RLN injury not always recognized intraoperatively. Dissection and identification of the RLN may be challenging due to patient factors such as a large goiter with retrosternal extension, Graves' disease, reoperative surgery, invasive thyroid cancer, a nonrecurrent laryngeal nerve, and extralaryngeal branching or other anatomic variability of the RLN [34].

A transected nerve can be reapproximated primarily with end-to-end epineural repair using 7.0 nylon suture [35] When a primary repair is not feasible, a nerve graft using the ansa cervicalis can be performed. The ipsilateral ansa cervicalis is mobilized from the strap muscle, transected distally, and anastomosed to the distal transected end of the RLN. This is important not to restore vocal cord mobility, but to maintain vocalis muscle tone, which will help to enhance the quality of the voice postoperatively [6]. This has been shown to improve symptoms and phonatory function at 9 months after surgery [35].

If VFD is known or suspected after thyroidectomy, the patient should be closely monitored after extubation, watching for altered respiration, stridor, and aspiration of secretions. The patient's symptoms and suspicion for unilateral or bilateral VFD dictates the level of intervention needed postoperatively, which may include simple observation, supplemental oxygen, racemic epinephrine, humidified oxygen, steroids, continuous intubation or reintubation, and rarely tracheostomy [6].

Voice changes are common after thyroidectomy. Hoarseness due to vocal fold edema from intubation usually improves within a few days. If a patient has persistent hoarseness, coughing with liquids, or concern for RLN injury during thyroidectomy, further evaluation is warranted. Postoperative RLN injury can be transient or permanent, which is defined by lack of recovery at 1 year after the index operation. The median recovery time after transient injury is 8 weeks [34]. Early referral to a laryngologist and early intervention (<3 months after thyroidectomy) is important for patients with presumed RLN injury, because it can result in improved voice outcomes [6, 36]. Speech therapy, cord medialization, and arytenoidectomy may have a role in helping to improve the patient's quality of life after RLN injury.

10.7.3 Hypocalcemia and Hypoparathyroidism

Transient hypocalcemia is a common complication after thyroidectomy, occurring in 19–38% of patients, with a median incidence of 27% [6, 31]. Hypocalcemia is defined as a serum calcium level below the lower limit of normal. Patients with mild hypocalcemia may be asymptomatic, while those with more severe hypocalcemia may experience acral and/or perioral numbness and tingling. Severe hypocalcemia can also manifest with muscle cramps, trismus, seizures, tetany, laryngospasm, bronchospasm, and cardiac dysrhythmias [37]. On physical exam, a Chvostek or Trousseau sign can be elicited in patients with hypocalcemia. A Chvostek sign is movement of the ipsilateral upper lip that occurs after tapping the skin of the face over the zygomatic branch of the facial nerve (approximately 2 cm anterior to the external auditory meatus). A Trousseau sign is carpopedal spasm induced by ischemia that occurs when a sphygmomanometer cuff on the patient's arm is inflated above the systolic blood pressure for 3 min.

Transient hypoparathyroidism after thyroidectomy is defined as hypocalcemia in combination with reduced PTH levels lasting less than 6 months postoperatively. Permanent hypoparathyroidism is defined by a requirement for calcium and/or calcitriol supplementation with a low or undetectable PTH level more than 6 months after thyroidectomy. Rates of permanent hypoparathyroidism after thyroidectomy range from 0% to 5%, with a median rate of 1% [6, 31].

Patients at increased risk of postthyroidectomy hypocalcemia due to hypoparathyroidism include those operated on for Graves' disease, concurrent central neck dissection, large or substernal goiter, reoperative thyroid surgery, inadvertent removal of a parathyroid gland, pediatric patients, and patients with malabsorptive conditions [6, 37]

Evaluation for postthyroidectomy hypocalcemia includes questioning the patient about symptoms of hypocalcemia, physical examination for a Chvostek sign or a Trousseau sign, and measurement of serum calcium. Some surgeons also routinely measure intact PTH levels to help guide the postoperative management of hypocalcemia. Additional laboratory studies, such as magnesium, phosphorus, albumin, or ionized calcium, may be of value in patients with more severe hypocalcemia or when hypocalcemia is difficult to correct.

The mainstay of therapy for postthyroidectomy hypocalcemia is calcium supplementation. Depending on the severity of hypocalcemia, 500–1000 mg of elemental calcium may be given orally 2–4 times per day. Calcitriol is added for patients with symptomatic hypocalcemia and patients with persistent hypocalcemia despite oral supplementation, at a dose of 0.25 to 0.5 mcg twice daily. Calcium gluconate mixed in saline can be administered intravenously over several hours in patients with severe hypocalcemia, symptomatic hypocalcemia, or refractory hypocalcemia. Additional interventions to treat severe hypocalcemia may include correction of hypomagnesium; addition of thiazide diuretics and avoidance of loop diuretics; administration of calcium supplements with food for better absorption in an acidic environment; and, if possible, avoidance of proton pump inhibitors and H2 blockers [38]. Preoperative patient education and postoperative communication with the patient is important to effectively manage transient hypocalcemia symptoms and minimize the need for readmission.

Answers

1. (d); 2. (d); 3. (a); 4. (b); 5. (e); 6. (a); 7. (a); 8. (e); 9. (d); 10. (e)

References

1. Sosa JA, Hanna JW, Robinson KA, Lanman RB. Increases in thyroid nodule fine-needle aspirations, operations, and diagnoses of thyroid cancer in the United States. Surgery. 2013;154(6):1420–6; discussion 6–7.

2. Roman BR, Randolph GW, Kamani D. Conventional thyroidectomy in the treatment of primary thyroid cancer. Endocrinol Metab Clin N Am. 2019;48(1):125–41.
3. Gan T, Randle RW. The role of surgery in autoimmune conditions of the thyroid. Surg Clin North Am. 2019;99(4):633–48.
4. Bobanga ID, McHenry CR. Treatment of patients with Graves' disease and the appropriate extent of thyroidectomy. Best Pract Res Clin Endocrinol Metab. 2019;33(4):101319.
5. Sinclair CF, Bumpous JM, Haugen BR, Chala A, Meltzer D, Miller BS, et al. Laryngeal examination in thyroid and parathyroid surgery: an American Head and Neck Society consensus statement: AHNS Consensus Statement. Head Neck. 2016;38(6):811–9.
6. Patel KN, Yip L, Lubitz CC, Grubbs EG, Miller BS, Shen W, et al. Executive summary of the American Association of Endocrine Surgeons guidelines for the definitive surgical management of thyroid disease in adults. Ann Surg. 2020;271(3):399–410.
7. McHenry CR. Thyroidectomy. In: Carty SE, editor. Atlas of endocrine surgical techniques. New Dehli: Jaypee Brothers Medical Publishers (P) Ltd; 2017. p. 13–24.
8. Barczyński M, Konturek A, Cichoń S. Randomized clinical trial of visualization versus neuromonitoring of recurrent laryngeal nerves during thyroidectomy. Br J Surg. 2009;96(3):240–6.
9. Yang S, Zhou L, Lu Z, Ma B, Ji Q, Wang Y. Systematic review with meta-analysis of intraoperative neuromonitoring during thyroidectomy. Int J Surg. 2017;39:104–13.
10. Dralle H, Sekulla C, Haerting J, Timmermann W, Neumann HJ, Kruse E, et al. Risk factors of paralysis and functional outcome after recurrent laryngeal nerve monitoring in thyroid surgery. Surgery. 2004;136(6):1310–22.
11. Lombardi CP, Carnassale G, Damiani G, Acampora A, Raffaelli M, De Crea C, et al. "The final countdown": Is intraoperative, intermittent neuromonitoring really useful in preventing permanent nerve palsy? Evidence from a meta-analysis. Surgery. 2016;160(6):1693–706.
12. Brajcich BC, McHenry CR. The utility of intraoperative nerve monitoring during thyroid surgery. J Surg Res. 2016;204(1):29–33.
13. Randolph GW, Dralle H, Abdullah H, Barczynski M, Bellantone R, Brauckhoff M, et al. Electrophysiologic recurrent laryngeal nerve monitoring during thyroid and parathyroid surgery: international standards guideline statement. Laryngoscope. 2011;121(Suppl 1):S1–16.
14. Moalem J. Thyroidectomy – standard. In: Clark O, Duh Q-Y, Kebebew E, Gosnell JE, Shen WT, editors. Textbook of endocrine surgery. 3rd ed. New Delhi: Jaypee Brothers Medical Publishers (P) Ltd; 2016. p. 339–47.
15. Snyder SK, Hamid KS, Roberson CR, Rai SS, Bossen AC, Luh JH, et al. Outpatient thyroidectomy is safe and reasonable: experience with more than 1,000 planned outpatient procedures. J Am Coll Surg. 2010;210(5):575–82, 82–4.
16. Rosenbaum MA, Haridas M, McHenry CR. Life-threatening neck hematoma complicating thyroid and parathyroid surgery. Am J Surg. 2008;195(3):339–43; discussion 43.
17. Balentine CJ, Sippel RS. Outpatient thyroidectomy: is it safe? Surg Oncol Clin N Am. 2016;25(1):61–75.
18. McHenry CR. "Same-day" thyroid surgery: an analysis of safety, cost savings, and outcome. Am Surg. 1997;63(7):586–9; discussion 89–90.
19. Brady JT, Dreimiller A, Miller-Spalding S, Gesang T, Sehgal AR, McHenry CR. Are narcotic pain medications necessary after discharge following thyroidectomy and parathyroidectomy? Surgery. 2020;169(1):202–8.
20. Orloff LA, Wiseman SM, Bernet VJ, Fahey TJ, Shaha AR, Shindo ML, et al. American Thyroid Association statement on postoperative hypo-

parathyroidism: diagnosis, prevention, and management in adults. Thyroid. 2018;28(7):830–41.
21. Oltmann SC, Brekke AV, Schneider DF, Schaefer SC, Chen H, Sippel RS. Preventing postoperative hypocalcemia in patients with Graves disease: a prospective study. Ann Surg Oncol. 2015;22(3):952–8.
22. Burmeister LA, Goumaz MO, Mariash CN, Oppenheimer JH. Levothyroxine dose requirements for thyrotropin suppression in the treatment of differentiated thyroid cancer. J Clin Endocrinol Metab. 1992;75(2):344–50.
23. Jin J, Allemang MT, McHenry CR. Levothyroxine replacement dosage determination after thyroidectomy. Am J Surg. 2013;205(3):360–3; discussion 3–4.
24. Elfenbein DM, Schaefer S, Shumway C, Chen H, Sippel RS, Schneider DF. Prospective intervention of a novel levothyroxine dosing protocol based on body mass index after thyroidectomy. J Am Coll Surg. 2016;222(1):83–8.
25. Haugen BR, Alexander EK, Bible KC, Doherty GM, Mandel SJ, Nikiforov YE, et al. 2015 American Thyroid Association Management Guidelines for adult patients with thyroid nodules and differentiated thyroid cancer: the American Thyroid Association Guidelines Task Force on thyroid nodules and differentiated thyroid cancer. Thyroid. 2016;26(1):1–133.
26. McHenry CR, Slusarczyk SJ. Hypothyroidisim following hemithyroidectomy: incidence, risk factors, and management. Surgery. 2000;128(6):994–8.
27. Lee DY, Seok J, Jeong WJ, Ahn SH. Prediction of thyroid hormone supplementation after thyroid lobectomy. J Surg Res. 2015;193(1):273–8.
28. Stoll SJ, Pitt SC, Liu J, Schaefer S, Sippel RS, Chen H. Thyroid hormone replacement after thyroid lobectomy. Surgery. 2009;146(4):554–8; discussion 58–60.
29. Jeannon JP, Orabi AA, Bruch GA, Abdalsalam HA, Simo R. Diagnosis of recurrent laryngeal nerve palsy after thyroidectomy: a systematic review. Int J Clin Pract. 2009;63(4):624–9.
30. Dehal A, Abbas A, Hussain F, Johna S. Risk factors for neck hematoma after thyroid or parathyroid surgery: ten-year analysis of the nationwide inpatient sample database. Perm J. 2015;19(1):22–8.
31. Edafe O, Antakia R, Laskar N, Uttley L, Balasubramanian SP. Systematic review and meta-analysis of predictors of post-thyroidectomy hypocalcaemia. Br J Surg. 2014;101(4):307–20.
32. Fan C, Zhou X, Su G, Zhou Y, Su J, Luo M, et al. Risk factors for neck hematoma requiring surgical re-intervention after thyroidectomy: a systematic review and meta-analysis. BMC Surg. 2019;19(1):98.
33. Wu K, Kim S, Rajasingham SJ, Bruni I, Fung K, Roth KE. Simulation of urgent airway management in a postthyroidectomy hematoma. MedEdPORTAL. 2019;15:10802.
34. Joliat GR, Guarnero V, Demartines N, Schweizer V, Matter M. Recurrent laryngeal nerve injury after thyroid and parathyroid surgery: incidence and postoperative evolution assessment. Medicine (Baltimore). 2017;96(17):e6674.
35. Gurrado A, Pasculli A, Pezzolla A, Di Meo G, Fiorella ML, Cortese R, et al. A method to repair the recurrent laryngeal nerve during thyroidectomy. Can J Surg. 2018;61(4):278–82.
36. Chandrasekhar SS, Randolph GW, Seidman MD, Rosenfeld RM, Angelos P, Barkmeier-Kraemer J, et al. Clinical practice guideline: improving voice outcomes after thyroid surgery. Otolaryngol Head Neck Surg. 2013;148(6 Suppl):S1–37.

37. Kazaure HS, Sosa JA. Surgical hypoparathyroidism. Endocrinol Metab Clin N Am. 2018;47(4):783–96.
38. Mejia M, Gonzalez-Devia D, Fierro F, Tapiero M, Rojas L. Hypocalcemia posthyroidectomy: prevention, diagnosis and management. J Transl Sci. 2018;4 https://doi.org/10.15761/JTS.1000212.

Neck Dissection: Indications, Extension, Operative Technique

Marco Raffaelli and Amy Y. Chen

Contents

A. L. Shifrin et al. (eds.), *Endocrine Surgery Comprehensive Board Exam Guide*,
https://doi.org/10.1007/978-3-030-84737-1_11

Case Presentation

An 18-year-old female, whose previous medical history was characterized by a Hashimoto thyroiditis and euthyroidism, underwent neck ultrasonography that showed a 15-mm suspicious nodule on the right thyroid lobe (TI-RADS 5) 8 months before consultation. Due to limitations related to the COVID-19 pandemic, she underwent ultrasound-guided fine needle aspiration cytology 5 months later. Cytological result demonstrated a papillary thyroid carcinoma of the right thyroid lobe (TIR5 – Bethesda VI).

Preoperative ultrasound performed at first surgical consultation showed an 18-mm right nodule with bilateral suspicious cervical lymph nodes. Fine needle aspiration cytology showed a metastasis of papillary thyroid carcinoma in a right lateral lymph node (level III, largest diameter 20 mm) and reactive changes in a 9-mm left lateral lymph node (level IIa).

Laboratory results showed normal calcitonin of 0.5 pg/mL in the context of functional euthyroidism, characterized by an fT3 level of 3.44 pg/mL, an fT4 level of 14.8 pg/mL, and a TSH of 2.31 μUI/mL. Furthermore, calcium was 9.2 mg/dL, parathormone level was 27.8 pg/mL, and vitamin D was 30.8 ng/mL.

She was scheduled for surgery. An intraoperative frozen section examination of left level IIa lateral neck nodes showed presence of metastases of papillary thyroid carcinoma, and she underwent total thyroidectomy plus central neck (level VI–VII) and bilateral lateral neck dissection (levels II–III–IV–Vb). The postoperative course was uneventful, in particular no hypocalcemia, no laryngeal nerve injury, no lymphatic leak, and no other complications occurred.

Final histology showed a multifocal papillary thyroid carcinoma (diffuse sclerosing variant) and confirmed central and bilateral lateral lymph node metastases (pT1bm, pN1b-TNM/AJCC 8th ed. 2017).

Two months after surgery she underwent ^{131}I treatment (150 mCi). Post-treatment whole body scan was negative for local residual disease and distant metastases. Stimulated serum thyroglobulin (TSH 45 μUI/mL) was 0.6 ng/mL, and neck ultrasound confirmed absence of structural residual and/or recurrent disease.

11

Questions

1. In case of diagnosis of papillary thyroid carcinoma with central and unilateral lateral neck nodal metastases, which of the following is indicated?
   - I. Thyroid lobectomy is mandatory.
   - II. Total thyroidectomy plus bilateral neck dissection is mandatory.
   - III. Thyroid lobectomy plus ipsilateral central neck dissection is mandatory.
   - IV. Total thyroidectomy is mandatory.
   - V. Central neck dissection is mandatory.
   - VI. Unilateral lateral neck dissection is mandatory.
     - (a) I and VI
     - (b) II
     - (c) IV, V, and VI
     - (d) III

2. If the ultrasound demonstrated a thyroid hypoechoic nodule of 18 mm in its maximum diameter with irregular margins and internal microcalcifications, which of the following is indicated?
   (a) Fine needle aspiration biopsy is always indicated.
   (b) Fine needle aspiration biopsy is never indicated.
   (c) Fine needle aspiration biopsy can be useful only when a compressive symptomatology is present.
   (d) Fine needle aspiration biopsy can provide useful information only in presence of extracapsular extension by the nodule.
3. In case of medullary thyroid carcinoma without evidence of lateral neck nodal metastases, which of the following is indicated?
   I. Level III and IV dissection is indicated.
   II. Total thyroidectomy is mandatory.
   III. Central neck dissection is mandatory.
   IV. Level II–V dissection is mandatory.
   V. Level II dissection on the side of the tumor is indicated.
   VI. Unilateral lateral neck dissection is mandatory.
      (a) I and II
      (b) II and III
      (c) I and V
      (d) IV and VI
4. Selective lateral neck dissection includes the following:
   I. Removal of lymph nodes from levels I to V and resection of the internal jugular vein
   II. Removal of lymph nodes from levels II to IV and the spinal accessory nerve
   III. Removal of nodal basins (levels I–V) with preservation of spinal accessory nerve
   IV. Removal of less than all five lateral neck nodal levels
   V. Preservation of spinal accessory nerve
   VI. Preservation of internal jugular vein
      (a) I and III
      (b) II
      (c) V and VI
      (d) IV, V, and VI
5. In the treatment of thyroid carcinoma "ipsilateral central neck dissection" includes:
   I. Contralateral node picking
   II. Removal of mid-jugular nodes on the side of the tumor
   III. Lateral neck dissection on the side of the tumor
   IV. Removal of prelaryngeal lymph nodes
   V. Removal of pretracheal lymph nodes
   VI. Removal of paratracheal lymph nodes on the side of the tumor
      (a) II and III
      (b) III and VI
      (c) IV, V, and VI
      (d) II

6. Regarding the treatment of papillary thyroid carcinoma, "cN0" means:
   I. Lymph node dissection is required.
   II. The absence of preoperative evidence at ultrasound examination of lymph node involvement.
   III. Final histology showed no lymph node metastases.
   IV. The absence of clinical preoperative evidence of lymph node involvement.
   V. There is clinical evidence of lateral neck lymph node involvement.
   VI. The absence of intraoperative evidence of macroscopic lymph node involvement.
      (a) II, IV, and VI
      (b) III and VI
      (c) I and III
      (d) V and VI
7. Are there unequivocal risk factors for occult lymph node metastases in the central neck compartment in patients affected by papillary thyroid carcinoma?
   I. No
   II. Yes, in particular age >45 years
   III. Yes, in particular female sex
   IV. Yes, in particular estimated thyroid volume >100 mL
   V. Yes, in particular male sex
   VI. Yes, in particular age ≤ 45 years
      (a) I
      (b) II and III
      (c) IV and V
      (d) V and VI
8. "Ipsilateral central neck dissection" is a valid treatment option in clinically unifocal cN0 papillary thyroid carcinoma but:
   (a) It reduces the overall survival.
   (b) It carries the risk of contralateral occult lymph node metastases being overlooked.
   (c) It increases the risk of hypoparathyroidism when compared with bilateral central neck dissection.
   (d) It decreases the accuracy of staging when compared with total thyroidectomy with bilateral central neck dissection.
9. Frozen section examination on the "ipsilateral central neck nodes" in the treatment of clinically unifocal cN0 papillary thyroid carcinoma:
   (a) Has an overall accuracy of 100%
   (b) Increases the disease-specific overall survival
   (c) Decreases the postoperative complications of total thyroidectomy
   (d) Allows an intraoperative decision-making approach regarding the extension of central neck dissection

11.1 Introduction

Lymph node involvement is common in patients with thyroid carcinoma. It may negatively affect recurrence rate and survival [1–4].

Lymph node neck dissections are technically demanding, and sometimes challenging operations associated with several possible complications, as several anatomic structures are at risk. The trachea, esophagus, laryngeal nerves, and parathyroid glands are extensively exposed during central neck dissection (CND). Moreover, when a lateral neck dissection (LND) is performed, the internal jugular vein (IJV), common carotid artery (CCA), vagus (VN), hypoglossal, spinal accessory (SAN) and phrenic nerves, sympathetic trunk, brachial plexus, and thoracic duct are at risk of injury.

Knowledge of surgical techniques, anatomic landmarks, nomenclatures, and classifications is essential to offer the most appropriate surgery, but also to obtain homogeneous data to evaluate and compare literature results [5, 6].

Inadequate lymph node surgery is the main cause of recurrent or persistent thyroid cancer [7] since recurrent disease in lymph nodes accounts for 60–75% of all neck recurrences [4, 8].

Lymph node metastases to the regional lymph nodes occur approximately in 30–80% of patients with papillary thyroid carcinoma (PTC) [9, 10]; nodal metastases from follicular thyroid carcinoma (FTC) are quite rare (1–8% of the patients) [11]. Metastases to regional lymph nodes in medullary thyroid carcinoma (MTC) have been reported in 34–81% of the patients [12–14].

Clinical evaluation and preoperative workup is of utmost importance to plan the correct initial surgical procedure, balancing complete oncological removal of tumor and nodal disease while minimizing the complication rate.

An accurate ultrasound evaluation, ideally performed by the surgeon him/herself [15], is essential in the evaluation of the thyroid tumor and of the nodal status. Loss of fatty hilum, calcifications, peripheral vascularity, hyperechogenicity, rounded rather than oval shape, cystic changes, and large size are all characteristics of lymph nodes suspicious for nodal metastases at ultrasound [4]. Pre-operative fine needle aspiration cytology confirms in many cases the suspicion of nodal involvement. Thyroglobulin measurement in the washing fluid of the fine needle aspirate can be helpful in the diagnosis of node positive (N1) differentiated thyroid carcinoma (DTC), especially in case of cystic lateral neck masses where aspiration cytology is often paucicellular [4]. Similarly, calcitonin measurement in the washing fluid of fine-needle aspirates is able to detect central and/or lateral neck metastasis of MTC [16, 17]. In selected cases, cross-sectional imaging studies (computed tomography, CT, or magnetic resonance imaging, MRI) with intravenous contrast could be helpful in the identification of tracheal/esophageal involvement and nodal involvement, especially in the upper mediastinum and in the retropharyngeal and parapharyngeal spaces [1, 4].

While macroscopic nodal disease and extranodal extension are well-recognized risk factors impacting prognosis in thyroid carcinomas, occult microscopic nodal disease seems to have no influence on survival and a limited impact on recurrence [2].

On the other hand, not all occult nodal disease is microscopic (<2 mm) nodal disease.

Therapeutic central with/without LND is mandatory in all patients with thyroid carcinoma and clinical evidence of central and/or lateral nodal involvement [1, 3, 4, 8, 18, 19].

The role of prophylactic CND in patients with clinically node negative (cN0) thyroid carcinoma remains a matter of debate [1, 2, 4, 8, 18–23]. It is strongly indicated in patients with MTC and encouraged in those with advanced primary DTC (T3, T4) [1, 3, 4, 8, 18, 19].

With regard to LND, current evidence supports no role for prophylactic LND in patients with DTC in the absence of any pre- or intraoperative evidence of lateral neck nodal metastases [1, 4, 8, 18, 19]. Some debate still exists with regard to the possible role of prophylactic LND in patients with MTC [1, 3, 8, 18].

Another important point is the surgical technique. Neck dissection has to be considered one of the most challenging (complicated) surgeries of the human body [24]. After the initial description by G. Crile in 1906 of a series of patients who successfully underwent radical neck dissection (RND) [25], (i.e., the removal of neck nodes *en bloc* with IJV, sternocleidomastoid muscle (SCM), and SAN), several modifications have been proposed over the last century to maximize functional outcomes. However, two main concepts have highly influenced the surgical approach to the neck nodal disease over the last seven decades. First of all, the understanding that the cervical lymph nodes are without exception contained in the spaces defined by the muscular fasciae and vascular aponeuroses. As a consequence, in the absence of direct muscular, vascular and/or nervous invasion, neck dissection can be safely achieved by removing the fascial covering *en bloc* with the fibrofatty tissue containing the lymph nodes, while preserving muscular, vascular, and nervous structures [26]. The crucial point is the fascial compartmentalization of the neck: the "wrapping cloth" (i.e., the whole aponeurotic system) can be removed in one piece together with the packing material (i.e., the cellular and fat tissue contained therein), while preserving important and non-affected structures [26]. The second aspect is that different head and neck tumors involve different levels of neck nodes. Therefore, neck dissection for a specific tumor may be limited to a group/groups of lymph node at higher risk of being affected, in the absence of overt involvement of other groups. Consequently, neck lymph nodes have been grouped in levels

(I–VI) by a Committee for Head and Neck Surgery and Oncology of the American Academy of Otolaryngology-Head and Neck Surgery (AAO-HNS), with the specific aim to standardize the nomenclature and the reporting system of neck dissections (see below).

Since both the discussed aspects represent the rationale for the current approach to neck dissection, the detailed knowledge of the anatomical basis and of the nomenclature are of utmost importance.

11.2 Applied Anatomy

The thyroid has an extensive lymphatic drainage, which may flow in a variety of directions [27]. The intraglandular lymphatic connections are extensive and enable lymphatic drainage from one lobe to the other through a complex of intrathyroidal and pericapsular nodes [27]. The major lymph vessels running efferently follow the branches of the thyroid arteries and veins in three main directions: superiorly, laterally, and inferiorly. The upper thyroid region is drained by the superior thyroid vessels into the upper jugular nodes. From the isthmus, the lymphatic vessels run to prelaryngeal, or Delphian, nodes, which are connected to the upper jugular nodes. Lateral lymph vessels follow the medial thyroid vein to the mid- and lower jugular nodes. The lower lymphatic drainage is directed to the pretracheal and paratracheal nodes and to the lower jugular chain.

The central compartment (defined as level VI and VII; see below) is typically the first site for lymph node metastases [5]. One exception can occur when the primary tumor is located in the upper pole and lymph node metastases may "skip" the central compartment, to be initially found in the lateral compartment only [28]. Unusual and rare sites for thyroid carcinoma nodal metastases include retropharyngeal, parapharyngeal, retrocarotid, sublingual, axillary, and intraparotid locations, as well as nodal involvement at level of thyrohyoid membrane and/or superficial to the strap muscles [29].

▪▪ Cervical fascial planes

In spite of some disagreements about the definitions and the limits of the cervical fascial planes in anatomic textbooks and published papers [26, 30, 31], classically four different fascial layers have been described in the neck: the superficial cervical fascia (SCF) and the deep cervical fascia (DCF). The last further recognizes three more different layers: the superficial (SLDCF), the middle (MLDCF), and the deep layer of the DCF (DLDCF).

The SCF, variably recognized [30], is just underneath the dermis and is composed of loose connective tissue, fat, the platysma muscle, and small unnamed nerves and blood vessels.

The SLDCF is described as a definite sheath of fibrous tissue encircling the neck and extending between the face and pectoral regions. It splits in two layers and envelops two muscles (the trapezius and the sternocleidomastoid) and two glands (the parotid and the submandibular) and forms two spaces (the supraclavicular and the suprasternal). It attaches cranially to the hyoid bone where it merges with the MLDCF and inferiorly to the acromion of the scapula, the clavicle, and the sternum. The fascia remains split in two layers until it attaches to the sternum. Thus, the superficial layer attaches to the anterior surface of the sternum and the posterior layer to the posterior surface of the sternum. It forms the roof of the anterior and posterior cervical triangles and the midline raphe of the strap muscles.

The MLDCF splits into an anterior portion (muscular component) that envelops the strap muscles (sternohyoid, sternothyroid, thyrohyoid, omohyoid) and a posterior layer (visceral component) that includes both the pretracheal and buccopharyngeal fascia and envelops thyroid gland, larynx/trachea, and pharynx/esophagus [24, 30].

The DLDCF has two main subdivisions: the first comprised the prevertebral fascia spanning the tips of the transverse processes anterior to the vertebral bodies and extending from skull base to coccyx. It continues laterally and posteriorly as the scalenus fascia covering the scalene muscles, splenius capitis, and levator scapulae to attach to the spinous processes of the vertebrae. The other subdivision consisted of a layer of alar fascia lying anterior to the prevertebral fascia but posterior to the pharynx/esophagus and visceral fascia. It is described to pass anterolaterally to fuse with the carotid sheath and prevertebral fascia and extends inferiorly from the base of the skull to about the C7 vertebral level where it fuses with the visceral fascia.

All the layers of the DCF contribute to the carotid sheath, which includes the CCA, the IJV, and the VN.

The fibrofatty tissue encompassing the lymph nodes in the neck can thus be found in two main spaces in the neck, the central and the lateral, which are separated by the carotid sheath.

The lateral space of the neck on both sides is limited externally by the SLDCF and MLDCF, posteriorly by DLDCF, and medially by the carotid sheath. The lateral space of the neck is divided vertically on each side by (1) the transverse aponeurosis, which originates from around the internal jugular vein and carotid artery and runs in a lateral direction toward the external jugular vein; and (2) the sagittal aponeurosis which, starting from the carotid sheath, runs posteriorly to the scalenus group of muscles [26]. The cervical and brachial plexus, embryologically independent of the branchial apparatus, lies outside the space limited by this aponeurotic system. The same is true for the phrenic nerve. The cervical sympathetic chain, which also lies outside this space, is in close connection with it [26]. The hypoglossal nerve and the SAN run across this space for a part of their course. The VN runs in the narrow fissure between the venous and arterial divisions of the sagittal aponeurosis, which envelops the internal jugular vein and carotid artery, respectively. The thoracic duct crosses the lateral space of the neck at its lower end [26].

The central space is further divided into several compartments: the visceral space, enveloped by the visceral layer of the MLDCF, and the paravisceral space, bilateral, which the carotid sheath separates from the lateral space [32]. The sagittal aponeurosis divides it from the retrovisceral (prevertebral) space, outlined by the MLDCF and the alar fascia.

Because of such anatomical basis, lymph node dissection, in both the central and the lateral compartments, can be achieved satisfactorily when vessels, muscles, and glands are carefully stripped of their aponeurotic coverings, and when all aponeurotic septa are removed in one block together with their contents. The essential structures running in them should have been previously identified and dissected free [26, 32]. Such an approach, as discussed later, emphasize that lymph node dissection is not the one-by-one removal of (enlarged) lymph nodes in a certain region or of a certain group of nodes (*cherry picking*), rather a systematic and comprehensive dissection of lymph nodes containing fibrofatty tissue embedded and covered by the relative fascial layer(s).

11.2.1 Standardized Terminology in Neck Dissection

Since the 1930s, the locations of cervical lymph node groups have been designated using a system developed at the Memorial Sloan-Kettering Cancer Center in which groups of lymph nodes at various anatomic levels are described. This system, initially used for labeling of neck dissection specimens, has achieved worldwide acceptance, as it not only designates the anatomical location of groups of lymph nodes, but also reflects, rather consistently, the progress of spread of tumors at various locations through the neck, and indicates which levels are at greatest risk of involvement for early metastasis from tumors at various primary sites.

In order to standardize the definition and the approaches to the cervical nodes, the American Head and Neck Society Committee for Neck Dissection Classification and the American Academy of Otolaryngology Head and Neck Surgery, Committee for Head and Neck Surgery and Oncology, in 1988 began the process that resulted in the publication of the classification of the neck dissection [33] that, with subsequent modifications [34, 35] still constitute the basis for the understanding and the reporting of the surgical approach to the cervical lymph nodes.

The two main objectives of the AHNS/AAOHNS Committees were the definition of the level system to delineate the location of nodal disease in the neck and the definition of a standard nomenclature for neck dissection [34].

11.2.2 Levels of Cervical Lymph Nodes

The cervical nodes have been divided into six levels (I–VI) that have been widely accepted. Anatomical boundaries that have been defined for neck lymph node levels represent practical intraoperative landmarks during neck dissection, but also well-defined and readily visible radiological landmarks, useful to preoperatively evaluate the extent of neck nodal disease and plan the surgical resection [34].

Of note, especially when dealing with thyroid carcinoma, upper mediastinal nodes, below the sternal notch to the level of the innominate artery, may be involved and need to be removed. This group of nodes, which represent an extension of the paratracheal nodes in both sides and are reachable and removable trough a neck (collar incision) approach, are usually indicated as level VII and included in the central compartment dissection (see below) [5, 35].

The neck lymph node levels are identified as follow:

Level I: it includes *submental (Ia)* and *submandibular nodes (Ib)*. Level Ia (submental triangle), which is unpaired, is a midline level bounded by the anterior belly of the digastric muscle and the hyoid bone, inferiorly. The level Ib, containing the submandibular gland and its nodes, is defined by the body of the mandible superiorly, the anterior belly of the ipsilateral digastric muscle anteriorly, the posterior belly of the ipsilateral digastric muscle inferiorly, and the stylohyoid muscle posteriorly. Radiologically, the sagittal plane passing through the posterior border of the submandibular gland is used to define the boundary between the Ib and IIa levels (posterior boundary). During neck dissection it is useful to consider the fascia overlying the posterior aspect of the submandibular gland [36]. Level I is not usually involved in thyroid carcinomas and does not need to be routinely dissected, in the absence of overt/gross involvement [6]. The key structures that can be found and should be preserved at this level include the lingual nerve, hypoglossal nerve, submandibular duct, and facial artery and vein are all found in level I. The only significant structure found lateral to the posterior belly of the digastric is the facial vein. The *marginalis mandibulae* branch of the facial nerve can be found in the fascia overlying the submandibular gland superficial to the facial vessels [24].

Level II: it includes the *upper jugular nodes*, which are located by the upper third of the IJV. It extends from the skull base to a horizontal line defined by the inferior border of the body of the hyoid bone. The anterior border of level II is the stylohyoid muscle but conventionally by a line passing along the posterior border of the submaxillary gland (see above), and the posterior border is the posterior (lateral) border of the SCM. The SAN, which travels obliquely across this area, is used as a landmark to subdivide this group into IIb, the portion above and behind the nerve, and IIa, the portion that lays antero-inferiorly to it [34].

The key structure found during dissection is the SAN, which runs deep to the posterior digastric muscle and the occipital artery, superficially to the internal jugular vein. It often gives off a small branch to the trapezius prior to entering the sternocleidomastoid muscle [24].

Level III: it includes the *mid jugular nodes*. This level is bounded superiorly by a horizontal plane passing along the inferior border of the body of the hyoid bone, inferiorly by a horizontal plane passing along the inferior border of the cricoid cartilage, posteriorly (laterally) by the posterior margin of the SCM, and anteriorly (medially) by the lateral border of the sternohyoid muscle [34]. Since this last is not an easily visible landmark from a radiological point of view, it has been proposed that the medial border of the CCA could serve as an alternate radiological landmark [35]. However, it should be noted that from an anatomical and surgical point of view, the lateral border of the sternohyoid muscle with its investing fascia (muscular component of the MLDCF), which participates to the carotid sheath (see above), better defines the boundary between the anterior (central) and the lateral (or posterolateral) compartments of the neck (◘ Fig. 11.1). Indeed, as described above, it is the carotid sheath that anatomically divides the anterior and the lateral compartments of the necks, and it is formed by the coalescence of all the layers of the DCF. Such consideration has important consequences during neck dissection, since following the investing fascia of the sternohyoid muscle would allow to avoid to expose the CCA during LND and to enter the central (anterior) compartment [35, 36]. All these considerations are true for both the III (mid-jugular) and the IV (lower-jugular) lymph node levels.

Conversely, not removing the lymph nodes along the lateral border of the sternohyoid muscle, during dissection of the central compartment could result in an inadequate dissection.

In addition, in the first version of the classification [33], the anterior belly of the omohyoid muscle was chosen as the surgical boundary between the III and the IV levels. In the revised classification it crosses the III levels, and the lymph nodes underneath the anterior belly of the omohyoid muscle should be included in the III levels [35].

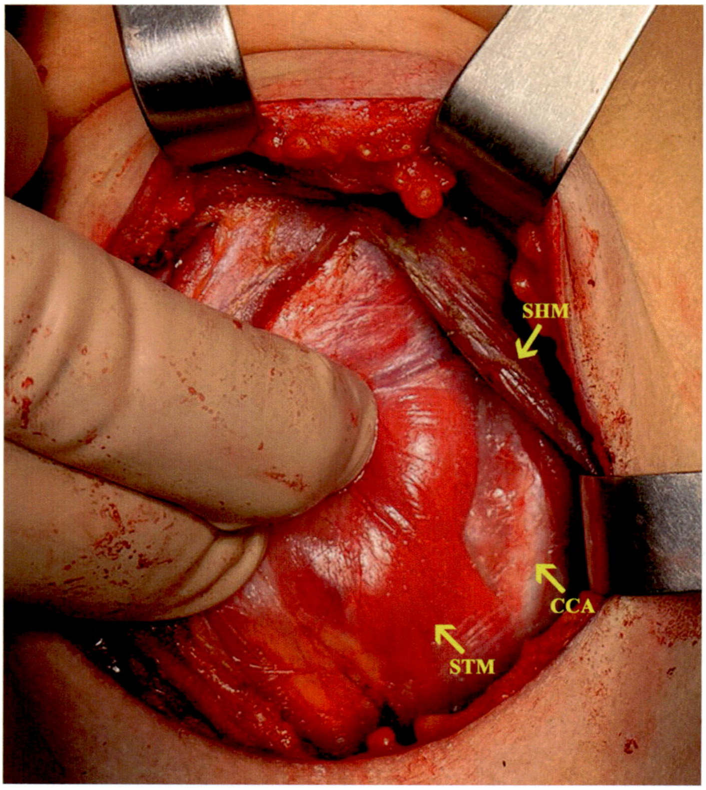

Fig. 11.1 Boundary between the anterior (central) and the lateral (or posterolateral) compartments of the neck: coalescence of the fascia covering lateral border of the sternothyroid muscle with the carotid sheet. SHM sternohyoid muscle, CCA common carotid artery, STM sternothyroid muscle

The key structures encountered during dissection at this level are the anterior belly and the intermediate tendon of the omohyoid muscle, the cervical rootlets, and the phrenic nerve which runs superficial to the anterior scalene muscle beneath the DLDCF.

Level IV: it includes the lower jugular nodes which are located between a plane passing along the inferior border of the cricoid cartilage superiorly and the clavicle inferiorly. The anterior (medial) and the posterior (lateral) boundaries of the level IV are represented, as for level III, by the sternohyoid muscle and the posterior border of the SCM, respectively (see above). The key structures which are encountered during dissection are the thoracic duct (more commonly seen in the left neck), the transverse cervical artery, phrenic nerve, and anterior scalene muscle, as well as the confluence of the IJV and the subclavian veins (Pirogoff's trunk). The lung apices may also be present at the inferior aspect of level IV.

Level V: it includes the posterior triangle of the neck. It is bounded anteriorly by the posterior border of the SCM, posteriorly by the anterior border of the trapezius muscle, superiorly by the convergence of the SCM, and the trapezius muscle and inferiorly by the clavicle [33]. This level is furtherly subdivided by a plane passing along the inferior border of the cricoid cartilage into level Va, superiorly, and level Vb, inferiorly [34]. The superior subgroup, level Va, primarily contains the spinal accessory nodes, and the SAN. Level Vb contains the transverse cervical and supraclavicular nodes. As a consequence, in order to reduce the risk of inadvertent SAN injury, dissection of level Va is usually not recommended in neck dissection for thyroid carcinoma (see below). Besides SAN, key structures encountered during dissection of this level are the posterior belly of the omohyoid muscle, the brachial plexus, and the confluence of external and anterior jugular veins.

Level VI–VII (central compartment): this group of nodes includes the lymph nodes of the anterior cervical compartment (level VI) and the superior mediastinal nodes that can be reached via cervical incision (previously reported as level VII), more commonly reported as central compartment.

The boundaries of the anterior compartment (level VI) are defined superiorly by the hyoid bone, inferiorly by the sternal notch, laterally by the medial aspect of the carotid sheath. Superior mediastinal nodes (Level VII lymph nodes) that are removable by a trans-cervical approach are those associated with the brachiocephalic vein and innominate artery. The boundaries of the level VII are the suprasternal notch superiorly, the medial aspect of the carotid sheath laterally, and the innominate artery on the right (at its point of tracheal crossing) and the corresponding axial plane on the left [5, 37]. Consequently, the central neck compartment is bounded superiorly by the hyoid bone, laterally by the medial aspect of the carotid sheath, inferiorly by point where the innominate artery crosses the trachea on the right and the corresponding axial plane on the left, anteriorly by the SLDCF, and posteriorly by the DLDCF [5, 37].

However, it should be noted that if the boundary between the anterior (central) and the lateral (posterolateral) compartments of the neck is represented by the lateral border of the sternothyroid muscle and its fascial insertion over the carotid sheath, as reported above (level III), the same boundary should be used as lateral limit of the central compartment, instead of the medial border of the carotid sheath [33].

Mediastinal lymph nodes located inferior to the innominate artery and caudal to the brachiocephalic vein are rarely involved in patients with existing central compartment lymph node metastases, usually cannot be removed by a transcervical approach, and should be reported as a separate level (mediastinal lymph node below the innominate artery) [35, 37].

According to their anatomical locations, the lymph nodes of the central compartment are conventionally subdivided in prelaryngeal (Delphian), pretracheal, and left and right paratracheal lymph nodes [37]. Thyroid cancer often metastasizes to the lymph nodes in these four groups. It should be underlined once more that it is a conventional subdivision based on the anatomical position of the groups of lymph nodes, rather than a true anatomical subdivision. No fascial plane divides these groups of lymph nodes.

The retropharyngeal and retroesophageal lymph nodes deeper with respect to the sagittal fascia and not included in the visceral layer of the MLDCF (see above) are rarely involved and are outside the boundary of the central compartment, as delimited by the fascial planes.

The majority of the central region lymph nodes are inferior to the larynx. Upper pole tumors may occasionally metastasize to the paralaryngopharyngeal lymph nodes coursing along the superior thyroid vessels very close to the investing layers of the sternohyoid and omohyoid muscles, fascial layers that should consequently be removed in order to achieve adequate clearance. Sometimes the mediastinal lymph nodes inferior to the innominate artery can also be involved [5].

The *prelaryngeal (Delphian) lymph nodes* are localized in the fibrofatty tissue medial to the thyrohyoid muscle on both sides and bordered caudally by the upper edge of the thyroid isthmus and cranially by the hyoid bone [36]. The *pretracheal lymph nodes* are localized in the fibrofatty tissue on the anterior aspect of the trachea between the two edges of the trachea and bordered cranially by the lower edge of the isthmus and caudally by a line drawn from the intersection point between the innominate artery and the trachea. The *paratracheal lymph nodes* are embedded in the fibrofatty tissue contained in the trapezoidal compartment bordered cranially by the line passing through the lower edge of the cricoid cartilage, caudally by the line where the innominate artery crosses over the trachea on the right, the projection of this point on the axial plane on the left, laterally by the carotid sheath (or the lateral border of the sternothyroid muscle), medially by the ipsilateral lateral edge of the trachea, anteriorly by the muscular component of the MLDCF, and posteriorly by the sagittal aponeurosis. Due to the obliquus course of the right inferior laryngeal nerve (ILN) from behind the right subclavian artery to its laryngeal entry point, the right paratracheal region is further subdivided in two different areas by a plane passing through the right ILN: the posterolateral and the anterio-medial. That has important consequence during central neck dissection, since to obtain adequate clearance of the central compartment the lymph nodes both anteriorly and posteriorly to the ILN have to be removed. That requires a mobilization of the ILN in order to mobilize the fibrofatty tissue on the posterolateral area, transposing it antero-medially passing behind the ILN [37]. That is not true in the case of non-recurrent ILN [38]. On the left side the course of the ILN is more vertical from behind the aortic arch, along the tracheoesophageal groove. Thus, on the left side, the paratracheal lymphatic tissue is located anterolateral to the

ILN and esophagus. In this context, mobilization of ILN is not necessary when left paratracheal lymphatic dissection is performed [37].

11.3 Classification of Neck Dissections

Following the consensus statement of the working group of the American Thyroid Association (ATA) with participation from the American Association of Endocrine Surgeons (AAES), AAO-HNS, and American Head and Neck Society (AHNS) [5, 37], CND has been defined as the comprehensive removal of the pretracheal and prelaryngeal lymph nodes, along with at least one paratracheal nodal basin [5, 37]. The CND can be unilateral or bilateral if only one or both the paratracheal nodal basins are dissected and removed [5, 37].

The nomenclature of the LND follows the indications of the committee of the AHNS and the AO-HNS in 1991 [33] and subsequently updated in 2002 and 2008 [34, 35].

RND includes the removal of lymph nodes from levels I to V with *en bloc* resection of the IJV, SAN, and SCM [6, 34, 35]. This procedure, initially described by G. Crile [25] in 1906, rarely is indicated in patients with thyroid carcinoma.

Owing to the high morbidity and anatomical deformity due to RND, in 1963, O. Suarez [26, 39] and, subsequently, Bocca and Pignataro [26] and Gavilan et al. [40–42] described a modified RND (MRND) as functional neck dissection [26, 43] in which satisfactory oncological results could be obtained, while preserving key anatomical structures, i.e., SAN, IJV, and SCM, using a fascial dissection technique.

In 1989, Medina divided MRND into three types [44]. In type I, only SAN is preserved, in type II SAN and IJV, and in type III IJV, SAN, and SCM are all preserved. In addition, RND and MRND were divided into type A if all lymph nodes of levels I–V were all removed and type B if levels II–V were removed [44].

The study group of the AAO-HNS defined MRD as the comprehensive removal of all the levels included in the RND (levels I–V) with preservation of one or more of the nonlymphatic structures removed in the RND (SAN, IJV, SCM) [34, 35]. Preserved structures should be specifically named in the report (i.e., MRND with preservation of SAN) [35].

Alternate terms that have been used to refer to MRND in the published literature are total neck dissection, as proposed by the Japan Neck Dissection Study Group [45, 46], functional neck dissection [32, 42, 47, 48], and comprehensive neck dissection [35, 49, 50]. However, such terms are not widely accepted in the English literature, and their use has been discouraged or not recommended by the Neck Dissection Classification Committee of the AHNS [35].

The term selective neck dissection (SND) encompasses all the neck dissections in which there is the preservation of 1 or more of the lymph node levels routinely removed in RND. Dissection is thus directed by the patterns of lymphatic drainage of the primary tumor. In the 1991 classification of the AAO-HNS committee, four subtypes of SND were recognized (supraomohyoid, levels I, II, and III; lateral, levels II, III, and IV; posterolateral, levels II, III, IV, and V; anterior, level VI) [33], while in the revised consensus of the AAO-HNS committee such subtypes were abandoned, and it was suggested to report in parentheses next to SND the removed lymph node levels with roman numbers [i.e., SND (III–IV)], in order to avoid confusion and to encompass all the possible dissections [34]. SND (IIa, III, IV, and Vb) is the most commonly used in the management of lateral neck metastasis of thyroid carcinoma [(i.e., SND (IIa, III, IV, and Vb)].

The term extended radical neck dissection (ERND) refers to the removal of one or more additional lymph node groups or non-lymphatic structures, or both, routinely not removed in RND [34, 35]. Examples of additional lymph node groups include superior mediastinal, parapharyngeal, retropharyngeal, periparotid, postauricular, suboccipital, and buccinator. Examples of other non-lymphatic structures include CCA, hypoglossal nerve, VN, paraspinal muscles, and other neural, osseous, cutaneous, muscular, or vascular structures. All additional lymphatic and/or non-lymphatic structure(s) to be removed should be identified in parentheses [34].

Current accepted classification of neck dissections is reported in ◘ Table 11.1.

◘ **Table 11.1** Classification of neck dissections

Bilateral central neck dissection	Removal of the prelaryngeal, pretracheal, and both the right and left paratracheal nodal basins (levels VI and VII)
Unilateral/ ipsilateral central neck dissection	Removal of the prelaryngeal, pretracheal, and one paratracheal nodal basin (ipsilateral to primary tumor)
Radical neck dissection	Removal of levels I–V and resection of the internal jugular vein, the spinal accessory nerve, and the sternocleidomastoid muscle
Modified radical dissection	Removal of levels I–V, with preservation of one or more of the following non-lymphatic structures: spinal accessory nerve, internal jugular vein, or sternocleidomastoid muscle
Selective lateral neck dissection	Removal of less than all five lateral neck nodal levels, while preserving spinal accessory nerve, internal jugular vein, and sternocleidomastoid muscle. Removed lymph node levels have to be specified
Extended radical neck dissection	Removal of one or more additional lymph node groups or non-lymphatic structures, or both, routinely not removed in Radical Neck Dissection (parapharyngeal, retropharyngeal, periparotid, postauricular, suboccipital, and buccinators nodes/carotid artery, hypoglossal nerve, vagus nerves, paraspinal muscles, etc.). Additional removed lymph nodes and/or non-lymphatic structure have to be specified

In order to further reduce the possibility of confusion, misinterpretation, and redundancy of terms with respect to neck dissection, more recently an international group of experts has proposed a further revision of the classification of the neck dissections [51]. Three main aspects are needed to categorize the extent of the dissection: (1) the abbreviations "ND" should be used to represent the term neck dissection and applied as the first component of the description. A prefix should be included to denote the side of the neck upon which the dissection has been performed using the abbreviation L for left and R for right. If bilateral, both sides must be classified independently; (2) the second component of the description should be the neck levels and/or sublevels removed, designated with Roman numbers, in ascending order. For levels in which subdivision is applicable (such as I, II, V), the level is stated without a subdivision to indicate that the entire level (both a and b) was removed. If a sublevel is named, it means that the remaining sublevel was preserved; (3) the third component of the description should be the non-lymphatic structures removed, each identified using specified acronyms (symbols), all of which have been universally accepted.

For example, a left RND could be indicated as "L ND (I–V SCM, IJV, CN XI)" [51].

Subclassification into therapeutic and elective or prophylactic neck dissection refers to the indication for surgery but does not specify the extent of the dissection [1].

The term therapeutic neck dissection is used when cervical metastases are demonstrated pre- or intra-operatively. The term prophylactic, or elective, neck dissection is used when neck dissection is done for potential subclinical cervical metastases, not demonstrated at preoperative work up, intraoperative inspection, and/or intraoperative frozen section examination [1].

11.4 Central Neck Dissection: Indications and Extension

Current evidences endorse CND associated to total thyroidectomy in all the patients with clinical (pre- or intraoperative) evidence of central neck nodal involvement both for DTC (follicular cell-derived thyroid carcinomas – PTC and FTC) and MTC (C-cell carcinoma) [1, 3, 8, 18, 19, 52].

In order to reduce the complication rate (namely, ILN injury and parathyroid dysfunction) associated with bilateral CND, it has been proposed, in patients with DTC, in the presence of lymph node involvement clinically limited to only one paratracheal nodal basin, to limit the extension of CND (unilateral CND) [37]. However, if CND at the time of the initial thyroid surgery in clinically node positive PTC has the main role to comprehensively remove all the nodal metastatic disease, reducing the risk of persistent and/or recurrent disease, it is important to underline that the ipsilateral nodal involvement is one of the main risk factors for contralateral nodal disease [53, 54]. Contralateral occult nodal disease is indeed found in about 25% of the cases with nodal disease clinically limited to only one paratracheal region [55, 56]. Moreover, patients with clinical node involvement, >5 involved nodes and extranodal invasion are at higher risk of recurrence [57]. Therefore, patient with clinical central neck nodal involvement would probably benefit of a more aggressive approach (i.e., bilateral CND) if the potential benefits are not outweighed by the risk of complications. The extent of CND should then be adjusted on the surgeon's judgment balancing the safety of the procedure and the risk of recurrence and consequent eventual need of reoperation [37]. Indeed, even if it has been reported that in experienced hands reoperative CND can be as safe as primary surgery [58], it should be considered that reoperative surgical procedures are usually more challenging and at increased risk of complications, because of scar and altered anatomy [1]. Since in MTC lymph node metastases are present in the vast majority of patients at diagnosis and are not apparent by pre- or intraoperative assessment and no effective adjuvant treatment is available and indicated, prophylactic bilateral CND associated to total thyroidectomy is recommended in all the patients who undergo initial surgery for MTC [1, 3, 8, 18]. It has been recently proposed a more conservative approach, including unilateral thyroid resection instead of total thyroidectomy and bilateral CND for sporadic intrathyroidal MTC not showing desmoplasia at frozen section evaluation (FSE) [59], basing on the assumption that the absence of desmoplastic stromal reaction is correlated with the absence of lymph node involvement [60].

In patients with clinically node negative (cN0) DTC the role of prophylactic CND (pCND) remains controversial and matter of debate [1, 2, 8, 18–21, 23, 52].

pCND is associated with lower postoperative serum thyroglobulin; it allows to improve accuracy in staging and to reduce the risks of reoperation for recurrence [2].

In addition, the assessment of central compartment nodal status is particularly challenging with currently available diagnostic tools. Indeed, it has been demonstrated that neck ultrasonography, which can reliably diagnose lymph node metastases in the lateral neck compartments, has a poor sensitivity for the detection of the central neck nodal involvement [61]. The sensitivity of ultrasonography in detecting abnormal lymph nodes varies from 25% to 60% for the central neck and 70–95% for the lateral neck [62, 63]. One of the main factors influencing sensitivity is the expertise of the evaluating physician [1]. CT, MRI, and Positron Emission Tomography (PET) may give additional details, but they are indicated only in selected cases

[1, 37] and the sensitivity in detecting central nodal disease is relatively low (30–40%) [64]. Surgeon-performed ultrasonography, useful for mapping and planning the operative procedure, has been demonstrated to be more accurate in detecting lymph node involvement and associated with lower local recurrence rates compared to radiologist-performed ultrasonography, especially if performed just prior surgical incision with optimized patient's position under general anesthesia [15, 65, 66].

Conversely, one of the main arguments against pCND is the higher risk of complications, in the absence of unequivocal benefits [1, 2, 8, 18, 19, 52, 67]. In order to reduce postoperative morbidity, proponents of pCND would favor unilateral dissection that has complications rate similar to total thyroidectomy alone, while maintaining the accuracy in staging of bilateral pCND in clinical unifocal disease [67, 68].

In addition, the recurrence rate following total thyroidectomy alone is quite low (<5%) [57], and the prognostic impact of small volume lymph node involvement has been reduced by the current staging system (ATA Risk stratification, 8th Edition of AJCC TNM Staging) [1, 69].

Multifocal disease and extracapsular tumor invasion have been suggested as potential risk factors for occult nodal metastases [8, 20, 70, 71]. Possible risk factors included also age, sex, tumor size, and aggressive pathological variants [8, 20, 70, 71]. The available studies on this topic report discordant results, probably because of the heterogeneous patients' populations concerning operative and clinicopathologic features (prophylactic vs therapeutic central neck dissection, clinical unifocal vs clinical multifocal carcinomas, unilateral vs bilateral CND) source of uncontrolled bias [20]. None of the current molecular markers, including B-type RAF (BRAF) rearrangements, have been so far demonstrated to be strong independent prognostic indicators. Therefore they should not drive the decision to perform or not a pCND [37].

In definitive, to date there are no evidence to suggest unequivocal pre-operatively available clinical parameter as a reliable predictor of nodal disease in clinically node negative patients.

Basing on the previous considerations, most of the authors currently agree that pCND is generally not indicated in DTC [72]. Current guidelines [1, 4] and positional statements [37] suggest, instead, a selective approach to pCND in larger and locally more advanced tumor (T3 and T4) or in case of evidence of lateral neck nodal involvement (N1b). However, such kind of recommendation is mainly based on expert opinion, rather than on high level evidence [1].

Other selective approaches to pCND aim to intraoperatively evaluate central neck nodal status, assuming that an enlarged lymph node does not necessarily mean a metastasized node and that a normal-appearing node can harbor non-microscopic (>2 mm) metastasis [55, 56]. Indeed, intraoperative surgeon's judgment has a limited role in detecting occult central neck nodal disease [73].

Among these selective approaches, the sentinel lymph node biopsy technique has been proposed as an alternative to elective lymph node dissection in patients with clinically node negative (cN0) disease, theoretically allowing a histological staging of the lymphatic drainage without excising the whole lymphatic basin [74]. Vital blue dyes, radioisotopes, and the combination of both techniques are used in PTC patients [74, 75]. The results reported are variable and high-level evidence is lacking. Consequently, sentinel node biopsy for cN0 DTC has to be considered investigational [1].

FSE of central neck nodes is an important intraoperative adjunct to determine if CND is needed and has also been used to guide the need for bilateral CND, because of the high specificity and accuracy in detecting occult nodal involvement [1]. Delphian lymph node biopsy is able to predict other central neck nodal disease, but with a low sensitivity (35%) [76, 77].

It has been suggested that FSE on the ipsilateral central neck nodes can be used to intraoperatively assess the ipsilateral nodal status in clinically unifocal PTC and to subsequently modulate the extension of the prophylactic CND ensuring bilateral CND in case of positive FSE [55, 56]. The reported sensitivity, specificity, and overall accuracy of FSE are 80.7%, 100%, 90%, respectively, in detecting occult ipsilateral central neck metastases in clinically unifocal cN0 PTC [55, 56]. Most of the false negative results are observed in case of micrometastases, which are usually of negligible clinical significance [78]. Accuracy of N staging and short-term oncologic outcome seems comparable with those of patients with clinically unifocal cN0 PTC who underwent prophylactic bilateral CND [55].

FSE evaluation of prophylactically removed ipsilateral central neck nodes has been recently proposed also to guide the extent of thyroidectomy in patients eligible for thyroid lobectomy [79, 80]. In such protocol, ipsilateral pCND is performed at the time of lobectomy and sent for FSE. If central neck node metastases are found at FSE, completion thyroidectomy and contralateral paratracheal dissection is suggested, to reduce the risk of persistent/recurrent disease [79, 80].

In summary, bilateral CND is indicated at first time surgery in MTC, both with a therapeutic and prophylactic intent. A CND is indicated in clinically node positive DTC. Bilateral CND should be performed in case of bilateral paratracheal nodal basins macroscopic involvement. Unilateral CND could be considered adequate in the case of unilateral paratracheal involvement, even if it implies the risk of overlooking contralateral occult nodal disease. Given the lack of feasibility for a well-designed, adequately powered randomized clinical study on pCND [81] and the subsequent lack of high level evidences, the role of pCND in DTC remains controversial, although most of the guidelines and expert opinions are against, because of the increased risk of complications and the absence of clear-cut oncologic advantages [2]. Overall, basing on current evidences, whether prophylactic CND for PTC is performed or not during initial thyroidectomy should depend on tumor and patient characteristics and surgeon expertise [1].

11.4.1 Lateral Neck Dissection: Indications and Extension

In patients with DTC LND should be performed only with therapeutic intent for known disease and not for prophylactic purpose [1, 2, 6, 8, 18, 19, 52].

Indeed, it has been reported that prophylactic SND dissection (levels III and IV) yields occult nodal disease in 8–23% of patients that is a much lower rate with respect to central compartment involvement. In addition, accuracy of imaging studies (ultrasound) in detecting lateral neck node metastases is much higher than in the central compartment evaluation [82]. Furthermore, prophylactic LND results in high risk of surgical complications [83], and there is no evidence to indicate that prophylactic lateral neck dissection has clinical benefits in terms of survival or loco-regional control [83, 84].

In patients with MTC, guidelines recommend therapeutic uni- or bilateral LND in case of clinical evidence of lateral neck nodal metastases [1, 3, 8, 18, 85, 86].

Contrary to DTC, the role and indications of prophylactic LND in sporadic MTC without clinical evidence of lateral neck nodal metastases is debated [1, 3, 8, 18].

Several clinical and pathologic characteristics, including tumor size [87], serum calcitonin levels [18, 86], number of central neck nodes metastases [14], and the presence of stromal desmoplasia on tumor FSE [60, 88] have been investigated as potential risk factors for lateral neck metastases. No uniform conclusions have been derived, and the attitude toward the need/indication of prophylactic unilateral or bilateral LND in patients with MTC is still controversial.

In such context, the proposed approaches range from prophylactic bilateral LND (in the case of palpable tumors and/or central neck metastases and/or high serum calcitonin levels – >200 pg/mL) [12, 18, 86] to prophylactic ipsilateral LND (in the case of palpable tumors and/or moderately increased serum calcitonin levels – 20–200 pg/mL) [3].

Since persistent disease should be the unique source of increased calcitonin levels in patients with MTC, intraoperative calcitonin monitoring with or without provocative tests (high-dose calcium or pentagastrin stimulation tests) has been investigated in recent years, but the reported evidence are not unequivocal and not reliably applicable in the clinical practice [89, 90].

The optimal extension of LND in patients with thyroid carcinoma is still debated. Several approaches to lateral neck node dissection have been proposed raging from "cherry picking" to MRND [91–93]. Nodal metastases in level I are rare (<10%), and recurrence is also rare (<1%) if not dissected at initial SND [94–96]. It has been demonstrated that levels III and IV are the most common sites for lateral neck node metastases [92, 94, 95]. Thus, SND of levels III and IV could seem adequate in the treatment of regionally metastatic PTC, especially when there is no suspicion of lymph node metastases in the other levels or when multilevel aggressive neck metastases are not found [91, 95]. Conversely, it has been demonstrated that the rate of involvement of lymph nodes in levels II and V is quite similar to that of levels III and IV in patients undergoing LND [97]. Omitting the dissection of the levels II and V during therapeutic LND carries the potential risk to miss metastatic lymph nodes in two-thirds and one-fifth of the pN1b patients, respectively [97, 98].

To reduce the risk of injury to spinal accessory nerve and given the low likelihood of nodal involvement, level IIb should be dissected only in the presence of proven or suspected nodal metastases (similarly to level I) or if level IIa is positive, and similarly level Va is only dissected when it has clinically or ultrasound apparent nodal metastases [1, 2, 6, 98].

Consequently, SND, including levels IIa–III–IV–Vb, is considered the standard treatment for patients with DTC and MTC scheduled for LND [1–3, 8, 18, 19, 52, 72].

RND and ERND should be reserved to more aggressive and locally advanced cases in which a functional compartment oriented SND is not feasible or not allow adequate clearance. However, the sequelae and the risk of complications of such extended resection should be balanced with the possible benefits in each case, preferably by multidisciplinary discussion.

In summary, comprehensive compartment oriented SND is indicated in patients with lateral neck nodal metastasis of thyroid carcinoma. In the absence of lymph node involvement at levels I, IIb, and Va, SND should include levels IIa, III, IV, and Vb, balancing the risks of complication and of recurrent/persistent disease.

Prophylactic LND is not indicated in patients with DTC, but it can be considered in patients with MTC, basing on preoperative serum calcitonin levels and tumor size.

11.5 Operative Procedure

Neck dissections have been described as one of the most complicated surgeries of the human body [24]. Both if performed at the time of thyroidectomy or as a revisional surgery, CND and LND should comprehensively remove fibrofatty tissue in the target compartments, ensuring complete oncological removal of all nodal disease, while preserving anatomical integrity and function of non-lymphatic structures.

Adequate knowledge of applied anatomy and surgical experience, as well as surgical planning, are of utmost importance to accomplish a safe and radical operation.

Therefore, patients should be better operated in high volume centers by experienced surgeons [93].

11.5.1 Planning the Surgical Procedure

The operation should be adequately planned, by accurate preoperative evaluation, including patient history and lymph node mapping. If needed, second-line cross sectional imaging studies (CT, MRI, and PET scan) can be selectively used with this purpose [1]. However, in most of the cases, preoperative ultrasound lymph node mapping, integrated with fine-needle aspiration biopsy of suspiciously enlarged lymph nodes, is adequate for preoperative workup. As reported above, surgeon performed ultrasonography could improve the accuracy in detecting nodal disease. In the cases in which there is no cytologically/histologically proven nodal disease, FSE of suspiciously enlarged nodes can enable definitive intraoperative diagnosis, reducing the need for further operations for persistent/recurrent disease [15].

Besides lymph node mapping in all the patients with thyroid carcinoma, it is of utmost importance to preoperatively evaluate ILNs function, by means of direct laryngoscopy. Preoperative vocal fold paralysis may indicate gross invasion by the tumor and/or lymph node metastasis or surgical injury during previous operations. The affected nerve can be confidently resected in similar scenarios in order to achieve adequate oncological resection. On the contrary, if normal vocal folds motility is demonstrated at preoperative workup, any effort should be made to preserve anatomic integrity and function of the ILN, even in the presence of macroscopic invasion by the tumor itself or by metastatic nodes with extranodal growth pattern, at least in DTC. However, in such challenging settings, every effort should be made to remove all gross disease, while preserving ILN function. The benefits of preserving a functioning nerve should be always weighed against the risks of leaving structural disease, especially when facing aggressive histopathological variants of follicular cells derived tumors, less prone to respond to adjuvant treatment (i.e., radioiodine treatment), or MTC.

Beyond ILN function, in selected cases (bulky tumors, tumors showing an unexpected rapid growth, signs and symptom of local invasion – i.e., dysphonia, dysphagia, dyspnea, suspicious findings at preoperative ultrasonography), additional cross-sectional imaging studies (CT, MRI scan) should be performed to confirm/exclude invasion of adjacent organs/structures, including esophagus, trachea, larynx, vessels, or the presence of lymph node metastases in unusual site (i.e., retropharyngeal, retroesophageal basins). In suspicious cases, esophagogastroduodenoscopy and/or endotracheal endoscopy can be used to preoperatively confirm/exclude local invasion.

11.5.2 Intraoperative Surgical Adjuncts

In recent years, several innovative technologies, materials, and techniques have been proposed as intraoperative surgical adjuncts for thyroidectomy and neck dissections.

The use of magnification technique (surgical loupes or surgical microscope) has been investigated, but current evidences suggest no clear advantages in preventing laryngeal nerves injuries or hypoparathyroidism when compared with direct vision in thyroid surgery [99].

Energy-based vessel-sealing devices (ultrasonic devices, electrothermal bipolar devices, and hybrid systems) have been introduced as adjuncts to titanium clips, electrocautery, and knot-tying to improve surgical dissection and hemostasis showing safety and efficacy in several reports, while reducing operative time, but with no clear advantages in terms of reducing complications rate [100–104].

Moreover, topical hemostatic agents have been investigated in achieving hemostasis either passively, via contact activation of the intrinsic coagulation pathway, or actively, by including thrombin and/or fibrinogen to produce a fibrin seal, albeit discordant results are reported in preventing postoperative bleeding in thyroid surgery [105]. Moreover, the use of topical hemostatic agents (cyanoacrylate adhesives or fibrin glue) has been suggested to prevent, and in some experiences to control, chyle leak after neck dissections, although some reports have underlined how they are not effective and may render more challenging reoperation for chyle fistulas [106].

The use of intraoperative intermittent and continuous nerve monitoring has been extensively investigated to intraoperatively assess recurrent laryngeal nerves functional integrity [107, 108]. Its use does not replace an appropriate and meticulous surgical technique and knowledge of ILN anatomy and its variation. Several papers do support the use of intraoperative nerve monitoring in thyroid cancer surgery especially in patients with locally advanced disease and/or massive central neck nodal involvement, in reoperative cases, and in case of previous documented vocal cord paralysis [107, 109, 110]. Moreover, the use of intraoperative nerve monitoring has been proposed to intraoperatively assess integrity of external branch of superior laryngeal nerve (EBSLN) during thyroidectomy [111], and SAN and marginal mandibular nerve integrity during LND [112, 113]. Use of intraoperative nerve monitoring can also be helpful in knowing when to stage thyroidectomy, and/or neck dissection, if there is a loss of signal of the RLN.

Because it can be difficult to differentiate benign parathyroid tissue from pathology lymph nodes, intraoperative techniques aiming to better identify and preserve parathyroid tissue have been described, including methylene blue injection, near-infrared fluorescence imaging, and indocyanine green [114].

11.5.3 Surgical Technique

Regardless of the surgeon's preferred technique and the surgical adjuncts used, lymph node dissection for thyroid carcinoma should include a comprehensive, ideally *en bloc*, removal of all the target nodal basins: prelaryngeal, pretracheal, and paratracheal lymph nodes in CND and levels IIa–Vb in LND. Dissection of additional nodal groups (i.e., retropharyngeal, retroesophageal, level I, level IIb, and level Va) is selectively needed on the basis of the dissemination of nodal disease (see above).

To achieve an adequate and comprehensive clearance of the target basins, the surgeon should follow the planes of coalescence of different fascial layers, which are avascular and allow to remove the target nodes *en bloc* with their investing fascial layers. This is the well-known principle of the fascial dissection, theorized for LND by O. Suarez and worldwide diffused by Bocca and Pignataro [26] and Gavilan et al. [40, 42, 115]. Even though this concept was primarily developed for LND dissection, it is applicable also for CND, owing the fascial envelopments of the central (anterior) compartment, as described above.

When neck dissection is performed at the time of thyroidectomy, the central compartment should ideally be removed *en bloc* with the thyroid gland, in order to respect the principles of oncologic resection. When LND is planned and performed at the same time of thyroidectomy and/or CND, it is preferred to accomplish LND first, to reduce the risk that traction on an empty thyroid bed (central compartment) could cause inadvertent injury of ILN and/or parathyroid glands, which are no longer protected by adjacent structures. For this reason, in the present chapter, the operative technique of LND will be discussed first.

En bloc resection of lateral and central compartment is not suitable, since the central and the lateral compartment are separated by the carotid sheath. Only in the case of RND or ERND for locally advanced tumors invading structures included in the carotid sheath *en bloc* resection of the lateral and the central compartment could be feasible and advisable.

11.5.3.1 Patient's Preparation and Positioning

General anesthesia with oro-tracheal intubation is needed. Nerve-monitoring endotracheal tube is preferred. The patient is in supine position with the neck slightly hyperextended, by means of a shoulder roll (◘ Fig. 11.2). Following confirmation of the integrity of the nerve monitoring system, the patients is prepared and draped in the usual way. The trapezoidal operative field should include the chin, the inferior margin of the mandible and the earlobe cranially, the anterior margin of the trapezius muscle laterally, and the sternal notch and the clavicle caudally (◘ Fig. 11.2).

In the case of LND, the head of the patients should be rotated on the opposite side to maximize exposure. During such maneuver it is important to avoid any dislodgment of the orotracheal tube and of its electrodes for intraoperative nerve monitoring.

11.5.3.2 Skin Incision and Flap Elevation

In conventional procedure, a 4–5-cm collar incision about 2 fingers above the sternal notch, ideally in a natural neck crease, is usually adequate to provide access and good exposure for total thyroidectomy and CND. In the case of LND, incision should be prolonged on the side(s) of the dissection (◘ Figs. 11.2b and 11.3a). The horizontal skin incision should be prolonged until the posterior third/posterior margin of the ipsilateral SCM (◘ Fig. 11.3a). The extended collar incision can offer adequate exposure for neck dissections required in thyroid carcinoma. Other, less cosmetically favorable incisions (J shaped, U shaped, inverted T shaped), prolonged vertically to the mastoid area, are almost never required.

Monopolar cautery is used to elevate subplatysmal flap (◘ Fig. 11.3b), preserving the SLDCF, preserving the external and the anterior jugular veins and the greater auricular nerve.

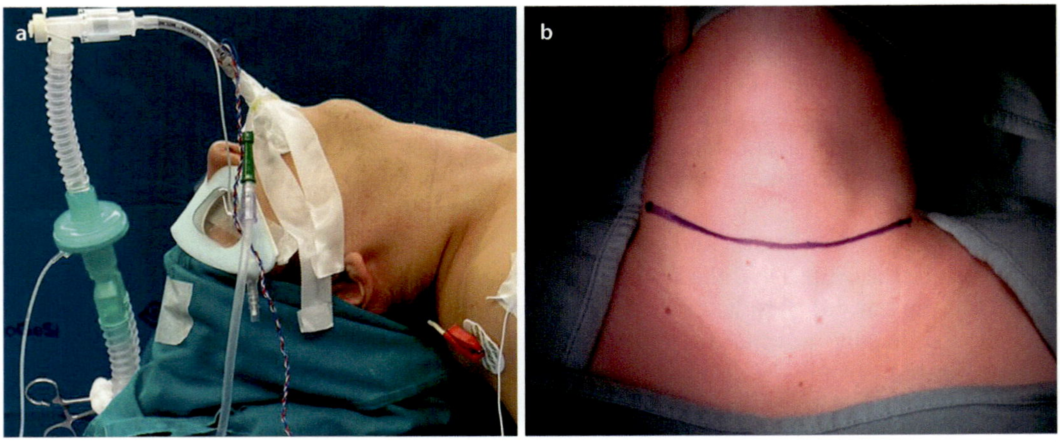

◘ **Fig. 11.2** **a** Position: patient in supine position with the neck slightly hyperextended. **b** Incision: A collar incision about 2 fingers above the sternal notch

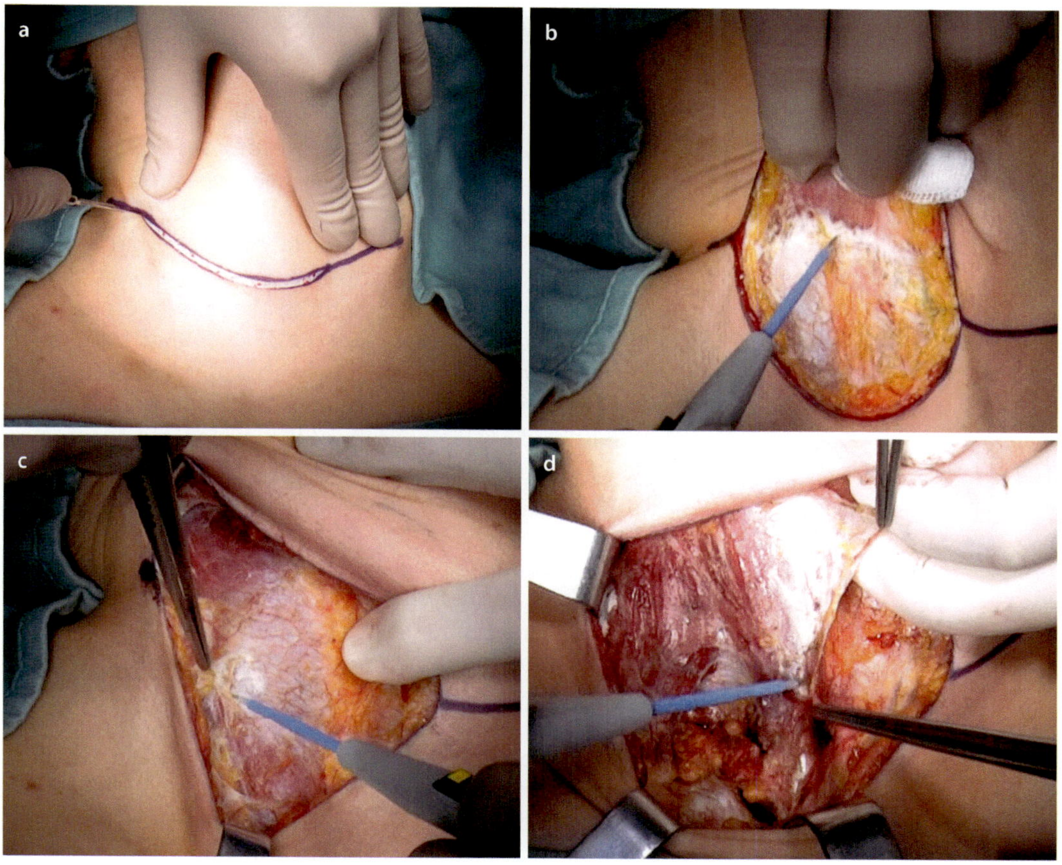

Fig. 11.3 **a** Skin incision should be prolonged on the side of the planned lateral neck dissection; **b** subplatysmal flap; **c** vertical incision of the superficial layer of the deep cervical fascia close to the posterior border of the sterno-cleidomastoid muscle; **d** the fibrofatty tissue contained between the two heads of the sternocleidomastoid muscle is dissected away, and the superficial layer of the deep cervical fascia detached from its infero-anterior attachments at the level of the sternum and the medial third of the clavicle

The flap should be extended cranially to expose the hyoid bone in the midline and the submaxillary gland laterally, if a LND is planned. Inferiorly the flap is elevated to the sternal notch in the midline and the clavicle laterally. The posterior border of the SCM should be exposed as well, if a LND is planned.

11.5.3.3 Selective Lateral Neck Dissection: Levels II–Vb

It should be underlined that the sequence of the steps usually reflects the operating surgeon's preference and experience (i.e., lateral to medial dissection, medial to lateral, clockwise, etc.). Usually, a medial to lateral approach is used by general and endocrine surgeons, while a lateral to medial approach is usually preferred by Head and Neck surgeons. Every approach has its own advantage(s). A combination of both a lateral to medial and medial to lateral approaches can be useful, depending on the step of the procedure and the individual patients and tumor to be treated.

What is of utmost importance is the comprehensive removal of all the fibrofatty tissue *en bloc* and embedded within the investing fascial planes.

1. ***Unwrapping the SCM***. The dissection usually starts with vertical incision of the SLDCF investing the SCM along all the length of the SCM itself. The incision is preferably close to the posterior border of the SCM (◘ Fig. 11.3c). At this point the SCM should be completely enwrapped. Most surgeons usually prefer to first proceed with subfascial dissection toward the anterior margin of the muscle. However, it could be preferable to prepare the dissection of the subclavicular triangle first, proceeding with a posterolateral direction. The incised fascia is then elevated by means of forceps and retracted posterolaterally at the level of the distal third of the SCM. Dissection is achieved by means of monopolar electrocautery or bipolar scissors, in order to avoid any minimal bleeding.

   The fibrofatty tissue contained between the two heads of the SCM is dissected away, *en bloc*, and the SLDCF detached from its infero-anterior attachments at the level of the sternum and the medial third of the clavicle (◘ Fig. 11.3d). Once reached the posterior border of the SCM, dissection of the fascia proceeds anteriorly along the posterior aspect of the distal third of the muscle, which is retracted antero-medially allowing progressive dissection of the fascial covering (◘ Fig. 11.4a). The posterior belly of the omohyoid muscle is then identified and enwrapped of its fascial coating, from its intermediate tendon, until the crossing with the trapezius muscle (◘ Fig. 11.4b, c). Unwrapping the omohyoid muscle, which will be continued anteriorly during the anterior dissection, it is essential to preserve the muscle and to obtain adequate exposure, especially during supraclavicular triangle dissection. In addition, it should be underlined that omohyoid muscle is embedded by the MLDCF that should be removed *en bloc* to ensure adequate clearance.

   Once achieved dissection of the posterior belly of the omohyoid muscle the SLDCF is detached inferiorly from the clavicle, posteriorly from the trapezius muscle. The clavicle and the trapezius muscle are exposed (◘ Fig. 11.4c). Dissection is continued upward along the anterior margin of the trapezius muscle, until exposure of the externa jugular vein, that can be ligated but also preserved. If preservation of the external jugular vein is chosen, it should be freed from investing fibrofatty tissue (◘ Fig. 11.4d). At this point, superficial dissection of the supraclavicular triangle is completed. A small gauze may be left at this level.

   From here dissection progresses anteriorly. The SLDCF is detached along the anterior aspect of the SMC. When dissection reaches the anterior border of the SCM, the mus-

11

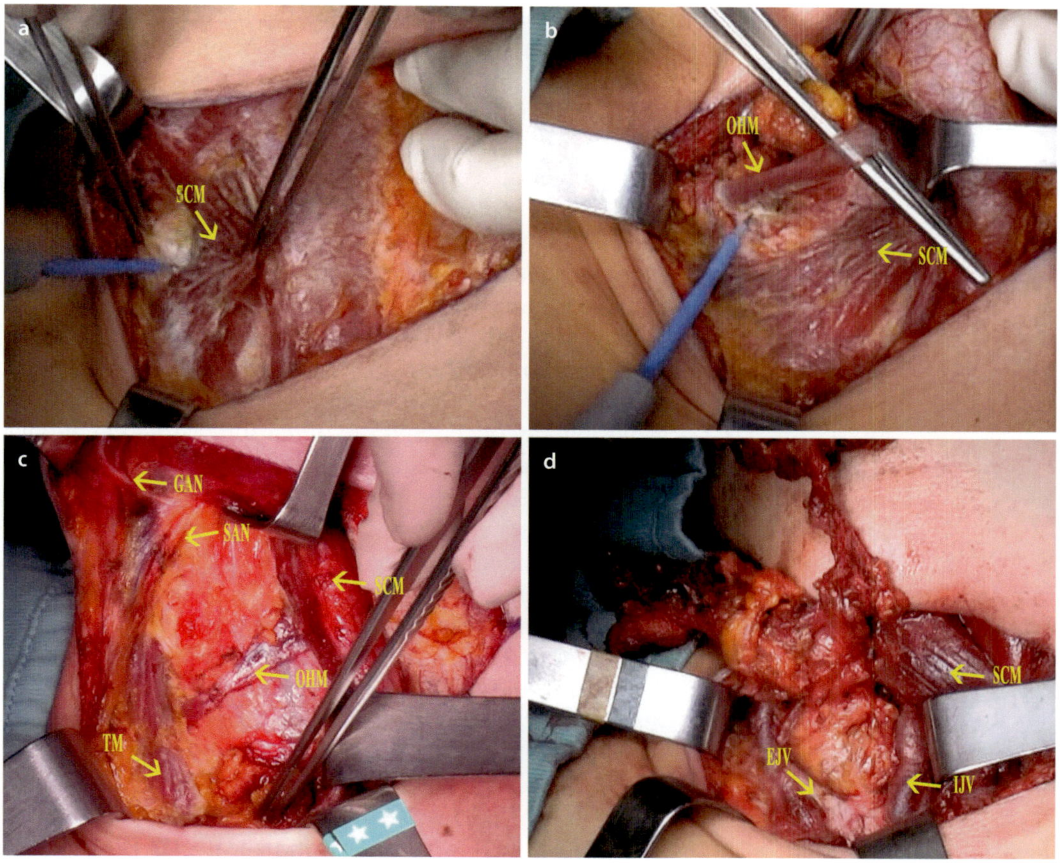

Fig. 11.4 **a** Dissection of the fascia along the posterior aspect of the distal third of the sternocleidomastoid muscle, which is retracted antero-medially allowing progressive dissection of the fascial covering; **b** the posterior belly of the omohyoid muscle is enwrapped of its fascial coating, from its intermediate tendon, until the crossing with the trapezius muscle; **c** superficial dissection of the supraclavicular triangle; **d** completing the supraclavicular triangle dissection. SCM sternocleidomastoid muscle, OHM omohyoid muscle, GAN great auricular nerve, SAN spinal accessory nerve, TM trapezius muscle, EJV external jugular vein, IJV internal jugular vein

cle is retracted posteriorly to continue dissection underneath, over its medial aspect, starting from the caudal portion upward, aiming to free the fascial covering from the posterior border of the SCM. Inferiorly, the dissection reaches the previously dissected supraclavicular triangle, as evidenced by the identification of the gauze left at that level.

Dissection over the medial surface of the SCM is then continued, allowing complete mobilization of the SCM. When dissection reaches the cranial third of the muscle, it should be paid special attention to the SAN that enters the muscle, approximately at the junction of its upper and middle thirds. In order to reduce the risk of SAN injury, it could be preferable to stop posterior dissection before reaching such dangerous area. Dissection can be more safely accomplished after dissection of the submandibular triangle and identification of the SAN in its proximal tract below the posterior belly of the digastric muscle.

In summary, the first step of the procedure consists of the complete unwrapping of the SCM and of the inferior belly of the omohyoid muscle and the dissection of the SLDCF from its clavicular and sternal attachments and from the anterior border of the trapezius muscle. Below the Erb's point dissection is accomplished posterior to the SCM, in the upper two thirds dissection is accomplished anterior to the SCM.

2. ***Preparing the submandibular triangle*** – At this point the SLDCF is incised along the inferior margin of the submaxillary gland. The gland is then retracted upward in order to expose the cranial boundary of the dissection represented by the posterior belly of the digastric muscle and the stylohyoid muscle. In the SND required for thyroid carcinoma section of the facial vein is unnecessary. However, it should be unwrapped of the investing fascial layer, since small lymph nodes may be missed along its posterior aspect, below the inferior margin of the submaxillary gland (◘ Fig. 11.5).
3. ***Dissecting the medial boundary*** – At this point the dissection of the SLDCF is continued along the lateral margin of the sternohyoid muscle by preserving the anterior jugular veins. The SLDCF is dissected away from the antero-lateral aspect of the sternohyoid muscle. That allows to expose the medial border of the LND, which is represented by the coalescence of the fascia covering lateral border of the sternothyroid muscle with the carotid sheath (◘ Fig. 11.6a). Proceeding in a posterolateral direction, the superior belly

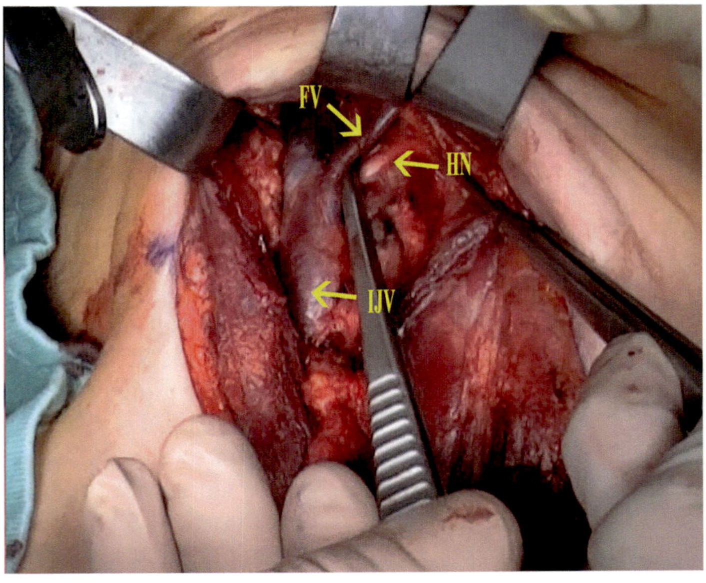

◘ **Fig. 11.5** Submaxillary gland and posterior belly of the digastric muscle are retracted upward, the hypoglossal nerve is identified and preserved, and the facial vein is unwrapped of the investing fascial layer. FV facial vein, HN hypoglossal nerve, IJV internal jugular vein

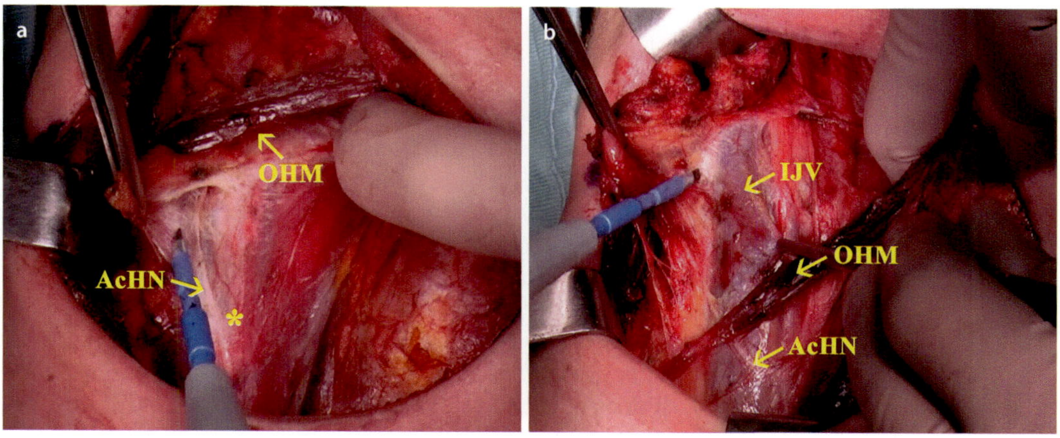

Fig. 11.6 **a** The superior belly of the omohyoid muscle is unwrapped of its investing fascia; the medial border of the lateral neck dissection is exposed; **b** the neuro-vascular bundle is unwrapped, caudal to cranial, until to reach the sagittal aponeurosis, posterior to the neurovascular bundle, and, consequently, the avascular plane of coalescence with the deep layer of the deep cervical fascia. OHM omohyoid muscle, AcHN *ansa cervicalis* hypoglossal nerve, * medial border of the lateral neck dissection represented by the coalescence of the fascia covering lateral border of the sternothyroid muscle with the carotid sheet, IJV internal jugular vein

of the omohyoid muscle is identified, and completely unwrapped of its investing fascia. That allows for a complete the mobilization of the muscle, very useful for further steps of the dissection, and for a complete exposure of the carotid sheath and neuro-vascular bundle of the neck. By retracting posterolaterally the medial border of the dissected SLDCF, the neuro-vascular bundle is unwrapped, caudal to cranial, until to reach the sagittal aponeurosis, posterior to the neurovascular bundle, and, consequently, the avascular plane of coalescence with the DLDCF (Fig. 11.6b). It should be paid attention to preserve the descending branch of the *ansa cervicalis* that should be followed upward till its origin from the hypoglossal nerve. Moreover, during the most posterior part of the dissection, its ascending branch should be preserved as well, since it represents an important landmark for the deepest plan of dissection. During this step of the dissection, it is usually unnecessary to ligate facial, lingual, and thyroid artery and veins, but they should be completely freed from the investing fascia.

In the caudal portion of the field, the IJV has to be freed till the confluence with subclavian vein (Pirogoff's trunk), eventually preserving also the external and anterior jugular veins. At this level, it should be paid attention to avoid injury of the thoracic duct on the left and the right lymphatic duct (if present) at their confluence on the Pirogoff's trunk.

Finally, it should be kept in mind that dissecting behind the neuro-vascular bundle may result in inadvertent injury of the sympathetic chain, and subsequent Horner's syndrome.

4. ***Dissecting level II*** – Proceeding upward, the fascia is incised along the posterior belly of the digastric muscle. Countertraction by the assistant over the upper most portion of CCA facilitates the identification of the hypoglossal nerve (◘ Fig. 11.5), following the descending branch of the *ansa cervicalis*. Dissection over the fascial plane is then continued laterally, to complete the dissection of the anterior and lateral aspect of the IJV. At this point, while superomedially retracting the posterior belly of the digastric muscle and latero-inferiorly the SCM muscle, the SAN is exposed between the SCM and the IJV. The SAN has then to be completely dissected from its surrounding tissue, since it does not follow a fascial plane, but it crosses the intrafascial tissue and it is completely embedded by lymph nodes containing fibrofatty tissue. In the absence of gross involvement of such lymph nodes, it would be enough to dissect the tissue anterior to the nerve (IIa dissection) (◘ Fig. 11.7a). In the case where a level IIb dissection is needed, the SAN must be gently displaced to dissect the fibrofatty tissue cranial and posterior. Then the dissected IIb tissue has to be passed behind the nerve to be removed *en bloc* with the remaining specimen. Thus, in level IIb dissection the splenius capitis and the levator scapulae muscles represent the most posterior aspect of the dissection in the cranial part of the operative field (◘ Fig. 11.7b).
5. ***Level III and IV dissection*** – At this point while the SCM in retracted laterally and the vascular bundle medially, downward retraction of the specimen allows to complete the dissection of the posterior boundary along the plane of coalescence of the SLDCF and DLDCF, by preserving the roots of the cervical plexus (level III). The specimen is then

11

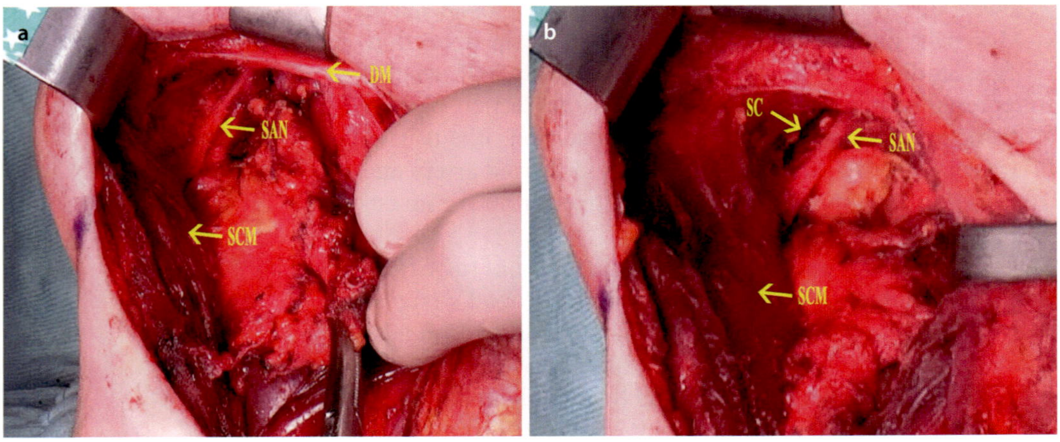

◘ **Fig. 11.7** **a** The spinal accessory nerve is exposed between the sternocleidomastoid muscle and the internal jugular vein; IIa dissection includes the fibrofatty tissue anterior to the nerve; **b** IIb dissection includes the fibrofatty tissue cranial and posterior to the spinal accessory nerve. Splenius capitis and the levator scapulae muscles represent most posterior aspect of the dissection in the cranial part of the operative field. DM digastric muscle, SAN spinal accessory nerve, SCM sternocleidomastoid muscle, SC splenius capitis

passed behind the omohyoid muscle, and dissection continued downward (level IV). Following the fascial plane preserves the integrity of the phrenic nerve and thyrocervical trunk. However, infrascalenic nodes can be safely removed *en bloc*, after identifying the phrenic nerve. Small vascular branches arising from the thyrocervical trunk have to be ligated. Preserving the thyrocervical trunk, it is of utmost importance to reduce the risk of postoperative hypoparathyroidism. The utmost care of the thoracic duct as it emerges posterior to the inferior IJ is essential when one is dissecting in low level IV. The thoracic duct should be identified and ligated. No evidence of chylous fistula should be confirmed prior to closure.

In summary during this step, since both the lateral and the medial border have been already prepared, it is possible to safely dissect the posterior aspect along the DLDCF that should not be violated.

6. ***Completing level Vb dissection (supraclavicular)*** – At this point in time the SCM is retracted medially, and the specimen passed behind and transposed posterolaterally. The dissection follows along the superior aspect of the subclavian vein, exposing posteriorly the brachial plexus (◘ Figs. 11.4d and 11.8). Then, the dissection is completed along the anterior margin of the trapezius muscle and the specimen removed.

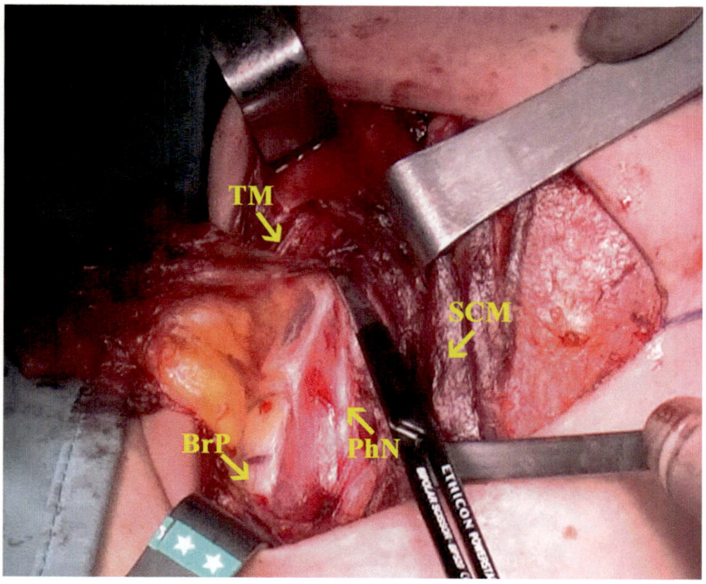

◘ **Fig. 11.8** Completing level Vb dissection/supraclavicular triangle. TM trapezius muscle, SCM sternocleidomastoid muscle, PhN phrenic nerve, BrP brachial plexus

11.5.3.4 Central Neck Dissection (Level VI–VII)

1. *Strap muscles dissection* (◘ Fig. 11.9) – The strap muscles are separated along the midline, as extensively as possible from the hyoid bone to the sternal notch. In order to obtain an adequate clearance, especially in large infiltrating tumors and/or bulky lymph node metastases, *en bloc* resection of the sternothyroid muscles can be preferable. In such cases, the posterior aspect of the sterno-hyoid muscle should be completely freed from the anterior aspect of the ipsilateral sternothyroid and thyrohyoid muscles, in order to be completely mobilized. After that, the sternohyoid muscle is sectioned at its proximal (thyroid cartilage) and distal (sternal) insertions. If needed or preferred, the SLDCF, in its anterior portion, covering the strap muscles, can be removed *en bloc* with the central compartment. It is sectioned cranially at the level of the hyoid bone and caudally at the level of the sternal notch. Then the sternohyoid muscles are unwrapped from lateral to medial. When the dissection reaches the

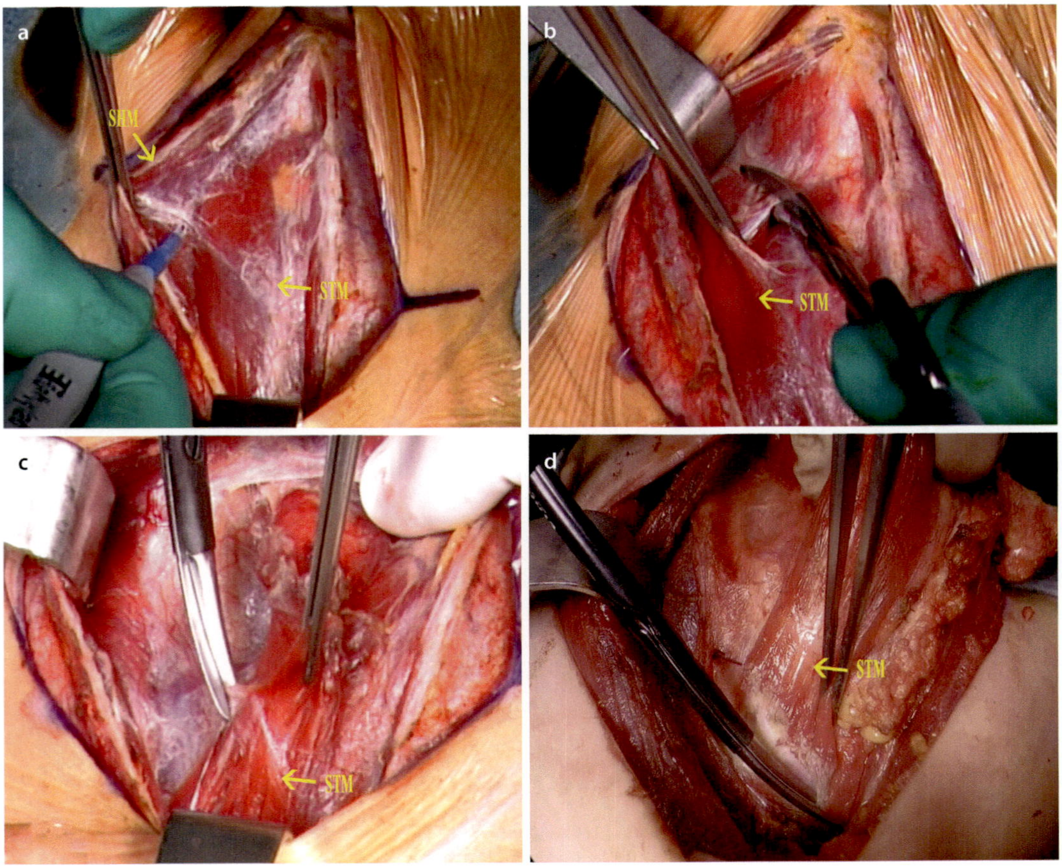

◘ **Fig. 11.9** Strap muscles dissection – The posterior aspect of the sterno-hyoid muscle should be completely freed from the anterior aspect of the ipsilateral sternothyroid and thyrohyoid muscles; after that, the sternohyoid muscle is sectioned at its proximal (thyroid cartilage) and distal (sternal) insertions. SHM sternohyoid muscle, STM sternothyroid muscle

medial border of the sternohyoid muscles on each side, it changes direction and the posterior aspect of the sternohyoid muscles is dissected as described above, leaving the fascial envelopment connected along the median raphe with the sternothyroid muscles and the "content" of the central compartment.

2. *Dissection of the lateral boundary (Exposure of the CCA)* – The dissection, using both monopolar or bipolar cautery, follows the lateral margin of the sternothyroid muscle, along the carotid sheath (◘ Fig. 11.1). Complete exposure should be obtained from the thyroid cartilage to the innominate trunk on the right side and as low as possible on the left side, depending on patient' morphotype, but at least to the plane corresponding to the level where the innominate trunk crosses the trachea on the right side.
3. *Identification of the ILN and paratracheal dissection* – If total thyroidectomy is associated, after the section of the vessels of the upper pole (see ► Chap. 10), the thyroid lobe is retracted medially, to expose the tracheoesophageal groove. The ILN is usually identified where it crosses the inferior thyroid artery or its branches, possibly using intraoperative nerve monitoring to confirm correct identification. On the right side, the nerve should be dissected from the surrounding fibrofatty tissue in all along its cervical course from its origin behind the subclavian artery to its entrance into the larynx. After that the sagittal aponeurosis posterior to the carotid sheath should be incised and the posterolateral fibrofatty tissue dissected from lateral to medial along the lateral aspect of the ILN, preserving the small sympathetic-inferior laryngeal nerve connecting branches [116]. Then, the posterior aspect of the nerve is freed from the fibrofatty tissue. ILN is cautiously anterolaterally displaced, and the posterolateral portion of the paratracheal nodes are transposed behind it medially (◘ Fig. 11.10). At this point dissection continues in the antero-medial portion of the paratracheal nodes, exposing the antero-lateral aspect of the esophagus and the lateral aspect of the trachea. In most of the cases, the infero-lateral part of the dissected field may expose the apex of the ipsilateral lung. On the left side, the nerve is similarly identified where it crossed the inferior thyroid artery and followed in a caudal direction as deep as possible in the upper mediastinum. At this point the sagittal aponeurosis is incised behind the carotid sheath. By lateral to antero-medial retraction, the lymph node containing fibrofatty tissue is completely freed along the antero-lateral aspect of the ILN, exposing the esophagus and the lateral margin of the trachea. Any effort should be done to preserve the superior parathyroid glands (◘ Figs. 11.10d and 11.11) (see ► Chap. 10). For re-operative central node dissection,

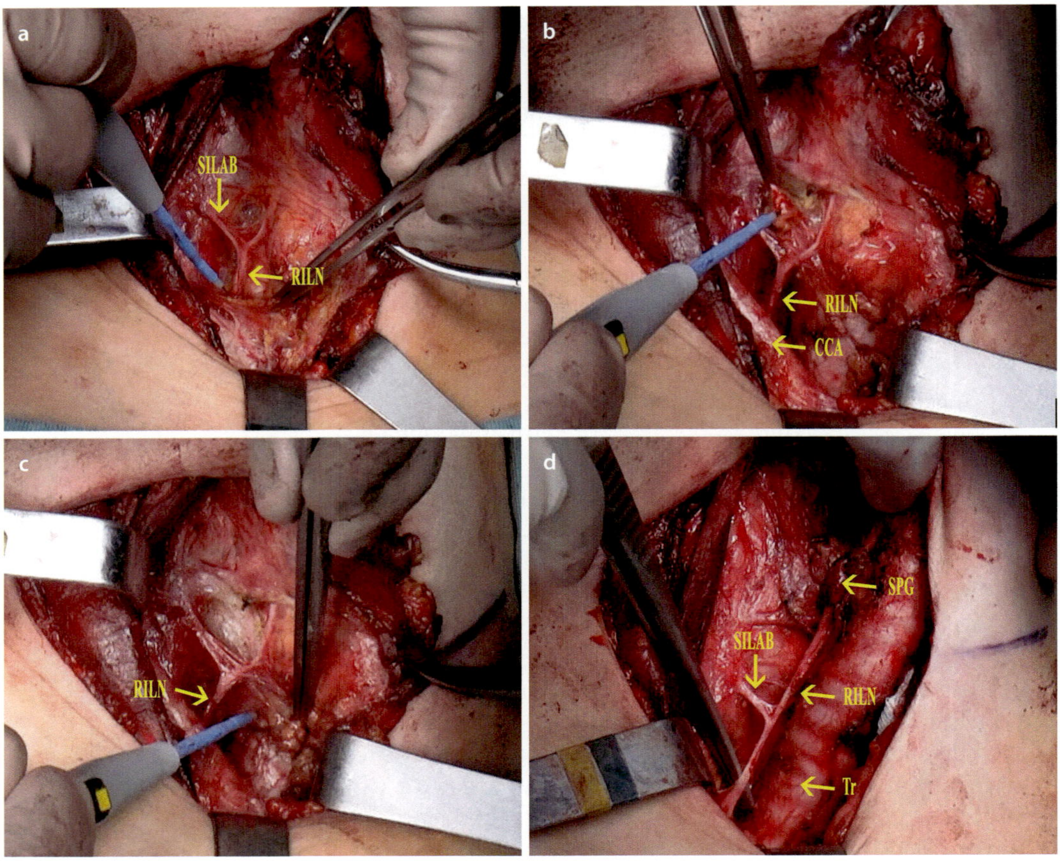

Fig. 11.10 Identification of the right inferior laryngeal nerve and paratracheal dissection – On the right side the nerve should be dissected from the surrounding fibrofatty tissue all along its cervical course from its origin behind the subclavian artery to its entrance into the larynx. The sagittal aponeurosis should be incised and the posterolateral fibrofatty tissue dissected from lateral to medial along the lateral aspect of the inferior laryngeal nerve, preserving the sympathetic-inferior laryngeal nerve anastomotic branches. Then, the posterolateral portion of the paratracheal nodes is transposed behind it medially. SILAB sympathetic inferior laryngeal anastomotic branch, RILN right inferior laryngeal nerve, CCA common carotid artery, SPG superior parathyroid gland, Tr trachea

it is essential to dissect posterior to the laryngeal nerve as it is in this region that recurrent/ persistent pathologic central lymph nodes are found.

4. *Pretracheal dissection* – Just below the sternothyroid muscle, it is possible to identify the thymus. It should be explored for identifying intrathymic parathyroid glands which are often encountered or used as a landmark for the identification of inferior parathyroid gland embedded in the thyrothymic tract. The thymus, and the eventually identified inferior parathyroid gland, in the absence of overt involvement by the tumor or nodal disease, should be preserved, since it lies in an anatomical plane anterior to the pretracheal nodes, in order to preserve inferior parathyroid glands viability (Fig. 11.11). After that the most inferior portion of the central compartment (upper mediastinal nodes) is dissected from the antero-superior aspect of the innominate

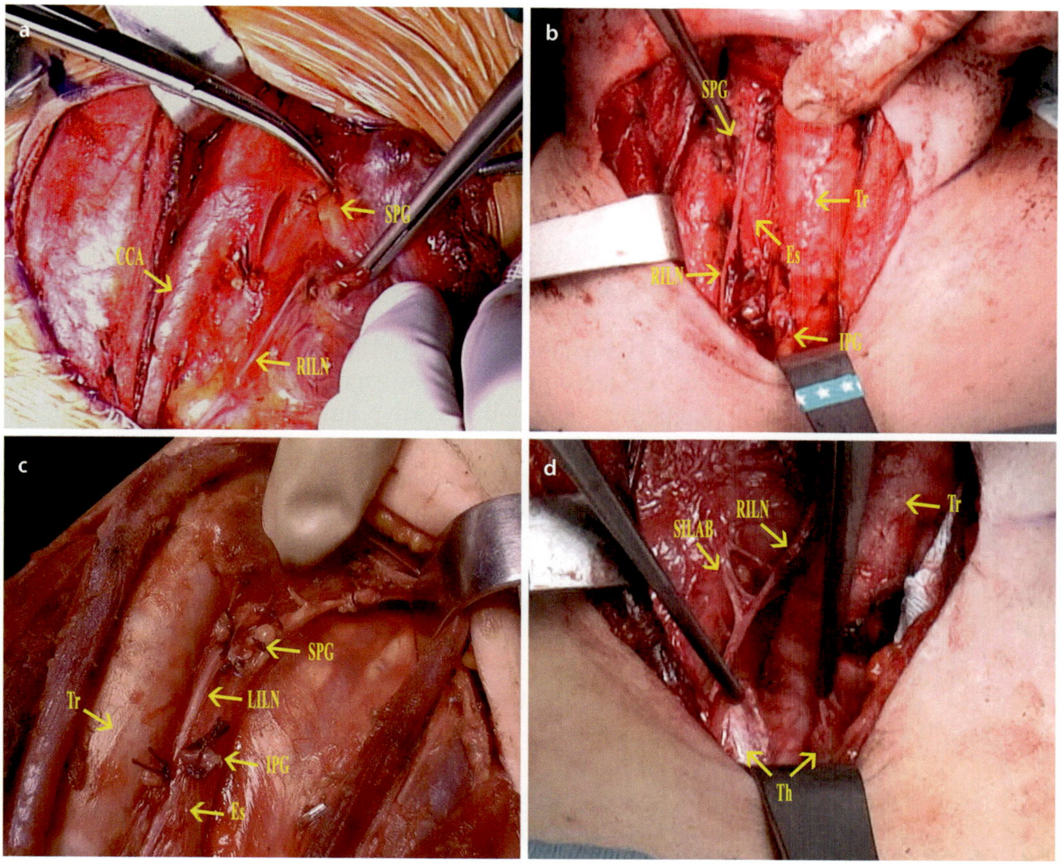

Fig. 11.11 Parathyroid preservation during central neck dissection – During central neck dissection any effort should be done to preserve the superior parathyroid glands. The thymus should be explored for identifying intrathymic parathyroid glands or using it as a landmark for the identification of inferior parathyroid gland embedded in the thyrothymic tract. SPG superior parathyroid gland, CCA common carotid artery, RILN right inferior laryngeal nerve, Tr trachea, Es esophagus, IPG inferior parathyroid gland, LILN left inferior laryngeal nerve, SILAB sympathetic inferior laryngeal anastomotic branch, Th thymus

trunk, exposing the right brachiocephalic vein. Dissection is continued upward dissecting the fibrofatty tissue embedded in the visceral portion of the MLDCF from tracheal fascia.

5. *Prelaryngeal (Delphian) nodes* – Dissection then continues, en bloc with the thyroid gland and/or the resected sternothyroid muscles, in the prelaryngeal compartment, paying attention to avoid injury of the cricothyroid muscle, cricothyroid membrane, and thyroid cartilage, along with the pyramidal lobe in the case of synchronous thyroidectomy. Dissection should be continued extensively upward in order to expose the hyoid bone.
6. *Unilateral* vs *bilateral dissection* – If unilateral dissection is accomplished, it should be stopped at the lateral margin of the trachea on the contralateral side. If bilateral CND dissection is required, dissection continues in the contralateral paratracheal basin.

7. *Wound closure* – After checking the hemostasis and lymphatic leak, the sternohyoid muscles are re-approximated along the midline. The wound is closed with subcuticular running suture. Suction drains may be left inside.

11.5.4 Alternate Operative Approaches (Minimally Invasive, Remote Access, and Radio-Guided Procedures)

Even though the conventional approach to CND and LND via cervical incision remains the standard approach, in recent years numerous minimally invasive and remote access procedures approaches have been described [47, 117–122].

Among cervical minimally invasive approaches, video-assisted CND has been proposed and validated in selected preoperative cN0 low-risk papillary thyroid carcinoma in case of intraoperative evidence of enlarged/suspicious central neck nodes during video-assisted thyroidectomy [118] and in *RET* mutation carriers [123]. Nonetheless, overt lymph node involvement remains a contraindication for video-assisted approach, and conversion to conventional approach is mandatory when an accurate node clearance cannot be obtained using the video-assisted approach [124].

Supported by the results of video-assisted approach for selected cases of DTC and encouraged by the results of video-assisted CND, a preliminary experience showing only the feasibility of the technique, a video-assisted approach to LND has been described for selected low-risk PTC with lateral neck nodal metastases <2 cm, without evidence of great vessels involvement [47], but it remained a feasibility study with no further diffusion.

Among remote approaches for ND, endoscopic and robot-assisted techniques have been evaluated including transaxillary, retroauricular, modified facelift, and trans-oral approaches [119–122]. Preliminary results demonstrated the feasibility and safety of such alternate approaches, but high level evidences and data on long-term outcomes are lacking and they haven't so far gained wide diffusion worldwide and, in most cases, remained limited to the authors' experience [1]. To date alternate approaches for ND are to be considered investigational [1].

Radio-guided surgery has been investigated for possible utilization in patients with iodine avid recurrent disease to achieve targeted resection in patients previously undergone comprehensive ND, aiming to ensure the completeness of the resection of iodine avid tissue [125]. In limited experiences radionuclide occult lesion localization, by injecting 0.5 mCi Tc-99m macro-aggregate albumin into the lesion under ultrasound guidance (USG), has been used as an adjunct for targeted removal of recurrent or persistent nodal disease [126].

11.5.5 Knowing and Avoiding Complications of ND

CDN and LND increase both intra- and postoperative complication rates when compared with thyroidectomy alone [78, 127, 128].

Knowledge, prevention, and management of complications that could occur during neck dissections are essential for a proper care of thyroid cancer patients.

Complications related to ND include nerve complications, hematoma and vascular complications, hypoparathyroidism, chyle fistula, pneumothorax, and wound complications.

Nerve complications include great auricular nerve, cervical sensory nerves, facial nerve, lingual nerve, hypoglossal nerve, SAN, sympathetic nerves, phrenic nerve, brachial plexus, VN, external branch of superior laryngeal nerve, and ILN injuries.

The great auricular nerve emerges from beneath the posterior border of the SCM in the upper half of level V of the neck; it travels across the lateral surface of the SCM toward the auricle. Sacrifice of this nerve during ND leads to a sensory deficit of the auricle that usually diminishes with time. Ear lobule numbness, however, tends to persist [129].

Injuries to the cervical and marginal mandibular branches of the facial nerve may occur during ND. The cervical branch of the facial nerve innervates the platysma muscle, and its sacrifice does not usually produce clinically significant deficits. The marginal mandibular nerve is encountered when approaching level I of the neck and its injury results in asymmetry of the lower lip at rest with inability to depress the lip during facial expression. During the dissection, elevating the submandibular fascia inferiorly on the gland adequately protects the nerve [130].

In the case of level I lymph node dissection and/or concomitant submandibular gland excision, injury of the lingual nerve may occur. Clinically, injury results in loss of taste and sensation from the ipsilateral anterior two-thirds of the tongue.

Hypoglossal nerve injury is a rare complication of LND [131]. The nerve is susceptible to injury during dissection of levels I and II. The deficits from hypoglossal injury include ipsilateral tongue weakness, deviation of the tongue toward the affected side with tongue protrusion, and difficulty with speech and swallowing.

Shoulder dysfunction has been reported in up to 30–40% of patients undergoing LND, even when the SAN is anatomically preserved [132, 133]. SAN injury results in shoulder drooping, aberrant scapular rotation, inability to fully abduct the shoulder, and a dull ache secondary to atrophy of the trapezius muscle and adhesive capsulitis of the glenohumeral joint [132, 133].

In several cases, atrophy and stiffness of the SCM may occur after vigorous and protracted retraction, and they might be mistaken for SAN injury [132, 134].

Physical therapy and postoperative shoulder rehabilitation have positive effects on quality of life in selected patients. Low-dose botulin toxin injection in the territory of the nerve was proved effective in managing the condition in some patients [135].

The cervical sympathetic chain consists of two to four ganglia with a connecting neural trunk that runs parallel and posteromedial to the carotid sheath. Loss of sympathetic innervation results in Claude-Bernard-Horner syndrome (ptosis, miosis, and anhidrosis). The manifestations of partial losses vary depending on the location of the injury in relation to the ganglia. In order to reduce the risk of this complication, attention should be paid in dissecting behind the neuro-vascular bundle.

Phrenic nerve paralysis is considered a rare complication of LND. Injury to the phrenic nerve leads to ipsilateral hemidiaphragm elevation, with or without mediastinal shift on chest radiograph, and symptoms such as cough, chest pain, or abdominal discomfort mediated by the somatic afferents. The paresis is generally transient and without sequelae. Preserving the fascial layer over the nerve and anterior scalene muscle during level IV dissection is the primary method for prevention of injury.

Brachial plexus injury is rarely reported after neck dissection. The roots lie between the anterior and middle scalene muscles, the trunks in the posterior triangle, the divisions behind the clavicle, and the cords in the axilla. The plexus is involved with the motor and sensory function of the shoulder down to the fingertips. Injuries to this plexus can lead to significant deficits in quality of life [136, 137]. Dissecting above the DLDCF allows to avoid any injury.

Injury to the main trunk of the VN may occur during dissection of level III and IV lymph nodes and eventual ligation of the IJV in the inferior neck or at the skull base. High VN injuries result in significant dysphonia from vocal fold paralysis, dysphagia, and sensory loss.

For complications related to injury to ILN, EBSLN please refer to ▶ Chap. 10.

Hematoma occurs in approximately 1% of neck dissections. A hematoma within the central neck after thyroidectomy and/or neck dissection can sufficiently impede the venous and lymphatic outflow of the larynx, causing life-threatening airway problems [109, 138]. In case of compressive hematoma, bedside evacuation of the hematoma may be necessary. At the time of surgical re-exploration, attention to the structures at risk remains of paramount importance, as always. Gentle irrigation and clot evacuation, as well as blind clamping of vessels, are mandatory to avoid further complications. Saline solution is useful in cleaning the operative field and identifying any source of bleeding.

The use of hemostatic agents (i.e., oxidized cellulose, fibrin sealant, etc.) may be useful in selected cases to facilitate hemostasis by mechanical pressure and promoting coagulum formation, thus resulting in reducing capillary ooze, wound collection, and drainage [105].

In rare cases, intraoperative injuries to the common carotid could occur and generally require primary vascular repair, and vascular surgery consultation is highly recommended. Acute postoperative carotid artery rupture has been described: this rare but life-threating condition is generally subsequent to wound necrosis and infection, salivary fistula, prior radiation therapy, and tumor involvement of the arterial wall.

Finally, other vascular complications following neck dissections include postoperative thrombosis and hemorrhage of intraoperatively preserved IJV. Many IJV postoperative thromboses result in a recanalization of the vessel with reestablishment of the patency after adequate anticoagulant therapy [139]. IJV ligation should be avoided if possible since in case of bilateral neck dissection it is demonstrated that the preservation of at least one IJV is beneficial to avoid facial or laryngeal edema, intracranial pressure elevations, and stroke [140].

Hypoparathyroidism and hypocalcemia are the most common complications following thyroidectomy and neck dissection [141] (see ► Chap. 10).

The best way to avoid parathyroid damage is to clearly know the embryology and the surgical anatomy of the glands and their blood supply and make every effort to preserve them avoiding removal or devascularization of parathyroid tissue or to perform an auto-transplant of de-vascularized or inadvertently removed normal parathyroid glands [109].

The incidence of parathyroid gland injury is related to the extent of the operation and to surgeon's experience.

Some technical aspects have a crucial role in parathyroid glands preservation.

First of all, a bloodless surgical field is essential, since any bleeding could determine an alteration of the colors that is essential for parathyroid identification.

Given the high variety of inferior parathyroid location, missing identification of one or two inferior parathyroids does not mean inadvertent removal: the gland(s) can be located cephalad or caudal (i.e., intrathymic) to the site of dissection. Conversely, not identifying a superior parathyroid gland can signify inadvertent removal, since it is usually located on the posterior aspect of the thyroid lobe, close to the point where the ILN enters the larynx.

During lateral neck dissection, it is of the utmost importance to preserve the thyrocervical trunk to preserve parathyroid vascularization from branches of inferior thyroid artery.

Moreover, intraoperative techniques aiming to better identify and preserve parathyroid tissue have been described, including methylene blue injection, near-infrared fluorescence imaging, and indocyanine green [114], but to date no technique or technology is able to replace a meticulous surgical approach based on detailed knowledge of embryology and anatomy of the parathyroid glands and their blood supply.

Several postoperative protocols have been proposed and validated for the management of symptomatic and asymptomatic hypocalcemia and/or clinical or relative hypoparathyroidism. Routine or selective oral calcium and calcitriol supplementation results effective in the majority of the cases [142–145]. Intravenous calcium administration should be considered in case of severe symptomatic hypocalcemia or in case of symptoms progression (paresthesias, numbness, tingling, cramps, etc.) despite oral calcium and calcitriol therapy (see ▶ Chap. 10).

Chyle leak may complicate neck dissection in 1–8% of the cases [146, 147]. Chyle leak occurs in the majority of the cases after left neck dissections, but it is important to remember that up to 25% of chyle leaks occurs on the right side [146, 147]. The thoracic duct consists of a plexus of tributaries and terminal ducts, each of which can create a chyle fistula if transected or incompletely ligated.

Intraoperative suspicion of chyle leak during any lower neck dissection should be investigated. In case of intraoperatively identified chyle leak, gentle exploration and meticulous ligation of the duct and identifiable branches with nonabsorbable sutures are recommended. Postoperative leaks are usually discovered with resumption of feeding. Most are easily diagnosed clinically by observing a change in the character of the drain output from serosanguinous to milky. Conservative management with use of a long-acting analog of the hormone somatostatin (subcutaneous octreotide) and low-fat diet, closed drainage to promote adherence of skin flaps, and/or pressure dressings may be sufficient to promote spontaneous closure of most fistulas [148]. Cases of persistent leak after conservative management and/or high-output leaks (>500 mL/24 hours) require operative intervention and ligation of the duct and identifiable branches. Most recently the role of lymphangiography and percutaneous embolization of the thoracic duct has been shown to be feasible and effective in chyle leaks [149]. Video-assisted thoracoscopic ligation of the thoracic duct has been recommended by some as the preferred treatment of chyle leaks [150].

In rare cases a leak originating in the neck or retrograde pressure formation from cervical thoracic duct ligation leads to extravasation or mediastinal propagation of the chyle leak (chylothorax) [151]. In such cases, thoracentesis or thoracostomy tube drainage is indicated, and, rarely, operative intervention via thoracoscopic or open thoracotomy approaches is necessary to identify the leak and ligate the thoracic duct in the chest.

Pleural injury during dissections at the base of the neck can lead to pneumothorax. Thoracostomy tube placement is required. Chest radiographs after neck dissection could be considered in selected cases (changes in ventilator status, decreased breath sounds on chest auscultation, extensive dissection at the base of the neck for gross nodal involvement) to exclude pneumothorax [152].

Extensive dissection at the pharyngoesophageal junction for infiltrative thyroid tumors or parotid leaks may cause salivary fistula after neck surgery. Conservative management with antibiotics and closed drainage is usually successful. In selected cases salivary gland botulinum toxin injection improves the closure of the fistula [153].

Wound complications following neck surgery include dehiscence and flap necrosis, seroma, wound infection, and lymphedema.

Wound dehiscence and flap necrosis is quite rare in case of correct surgical technique and adequate subplatysmal flap, but its incidence is increased in case of excision of previous skin scars or excision of skin *en bloc* with underlying involved fascial/muscular/vascular/lymphatic structures increasing tension on the skin closure. Other reported risk factors include previous neck irradiation and poor microvasculature secondary to tobacco use, malnutrition, and diabetes mellitus [154].

Seroma is the collection of serous fluid in the space between cervical skin flaps, and underlying structures could be subsequent to division of lymphatic and adipose tissue during neck dissections. Early drain removal, incorrect drain placement, or drain failure could cause seromas. Self-reabsorption is observed in the majority of small seromas; needle aspiration or drain replacement is indicated in selected cases avoiding flap necrosis or infection.

Wound infection is quite rare in case of neck dissection for thyroid carcinomas and could be subsequent to seroma and/or hematoma formation. Collections must be completely drained, wounds should be cultured, and adequate antibiotics therapy should be used according to the potential or confirmed pathogens.

Lymphedema can be subsequent to stagnation of lymphatic fluid and may develop externally in the superficial layers and/or internally within the mucosa, submucosa, and muscles of the upper aerodigestive tract. Neck stiffness, limitations in motion, pain, dysphagia, hearing impairment, and, rarely, airway compromise may be observed. Referrals to certified lymphedema therapists should be recommended in selected cases with decreased quality of life [155].

Postoperative wound infection or inadequate skin closure techniques may lead to the development of a *keloid* (hypertrophic scar). Neck lift and midline platysmoplasty can be considered in selected cases [156].

Answers to the Questions

1. (c); 2. (a); 3. (b); 4. (d); 5. (c); 6. (a); 7. (a); 8. (b); 9. (d)

References

1. Patel KN, Yip L, Lubitz CC, Grubbs EG, Miller BS, Shen W, et al. The American Association of Endocrine Surgeons guidelines for the definitive surgical management of thyroid disease in adults. Ann Surg. 2020;271:E21–93.
2. Asimakopoulos P, Shaha AR, Nixon IJ, Shah JP, Randolph GW, Angelos P, et al. Management of the neck in well-differentiated thyroid cancer. Curr Oncol Rep. 2021;23(1):1–2.
3. Wells SA, Asa SL, Dralle H, Elisei R, Evans DB, Gagel RF, et al. Revised American thyroid association guidelines for the management of medullary thyroid carcinoma. Thyroid. 2015;25:567–610.
4. Haugen BR, Alexander EK, Bible KC, Doherty GM, Mandel SJ, Nikiforov YE, et al. 2015 American Thyroid Association management guidelines for adult patients with thyroid nodules and differentiated thyroid cancer: the American Thyroid Association guidelines task force on thyroid nodules and differentiated thyroid cancer. Thyroid. 2016;26:1–133.
5. Carty SE, Cooper DS, Doherty GM, Duh QY, Kloos RT, Mandel SJ, et al. Consensus statement on the terminology and classification of central neck dissection for thyroid cancer. Thyroid. 2009;19:1153–8.
6. Stack BC, Ferris RL, Goldenberg D, Haymart M, Shaha A, Sheth S, et al. American Thyroid Association consensus review and statement regarding the anatomy, terminology, and rationale for lateral neck dissection in differentiated thyroid cancer. Thyroid. 2012;22:501–8.
7. Kouvaraki MA, Lee JE, Shapiro SE, Sherman SI, Evans DB. Preventable reoperations for persistent and recurrent papillary thyroid carcinoma. Surgery. 2004;136:1183–91.
8. Perros P, Boelaert K, Colley S, Evans C, Evans RM, Gerrard Ba G, et al. Guidelines for the management of thyroid cancer. Clin Endocrinol. 2014;81:1–122.
9. Shaha AR, Shah JP, Loree TR. Patterns of nodal and distant metastasis based on histologic varieties in differentiated carcinoma of the thyroid. Am J Surg. 1996;172:692–4.
10. Roh JL, Park JY, Park CI. Total thyroidectomy plus neck dissection in differentiated papillary thyroid carcinoma patients: pattern of nodal metastasis, morbidity, recurrence, and postoperative levels of serum parathyroid hormone. Ann Surg. 2007;245:604–10.
11. Alfalah H, Cranshaw I, Jany T, Arnalsteen L, Leteurtre E, Cardot C, et al. Risk factors for lateral cervical lymph node involvement in follicular thyroid carcinoma. World J Surg. 2008;32:2623–6.
12. Scollo C, Baudin E, Travagli JP, Caillou B, Bellon N, Leboulleux S, et al. Rationale for central and bilateral lymph node dissection in sporadic and hereditary medullary thyroid cancer. J Clin Endocrinol Metab. 2003;88:2070–5.
13. Cohen MS, Moley JF. Surgical treatment of medullary thyroid carcinoma. J Intern Med. 2003;253:616–26.
14. Machens A, Hinze R, Thomusch O, Dralle H. Pattern of nodal metastasis for primary and reoperative thyroid cancer. World J Surg. 2002;26:22–8.
15. Monteiro R, Han A, Etiwy M, Swearingen A, Krishnamurthy V, Jin J, et al. Importance of surgeon-performed ultrasound in the preoperative nodal assessment of patients with potential thyroid malignancy. Surgery. 2018;163:112–7.
16. De Crea C, Raffaelli M, Maccora D, Carrozza C, Canu G, Fadda G, et al. Dosaggio della calcitonina nel liquido di lavaggio dell'agoaspirato vs.

esame citologico nella diagnosi del carcinoma midollare della tiroide primitivo o metastatico. Acta Otorhinolaryngol Ital. 2014;34:399–405.
17. Marques B, Cunha N, Martins RG, Elvas AR, Couto J, Santos J, et al. Lymph node metastases of medullary thyroid cancer: role of calcitonin in the washout fluid of fine-needle aspiration. Int J Endocrinol. 2020;2020:1–6.
18. Dralle H, Musholt TJ, Schabram J, Steinmüller T, Frilling A, Simon D, et al. German Association of Endocrine Surgeons practice guideline for the surgical management of malignant thyroid tumors. Langenbeck's Arch Surg. 2013;398:347–75.
19. Pacini F, Basolo F, Bellantone R, Boni G, Cannizzaro MA, De Palma M, et al. Italian consensus on diagnosis and treatment of differentiated thyroid cancer: joint statements of six Italian societies. J Endocrinol Investig. 2018;41:849–76.
20. Sancho JJ, Lennard TWJ, Paunovic I, Triponez F, Sitges-Serra A. Prophylactic central neck disection in papillary thyroid cancer: a consensus report of the European Society of Endocrine Surgeons (ESES). Langenbeck's Arch Surg. 2014;399:155–63.
21. Barczyński M, Konturek A, Stopa M, Nowak W. Prophylactic central neck dissection for papillary thyroid cancer. Br J Surg. 2013;100:410–8.
22. Park JP, Roh JL, Lee JH, Baek JH, Gong G, Cho KJ, et al. Risk factors for central neck lymph node metastasis of clinically noninvasive, node-negative papillary thyroid microcarcinoma. Am J Surg. 2014;208:412–8.
23. Lang BHH, Ng SH, Lau LLH, Cowling BJ, Wong KP, Wan KY. A systematic review and meta-analysis of prophylactic central neck dissection on short-term locoregional recurrence in papillary thyroid carcinoma after total thyroidectomy. Thyroid. 2013;23:1087–98.
24. Skandalakis LJ, Skandalakis JE, Skandalakis PN. Surgical anatomy and technique. Surg Anat Tech. 2009;71(8):954–71.
25. Crile G. Excision of cancer of the head and neck: with special reference to the plan of dissection based on one hundred and thirty-two operations. J Am Med Assoc. 1906;XLVII:1780–6.
26. Bocca E, Pignataro O. A conservation technique in radical neck dissection. Ann Otol Rhinol Laryngol. 1967;76:975–87.
27. Russell WO, Ibanez ML, Clark RL, White EC. Thyroid carcinoma. Classification, intraglandular dissemination, and clinicopathological study based upon whole organ sections of 80 glands. Cancer. 1963;16:1425–60.
28. Qiu Y, Fei Y, Liu J, Liu C, He X, Zhu N, et al. Prevalence, risk factors and location of skip metastasis in papillary thyroid carcinoma: a systematic review and meta-analysis. Cancer Manag Res. 2019;11:8721–30.
29. Ranganath R, Dhillon VK, Shaear M, Rooper L, Russell JO, Tufano RP. Unusual locations for differentiated thyroid cancer nodal metastasis. World J Otorhinolaryngol – Head Neck Surg. 2020;6:176–81.
30. Guidera AK, Dawes PJD, Stringer MD. Cervical fascia: a terminological pain in the neck. ANZ J Surg. 2012;82:786–91.
31. Guidera AK, Dawes PJD, Fong A, Stringer MD. Head and neck fascia and compartments: no space for spaces. Head Neck. 2014;36:1058–68.
32. Calearo CV, Teatini G. Functional neck dissection: anatomical grounds, surgical technique, clinical observations. Ann Otol Rhinol Laryngol. 1983;92:215–22.
33. Robbins KT, Medina JE, Wolfe GT, Levine PA, Sessions RB, Pruet CW. Standardizing neck dissection terminology: official report of the Academy's Committee for Head and Neck Surgery and Oncology. Arch Otolaryngol Neck Surg. 1991;117:601–5.
34. Thomas Robbins K, Clayman G, Levine PA, Medina J, Sessions R, Shaha A, et al. Neck dissection classification update: revisions proposed by the American Head and Neck Society and the American Academy of Otolaryngology-Head and Neck Surgery. Arch Otolaryngol – Head Neck Surg. 2002;128:751–8.

35. Robbins KT, Shaha AR, Medina JE, Califano JA, Wolf GT, Ferlito A, et al. Consensus statement on the classification and terminology of neck dissection. Arch Otolaryngol – Head Neck Surg. 2008;134:536–8.
36. Uludağ M. The standards and definitions in neck dissections of differentiated thyroid cancer. SiSli Etfal Hastan Tip Bul/Med Bull Sisli Hosp. 2018;52(3):149.
37. Agrawal N, Evasovich MR, Kandil E, Noureldine SI, Felger EA, Tufano RP, et al. Indications and extent of central neck dissection for papillary thyroid cancer: an American Head and Neck Society Consensus Statement. Head Neck. 2017;39:1269–79.
38. Pradhan R, Agarwal A, Lombardi CP, Raffaelli M. Applied embryology of the thyroid and parathyroid glands. In: Randolph GW, editor. Surgery of the thyroid and parathyroid glands. 3rd ed. Philadelphia: Elsevier Inc; 2021. p. 15–25.e4.
39. Ferlito A, Rinaldo A. Osvaldo Suárez: often-forgotten father of functional neck dissection (in the non-Spanish-speaking literature). Laryngoscope. 2004;114:1177–8.
40. Gavilán J, Herranz J, Gavilán C. Functional neck dissection. Otolaryngol Head Neck Surg. 1995;112:P73.
41. Gavilán J, Herranz J, Martín L. Functional neck dissection: the Latin approach. Oper Tech Otolaryngol – Head Neck Surg. 2004;15:168–75.
42. Gavilán J, Moñux A, Herranz J, Gavilán J. Functional neck dissection: surgical technique. Oper Tech Otolaryngol – Head Neck Surg. 1993;4:258–65.
43. Ferlito A, Robbins KT, Silver CE, Hasegawa Y, Rinaldo A. Classification of neck dissections: an evolving system. Auris Nasus Larynx. 2009;36:127–34.
44. Medina JE. A rational classification of neck dissections. Otolaryngol Neck Surg. 1989;100:169–76.
45. Hasegawa Y, Saikawa M, Miyazaki M, Hayasaki K, Sugasawa M, Asakage T, et al. A new classification and nomenclature system for neck dissections: a proposal by the Japan Neck Dissection Study Group (JNDSG). Toukeibu Gan. 2005;31:71–8.
46. Hasegawa Y, Saikawa M. Update on the classification and nomenclature system for neck dissection: revisions proposed by the Japan Neck Dissection Study Group. Int J Clin Oncol. 2010;15(1):5–12.
47. Lombardi CP, Raffaelli M, Princi P, De Crea C, Bellantone R. Minimally invasive video-assisted functional lateral neck dissection for metastatic papillary thyroid carcinoma. Am J Surg. 2007;193:114–8.
48. Goodger NM. Functional and selective neck dissection. Br J Oral Maxillofac Surg. 2003;41:208.
49. Andersen PE, Shah JP, Cambronero E, Spiro RH. The role of comprehensive neck dissection with preservation of the spinal accessory nerve in the clinically positive neck. Am J Surg. 1994;168:499–502.
50. Hillel AT, Fakhry C, Pai SI, Williams MF, Blanco RGF, Zinreich ES, et al. Selective versus comprehensive neck dissection after chemoradiation for advanced oropharyngeal squamous cell carcinoma. Otolaryngol – Head Neck Surg. 2009;141:737–42.
51. Ferlito A, Robbins KT, Shah JP, Medina JE, Silver CE, Al-Tamimi S, et al. Proposal for a rational classification of neck dissections. Head Neck. 2011;33:445–50.
52. Haugen BR, Alexander EK, Bible KC, Doherty GM, Mandel SJ, Nikiforov YE, et al. 2015 American Thyroid Association management. Thyroid. 2016;26:1–133.
53. Koo BS, Choi EC, Yoon YH, Kim DH, Kim EH, Lim YC. Predictive factors for ipsilateral or contralateral central lymph node metastasis in unilateral papillary thyroid carcinoma. Ann Surg. 2009;249:840–4.
54. Liu N, Yang Y, Chen B, Li L, Zeng Q, Sheng L, et al. The extent of therapeutic central compartment neck dissection in unilateral ct1n1a or ct2n1a papillary thyroid carcinoma. Cancer Manag Res. 2020;12: 12801–9.

55. Raffaelli M, De Crea C, Sessa L, Fadda G, Bellantone C, Lombardi CP. Ipsilateral central neck dissection plus frozen section examination versus prophylactic bilateral central neck dissection in cN0 papillary thyroid carcinoma. Ann Surg Oncol. 2015;22:2302–8.
56. Raffaelli M, De Crea C, Sessa L, Giustacchini P, Bellantone R, Lombardi CP. Can intraoperative frozen section influence the extension of central neck dissection in cN0 papillary thyroid carcinoma? Langenbeck's Arch Surg. 2013;398:383–8.
57. Randolph GW, Duh QY, Heller KS, Livolsi VA, Mandel SJ, Steward DL, et al. The prognostic significance of nodal metastases from papillary thyroid carcinoma can be stratified based on the size and number of metastatic lymph nodes, as well as the presence of extranodal extension. Thyroid. 2012;22:1144–52.
58. Lombardi CP, Raffaelli M, De Crea C, Sessa L, Bellantone R. Morbidity of central neck dissection: primary surgery vs reoperation. Results of a case-control study. Langenbeck's Arch Surg. 2014;399:747–53.
59. Lorenz K, Machens A, Siebolts U, Dralle H. Extent of resection in intra-thyroidal medullary thyroid cancer. Chirurg. 2020;91:1017–24.
60. Koperek O, Scheuba C, Cherenko M, Neuhold N, De Micco C, Schmid KW, et al. Desmoplasia in medullary thyroid carcinoma: a reliable indicator of metastatic potential. Histopathology. 2008;52:623–30.
61. Zhao H, Li H. Meta-analysis of ultrasound for cervical lymph nodes in papillary thyroid cancer: diagnosis of central and lateral compartment nodal metastases. Eur J Radiol. 2019;112:14–21.
62. Choi JS, Kim J, Kwak JY, Kim MJ, Chang HS, Kim EK. Preoperative staging of papillary thyroid carcinoma: comparison of ultrasound imaging and CT. Am J Roentgenol. 2009;193:871–8.
63. Hwang HS, Orloff LA. Efficacy of preoperative neck ultrasound in the detection of cervical lymph node metastasis from thyroid cancer. Laryngoscope. 2011;121:487–91.
64. Jeong HS, Baek CH, Son YI, Choi JY, Kim HJ, Ko YH, et al. Integrated 18F-FDG PET/CT for the initial evaluation of cervical node level of patients with papillary thyroid carcinoma: comparison with ultrasound and contrast-enhanced CT. Clin Endocrinol (Oxf). 2006;65:402–7.
65. Al-Azawi D, Mann GB, Judson RT, Miller JA. Endocrine surgeon-performed US guided thyroid FNAC is accurate and efficient. World J Surg. 2012;36:1947–52.
66. Kumbhar SS, O'Malley RB, Robinson TJ, Maximin S, Lalwani N, Byrd DR, et al. Why thyroid surgeons are frustrated with radiologists: lessons learned from pre- and postoperative US. Radiographics. 2016;36: 2141–53.
67. Raffaelli M, De Crea C, Sessa L, Giustacchini P, Revelli L, Bellantone C, et al. Prospective evaluation of total thyroidectomy versus ipsilateral versus bilateral central neck dissection in patients with clinically node-negative papillary thyroid carcinoma. Surgery (United States). 2012;152:957–64.
68. Calò PG, Conzo G, Raffaelli M, Medas F, Gambardella C, De Crea C, et al. Total thyroidectomy alone versus ipsilateral versus bilateral prophylactic central neck dissection in clinically node-negative differentiated thyroid carcinoma. A retrospective multicenter study. Eur J Surg Oncol. 2017;43:126–32.
69. Tuttle RM, Haugen B, Perrier ND. The updated AJCC/TNM staging system for differentiated and anaplastic thyroid cancer, 8th edition: what changed and why? Thyroid. 2017;27:751–6.
70. Raffaelli M, De Crea C, Sessa L, Fadda G, Lombardi CP, Bellantone R. Risk factors for central neck lymph node metastases in follicular variant vs. classic papillary thyroid carcinoma. Endocrine. 2018;62: 64–70.
71. Sessa L, Lombardi CP, De Crea C, Tempera SE, Bellantone R, Raffaelli M. Risk factors for central neck lymph node metastases in micro- versus

macro- clinically node negative papillary thyroid carcinoma. World J Surg. 2018;42:623–9.
72. Asimakopoulos P, Nixon IJ, Shaha AR. Differentiated and medullary thyroid cancer: surgical management of cervical lymph nodes. Clin Oncol. 2017;29:283–9.
73. Scherl S, Mehra S, Clain J, Dos Reis LL, Persky M, Turk A, et al. The effect of surgeon experience on the detection of metastatic lymph nodes in the central compartment and the pathologic features of clinically unapparent metastatic lymph nodes: what are we missing when we don't perform a prophylactic dissection of cent. Thyroid. 2014;24:1282–8.
74. Garau LM, Rubello D, Morganti R, Boni G, Volterrani D, Colletti PM, et al. Sentinel lymph node biopsy in small papillary thyroid cancer: a meta-analysis. Clin Nucl Med. 2019;44:108–18.
75. Garau LM, Rubello D, Muccioli S, Boni G, Volterrani D, Manca G. The sentinel lymph node biopsy technique in papillary thyroid carcinoma: the issue of false-negative findings. Eur J Surg Oncol. 2020;46:967–75.
76. Iyer NG, Shaha AR, Ferlito A, Robbins KT, Medina JE, Silver CE, et al. Delphian node metastasis in head and neck cancers – Oracle or myth? J Surg Oncol. 2010;102:354–8.
77. Kim WW, Yang SI, Kim JH, Choi YS, Park YH, Kwon SK. Experience and analysis of Delphian lymph node metastasis in patients with papillary thyroid carcinoma. World J Surg Oncol. 2012;10:1–7.
78. De Crea C, Raffaelli M, Sessa L, Lombardi CP, Bellantone R. Surgical approach to level VI in papillary thyroid carcinoma: an overview. Updat Surg. 2017;69:205–9.
79. Raffaelli M, Sessa L, De Crea C, Fadda G, Princi P, Rossi ED, et al. Is it possible to intraoperatively modulate the extent of thyroidectomy in small papillary thyroid carcinoma? Surgery. 2021;169:77–81.
80. Raffaelli M, De Crea C, Sessa L, Tempera SE, Fadda G, Pontecorvi A, et al. Modulating the extension of thyroidectomy in patients with papillary thyroid carcinoma pre-operatively eligible for lobectomy: reliability of ipsilateral central neck dissection. Endocrine. 2020;72(2):437–44.
81. Carling T, Carty SE, Ciarleglio MM, Cooper DS, Doherty GM, Kim LT, et al. American Thyroid Association design and feasibility of a prospective randomized controlled trial of prophylactic central lymph node dissection for papillary thyroid carcinoma. Thyroid. 2012;22:237–44.
82. Lee YJ, Kim DW, Park HK, Kim DH, Jung SJ, Oh M, et al. Pre-operative ultrasound diagnosis of nodal metastasis in papillary thyroid carcinoma patients according to nodal compartment. Ultrasound Med Biol. 2015;41:1294–300.
83. Hartl DM, Leboulleux S, Al Ghuzlan A, Baudin E, Chami L, Schlumberger M, et al. Optimization of staging of the neck with prophylactic central and lateral neck dissection for papillary thyroid carcinoma. Ann Surg. 2012;255:777–83.
84. Ito Y, Miyauchi A, Kudo T, Kihara M, Fukushima M, Miya A. The effectiveness of prophylactic modified neck dissection for reducing the development of lymph node recurrence of papillary thyroid carcinoma. World J Surg. 2017;41:2283–9.
85. Gimm O. Extent of surgery in clinically evident but operable MTC – when is central and/or lateral lympadenectomy indicated? Thyroid Res. 2013;6(1):1–5.
86. Dralle H, Machens A. Surgical management of the lateral neck compartment for metastatic thyroid cancer. Curr Opin Oncol. 2013;25:20–6.
87. Moley JF, DeBenedetti MK. Patterns of nodal metastases in palpable medullary thyroid carcinoma: recommendations for extent of node dissection. Ann Surg. 1999;229:880–8.
88. Dralle H, Machens A. Surgical approaches in thyroid cancer and lymph-node metastases. Best Pract Res Clin Endocrinol Metab. 2008;22:971–87.
89. De Crea C, Raffaelli M, Milano V, Carrozza C, Zuppi C, Bellantone R, et al. Intraoperative high-dose calcium stimulation test in patients with

sporadic medullary thyroid carcinoma is highly accurate in predicting lateral neck metastases. Surgery (United States). 2016;159(1):70–7.
90. Scheuba C, Bieglmayer C, Asari R, Kaczirek K, Izay B, Kaserer K, et al. The value of intraoperative pentagastrin testing in medullary thyroid cancer. Surgery. 2007;141:166–72.
91. Park JY, Koo BS. Individualized optimal surgical extent of the lateral neck in papillary thyroid cancer with lateral cervical metastasis. Eur Arch Oto-Rhino-Laryngol. 2014:1355–60.
92. Merdad M, Eskander A, Kroeker T, Freeman JL. Predictors of level II and Vb neck disease in metastatic papillary thyroid cancer. Arch Otolaryngol – Head Neck Surg. 2012;138:1030–3.
93. Raffaelli M, De Crea C, Sessa L, Tempera SE, Belluzzi A, Lombardi CP, et al. Risk factors for local recurrence following lateral neck dissection for papillary thyroid carcinoma. Endocrine. 2019;63:310–5.
94. Eskander A, Merdad M, Freeman JL, Witterick IJ. Pattern of spread to the lateral neck in metastatic well-differentiated thyroid cancer: a systematic review and meta-analysis. Thyroid. 2013;23:583–92.
95. Caron NR, Tan YY, Ogilvie JB, Triponez F, Reiff ES, Kebebew E, et al. Selective modified radical neck dissection for papillary thyroid cancer – is level I, II and V dissection always necessary? World J Surg. 2006;30:833–40.
96. Eskander A, Merdad M, Irish JC, Hall SF, Groome PA, Freeman JL, et al. Volume-outcome associations in head and neck cancer treatment: a systematic review and meta-analysis. Head Neck. 2014;36:1820–34.
97. Javid M, Graham E, Malinowski J, Quinn CE, Carling T, Udelsman R, et al. Dissection of levels II through v is required for optimal outcomes in patients with lateral neck lymph node metastasis from papillary thyroid carcinoma. J Am Coll Surg. 2016;222:1066–73.
98. Khafif A, Medina JE, Robbins KT, Silver CE, Weber RS, Rinaldo A, et al. Level V in therapeutic neck dissections for papillary thyroid carcinoma. Head Neck. 2013;35(4):605–7.
99. Sapalidis K, Papanastasiou A, Fyntanidou V, Aidoni Z, Michalopoulos N, Katsaounis A, et al. Comparison between magnification techniques and direct vision in thyroid surgery: a systematic review and meta-analysis. Medicina. 2019;55(11):725.
100. Verma RK, Mathiazhagan A, Panda NK. Neck dissection with harmonic scalpel and electrocautery? A randomised study. Auris Nasus Larynx. 2017;44:590–5.
101. Suzuki K, Shimizu M, Sakagami T, Yagi M, Fujisawa T, Sawada S, et al. A comparison of short-term outcomes of neck dissection for head and neck cancers using Thunderbeat™, LigaSure™ or treatment without an energy-based device: a case controlled study. Int J Surg. 2018;58:60–4.
102. Revelli L, Damiani G, Bianchi CBNA, Vanella S, Ricciardi W, Raffaelli M, et al. Complications in thyroid surgery. Harmonic scalpel, harmonic focus versus conventional hemostasis: a meta-analysis. Int J Surg. 2016;28:S22–32.
103. Lombardi CP, Raffaelli M, Cicchetti A, Marchetti M, De Crea C, Di Bidino R, et al. The use of "harmonic scalpel" versus "knot tying" for conventional "open" thyroidectomy: results of a prospective randomized study. Langenbeck's Arch Surg. 2008;393:627–31.
104. Miccoli P, Materazzi G, Fregoli L, Panicucci E, Kunz-Martinez W, Berti P. Modified lateral neck lymphadenectomy: prospective randomized study comparing harmonic scalpel with clamp-and-tie technique. Otolaryngol – Head Neck Surg. 2009;140:61–4.
105. Polychronidis G, Hüttner FJ, Contin P, Goossen K, Uhlmann L, Heidmann M, et al. Network meta-analysis of topical haemostatic agents in thyroid surgery. Br J Surg. 2018;105:1573–82.
106. Delaney SW, Shi H, Shokrani A, Sinha UK. Management of chyle leak after head and neck surgery: review of current treatment strategies. Int J Otolaryngol. 2017.2017:1–12.

107. Wu CW, Dionigi G, Barczynski M, Chiang FY, Dralle H, Schneider R, et al. International Neuromonitoring Study Group guidelines 2018: part II: optimal recurrent laryngeal nerve management for invasive thyroid cancer—incorporation of surgical, laryngeal, and neural electrophysiologic data. Laryngoscope. 2018;128:S18–27.
108. Kandil E, Mohsin K, Murcy MA, Randolph GW. Continuous vagal monitoring value in prevention of vocal cord paralysis following thyroid surgery. Laryngoscope. 2018;128:2429–32.
109. Lombardi CP, Raffaelli M, De Crea C, Traini E, Oragano L, Sollazzi L, et al. Complicanze in chirurgia tiroidea. Minerva Chir. 2007;62: 395–408.
110. Cirocchi R, Arezzo A, D'Andrea V, Abraha I, Popivanov GI, Avenia N, et al. Intraoperative neuromonitoring versus visual nerve identification for prevention of recurrent laryngeal nerve injury in adults undergoing thyroid surgery. Cochrane Database Syst Rev. 2019;(1):CD012483.
111. Naytah M, Ibrahim I, da Silva S. Importance of incorporating intraoperative neuromonitoring of the external branch of the superior laryngeal nerve in thyroidectomy: a review and meta-analysis study. Head Neck. 2019;41:2034–41.
112. Lee CH, Huang NC, Chen HC, Chen MK. Minimizing shoulder syndrome with intra-operative spinal accessory nerve monitoring for neck dissection. Acta Otorhinolaryngol Ital. 2013;33:93–936.
113. Tirelli G, Bergamini PR, Scardoni A, Gatto A, Boscolo Nata F, Marcuzzo AV. Intraoperative monitoring of marginal mandibular nerve during neck dissection. Head Neck. 2018;40:1016–23.
114. Barbieri D, Indelicato P, Vinciguerra A, Di Marco F, Formenti AM, Trimarchi M, et al. Autofluorescence and indocyanine green in thyroid surgery: a systematic review and meta-analysis. Laryngoscope. 2020;131(7):1683–92.
115. Ferlito A, Rinaldo A, Silver CE, Shah JP, Suárez C, Medina JE, et al. Neck dissection: then and now. Auris Nasus Larynx. 2006;33:365–74.
116. Raffaelli M, Iacobone M, Henry JF. The "false" nonrecurrent inferior laryngeal nerve. Surgery. 2000;128:1082–7.
117. Bellantone R, Lombardi CP, Raffaelli M, Boscherini M, Alesina PF, Princi P. Central neck lymph node removal during minimally invasive video-assisted thyroidectomy for thyroid carcinoma: a feasible and safe procedure. J Laparoendosc Adv Surg Tech – Part A. 2002;12:181–5.
118. Lombardi CP, Raffaelli M, De Crea C, Sessa L, Rampulla V, Bellantone R. Video-assisted versus conventional total thyroidectomy and central compartment neck dissection for papillary thyroid carcinoma. World J Surg. 2012;36:1225–30.
119. Sukato DC, Ballard DP, Abramowitz JM, Rosenfeld RM, Mlot S. Robotic versus conventional neck dissection: a systematic review and meta-analysis. Laryngoscope. 2019;129:1587–96.
120. Yan HC, Xiang C, Wang Y, Wang P. Scarless endoscopic thyroidectomy (SET) lateral neck dissection for papillary thyroid carcinoma through breast approach: 10 years of experience. Surg Endosc. 2020;35(7):3540–6.
121. Tae K, Kim KH. Transoral robotic selective neck dissection for papillary thyroid carcinoma: dissection of levels III and IV. Head Neck. 2020;42:3084–8.
122. Ngo DQ, Tran TD, Le DT, Ngo QX, Van Le Q. Transoral endoscopic modified radical neck dissection for papillary thyroid carcinoma. Ann Surg Oncol. 2021;28(5):2766.
123. Miccoli P, Elisei R, Donatini G, Materazzi G, Berti P. Video-assisted central compartment lymphadenectomy in a patient with a positive RET oncogene: initial experience. Surg Endosc Other Interv Tech. 2007;21:120–3.
124. Bellantone R, Raffaelli M, De Crea C, Sessa L, Traini E, Princi P, et al. Video-assisted thyroidectomy for papillary thyroid carcinoma: oncologic outcome in patients with follow-up ≥ 10 years. World J Surg. 2018;42:402–8.

125. Salvatori M, Rufini V, Reale F, Gajate AMS, Maussier ML, Revelli L, et al. Radio-guided surgery for lymph node recurrences of differentiated thyroid cancer. World J Surg. 2003;27:770–5.
126. Dalcı K, Topal U, Ünal AG, Eray İC, Yalav O, Güney İB, et al. Is radioguided occult lesion localization (ROLL) an effective and reliable method in thyroid cancer and parathyroid redo surgery? Ann Ital Chir. 2020;91:166–72.
127. Rocke DJ, Mulder H, Cyr D, Kahmke R, Lee WT, Puscas L, et al. The effect of lateral neck dissection on complication rate for total thyroidectomy. Am J Otolaryngol – Head Neck Med Surg. 2020;41:102421.
128. Al-Qurayshi Z, Sullivan CB, Pagedar N, Randolph G, Kandil E. Prevalence of major structures injury in thyroid and neck surgeries: a national perspective. Gland Surg. 2020;9:1924–32.
129. Ryan WR, Fee WE. Long-term great auricular nerve morbidity after sacrifice during parotidectomy. Laryngoscope. 2009;119:1140–6.
130. Murthy SP, Paderno A, Balasubramanian D. Management of the marginal mandibular nerve during and after neck dissection. Curr Opin Otolaryngol Head Neck Surg. 2019;27:104–9.
131. Prim MP, De Diego JI, Verdaguer JM, Sastre N, Rabanal I. Neurological complications following functional neck dissection. Eur Arch Oto-Rhino-Laryngol. 2006;263:473–6.
132. Salerno G, Cavaliere M, Foglia A, Pellicoro DP, Mottola G, Nardone M, et al. The 11th nerve syndrome in functional neck dissection. Laryngoscope. 2002;112:1299–307.
133. Larsen MH, Lorenzen MM, Bakholdt V, Sørensen JA. The prevalence of nerve injuries following neck dissections – a systematic review and meta-analysis. Dan Med J. 2020;67:1–15.
134. Gane EM, Michaleff ZA, Cottrell MA, McPhail SM, Hatton AL, Panizza BJ, et al. Prevalence, incidence, and risk factors for shoulder and neck dysfunction after neck dissection: a systematic review. Eur J Surg Oncol. 2017;43:1199–218.
135. Wittekindt C, Liu WC, Preuss SF, Guntinas-Lichius O. Botulinum toxin A for neuropathic pain after neck dissection: a dose-finding study. Laryngoscope. 2006;116:1168–71.
136. Ferreira SR, Martins RS, Siqueira MG. Correlação entre a recuperação motora funcional e as atividades de vida diária após cirurgia do plexo braquial. Arq Neuropsiquiatr. 2017;75:631–4.
137. Monteiro MJ, Altman K, Khandwala A. Injury to the brachial plexus in neck dissections. Br J Oral Maxillofac Surg. 2010;48:197–8.
138. Shandilya M, Walshe P, Timon C, Kieran S. Cervical haematoma after thyroid surgery: management and prevention. Ir Med J. 2006;99:266–8.
139. Harada H, Omura K, Takeuchi Y. Patency and caliber of the internal jugular vein after neck dissection. Auris Nasus Larynx. 2003;30:269–72.
140. Weiss KL, Wax MK, Haydon RC, Kaufman HH, Hurst MK. Intracranial pressure changes during bilateral radical neck dissections. Head Neck. 1993;15:546–52.
141. Orloff LA, Wiseman SM, Bernet VJ, Fahey TJ, Shaha AR, Shindo ML, et al. American Thyroid Association statement on postoperative hypoparathyroidism: diagnosis, prevention, and management in adults. Thyroid. 2018;28:830–41.
142. Bellantone R, Lombardi CP, Raffaelli M, Boscherini M, Alesina PF, De Crea C, et al. Is routine supplementation therapy (calcium and vitamin D) useful after total thyroidectomy?. Surgery. 2002;132(6):1109–13.
143. Shoback DM, Bilezikian JP, Costa AG, Dempster D, Dralle H, Khan AA, et al. Presentation of hypoparathyroidism: Etiologies and clinical features. J Clin Endocrinol Metab. 2016;101:2300–12.
144. Raffaelli M, De Crea C, Carrozza C, D'Amato G, Zuppi C, Bellantone R, et al. Combining early postoperative parathyroid hormone and serum calcium levels allows for an efficacious selective post-thyroidectomy supplementation treatment. World J Surg. 2012;36:1307–13.

145. Raffaelli M, De Crea C, D'Amato G, Moscato U, Bellantone C, Carrozza C, et al. Post-thyroidectomy hypocalcemia is related to parathyroid dysfunction even in patients with normal parathyroid hormone concentrations early after surgery. Surgery. 2016;159:78–85.
146. Roh JL, Kim DH, Park CIL. Prospective identification of chyle leakage in patients undergoing lateral neck dissection for metastatic thyroid cancer. Ann Surg Oncol. 2008;15:424–9.
147. Campisi CC, Boccardo F, Piazza C, Campisi C. Evolution of chylous fistula management after neck dissection. Curr Opin Otolaryngol Head Neck Surg. 2013;21:150–6.
148. Nussenbaum B, Liu JH, Sinard RJ. Systematic management of chyle fistula: The Southwestern experience and review of the literature. Otolaryngol – Head Neck Surg. 2000;122:31–8.
149. Scorza LB, Goldstein BJ, Mahraj RP. Modern management of chylous leak following head and neck surgery: a discussion of percutaneous lymphangiography-guided cannulation and embolization of the thoracic duct. Otolaryngol Clin N Am. 2008;41:1231–40.
150. Abdel-Galil K, Milton R, McCaul J. High output chyle leak after neck surgery: the role of video-assisted thoracoscopic surgery. Br J Oral Maxillofac Surg. 2009;47:478–80.
151. Merki V, Pichler J, Giger R, Mantokoudis G. Chylothorax in thyroid surgery: a very rare case and systematic review of the literature. J Otolaryngol Head Neck Surg. 2016;45:1–8.
152. Lee SW, Cho SH, Lee JD, Lee JY, Kim SC, Koh YW. Bilateral pneumothorax and pneumomediastinum following total thyroidectomy with central neck dissection. Clin Exp Otorhinolaryngol. 2008;1:49.
153. Marchese-Ragona R, Marioni G, Restivo DA, Staffieri A. The role of botulinum toxin in postparotidectomy fistula treatment. A technical note. Am J Otolaryngol – Head Neck Med Surg. 2006;27:221–4.
154. Davidson BJ, Newkirk KA, Harter KW, Picken CA, Cullen KJ, Sessions RB. Complications from planned, posttreatment neck dissections. Arch Otolaryngol – Head Neck Surg. 1999;125:401–5.
155. Deng J, Murphy BA, Dietrich MS, Wells N, Wallston KA, Sinard RJ, et al. Impact of secondary lymphedema after head and neck cancer treatment on symptoms, functional status, and quality of life. Head Neck. 2013;35:1026–35.
156. Ducic Y, Hilger PA. The use of unilateral deep plane neck lifting to improve the aesthetic appearance of the neck dissection deformity. Am J Otolaryngol Head Neck Med Surg. 2000;21:202–6.

Parathyroid

Contents

Parathyroid Glands: Anatomy, Physiology, Pathophysiology, and Ultrasound

Marika D. Russell and Gregory W. Randolph

Contents

A. L. Shifrin et al. (eds.), *Endocrine Surgery Comprehensive Board Exam Guide*,
https://doi.org/10.1007/978-3-030-84737-1_12

Questions

1. Which of the following statements regarding parathyroid embryologic development are correct?
   1. Parathyroid gland development occurs between the 5th and 12th weeks of gestation.
   2. The superior parathyroid glands develop from ventral aspect of the 4th branchial pouches and descend with the ultimobranchial bodies.
   3. The inferior parathyroid glands develop from the ventral aspect of the 3rd branchial pouches and descend with the thymus.
   4. The timing of separation of the PIII from the thymus determines the location of the inferior parathyroid glands.
      (a) Only (1) and (2) are correct.
      (b) Only (1), (2), and (3) are correct.
      (c) Only (1) and (4) are correct.
      (d) All are correct.
2. Which of the following statements about parathyroid gland anatomy are correct?
   1. The superior parathyroid glands are more constant in their position relative to the thyroid.
   2. The arterial blood supply for the superior parathyroid most commonly derives from the superior thyroid artery.
   3. The inferior parathyroid gland has a wider normal distribution than the superior parathyroid gland owing to its longer migration path.
   4. Symmetry of the inferior parathyroid glands is uncommonly seen within the same subjects.
      (a) Only (1), (2), and (3) are correct.
      (b) Only (1), (3), and (4) are correct.
      (c) Only (1) and (3) are correct.
      (d) All are correct.
3. Which of the following statements regarding ectopic parathyroid gland anatomy are correct?
   1. Major ectopic locations of the superior parathyroid gland are common.
   2. Intrathyroidal parathyroid glands are always inferior glands.
   3. Supernumerary ectopic glands identified within the vagus nerve have been reported.
   4. Acquired ectopia refers to migration of pathologically enlarged gland.
      (a) Only (2), (3), and (4) are correct.
      (b) Only (3) and (4) are correct.
      (c) None are correct.
      (d) All are correct.

4. Which of the following statements regarding parathyroid physiology are correct?
   1. Parathyroid glands are comprised primarily of chief cells, which secrete PTH, and oxyphil cells.
   2. Magnesium is essential for PTH synthesis and secretion.
   3. Familial hypocalciuric hypercalcemia is caused by a gain of function mutation of the CaSR.
   4. In hypercalcemia, the CaSR promotes PTH degradation and inhibits parathyroid cellular proliferation.
      (a) Only (1), (2), and (4) are correct.
      (b) Only (1), (2), and (3) are correct.
      (c) Only (1) and (2) are correct.
      (d) All are correct.
5. Which of the following statements about PTH are correct?
   1. PTH is an 84-amino acid polypeptide with a short half-life of 3 to 4 minutes.
   2. PTH principally acts on bone and the kidneys.
   3. PTH may have either a catabolic or anabolic effect on bone.
   4. PTH promotes conversion of 25-hydroxyvitamin D (25(OH)D) to 1,25-dihydroxyvitamin D ($1,25(OH)_2D$) in the kidney.
      (a) Only (1), (2), and (3) are correct.
      (b) Only (1), (3), and (4) are correct.
      (c) Only (2), (3), and (4) are correct.
      (d) All are correct.
6. Which of the following statements regarding primary hyperparathyroidism (PHPT) are correct?
   1. PTH levels are always elevated above the normal range.
   2. Most patients with PHPT are symptomatic.
   3. A single gland adenoma is the most common cause of PHPT.
   4. Normohormonal and normocalcemic variants of PHPT are more likely to present with multiglandular disease.
      (a) Only (1), (3), and (4) are correct.
      (b) Only (2), (3), and (4) are correct.
      (c) Only (3) and (4) are correct.
      (d) Only (1), (2), and (3) are correct.
7. The following are inherited disorders of hyperparathyroidism:
   1. Familial hypercalcemic hypocalciuria
   2. MEN 1
   3. Hyperparathyroidism-jaw tumor syndrome
   4. Autoimmune polyglandular syndrome type 1
      (a) Only (1), (2), and (4) are correct.
      (b) Only (1), (2), and (3) are correct.
      (c) Only (1) and (2) are correct.
      (d) All are correct.

8. Which of the following statements regarding secondary hyperparathyroidism (SHPT) in chronic kidney disease (CKD) are correct?
   1. Hypocalcemia results from increased phosphate retention.
   2. There is decreased renal production of $1,25(OH)_2D$.
   3. Hyperphosphatemia directly stimulates PTH synthesis.
   4. Skeletal PTH resistance contributes to increased secretion of PTH.
      (a) Only (2), (3), and (4) are correct.
      (b) Only (1), (2), and (4) are correct.
      (c) Only (1), (3), and (4) are correct.
      (d) All are correct.
9. Which of the following are appropriate medical therapies for the treatment of SHPT in chronic kidney disease?
   1. Calcimimetic agents
   2. Vitamin D
   3. Diuretics
   4. Phosphate binders
      (a) Only (1), (2), and (4) are correct.
      (b) Only (2), (3), and (4) are correct.
      (c) Only (1) and (4) are correct.
      (d) Only (2) and (4) are correct.
10. Which of the following statements regarding hypoparathyroidism are correct?
    1. Hypoparathyroidism is most often iatrogenic in etiology.
    2. Riedel's thyroiditis may be present with hypoparathyroidism.
    3. Hypomagnesemia results in decreased PTH synthesis and secretion.
    4. Hypermagnesemia results in PTH suppression.
       (a) Only (1), (2), and (3) are correct.
       (b) Only (1), (2), and (4) are correct.
       (c) Only (1), (3), and (4) are correct.
       (d) All are correct.
11. Which of the following statements about parathyroid ultrasonography are correct?
    1. Normal parathyroid glands can be visualized with high-resolution US.
    2. The classic appearance of a parathyroid adenoma is a well-circumscribed hyperechoic nodule.
    3. Nodularity of the parathyroid gland can be appreciated in patients with longstanding SHPT.
    4. Ultrasound is limited in evaluation of the retropharyngeal and retroesophageal spaces.
       (a) Only (1), (3), and (4) are correct.
       (b) Only (2), (3), and (4) are correct.
       (c) Only (3) and (4) are correct.
       (d) Only (2) and (4) are correct.

12.1 Introduction

The parathyroid glands are typically comprised of four small glands located posterior to the thyroid, though their location, size, and shape may vary widely. The location of the parathyroid glands is derived from their embryologic development. As such, familiarity with embryologic development patterns is critical to successful surgical identification and management. The parathyroid glands maintain calcium homeostasis and must be meticulously managed along with their blood supply in order to preserve their physiologic function. Hypoparathyroidism, as can occur after thyroidectomy with devascularization of the parathyroid glands or inadvertent parathyroidectomy, may be associated with severe, life-threatening hypocalcemia [1]. Similarly, careful preoperative evaluation and surgical strategy must be employed when performing parathyroidectomy for hyperparathyroidism; reoperative parathyroidectomy after failed surgery is complex and carries additional surgical risk [2]. To optimize outcomes in thyroid and parathyroid surgery, the surgeon must have an appreciation for parathyroid function and be skilled in the identification and surgical manipulation of the parathyroid glands. This chapter will review the elements of parathyroid anatomy and physiology fundamental to this task.

12.2 Parathyroid Anatomy

12.2.1 Embryologic Development

The paired superior and inferior parathyroid glands develop from the third and fourth branchial pouches between the 5th and 12th weeks of gestation [3] (◘ Fig. 12.1). The inferior parathyroid glands derive from the dorsal aspect of the third branchial pouches and are thus designated as parathyroid III (P III). The thymus originates from the ventral aspect of the same pouch and descends caudally in close association with the P III as the *parathymus complex* [4]; during this migration, the P III separate from the thymic lobes, which continue to the anterior mediastinum. The relatively long descent of the P III and variable timing of separation from the thymus yields variability in the final anatomic position of the inferior parathyroid glands [5]. Separation may occur at the level of the inferior thyroid pole or along the course of the thyrothymic ligament, a vestigial structure derived from the previous connection of these two structures.

The superior parathyroid glands arise from the dorsal aspect of the fourth branchial pouches (P IV). The ventral aspect of these pouches is believed to fuse with the rudimentary fifth pouches to form the ultimobranchial bodies. The P

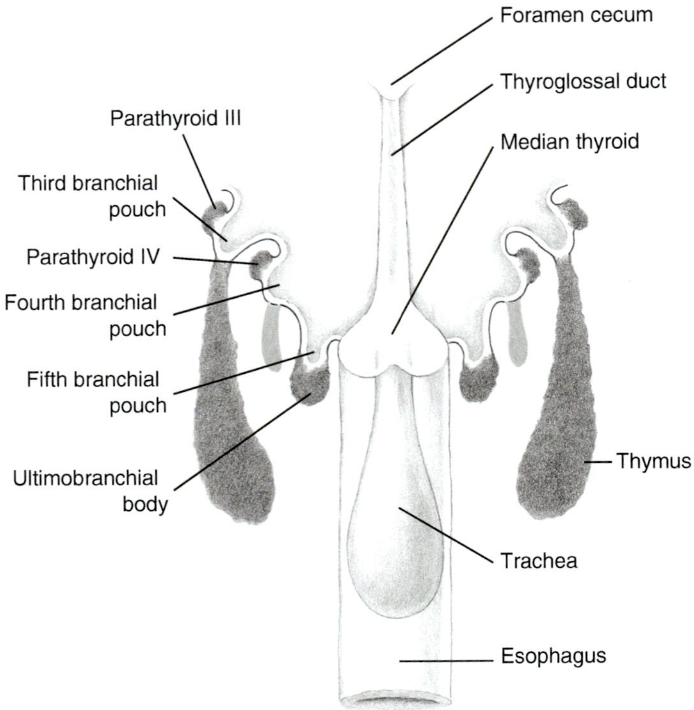

Fig. 12.1 Schematic view of the primitive pharynx in an 8–10 mm embryo (*from Surgery of the Thyroid and Parathyroid Glands, 3rd ed., Randolph GW, editor; reprinted with permission*)

IV follow the migration of the ultimobranchial bodies, which descend a relatively limited path toward the lateral thyroid region, ultimately giving rise to the parafollicular-C cells of the thyroid. The P IV separate from the ultimobranchial bodies as the median and lateral thyroid elements fuse and incorporate the ultimobranchial bodies. This separation event determines the final anatomic position of the superior parathyroid glands relative to the thyroid [4].

12.2.2 Normal Parathyroid Gland Anatomy

Parathyroid glands may assume a variety of shapes, including oval, teardrop, flattened, spherical, or bi-lobed. Average size ranges from 3 to 8 mm in length and 2 to 4 mm in width, with each gland weighing 30 to 60 mg [6, 7]. Parathyroid glands are soft and pliable in consistency, ranging in color from reddish-brown to yellow-tan. Their color and consistency distinguish them from the firmer and darker thyroid tissue; an experienced surgeon should be able to appreciate this difference on gross inspection.

The position of the parathyroid glands derives from their embryologic development. As a result of limited embryologic

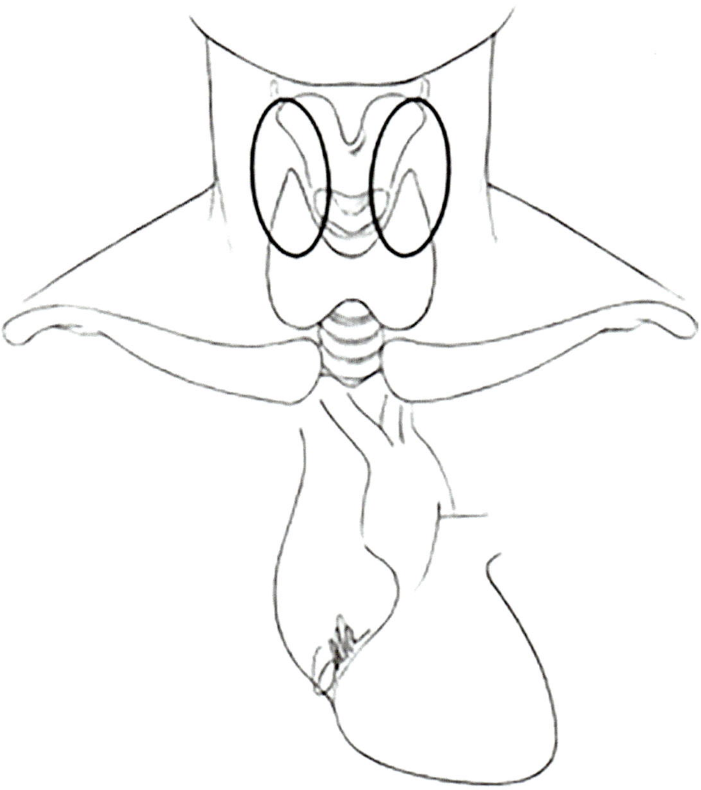

Fig. 12.2 The area of distribution for the superior parathyroid glands is limited by their relatively short embryonic migration path (*from Surgery of the Thyroid and Parathyroid Glands, 3rd ed., Randolph GW, editor; reprinted with permission*)

migration, the superior parathyroid glands are fairly constant in their position relative to the thyroid (Fig. 12.2). In over 80% of cases, they can be found on the posterior aspect of the thyroid lobe, near the cricothyroid joint approximately 1 cm above the intersection of the recurrent laryngeal nerve and the inferior thyroid artery [6, 8]. In 20% of subjects the superior parathyroid is intimately associated with the perithyroidal fascia and closely tethered to the thyroid, but in most cases, the superior parathyroid is enveloped in a pocket of fatty tissue, rendering it freely mobile [4, 6]. The arterial blood supply for the superior parathyroid derives from the inferior thyroid artery in 80% of subjects; in the remainder, the gland is supplied from a posterior branch of the superior thyroid artery or from an anastomotic branch between the superior and inferior thyroid arteries [9, 10].

The normal distribution of the inferior parathyroid glands is wider, owing to their longer embryologic migration path (Fig. 12.3). In about half of cases, the inferior parathyroid is located at the level of the inferior thyroid lobe, on the anterior or posterolateral surface. In about a quarter of cases, it is

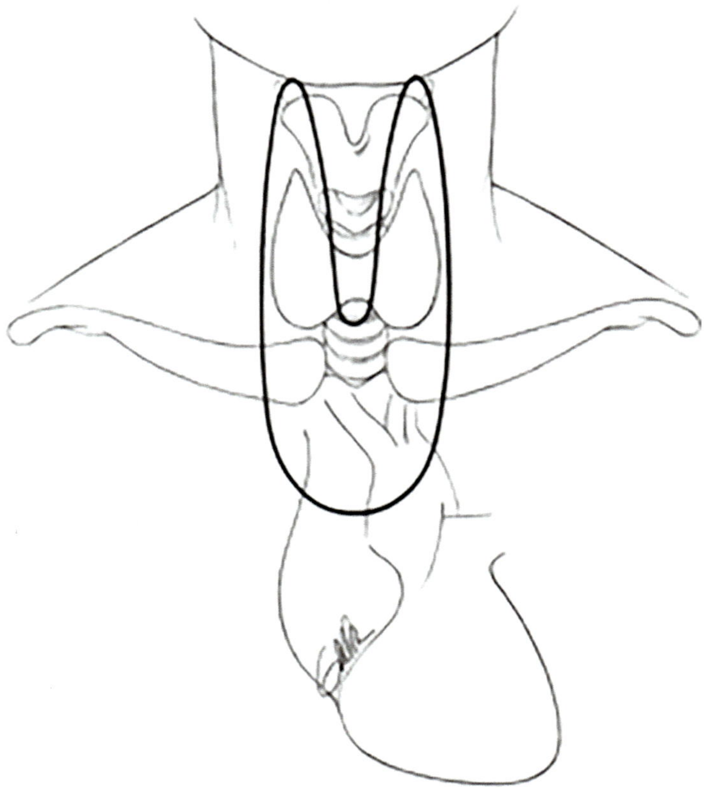

Fig. 12.3 The area of distribution of the inferior parathyroid glands is wide, extending from the angle of the mandible to the pericardium (*from Surgery of the Thyroid and Parathyroid Glands, 3rd ed., Randolph GW, editor; reprinted with permission)*

located along the thyrothymic ligament or within thymic tongue at the thoracic inlet; occasionally it is located within a crease of the thyroid lobe. Because the inferior and superior glands cross paths during embryologic migration, the inferior gland may on occasion be located cranial to the superior gland, or the two glands may be found in close apposition [9]. The inferior parathyroid gland is typically situated within a pocket of thymic derived fatty tissue but may be closely adherent to the thyroid capsule [4, 6, 8]. Its arterial blood supply originates from the inferior thyroid artery; in rare cases where the inferior thyroid artery is absent, it is supplied by a branch of the superior thyroid artery [9, 10].

While the location of glands may vary considerably, there is often symmetry within individual subjects. Symmetry of the superior and inferior glands is seen in approximately 80% and 70% subjects, respectively, with relative symmetry of all four glands seen in 60% of subjects [8]. The most common form of asymmetry occurs when only one gland is located in the thymus [4].

12.2.3 Ectopic Parathyroid Gland Anatomy

Descent of the parathymus complex during embryologic migration begins at the angle of the mandible, with the thymus extending to the pericardium; anomalies of P III migration can result in ectopia of the inferior parathyroid glands anywhere along this path. The undescended P III is estimated to occur in just 1–2% of subjects but may represent up to 22% of missed adenomas undergoing reoperation [11, 12]. The undescended inferior gland may be found above the hyoid beneath the angle of the mandible, or may be positioned in the carotid sheath, often adjacent to the carotid bifurcation, sometimes situated within a small pad of thymic tissue. In these instances, the vascular supply for the gland originates from the superior thyroid artery [4, 11].

Delay of P III separation from the thymus, on the other hand, may result in migration of the PIII into the chest. In approximately 4–5% of subjects, the inferior parathyroid gland is located within or adjacent to the retrosternal thymus, and may be in contact with the brachiocephalic vein or ascending aorta [4]. Rarely, ectopia may occur adjacent to the pleura or pericardium [13]. In instances where the ectopic gland rests below the level of the brachiocephalic vein and aortic arch, the blood supply is anomalous and typically derived from the internal mammary artery, though it may arise from a thymic artery or direct branch of the aorta [14].

Major ectopic locations of the superior parathyroid gland are rare but may result from failure of descent or laterally directed descent resulting in a location adjacent to the carotid artery. More commonly, the superior parathyroid gland may be found at or above the superior pole of the thyroid (1–2%) or in the retropharyngeal or retroesophageal space (1–4%) [4, 6, 8]. In the rare case where the P IV fails to separate during its downward migration, the superior parathyroid gland may develop within the pyriform sinus [15].

Ectopic glands may be found within the thyroid parenchyma with an estimated incidence of 0.5–4% [6, 8, 15, 16]. A true intrathyroidal parathyroid gland is surrounded by thyroid parenchyma and should be differentiated from a gland within the thyroid capsule or buried within a thyroid crease [4, 9]. The etiology of this phenomenon is not well understood; while it would appear that the P IV might become incorporated into the thyroid with the ultimobranchial body, several authors have found intrathyroidal glands to be primarily inferior glands based on their lower one-third intrathyroidal position [16–18]. Still, it is generally accepted that intrathyroidal glands may be inferior, superior, or even supernumerary (see discussion of supernumerary glands below) [4, 9].

In some cases, acquired ectopia may result from migration of pathologically enlarged glands. The force of gravity in combination with repetitive movement of the pharynx and larynx and favorable tissue planes is thought to contribute to downward migration, especially of superior glands [17]. Enlarged superior glands often migrate into the superior posterior mediastinum, following along the course of the esophagus. Indeed, 40% of superior parathyroid adenomas are found in posterior locations including retropharyngeal, paraesophageal, or retroesophageal positions [17]. Acquired ectopia of the inferior parathyroid glands is much less common, likely because adjacent structures and tissue planes are less conducive to displacement [4].

12.2.4 Supernumerary Glands

Autopsy studies of patients without parathyroid disease have suggested that fewer than four glands are present in up to 6% of subjects, though failure to account for all glands cannot be excluded as an explanation for this finding [4, 6]. On the other hand, autopsy series have reported more than four glands in 5–13% of subjects [8, 19]. Operative series of patients with renal disease and diffuse parathyroid hyperplasia have reported a much higher incidence, up to 30%, though it is possible these findings represent hyperplasia of small ectopic migratory rests and not true supernumerary glands [4, 20, 21]. Most supernumerary glands are identified within the thymus or thyrothymic ligament, though may be found in ectopic positions including within the thyroid, carotid sheath, or in retroesophageal or mediastinal locations [20]. Exceptional ectopic positions of hyperfunctional supernumerary glands have been described, including locations within the aortopulmonary window and deep within the middle mediastinum [22–24]. Several published reports have described hyperfunctioning parathyroid gland within the vagus nerve or its epineurium [25–27]. The etiology of this latter finding is not known, though it has been hypothesized that embryologic parathyroid tissue derived from the third branchial pouch separates and becomes embedded in the embryologic vagus nerve, which originates from the third and fourth branchial arches [28].

12.3 Parathyroid Physiology

The principal function of the parathyroid glands is secretion of parathyroid hormone (PTH) which serves to regulate calcium homeostasis. The parathyroid gland is comprised primarily of chief cells, which synthesize and secrete PTH, and oxyphil cells

[29]. The function of oxyphil cells is not well understood, though they are believed to produce additional regulatory factors and may be derived from chief cells [30]. An increased preponderance of oxyphil cells has been noted in patients with chronic renal failure [30, 31]. Oxyphil cells are larger than chief cells and contain abundant mitochondria; notably, the radioisotope utilized in sestamibi scans is retained in mitochondria and thus the sensitivity of the sestamibi scan is dependent on the relative concentration of oxyphil cells [32].

Chief cells contain calcium-sensing receptors (CaSR) within the cell membrane which "sense" extracellular calcium levels and alter the secretion of PTH through a G-protein mediated pathway [33]. Low levels of circulating calcium stimulate secretion of PTH; hypercalcemia suppresses release of PTH. Additionally, when calcium levels are elevated, the CaSR promotes PTH degradation and inhibits parathyroid cellular proliferation [34]. Magnesium also binds to the CaSR and is required for PTH synthesis and secretion [35]. Inactivating mutations in the CaSR gene lead to the disorder known as familial hypocalciuric hypercalcemia (FHH). This condition is characterized by general calcium hypo-sensitivity with elevated or unsuppressed PTH, hypercalcemia, and inappropriately low urinary excretion of calcium [36].

PTH is an 84-amino acid polypeptide with a short half-life of approximately 3–4 minutes. The principal target organs of PTH are bone and the kidneys. In bone, PTH has either a catabolic or anabolic effect, depending on the level and timing of its signal. Low intermittent doses of PTH promote bone formation through stimulation of osteoblasts, whereas prolonged PTH stimulates bone resorption and demineralization. Under physiologic conditions, PTH supports bone formation; during periods of hypocalcemia, bone resorption serves to restore normal serum calcium levels [35]. In the kidney, PTH promotes calcium and magnesium reabsorption and phosphate excretion via conversion of 25-hydroxyvitamin D (25(OH)D) to its active form, 1,25-dihydroxyvitamin D ($1,25(OH)_2D$). Activation of 25(OH)D also indirectly facilitates uptake of calcium in the intestine [37].

12.4 Parathyroid Pathophysiology

Derangements in parathyroid gland function may occur as disorders of hyperfunction or hypofunction. Disorders of hyperparathyroidism occur as primary, secondary, or tertiary states and often require surgical intervention. These disorders are briefly reviewed here; more extensive discussion is provided in the ensuing chapters.

12.4.1 Hyperparathyroidism

12.4.1.1 Primary Hyperparathyroidism

Primary hyperparathyroidism (PHPT) is due to abnormal, autonomous secretion of PTH from one or more parathyroid glands. The disease is classically characterized by hypercalcemia and levels of PTH that are abnormally high or inappropriately elevated for the level of hypercalcemia present. Distinct phenotypes of PHPT are now recognized, including symptomatic, asymptomatic, and normocalcemic PHPT. Normohormonal PHPT has also been described as a unique clinical entity [38]. Symptoms of PHPT may be due to the hypercalcemia itself (including anorexia, nausea, vomiting, dehydration, fatigue, and altered mental status) or related to effects on target organs, including nephrolithiasis, proximal muscle weakness, or skeletal fractures [39]. Since the development of widespread biochemical screening in the 1970s, overt symptomatic manifestations of PHPT are less commonly seen, and the asymptomatic form is predominant [39, 40]. Normocalcemic PTHP is characterized by elevated PTH with persistently normal levels of serum calcium and may occur in symptomatic or asymptomatic forms [39, 40]. Normohormonal PHPT is a less well-characterized disorder marked by a normal PTH level with increased serum calcium. This phenotype often presents a diagnostic challenge owing to mild biochemical derangements and fewer presenting symptoms [38].

PHPT most commonly presents as a sporadic disease with uniglandular involvement; a singular parathyroid adenoma accounts for 80% to 85% of cases of PHPT. The disease has a higher prevalence in women and tends to present in the fourth decade of life [41]. Sporadic development of a parathyroid adenoma is thought to occur through stepwise acquired mutations resulting in the emergence of a neoplastic clone within the parathyroid gland [42].

Multiglandular disease is seen in approximately 15–20% of patients and commonly presents as asymmetric four-gland hyperplasia, though multiple parathyroid adenomas are a well-recognized phenomenon occurring in 2–5% of cases [41, 43]. Normohormonal and normocalcemic variants of PHPT are more likely to present with multiglandular disease and milder biochemical abnormalities [38, 44, 45].

Inherited disorders of PHPT include multiple endocrine neoplasia (MEN) syndromes, familial isolated hyperparathyroidism, hyperparathyroidism-jaw tumor syndrome, and familial hypocalciuric hypercalcemia. This latter disorder, as previously noted, is caused by an inactivating mutation in the CaSR and presents with mild hypercalcemia when present in a heterozygous form. When inactivating mutations of the CaSR are inherited in a homozygous form, neonatal severe hypercalcemia develops and may be life-threatening if not promptly recognized [40, 41].

Parathyroid carcinoma is a rare cause of primary hyperparathyroidism, accounting for less than 0.5% of cases of PHPT [40]. The disease manifests with markedly elevated levels of PTH and calcium. While the etiology is unknown, there is no evidence to suggest that parathyroid carcinoma arises from malignant transformation of a benign adenoma.

12.4.1.2 Secondary and Tertiary Hyperparathyroidism

Secondary hyperparathyroidism (SHPT) refers to the situation in which hyperfunction of the parathyroid glands develops as a result of chronic hypocalcemia. This condition is typically associated with progressive renal disease, though may be associated with prolonged lithium therapy, vitamin D deficiency, and gastrointestinal malabsorption disorders [31]. Chronic kidney disease (CKD) is characterized by phosphate retention and decreased renal production of 1,25$(OH)_2$D, resulting in low levels of serum calcium. Moreover, hyperphosphatemia acts directly on parathyroid cells to stimulate PTH synthesis and secretion and parathyroid cell proliferation. Downregulation of the CaSR and the vitamin D receptor (VDR) in parathyroid cells increases PTH secretion, as does skeletal resistance to PTH mediated by decreased expression of the PTH receptor on osteoblasts [31].

SHPT is characterized by asymmetric parathyroid enlargement with varying degrees of hyperplasia and nodularity [46]. It has been hypothesized that early hyperplasia of parathyroid cells represents polyclonal proliferation; later development of regions of nodularity correspond to areas of monoclonal proliferation. The eventual dominance of one nodule with the greatest proliferative ability generates a single nodule within the gland, akin to the development of a parathyroid adenoma [46].

Medical treatment of SHPT involves administration of phosphate binders, vitamin D or VDR agonists, and calcimimetic agents. Surgical treatment is typically reserved for cases of severe SHPT or medically refractory disease. It has been suggested that development of nodular hyperplasia is associated with poor response to medical treatment [46].

SHPT usually resolves within 6–12 months after renal transplantation; the persistence of hyperparathyroidism after renal transplantation is termed tertiary hyperparathyroidism (THPT). THPT manifests with hypercalcemia, hypophosphatemia, and moderately elevated levels of PTH. Recently, treatment with cinacalcet, a calcimimetic agent, has been shown to be effective in the treatment of TPHP [47, 48]. Surgical treatment may be indicated for persistent hypercalcemia or effects on target organs, or where a single enlarged gland is identified [31].

12.4.2 Hypoparathyroidism

Hypoparathyroidism is most often iatrogenic in etiology. Inadvertent removal of the parathyroid glands or damage to their blood supply during total thyroidectomy is the most common cause of temporary, or less frequently, permanent hypoparathyroidism [42]. Other acquired forms of hypoparathyroidism are less common. Riedel's thyroiditis is a rare inflammatory condition of the thyroid marked by dense progressive fibrosis extending outside the thyroid capsule. Involvement of the parathyroid glands may lead to hypoparathyroidism in a subset of these cases [49]. Acquired autoimmune hypoparathyroidism mediated by antibodies which functionally activate the CaSR has also been described [50]. Magnesium imbalance may cause a reversible hypoparathyroidism. Magnesium is essential in PTH synthesis and secretion; hypomagnesemia as seen with chronic alcoholism may cause parathyroid hypofunction. Moreover, magnesium, like calcium, binds to and stimulates the CaSR; thus, hypermagnesemia due to parenteral administration or resulting from renal insufficiency may activate the CaSR and suppress PTH release [51].

Uncommonly, hypoparathyroidism is the result of a congenital or inherited disorder. DiGeorge syndrome and other related disorders caused by a deletion or rearrangement of chromosome 22q11.2 involve embryologic defects in the third, fourth, and fifth branchial pouches leading to hypoplasia or agenesis of the parathyroid glands, in addition to several other facial and cardiac anomalies [52]. Other rare genetic syndromes associated with hypoparathyroidism have been described. Hypoparathyroidism-deafness-renal dysplasia (HDR) syndrome results from a mutation in *GATA3*, a transcription factor important in the embryologic development of the parathyroid gland, inner ear, and kidneys [53]. Autoimmune polyglandular syndrome type 1 is an inherited disorder associated with multiple autoimmune endocrinopathies including hypoparathyroidism, as well as ectodermal dystrophies and chronic mucocutaneous candidiasis [54]. Familial hypocalcemic hypercalciuria is an inherited disorder characterized by a *gain of function* mutation in the CaSR gene. This manifests with oversensitivity to calcium, causing suppression of PTH secretion with resultant hypocalcemia and inappropriately elevated urinary excretion of calcium [55]. Cases of familial isolated hypoparathyroidism marked by agenesis of the parathyroid glands or synthesis of a defective PTH molecule have also been described [42].

Hypocalcemia resulting from hypoparathyroidism may range from mild to severe, with variable symptomatology. Severe hypocalcemia may present with fatigue, confusion, paresthesias, and muscle cramping or twitching. Laryngospasm, bronchospasm, or seizures may occur. Cardiac dysfunction manifested by a prolonged QTc interval may be seen; in rare cases, congestive heart failure may develop [51]. Treatment involves oral repletion of calcium; intravenous calcium repletion may be indicated for acutely symptomatic or severe cases. Vitamin D supplementation (ergocalciferol or cholecalciferol) should be initiated. Calcitriol (1,25(OH)$_2$D3), the active metabolite of vitamin D, may be administered and is effective in increasing serum calcium levels within a few days [56].

12.5 Parathyroid Ultrasound

Because of their small size, normal parathyroid glands generally cannot be appreciated on ultrasound (US). On the other hand, pathologically enlarged parathyroid glands have a characteristic appearance on grayscale imaging and may be readily detected (◘ Fig. 12.4). The characteristic appearance of a parathyroid adenoma is of a hypoechoic, homogenous, well-circumscribed ovoid structure, though a variety of shapes may be seen and the degree of hypoechogenicity may be variable. Parathyroid adenomas are typically vascular and have a polar blood vessel, most often a branch of the inferior thyroid artery, which terminates near the capsule in the gland. This latter finding may be useful in differentiating a parathyroid adenoma from reactive lymphadenopathy, as is often seen with autoimmune thyroiditis [57]. Hyperplastic parathyroid glands warranting surgical excision can be readily appreciated and similarly appear as hypoechoic ovoid structures. In longstanding SHPT or THPT, nodularity of the gland may generate the appearance of irregular borders. Calcifications within the gland may also be seen [57].

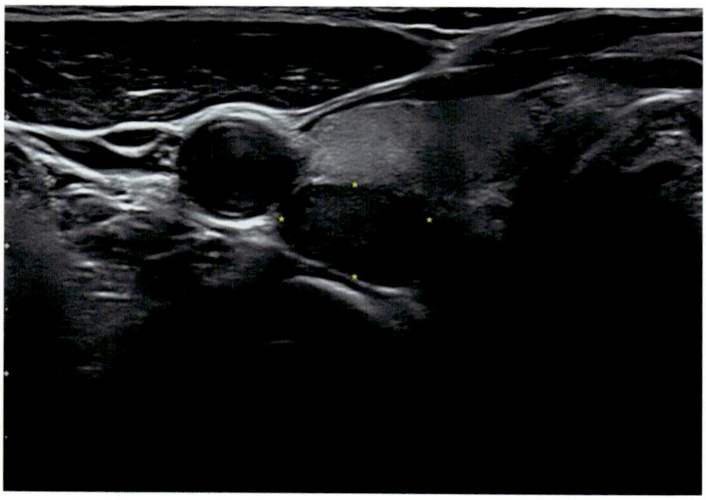

◘ **Fig. 12.4** Ultrasound image of a right superior parathyroid adenoma, which appears as a hypoechoic, well-circumscribed ovoid nodule posterior to the thyroid gland

High-resolution US is a highly useful surgical planning tool and the preferred initial method of localization in the evaluation of parathyroid adenoma [58]. Surgeon-performed US has been shown to be more sensitive than sestamibi for localization to the correct side and quadrant [59]. When localizing enlarged parathyroid glands, the examiner directs attention to the regions posterior and inferior to the thyroid gland. As noted above, the superior parathyroid gland is typically encountered on the posterior aspect of the mid-portion of the thyroid gland. The inferior parathyroid is often identified just inferior or posterior to the lower pole of the thyroid gland. When an enlarged gland is not identified in an expected location, ectopia should be suspected. Ectopic glands located above the superior pole, in the carotid sheath, or within the thyroid parenchyma can be readily appreciated on US. However, ectopic glands located within the retroesophageal or retroesophageal space may be difficult to visualize, as US is limited in these areas. Similarly, ectopic glands located in the mediastinum cannot be visualized with neck US.

Answers

1. (c); 2. (c); 3. (b); 4. (a); 5. (d); 6. (c); 7. (b); 8. (d); 9. (a); 10. (d); 11. (c)

References

1. Kazaure HS, Zambeli-Ljepovic A, Oyekunle TM, Roman SA, Sosa JAM, Stang MT, et al. Severe hypocalcemia after thyroidectomy: an analysis of 7366 patients. Ann Surg.
2. Stack BC, Tolley NS, Bartel TB, Bilezikian JP, Bodenner D, Camacho P, et al. AHNS series: do you know your guidelines? Optimizing outcomes in reoperative parathyroid surgery: definitive multidisciplinary joint consensus guidelines of the American Head and Neck Society and the British Association of Endocrine and Thyroid Surgeons. Head Neck. 2018;40(8):1617–29.
3. Zajac JD, Danks JA. The development of the parathyroid gland: from fish to human. Curr Opin Nephrol Hypertens. 2008;17(4):353–6.
4. Pradhan R, Agarwal A, Lombardi CP, Raffaelli M. Applied embryology of the thyroid and parathyroid glands. In: Randolph GW, editor. Surgery of the thyroid and parathyroid glands. 3rd ed. Elsevier; 2021. p. 15–25.e4.
5. Peissig K, Condie BG, Manley NR. Embryology of the parathyroid glands. Endocrinol Metab Clin N Am. 2018;47(4):733–42.
6. Wang C. The anatomic basis of parathyroid surgery. Ann Surg. 1976;183(3):271–5.
7. Mohebati A, Shaha AR. Anatomy of thyroid and parathyroid glands and neurovascular relations. Clin Anat N Y N. 2012;25(1):19–31.
8. Akerström G, Malmaeus J, Bergström R. Surgical anatomy of human parathyroid glands. Surgery. 1984;95(1):14–21.
9. Palestini N. Surgical anatomy of the parathyroid glands. In: Gasparri G, Camandona M, Palestini N, editors. Primary, secondary and tertiary hyperparathyroidism: diagnostic and therapeutic updates. Springer; 2015.

10. Delattre JF, Flament JB, Palot JP, Pluot M. Variations in the parathyroid glands. Number, situation and arterial vascularization. Anatomical study and surgical application. J Chir (Paris). 1982;119(11):633–41.
11. Edis AJ, Purnell DC, van Heerden JA. The undescended "parathymus". An occasional cause of failed neck exploration for hyperparathyroidism. Ann Surg. 1979;190(1):64–8.
12. Fraker DL, Doppman JL, Shawker TH, Marx SJ, Spiegel AM, Norton JA. Undescended parathyroid adenoma: an important etiology for failed operations for primary hyperparathyroidism. World J Surg. 1990;14(3):342–8.
13. Wheeler MH. Clinical anatomy, developmental aberrations and endocrinology. In: Arora A, Tolley N, Tuttle RM, editors. Practical manual of thyroid and parathyroid disease. Wiley; 2009.
14. Doppman JL, Marx SJ, Brennan MF, Beazley RM, Geelhoed G, Aurbach GD. The blood supply of mediastinal parathyroid adenomas. Ann Surg. 1977;185(4):488–90.
15. Fukumoto A, Nonaka M, Kamio T, Kamura E, Ozu C, Baba S, et al. A case of ectopic parathyroid gland hyperplasia in the pyriform sinus. Arch Otolaryngol Head Neck Surg. 2002;128(1):71–4.
16. Wheeler MH, Williams ED, Wade JS. The hyperfunctioning intrathyroidal parathyroid gland: a potential pitfall in parathyroid surgery. World J Surg. 1987;11(1):110–4.
17. Thompson NW, Eckhauser FE, Harness JK. The anatomy of primary hyperparathyroidism. Surgery. 1982;92(5):814–21.
18. Proye C, Bizard JP, Carnaille B, Quiévreux JL. Hyperparathyroidism and intrathyroid parathyroid gland. 43 cases. Ann Chir. 1994;48(6):501–6.
19. Lappas D, Noussios G, Anagnostis P, Adamidou F, Chatzigeorgiou A, Skandalakis P. Location, number and morphology of parathyroid glands: results from a large anatomical series. Anat Sci Int. 2012;87(3):160–4.
20. Pattou F, Combemale F, Fabre S, Carnaille B, Decoulx M, Wemeau JL, et al. Hypocalcemia following thyroid surgery: incidence and prediction of outcome. World J Surg. 1998;22(7):718–24.
21. Numano M, Tominaga Y, Uchida K, Orihara A, Tanaka Y, Takagi H. Surgical significance of supernumerary parathyroid glands in renal hyperparathyroidism. World J Surg. 1998;22(10):1098–102; discussion 1103.
22. McHenry C, Walsh M, Jarosz H, Henkin R, Tope J, Lawrence AM, et al. Resection of parathyroid tumor in the aorticopulmonary window without prior neck exploration. Surgery. 1988;104(6):1090–4.
23. Arnault V, Beaulieu A, Lifante J-C, Sitges Serra A, Sebag F, Mathonnet M, et al. Multicenter study of 19 aortopulmonary window parathyroid tumors: the challenge of embryologic origin. World J Surg. 2010;34(9):2211–6.
24. Curley IR, Wheeler MH, Thompson NW, Grant CS. The challenge of the middle mediastinal parathyroid. World J Surg. 1988;12(6):818–24.
25. Buell JF, Fraker DL, Doppman JL, Shawker TH, Skarulis MC, Spiegel AM, et al. High cervical intravagal hypercellular parathyroid gland as the etiology of severe persistent primary hyperparathyroidism. Am Surg. 1995;61(11):943–6.
26. Pawlik TM, Richards M, Giordano TJ, Burney R, Thompson N. Identification and management of intravagal parathyroid adenoma. World J Surg. 2001;25(4):419–23.
27. Henry JF, Defechereux T, Raffaelli M, Lubrano D, Iacobone M. [Supernumerary ectopic hyperfunctioning parathyroid gland: a potential pitfall in surgery for sporadic primary hyperthyroidism]. Ann Chir. 2000;125(3):247–52.
28. Takimoto T, Okabe Y, Ito M, Umeda R. Intravagal parathyroid adenoma. J Laryngol Otol. 1989;103(7):704–6.

29. Isono H, Shoumura S, Emura S. Ultrastructure of the parathyroid gland. Histol Histopathol. 1990;5(1):95–112.
30. Ritter CS, Haughey BH, Miller B, Brown AJ. Differential gene expression by oxyphil and chief cells of human parathyroid glands. J Clin Endocrinol Metab. 2012;97(8):E1499–505.
31. Tominaga Y. Surgical management of secondary and tertiary hyperparathyroidism. In: Randolph GW, editor. Surgery of the thyroid and parathyroid glands. 3rd ed. Elsevier; 2021. p. 564–575.e4.
32. Carpentier A, Jeannotte S, Verreault J, Lefebvre B, Bisson G, Mongeau CJ, et al. Preoperative localization of parathyroid lesions in hyperparathyroidism: relationship between technetium-99m-MIBI uptake and oxyphil cell content. J Nucl Med. 1998;39(8):1441–4.
33. Tu C-L, Chang W, Shoback DM. Chapter 23 – Biology of the extracellular calcium-sensing receptor. In: Bilezikian JP, Martin JT, Clemens TL, Rosen CJ, editors. Principles of bone viology. 4th ed. Elsevier Health Sciences; 2020. p. 539–71.
34. Brown EM. Role of the calcium-sensing receptor in extracellular calcium homeostasis. Best Pract Res Clin Endocrinol Metab. 2013;27(3):333–43.
35. Shifrin A. Brief overview of calcium, vitamin D, parathyroid hormone metabolism, and calcium-sensing receptor function. In: Shifrin AL, editor. Advances in treatment and management in surgical endocrinology. Elsevier; 2020. p. 63–70.
36. Christensen SE, Nissen PH, Vestergaard P, Mosekilde L. Familial hypocalciuric hypercalcaemia: a review. Curr Opin Endocrinol Diabetes Obes. 2011;18(6):359–70.
37. Nussey S, Whitehead S. The parathyroid glands and vitamin D. In: Endocrinology: an integrated approach. BIOS Scientific Publishers; 2001.
38. Applewhite MK, White MG, Tseng J, Mohammed MK, Mercier F, Kaplan EL, et al. Normohormonal primary hyperparathyroidism is a distinct form of primary hyperparathyroidism. Surgery. 2017;161(1):62–9.
39. Bilezikian JP. Primary hyperparathyroidism. J Clin Endocrinol Metab. 2018;103(11):3993–4004.
40. Silverberg SJ, Bilezikian JP. Primary hyperparathyroidism: pathophysiology, surgical indications, and preoperative workup. In: Randolph GW, editor. Surgery of the thyroid and parathyroid glands. 3rd ed. Elsevier; 2021. p. 486–493.e2.
41. Ahadi MS, Gill AJ. Surgical pathology of the parathyroid glands. In: Randolph GW, editor. Surgery of the thyroid and parathyroid glands. 3rd ed. Elsevier; 2021. p. 597–604.e6.
42. Marx SJ. Hyperparathyroid and hypoparathyroid disorders. N Engl J Med. 2000;343(25):1863–75.
43. Kebebew E, Hwang J, Reiff E, Duh Q-Y, Clark OH. Predictors of single-gland vs multigland parathyroid disease in primary hyperparathyroidism: a simple and accurate scoring model. Arch Surg Chic Ill 1960. 2006;141(8):777–82; discussion 782.
44. Lim JY, Herman MC, Bubis L, Epelboym I, Allendorf JD, Chabot JA, et al. Differences in single gland and multigland disease are seen in low biochemical profile primary hyperparathyroidism. Surgery. 2017;161(1):70–7.
45. Schneider DF, Burke JF, Ojomo KA, Clark N, Mazeh H, Sippel RS, et al. Multigland disease and slower decline in intraoperative PTH characterize mild primary hyperparathyroidism. Ann Surg Oncol. 2013;20(13):4205–11.
46. Tominaga Y, Tanaka Y, Sato K, Nagasaka T, Takagi H. Histopathology, pathophysiology, and indications for surgical treatment of renal hyperparathyroidism. Semin Surg Oncol. 1997;13(2):78–86.
47. Paschoalin RP, Torregrosa J-V, Sánchez-Escuredo A, Barros X, Durán CE, Campistol JM. Cinacalcet treatment for stable kidney transplanta-

tion patients with hypercalcemia due to persistent secondary hyperparathyroidism: a long-term follow-up. Transplant Proc. 2012;44(9):2588–9.
48. López V, Toledo R, Sola E, Gutiérrez C, Sujan S, Rodríguez MA, et al. Treatment with cinacalcet in 29 kidney transplant patients with persistent hyperparathyroidism. Transplant Proc. 2009;41(6):2394–5.
49. Fatourechi MM, Hay ID, McIver B, Sebo TJ, Fatourechi V. Invasive fibrous thyroiditis (riedel thyroiditis): the Mayo clinic experience, 1976–2008. Thyroid. 2011;21(7):765–72.
50. Brown EM. Anti-parathyroid and anti-calcium sensing receptor antibodies in autoimmune hypoparathyroidism. Endocrinol Metab Clin N Am. 2009;38(2):437–45, x.
51. Shoback D. Clinical practice. Hypoparathyroidism. N Engl J Med. 2008;359(4):391–403.
52. Kobrynski LJ, Sullivan KE. Velocardiofacial syndrome, DiGeorge syndrome: the chromosome 22q11.2 deletion syndromes. Lancet Lond Engl. 2007;370(9596):1443–52.
53. Lindstrand A, Malmgren H, Verri A, Benetti E, Eriksson M, Nordgren A, et al. Molecular and clinical characterization of patients with overlapping 10p deletions. Am J Med Genet A. 2010;152A(5):1233–43.
54. Björses P, Halonen M, Palvimo JJ, Kolmer M, Aaltonen J, Ellonen P, et al. Mutations in the AIRE gene: effects on subcellular location and transactivation function of the autoimmune polyendocrinopathy-candidiasis-ectodermal dystrophy protein. Am J Hum Genet. 2000;66(2):378–92.
55. Pearce SH, Williamson C, Kifor O, Bai M, Coulthard MG, Davies M, et al. A familial syndrome of hypocalcemia with hypercalciuria due to mutations in the calcium-sensing receptor. N Engl J Med. 1996;335(15):1115–22.
56. Al-Azem H, Khan AA. Hypoparathyroidism. Best Pract Res Clin Endocrinol Metab. 2012;26(4):517–22.
57. Shindo M. Parathyroid ultrasonography. In: Orloff LA, editor. Head and neck ultrasonography: essential and extended applications. 2nd ed. Plural Publishing; 2017. p. 137–53.
58. Zafereo M, Yu J, Angelos P, Brumund K, Chuang HH, Goldenberg D, et al. American Head and Neck Society Endocrine Surgery Section update on parathyroid imaging for surgical candidates with primary hyperparathyroidism. Head Neck. 2019;41(7):2398–409.
59. Steward DL, Danielson GP, Afman CE, Welge JA. Parathyroid adenoma localization: surgeon-performed ultrasound versus sestamibi. Laryngoscope. 2006;116(8):1380–4.

Diagnosis and Surgical Management of Primary Hyperparathyroidism

Alexander L. Shifrin and David J. Terris

Contents

A. L. Shifrin et al. (eds.), *Endocrine Surgery Comprehensive Board Exam Guide*,
https://doi.org/10.1007/978-3-030-84737-1_13

Case Presentation

Patient Primary hyperparathyroidism (PHPT) patient history is a 53-year-old female who presented with incidental findings of elevated calcium level on a routine blood test. She reported no significant complaints besides symptoms of tiredness and fatigue. Past medical history was significant for the absence of kidney stones or fractures. She mentioned that she was treated for acne with radiation to her face in her early teenage years. No family history of cancer or hypercalcemia. No significant comorbidities. Medication includes only multivitamin which contains 500 mg of calcium daily. Prior surgery included cholecystectomy. On physical examination, vital signs are within normal range, no other abnormalities detected. She presented with laboratory data from the last 4 years which includes several total calcium measurements ranging between 10.4 mg/dL (2.75 mmol/L) and 11.2 mg/dL (2.85 mmol/L) (normal 8.5–10.2 mg/dL and 2.2 to 2.7 mmol/L, resp.), ionized calcium level 6.5 mg/dL (1.45 mmol/L) (normal 4.64–5.28 mg/dL and 1.14–1.34 mmol/L, resp.), PTH level on two occasions was 85 pg/mL (8.5 pmol/l) and 125 pg/mL (12.5 pmol/l) (normal 25–65 pg/mL and 1.6–6.9 pmol/L, resp.). Creatinine level was 0.95 mg/dL (84 μmol/L) (normal 0.6–1.0 mg/dL and 45–90 μmol/L, resp.), glomerular filtration rate (GFR) was 90 mL/min/1.73 m^2 (normal above 60 mL/min/1.73 m^2), phosphorus level was within normal range, and vitamin D25OH level was 15 ng/mL (37.5 nmol/L) (normal above 50 ng/mL and 125 nmol/L, resp.).

13

Questions

1. What are criteria to establish the diagnosis of primary hyperparathyroidism?
   1. Findings of a parathyroid adenoma on CT scan or neck ultrasound
   2. History of kidney stones and findings of a parathyroid adenoma on sestamibi scan
   3. Findings of normal serum calcium level and high serum PTH level
   4. Elevated 24-hour urine calcium level
   5. Findings of elevated serum calcium and PTH levels
      (a) Only (1) and (2) and (3) are correct.
      (b) Only (3) and (5) are correct.
      (c) Only (4) and (5) are correct.
      (d) Only (2) and (4) and (5) are correct.
      (e) All are correct.
2. In which of the following would you establish the diagnosis of primary hyperparathyroidism?
   1. Elevation of both serum calcium and serum PTH levels
   2. Elevation of serum PTH but high normal serum calcium level
   3. Elevation of serum calcium but high normal serum PTH level
   4. Elevation of serum PTH level, normal serum calcium but elevation of ionized calcium level
      (a) Only (1) and (2) and (3) are correct.
      (b) Only (1) and (2) and (4) are correct.
      (c) Only (1) and (3) and (4) are correct.
      (d) Only (2) and (3) and (4) are correct.
      (e) All are correct.

3. In which of the following would you establish the diagnosis of normohormonal primary hyperparathyroidism?
    1. Elevation of both serum calcium and serum PTH levels
    2. Elevation of serum PTH but high normal serum calcium level
    3. Elevation of serum calcium but high normal serum PTH level
    4. Elevation of serum PTH level, normal serum calcium but elevation of ionized calcium level
        (a) Only (1) and (2) and (3) are correct.
        (b) Only (1) and (2) and (4) are correct.
        (c) Only (3) is correct.
        (d) Only (1) and (2) are correct.
        (e) All are correct.
4. In which of the following would you establish the diagnosis of normocalcemic primary hyperparathyroidism?
    1. Elevation of both serum calcium and serum PTH levels
    2. Elevation of serum PTH but high normal serum calcium level
    3. Elevation of serum calcium but high normal serum PTH level
    4. Elevation of serum PTH level, normal serum calcium but elevation of ionized calcium level
        (a) Only (1) and (2) and (3) are correct.
        (b) Only (1) and (2) and (4) are correct.
        (c) Only (2) and (4) are correct.
        (d) Only (2) is correct.
        (e) All are correct.
5. What are recommendations for surgical management of asymptomatic PHPT based on the Summary Statement from the Fourth International Workshop?
    1. Serum calcium 1.0 mg/dL (0.25 mmol/L) above upper limit of normal
    2. Presence of osteoporosis defined as BMD by DEXA scan, a T-score of less than −2.5 at lumbar spine, total hip, femoral neck, or distal 1/3 of the radius
    3. Presence of vertebral fracture by imaging studies such as x-ray, CT scan, MRI, or Vertebral Fracture Assessment (VFA) by the DEXA scan
    4. 24-h urine for calcium above 400 mg/d (10 mmol/d)
    5. Presence of nephrolithiasis or nephrocalcinosis by x-ray, ultrasound, or CT scan
    6. Individuals less than 50 years of age
        (a) Only (1) and (2) and (3) are correct.
        (b) Only (1) and (2) and (4) and (5) are correct.
        (c) Only (1) and (3) and (4) are correct.
        (d) Only (2) and (3) and (4) and (5) are correct.
        (e) All are correct.

6. What statements regarding preoperative management of her calcium supplementation and vitamin D level are correct?
   1. Preoperative dietary calcium intake should be restricted, and her daily calcium supplementation should be stopped to prevent worsening of hypercalcemia.
   2. If daily dietary calcium intake is lower than 450 mg a day, she can continue daily calcium supplementation.
   3. Her low vitamin D level should be repleted by giving her the regiment of small doses of vitamin D such as 600–1000 IU of cholecalciferol to achieve the goal of the serum 25-OH vitamin D level in between 50 and 75 nmol/L.
   4. Her vitamin D supplementation should not be performed at this time, but should be postponed until after the surgery to prevent uncontrollable increase of preoperative serum calcium level and urinary calcium excretion that could result in the development of kidney stones.
      (a) Only (1) and (4) are correct.
      (b) Only (1) and (3) are correct.
      (c) Only (2) and (4) are correct.
      (d) Only (2) and (3) are correct.
      (e) All are correct.
7. Which statement(s) regarding PHPT is correct?
   1. About 85% of the patients with PHPT will have findings of a single adenoma.
   2. About 10% of patients with PHPT may have one of the familial syndromes such as MEN type 1, MEN 2, or other familial endocrine syndromes.
   3. Conservative follow-up for patients with normocalcemic PHPT showed that about 20% of them will become hypercalcemic.
   4. 15-years follow-up for patients who do not meet criteria for parathyroidectomy showed that after nonsurgical observation 40% of patients develop at least one indication for the surgery.
      (a) Only (1) and (2) and (3) are correct.
      (b) Only (1) and (2) and (4) are correct.
      (c) Only (1) and (3) and (4) are correct.
      (d) Only (2) and (3) and (4) are correct.
      (e) All are correct.
8. At what age MEN 1 and MEN 2 mutational analyses are indicated in patient with PHPT based on current guidelines?
   1. 10 years of age
   2. 20 years of age
   3. 30 years of age
   4. 40 years of age

   - (a) Only (1) and (2) and (3) are correct.
   - (b) Only (2) and (3) and (4) are correct.
   - (c) Only (3) and (4) are correct.
   - (d) Only (4) is correct.
   - (e) All are correct.

9. What is the best and the most cost-effective strategy to localize a solitary parathyroid adenoma?
   1. Sestamibi scan
   2. Neck ultrasound
   3. 4D CT scan
   4. Spect CT sestamibi scan
   5. Ultrasound plus Spect CT sestamibi scan
      - (a) Only (1) and (2) are correct.
      - (b) Only (1) and (3) are correct.
      - (c) Only (2) and (3) are correct.
      - (d) Only (5) is correct.
      - (e) All are correct.
10. Which patient with PHPT would have high likelihood of multiglandular parathyroid hyperplasia?
    1. Patient with history of radiation exposure to the neck during childhood
    2. Patient with long history of Lithium therapy
    3. Patient with history of MEN 1 syndrome
    4. Patient with history of MEN 2 syndrome
    5. Patient with truly negative Spect CT sestamibi scan
    6. Patient presented with normohormonal PHPT
       - (a) Only (2) and (3) and (4) are correct.
       - (b) Only (2) and (3) and (5) and (6) are correct.
       - (c) Only (1) and (3) and (4) and (6) are correct.
       - (d) Only (2) and (3) and (4) and (6) are correct.
       - (e) All are correct.
11. Taking in consideration that this patient has no history of kidney stones and no family history of hypercalcemia, but she mentioned that she was treated for acne with radiation to her face in early teenager years, which of the following is correct?
    1. Order bone density (DEXA) study, if no osteoporosis is present, then conservative follow-up is recommended since there are no complications of PHPT, unless patient wants to have a surgery.
    2. Advise patient to have parathyroidectomy.
    3. Perform neck ultrasound and order Spect CT sestamibi scan.
    4. Advise patient that she may have parathyroid hyperplasia due to prior history of radiation exposure.
    5. Advise patient that even with findings of one parathyroid gland, future recurrence is possible due to prior history of radiation exposure.
       - (a) Only (1) and (2) and (3) are correct.
       - (b) Only (2) and (3) and (4) and (5) are correct.

(c) Only (1) and (3) and (4) are correct.
(d) Only (2) and (3) and (5) are correct.
(e) All are correct.

12. What statements are correct regarding PTH and calcium kinetics?
    1. PTH half-life after the adenoma removal is approximately 3 to 4 minutes.
    2. Calcium measurements are not beneficial during the parathyroidectomy because ionized calcium level started to decrease only at 30 min after the adenoma removal.
    3. PTH elimination is proportional to its initial preoperative plasma concentration. Usually, the lowest drop of PTH level occurs at five hours after the adenoma removal.
    4. PTH levels start to increase after parathyroidectomy again at postoperative day 2.
    (a) Only (1) and (2) and (3) are correct.
    (b) Only (1) and (2) and (4) are correct.
    (c) Only (1) and (3) and (4) are correct.
    (d) Only (2) and (3) and (4) are correct.
    (e) All are correct.

13. What are the best criteria for intraoperative PTH monitoring to achieve a long-term cure?
    1. Drop of PTH level more than 50% from pre-excision (T baseline) and stimulation (during the manipulation of the gland) (T-0) levels at 5 and 10 minutes after the excision of the parathyroid adenoma
    2. Drop of PTH level more than 50% from pre-excision (T baseline) and stimulation (T-0) levels at 5 and 10 minutes and to the level of below 40 pg/mL (4.2 pmol/L) (normal 25–65 pg/mL and 1.6–6.9 pmol/L, resp.) after the excision of the parathyroid adenoma
    3. Drop of PTH level more than 50% from pre-excision (T baseline) and stimulation (T-0) levels at 1 hour after the excision of the parathyroid adenoma
    4. Drop of PTH level from 80 pg/mL (8.4 pmol/L) (normal 25–65 pg/mL and 1.6–6.9 pmol/L, resp.) at pre-excision (T baseline) and stimulation (T-0) 120 pg/mL (12.7 pmol/L) (normal 25–65 pg/mL and 1.6–6.9 pmol/L, resp.) levels to below 40 pg/mL (4.2 pmol/L) (normal 25–65 pg/mL and 1.6–6.9 pmol/L, resp.) at 10 minutes after the excision of the parathyroid adenoma
    (a) Only (1) and (2) and (3) are correct.
    (b) Only (1) and (2) and (4) are correct.
    (c) Only (1) and (3) and (4) are correct.
    (d) Only (2) and (4) are correct.
    (e) All are correct.

14. Which statements are correct regarding utilization of intra-operative parathyroid hormone (IOPTH) monitoring?
    1. Operative failure of minimally invasive surgical approach utilizing IOPTH monitoring related to the surgeons' misinterpretation of the IOPTH result and the failure to identify all abnormal parathyroid glands rather than IOPTH results itself.
    2. Bilateral parathyroid exploration could be considered in perioperative planning of patients with either normohormonal or normocalcemic PHPT.
    3. There is no difference in recurrence rate between minimally invasive (focused) approach utilizing IOPTH monitoring in patients with localized adenoma preoperatively and open four glands exploration approach.
    4. Minimally invasive parathyroidectomy can achieve a cure rate in up to 97–99% of patients when IOPTH monitoring is used.
        (a) Only (1) and (2) and (3) are correct.
        (b) Only (1) and (2) and (4) are correct.
        (c) Only (1) and (3) and (4) are correct.
        (d) Only (2) and (3) and (4) are correct.
        (e) All are correct.

15. Benefits of minimally invasive (focused) approach utilizing IOPTH monitoring are:
    1. To minimize the risk of complications, compare to more extensive exploratory surgery
    2. To decrease postoperative pain and discomfort
    3. To decrease surgical operative time
    4. To obtain the best cosmetic result
        (a) Only (1) and (2) and (3) are correct.
        (b) Only (1) and (2) and (4) are correct.
        (c) Only (1) and (3) and (4) are correct.
        (d) Only (2) and (3) and (4) are correct.
        (e) All are correct.

16. Which statements regarding surgical management of patient with PHPT are correct?
    1. Parathyroidectomy is indicated for all symptomatic patients and should be considered for most asymptomatic patients.
    2. Parathyroidectomy is more cost-effective in younger patients than observation or pharmacologic therapy.
    3. Parathyroidectomy is recommended regardless of the results of preoperative localizing studies for all patients who have met the surgical criteria.
    4. Minimally invasive parathyroidectomy using intraoperative PTH monitoring can achieve cure rate similar to open bilateral neck exploration in up to 99% of patients.

(a) Only (1) and (2) and (3) are correct.
(b) Only (1) and (2) and (4) are correct.
(c) Only (1) and (3) and (4) are correct.
(d) Only (2) and (3) and (4) are correct.
(e) All are correct.

17. What PTH level following parathyroidectomy increases the risk for symptomatic postoperative hypocalcemia?
    1. 10 pg/mL (1.06 pmol/L)
    2. 20 pg/mL (2.12 pmol/L)
    3. 30 pg/mL (3.18 pmol/L)
    4. 50 pg/mL (4.24 pmol/L)
       (a) Only (1) and (2) and (3) are correct.
       (b) Only (1) and (2) are correct.
       (c) Only (1) is correct.
       (d) Only (2) and (3) and (4) are correct.
       (e) All are correct.
18. What surgical steps can be undertaken to find an ectopic superior parathyroid gland adenoma?
    1. Dissect lower pole of the thyroid lobe in the plane to the RLN.
    2. Look at the intrathyroidal location at the inferior pole of the thyroid lobe.
    3. Look in the carotid sheath at the level of carotid bifurcation and above the bifurcation at the level of the skull base.
    4. Dissect down into paraesophageal, retroesophageally, retrolaryngeal, or retrotracheal space.
       (a) Only (1) and (4) are correct.
       (b) Only (1) and (2) are correct.
       (c) Only (1) and (3) and (4) are correct.
       (d) Only (4) is correct.
       (e) All are correct.
19. What surgical steps can be undertaken to locate an ectopic inferior parathyroid gland?
    1. Dissect deep under tubercle of Zuckerkandl.
    2. Dissect along and into the thyrothymic ligament or posterior thymus.
    3. Dissect a plane deep and posterior to the recurrent laryngeal nerve along the esophagus toward the posterior mediastinum.
    4. Dissect lateral to the recurrent laryngeal nerve along the medial border of the common carotid artery into the carotid sheath.
       (a) Only (1) and (4) are correct.
       (b) Only (2) is correct.
       (c) Only (1) and (3) and (4) are correct.
       (d) Only (4) is correct.
       (e) All are correct.

20. Following successful parathyroidectomy, the patient may expect:
    1. Bone mineral density will improve as early as 6 months after the parathyroidectomy.
    2. Quality of life may improve after the successful parathyroidectomy based on two scoring systems, PAS and SF-36.
    3. Since both scoring systems (PAS and SF-36) are easy to quantify, showing patients improvement after the parathyroidectomy in 6 months to up to 10 years after the surgery, they can be used as a part of the workup to recommend surgery in patients with PHPT.
    4. Despite the fact that nephrolithiasis risk decreases following parathyroidectomy, surgery has not been shown to improve renal function.
        (a) Only (1) and (2) and (3) are correct.
        (b) Only (1) and (2) and (4) are correct.
        (c) Only (1) and (3) and (4) are correct.
        (d) Only (2) and (3) and (4) are correct.
        (e) All are correct.
21. A 32-year-old female at her eighth week of pregnancy was found to have elevated calcium level 10.4 (2.59 mmol/L) and 10.8 mg/dL (2.69 mmol/L). She has no symptoms, no history of kidney stones. Which statements are correct regarding the management of pregnant patient who was diagnosed with PHPT?
    1. PHPT may have serious consequences to the mother and to the fetus if it remains unrecognized and untreated.
    2. PHPT remains undiagnosed during pregnancy in up to 80% of cases due to physiological changes that may mask gestational hypercalcemia.
    3. If clinically necessary, sestamibi scan can be safely used during pregnancy.
    4. Ultrasound scan can be safely used during pregnancy.
        (a) Only (1) and (2) and (4) are correct.
        (b) Only (1) and (2) and (3) are correct.
        (c) Only (1) and (3) and (4) are correct.
        (d) Only (2) and (3) and (4) are correct.
        (e) All are correct.
22. Which statements regarding the management of the pregnant patient with PHPT are correct?
    1. Management of PHPT during pregnancy should be individualized based on symptoms and severity of hypercalcemia.
    2. Bisphosphonates do not cross the placenta and appear to be safe during the pregnancy.

3. Calcitonin and Cinacalcet cross the placenta and are contraindicated during the pregnancy.
4. In case of a mild form of PHPT in an asymptomatic patient, the risk of maternal and obstetrical complications is low and patients can be safely managed conservatively during the pregnancy, and parathyroidectomy can be delayed until after the delivery.
5. In cases of severe hypercalcemia when calcium level is above 11 mg/dL (2.74 mmol/L), or in symptomatic patient, the risk of preeclampsia and preterm delivery is high, and parathyroidectomy is indicated which should be performed in the second trimester.
   (a) Only (1) and (4) and (5) are correct.
   (b) Only (2) and (4) and (5) are correct.
   (c) Only (1) and (3) and (5) are correct.
   (d) Only (2) and (3) and (4) are correct.
   (e) All are correct.

13.1 Introduction

Primary hyperparathyroidism (PHPT) is defined by persistent elevation of serum calcium level with corresponding elevation of serum parathyroid hormone (PTH) level. Etiology of PHPT is mostly idiopathic due to autonomous overproduction of PTH by the abnormal parathyroid gland or glands. Normocalcemic PHPT is defined as an elevation of serum PTH level but inappropriately normal serum total and ionized calcium levels, when secondary causes are excluded such as vitamin D deficiency, primary hypercalciuria, chronic kidney disease, calcium malabsorption, and medications that can cause elevation of the PTH level (thiazides, lithium, anticonvulsants, bisphosphonates, and denosumab) [1]. Normohormonal PHPT is defined by inappropriately normal non-suppressed serum PTH level and high serum calcium level. Follow-up of patients with normocalcemic PHPT showed that in approximately 4 years, 22% of them will become hypercalcemic [1–4]. Approximately 85% of patients with PHPT will have a single parathyroid adenoma, and 15% of the patients will have either double adenoma or hyperplasia. Diagnosis of Asymptomatic Primary Hyperparathyroidism: Proceedings of the Fourth International Workshop reported that more than 10% of patients with PHPT will have a mutation in 1 of 11 genes (MEN1, RET, CDKN1A, CDKN1B, CDKN2B, CDKN2C, CASR, CDC73, GNA11, AP2S1, and PTH) and may have familial syndromes such as multiple endocrine neoplasia (MEN) type 1, MEN 2, MEN 3, MEN 4, hyperparathyroidism jaw-tumor syndrome (HPT-JT), familial isolated hyperparathyroidism (FIHPT), neonatal severe PHPT (NSPHPT), Familial Hypocalciuric Hypercalcemia (FHH) type 1, FHH 2, FHH 3, and nonsyndromic PHPT (nsPHPT) [5–8].

13.2 Diagnosis of PHPT

Diagnosis of PHPT is biochemical and established by measuring of serum total and ionized calcium levels, and parathyroid hormone (PTH) level. Additional measurements include vitamin D25-OH level, phosphate, creatinine levels, glomerular filtration rate (GFR), alkaline phosphatase activity, and 24-hr urine calcium level [1, 5, 6]. The measurement of Bone Mineral Density (BMD) by DEXA scan should be included to evaluate for the presence of osteoporosis in the lumbar spine, femoral hip, and the wrist. Imaging studies may be ordered to evaluate for the presence of nephrolithiasis, such as kidney ultrasonography, abdominal X-ray, or abdominal CT scan [1], and to evaluate for possible bone stress fractures [1–4]. The patients with hyperparathyroidism who are less than 40 years of age, patients with positive family history for familial syndromes, the presence of multiglandular disease, and findings of parathyroid carcinoma or atypical adenoma should be considered for genetic testing [1, 5].

13.3 Indications for Surgical Treatment of PHPT

The Fourth International Workshop for the Management of Asymptomatic PHPT and the American Association of Endocrine Surgeons (AAES) Guidelines for Definitive Management of Primary Hyperparathyroidism have established the following criteria for surgical treatment of PHPT [1, 5, 6]:

1. Serum calcium 1.0 mg/dL (0.25 mmol/L) above upper limit of normal
2. Presence of osteoporosis defined as BMD by DEXA scan as T-score of less than −2.5 at lumbar spine, total hip, femoral neck, and especially, distal 1/3 of the radius (Z-scores should be used instead of T-scores in premenopausal women and men younger than 50 years of age)
3. Presence of vertebral fracture by imaging studies such as X-ray, CT scan, MRI, or Vertebral Fracture Assessment (VFA) by the DEXA scan
4. 24-h urine for calcium above 400 mg/d (10 mmol/d) and increased kidney stone risk by biochemical stone risk analysis
5. Presence of nephrolithiasis or nephrocalcinosis by X-ray, ultrasound, or CT scan
6. Individuals less than 50 years of age

In addition to above criteria, the improved outcomes have been shown in all patients with asymptomatic PHPT who underwent a curative parathyroidectomy. Parathyroidectomy was more cost-effective than observation or pharmacologic therapy [5]. Therefore, the American Association of Endocrine Surgeons Guidelines for Definitive Management of Primary Hyperparathyroidism stated that parathyroidectomy is indicated for all symptomatic patients and should be considered for most asymptomatic patients, even those who do not meet criteria for surgery [5].

13.4 Preoperative Radiological Studies and Surgical Treatment of PHPT

Radiological localization is important to help with localization of parathyroid adenoma in order to perform minimally invasive surgical approach. Minimally invasive surgical approach helps to decrease surgical time and the rate of complications, and to avoid extensive neck dissection. Radiological studies should not be used to establish the diagnosis of PHPT. The finding of the parathyroid adenoma on radiological studies does not serve as an indication for the parathyroidectomy, unless biochemical diagnosis of primary hyperparathyroidism has been established and the patient met the above-mentioned criteria. Diagnosis of PHPT should be established based on biochemical values of serum calcium and PTH levels. When parathyroid adenoma is not localized by any imaging studies, but surgical criteria are met, the patient is still a candidate for parathyroid exploration [5].

Out of all radiological studies, neck ultrasound is the safest and the least expensive imaging study for preoperative localization of parathyroid adenoma with no risk of radiation exposure. It was recommended that ultrasound should always be performed prior to a parathyroidectomy for operative planning of all patients with PHPT. Neck ultrasound is helpful not only in preoperative localization of parathyroid adenoma but also in evaluation of the thyroid gland, and visualization of the soft tissue of the neck. Findings of thyroid nodules or neck lymph nodes may change preoperative and operative plans. Thyroid nodules and lymph nodes that show worrisome features and sizes may require preoperative evaluation by fine needle aspiration biopsy (FNA). If the thyroid is very large and multinodular, and/or FNA biopsy will show findings suspicious for the cancer (Bethesda category V) or a diagnosis of the cancer (Bethesda category VI), the surgical procedure may be changed to include thyroidectomy or thyroid lobectomy.

It has been shown that the neck ultrasound is more sensitive when performed by the surgeon. When high-resolution neck ultrasound was interpreted by radiologists, the sensitivity was reported between 51 and 89%, while surgeons-performed ultrasonography correctly identified a parathyroid adenoma in 74–90% of patients with a sensitivity 87% and specificity 88% [9–11].

The second study which is recommended to use for preoperative localization of parathyroid adenoma is dual-isotope subtraction single-photon emission computed tomography-computed tomography scan (SPECT-CT) that showed superior result compared with the regular sestamibi scan. Recent study showed that the sensitivity of the SPECT-CT scan was 95%, and specificity 89% for the detection and localization of a parathyroid adenoma. The positive predictive value was estimated to be 97% and the negative predictive value to be 83%. The accuracy of the technique was reported from 80% to 94% in detecting parathyroid adenoma and 92% in accurate localization to the appropriate gland and not only the laterality [1, 9, 12]. Similar to ultrasonography, sestamibi images should always be interpreted by the surgeon preoperatively. Sensitivity of technetium-99 m sestamibi scan is shown to be between 39% and 90% if the study is interpreted by the radiologist [10]. Preoperative assessment of the sestamibi scan by the surgeon, looking for subtleties or "shadows," may lead to the finding of parathyroid adenoma in imaging studies that were initially described as "negative" by the radiologist. Surgeons' evaluation of the "negative" sestamibi study reported findings 41% subtleties or "shadows," and evaluation of "indeterminate" sestamibi study reported findings of 76% subtleties or "shadows." In this group of patients, 91% underwent successful minimally invasive parathyroidectomy with a curative rate of 99% [13].

When the patient is presented with a truly negative sestamibi scan, then the likelihood of intraoperative findings of multiglandular disease is much higher [14]. When preoperative sestamibi scan shows persistent uptake on one side, but preoperative US failed to localize the adenoma, then the patient more likely has posteriorly located upper parathyroid gland adenoma [15]. It is important to know in planning for surgery if the patient had a history of lithium therapy or radiation exposure. Patients treated with lithium will most likely have multiglandular disease with an asymmetrical hyperplasia rather than a single adenoma. Therefore, the preoperative imaging studies could be misleading by showing only a single adenoma. Bilateral neck exploration is therefore recommended [16]. In contrast, the patient with radiation exposure (especially radioactive iodine ablation for Graves' disease) will most likely present with a single adenoma, but metachronous disease may develop several years after a successful parathyroidectomy.

Therefore, lifelong follow-up is essential which is usually done by an endocrinologist [17].

If a patient with PHPT presents with negative sestamibi scan and ultrasonography, or in patients that present with persistent or recurrent disease, four-dimensional computed tomography (4D CT) scan or thin-cut CT scan (2.5 mm cuts) can show superior results in localization of difficult to find parathyroid adenomas. Patients with negative preoperative sestamibi scans who subsequently had thin-cut CT scans had 85% sensitivity and 94% specificity for correctly lateralizing the side of the adenoma. Thin-cut CT scan also had 66% sensitivity and 89% specificity for predicting the exact location of the diseased gland [18]. Utilizing combination of different modalities, such as 4D CT scan and ultrasonography, helps maximize success of the minimally invasive approach in patients with PHPT [11, 19]. Patients who have precise localization of the parathyroid adenoma by preoperative 4D CT scan have less extensive surgical exploration directed to the parathyroid adenoma rather than the four-gland exploration. As a result of that, they have lower length of stay compared to those patients who did not have precise localization [20].

The cost of the healthcare became a significant burden not only to the patient but for healthcare systems. To assess cost utility, the analyses were performed to determine the best diagnostic and the least expensive diagnostic tests for preoperative localization of the parathyroid adenoma. While the least expensive test was an ultrasound, the most cost-effective strategy to localize a parathyroid adenoma was an ultrasound followed by the SPECT CT sestamibi scan plus/minus 4D-CT scan or ultrasound followed by 4D-CT scan. Ultrasound followed by 4D-CT scan was the least expensive strategy with an estimated cost reported as $5901 [11, 21]. The least cost-effective study was SPECT CT sestamibi alone [22]. The sensitivity and specificity of combination of both studies, ultrasound and SPECT CT sestamibi scan, were reported between 91% and 96% in localization of parathyroid adenoma [9]. Positive predictive value of SPECT CT was greater than 90% with accuracy at about 83%. It was also more accurate (36%) in predicting multiglandular disease [23, 24]. The risk of radiation exposure should be considered prior to ordering imaging studies. Sestamibi scan is contraindicated during the pregnancy and should be used very cautiously in children [25, 26].

13.5 Preoperative Management

Calcium intake influences PTH levels in patients with PHPT. If dietary calcium intake will be restricted, the urinary calcium excretion will also decrease which will lower the risk of kidney stones. However calcium restriction will increase PTH levels with worsening of bone demineralization in patients with PHPT and further increases of calcium load to the kidneys. Studies of patients with PHPT and supplementation of calcium by giving 500 mg oral calcium daily for those with <450 mg of daily calcium intake, compared to those patients with an intake >450 mg without supplementation, showed a significant decrease in PTH levels and an increase in femoral neck bone mineral density. Therefore the recommendation was made not to restrict dietary calcium intake in patients with asymptomatic PHPT but rather provide some calcium supplementation under close monitoring [5, 27, 28].

If a patient with PHPT presents with low vitamin D level, the vitamin D depletion was associated with elevation of PTH level and more severe PHPT. Repletion of vitamin D was associated with reductions in serum PTH levels. Some patients may experience increased serum calcium levels and increased urinary calcium excretion. Therefore the recommendation was made to replenish vitamin D in patients with asymptomatic PHPT to prevent postoperative hypocalcemia due to the hungry bone syndrome but under close monitoring. Regimen of vitamin D repletion should include smaller doses of vitamin D such as 600–1000 IU of cholecalciferol to achieve the goal of the serum 25OHD levels to >50 ng/mL (125 nmol/L) and up to 75 ng/mL (187.5 nmol/L) [28].

13.6 Intraoperative PTH Monitoring

Intraoperative PTH (IOPTH) measurement became the gold standard approach for minimally invasive parathyroidectomy. The goal of the IOPTH assessment is to achieve an instant intraoperative conformation of biochemical cure of hyperparathyroidism. It allows the performance of targeted parathyroidectomy directed toward the removal of a single parathyroid adenoma rather than the need for a bilateral neck exploration [29–32]. The rationale to perform an intraoperative PTH measurement is the development of a new generation of PTH assay with two monoclonal antibodies specific for the N- and C-terminal regions of the hormone (1–84)PTH, while earlier assays were directed to either N-terminal, midregion, or C-terminal [33]. Current assay allows the measurement of PTH levels very quickly during the surgery because the half-life of PTH is approximately 3 to 4 minutes compared to the calcium measurements which is not beneficial during the parathyroidectomy because ionized calcium level starts to decrease only at 30 min after the adenoma removal. PTH elimination is proportional to its initial plasma concentration with the lowest drop of PTH level occurring at 5 hours after the adenoma removal. PTH levels subsequently start to increase again at postoperative day 2 [33, 34]. The most common established protocol for the IOPTH assay is the 50% drop in PTH level at 5 and 10 minutes after the excision of the parathyroid adenoma [35–37]. It has been shown that using this timing accurately predicts operative success or failure in 96.3% of patients. Some authors also recommended to use additional measurements of IOPTH level at 20 minutes after the parathyroidectomy, which showed 97.3% operative success rate [38]. Therefore, the ideal time points for IOPTH measurements are the following: Tb, at baseline (before the parathyroidectomy); at the T0, during the parathyroid adenoma manipulation; T5, at 5 minutes after the adenoma removal; T10, at 10 minutes after the adenoma removal; T20 can be added if IOPTH levels are decreasing slowly as seen in the case of very high initial preoperative PTH level.

Earlier data on IOPTH measurements established that the goal of 50% IOPTH levels drop was enough to achieve the biochemical cure, even if final IOPTH levels were still above the upper limit of normal [39]. More recent data have shown that in addition to 50% IOPTH level drop, it is optimal if it falls into the normal range. It was therefore recommended to achieve the goal of IOPTH level less than 40 pg/mL (4.24 pmol/L). The study of patients 2 years after the parathyroidectomy has shown that patients with final IOPTH level less than 40 pg/mL (4.24 pmol/L) had lower rate of persistence and recurrence compared to patients with IOPTH level between 40 and 59 pg/mL (4.24 and 6.25 pmol/L). The patients with a final IOPTH level between 41 and 65 pg/mL (4.35 and 6.89 pmol/L) have a higher likelihood of persistent disease due to not identifying an additional parathyroid adenoma or hyperplasia. Patients with final IOPTH ≥60 pg/mL were reported to have recurrence rate of 5.9%, and persistence rate of 5.4% as compared to patients with IOPTH level <40 pg/mL (< 4.24 pmol/L) which had recurrence rate of 1.3% and the lowest persistence rate of 0.2% [40–42]. In addition, IOPTH level drop greater than 70% was protective against the recurrence [43].

It is important to look for multiglandular disease in patients with normocalcemic or normohormonal PHPT, and relying only on the IOPTH levels may not be sufficient. Patients presented with normocalcemic PHPT may have a chance of about 10% to have multigland disease, and patients presented with normohormonal PHPT may have up to 58% chance of multigland disease. Therefore, bilateral parathyroid exploration could be considered in perioperative planning [44, 45]. Patients with normohormonal PHPT most often had a negative sestamibi scan compared to classic PHPT (18.3% vs. 4.8%). Cure rate for normohormonal PHPT was 88% compared to 96% in the classic group. Patients with normohormonal PHPT with PTH ≤55 pg/mL (≤5.83 pmol/L) had 83% cure rate, and those with PTH 56–65 pg/mL (5.93–6.89 pmol/L) had cure rate of 96% [46]. The major cause of operative failure of minimally invasive surgical approach utilizing IOPTH monitoring was not the failure of IOPTH technique itself, but rather the surgeons' misinterpretation of the IOPTH result and the failure to identify all abnormal parathyroid glands [47].

13.7 Surgical Approach

Minimally invasive parathyroidectomy is defined as a focused resection of the single parathyroid gland adenoma performed through a small incision with minimal surgical dissection. It is possible since 85% of the patients with PHPT will have a single parathyroid adenoma. The goal of minimally invasive surgery is to achieve a biochemical cure with minimal surgical trauma which facilitates faster recovery, minimizes postoperative pain, and reduces the size of the incision with good cosmetic result [5, 48–50].

Minimally invasive approach showed no differences in recurrence compared to open technique [51]. Parathyroidectomy is recommended regardless of the results of preoperative localizing studies for all patients who have met surgical criteria. Minimally invasive parathyroidectomy can achieve cure rate in up to 97–99% of patients when IOPTH monitoring is used [5].

Accurate localization of parathyroid adenoma helps to achieve the following goals by using the minimally invasive approach: to minimize the risk of complications secondary to more extensive exploratory surgery, to decrease postoperative pain and discomfort, to decrease surgical operative time, and to obtain the best cosmetic result.

The recurrence rate after minimally invasive approach is similar to bilateral standard open neck exploration (2.5% vs. 2.1%) [43, 51].

The concept of minimal dissection is especially important when we encounter the recurrent or persistent disease that was reported to occur in 2.5–5% of patients with PHPT [24, 48]. Patients who were presented for reoperative surgery with persistent or recurrent disease after initial standard four-glands neck exploration had complication rates of 44% which are significantly higher compared to 15% of patients with an initial minimally invasive parathyroidectomy [52].

Several recent guidelines on the management of asymptomatic PHPT have established indications for surgery [1, 5]. In addition, 15-year follow-up data showed that after non-surgical observation 40% of patients develop at least one indication for the surgery [53].

The benefits include a targeted surgical approach to the parathyroid adenoma, and the ability to perform a neck exploration with possible thyroid lobectomy without the need to convert to a standard open procedure. This allows for cosmetically pleasing and curative results [54, 55].

Looking at the long-term recurrence risk after a parathyroidectomy, a retrospective study reported a 10-year recurrence rate of 14.8% with median recurrence time of 6.3 years. Forty-one percent of recurrences were detected by 5 years, 65.5% by 10 years, and 34.5% at more than 10 years after the initial parathyroidectomy [43]. Another retrospective study reported the outcome of 1371 patients after a parathyroidectomy over the period of more than 10 years. Recurrence rate was dependent on final IOPTH values. With an IOPTH drop of less than 40 pg/mL (4.24 pmol/L) 1 year recurrence rate was 0.5%, 2 years recurrence rate was 1.5%, and 5 years recurrence rate was 4.3%. In contrast, with IOPTH level above 60 pg/mL (6.36 pmol/L), recurrence rate at 1 year was 3.7%, at 2 years was 9.5%, and at 5 years was 25.2% [42].

13.8 PHPT During Pregnancy

Prevalence of PHPT during pregnancy was reported between 0.15% and 1.4%. PHPT may have serious consequences to the mother and to the fetus if it remains unrecognized or untreated. In up to 80% of patients, it is not recognized due to physiological changes during pregnancy that mask gestational PHPT, such as hemodilution related to intravascular fluid expansion, hypoalbuminemia, increased glomerular filtration rate resulting in hypercalciuria, and transplacental transfer of calcium. Clinical presentation of PHPT may range from hyperemesis, lethargy, hypertension, thirst, abdominal pain, depression, constipation, bone fracture, maternal heart rhythm disorders, maternal hypertension to preeclampsia, nephrolithiasis, pancreatitis, hyperemesis gravidarum, and hypercalcemic crisis. Because the understanding of this concept and standard monitoring of all pregnant patients in developed countries, the presentation of PHPT during pregnancy is very mild, and it is diagnosed in earlier stages [25, 56–62]. As it was mentioned earlier, sestamibi scan is contraindicated during pregnancy due to radiation exposure risk to the fetus [25, 26]. Ultrasound is the only diagnostic option since it carries no risk of radiation exposure and is easy to perform [25]. Management of PHPT during pregnancy should be individualized based on symptoms and severity of hypercalcemia. Parathyroidectomy is indicated in symptomatic patients and patients with severe hypercalcemia, when calcium level is elevated above 11 mg/dL (2.74 mmol/L). Parathyroidectomy should be performed only in the second trimester to prevent miscarriage and anesthetic drugs exposure in the first trimester or spontaneous delivery in the third trimester [62]. Mild form of PHPT causes low risk of maternal and obstetrical complications; therefore the patients can be managed conservatively, and parathyroidectomy can be deferred until after the delivery. Some medications, such as bisphosphonates, are contraindicated during pregnancy [63]. Calcitonin showed limited data and poor effectiveness, but it does not cross the placenta and appears to be safe [64]. Cinacalcet has shown good results in several studies, although safety data are limited [65, 66]. Recent paper published by Rigg et al. retrospectively reviewed data of 28 pregnant patients with PHPT (22 managed medically and 6 surgically by elective parathyroidectomies) showed that 30% of those who were managed medically developed preeclampsia, and 66% managed medically had preterm deliveries [67].

13.9 Location of Ectopic Parathyroid Glands

Since embryological development of the inferior parathyroid glands is closely related to the thymus, both derived from the third pharyngeal pouch, the location of the inferior parathyroid glands usually can be found within the proximity to the inferior pole of the thyroid lobe: inferiorly, laterally, or posteriorly [68]. The inferior parathyroid gland can be found in the superior horn of the thymus or thyrothymic ligament in about 25% cases [69]. It could be medial to the inferior pole on the trachea in 8% or lateral in about 12% [70].

Ectopic location of the inferior parathyroid gland is related to the failure of the gland to detach from the thymus. They could be found anywhere along the line of descent of the thymus. Ectopic migration of parathyroid gland could be either high or low.

From undescended or incompletely descended (1% of cases), much higher in the neck at the level of angle of mandible, such as at the level or above the carotid bifurcation; 2–3 cm lateral to or above the superior pole of the thyroid lobe; in proximity to the submandibular salivary gland (that makes it very difficult to evaluate by sestamibi scan which usually shows persistent uptake at the salivary glands); intrathyroidal (1% of cases); to excessively descended, in about 3% cases can be found very low in the upper chest at the level of aortic arch, below it, or at pericardium [69, 71].

Surgical steps can be undertaken to locate a missing inferior parathyroid gland: dissect lower pole of the thyroid lobe in the plane to the RLN, dissect along and into the thyrothymic ligament or posterior thymus; look into the intrathyroidal location at the inferior pole of the thyroid lobe; look for undescended lower gland in the carotid sheath at the level of carotid bifurcation and above the bifurcation at the level of the skull base [72].

Superior parathyroid glands originated from dorsal wing of the fourth pharyngeal pouch and migrate down a shorter distance compared to inferior glands that makes an ectopic location more predictable [72]. Ectopic superior parathyroid glands can be found between the thyroid gland and carotid artery, or adjacent to the carotid artery. Superior parathyroid gland also could be intrathyroidal but less likely than inferior. The surgical steps that could be undertaken to locate a missing superior parathyroid gland include as follows: mobilize the superior pole of the thyroid lobe with rotation of the thyroid medially, looking superiorly, medially or posteriorly to the upper pole of the thyroid lobe; dissect deep under tubercle of Zuckerkandl; dissect a plane deep and posterior to the recurrent laryngeal nerve along the esophagus toward the posterior mediastinum; dissect down paraesophageal or retroesophageally; dissect lateral to the recurrent laryngeal nerve along the medial border of the common carotid artery; dissect into the carotid sheath caudally; dissect deep to the inferior thyroid artery; dissect into retrolaryngeal retrotracheal space [71, 72].

13.10 Prediction and Treatment of Postoperative Hypocalcemia

Complications of parathyroid surgery include hypocalcemia and recurrent laryngeal nerve injury. Collaborative Endocrine Surgery Quality Improvement Program (CESQIP) data from 2014 to 2017 showed that hypocalcemia develops in 2.4% of patients after first time parathyroidectomy, and in 10.5% of patients after remedial parathyroidectomy [73]. Temporary hypoparathyroidism and hungry bone syndrome can develop in 1.8–42% of patients after parathyroidectomy [74, 75]. The rate of permanent hypoparathyroidism is reported in up to 3.6% of patients after initial surgery, and the rate increases in patients having bilateral neck exploration [5]. To predict development of hypocalcemia, immediate postoperative PTH level can be measured and be predictive of the development of postoperative hypocalcemia symptoms [76]. A study of patients after a thyroidectomy showed that there was no statistically significant difference in predicting postoperative hypocalcemia when PTH levels were measured at 1 hour after the surgery versus at 24 hours after the surgery [77]. Another study of patients after a thyroidectomy showed that PTH levels less than 10 pg/mL (1.06 pmol/L) at 4 hours after the surgery accurately predict postoperative drop of serum calcium level below 8.02 mg/dL (2.0 mmol/L) [78]. Intraoperative or early postoperative intact PTH levels less than 15 pg/mL (1.59 pmol/L) increase the risk for symptomatic postoperative hypocalcemia. The reduction of the IOPTH level by 85% is predictive of the development of post-parathyroidectomy hypocalcemia in patients with PHPT [79]. An intact PTH level measured on postoperative day 1 after the parathyroidectomy showed the highest ability to predict temporary hypoparathyroidism, but not hungry bone syndrome. The best time for the evaluation of hungry bone syndrome is between postoperative day 5 and 7. Most centers perform the parathyroidectomy on an outpatient basis as a same day surgery; therefore delayed assessment of PTH level is not always possible prior to patient discharge from the hospital. Since development of hungry bone syndrome is difficult to predict and in order to prevent postoperative hypocalcemia, a routine, empiric, prophylactic postoperative administration of oral calcium with vitamin D is recommended to avoid development of symptoms in the early postoperative period [5, 76, 80]. It also appeared to be the most cost-effective approach. Recent statement of the American Association of Clinical Endocrinologists and American College of Endocrinology recommended routine, prophylactic treatment with oral calcium with or without calcitriol for all patients after a parathyroidectomy to prevent transient hypocalcemia [81]. If a IOPTH value measured at 20 minutes or longer after the parathyroidectomy is >15 pg/mL (1.59 pmol/L), the patient can be discharged home on a prophylactic oral calcium dose of between 500 mg and 1000 mg 3 times a day. If IOPTH level < 15 pg/mL (<1.59 pmol/L), calcitriol at dose 0.5 to 1.0 mcg twice a day should be started in addition to calcium and, possibly, magnesium supplementation. Patients also can be observed in the hospital overnight. In order for calcitriol to be effective, it may take up to 72 hours. For patients who develop severe symptoms of postoperative hypocalcemia, intravenous calcium is administered as 1–2 gram boluses in 50 mL of 5% dextrose infused over 20 minutes. If symptoms of severe hypocalcemia persist despite supplementation, then an intravenous calcium infusion of a solution composed of 11 grams of calcium gluconate added to normal saline or 5% dextrose water, to provide a final volume of 1000 mL, is administered at 50 mL/hour intravenous infusion rate and adjusted to maintain the calcium level in the low normal range [81, 82].

13.11 Postoperative Follow-Up

Postoperative follow-up should include measurements of calcium and PTH level shortly after the surgery and in 6 months after the parathyroidectomy. Persistent PHPT is defined as a failure to achieve normocalcemia within 6 months of parathyroidectomy, while recurrent PHPT is defined by the recurrence of hypercalcemia after a normocalcemic interval at more than 6 months after the parathyroidectomy [5]. When a diagnosis of persistent or recurrent PHPT is established, the patient should be re-evaluated with confirmatory biochemical tests to confirm the diagnosis of PHPT, and then assess to determine indications for surgery. Prior surgical records should be obtained and reviewed, new imaging studies should be obtained, and RLN function should be evaluated prior to surgery [5].

13.12 Long-Term Effect of Parathyroidectomy in Patients with PHPT

Successful parathyroidectomy will result in normalization of bone resorption markers within hours of surgery, with subsequent more gradual increase in bone mineral density as early as 6 months post parathyroidectomy at the lumbar spine and hip, and the distal 1/3 radius [83]. Parathyroidectomy was also associated with a 64% reduction in the absolute risk of hip fractures [50, 84, 85]. Despite the fact that nephrolithiasis risk decreases following parathyroidectomy, it has not been shown to improve renal function [53, 86].

Several studies have shown a positive effect of parathyroidectomy on left ventricular mass index, a predictor of cardiovascular mortality. They reported that the highest preoperative PTH levels were associated with the greatest improvements. The clinical significance of the left ventricular mass improvement is unclear; therefore the Proceedings of the Fourth International Workshop suggested that there are no data to support that cardiovascular evaluation should be part of the workup of PHPT, or that surgery should be undertaken to improve cardiovascular markers or function [83, 87, 88].

Quality of life of patients with PHPT have been studied as well, but most of the neurocognitive complaints are nonspecific and symptoms can be difficult to quantify. Several assessment scoring systems have been developed: the PAS (parathyroid assessment of symptoms) score, the PHPQoL (primary hyperparathyroidism quality of life) score, and SF-36. SF36 quality of life scale scores include vitality, physical functioning, body pain, general health, role physical, role emotional, role social, and role mental health. The PAS scores include feeling tired, feeling thirsty, mood swings, joint pains, irritability, feeling blue, feeling weak, itchy, forgetful, headache, abdominal pain, bone pain, and ability to move off chair. Based on those two scoring systems, the follow-up studies of patients with PHPT at 6 months and 12 months after a successful parathyroidectomy showed improvement of the quality of life that appeared to be stable for at least 10 years after the surgery [89–94].

Answers to the Questions

1. (b); 2. (e); 3. (c); 4. (d); 5. (e); 6. (d); 7. (e); 8. (e); 9. (d); 10. (b); 11. (d); 12. (e); 13. (d); 14. (e); 15. (e); 16. (e); 17. (c); 18. (d); 19. (b); 20. (b); 21. (a); 22. (a)

References

1. Bilezikian JP Brandi ML, Eastell R, Silverberg SJ, Udelsman R, Marcocci C, Potts JT Jr. Guidelines for the management of asymptomatic primary hyperparathyroidism: summary statement from the Fourth International Workshop. J Clin Endocrinol Metab. 2014;99(10):3561–9.
2. Jolobe OM. Normal ionized serum calcium is a prerequisite for characterization of normocalcemic primary hyperparathyroidism. Am J Med Sci. 2012;343(6):512.
3. Babwah F, Buch HN. Normocalcaemic primary hyperparathyroidism: a pragmatic approach. J Clin Pathol. 2018;71(4):291–7.
4. Bilezikian JP, Silverberg SJ. Normocalcemic primary hyperparathyroidism. Arq Bras Endocrinol Metabol. 2010;54(2):106–9.
5. Wilhelm SM, Wang TS, Ruan DT, Lee JA, Asa SL, Duh QY, Doherty GM, Herrera MF, Pasieka JL, Perrier ND, Silverberg SJ, Solórzano CC, Sturgeon C, Tublin ME, Udelsman R, Carty SE. The American Association of Endocrine Surgeons Guidelines for Definitive Management of Primary Hyperparathyroidism. JAMA Surg. 2016;151(10):959–68.
6. Udelsman R, Åkerström G, Biagini C, Duh QY, Miccoli P, Niederle B, Tonelli F. The surgical management of asymptomatic primary hyperparathyroidism: proceedings of the Fourth International Workshop. J Clin Endocrinol Metab. 2014;99(10):3595–606.
7. Eastell R, Brandi ML, Costa AG, D'Amour P, Shoback DM, Thakker RV. Diagnosis of asymptomatic primary hyperparathyroidism: proceedings of the Fourth International Workshop. J Clin Endocrinol Metab. 2014;99(10):3570–9.
8. Bilezikian JP, Cusano NE, Khan AA, Liu JM, Marcocci C, Bandeira F. Primary hyperparathyroidism. Nat Rev Dis Primers. 2016;2:16033.
9. Arora S, Balash PR, Yoo J, Smith GS, Prinz RA. Benefits of surgeon-performed ultrasound for primary hyperparathyroidism. Langenbeck's Arch Surg. 2009;394(5):861–7.
10. Deutmeyer C, Weingarten M, Doyle M, Carneiro-Pla D. Case series of targeted parathyroidectomy with surgeon-performed ultrasonography as the only preoperative imaging study. Surgery. 2011;150(6):1153–60.
11. Solorzano CC, Carneiro-Pla D. Minimizing cost and maximizing success in the preoperative localization strategy for primary hyperparathyroidism. Surg Clin North Am. 2014;94(3):587–605.
12. Keidar Z, Solomonov E, Karry R, Frenkel A, Israel O, Mekel M. Preoperative [99mTc]MIBI SPECT/CT interpretation criteria for localization of parathyroid adenomas-correlation with surgical findings. Mol Imaging Biol. 2017;19(2):265–70.
13. Neychev VK, Kouniavsky G, Shiue Z, Udall DN, Somervell H, Umbricht CB, Zeiger MA. Chasing "shadows": discovering the subtleties of sestamibi scans to facilitate minimally invasive parathyroidectomy. World J Surg. 2011;35(1):140–6.
14. Thier M, Daudi S, Bergenfelz A, Almquist M. Predictors of multiglandular disease in primary hyperparathyroidism. Langenbeck's Arch Surg. 2018;403(1):103–9.
15. Harari A, Mitmaker E, Grogan RH, Lee J, Shen W, Gosnell J, Clark O, Duh QY. Primary hyperparathyroidism patients with positive preoperative sestamibi scan and negative ultrasound are more likely to have posteriorly located upper gland adenomas (PLUGs). Ann Surg Oncol. 2011;18(6):1717–22.
16. Skandarajah AR, Palazzo FF, Henry JF. Lithium-associated hyperparathyroidism: surgical strategies in the era of minimally invasive parathyroidectomy. World J Surg. 2011;35(11):2432–9.
17. Ippolito G, Palazzo FF, Sebag F, Henry JF. Long-term follow-up after parathyroidectomy for radiation-induced hyperparathyroidism. Surgery. 2007;142(6):819–22; discussion 822.e1.

18. Harari A, Zarnegar R, Lee J, Kazam E, Inabnet WB 3rd, Fahey TJ 3rd. Computed tomography can guide focused exploration in select patients with primary hyperparathyroidism and negative sestamibi scanning. Surgery. 2008;144(6):970–6; discussion 976–9.
19. Shifrin A, Thind P, Neistadt D eds. Atlas of Parathyroid Imaging and Pathology. Publisher: Springer Inc. 1st Edition, 2020, Hardcover, 120 pages, ISBN-10: 3030409589; ISBN-13: 978-3030409586.
20. Abbott DE, Cantor SB, Grubbs EG, Santora R, Gomez HF, Evans DB, Lee JE, Vu T, Perrier ND. Outcomes and economic analysis of routine preoperative 4-dimensional CT for surgical intervention in de novo primary hyperparathyroidism: does clinical benefit justify the cost? J Am Coll Surg. 2012;214(4):629–37; discussion 637–9.
21. Lubitz CC, Stephen AE, Hodin RA, Pandharipande P. Preoperative localization strategies for primary hyperparathyroidism: an economic analysis. Ann Surg Oncol. 2012;19(13):4202–9.
22. Wang TS, Cheung K, Farrokhyar F, Roman SA, Sosa JA. Would scan, but which scan? A cost-utility analysis to optimize preoperative imaging for primary hyperparathyroidism. Surgery. 2011;150(6):1286–94.
23. McCoy KL, Ghodadra AG, Hiremath TG, Albarano A, Joyce JM, Yip L, Carty SE. Muthukrishnan A Sestamibi SPECT/CT versus SPECT only for preoperative localization in primary hyperparathyroidism: a single institution 8-year analysis. Surgery. 2018;163(3):643–7.
24. Madorin CA, Owen R, Coakley B, Lowe H, Nam K-H, Weber K, Kushnir L, Rios J, Genden E, Pawha PS, Inabnet WB. Comparison of radiation exposure and cost between dynamic computed tomography and sestamibi scintigraphy for preoperative localization of parathyroid lesions. JAMA Surg. 2013;148(6):500–3.
25. McMullen TP, Learoyd DL, Williams DC, Sywak MS, Sidhu SB, Delbridge LW. Hyperparathyroidism in pregnancy: options for localization and surgical therapy. World J Surg. 2010;34(8):1811–6.
26. Azarbar S, Salardini A, Dahdah N, Lazewatsky J, Sparks R, Portman M, Crane PD, Lee ML, Zhu Q. A phase I-II, open-label, multicenter trial to determine the dosimetry and safety of 99mTc-sestamibi in pediatric subjects. J Nucl Med. 2015;56(5):728–3.
27. Jorde R, Szumlas K, Haug E, Sundsfjord J. The effects of calcium supplementation to patients with primary hyperparathyroidism and a low calcium intake. Eur J Nutr. 2002;41:258–63.
28. Marcocci C, Bollerslev J, Aziz Khan A, Shoback D. Medical Management of Primary Hyperparathyroidism: Proceedings of the Fourth International Workshop on the Management of Asymptomatic Primary Hyperparathyroidism. J Clin Endocrinol Metabol. 2014;99(10):3607–18.
29. Irvin GL 3rd, Dembrow VD, Prudhomme DL. Operative monitoring of parathyroid gland hyperfunction. Am J Surg. 1991;162(4):299–302.
30. Irvin GL 3rd, Dembrow VD, Prudhomme DL. Clinical usefulness of an intraoperative "quick parathyroid hormone" assay. Surgery. 1993;114(6):1019–22; discussion 1022–3.
31. Irvin GL 3rd, Deriso GT 3rd. A new, practical intraoperative parathyroid hormone assay. Am J Surg. 1994;168(5):466–8.
32. Carneiro-Pla D. Contemporary and practical uses of intraoperative parathyroid hormone monitoring. Endocr Pract. 2011;17 Suppl 1:44–53.
33. Bieglmayer C, Prager G, Niederle B. Kinetic analyses of parathyroid hormone clearance as measured by three rapid immunoassays during parathyroidectomy. Clin Chem. 2002;48(10):1731–8.
34. Maier GW, Kreis ME, Renn W, Pereira PL, Häring HU, Becker HD. Parathyroid hormone after adenectomy for primary hyperparathyroidism. A study of peptide hormone elimination kinetics in humans. J Clin Endocrinol Metab. 1998;83(11):3852–6.

35. Carneiro DM, Irvin GL 3rd. New point-of-care intraoperative parathyroid hormone assay for intraoperative guidance in parathyroidectomy. World J Surg 2002;26(8):1074–7.
36. Carneiro-Pla D. Recent findings in the use of intraoperative parathyroid hormone monitoring in parathyroid disease. Curr Opin Oncol. 2009;21(1):18–22.
37. Trinh G, Noureldine SI, Russell JO, Agrawal N, Lopez M, Prescott JD, Zeiger MA, Tufano RP. Characterizing the operative findings and utility of intraoperative parathyroid hormone (IOPTH) monitoring in patients with normal baseline IOPTH and normohormonal primary hyperparathyroidism. Surgery. 2017;161(1):78–86.
38. Calò PG, Pisano G, Loi G, Medas F, Barca L, Atzeni M, Nicolosi A. Intraoperative parathyroid hormone assay during focused parathyroidectomy: the importance of 20 minutes measurement. BMC Surg. 2013;13:36.
39. Carneiro-Pla DM, Solorzano CC, Lew JI, Irvin GL 3rd. Long-term outcome of patients with intraoperative parathyroid level remaining above the normal range during parathyroidectomy. Surgery. 2008;144(6):989–93; discussion 993–4.
40. Wharry LI, Yip L, Armstrong MJ, Virji MA, Stang MT, Carty SE, McCoy KL. The final intraoperative parathyroid hormone level: how low should it go? World J Surg. 2014;38(3):558–63.
41. Rajaei MH, Bentz AM, Schneider DF, Sippel RS, Chen H, Oltmann SC. Justified follow-up: a final ioPTH over 40 pg/mL is associated with an increased risk of persistence and recurrence in primary hyperparathyroidism. Ann Surg Oncol. 2015;22(2):454–9.
42. Rajaei MH, Bentz AM, Schneider DF, Sippel RS, Chen H, Oltmann SC. Justified follow-up: a final intraoperative parathyroid hormone (ioPTH) Over 40 pg/mL is associated with an increased risk of persistence and recurrence in primary hyperparathyroidism. Ann Surg Oncol. 2015;22(2):454–9.
43. Lou I, Balentine C, Clarkson S, Schneider DF, Sippel RS, Chen H. How long should we follow patients after apparently curative parathyroidectomy? Surgery. 2017;161(1):54–61.
44. Trinh G, Rettig E, Noureldine SI, Russell JO, Agrawal N, Mathur A, Prescott JD, Zeiger MA. Tufano RP surgical management of normocalcemic primary hyperparathyroidism and the impact of intraoperative parathyroid hormone testing on outcome. Otolaryngol Head Neck Surg. 2018;159(4):630–7.
45. Javid M, Callender G, Quinn C, Carling T, Donovan P, Udelsman R. Primary hyperparathyroidism with normal baseline intraoperative parathyroid hormone: a challenging population. Surgery. 2017;161(2):493–8.
46. Orr LE, McKenzie TJ, Thompson GB, Farley DR, Wermers RA, Lyden ML. Surgery for primary hyperparathyroidism with normal non-suppressed parathyroid hormone can be both challenging and successful. World J Surg. 2018;42(2):409–14.
47. Lee S, Ryu H, Morris LF, Grubbs EG, Lee JE, Harun N, Feng L, Perrier ND. Operative failure in minimally invasive parathyroidectomy utilizing an intraoperative parathyroid hormone assay. Ann Surg Oncol. 2014;21(6):1878–83.
48. Starker L, Fonseca A, Carling T, Udelsman R. Minimally Invasive Parathyroidectomy. International Journal of Endocrinology. 2011;206502:1–8.
49. Henry JF. Minimally invasive thyroid and parathyroid surgery is not a question of length of the incision. Langenbeck's Arch Surg. 2008;393(5):621–6.
50. Stephen AE, Mannstadt M, Hodin RA. Indications for surgical management of hyperparathyroidism: a review. JAMA Surg. 2017;152(9):878–82.

51. Schneider D, Mazeh H, Chen H, Sippel R. Predictors of recurrence in primary hyperparathyroidism: an analysis of 1,386 cases. Ann Surg. 2014;259(3):563–8.
52. Morris LF, Lee S, Warneke CL, Abadin SS, Suliburk JW, Romero Arenas MA, Lee JE, Grubbs EG, Perrier ND. Fewer adverse events after reoperative parathyroidectomy associated with initial minimally invasive parathyroidectomy. Am J Surg. 2014;208(5):850–5.
53. Walker MD, Silverberg SJ. Primary hyperparathyroidism. Nat Rev Endocrinol. 2018;14(2):115–25.
54. Fouquet T, Germain A, Zarnegar R, Klein M, De Talance N, Claude Mayer J, Ayav A, Bresler L, Brunaud L. Totally endoscopic lateral parathyroidectomy: prospective evaluation of 200 patients. ESES 2010 Vienna presentation. Langenbeck's Arch Surg. 2010;395(7):935–40.
55. Bakkar S, Matteucci V, Corsini C, Pagliaro S, Miccoli P. Less is more: time to expand the indications for minimally invasive video-assisted parathyroidectomy. J Endocrinol Investig. 2017;40(9):979–83.
56. Stringer K, Gough J, Gough I. Primary hyperparathyroidism during pregnancy: management by minimally invasive surgery based on ultrasound localization. ANZ J Surg. 2017;87(10):E134–7.
57. Dochez V, Ducarme G. Primary hyperparathyroidism during pregnancy. Arch Gynecol Obstet. 2015;291(2):259–63.
58. Dahlman T, Sjoberg HE, Bucht E. Calcium homeostasis in normal pregnancy and puerperium. A longitudinal study. Acta Obstet Gynecol Scand. 1994;73(5):393–8.
59. Kamenický P, Lecoq AL, Chanson P. Primary hyperparathyroidism in pregnancy. Ann Endocrinol (Paris). 2016;77(2):169–71.
60. Hosking DJ. Calcium homeostasis in pregnancy. Clin Endocrinol. 1996;45(1):1–6.
61. Hirsch D, Kopel V, Nadler V, Levy S, Toledano Y, Tsvetov G. Pregnancy outcomes in women with primary hyperparathyroidism. J Clin Endocrinol Metab. 2015;100(5):2115–22.
62. Abood A, Vestergaard P. Pregnancy outcomes in women with primary hyperparathyroidism. Eur J Endocrinol. 2014;171(1):69–76.
63. Djokanovic N, Klieger-Grossmann C, Koren G. Does treatment with bisphosphonates endanger the human pregnancy? J Obstet Gynaecol Can. 2008;30(12):1146–8.
64. Krysiak R, Wilk M, Okopien B. Recurrent pancreatitis induced by hyperparathyroidism in pregnancy. Arch Gynecol Obstet. 2011;284(3):531–4.
65. Edling KL, Korenman SG, Janzen C, Sohsman MY, Apple SK, Bhuta S, Yeh MW. A pregnant dilemma: primary hyperparathyroidism due to parathyromatosis in pregnancy. Endocr Pract. 2014;20(2):e14–7.
66. Vera L, Oddo S, Di Iorgi N, Bentivoglio G, Giusti M. Primary hyperparathyroidism in pregnancy treated with cinacalcet: a case report and review of the literature. J Med Case Rep. 2016;10:361.
67. Rigg J, Gilbertson E, Barrett HL, Britten FL, Lust K. Primary hyperparathyroidism in pregnancy: maternofetal outcomes at a quaternary referral obstetric hospital, 2000 through 2015. J Clin Endocrinol Metab. 2019;104(3):721–9.
68. Fancy T, Gallagher D 3rd, Hornig JD. Surgical anatomy of the thyroid and parathyroid glands. Otolaryngol Clin N Am. 2010;43(2):221–7.
69. Akerström G, Malmaeus J, Bergström R. Surgical anatomy of human parathyroid glands. Surgery. 1984;95(1):14–21.
70. Bruining HA, Birkenhäger JC, Ong GL, Lamberts SW. Causes of failure in operations for hyperparathyroidism. Surgery. 1987;101(5):562–5.
71. Randolph GW. Surgery of the thyroid and parathyroid glands. Saunders; 2nd, 2012. ISBN-10: 9781437722277.
72. Cheatem D, Sturgeon C. Chapter 60 – Technique of parathyroidectomy. In: Clark O, Duh Q-Y, Kebebew E, Gosnell J, Shen W, editors. Textbook of endocrine surgery. 3rd ed. Jaypee; 2016.

73. Kazaure HS, Thomas S, Scheri RP, Stang MT, Roman SA, Sosa JA. The devil is in the details: assessing treatment and outcomes of 6,795 patients undergoing remedial parathyroidectomy in the Collaborative Endocrine Surgery Quality Improvement Program. Surgery. 2018. pii: S0039-6060(13)30526-9.
74. Allendorf J, DiGorgi M, Spanknebel K, Inabnet W, Chabot J, Logerfo P. 1112 consecutive bilateral neck explorations for primary hyperparathyroidism. World J Surg. 2007;31(11):2075–80.
75. Mittendorf EA, Merlino JI, McHenry CR. Post-parathyroidectomy hypocalcemia: incidence, risk factors, and management. Am Surg. 2004;70(2):114–9; discussion 119–20.
76. Kaderli RM, Riss P, Geroldinger A, Selberherr A, Scheuba C, Niederle B. Primary hyperparathyroidism: dynamic postoperative metabolic changes. Clin Endocrinol. 2018;88(1):129–38.
77. Yetkin G, Citgez B, Yazici P, Mihmanli M, Sit E, Uludag M. Early prediction of post-thyroidectomy hypocalcemia by early parathyroid hormone measurement. Ann Ital Chir. 2016;87:417–21.
78. Barczyński M, Cichoń S, Konturek A. Which criterion of intraoperative iPTH assay is the most accurate in prediction of true serum calcium levels after thyroid surgery? Langenbeck's Arch Surg. 2007;392(6):693–8.
79. Crea N, Pata G, Casella C, Cappelli C, Salerni B. Predictive factors for postoperative severe hypocalcaemia after parathyroidectomy for primary hyperparathyroidism. Am Surg. 2012;78(3):352–8.
80. Orloff LA, Wiseman SM, Bernet VJ, Fahey TJ 3rd, Shaha AR, Shindo ML, Snyder SK, Stack BC Jr, Sunwoo JB, Wang MB. American Thyroid Association Statement on Postoperative Hypoparathyroidism: Diagnosis, Prevention, and Management in Adults. Thyroid. 2018;28(7):830–41.
81. Stack BC Jr, Bimston DN, Bodenner DL, Brett EM, Dralle H, Orloff LA, Pallota J, Snyder SK, Wong RJ, Randolph GW. American Association of Clinical Endocrinologists and American College of Endocrinology Disease State Clinical Review: Postoperative Hypoparathyroidism – Definitions and Management. Endocr Pract. 2015;21(6):674–85.
82. Campbell S, Corrigan T, Bilezikian J, Shifrin A. in 1. "Endocrine Emergencies". Editor: Alexander Shifrin. Chapter 11. "Hypocalcemic crisis: acute postoperative management". Publisher: Elsevier Inc, 1st Edition, Hardcover, 352 pages. ISBN-13: 9780323760973; ISBN-10: 032376097X. Published Date: 15th July 2021.
83. Silverberg SJ, Clarke BL, Peacock M, Bandeira F, Boutroy S, Cusano NE, Dempster D, Lewiecki EM, Liu JM, Minisola S, Rejnmark L, Silva BC, Walker MD, Bilezikian JP. Current issues in the presentation of asymptomatic primary hyperparathyroidism: proceedings of the Fourth International Workshop. J Clin Endocrinol Metab. 2014;99(10):3580–94.
84. Cusano NE, Rubin MR, Silva BC, Tay YD, Williams JM, Agarwal S, Omeragic B, Guo XE, Bilezikian JP. Skeletal microstructure and estimated bone strength improve following parathyroidectomy in primary hyperparathyroidism. J Clin Endocrinol Metab. 2018;103(1):196–205.
85. Lee D, Walker MD, Chen HY, Chabot JA, Lee JA, Kuo JH. Bone mineral density changes after parathyroidectomy are dependent on biochemical profile. Surgery. 2019;165(1):107–13.
86. Khan AA, Hanley DA, Rizzoli R, Bollerslev J, Young JE, Rejnmark L, Thakker R, D'Amour P, Paul T, Van Uum S, Shrayyef MZ, Goltzman D, Kaiser S, Cusano NE, Bouillon R, Mosekilde L, Kung AW, Rao SD, Bhadada SK, Clarke BL, Liu J, Duh Q, Lewiecki EM, Bandeira F, Eastell R, Marcocci C, Silverberg SJ, Udelsman R, Davison KS, Potts JT Jr, Brandi ML, Bilezikian JP. Primary hyperparathyroidism: review and recommendations on evaluation, diagnosis, and management. A Canadian and international consensus. Osteoporos Int. 2017;28(1):1–19.

87. Pepe J, Cipriani C, Sonato C, Raimo O, Biamonte F, Minisola S. Cardiovascular manifestations of primary hyperparathyroidism: a narrative review. Eur J Endocrinol. 2017;177(6):R297–308.
88. McMahon DJ, Carrelli A, Palmeri N, Zhang C, DiTullio M, Silverberg SJ, Walker MD. Effect of parathyroidectomy upon left ventricular mass in primary hyperparathyroidism: a meta-analysis. J Clin Endocrinol Metab. 2015;100(12):4399–407.
89. Ejlsmark-Svensson H, Sikjaer T, Webb SM, Rejnmark L, Rolighed L. Health-related quality of life improves 1 year after parathyroidectomy in primary hyperparathyroidism: a prospective cohort study. Clin Endocrinol. 2019;90(1):184–91.
90. Pasieka JL, Parsons L, Jones J. The long-term benefit of parathyroidectomy in primary hyperparathyroidism: a 10-year prospective surgical outcome study. Surgery. 2009;146(6):1006–13.
91. Mihai R, Sadler GP. Pasieka's parathyroid symptoms scores correlate with SF-36 scores in patients undergoing surgery for primary hyperparathyroidism. World J Surg. 2008;32(5):807–14.
92. Greutelaers B, Kullen K, Kollias J, Bochner M, Roberts A, Wittert G, Pasieka J, Malycha P. Pasieka Illness Questionnaire: its value in primary hyperparathyroidism. ANZ J Surg. 2004;74(3):112–5.
93. Shah-Becker S, Derr J, Oberman BS, Baker A, Saunders B, Carr MM, Goldenberg D. Early neurocognitive improvements following parathyroidectomy for primary hyperparathyroidism. Laryngoscope. 2018;128(3):775–80.
94. Brito K, Edirimanne S, Eslick GD. The extent of improvement of health-related quality of life as assessed by the SF36 and Paseika scales after parathyroidectomy in patients with primary hyperparathyroidism–a systematic review and meta-analysis. Int J Surg. 2015;13:245–9.

Renal Hyperparathyroidism

Martin Almquist and Cornelia Dotzenrath

Contents

A. L. Shifrin et al. (eds.), *Endocrine Surgery Comprehensive Board Exam Guide*,
https://doi.org/10.1007/978-3-030-84737-1_14

Case

A 57-year-old man who had been undergoing chronic hemodialysis for 6 years was listed for kidney transplantation. He presented with bone pain, symptoms of weakness, tiredness, and nausea. He had a history of cardiac bypass operation 3 years ago.

He was treated for arterial hypertension. Further medication included sevelamer and calcium carbonate as phosphate binders and cinacalcet as calcimimetic. Paricalcitol was stopped because of elevated calcium phosphate product.

His laboratory findings were the following:

- Ca 2.3 mmol/l (normal range 2.1–2.6)
- iPTH 1250 pg/ml (normal range 15–65)
- P 4.5 mmol/l (normal range 0.84–1.45)
- Vitamin D 25-OH 10 ng/ml (normal range >37.5).

Questions

1. Which therapy would you suggest for this patient?
   1. Increase dose of cinacalcet
   2. Add cholecalciferol
   3. Waiting for kidney transplantation and no change of the medical treatment
   4. Parathyroid operation
   5. Switch from cinacalcet to etelcalcetide (iv)
      (a) Only (1) and (2) and (3) are correct.
      (b) Only (1) and (3) and (5) are correct.
      (c) Only (1) and (2) and (4) are correct.
      (d) (4) and (5) are correct.
      (e) All are correct.
2. What are the indications for operation in renal hyperparathyroidism?
   1. Resistance to medical treatment
   2. Hypocalcemia
   3. PTH >800 pg/ml
   4. Hypercalcemia
   5. Calciphylaxis
      (a) Only (1) and (2) and (3) are correct.
      (b) Only (1) and (3) and (5) are correct.
      (c) Only (1) and (2) and (4) are correct.
      (d) (1) and (3) and (4) and (5) are correct.
      (e) All are correct.
3. Which factors play a role in the pathophysiology of renal hyperparathyroidism?
   1. Phosphate
   2. Vitamin D
   3. PTH
   4. Fibroblast growth factor 23
   5. Alpha-Klotho

(a) Only (1) and (2) and (3) are correct.
(b) Only (1) and (3) and (5) are correct.
(c) Only (1) and (2) and (4) are correct.
(d) (2) and (3) and (4) and (5) are correct.
(e) All are correct.

4. Complications of renal hyperparathyroidism are:
   1. Kidney stones
   2. Vascular calcification
   3. Bone disease
   4. Pruritus
   5. Tissue calcification
      (a) Only (1) and (2) and (3) are correct.
      (b) Only (1) and (3) and (5) are correct.
      (c) Only (1) and (2) and (4) are correct.
      (d) (2) and (3) and (4) and (5) are correct.
      (e) All are correct.
5. What are medical treatment options for renal hyperparathyroidism
   1. Phosphate binders
   2. Supplementation with calciferol
   3. Calcimimetics
   4. Diuretics
   5. Calcium supplementation
      (a) Only (1) and (2) and (3) are correct.
      (b) Only (1) and (3) and (5) are correct.
      (c) Only (1) and (2) and (4) are correct.
      (d) (1) and (2) and (3) and (4) are correct.
      (e) All are correct.
6. Phosphate binders in the treatment of renal hyperparathyroidism are:
   1. Paricalcitol
   2. Lanthanum carbonate
   3. Ferric citrate
   4. Calcium carbonate
   5. Sevelamer
      (a) Only (1) and (2) and (3) are correct.
      (b) Only (1) and (3) and (5) are correct.
      (c) Only (1) and (2) and (4) are correct.
      (d) (2) and (3) and (4) and (5) are correct.
      (e) All are correct.
7. Which statements regarding cinacalcet are correct?
   1. Cinacalcet reduces the PTH level.
   2. Cinacalcet reduces the risk of death.
   3. Cinacalcet reduces the risk of cardiovascular disease.
   4. Cinacalcet reduces the risk of fractures.
   5. Cinacalcet reduces gastrointestinal symptoms like nausea.
      (a) Only (1) and (2) and (3) are correct.
      (b) Only (1) and (3) and (5) are correct.

(c) Only (1) and (2) and (4) are correct.
(d) (2) and (3) and (4) and (5) are correct.
(e) All are correct.

8. Which statements regarding renal hyperparathyroidism are correct?
   1. Adynamic bone disease is an indication for operation.
   2. The drop of intraoperative PTH is slower in renal hyperparathyroidism than in primary hyperparathyroidism.
   3. Supernumerary glands play a role in renal hyperparathyroidism.
   4. Recurrent disease is common in renal hyperparathyroidism due to the natural course of the disease.
   5. Kidney transplantation is the best therapy.
      (a) Only (1) and (2) and (3) are correct.
      (b) Only (1) and (3) and (5) are correct.
      (c) Only (1) and (2) and (4) are correct.
      (d) (2) and (3) and (4) and (5) are correct.
      (e) All are correct.
9. What statement(s) regarding preoperative management in renal hyperparathyroidism is(are) correct?
   1. Preoperative laryngoscopy should be performed.
   2. Preoperative ultrasound of the thyroid should be performed.
   3. A preoperative MIBI scan should be performed.
   4. Localization procedures are not mandatory in primary operation.
   5. Localization procedures should be performed in recurrent disease.
      (a) Only (1) and (2) and (3) are correct.
      (b) Only (1) and (3) and (5) are correct.
      (c) Only (1) and (2) and (4) and (5) are correct.
      (d) (1) and (2) and (3) and (5) are correct.
      (e) All are correct.
10. Which operative procedures are advisable in this patient (more than 1 choice)?
    1. Subtotal parathyroidectomy
    2. Subtotal parathyroidectomy with transcervical thymectomy
    3. Total parathyroidectomy with autotransplantation and with transcervical thymectomy
    4. Total parathyroidectomy without autotransplantation
    5. Removal of enlarged parathyroid glands
       (a) Only (1) and (2) and (3) are correct.
       (b) Only (1) and (3) and (5) are correct.
       (c) Only (1) and (2) and (4) are correct.
       (d) (1) and (2) and (3) and (4) are correct.
       (e) All are correct.

11. Which statement(s) regarding the operative strategy is(are) correct?
    1. Leaving too much parathyroid tissue increases the risk of recurrence.
    2. Leaving too little parathyroid tissue increases the risk of permanent hypocalcemia.
    3. The optimal level of postoperative PTH is unknown.
    4. A postoperative PTH level between 100 and 600 pg/ml seems to be associated with the lowest risk of mortality.
    5. Intraoperative PTH should be measured no earlier than 20 minutes post-resection.
        (a) Only (1) and (2) and (3) are correct.
        (b) Only (1) and (3) and (5) are correct.
        (c) Only (1) and (2) and (4) are correct.
        (d) (2) and (3) and (4) and (5) are correct.
        (e) All are correct.
12. If less than four parathyroid glands are found intraoperatively, what would you suggest to do:
    1. Autotransplantation of parathyroid tissue and termination of the operation
    2. Transcervical thymectomy
    3. Intraoperative PTH
    4. Venous sampling for ioPTH from the right and the left jugular vein
    5. Sternotomy
        (a) Only (1) and (2) and (3) are correct.
        (b) Only (1) and (3) and (5) are correct.
        (c) Only (1) and (2) and (4) are correct.
        (d) (2) and (3) and (4) are correct.
        (e) All are correct.

14.1 Introduction

Hyperparathyroidism (HPT) secondary to chronic kidney disease (CKD) is common in patients with chronic renal failure [1]. In this chapter, this condition is referred to throughout as *renal hyperparathyroidism (rHPT)*. Renal hyperparathyroidism is associated with decreased quality of life, increased risk of skeletal and cardiovascular complications, and mortality. Most patients with rHPT can be successfully managed medically, but some patients require surgery to control their hyperparathyroidism. Surgery with parathyroidectomy (PTX) cannot cure rHPT but will usually lead to markedly decreased levels of parathyroid hormone (PTH) and improved outcomes for patients with rHPT [1]. PTX should, in the vast majority of patients with rHPT, be performed as a bilateral, four-gland exploration. The endocrine surgeon performing parathyroid surgery in patients with rHPT thus must be familiar with the pathophysiology and the aspects of surgical and medical treatment, including their complications, of rHPT, and parathyroid embryology and anatomy, including variations. In this chapter, the conditions that cause parathyroid hyperplasia and autonomous production of parathyroid hormone (PTH) are outlined; indications and surgical technique are discussed, together with preoperative investigations and postoperative management.

14.2 Clinical Presentation

In most developed countries, patients with end-stage CKD are managed by nephrologists, i.e., internal medicine physicians specialized in kidney care. Almost all patients with CKD have rHPT to some extent, and the endocrine surgeon will usually only become involved once medical treatment can no longer control rHPT [1]. Hence, the common clinical presentation for the endocrine surgeon is that of a referral from the nephrologist for parathyroidectomy (PTX). In some units, patients are presented by the nephrologist to a multidisciplinary group, where endocrine surgeons, nephrologists, and kidney transplant surgeons discuss patients together.

Commonly, patients with rHPT referred for PTX suffer from the effects of long-standing renal disease; they also can have other complications to the underlying condition causing renal failure, such as hypertension or diabetes mellitus. Thus, patients with rHPT often have multiple comorbidities that have to be addressed before accepting and scheduling the patient for surgery. More detailed workup to establish whether the patient is fit for surgery, especially regarding the cardiopulmonary system, might be indicated.

Patients with rHPT referred for PTX usually have high levels of PTH, together with normal or high levels of calcium and phosphate. Apart from these laboratory manifestations, patients can also exhibit symptoms such as pruritus and thirst. Further symptoms are listed in ▶ Box 14.1. As rHPT becomes more pronounced, muscle weakness and fatigue are common. Vascular calcification and osteodystrophy can occur already during the early stages of CKD and progress as glomerular filtration rate (GFR) declines [2]. With advanced rHPT, patients can experience mood swings, conjunctivitis, as well as bone and joint pain. Late manifestations include soft tissue calcifications (◘ Fig. 14.1), brown tumors in the skeleton and calciphylaxis, and a severe, painful deposition of calcium salts in soft tissues [3].

Box 14.1 Some signs and symptoms in rHPT (Adapted from Pasieka et al. [118])

- Pruritus
- Thirst
- Headaches
- Muscle weakness

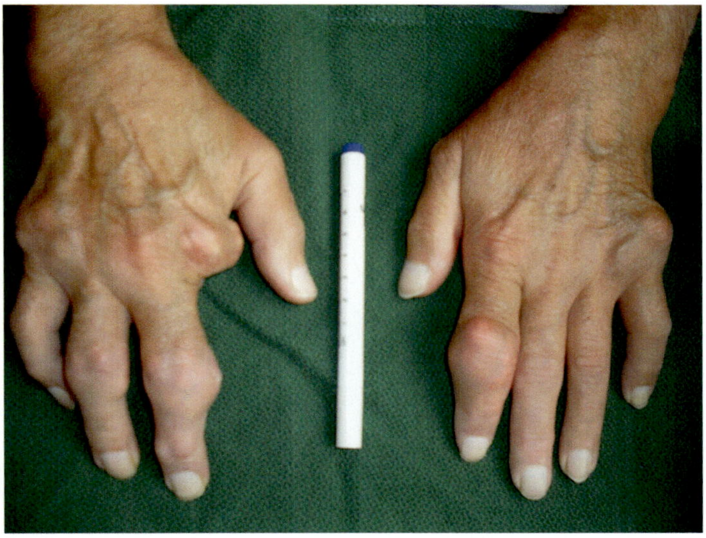

Fig. 14.1 Tissue calcifications in a patient with rHPT

- Bone pain
- Joint pain
- Tiring easily
- Abdominal pain
- Mood swings and/or depression
- Conjunctivitis – red eye syndrome
- Vascular calcification
- Osteodystrophy
- Brown tumors in the mandible
- Brown tumors in the bones of the extremities
- Low bone mineral density
- Fragility fractures

14.3 Natural History

14.3.1 Chronic Kidney Disease (CKD)

Chronic kidney disease, CKD, is defined as abnormalities of kidney structure or function, present for more than 3 months, with implications for health [4]. CKD ranges from a mild asymptomatic decrease in renal function that remains stable for decades to a rapidly decreasing renal function with multiple complications and finally renal failure. Renal failure affects almost all organs in the human body, and patients with ESRD have 10–20 times increased mortality compared to the general population [5]. The main cause of this increased mortality is cardiovascular disease, but patients with renal failure also develop bone disease. The complex relation between vascular

Table 14.1 Chronic kidney disease, CKD, is defined as abnormalities of kidney structure or function, present for >3 months, with implications for health

GFR stages in CKD	GFR (ml/min/1.73 m^2)	Terms
1*	≥ 90	Normal
2*	60–89	Normal to mildly decreased
3a	45–59	Mildly to moderately decreased
3b	30–44	Moderately to severely decreased
4	15–29	Severely decreased
5	< 15	Kidney failure

Abbreviations: *CKD* chronic kidney disease, *GFR* glomerular filtration rate, * in the absence of kidney damage neither of the categories qualifies as CKD

calcifications, bone, and kidney has led the international group *Kidney Disease Improving Global Outcomes* (KDIGO) to formulate clinical guidelines for the management of Chronic Kidney Disease – Mineral and Bone Disorder (CKD-MBD) [2].

Renal hyperparathyroidism, rHPT, with increasing levels of parathyroid hormone (PTH) and parathyroid gland hyperplasia, is a major part of CKD-MBD and develops in all patients with CKD as renal function deteriorates [2]. CKD is divided into five stages based on glomerular filtration rate (GFR) [4], ranging from stage 1 where the GFR is >90 ml/min/1.73m^2 to stage 5 where GFR is <15 ml/min/1.73m^2 (see Table 14.1). In a recent review, the global prevalence of CKD stages 3–5 was about 10% [6]. Thus, CKD is common, and with an aging population, it is a growing global problem [7]. Both death and disability-adjusted life years lost due to CKD are increasing [8]. The medical costs attributable to CKD are substantial and increase as disease severity worsens, particularly if renal replacement therapy (RRT) has to be initiated [9]. Renal hyperparathyroidism worsens outcomes in patients with CKD, especially regarding vascular and bone-related outcomes, but it also leads to shorter life expectancy [10].

14.3.2 FGF23, Klotho

A central hormone in rHPT is fibroblast growth factor 23 (FGF23). This hormone is produced by osteoblasts and osteocytes and is the major phosphate regulatory hormone [11]. FGF23 is induced by high levels of phosphate, active vitamin D, and PTH [12, 13] and increases early in CKD [11]. FGF23 binds to its receptor, FGF Receptor 1 (FGFR1), which requires a co-receptor, α-klotho, to function [14]. α-Klotho is expressed in the kidney and parathyroid tissue [15]. FGF23 decreases the phosphate reuptake in the distal tubule and thus lowers blood levels of phosphate [16]. FGF23 also downregulates 1-α-hydroxylase and upregulates D-24-hydroxylase in the kidney with the net effect of lower levels of active vitamin D and lower uptake of phosphate in the intestines [17].

FGF23 has two key effects on calcium-phosphate-vitamin D homeostasis: it suppresses the activation of vitamin D in the proximal tubules, functioning as a counterregulatory hormone for 1,25 dihydroxivitamin D_3 (calcitriol) and it suppresses the reabsorption of phosphate, thus inducing phosphaturia. In the course of progressive renal failure FGF23 increases first, followed by a decrease in 1, 25 dihydroxivitamin D_3 after which levels of parathyroid hormone increase. Finally, plasma phosphate further stimulates hyperparathyroidism [11, 18].

14.3.3 Phosphate Retention

A positive phosphate balance is another central factor in the development of rHPT. With declining renal function, the ability to maintain mineral homeostasis is impaired, both by a reduced capacity to filter phosphate due to loss of renal function and by the disturbed function of the bone. In CKD, various types of bone disease occur, all characterized by excessive bone resorption compared to formation [19]. This occurs early in CKD and reduces the capacity for the skeleton to buffer phosphate load. Instead, the skeleton contributes to hyperphosphatemia [20]. The positive phosphate balance leads to elevated levels of FGF23. Phosphate also stimulates the release of PTH. The phosphaturic actions of PTH together with FGF23 keep phosphate levels regulated in early CKD [16]. Phosphate levels in the blood remain normal until CKD stages 4–5 when hyperphosphatemia is common [21]. This is due to the loss of functioning nephrons and because tubular reabsorption is already maximally inhibited by FGF23 and PTH. In CKD, due to bone disease, the phosphate reservoir is shifted to soft tissue (e.g., vasculature), a process that is driven by multiple bone-specific signaling pathways, many of them directly activated by phosphate itself [20]. Long-lasting hyperphosphatemia thus leads to vascular calcifications [22] and is a central element of the development of CKD-MBD and rHPT (see also ◘ Fig. 14.2).

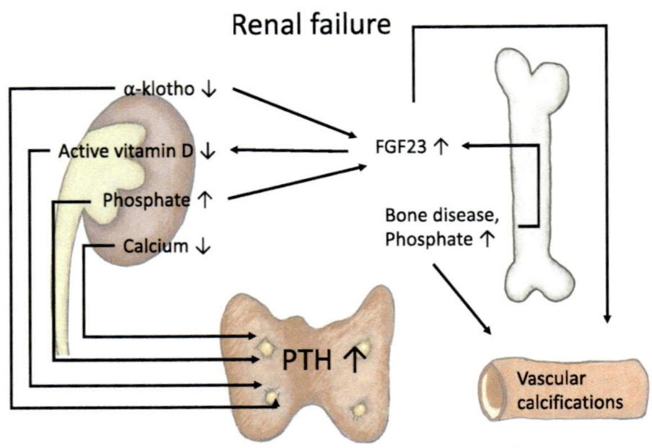

ANTI-proliferation factors:	PRO-proliferation factors:	Severe proliferation:
High levels of active vitamin D Hypercalcemia Hypophosphatemia	Low levels of active vitamin D Hypocalcemia Hyperphosphatemia	Loss of VDR, CaSR, α-klotho = no negative feedback

Fig. 14.2 Schematic illustration of pathophysiology in rHPT

14.3.4 Vitamin D and Calcium

Vitamin D plays an important role in mineral homeostasis. Native vitamin D (25-hydroxyvitamin-D) is activated in the kidney via 1- α-hydroxylase [23] to the active form 1,25-dihydr oxyvitamin-D. Activated vitamin D acts via the vitamin D receptor (VDR) in the intestines to stimulate calcium and phosphate uptake [24]. In the parathyroid gland, activation of vitamin D-receptors leads to reduced production and release of PTH and suppression of parathyroid gland proliferation [25]. The elevated levels of FGF23 in early CKD contribute to low levels of activated vitamin D, and later on, loss of nephrons also contributes to a deficiency of active vitamin D [21]. Patients with CKD also have low levels of native vitamin D due to albuminuria, low exposure to sunlight, and poor dietary intake [26]. The result of vitamin D deficiency is hypocalcemia. In late CKD, both high phosphate and vitamin D deficiency leads to hypocalcemia which is the most potent stimulator of PTH release via the calcium-sensing receptor in the parathyroid gland (CaSR) [27]. Apart from other effects of PTH described earlier, the most potent effect is to increase serum calcium levels by enhancing renal tubular calcium reabsorption, stimulating net bone resorption, and increasing the production of activated vitamin D (1,25(OH)2D3) [28]. Low levels of active vitamin D also directly result in PTH release and parathyroid cell proliferation.

14.3.5 Parathyroid Gland Hyperplasia

The leading factors for parathyroid gland hyperplasia are active vitamin D, calcium, and phosphate. Transforming growth factor-alpha (TGF-α) is a potent proliferative agent for parathyroid cells via the activation of the epidermal growth factor receptor (EGFR). Activation of EGFR both leads to the proliferation of parathyroid cells and lesser expression of VDR [29]. The anti-proliferation pathway is mediated via cyclin-dependent kinase inhibitor p21 and also reduced expression of TGF-α. Both active vitamin D and high levels of calcium inhibit parathyroid cell proliferation through this pathway [30, 31]. Thus, low levels of active vitamin D in CKD contribute to parathyroid cell proliferation [32]. In uremic rats, high dietary intake of phosphate increases TGF-α, and low dietary intake of phosphate enhances the expression of p21 independent of vitamin D, which is why phosphate also contributes to parathyroid cell proliferation [33]. In early CKD, the parathyroid gland often shows polyclonal proliferation, and in late CKD, monoclonal/nodular proliferation is more common. However, different pathological changes often coexist in the same parathyroid gland [34]. With more severe rHPT, the expression of VDR CaSR and α-klotho is reduced [35–37].

14.3.6 Tertiary Hyperparathyroidism

Long-standing CKD with rHPT leads to polyclonal and eventually monoclonal proliferation of parathyroid tissue with a loss of regulatory receptors [38]. This condition of autonomous parathyroid gland function is sometimes referred to as tertiary hyperparathyroidism and is characterized by high levels of PTH in the presence of persistent hypercalcemia [39]. A histological finding of severe hyperplasia together with high levels of parathyroid hormone and persistent hypercalcemia and hyperphosphatemia in patients with rHPT is associated with failure to respond to medical treatment [40]. Tertiary (autonomous) HPT is a complication of long-term CKD and can persist after successful renal transplantation. Two years after renal transplantation, an incidence of about 30% has been reported [41]. However, the term tertiary HPT has also been defined as persistent HPT after renal transplantation [42]. In reality, there is a gradual increase of autonomy in the parathyroid glands with increasing time of CKD, and even if renal transplantation ameliorates rHPT, it never corrects it completely.

14.4 Diagnosis

The diagnosis of rHPT is a process. Initially plasma calcium (low to normal), phosphate (elevated), PTH (elevated), and vitamin D (low) is sufficient for the diagnosis of rHPTH. Moreover, in patients with evidence of CKD-MBD or osteoporosis, monitoring of bone mineral density with dual-energy X-ray absorptiometry (DEXA) is recommended (KDIGO). As long as rHPT can be controlled with medical therapy, further investigations are generally not required. However, when PTH, plasma calcium, and phosphate no longer can be controlled, further investigation is necessary. Firstly, patient symptoms should be explored to guide the extent of the investigation. If the nephrologist is convinced that the patient has rHPT resistant to medical treatment, contact with an endocrine surgeon should be established.

14.5 Non-surgical Treatment

14.5.1 Medical

Most patients with rHPT are treated medically; only a minority require surgery. Medical treatment options are summarized in ◘ Table 14.2. The surgeon needs to have a general understanding of the medical treatment options, to be able to make balanced decisions on when and whom to operate.

14.5.1.1 Vitamin D

The first line of treatment is supplementation with vitamin D (calciferol), which is recommended in non-dialysis patients with CKD stages 3a to 5 [2, 43]. In a recent randomized controlled trial in patients with CKD stages 3 and 4, 12 weeks of supplementation with cholecalciferol resulted in a decrease in PTH with stable levels of plasma calcium [44].

14.5.1.2 Control of Calcium and Phosphate

Restriction of Dietary Intake

As plasma phosphate begins to rise, phosphate intake restriction is recommended. This can be difficult. Dietary protein restriction leads to lower phosphate intake and can be used for patients not yet on dialysis. Patients on dialysis need extra protein, which makes phosphate restriction more complicated. Thus, most patients will require treatment with phosphate binders.

Treatment with Phosphate Binders

Phosphate binders are central in the treatment of hyperphosphatemia. Phosphate levels are positively associated with mortality [45, 46]. Modern phosphate binders, such as sevelamer hydrochloride and lanthanum carbonate are effective and safe [47]. Phosphate control is an important priority in patients with CKD and levels should be maintained within the normal range [2].

Table 14.2 An overview of medical treatment options for renal HPT. Begin treatment options by using medication in the left column and proceed toward the right as the severity of the condition progresses

Vitamin D	Restriction of phosphate intake	Phosphate binders	Non-selective vitamin D receptor activators	Selective vitamin D receptor activators	Calcimimetics
Ergocalciferol	Avoid processed foods	Sevelamer hydrochloride	Calcitriol	Paricalcitol	Cinacalcet
Cholecalciferol	Avoid drinks with high phosphate	Lanthanum carbonate	Alfacalcidol	Maxacalcitol	Etelcalcetide (only iv administration)
	Avoid certain foods with high phosphate content	Ferric citrate	Doxercalciferol		
		Sucroferric oxyhydroxide			
		Calcium carbonate			

Active Vitamin D Analogs

The active vitamin D analogs bind to vitamin D receptors in many tissues such as the parathyroid gland and the intestine. They decrease levels of PTH but can cause hypercalcemia [48].

Calcimimetics

In 2002, cinacalcet was shown to successfully lower PTH in patients on hemodialysis [49]. A randomized controlled trial in 2004 showed that cinacalcet decreased PTH, calcium, and phosphate levels in patients on hemodialysis [50]. Similar positive results were also reported in patients with CKD stages 3–4 [51]. The introduction of cinacalcet carried high hopes and was thought of as a "medical parathyroidectomy." Disappointingly, cinacalcet has not been as effective as initially expected. In an observational study using data from a French registry, cinacalcet did not lower PTH values compared with patients without the treatment [52]. Further, cinacalcet treatment did not reduce the risk of death or major cardiovascular events in the EVOLVE trial, a large, double-blind, multi-center randomized trial (RCT) [53]. However, cinacalcet decreased rates of bone formation, and some biochemical markers of high-turnover bone disease as PTH was reduced, with 26% of the patients achieving normal bone histology after 12 months of treatment [54]. Cinacalet has some unwanted side effects. All studies report that hypocalcemia, nausea, and vomiting are frequent and difficult side effects in patients treated with cinacalcet [50, 52, 53], and these symptoms often cause the patient to stop treatment.

The latest calcimimetic, etelcalcetide, is administered intravenously. In an RCT in hemodialysis patients, the effects of etelcalcetide on PTH were found to be non-inferior to cinacalcet [55]. The frequency of nausea and vomiting was similar in both treatment groups, but the etelcalcetide group was more likely to experience hypocalcemia compared with the cinacalcet group [55].

14.5.2 Renal Transplantation

Renal transplantation offers the best outcomes for patients with CKD needing renal replacement therapy [56]. Mortality and morbidity are much lower, and quality of life higher, than with dialysis [56].

RHPT also improves after renal transplantation [57]. After successful renal transplantation, the mineral homeostasis changes completely. The remaining high FGF23 and PTH increase the secretion of phosphate in the urine, resulting in hypophosphatemia [58]. Levels of FGF23 decrease, and the expression of α-klotho increases after transplantation [59]. Levels of vitamin D and calcium increase [60]. Hypercalcemia in the first one to six months is common and is associated with high levels of PTH [61]. Levels of PTH accumulate during ESRD, and a rapid decrease in PTH is seen immediately after transplantation. Thereafter, levels of PTH keep decreasing slowly and stabilize after the first 6 months [57]. However, the majority of patients still have PTH levels above the reference range 1 year after transplantation [62]. Risk factors for post-transplant rHPT are pre-transplant levels of PTH and calcium, time spent on dialysis before transplantation, and nodular hyperplasia of the parathyroid glands [63]. Cardiovascular disease is the leading cause of death in renal transplant recipients [64], and some data support an association with rHPT [65, 66]. Bone disease after renal transplantation can be both due to rHPT but also to factors specific to transplantation such as corticosteroids and immunosuppressive agents [67, 68].

14.6 Surgical Treatment: Parathyroidectomy

14.6.1 Indications

As stated above, rHPT is initially a physiologic adaptation to the decreasing renal function. However, with time, hyperparathyroidism becomes deleterious, increasing the risk for cardiovascular and skeletal disease, and can lead to shortened survival in patients with CKD [1]. Most patients are successfully managed medically, as outlined above. However, in a small but important subset of patients, medical treatment cannot control rHPT. In these patients, surgical treatment with parathyroidectomy (PTX) is an option. KDIGO CKD-MBD guidelines state that PTX is indicated in "patients with ESRD and severe HPT who fail to respond to pharmacological treatment" [2]. The European Society of Endocrine Surgeons in 2015 stated that "PTX is an option in any patient with rHPT, but that in most patients, the condition can be managed medically." Specifically, PTX would be indicated when "medical treatment fails to correct metabolic parameters – PTH>85 pmol/l, hypercalcemia and hyperphosphatemia" [69].

No RCTs compare PTX to medical treatment. Hence, guideline recommendations rely on data from observational studies. Given the heterogeneity of patients with rHPT, the differences in types of dialysis, whether patients had or had not previously received a renal transplant, differences in medication, etc., it has been hard to define specific indications for surgery in a given patient. Indications likely differ according to sex, age, and type of underlying renal disease, whether the patient has a functioning transplant or the patient's chance of receiving a transplant.

Epidemiologic studies indicate that parathyroidectomy rates decreased in the first years after the introduction of calcimimetics but have since risen again [70]. They also point to regional differences within and between countries, probably due to different access to nephrologists and/or endocrine surgeons, and to different therapy strategies between institutions. Multiple regression models suggest that women, younger patients, and non-diabetic patients have a greater probability of undergoing PTX [70].

There is also evidence that PTX is associated with reduced risk of fractures [71], cardiovascular disease [72], and mortality [73]. Further, studies show improved quality of life after PTX [74]. PTX is also more cost-efficient than calcimimetics in most patients with ESRD [75]. However, morbidity and even mortality after PTX are not insignificant [76, 77]; hence, in all patients, surgical risk must be weighed against potential long-term improvement in outcomes.

Even if most of these studies tried to adjust for confounders, a selection bias cannot be completely ruled out. Patients that are referred for parathyroidectomy are healthier and have a better prognosis than patients who do not get referred for surgery. Unfortunately, it is unlikely that an RCT comparing medical treatment to PTX will ever be performed, given the large number of centers that would be needed to perform such a study.

14.6.1.1 Is There an Absolute Threshold of PTH When PTX Is Indicated?

In patients on dialysis, according to KDIGO, PTH levels should be maintained between 2 and 9 times the upper normal limit, corresponding to approximately between 15 and 55 pmol/L [2]. Although not explicitly stated in the guidelines, if medical treatment fails to keep PTH in this range, this value, 55 pmol/L, could be used as an indication for PTX. Other authors recommend PTX only at higher levels, 80–100 pmol/L [69, 78]. Published series report mean preoperative PTH levels ranging from 87 pmol/L [79] to 233 pmol/L [80]. Thus, there is no clear, absolute threshold of PTH levels where surgery is indicated.

14.6.1.2 Are There Other Specific, Absolute Indications for PTX, Apart from PTH Levels?

Calciphylaxis has by many been reported as an absolute indication for PTX [3], although this has also been disputed [81].

14.6.1.3 Should PTX Be Performed Before or After Renal Transplantation?

Whether to perform PTX or not is also influenced by potential future or previous renal transplantation. As discussed above, renal transplantation can be expected to ameliorate some but not all renal hyperparathyroidism. Some studies showed no difference in outcome [82], whereas others found better outcomes if PTX was performed before renal transplantation [83].

14.6.1.4 What, Exactly, Constitutes "Medical Failure"?

This is not exactly defined [2]. Patients with CKD are complex; they can have many comorbidities; the number of pills needed to compensate for the failing kidney and treat any underlying disease can be staggering [1]. Non-compliance is a common problem, often due to side effects [2]. Costs of treatment also need to be taken into consideration [75]. Thus, whether rHPT can be controlled medically or not has to be evaluated in each patient. In most settings, a specialized nephrologist is responsible for the patient and makes this evaluation. Accepted and pragmatic indications for PTX in rHPT are summarized in ▶ Box 14.2.

Box 14.2 Indications for operation in renal hyperparathyroidism

- Hypercalcemia
  - Spontaneous
  - Drug induced
  - Persistent after kidney transplantation
- Severe renal osteopathy (radiologically or histologically proven)
- Vascular or tissue calcification[a]
- Calciphylaxis[a]
- Drug resistant hyperphosphatemia[a]
- Drug resistant pruritus

[a]Under the condition that PTH is >800 pg/ml (88 pmol/l) and medical treatment failed or PTH is >100 and <800 pg/ml and adynamic bone disease is excluded; contraindication is adynamic bone disease

14.6.2 Surgical Technique

In almost all patients, PTX for rHPT should be conducted as a classical, bilateral, four-gland exploration [69] (◻ Figs. 14.3 and 14.4). Details of how to perform this operation are covered in other chapters. It has to be emphasized, that to perform parathyroid surgery successfully, the surgeon needs a detailed knowledge of parathyroid embryology and anatomy and its variations [84].

PTX is performed as either subtotal PTX, where the aim is to keep parathyroid tissue corresponding to one normal gland, or total parathyroidectomy, aiming at removing all parathyroid

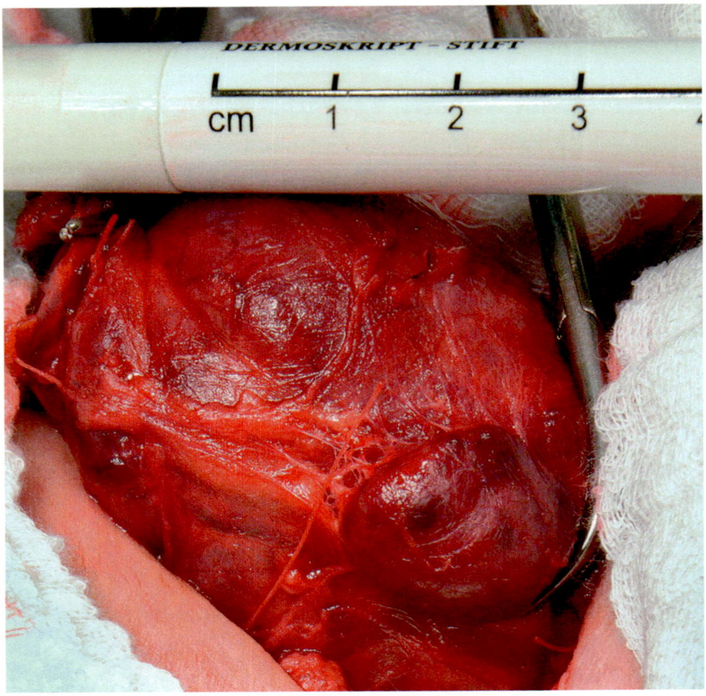

■ **Fig. 14.3** Right lower parathyroid gland in a patient with rHPT

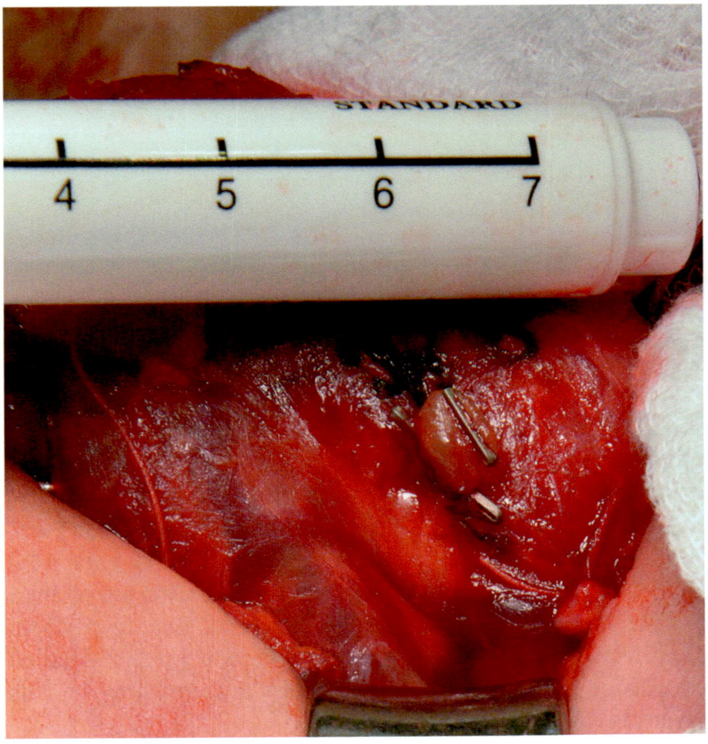

■ **Fig. 14.4** Partially resected right lower parathyroid gland in a patient with rHPT

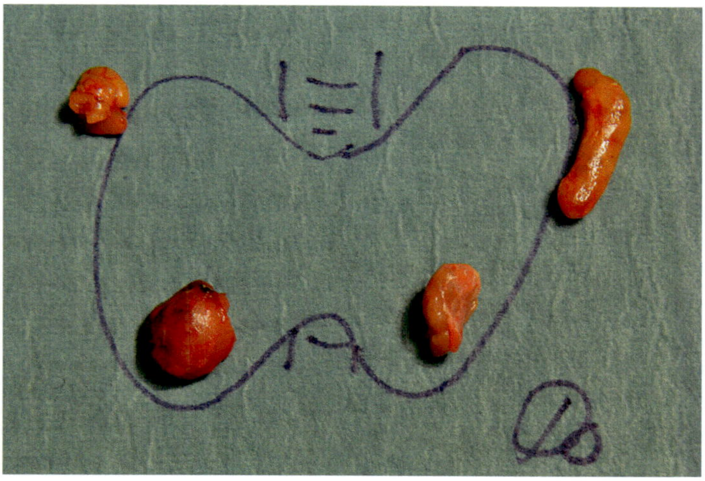

Fig. 14.5 Removed parathyroid glands

tissue (Fig. 14.5). PTX is usually performed with open surgery through a Kocher cervical incision in general anesthesia [69], although there have been reports on minimally invasive PTX [85–87]. Subtotal and total PTX can both be combined with transcervical thymus resection and/or parathyroid autotransplantation (AT). However, subtotal PTX is normally not combined with AT, and total parathyroidectomy without AT is often performed without thymus resection. The lower parathyroids are often found in or close to the thymus, and nests of parathyroid tissue are also often found in normal thymic tissue. Hence, many authors recommend performing transcervical thymectomy together with PTX [69, 88].

There has been a debate among endocrine surgeons as to whether less (subtotal/focused) or more (total) radical surgery is optimal in rHPT. Large population-based studies [89] and a meta-analysis [90] could not find any difference in long-term outcomes such as the risk of fracture, cardiovascular disease, and mortality between the two procedures. Furthermore, there has been a misunderstanding in that some authors believe that rHPT can be cured [91], analogous to primary HPT (pHPT), which has very high cure rates with the resection of one or more parathyroid glands [92]. However, pHPT and rHPT are different entities. It is evident from the discussion above that rHPT also persists even in mild renal dysfunction, even if the patient receives a renal transplant [93]. Hence, PTX cannot cure rHPT. Instead, PTX aims to reduce the amount of parathyroid tissue to such an extent that an optimal level of PTH post-PTX is achieved. This is similar to the situation in hereditary pHPT, e.g., multiple endocrine neoplasia type 1 (MEN1), which also cannot be cured, and where surgery aims to give the patient as many years with normocalcemia as possible [94].

The optimal level of PTH after PTX for rHPT is unknown. Probably, profound hypoparathyroidism is just as detrimental as severe hyperparathyroidism [78]– in patients with rHPT, as we have seen above, the initial adaptation of the parathyroids is physiologic, helping the body get rid of excess phosphate not cleared by the kidneys. Hence, leaving too little viable parathyroid tissue is suboptimal. On the other hand, leaving too much increases the risk of reoperation, due to persistent/recurrent disease. Thus, the question for the endocrine surgeon is not how much to remove, but how much to leave behind. Support for this concept comes from studies examining the correlation between PTH levels and long-term outcomes in patients with ESRD. Thus, a report from the DOPPS study in 2008 showed that PTH levels between 10 pmol/L and 60 pmol/L were associated with the lowest risk of mortality [45]. The same authors re-examined this issue and in 2015 reported similar findings [95]. In their multivariate analysis, patients in the reference group with levels of PTH between 15 and 30 pmol/L had the lowest mortality risk [95]. Data also show that PTH levels vary significantly after both subtotal and total PTX [89, 91].

14.6.2.1 Intraoperative Measurement of Parathyroid Hormone (ioPTH)

In primary HPT, intraoperative measurement of PTH (ioPTH) helps the surgeon to determine if there is more hyperfunctioning tissue left after resection or whether the operation can be terminated. There have been numerous studies investigating whether ioPTH also assists the surgeon performing PTX for rHPT [80, 96–104]. Most, but not all, of these studies indicate that there is a correlation between levels of ioPTH and postoperative PTH and that ioPTH helps determine the extent of PTX. Since PTH is cleared by the kidneys, the half-life of PTH, and hence the time needed to wait for a drop in intraoperative PTH, is longer after PTX for renal HPT. Probably, PTH should be measured no earlier than 15–20 minutes post-resection. Different criteria on the optimal level of ioPTH post-resection have been proposed, but there is no consensus on what level of ioPTH yields the best outcomes.

14.6.2.2 Preoperative Localization

The outcome of PTX is highly dependent on the skills and experience of the surgeon. In experienced hands, the main cause of persistent or recurrent rHPT after PTX is the inability to localize ectopic parathyroid glands [105]. From a surgical point of view, a distinction exists between minor ectopy (such as in the thyrothymic horn and upper anterior mediastinum, or beneath thyroid capsule) and major ectopy (such as low mediastinal, retro esophageal, above the level of the hyoid, in the carotid sheath, or within the thyroid parenchyma – truly intrathyroidal) [106]. Ectopic and/or supernumerary glands are common in rHPT [69] and the surgeon must identify all parathyroid glands. The experienced surgeon will usually find all

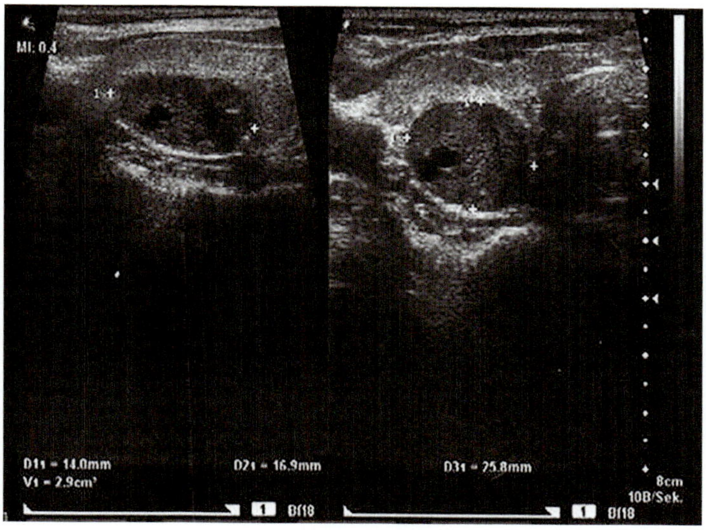

Fig. 14.6 Ultrasound of hyperplastic parathyroid remnant 13 years after subtotal parathyroidectomy. (With kind approval of Dr. M. Tosch, head of department of nuclear medicine, Helios university hospital, Wuppertal)

non-ectopic glands; preoperative localization should therefore positively and accurately localize all ectopic parathyroid glands. Similar to primary HPT, preoperative imaging, with modalities such as ultrasonography, 99-Technetium sestamibi scintigraphy, and four-dimensional computed tomography (4D-CT), has been evaluated but has not been shown to have greater accuracy in finding all parathyroid glands than traditional surgical exploration. A meta-analysis [107] reported that the sensitivity of the 99mTc-sestamibi scan in secondary HPT was only 58%. It was concluded that 99mTc-sestamibi is not a first-line diagnostic imaging method before PTX for rHPT. The sensitivity of ultrasound for the detection of enlarged parathyroid glands has been reported to be 46–81% in patients with secondary HPT [108–110]. The combination of ultrasound with 99mTc-sestamibi SPECT/CT had a higher sensitivity than US or 99mTc-sestamibi SPECT/CT alone [110]. Most authors thus conclude that ultrasound and sestamibi scintigraphy offer little benefit in localizing ectopic glands and rarely change the conduct of a standard four-gland exploration [38, 111, 112], although ESES recommended ultrasound pre-PTX, also to rule out co-existing thyroid disease [69]. However, some authors have found that SPECT-CT offers useful information [106]. On the contrary, in the setting of re-PTX, i.e. surgery for persistent or recurrent HPT after previous PTX, imaging studies are mandatory [69] (Figs. 14.6 and 14.7).

14.6.2.3 Intraoperative Angiography

A further issue complicating PTX is that it is difficult to be certain that the parathyroid tissue left in the neck at surgery is viable – unintentional devascularization of parathyroid glands

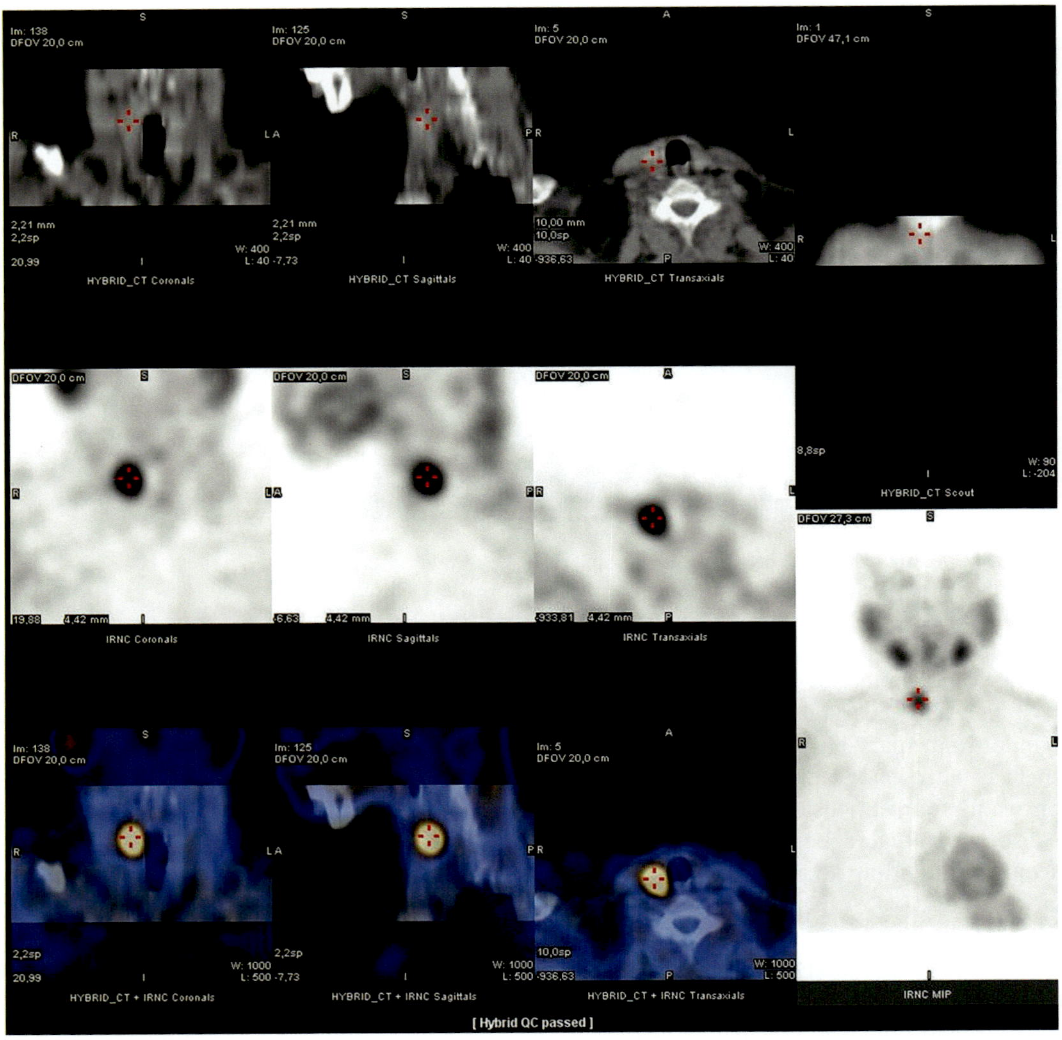

Fig. 14.7 Corresponding sestamibi scintigraphy of hyperplastic parathyroid remnant in a patient with recurrent disease 13 years after subtotal parathyroidectomy. (With kind approval of Dr. M. Tosch, head of department of nuclear medicine, Helios university hospital, Wuppertal)

is common, both during parathyroid and thyroid surgery. Recently, intraoperative angiography of the parathyroids using indocyanine green has shown great promise in aiding the surgeon to determine whether parathyroid glands are functioning or not [113]. Combined with ioPTH and possibly with cross-sectional imaging, these tools might enable the surgeon to deliver a more precise PTX, yielding an optimal postoperative level of PTH [114].

14.6.2.4 Surgical Complications

Risks of PTX include damage to the recurrent laryngeal nerve, bleeding, and infection. These risks are small in the hands of experienced surgeons, and nationwide studies have shown these complications to be rare [115]. However, complications related to abnormal mineral metabolism are common and expected.

14.6.2.5 Postoperative Management

Patients undergoing PTX for renal hyperparathyroidism are best managed by nephrologists perioperatively, with input from the endocrine surgeon if needed. Profound postoperative hypocalcemia is not uncommon and perhaps ameliorated with preoperative calcitriol loading [116]. Admissions to intensive care units for hypocalcemia and re-admissions due to mineral metabolism imbalances are common; protocols for postoperative care after PTX might reduce these [117].

14.7 Outcomes and Prognosis

Overall, patient outcome after PTX is mainly determined by whether the patient will receive renal transplantation or not. Chronic dialysis is associated with a markedly reduced lifespan; patients with renal transplants have an expected survival that is close to that of the normal population. Both patient and other factors are related to the chance of receiving a transplant; this is outside the scope of this chapter.

Regarding outcome after PTX, studies indicate that PTX diminishes the risk of fractures and is associated with better survival. As noted above, there is a significant risk of re-PTX after subtotal PTX; this risk is much lower after total PTX. However, studies also indicate that persistently low levels of PTH are associated with an increased risk of cardiovascular disease. No difference in survival has been established between total and subtotal PTX.

More research is needed to establish the exact indications for PTX, especially concerning its timing concerning renal transplantation. Knowledge of the optimal level of PTH after PTX for favorable long-term outcomes would also be useful, and application of modern tools (fluorescence, angiography) together with ioPTH to arrive at this level of PTH might be ways to improve outcomes in the future.

In conclusion, renal hyperparathyroidism develops early in renal failure, mainly as a consequence of reduced levels of vitamin D, hypocalcemia, diminished excretion of phosphate, and inability to activate vitamin D. RHPT is associated with increased morbidity and mortality. RHPT is a continuum and diagnosis depends on demonstrating elevated levels of parathyroid hormone, PTH. Treatment consists of supplying vitamin D, reducing phosphate intake, and treatment with active vitamin D analogs. In later stages, calcimimetics might be added. In rHPT, parathyroid glands grow and can become refractory to medical treatment. Patients with rHPT refractory to medical treatment should be considered for parathyroidectomy, PTX. A close collaboration between nephrologists, endocrinologists, and endocrine surgeons is required to achieve optimal outcomes. Risks of surgery are small but not negligible. Surgery should likely not be too radical, especially if the patient is a candidate for future renal transplantation. Subtotal or total parathyroidectomy with autotransplantation is recognized surgical options. Intraoperative measurement of PTH can be helpful; the value of preoperative imaging studies to localize parathyroid glands has not been established for PTX in rHPT.

Answers to Questions

1. (d); 2. (d); 3. (e); 4. (d); 5. (a); 6. (d); 7. (a); 8. (d); 9. (c); 10. (a); 11. (e); 12. (d)

Acknowledgments There is no conflict of interest that could be perceived as prejudicing the impartiality of the research reported. There were no sources of funding other than the authors' salaries. This research did not receive any specific grant from any funding agency in the public, commercial, or not-for-profit sector. Both authors contributed to the literature search, drafting of the manuscript, and critical review. There are no specific acknowledgments.

Sources of Support

There were no other sources of support than the authors' salaries.

Conflict of Interest

There are no financial or other relationships that might lead to any conflict of interest.

References

1. Almquist M, Isaksson E, Clyne N. The treatment of renal hyperparathyroidism. Endocr Relat Cancer. 2020;27(1):R21–34.
2. Kidney Disease: Improving Global Outcomes CKDMBDWG. KDIGO clinical practice guideline for the diagnosis, evaluation, prevention, and treatment of Chronic Kidney Disease-Mineral and Bone Disorder (CKD-MBD). Kidney Int Suppl. 2009;(113):S1–130.
3. McCarthy JT, El-Azhary RA, Patzelt MT, et al. Survival, risk factors, and effect of treatment in 101 patients with calciphylaxis. Mayo Clin Proc. 2016;91(10):1384–94.
4. Chapter 1: Definition and classification of CKD. Kidney Int Suppl (2011). 2013;3(1):19–62.
5. Foley RN, Parfrey PS, Sarnak MJ. Clinical epidemiology of cardiovascular disease in chronic renal disease. Am J Kidney Dis. 1998;32(5 Suppl 3):S112–9.
6. Hill NR, Fatoba ST, Oke JL, et al. Global prevalence of chronic kidney disease – a systematic review and meta-analysis. PLoS One. 2016;11(7):e0158765.
7. Coresh J, Selvin E, Stevens LA, et al. Prevalence of chronic kidney disease in the United States. JAMA. 2007;298(17):2038–47.

8. Jager KJ, Fraser SDS. The ascending rank of chronic kidney disease in the global burden of disease study. Nephrol Dial Transplant. 2017;32(suppl_2):ii121–8.
9. Honeycutt AA, Segel JE, Zhuo X, Hoerger TJ, Imai K, Williams D. Medical costs of CKD in the Medicare population. J Am Soc Nephrol. 2013;24(9):1478–83.
10. Young EW, Akiba T, Albert JM, et al. Magnitude and impact of abnormal mineral metabolism in hemodialysis patients in the Dialysis Outcomes and Practice Patterns Study (DOPPS). Am J Kidney Dis. 2004;44(5 Suppl 2):34–8.
11. Isakova T, Wahl P, Vargas GS, et al. Fibroblast growth factor 23 is elevated before parathyroid hormone and phosphate in chronic kidney disease. Kidney Int. 2011;79(12):1370–8.
12. Bon N, Frangi G, Sourice S, Guicheux J, Beck-Cormier S, Beck L. Phosphate-dependent FGF23 secretion is modulated by PiT2/Slc20a2. Mol Metab. 2018;11:197–204.
13. Meir T, Durlacher K, Pan Z, et al. Parathyroid hormone activates the orphan nuclear receptor Nurr1 to induce FGF23 transcription. Kidney Int. 2014;86(6):1106–15.
14. Kurosu H, Kuro OM. The Klotho gene family as a regulator of endocrine fibroblast growth factors. Mol Cell Endocrinol. 2009;299(1):72–8.
15. Lim K, Groen A, Molostvov G, et al. Alpha-klotho expression in human tissues. J Clin Endocrinol Metab. 2015;100(10):E1308–18.
16. Sneddon WB, Ruiz GW, Gallo LI, et al. Convergent signaling pathways regulate parathyroid hormone and fibroblast growth Factor-23 action on NPT2A-mediated phosphate transport. J Biol Chem. 2016;291(36):18632–42.
17. Shimada T, Hasegawa H, Yamazaki Y, et al. FGF-23 is a potent regulator of vitamin D metabolism and phosphate homeostasis. J Bone Miner Res. 2004;19(3):429–35.
18. Kuro OM. Klotho and endocrine fibroblast growth factors: markers of chronic kidney disease progression and cardiovascular complications? Nephrol Dial Transplant. 2019;34(1):15–21.
19. Drueke TB, Massy ZA. Changing bone patterns with progression of chronic kidney disease. Kidney Int. 2016;89(2):289–302.
20. Hruska KA, Mathew S, Lund R, Qiu P, Pratt R. Hyperphosphatemia of chronic kidney disease. Kidney Int. 2008;74(2):148–57.
21. Levin A, Bakris GL, Molitch M, et al. Prevalence of abnormal serum vitamin D, PTH, calcium, and phosphorus in patients with chronic kidney disease: results of the study to evaluate early kidney disease. Kidney Int. 2007;71(1):31–8.
22. Mathew S, Tustison KS, Sugatani T, Chaudhary LR, Rifas L, Hruska KA. The mechanism of phosphorus as a cardiovascular risk factor in CKD. J Am Soc Nephrol. 2008;19(6):1092–105.
23. Brunette MG, Chan M, Ferriere C, Roberts KD. Site of 1,25(OH)2 vitamin D3 synthesis in the kidney. Nature. 1978;276(5685):287–9.
24. Xue Y, Fleet JC. Intestinal vitamin D receptor is required for normal calcium and bone metabolism in mice. Gastroenterology. 2009;136(4):1317–27, e1311–1312.
25. Silver J, Naveh-Many T, Mayer H, Schmelzer HJ, Popovtzer MM. Regulation by vitamin D metabolites of parathyroid hormone gene transcription in vivo in the rat. J Clin Invest. 1986;78(5):1296–301.
26. Obi Y, Hamano T, Isaka Y. Prevalence and prognostic implications of vitamin D deficiency in chronic kidney disease. Dis Markers. 2015;2015:868961.
27. Brown EM, Gamba G, Riccardi D, et al. Cloning and characterization of an extracellular Ca(2+)-sensing receptor from bovine parathyroid. Nature. 1993;366(6455):575–80.
28. Pocotte SL, Ehrenstein G, Fitzpatrick LA. Regulation of parathyroid hormone secretion. Endocr Rev. 1991;12(3):291–301.

29. Arcidiacono MV, Sato T, Alvarez-Hernandez D, et al. EGFR activation increases parathyroid hyperplasia and calcitriol resistance in kidney disease. J Am Soc Nephrol. 2008;19(2):310–20.
30. Cordero JB, Cozzolino M, Lu Y, et al. 1,25-Dihydroxyvitamin D downregulates cell membrane growth- and nuclear growth-promoting signals by the epidermal growth factor receptor. J Biol Chem. 2002;277(41):38965–71.
31. Cozzolino M, Lu Y, Finch J, Slatopolsky E, Dusso AS. p21WAF1 and TGF-alpha mediate parathyroid growth arrest by vitamin D and high calcium. Kidney Int. 2001;60(6):2109–17.
32. Tokumoto M, Tsuruya K, Fukuda K, Kanai H, Kuroki S, Hirakata H. Reduced p21, p27 and vitamin D receptor in the nodular hyperplasia in patients with advanced secondary hyperparathyroidism. Kidney Int. 2002;62(4):1196–207.
33. Dusso AS, Pavlopoulos T, Naumovich L, et al. p21(WAF1) and transforming growth factor-alpha mediate dietary phosphate regulation of parathyroid cell growth. Kidney Int. 2001;59(3):855–65.
34. Basile C, Lomonte C, Vernaglione L, et al. A high body mass index and female gender are associated with an increased risk of nodular hyperplasia of parathyroid glands in chronic uraemia. Nephrol Dial Transplant. 2006;21(4):968–74.
35. Fukuda N, Tanaka H, Tominaga Y, Fukagawa M, Kurokawa K, Seino Y. Decreased 1,25-dihydroxyvitamin D3 receptor density is associated with a more severe form of parathyroid hyperplasia in chronic uremic patients. J Clin Invest. 1993;92(3):1436–43.
36. Lee HJ, Seo UH, Kim WY, Woo SU, Lee JB. Calcium-sensing receptor and apoptosis in parathyroid hyperplasia of patients with secondary hyperparathyroidism. J Int Med Res. 2013;41(1):97–105.
37. Komaba H, Goto S, Fujii H, et al. Depressed expression of Klotho and FGF receptor 1 in hyperplastic parathyroid glands from uremic patients. Kidney Int. 2010;77(3):232–8.
38. van der Plas WY, Noltes ME, van Ginhoven TM, Kruijff S. Secondary and tertiary hyperparathyroidism: a narrative review. Scand J Surg. 2019:1457496919866015.
39. Pitt SC, Sippel RS, Chen H. Secondary and tertiary hyperparathyroidism, state of the art surgical management. Surg Clin North Am. 2009;89(5):1227–39.
40. Tominaga Y, Matsuoka S, Sato T, et al. Clinical features and hyperplastic patterns of parathyroid glands in hemodialysis patients with advanced secondary hyperparathyroidism refractory to maxacalcitol treatment and required parathyroidectomy. Ther Apher Dial. 2007;11(4):266–73.
41. Shindo M, Lee JA, Lubitz CC, et al. The changing landscape of primary, secondary, and tertiary hyperparathyroidism: highlights from the American College of Surgeons Panel, "What's New for the Surgeon Caring for Patients with Hyperparathyroidism". J Am Coll Surg. 2016;222(6):1240–50.
42. Dulfer RR, Franssen GJH, Hesselink DA, Hoorn EJ, van Eijck CHJ, van Ginhoven TM. Systematic review of surgical and medical treatment for tertiary hyperparathyroidism. Br J Surg. 2017;104(7):804–13.
43. Goldsmith DJ. Pro: Should we correct vitamin D deficiency/insufficiency in chronic kidney disease patients with inactive forms of vitamin D or just treat them with active vitamin D forms? Nephrol Dial Transplant. 2016;31(5):698–705.
44. Westerberg PA, Sterner G, Ljunggren O, et al. High doses of cholecalciferol alleviate the progression of hyperparathyroidism in patients with CKD Stages 3–4: results of a 12-week double-blind, randomized, controlled study. Nephrol Dial Transplant. 2018;33(3):466–71.
45. Tentori F, Blayney MJ, Albert JM, et al. Mortality risk for dialysis patients with different levels of serum calcium, phosphorus, and PTH: the Dialysis Outcomes and Practice Patterns Study (DOPPS). Am J Kidney Dis. 2008;52(3):519–30.

46. Tentori F, Wang M, Bieber BA, et al. Recent changes in therapeutic approaches and association with outcomes among patients with secondary hyperparathyroidism on chronic hemodialysis: the DOPPS study. Clin J Am Soc Nephrol. 2015;10(1):98–109.
47. Patel L, Bernard LM, Elder GJ. Sevelamer versus calcium-based binders for treatment of hyperphosphatemia in CKD: a meta-analysis of randomized controlled trials. Clin J Am Soc Nephrol. 2016;11(2):232–44.
48. Zand L, Kumar R. The use of vitamin D metabolites and analogues in the treatment of chronic kidney disease. Endocrinol Metab Clin N Am. 2017;46(4):983–1007.
49. Goodman WG, Hladik GA, Turner SA, et al. The Calcimimetic agent AMG 073 lowers plasma parathyroid hormone levels in hemodialysis patients with secondary hyperparathyroidism. J Am Soc Nephrol. 2002;13(4):1017–24.
50. Block GA, Martin KJ, de Francisco AL, et al. Cinacalcet for secondary hyperparathyroidism in patients receiving hemodialysis. N Engl J Med. 2004;350(15):1516–25.
51. Charytan C, Coburn JW, Chonchol M, et al. Cinacalcet hydrochloride is an effective treatment for secondary hyperparathyroidism in patients with CKD not receiving dialysis. Am J Kidney Dis. 2005;46(1):58–67.
52. Brunaud L, Ngueyon Sime W, Filipozzi P, et al. Minimal impact of calcimimetics on the management of hyperparathyroidism in chronic dialysis. Surgery. 2016;159(1):183–91.
53. Investigators ET, Chertow GM, Block GA, et al. Effect of cinacalcet on cardiovascular disease in patients undergoing dialysis. N Engl J Med. 2012;367(26):2482–94.
54. Behets GJ, Spasovski G, Sterling LR, et al. Bone histomorphometry before and after long-term treatment with cinacalcet in dialysis patients with secondary hyperparathyroidism. Kidney Int. 2015;87(4):846–56.
55. Block GA, Bushinsky DA, Cheng S, et al. Effect of etelcalcetide vs cinacalcet on serum parathyroid hormone in patients receiving hemodialysis with secondary hyperparathyroidism: a randomized clinical trial. JAMA. 2017;317(2):156–64.
56. Ortiz A, Covic A, Fliser D, et al. Epidemiology, contributors to, and clinical trials of mortality risk in chronic kidney failure. Lancet. 2014;383(9931):1831–43.
57. Isaksson E, Sterner G. Early development of secondary hyperparathyroidism following renal transplantation. Nephron Clin Pract. 2012;121(1–2):c68–72.
58. Bhan I, Shah A, Holmes J, et al. Post-transplant hypophosphatemia: tertiary 'hyper-phosphatoninism'? Kidney Int. 2006;70(8):1486–94.
59. Kimura T, Akimoto T, Watanabe Y, et al. Impact of renal transplantation and nephrectomy on urinary soluble klotho protein. Transplant Proc. 2015;47(6):1697–9.
60. Reinhardt W, Bartelworth H, Jockenhovel F, et al. Sequential changes of biochemical bone parameters after kidney transplantation. Nephrol Dial Transplant. 1998;13(2):436–42.
61. Amin T, Coates PT, Barbara J, Hakendorf P, Karim N. Prevalence of hypercalcaemia in a renal transplant population: a single centre study. Int J Nephrol. 2016;2016:7126290.
62. Sprague SM, Belozeroff V, Danese MD, Martin LP, Olgaard K. Abnormal bone and mineral metabolism in kidney transplant patients–a review. Am J Nephrol. 2008;28(2):246–53.
63. Taweesedt PT, Disthabanchong S. Mineral and bone disorder after kidney transplantation. World J Transplant. 2015;5(4):231–42.
64. Kasiske BL, Guijarro C, Massy ZA, Wiederkehr MR, Ma JZ. Cardiovascular disease after renal transplantation. J Am Soc Nephrol. 1996;7(1):158–65.
65. Pihlstrom H, Dahle DO, Mjoen G, et al. Increased risk of all-cause mortality and renal graft loss in stable renal transplant recipients with hyperparathyroidism. Transplantation. 2015;99(2):351–9.

66. Bleskestad IH, Bergrem H, Leivestad T, Hartmann A, Goransson LG. Parathyroid hormone and clinical outcome in kidney transplant patients with optimal transplant function. Clin Transpl. 2014;28(4):479–86.
67. Julian BA, Laskow DA, Dubovsky J, Dubovsky EV, Curtis JJ, Quarles LD. Rapid loss of vertebral mineral density after renal transplantation. N Engl J Med. 1991;325(8):544–50.
68. Weisinger JR, Carlini RG, Rojas E, Bellorin-Font E. Bone disease after renal transplantation. Clin J Am Soc Nephrol. 2006;1(6):1300–13.
69. Lorenz K, Bartsch DK, Sancho JJ, Guigard S, Triponez F. Surgical management of secondary hyperparathyroidism in chronic kidney disease--a consensus report of the European Society of Endocrine Surgeons. Langenbeck's Arch Surg. 2015;400(8):907–27.
70. Akaberi S, Clyne N, Sterner G, et al. Temporal trends and risk factors for parathyroidectomy in the Swedish dialysis and transplant population – a nationwide, population-based study 1991–2009. BMC Nephrol. 2014;15:75.
71. Isaksson E, Ivarsson K, Akaberi S, et al. The effect of parathyroidectomy on risk of hip fracture in secondary hyperparathyroidism. World J Surg. 2017;41(9):2304–11.
72. Ivarsson KM, Akaberi S, Isaksson E, et al. Cardiovascular and cerebrovascular events after parathyroidectomy in patients on renal replacement therapy. World J Surg. 2019;
73. Ivarsson KM, Akaberi S, Isaksson E, et al. The effect of parathyroidectomy on patient survival in secondary hyperparathyroidism. Nephrol Dial Transplant. 2015;30(12):2027–33.
74. van der Plas WY, Dulfer RR, Engelsman AF, et al. Effect of parathyroidectomy and cinacalcet on quality of life in patients with end-stage renal disease-related hyperparathyroidism: a systematic review. Nephrol Dial Transplant. 2017;32(11):1902–8.
75. Narayan R, Perkins RM, Berbano EP, et al. Parathyroidectomy versus cinacalcet hydrochloride-based medical therapy in the management of hyperparathyroidism in ESRD: a cost utility analysis. Am J Kidney Dis. 2007;49(6):801–13.
76. Kestenbaum B, Andress DL, Schwartz SM, et al. Survival following parathyroidectomy among United States dialysis patients. Kidney Int. 2004;66(5):2010–6.
77. Ishani A, Liu J, Wetmore JB, et al. Clinical outcomes after parathyroidectomy in a nationwide cohort of patients on hemodialysis. Clin J Am Soc Nephrol. 2015;10(1):90–7.
78. El-Husseini A, Wang K, Edon AA, Sawaya BP. Parathyroidectomy-A last resort for hyperparathyroidism in dialysis patients. Semin Dial. 2017;30(5):385–9.
79. Matsuoka S, Tominaga Y, Sato T, et al. QuiCk-IntraOperative Bio-Intact PTH assay at parathyroidectomy for secondary hyperparathyroidism. World J Surg. 2007;31(4):824–31.
80. Zhang L, Xing C, Shen C, et al. Diagnostic accuracy study of intraoperative and perioperative serum intact PTH level for successful parathyroidectomy in 501 secondary hyperparathyroidism patients. Sci Rep. 2016;6:26841.
81. Nigwekar SU, Sprague SM. We do too many parathyroidectomies for calciphylaxis. Semin Dial. 2016;29(4):312–4.
82. van der Plas WY, El Moumni M, von Forstner PJ, et al. Timing of parathyroidectomy does not influence renal function after kidney transplantation. World J Surg. 2019;43(8):1972–80.
83. Schwarz A, Rustien G, Merkel S, Radermacher J, Haller H. Decreased renal transplant function after parathyroidectomy. Nephrol Dial Transplant. 2007;22(2):584–91.
84. Akerstrom G, Malmaeus J, Bergstrom R. Surgical anatomy of human parathyroid glands. Surgery. 1984;95(1):14–21.

85. Alesina PF, Hinrichs J, Kribben A, Walz MK. Minimally invasive video-assisted parathyroidectomy (MIVAP) for secondary hyperparathyroidism: report of initial experience. Am J Surg. 2010;199(6):851–5.
86. Sun Y, Cai H, Bai J, Zhao H, Miao Y. Endoscopic total parathyroidectomy and partial parathyroid tissue autotransplantation for patients with secondary hyperparathyroidism: a new surgical approach. World J Surg. 2009;33(8):1674–9.
87. Barbaros U, Erbil Y, Yildirim A, Saricam G, Yazici H, Ozarmagan S. Minimally invasive video-assisted subtotal parathyroidectomy with thymectomy for secondary hyperparathyroidism. Langenbeck's Arch Surg. 2009;394(3):451–5.
88. Schneider R, Bartsch DK, Schlosser K. Relevance of bilateral cervical thymectomy in patients with renal hyperparathyroidism: analysis of 161 patients undergoing reoperative parathyroidectomy. World J Surg. 2013;37(9):2155–61.
89. Isaksson E, Ivarsson K, Akaberi S, et al. Total versus subtotal parathyroidectomy for secondary hyperparathyroidism. Surgery. 2019;165(1):142–50.
90. Chen J, Zhou QY, Wang JD. Comparison between subtotal parathyroidectomy and total parathyroidectomy with autotransplantation for secondary hyperparathyroidism in patients with chronic renal failure: a meta-analysis. Horm Metab Res. 2015;47(9):643–51.
91. Burgstaller T, Selberherr A, Brammen L, Scheuba C, Kaczirek K, Riss P. How radical is total parathyroidectomy in patients with renal hyperparathyroidism? Langenbeck's Arch Surg. 2018;403(8):1007–13.
92. Bergenfelz AO, Jansson SK, Wallin GK, et al. Impact of modern techniques on short-term outcome after surgery for primary hyperparathyroidism: a multicenter study comprising 2,708 patients. Langenbeck's Arch Surg. 2009;394(5):851–60.
93. Lou I, Foley D, Odorico SK, et al. How well does renal transplantation cure hyperparathyroidism? Ann Surg. 2015;262(4):653–9.
94. Schreinemakers JM, Pieterman CR, Scholten A, Vriens MR, Valk GD, Rinkes IH. The optimal surgical treatment for primary hyperparathyroidism in MEN1 patients: a systematic review. World J Surg. 2011;35(9):1993–2005.
95. Tentori F, Zepel L, Fuller DS, et al. The DOPPS practice monitor for US dialysis care: PTH levels and management of mineral and bone disorder in US hemodialysis patients. Am J Kidney Dis. 2015;66(3):536–9.
96. Marcadis AR, Teo R, Ouyang W, Farra JC, Lew JI. Successful parathyroidectomy guided by intraoperative parathyroid hormone monitoring for primary hyperparathyroidism is preserved in mild and moderate renal insufficiency. Surgery. 2018;163(3):633–7.
97. El-Husseini A, Wang K, Edon A, et al. Value of intraoperative parathyroid hormone assay during parathyroidectomy in dialysis and renal transplant patients with secondary and tertiary hyperparathyroidism. Nephron. 2018;138(2):119–28.
98. Sohn JA, Oltmann SC, Schneider DF, Sippel RS, Chen H, Elfenbein DM. Is intraoperative parathyroid hormone testing in patients with renal insufficiency undergoing parathyroidectomy for primary hyperparathyroidism accurate? Am J Surg. 2015;209(3):483–7.
99. Freriks K, Hermus AR, de Sevaux RG, et al. Usefulness of intraoperative parathyroid hormone measurements in patients with renal hyperparathyroidism. Head Neck. 2010;32(10):1328–35.
100. Meyer SK, Zorn M, Frank-Raue K, Buchler MW, Nawroth P, Weber T. Clinical impact of two different intraoperative parathyroid hormone assays in primary and renal hyperparathyroidism. Eur J Endocrinol. 2009;160(2):275–81.
101. Haustein SV, Mack E, Starling JR, Chen H. The role of intraoperative parathyroid hormone testing in patients with tertiary hyperparathyroidism after renal transplantation. Surgery. 2005;138(6):1066–71; discussion 1071.

102. Weber T, Zeier M, Hinz U, Schilling T, Buchler MW. Impact of intraoperative parathyroid hormone levels on surgical results in patients with renal hyperparathyroidism. World J Surg. 2005;29(9):1176–9.
103. Seehofer D, Rayes N, Ulrich F, et al. Intraoperative measurement of intact parathyroid hormone in renal hyperparathyroidism by an inexpensive routine assay. Langenbeck's Arch Surg. 2001;386(6):440–3.
104. Lokey J, Pattou F, Mondragon-Sanchez A, et al. Intraoperative decay profile of intact (1–84) parathyroid hormone in surgery for renal hyperparathyroidism–a consecutive series of 80 patients. Surgery. 2000;128(6):1029–34.
105. Dotzenrath C, Cupisti K, Goretzki E, et al. Operative treatment of renal autonomous hyperparathyroidism: cause of persistent or recurrent disease in 304 patients. Langenbeck's Arch Surg. 2003;387(9–10):348–54.
106. Taieb D, Urena-Torres P, Zanotti-Fregonara P, et al. Parathyroid scintigraphy in renal hyperparathyroidism: the added diagnostic value of SPECT and SPECT/CT. Clin Nucl Med. 2013;38(8):630–5.
107. Caldarella C, Treglia G, Pontecorvi A, Giordano A. Diagnostic performance of planar scintigraphy using (9)(9)mTc-MIBI in patients with secondary hyperparathyroidism: a meta-analysis. Ann Nucl Med. 2012;26(10):794–803.
108. Sukan A, Reyhan M, Aydin M, et al. Preoperative evaluation of hyperparathyroidism: the role of dual-phase parathyroid scintigraphy and ultrasound imaging. Ann Nucl Med. 2008;22(2):123–31.
109. Li P, Liu Q, Tang D, et al. Lesion based diagnostic performance of dual phase (99m)Tc-MIBI SPECT/CT imaging and ultrasonography in patients with secondary hyperparathyroidism. BMC Med Imaging. 2017;17(1):60.
110. Yuan LL, Kan Y, Ma DQ, Yang JG. Combined application of ultrasound and SPECT/CT has incremental value in detecting parathyroid tissue in SHPT patients. Diagn Interv Imaging. 2016;97(2):219–25.
111. Alkhalili E, Tasci Y, Aksoy E, et al. The utility of neck ultrasound and sestamibi scans in patients with secondary and tertiary hyperparathyroidism. World J Surg. 2015;39(3):701–5.
112. Karipineni F, Sahli Z, Somervell H, et al. Are preoperative sestamibi scans useful for identifying ectopic parathyroid glands in patients with expected multigland parathyroid disease? Surgery. 2018;163(1):35–41.
113. Cui L, Gao Y, Yu H, et al. Intraoperative parathyroid localization with near-infrared fluorescence imaging using indocyanine green during total parathyroidectomy for secondary hyperparathyroidism. Sci Rep. 2017;7(1):8193.
114. Vidal Fortuny J, Guigard S, Diaper J, Karenovics W, Triponez F. Subtotal parathyroidectomy under indocyanine green angiography. Video Endocrinol. 2016;3(1)
115. van der Plas WY, Dulfer RR, Koh EY, et al. Safety and efficacy of subtotal or total parathyroidectomy for patients with secondary or tertiary hyperparathyroidism in four academic centers in the Netherlands. Langenbeck's Arch Surg. 2018;403(8):999–1005.
116. Alsafran S, Sherman SK, Dahdaleh FS, et al. Preoperative calcitriol reduces postoperative intravenous calcium requirements and length of stay in parathyroidectomy for renal-origin hyperparathyroidism. Surgery. 2019;165(1):151–7.
117. Walsh NJ, Caten AJ, White JJ, Terris DJ. Protocol driven outcomes in renal parathyroid surgery. Head Neck. 2019;41(4):880–4.
118. Pasieka JL, Parsons LL. A prospective surgical outcome study assessing the impact of parathyroidectomy on symptoms in patients with secondary and tertiary hyperparathyroidism. Surgery. 2000;128(4):531–9.

Diagnosis and Surgical Management of Parathyroid Carcinoma

Angelica Silva-Figueroa and Nancy D. Perrier

Contents

A. L. Shifrin et al. (eds.), *Endocrine Surgery Comprehensive Board Exam Guide*,
https://doi.org/10.1007/978-3-030-84737-1_15

Case Presentation

The patient is 37-year-old woman who presented with a 1-month evolution headache associated with dizziness and irritability. Her past medical history showed no nephrolithiasis or fractures. She mentioned that she suffered from depression 1 year ago. No family history of cancer or hypercalcemia was reported. Her medications include omeprazole (40 mg per day) and sertraline (100 μg per day). She is an active smoker with five cigarettes per day for the previous 10 years. On physical examination, vital signs were within normal limits, thyroid was palpable and irregular, and dry skin was noted. No other physical findings were detected. She presented her recent serum laboratory tests from a medical check-up (she has no results from before this latest examination), which indicate calcium 15.3 mg/dl (3.82 mmol/L; normal, 8.5–10.2 mg/dl and 2.2–2.7 mmol/L); PTH 492.5 pg/ml (52.2 pmol/L; normal, 25–65 pg/ml and 1.6–6.9 pmol/L); creatinine 0.95 mg/dl (84 μmol/L; normal, 0.6–1.0 mg/dl and 45–90 μmol/L); phosphorus level within the normal range; and vitamin D25IH 22 ng/ml (54.9 nmol/L; normal, above 50 ng/ml and 125 nmol/L). Neck US showed displacement of the thyroid gland anteriorly in the right retrothyroid region and a solid hypoechogenic mass, with some cystic areas, of 24 × 26 × 18 mm, with marked peripheral and central radial vascular flow on color Doppler.

Questions

1. Which of the following are clinical criteria for suspected PC?
   1. PTH raised 3–10 times the normal value.
   2. Palpable cervical mass.
   3. Age younger than 55 years.
   4. Severe hypercalcemia.
   5. Findings of a parathyroid neoplasm larger than 3 cm and irregular edges.
      (a) Only (1) and (2) and (3) are correct.
      (b) Only (3) and (5) are correct.
      (c) Only (4) and (5) are correct.
      (d) Only (2) and (4) and (5) are correct.
      (e) All are correct.

15

2. In which of the following cases would you establish the diagnosis of PC?
   1. Unequivocal vascular invasion.
   2. Regional metastasis.
   3. Distant metastasis.
   4. Elevation of both serum calcium and serum PTH levels.
   5. Findings of a parathyroid adenoma on CT scan or neck US.
      (a) Only (1) and (2) and (3) are correct.
      (b) Only (3) and (5) are correct.
      (c) Only (4) and (5) are correct.
      (d) Only (2) and (4) and (5) are correct.
      (e) All are correct.

3. Which statement(s) regarding PC is correct?
   1. PC has a worldwide incidence rate of 6%.
   2. The prevalence of nephrological disturbances in PC reaches 32–60%.
   3. Detection of palpable cervical mass on physical examination is infrequent.
   4. Non-functional PC represents less than 5% of PCs.
   5. Most PCs are sporadic but have been described in HPT-JT syndrome, MEN1, and MEN2A.
      (a) Only (1) and (2) and (3) are correct.
      (b) Only (3) and (5) are correct.
      (c) Only (4) and (5) are correct.
      (d) Only (2) and (4) and (5) are correct.
      (e) All are correct.
4. What US findings are suggestive of PC?
   1. Hyperechogenic parathyroid tumor.
   2. Extracapsular to local invasion.
   3. Parathyroid tumor soft and compressible on US.
   4. Calcifications.
   5. Intralesional vessels with radial distribution.
      (a) Only (1) and (2) and (3) are correct.
      (b) Only (3) and (5) are correct.
      (c) Only (4) and (5) are correct.
      (d) Only (2) and (4) and (5) are correct.
      (e) All are correct.
5. Which statements regarding the management of a patient with PC are correct?
   1. The initial step is hydration with saline solutions to control moderate to severe hypercalcemia.
   2. Bisphosphonates are drugs of choice before surgical intervention.
   3. Cinacalcet should be used rarely in unresectable PCs owing to its ineffectiveness to reduce hypercalcemia.
   4. In cases refractory to bisphosphonates, denosumab may be used.
      (a) Only (1) and (2) and (3) are correct.
      (b) Only (1) and (2) and (4) are correct.
      (c) Only (1) and (3) and (4) are correct.
      (d) Only (2) and (3) and (4) are correct.
      (e) All are correct.
6. Which statements regarding the surgical management of patients with PC are correct?
   1. Parathyroidectomy is indicated for all patients with PC.
   2. En bloc resection is the treatment of choice.
   3. Cervical dissection should be performed only in the presence of documented regional metastases.
   4. Preservation of the recurrent laryngeal nerve is recommended.
      (a) Only (1) and (2) and (3) are correct.
      (b) Only (1) and (2) and (4) are correct.

(c) Only (1) and (3) and (4) are correct.
(d) Only (2) and (3) and (4) are correct.
(e) All are correct.

7. Which statements regarding the surgical management of patients with PC are correct?
   1. PC should be removed entirely with negative margins.
   2. The ipsilateral thyroid and isthmus should be removed.
   3. Rupture of the PC capsule should be avoided.
   4. All macroscopically compromised tissues or organs should be resected.
      (a) Only (1) and (2) and (3) are correct.
      (b) Only (1) and (2) and (4) are correct.
      (c) Only (1) and (3) and (4) are correct.
      (d) Only (2) and (3) and (4) are correct.
      (e) All are correct.
8. Which statements regarding non-functional (NF) PC are correct?
   1. NF PC is characterized by normal or slightly elevated PTH and calcium.
   2. Most NF PC present with a locally advanced cervical mass.
   3. The median size described is 9 cm.
   4. It is considered a poor prognostic factor, with survival of fewer than 3 years.
      (a) Only (1) and (2) and (3) are correct.
      (b) Only (1) and (2) and (4) are correct.
      (c) Only (1) and (3) and (4) are correct.
      (d) Only (2) and (3) and (4) are correct.
      (e) All are correct.
9. Which statements regarding prognostic factors for PC are correct?
   1. Vascular invasion is one of the most potent risk factors for death, and recurrence is described in the literature.
   2. The presence of metastases in PC dramatically decreases the 5-year overall survival rate from 87% to 16%.
   3. The absence of parafibromin staining in PC is an indicator of risk for recurrence and metastasis.
   4. The staging system in PC includes vascular invasion.
      (a) Only (1) and (2) and (3) are correct.
      (b) Only (1) and (2) and (4) are correct.
      (c) Only (1) and (3) and (4) are correct.
      (d) Only (2) and (3) and (4) are correct.
      (e) All are correct.
10. What should be done when detecting elevated PTH and calcium levels after en bloc resection for PC?
    1. Multimodal imaging study, including US + MIBI + PET/CT, looking for local or distant metastases.

2. It can include US + MIBI + PET/CT.
3. An imaging test is not justified, because, in these cases, neck exploration should be performed promptly.
4. It can include US + full-body MIBI.
   (a) Only (1) and (2) and (3) are correct.
   (b) Only (1) and (2) and (4) are correct.
   (c) Only (1) and (3) and (4) are correct.
   (d) Only (2) and (3) and (4) are correct.
   (e) All are correct.

15.1 Introduction

Parathyroid carcinoma (PC) is an infrequent cause of sporadic primary hyperparathyroidism (PHPT), with a worldwide incidence range between 1% and 5% [1–4]. PC is typically a sporadic endocrinopathy but might manifest as a familial component of PHPT known as hyperparathyroidism-jaw tumor (HPT-JT)x hyperparathyroidism-jaw tumor (HPT-JT) syndrome. Rare case reports have noted the possibility that PC might be expressed as a manifestation of multiple endocrine neoplasia type 1 (MEN1) or multiple endocrine neoplasia type 2A (MEN2A) [5–13]. Unlike benign PHPT, PC occurrence is equal between genders and generally clinically manifests a decade before the age of presentation of benign PHPT [4, 14–16]. Typically, PC produces excessive parathormone (PTH) and causes moderate or severe hypercalcemia, which is associated with the classic renal, bone, cardiac, and neurocognitive disturbances of the natural evolution associated with PHPT [14, 17, 18]. It is rarely possible to detect a PC with normal serum calcium and PTH; this is called non-functional PC (NF PC) and is characterized by local signs of a cervical mass [19, 20]. The diagnosis of PC in clinical practice is challenging, as preoperative suspicion can arise owing to non-specific biochemical elevations of PTH and serum calcium, as well as images that are insufficient to enable distinguishing between a benign and a malignant parathyroid tumor [17, 21]. Commonly, PC diagnosis is rendered only after intraoperative suspicion is corroborated by histopathology with certain immunohistochemical stains that is suggestive of disease [22]. The unequivocal diagnosis occurs with local recurrence or distant metastases upon clinical follow-up to the first surgical intervention. By definition, treatment is en bloc resection of the PC with all adjacent tissues involved, achieving negative margins [23]. It is critical for physicians and surgeons to maintain a high level of suspicion of parathyroid malignancy during the management of all PHPTs but especially in patients who present with severe hypercalcemia or a large parathyroid mass, which might be detected by imaging or during surgical exploration when firmness or invasion is noted.

15.2 Clinical Presentation

Unlike PHPT, PC is distributed equally between the genders [4, 15–17, 24]. In most literature reports, the median age of PC presentation fluctuates between 45 and 62 years old [15, 17, 24–26]. The clinical manifestations of PC are similar to PHPT and are secondary to the effects of the excessive presence of PTH, hypercalcemia, and/or invasive mass of the functional parathyroid tumor.

Signs and Symptoms Classic advanced clinical presentation is characterized by signs and symptoms secondary to severe hypercalcemia with nephrocalcinosis, nephrolithiasis, renal function failure, fibrous osteitis cystic, subperiosteal resorption, diffuse osteopenia, and skull "salt and pepper" [27–29]. The prevalence of kidney disturbances in patients with PC is between 32% and 60%, with nephrolithiasis (56%) and kidney failure (84%) being the most frequent renal manifestations [18, 30, 31]. PC is frequently associated with symptomatic hypercalcemia represented by nausea, vomiting, constipation, abdominal pain, fatigue, polydipsia, polyuria, disorientation, neurocognitive deficit, and myopathies [32]. It is relatively frequent (34%–69%) to detect a palpable cervical mass on physical examination, and, in some cases, dysphonia or dysphagia occurs [1, 27, 29, 32–38]. Acute pancreatitis develops in only 15% of PC cases [28].

Laboratory Before routine testing of serum calcium levels in general medicine, which occurred between 1960 and 1990, severe hypercalcemia (>14 mg/dl) was detected in 39–75% of PC cases, and it was often associated with acute kidney failure, cardiac arrhythmias, or secondary coma [27–29]. In recent reviews, the median calcium range at diagnosis is 12–14 mg/dl, and only 15% of PC cases present with severe hypercalcemia [17]. Serum levels of PTH between 3 and 10 times the normal value [1, 2, 17, 33] are also typical. In some reports, high levels of plasma and urinary human chorionic gonadotropin (hCG) were detected, suggesting that an elevated urinary hCG is highly suggestive of PC [39–41]. Comparisons between PC and benign parathyroid tumors have identified significant differences in alkaline phosphatase levels, with values greater than 480 IU/L in PC [42, 43].

Imaging Studies Because preoperative detection of PC is uncommon, the imaging findings described below are related to the images commonly used in the study of a PHPT to inform the surgical approach in targeted cases and to rule out concomitant thyroid disease. The images are often useful to locate the parathyroid tumor but are not capable of categorically discriminating between benign adenomas and PCs, unless the presence of metastasis is detected.

Neck Ultrasound The classic ultrasound (US) description of PC is a cervical mass adjacent to the thyroid tissue. This mass is very firm on compression; is non-homogeneous; is hypoechoic, with irregular or lobed edges; and occasionally contains a cystic component [44–49]. The echogenicity described for PC in the US varies, and it is affected by factors such as bleeding or necrosis, regardless of tumor size. Local invasion, extracapsular extension, parathyroid tumors larger than 3 cm, calcifications, intralesion vessels with radial distribution, and detection of regional metastases are all considered sonographic elements of malignancy in parathyroid tumors [17, 21, 46, 50–52]. In a US analysis of 16 PCs, 95% (15) of cases presented with a depth/width ratio (D/W r) of 1 or more. By comparison, US evaluation of 61 benign adenomas identified only 3% (3) with a D/W r of 1 or more [46].

Technetium-99 mm Sestamibi Scintigraphy Technetium-99 mm sestamibi scintigraphy (Tc-99m MIBI) US is typically prioritized in the assessment of parathyroid tumors in PHPT, primarily to detect single-gland disease [53]. However, the exact mechanism of Tc-99m evaluation for PC is unknown. Increased in intralesion blood flow and elevated mitochondrial activity might contribute to uptake of the isotope in PC, but it is not possible to discriminate a PC from a parathyroid adenoma based on this characteristic [54, 55]. Moreover, because it allows whole-body scanning, this technique can be used for recurrent PC at the primary site, as well as to detect distant metastases [56–59].

Multiphase Four-Dimensional Computed Tomography and Magnetic Resonance Imaging Both multiphase four-dimensional computed tomography (4DCT) and magnetic resonance imaging (MRI) might provide information about the extension of PC to adjacent tissues and distant or recurrent disease; however, 4DCT alone has a low sensitivity to detect PC [60, 61]. Compared to parathyroid carcinomas and parathyroid adenomas, PCs are associated with a slower washout rate when early and late arterial phases are compared by 4DCT analysis (−17%, $P < 0.05$) [49, 62]. In another study, univariate and bivariate analyses revealed arterial phase enhancement as the best parameter to differentiate between PCs and parathyroid adenomas using 4DCT ($P = 0.008$). The best independent predictors of PC were short-to-long axis ratio ($P = 0.0037$ vs. 0.133) and peritumoral infiltration ($P = 0.0037$ vs. 0.117) [52].

A report that assessed the ability to localize PC using US, 4DCT, or Tc-99m MIBI in 20 PC detected individual diagnostic acuities for each imaging test of 80%, 82%, and 95%, respectively. Moreover, combining all three modalities increased diagnostic accuracy to 100%, and combining either US and 4DCT or US and Tc-99m resulted in 88% and 82% accuracy, respectively [49].

Positron Emission Tomography/Computed Tomography with 18-Fluorodeoxyglucose Scanning Case reports describe the use of positron emission tomography/computed tomography with 18-fluorodeoxyglucose (18FDG-PET/CT) scanning to assess locoregional PC and distant hypermetabolic disease as well as recurrent or persistent disease at the clinical follow-up after the first surgical intervention [60, 63–67].

18F-Choline PET/CT 18F-choline PET/CT (18FC-PET/CT) is a promising tool to localize parathyroid adenomas preoperatively [68]. Some reports have identified locoregional invasiveness and distant PC dissemination using this approach [69, 70]. In a study by Deandreis et al., 18FC-PET/CT was used in conjunction with 18FDG-PET/CT to detect associated metastatic lesions not captured by 18FC-PET/CT alone [69].

Although laboratory or imaging studies are not sufficient for a definitive PC diagnosis, positive findings in the serum, urinary, and imaging analyses described above lead to a high suspicion of PC preoperatively.

15.3 Non Functional PC

Of all PC tumors, fewer than 5% are non-functional [19, 71–74], which refers to tumors of the parathyroid gland that are hormonally inactive, leading to both serum calcium and PTH levels that remain normal or only slightly elevated [74, 75]. NF PCs are typically unique and sporadic, although there is one report each in the literature of a double NF PC and an NF PC in the context of MEN2A [13, 76]. Patients with NF PC often develop a more advanced neoplastic disease compared to functional PC and signs and symptoms of distant metastasis in the absence of serologic abnormalities [73, 77–79]. In the literature since the first case description in 1929 indicates that the median size of NF PC lesions is 5 cm (range, 1.4–11 cm) [19, 71, 73, 76–81]. NF PC can be detected radiologically by Tc-99m MIBI scanning, neck US, and neck MRI [78, 82]. NF PC is associated with a poor prognosis and requires extensive surgical approaches, and patient survival does not exceed 25 months. These poor clinical outcomes likely reflect the advanced state of NF PC at the time of diagnosis, in addition to probably more aggressive and undifferentiated tumor biology [3, 73].

15.4 Natural History

Most PCs have an indolent growth phenotype, and clinical manifestations are secondary to PTH-related hypercalcemia, which, unlike benign etiology cases, is usually moderate to severe. At the time of PC diagnosis, the median tumor size is 3 cm [2, 15–17, 21], and fewer than 10% of cases present with regional metastasis [3, 15, 17, 21, 24, 80, 83]. Between 5% and 15% of PCs present with distant metastasis at the time of diagnosis, in the following order of frequency: lung, bone, liver, brain, pericardium, and pancreas [3, 25]. In pre-1990 reports, PC was associated with a 25% rate of distant metastasis at diagnosis [1, 28].

The median time to PC recurrence after the first surgical intervention is 3 years, although the range for this can be as wide as 20 years [2, 14, 18, 21, 29, 30, 32, 84]. Patients with PC generally undergo at least two to three surgical procedures during their disease [1, 30]. PC has a progressive course associated with a high rate of relapse after the first therapeutic intervention. Both local (21%) and distant (28%) recurrences are common, and both local and distant lesions recur together at a frequency of 14% [15, 17, 85]. Recurrence ranges rates reach 33–78%, with a 5-year survival rate of 78–91% and a 10-year survival rate of 49–72% [4, 15–17, 21, 25, 30, 86–88]. Most PC patients with recurrent disease after the first surgical intervention will eventually die of cancer-related metabolic complications of uncontrollable hypercalcemia [1, 89, 90].

15.5 Diagnosis

Preoperative, intraoperative, and histopathological diagnosis is challenging, but it is crucial to maintain a high level of suspicion when the factors most commonly related to the clinical presentation of PC (▪ Table 15.1) are identified.

Intraoperative Findings The classic macroscopic description of PC is a solitary and spherical tumor larger than 3 cm, irregular, attached to adjacent planes, hard, and surrounded by a dense fibrous reaction, which gives it its characteristic grayish white color [27, 28, 32, 34, 59, 91–94]. Local invasiveness is a clear indicator of malignancy during surgical resection, and the infiltration to adjacent tissues can be minimal to massive involving the ipsilateral thyroid gland, strap muscles, esophagus, trachea, recurrent laryngeal nerve, and/or great vessels of the neck (e.g., internal jugular vein) [18, 27, 28, 59, 95–97].

It is essential to consider the suspicion level as low when there is no macroscopic invasiveness to the adjacent tissues during neck exploration. Owing to its rarity, in the largest North American case-cohort, fewer than 38% of patients with PC underwent complete resection of the tumor with concomitant removal of involved tissue [4, 16, 17, 24], unlike Asian groups, where the incidence of PC is higher than in North America, and radical resection exceeds 60% [1, 25].

Table 15.1 PC versus benign parathyroid tumor: Summary of typical features

	Parathyroid carcinoma	Benign parathyroid tumor
General		
Female: Male r	1:1	3.5:1
Average age (yr)	48–50	59–62
CDC73/HRPT2 gen linked	>20%	Exceptionally rare
Laboratory		
Serum calcium (mg/dl)	12–16	11–12
Severe hypercalcemia	15%	Infrequent
Parathormone (PTH) level	3 to 10 times the upper normal limit	1,5 to 2,5 times the upper normal limit
Clinically		
Tumor size >3 cm	Frequently	Rare
Palpable neck mass	34–69%	Rare
Dysphonia	1–14%	–
Renal disturbances	30–60%	<18%
Bone disturbances	30–50%	<5%
Intraoperative findings		
Local invasion	Yes	No
Parathyroid gland (neoplasm)	Firm and lobulated	Soft and oval
Parathyroid gland color on inspection	White, dark red, gray	Yellow, tan, peanut butter
US findings		
Calcifications	Yes	No
Depth-width ratio ≥1	Yes	No
Local invasion	Yes	No
Lymphadenopathy	Yes	No
Irregular margins	Yes	No
Histopatological findings		
Lymphovascular invasion	Yes	No
Perineural invasion	Yes	No
Minimal or gross tissue or organ invasion	Yes	No

(continued)

Table 15.1 (continued)

	Parathyroid carcinoma	Benign parathyroid tumor
Regional or distant metastasis	Yes	No
Ancillary biomarkers		
Parafibromin complete loss	Yes	Rare
Galectin-3 overexpression	Yes	No
High proliferation rate, Ki67	Yes	Rare
Outcomes		
Locoregional recurrence after first surgical intervention	33–78%	NA
5-year overall survival	78–92%	NA
10-year overall survival	49–72%	NA
Develop distant metastasis	10–28%	NA

Histopathological Diagnosis Histopathology should be performed when unequivocal invasion of soft tissues; muscles or other adjacent organs (e.g., thyroid and internal jugular vein); lymphovasculature; or the perineural region is observed or when the presence of regional or distant metastases is detected [98, 99]. Histologically, the identification of significant cell groups with pleomorphism, high mitotic rate, coagulative necrosis, macronucleoli, and increased cell proliferation represent high-grade PC [100–102].

The clinical diagnosis of PC is confirmatory with local, regional, or metastatic invasion. In some cases, primarily in low-grade PC without the presence of gross invasiveness, a histopathologic distinction is challenging, which is largely owing to the shared histopathological characteristics between PC and its benign or atypical counterparts, including fibrous bands, trabecular pattern, fibrotic capsule, mitotic figures, necrosis, or adherence to adjacent tissues [100, 101, 103, 104]. Because it is essential to standardize the diagnosis, the International Collaboration on Cancer Reporting recently created a universal collection template for diagnostic gross and histopathological criteria to facilitate the reporting of this rare disease throughout the world [105].

Ancillary Biomarkers Considering that parathyroid tumors share histopathological similarities that can make benign and malignant disease indistinguishable in clinical and intraoperative scenarios, immunohistochemical biomarker panels can be used to provide additional information that is useful to achieve a definitive diagnosis of parathyroid tumors [22]. Parafibromin (PF) is a nuclear protein encoded by the *CDC73* gene. Germline mutations of *CDC73* define HPT-JT syndrome, where the risk of PC reaches 15%. These mutations have been detected in more than 70% of sporadic PCs [7, 106, 107]. Owing to its high specificity, PF has been widely used in combination with other biomarkers to increase the sensitivity of immunohistochemical analysis [108–110]. Immunohistochemistry panels to diagnose PC include at least three of the following biomarkers to increase the diagnostic accuracy with regard to differentiating PC from other parathyroid identities in limited cohorts. Useful biomarkers include galectin-3, PGP9.5, Ki67, retinoblastoma, E-cadherin, and bcl2, among others [110–113].

Fine-Needle Aspiration Biopsy Fine-needle aspiration (FNA) biopsy is generally not recommended in cases of suspected PC [1, 28]. There are at least three compelling reasons for this recommendation. First, diagnosis of PC, even with the complete specimen, is already challenging; therefore, attempting diagnosis using FNA is prone to false negatives [55, 59, 62, 114]. Second, there is an established risk of dermal or subcutaneous spread upon rupturing of the PC capsule [96, 115], and, although the incidence of dissemination secondary to FNA in different cancer types is less than 0.005%, in PC, these events would affect the oncological prognosis [116, 117]. Third, FNA is not essential in the study of PHPT, and the only context in which FNA or core biopsy is recommended in the study of PC is before a radical surgical procedure when metastatic disease is suspected [59, 62, 118–121].

15.6 Treatment

15.6.1 Medical Treatment

The primary objective of clinical management of PC is to control serum calcium levels preoperatively and to correct all secondary metabolic alterations. Initial steps include hydration with saline solutions and then incorporation of specific drugs to control hypercalcemia [58, 122, 123]. Bisphosphonates, such as pamidronate and zoledronate, inhibit osteoclastic activity and are considered first-line treatment to control severe hypercalcemia, albeit slowly and temporarily [58, 122, 123]. In cases refractory to bisphosphonates, denosumab, which is a monoclonal antibody targeting receptor activator of nuclear factor kB ligand (RANKL), can be used to decrease bone resorption via osteoclastic activity for several months [124, 125]. In unresectable PCs, calcimimetics have shown some effectiveness to control hypercalcemia by binding to the calcium-sensing receptor (CASR) on parathyroid cells, which hypersensitizes the receptors to extracellular calcium [126–129]. Cinacalcet is a highly effective CASR modulator that has been shown to effectively reduce serum hypercalcemia in two-thirds of unresectable PC cases [15, 128, 129].

15.6.2 Surgical Treatment

Complete surgical resection is unequivocally the treatment of choice owing to its curative potential for PC [3, 18, 21, 28, 84, 130–132].

Primary PC Tumor En bloc surgical resection of the primary tumor should avoid capsular rupture while removing all compromised structures to ensure tumor-cell-free margins after the first surgical intervention [3, 16, 23, 80, 87, 91, 120, 133, 134]. By definition, en bloc resection consists of complete removal of the PC next to the ipsilateral thyroid lobe, isthmus, and compromised pre-thyroid muscles as well as central lymph node dissection [83, 135]. Dissection of the central cervical lymph node is not recommended in the absence of suspicion of regional disease. Although central cervical lymph node dissection is associated with a low rate of regional metastasis, all data regarding outcomes from this procedure are retrospective, and it is not clear that it improves survival outcomes or reduces the risk of recurrence; therefore, central cervical lymph node dissection is not recommended unless regional disease is suspected [84, 136]. One exception where central cervical lymph node dissection may be considered is in PC larger than 3 cm, owing to its higher probability of regionally metastatic disease [133]. Modified radical neck dissection and simple parathyroidectomy are not recommended [3, 83]. Preservation of the recurrent laryngeal nerve is recommended, and its sacrifice should be considered only in cases of obvious neoplastic involvement [1, 137]. Although initial resection might be extensive if surrounding structures are involved, the benefit is evident, as shown in ◘ Fig. 15.1.

Preoperative suspicion of PC, intraoperative recognition, and surgeon experience are highly relevant to achieving adequate initial surgical management [16, 25]. Incomplete resection is associated as one would expect with increased risk of recurrence, but any surgical resection, regardless of its extent, reduces the risk of death [16, 17, 24, 102, 132, 138, 139]. In cases of incomplete resection, complete en bloc resection is indicated to reduce recurrence and rule out distant disease, particularly in cases with extensive capsular, vascular, or perineural invasion, or when high PTH and calcium persist postoperatively [15, 97].

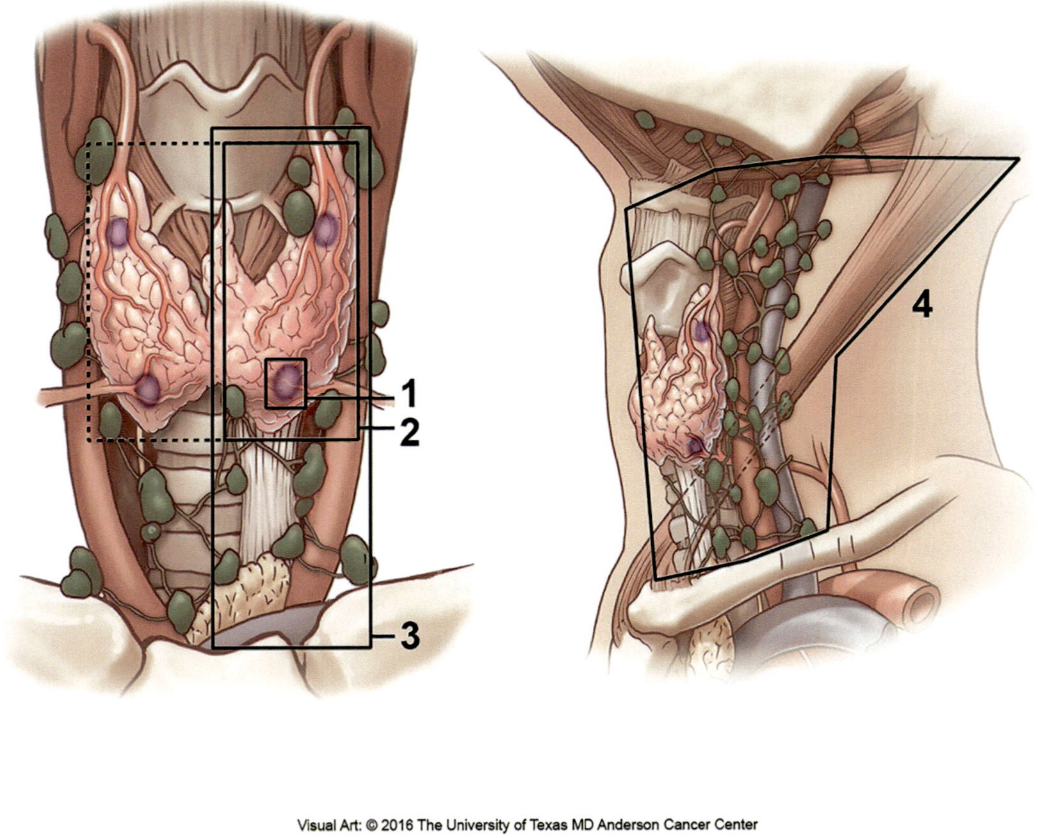

Fig. 15.1 Schematic of en bloc resection and its surgical derivations described in PC: (1) parathyroidectomy; (2) parathyroidectomy with lobectomy or thyroidectomy; (3) en bloc (ipsilateral level VI); and (4) compartment-oriented modified lateral neck dissection

In patients with *CDC73* or *MEN1* germline mutations who develop PC, bilateral cervical exploration, and en bloc resection of the identified PC are standard clinical management [15, 131].

Recurrences and Metastatic Disease It is important to identify the precise location of recurrent disease with multimodal imaging studies before subsequent operation [60, 121]. 4DCT, US, Tc-99m MIBI, PET/CT, and MRI can be used in combination to evaluate local and regional recurrence and distant metastases. FNA biopsy can be used for preoperative confirmation of distant metastatic lesions [1]. Neck recurrence should be treated with wide resection of the compromised area, including involved lymph nodes. Distant metastases should be resected if possible [1, 18, 31, 37, 97, 119, 133]. Even in the case of multiple surgical interventions, resection is rarely curative. Metastasectomies, in some cases, can normalize serum calcium levels for a period of time or make hypercalcemia more manageable with medical treatment [17, 60, 119, 121, 131, 140].

15.6.3 Chemotherapy

The use of chemotherapy appears in isolated reports in the context of recurrent or unresectable metastatic PC, but there is no standardized protocol for its use, and oncological benefit has not been demonstrated [24, 31, 32, 141, 142]. Regimens that have been reported include dacarbazine-based monotherapy or dacarbazine in combination with other chemotherapeutic drugs: fluorouracil, cyclophosphamide, methotrexate, lomustine, and doxorubicin [121].

It is essential to note the reports of relatively fast but temporary control of hypercalcemia by the tyrosine kinase inhibitor sorafenib in patients with recurrent or metastatic PC [15, 121, 143–145]. The latest advances in the systemic treatment of PC are focused on genomic sequencing to recognize mutations that might make tumors amenable to targeted therapies [145, 146].

15.6.4 Radiotherapy

Radiotherapy (RT) has been used historically in PC cases with unresectable residual disease, advanced disease, unresectable recurrence, or bone metastases where other therapeutic options are not possible [3, 89, 147–150]. However, no benefit of RT to overall survival has been demonstrated [4, 16, 31, 119, 121, 151, 152]. The consensus of treatment for recurrence is surgical resection, which, in the case of PC, is associated with multiple surgical risks involved; therefore, RT could be an option for those patients with recurrent disease who are not candidates for surgical re-intervention [87, 121, 151]. Limberg et al. recently published a multivariate analysis and inverse probability weighting adjustment of overall survival from the National Cancer Database Analysis of patients with PC who received RT [151]. In this cohort of 885 patients with PC, 14.2% underwent adjuvant RT owing to extensive regional disease, regional metastases, residual disease, or positive margins. The authors also confirmed that, according to both their multivariate analysis and inverse probability weighting assessment, RT offered no overall survival benefit to patients with PC [151].

15.7 Prognostic Factors

There is currently no validated staging system for PC, but multiple prognostic factors have been reported in the last decade that aim to stratify the risk of recurrence, progression, and death [15]. The most frequently reported prognostic factors associated with poor clinical outcomes include male gender, high calcium levels (>15 mg/dl), positive margins, advanced age (>65 years), and regional or distant metastases [16, 17, 23, 30, 37, 119, 133, 153]. In a retrospective series published in 2019, the effect of distant metastases in PC was evaluated, which demonstrated a 5-year overall survival rate of 16% in patients with metastatic PC versus 87% in patients with local or regional disease, and a death hazard ratio (HR) of 9.6 (95% confidence interval [CI], 4.2–22.3; $P < 0.0001$) [154].

One of the most highly predictive independent risk factors of death and distant metastasis, which is also associated with poor prognosis, is histopathological finding of unequivocal vascular invasion, which carries a four-fold higher risk of death or recurrence(s) at 5 years [17, 30, 155]. Also, a recent meta-analysis of immunostaining of PF in PC showed that the absence of PF staining is an indicator of recurrence/metastasis and death in patients with PC (HR = 2.73 and $P = 0.002$; HR = 2.54 and $P = 0.004$, respectively) [156].

15.8 Clinical Follow-Up

The clinical follow-up of patients with PC should be periodic and long term. Even in the absence of standardized guidelines, in the context of a high rate of recurrence in the 3 years after the first surgical intervention (primarily locoregional), serum calcium and PTH should be monitored every 6 months, and imaging follow-up (neck US or 4DCT) is also indicated. After the first 3 years, annual assessment of serum calcium and PTH is recommended to detect relapse [15, 31, 141]. More frequent clinical follow-up of PC patients with a high risk of relapse or death owing to the presence of the previously mentioned prognostic factors is also recommended [15, 17, 30]. For patients with NF PC, clinical follow-up should focus on periodic imaging.

Upon detection of rising serum calcium and PTH levels, systemic multimodal imaging study (US, MIBI, 4DCT, PET/CT, and MRI) is suggested, as no single image alone can detect recurrence, persistence, or distant metastasis [66, 152].

Answers to the Questions

1. (e); 2. (a); 3. (d); 4. (d); 5. (b); 6. (d); 7. (e); 8. (b); 9. (a); 10. (b)

References

1. Obara T, Fujimoto Y. Diagnosis and treatment of patients with parathyroid carcinoma: an update and review. World J Surg. 1991;15(6):738–44.
2. Favia G, Lumachi F, Polistina F, D'Amico DF. Parathyroid carcinoma: sixteen new cases and suggestions for correct management. World J Surg. 1998;22(12):1225–30. https://doi.org/10.1007/s002689900549.
3. Koea JB, Shaw JH. Parathyroid cancer: biology and management. Surg Oncol. 1999;8(3):155–65.

4. Lee PK, Jarosek SL, Virnig BA, Evasovich M, Tuttle TM. Trends in the incidence and treatment of parathyroid cancer in the United States. Cancer. 2007;109(9):1736–41. https://doi.org/10.1002/cncr.22599.
5. Howell VM, Haven CJ, Kahnoski K, Khoo SK, Petillo D, Chen J, et al. HRPT2 mutations are associated with malignancy in sporadic parathyroid tumours. J Med Genet. 2003;40(9):657–63.
6. Chen JD, Morrison C, Zhang C, Kahnoski K, Carpten JD, Teh BT. Hyperparathyroidism-jaw tumour syndrome. J Intern Med. 2003;253(6):634–42.
7. Cetani F, Pardi E, Borsari S, Viacava P, Dipollina G, Cianferotti L, et al. Genetic analyses of the HRPT2 gene in primary hyperparathyroidism: germline and somatic mutations in familial and sporadic parathyroid tumors. J Clin Endocrinol Metab. 2004;89(11):5583–91. https://doi.org/10.1210/jc.2004-0294.
8. Sharretts JM, Simonds WF. Clinical and molecular genetics of parathyroid neoplasms. Best Pract Res Clin Endocrinol Metab. 2010;24(3):491–502. https://doi.org/10.1016/j.beem.2010.01.003.
9. Mehta A, Patel D, Rosenberg A, Boufraqech M, Ellis RJ, Nilubol N, et al. Hyperparathyroidism-jaw tumor syndrome: results of operative management. Surgery. 2014;156(6):1315–24.; discussion 24–5. https://doi.org/10.1016/j.surg.2014.08.004.
10. Singh Ospina N, Sebo TJ, Thompson GB, Clarke BL, Young WF Jr. Prevalence of parathyroid carcinoma in 348 patients with multiple endocrine neoplasia type 1 – case report and review of the literature. Clin Endocrinol. 2016;84(2):244–9. https://doi.org/10.1111/cen.12714.
11. Christakis I, Busaidy NL, Cote GJ, Williams MD, Hyde SM, Silva Figueroa AM, et al. Parathyroid carcinoma and atypical parathyroid neoplasms in MEN1 patients; a clinico-pathologic challenge. The MD Anderson case series and review of the literature. Int J Surg. 2016;31:10–6. https://doi.org/10.1016/j.ijsu.2016.05.035.
12. Jenkins PJ, Satta MA, Simmgen M, Drake WM, Williamson C, Lowe DG, et al. Metastatic parathyroid carcinoma in the MEN2A syndrome. Clin Endocrinol 1997;47(6):747–51.
13. Alfaro JJ, Lamas C, Estrada J, Lucas T. MEN-2A syndrome and pulmonary metastasis. Postgrad Med J. 2002;78(915):51–2. https://doi.org/10.1136/pmj.78.915.51.
14. Obara T, Okamoto T, Kanbe M, Iihara M. Functioning parathyroid carcinoma: clinicopathologic features and rational treatment. Semin Surg Oncol. 1997;13(2):134–41.
15. Rodrigo JP, Hernandez-Prera JC, Randolph GW, Zafereo ME, Hartl DM, Silver CE, et al. Parathyroid cancer: an update. Cancer Treat Rev. 2020;86:102012. https://doi.org/10.1016/j.ctrv.2020.102012.
16. Asare EA, Sturgeon C, Winchester DJ, Liu L, Palis B, Perrier ND, et al. Parathyroid carcinoma: an update on treatment outcomes and prognostic factors from the National Cancer Data Base (NCDB). Ann Surg Oncol. 2015;22(12):3990–5. https://doi.org/10.1245/s10434-015-4672-3.
17. Talat N, Schulte KM. Clinical presentation, staging and long-term evolution of parathyroid cancer. Ann Surg Oncol. 2010;17(8):2156–74. https://doi.org/10.1245/s10434-010-1003-6.
18. Shane E. Clinical review 122: parathyroid carcinoma. J Clin Endocrinol Metab. 2001;86(2):485–93. https://doi.org/10.1210/jcem.86.2.7207.
19. Wilkins BJ, Lewis JS Jr. Non-functional parathyroid carcinoma: a review of the literature and report of a case requiring extensive surgery. Head Neck Pathol. 2009;3(2):140–9. https://doi.org/10.1007/s12105-009-0115-4.
20. Wang L, Han D, Chen W, Zhang S, Wang Z, Li K, et al. Non-functional parathyroid carcinoma: a case report and review of the literature. Cancer Biol Ther. 2015;16(11):1569–76. https://doi.org/10.1080/15384047.2015.1070989.
21. Hundahl SA, Fleming ID, Fremgen AM, Menck HR. Two hundred eighty-six cases of parathyroid carcinoma treated in the U.S. between

1985-1995: a National Cancer Data Base Report. The American College of Surgeons Commission on Cancer and the American Cancer Society. Cancer. 1999;86(3):538–44.

22. Erickson LA, Mete O. Immunohistochemistry in diagnostic parathyroid pathology. Endocr Pathol. 2018;29(2):113–29. https://doi.org/10.1007/s12022-018-9527-6.
23. Schulte KM, Talat N, Galata G, Gilbert J, Miell J, Hofbauer LC, et al. Oncologic resection achieving r0 margins improves disease-free survival in parathyroid cancer. Ann Surg Oncol. 2014;21(6):1891–7. https://doi.org/10.1245/s10434-014-3530-z.
24. Sadler C, Gow KW, Beierle EA, Doski JJ, Langer M, Nuchtern JG, et al. Parathyroid carcinoma in more than 1,000 patients: a population-level analysis. Surgery. 2014;156(6):1622–9.; discussion 9–30. https://doi.org/10.1016/j.surg.2014.08.069.
25. Wang P, Xue S, Wang S, Lv Z, Meng X, Wang G, et al. Clinical characteristics and treatment outcomes of parathyroid carcinoma: a retrospective review of 234 cases. Oncol Lett. 2017;14(6):7276–82. https://doi.org/10.3892/ol.2017.7076.
26. Marcocci C, Cetani F, Rubin MR, Silverberg SJ, Pinchera A, Bilezikian JP. Parathyroid carcinoma. J Bone Miner Res. 2008;23(12):1869–80. https://doi.org/10.1359/jbmr.081018.
27. Holmes EC, Morton DL, Ketcham AS. Parathyroid carcinoma: a collective review. Ann Surg. 1969;169(4):631–40.
28. Fujimoto Y, Obara T. How to recognize and treat parathyroid carcinoma. Surg Clin North Am. 1987;67(2):343–57.
29. Levin KE, Galante M, Clark OH. Parathyroid carcinoma versus parathyroid adenoma in patients with profound hypercalcemia. Surgery. 1987;101(6):649–60.
30. Silva-Figueroa AM, Hess KR, Williams MD, Clarke CN, Christakis I, Graham PH, et al. Prognostic scoring system to risk stratify parathyroid carcinoma. J Am Coll Surg. 2017; https://doi.org/10.1016/j.jamcollsurg.2017.01.060.
31. Christakis I, Silva AM, Kwatampora LJ, Warneke CL, Clarke CN, Williams MD, et al. Oncologic progress for the treatment of parathyroid carcinoma is needed. J Surg Oncol. 2016; https://doi.org/10.1002/jso.24407.
32. Wynne AG, van Heerden J, Carney JA, Fitzpatrick LA. Parathyroid carcinoma: clinical and pathologic features in 43 patients. Medicine (Baltimore). 1992;71(4):197–205.
33. Shane E, Bilezikian JP. Parathyroid carcinoma: a review of 62 patients. Endocr Rev. 1982;3(2):218–26. https://doi.org/10.1210/edrv-3-2-218.
34. Wang CA, Gaz RD. Natural history of parathyroid carcinoma. Diagnosis, treatment, and results. Am J Surg. 1985;149(4):522–7.
35. Fujimoto Y, Obara T, Ito Y, Kodama T, Nobori M, Ebihara S. Localization and surgical resection of metastatic parathyroid carcinoma. World J Surg. 1986;10(4):539–47. https://doi.org/10.1007/BF01655520.
36. Vieira JG, Ohe MN, Hauache OM, Oliveira UM, Delana JM, Goncalves A, et al. Parathyroid carcinoma. Arq Bras Endocrinol Metabol. 2005;49(5):811–5. https://doi.org/10.1590/s0004-27302005000500023.
37. Schaapveld M, Jorna FH, Aben KKH, Haak HR, Plukker JTM, Links TP. Incidence and prognosis of parathyroid gland carcinoma: a population-based study in The Netherlands estimating the preoperative diagnosis. Am J Surg. 2011;202(5):590–7.
38. Duan K, Mete O. Parathyroid carcinoma: diagnosis and clinical implications. Turk Patoloji Derg. 2015;31(Suppl 1):80–97. https://doi.org/10.5146/tjpath.2015.01316.
39. Stock JL, Weintraub BD, Rosen SW, Aurbach GD, Spiegel AM, Marx SJ. Human chorionic gonadotropin subunit measurement in primary hyperparathyroidism. J Clin Endocrinol Metab. 1982;54(1):57–63. https://doi.org/10.1210/jcem-54-1-57.

40. Rubin MR, Bilezikian JP, Birken S, Silverberg SJ. Human chorionic gonadotropin measurements in parathyroid carcinoma. Eur J Endocrinol. 2008;159(4):469–74. https://doi.org/10.1530/EJE-08-0169.
41. Gupta SP, Mittal A, Sathian B. Significance of HCG to distinguish parathyroid carcinoma from benign disease and in adding prognostic information: a hospital based study from Nepal. Asian Pac J Cancer Prev. 2013;14(1):325–7. https://doi.org/10.7314/apjcp.2013.14.1.325.
42. Chen Q, Kaji H, Nomura R, Sowa H, Yamauchi M, Tsukamoto T, et al. Trial to predict malignancy of affected parathyroid glands in primary hyperparathyroidism. Endocr J. 2003;50(5):527–34. https://doi.org/10.1507/endocrj.50.527.
43. Bae JH, Choi HJ, Lee Y, Moon MK, Park YJ, Shin CS, et al. Preoperative predictive factors for parathyroid carcinoma in patients with primary hyperparathyroidism. J Korean Med Sci. 2012;27(8):890–5. https://doi.org/10.3346/jkms.2012.27.8.890.
44. Kinoshita Y, Fukase M, Uchihashi M, Takenaka M, Hishikawa R, Nakada M, et al. Significance of preoperative use of ultrasonography in parathyroid neoplasms: comparison of sonographic textures with histologic findings. J Clin Ultrasound. 1985;13(7):457–60. https://doi.org/10.1002/jcu.1870130704.
45. Edmonson GR, Charboneau JW, James EM, Reading CC, Grant CS. Parathyroid carcinoma: high-frequency sonographic features. Radiology. 1986;161(1):65–7. https://doi.org/10.1148/radiology.161.1.3532184.
46. Hara H, Igarashi A, Yano Y, Yashiro T, Ueno E, Aiyoshi Y, et al. Ultrasonographic features of parathyroid carcinoma. Endocr J. 2001;48(2):213–7. https://doi.org/10.1507/endocrj.48.213.
47. Tamler R, Lewis MS, LiVolsi VA, Genden EM. Parathyroid carcinoma: ultrasonographic and histologic features. Thyroid. 2005;15(7):744–5. https://doi.org/10.1089/thy.2005.15.744.
48. Fakhran S, Branstetter BF, Pryma DA. Parathyroid imaging. Neuroimaging Clin N Am. 2008;18(3):537–49., ix. https://doi.org/10.1016/j.nic.2008.03.006.
49. Christakis I, Vu T, Chuang HH, Fellman B, Figueroa AMS, Williams MD, et al. The diagnostic accuracy of neck ultrasound, 4D-computed tomographyand sestamibi imaging in parathyroid carcinoma. Eur J Radiol. 2017;95:82–8. https://doi.org/10.1016/j.ejrad.2017.07.026.
50. Sidhu PS, Talat N, Patel P, Mulholland NJ, Schulte KM. Ultrasound features of malignancy in the preoperative diagnosis of parathyroid cancer: a retrospective analysis of parathyroid tumours larger than 15 mm. Eur Radiol. 2011;21(9):1865–73. https://doi.org/10.1007/s00330-011-2141-3.
51. Nam M, Jeong HS, Shin JH. Differentiation of parathyroid carcinoma and adenoma by preoperative ultrasonography. Acta Radiol. 2017;58(6):670–5. https://doi.org/10.1177/0284185116666418.
52. Takumi K, Fukukura Y, Hakamada H, Nagano H, Kumagae Y, Arima H, et al. CT features of parathyroid carcinomas: comparison with benign parathyroid lesions. Jpn J Radiol. 2019;37(5):380–9. https://doi.org/10.1007/s11604-019-00825-3.
53. Chen H, Mack E, Starling JR. A comprehensive evaluation of perioperative adjuncts during minimally invasive parathyroidectomy: which is most reliable? Ann Surg. 2005;242(3):375–80.; discussion 80–3. https://doi.org/10.1097/01.sla.0000179622.37270.36.
54. Kitapci MT, Tastekin G, Turgut M, Caner B, Kars A, Barista I, et al. Preoperative localization of parathyroid carcinoma using Tc-99m MIBI. Clin Nucl Med. 1993;18(3):217–9. https://doi.org/10.1097/00003072-199303000-00007.
55. Thompson SD, Prichard AJ. The management of parathyroid carcinoma. Curr Opin Otolaryngol Head Neck Surg. 2004;12(2):93–7.
56. Aso Y, Sato A, Tayama K, Takanashi K, Satoh H, Takemura Y. Parathyroid carcinoma with metastatic calcification identified by

technetium-99m methylene diphosphonate scintigraphy. Intern Med. 1996;35(5):392–5. https://doi.org/10.2169/internalmedicine.35.392.

57. Al-Sobhi S, Ashari LH, Ingemansson S. Detection of metastatic parathyroid carcinoma with Tc-99m sestamibi imaging. Clin Nucl Med. 1999;24(1):21–3. https://doi.org/10.1097/00003072-199901000-00005.

58. Rodgers SE, Perrier ND. Parathyroid carcinoma. Curr Opin Oncol. 2006;18(1):16–22.

59. Kassahun WT, Jonas S. Focus on parathyroid carcinoma. Int J Surg (London, England). 2011;9(1):13–9. https://doi.org/10.1016/j.ijsu.2010.09.003.

60. Kebebew E, Arici C, Duh QY, Clark OH. Localization and reoperation results for persistent and recurrent parathyroid carcinoma. Arch Surg. 2001;136(8):878–85.

61. Clark P, Wooldridge T, Kleinpeter K, Perrier N, Lovato J, Morton K. Providing optimal preoperative localization for recurrent parathyroid carcinoma: a combined parathyroid scintigraphy and computed tomography approach. Clin Nucl Med. 2004;29(11):681–4. https://doi.org/10.1097/00003072-200411000-00001.

62. Mohebati A, Shaha A, Shah J. Parathyroid carcinoma: challenges in diagnosis and treatment. Hematol Oncol Clin North Am. 2012;26(6):1221–38. https://doi.org/10.1016/j.hoc.2012.08.009.

63. Evangelista L, Sorgato N, Torresan F, Boschin IM, Pennelli G, Saladini G, et al. FDG-PET/CT and parathyroid carcinoma: review of literature and illustrative case series. World J Clin Oncol. 2011;2(10):348–54. https://doi.org/10.5306/wjco.v2.i10.348.

64. Neumann DR, Esselstyn CB, Siciliano D, MacIntyre WJ, Kohse LM, Licata AA. Preoperative imaging of parathyroid carcinoma by positron emission tomography. Ann Otol Rhinol Laryngol. 1994;103(9):741–5.

65. Neumann DR, Esselstyn CB, Kim EY. Recurrent postoperative parathyroid carcinoma: FDG-PET and sestamibi-SPECT findings. J Nucl Med. 1996;37(12):2000–1.

66. Gardner CJ, Wieshmann H, Gosney J, Carr HM, Macfarlane IA, Cuthbertson DJ. Localization of metastatic parathyroid carcinoma by 18F FDG PET scanning. J Clin Endocrinol Metab. 2010;95(11):4844–5. https://doi.org/10.1210/jc.2010-1479.

67. Arslan N, Rydzewski B. Detection of a recurrent parathyroid carcinoma with FDG positron emission tomography. Clin Nucl Med. 2002;27(3):221–2.

68. Cuderman A, Senica K, Rep S, Hocevar M, Kocjan T, Sever MJ, et al. (18)F-Fluorocholine PET/CT in primary hyperparathyroidism: superior diagnostic performance to conventional Scintigraphic imaging for localization of Hyperfunctioning parathyroid glands. J Nucl Med. 2020;61(4):577–83. https://doi.org/10.2967/jnumed.119.229914.

69. Deandreis D, Terroir M, Al Ghuzlan A, Berdelou A, Lacroix L, Bidault F, et al. (1)(8)Fluorocholine PET/CT in parathyroid carcinoma: a new tool for disease staging? Eur J Nucl Med Mol Imaging. 2015;42(12):1941–2. https://doi.org/10.1007/s00259-015-3130-6.

70. Morand GB, Helmchen BM, Steinert HC, Schmid C, Broglie MA. 18F-choline-PET in parathyroid carcinoma. Oral Oncol. 2018;86:314–5. https://doi.org/10.1016/j.oraloncology.2018.09.009.

71. Sieracki JC, Horn RC Jr. Nonfunctional carcinoma of the parathyroid. Cancer. 1960;13:502–6. https://doi.org/10.1002/1097--0142(196005/06)13:3<502::aid-cncr2820130312>3.0.co;2-r.

72. Ordonez NG, Ibanez ML, Samaan NA, Hickey RC. Immunoperoxidase study of uncommon parathyroid tumors. Report of two cases of nonfunctioning parathyroid carcinoma and one intrathyroid parathyroid tumor-producing amyloid. Am J Surg Pathol. 1983;7(6):535–42. https://doi.org/10.1097/00000478-198309000-00004.

73. Gao WC, Ruan CP, Zhang JC, Liu HM, Xu XY, Sun YP, et al. Nonfunctional parathyroid carcinoma. J Cancer Res Clin Oncol. 2010;136(7):969–74. https://doi.org/10.1007/s00432-009-0740-z.
74. Aldinger KA, Hickey RC, Ibanez ML, Samaan NA. Parathyroid carcinoma – a clinical-study of 7 cases of functioning and 2 cases of nonfunctioning parathyroid cancer. Cancer. 1982;49(2):388–97. https://doi.org/10.1002/1097-0142(19820115)49:2<388::Aid-Cncr2820490230>3.0.Co;2-F.
75. Klink BK, Karulf RE, Maimon WN, Peoples JB. Nonfunctioning parathyroid carcinoma. Am Surg. 1991;57(7):463–7.
76. Dikmen K, Bostanci H, Gobut H, Yildiz A, Ertunc O, Celik A, et al. Nonfunctional double parathyroid carcinoma with incidental thyroid micropapillary carcinoma: a rare case. Pan Afr Med J. 2017;27:241. https://doi.org/10.11604/pamj.2017.27.241.11503.
77. Messerer CL, Bugis SP, Baliski C, Wiseman SM. Normocalcemic parathyroid carcinoma: an unusual clinical presentation. World J Surg Oncol. 2006;4:10. https://doi.org/10.1186/1477-7819-4-10.
78. Nakamura Y, Kataoka H, Sakoda T, Horie Y, Kitano H. Nonfunctional parathyroid carcinoma. Int J Clin Oncol. 2010;15(5):500–3. https://doi.org/10.1007/s10147-010-0062-9.
79. Guo H, Mai R, Liu M, Peng H, Yang X, Wu M, et al. Nonfunctional parathyroid carcinoma after breast carcinoma. J Clin Oncol. 2013;31(9):e122–4. https://doi.org/10.1200/JCO.2012.44.7227.
80. Stephenson HU, Jr. Malignant tumors of the parathyroid glands; a review of the literature with report of a case. Arch Surg. 1950;60(2):247–66, illust. https://doi.org/10.1001/archsurg.1950.01250010265005.
81. Posada-Gonzalez M, Gomez-Ramirez J, Luque-Ramirez M, Guijarro M, Martin-Perez E, Rodriguez-Sanchez A, et al. Nonfunctional metastatic parathyroid carcinoma in the setting of multiple endocrine Neoplasia type 2A syndrome. Surg Res Pract. 2014;2014:731481. https://doi.org/10.1155/2014/731481.
82. Ashkenazi D, Elmalah I, Rakover Y, Luboshitzky R. Concurrent nonfunctioning parathyroid carcinoma and parathyroid adenoma. Am J Otolaryngol. 2006;27(3):204–6. https://doi.org/10.1016/j.amjoto.2005.01.006.
83. Schulte KM, Talat N, Miell J, Moniz C, Sinha P, Diaz-Cano S. Lymph node involvement and surgical approach in parathyroid cancer. World J Surg. 2010;34(11):2611–20. https://doi.org/10.1007/s00268-010-0722-y.
84. Kebebew E. Parathyroid carcinoma. Curr Treat Options in Oncol. 2001;2(4):347–54.
85. Sandelin K, Tullgren O, Farnebo LO. Clinical course of metastatic parathyroid cancer. World J Surg. 1994;18(4):594–9.
86. Sandelin K, Auer G, Bondeson L, Grimelius L, Farnebo LO. Prognostic factors in parathyroid cancer – a review of 95 cases. World J Surg. 1992;16(4):724–31.
87. Givi B, Shah JP. Parathyroid carcinoma. Clin Oncol (R Coll Radiol). 2010;22(6):498–507. https://doi.org/10.1016/j.clon.2010.04.007.
88. Ricci G, Assenza M, Barreca M, Liotta G, Paganelli L, Serao A, et al. Parathyroid carcinoma: the importance of high clinical suspicion for a correct management. Int J Surg Oncol. 2012;2012:649148. https://doi.org/10.1155/2012/649148.
89. Busaidy NL, Jimenez C, Habra MA, Schultz PN, El-Naggar AK, Clayman GL, et al. Parathyroid carcinoma: a 22-year experience. Head Neck. 2004;26(8):716–26.
90. Iacobone M, Lumachi F, Favia G. Up-to-date on parathyroid carcinoma: analysis of an experience of 19 cases. J Surg Oncol. 2004;88(4):223–8. https://doi.org/10.1002/jso.20152.
91. Cope O, Nardi GL, Castleman B. Carcinoma of the parathyroid glands: 4 cases among 148 patients with hyperparathyroidism. Ann Surg. 1953;138(4):661–71.

92. Mallette LE, Bilezikian JP, Ketcham AS, Aurbach GD. Parathyroid carcinoma in familial hyperparathyroidism. Am J Med. 1974;57(4):642–8. https://doi.org/10.1016/0002-9343(74)90018-7.
93. Lee JE. Predicting the presence of parathyroid carcinoma. Ann Surg Oncol. 2005;12(7):513–4. https://doi.org/10.1245/ASO.2005.03.904.
94. Fernandez-Ranvier GG, Khanafshar E, Jensen K, Zarnegar R, Lee J, Kebebew E, et al. Parathyroid carcinoma, atypical parathyroid adenoma, or parathyromatosis? Cancer. 2007;110(2):255–64. https://doi.org/10.1002/cncr.22790.
95. Dinnen JS, Greenwoood RH, Jones JH, Walker DA, Williams ED. Parathyroid carcinoma in familial hyperparathyroidism. J Clin Pathol. 1977;30(10):966–75.
96. Agarwal G, Dhingra S, Mishra SK, Krishnani N. Implantation of parathyroid carcinoma along fine needle aspiration track. Langenbeck's Arch Surg. 2006;391(6):623–6. https://doi.org/10.1007/s00423-006--0095-8.
97. Xue S, Chen H, Lv C, Shen X, Ding J, Liu J, et al. Preoperative diagnosis and prognosis in 40 parathyroid carcinoma patients. Clin Endocrinol. 2016; https://doi.org/10.1111/cen.13055.
98. Williams MD, DeLellis RA, Erickson LA, Gupta R, Johnson SJ, Kameyama K, et al. Pathology data set for reporting parathyroid carcinoma & atypical parathyroid neoplasm: recommendations from the International Collaboration on Cancer Reporting (ICCR). Hum Pathol. 2020; https://doi.org/10.1016/j.humpath.2020.07.008.
99. DeLellis RA, Larsson C, Arnold A, Lloy R, Bilezikian J, Mete O. Tumors of the parathyroid glands. In: Lloyd RV, Osamura RY, Kloppel G, Rosai J, editors. In WHO classification of tumors of endocrine organs. Lyon: IARC Press; 2017. pp 145–59.
100. Bondeson L, Sandelin K, Grimelius L. Histopathological variables and DNA cytometry in parathyroid carcinoma. Am J Surg Pathol. 1993;17(8):820–9.
101. Stojadinovic A, Hoos A, Nissan A, Dudas ME, Cordon-Cardo C, Shaha AR, et al. Parathyroid neoplasms: clinical, histopathological, and tissue microarray-based molecular analysis. Hum Pathol. 2003;34(1):54–64. https://doi.org/10.1053/hupa.2003.55.
102. Erovic BM, Goldstein DP, Kim D, Mete O, Brierley J, Tsang R, et al. Parathyroid cancer: outcome analysis of 16 patients treated at the Princess Margaret Hospital. Head Neck. 2013;35(1):35–9. https://doi.org/10.1002/hed.22908.
103. McKeown PP, McGarity WC, Sewell CW. Carcinoma of the parathyroid gland: is it overdiagnosed? A report of three cases. Am J Surg. 1984;147(2):292–8.
104. Okamoto T, Iihara M, Obara T, Tsukada T. Parathyroid carcinoma: etiology, diagnosis, and treatment. World J Surg. 2009;33(11):2343–54. https://doi.org/10.1007/s00268-009-9999-0.
105. Williams M, DeLellis R, Erickson L, Gupta R, Johnson S, Kameyama K, Natu S, Ng T, Perren A, Perrier N, Seethala R, Gill A. Parathyroid carcinoma & atypical parathyroid neoplasm histopathology reporting guide. International Collaboration on Cancer Reporting; Sydney, Australia; 2019.
106. Iacobone M, Carnaille B, Palazzo FF, Vriens M. Hereditary hyperparathyroidism–a consensus report of the European Society of Endocrine Surgeons (ESES). Langenbecks Arch Surg. 2015;400(8):867–86. https://doi.org/10.1007/s00423-015-1342-7.
107. Gill AJ, Clarkson A, Gimm O, Keil J, Dralle H, Howell VM, et al. Loss of nuclear expression of parafibromin distinguishes parathyroid carcinomas and hyperparathyroidism-jaw tumor (HPT-JT) syndrome-related adenomas from sporadic parathyroid adenomas and hyperplasias. Am J Surg Pathol. 2006;30(9):1140–9. https://doi.org/10.1097/01.pas.0000209827.39477.4f.

108. Juhlin CC, Nilsson IL, Lagerstedt-Robinson K, Stenman A, Branstrom R, Tham E, et al. Parafibromin immunostainings of parathyroid tumors in clinical routine: a near-decade experience from a tertiary center. Mod Pathol. 2019;32(8):1082–94. https://doi.org/10.1038/s41379-019-0252-6.
109. Kruijff S, Sidhu SB, Sywak MS, Gill AJ, Delbridge LW. Negative parafibromin staining predicts malignant behavior in atypical parathyroid adenomas. Ann Surg Oncol. 2014;21(2):426–33. https://doi.org/10.1245/s10434-013-3288-8.
110. Truran PP, Johnson SJ, Bliss RD, Lennard TW, Aspinall SR. Parafibromin, galectin-3, PGP9.5, Ki67, and cyclin D1: using an immunohistochemical panel to aid in the diagnosis of parathyroid cancer. World J Surg. 2014;38(11):2845–54. https://doi.org/10.1007/s00268-014-2700-2.
111. Kumari N, Chaudhary N, Pradhan R, Agarwal A, Krishnani N. Role of histological criteria and immunohistochemical markers in predicting risk of malignancy in parathyroid neoplasms. Endocr Pathol. 2016;27(2):87–96. https://doi.org/10.1007/s12022-016-9426-7.
112. Silva-Figueroa AM, Bassett R Jr, Christakis I, Moreno P, Clarke CN, Busaidy NL, et al. Using a novel diagnostic Nomogram to differentiate malignant from benign parathyroid neoplasms. Endocr Pathol. 2019;30(4):285–96. https://doi.org/10.1007/s12022-019-09592-3.
113. Hadar T, Shvero J, Yaniv E, Ram E, Shvili I, Koren R. Expression of p53, Ki-67 and Bcl-2 in parathyroid adenoma and residual normal tissue. Pathol Oncol Res. 2005;11(1):45–9. https://doi.org/10.1007/BF03032405.
114. Holmquist N. Fine-needle aspiration and parathyroid carcinoma. Diagn Cytopathol. 1986;2(2):179–80. https://doi.org/10.1002/dc.2840020218.
115. Spinelli C, Bonadio AG, Berti P, Materazzi G, Miccoli P. Cutaneous spreading of parathyroid carcinoma after fine needle aspiration cytology. J Endocrinol Investig. 2000;23(4):255–7. https://doi.org/10.1007/BF03343718.
116. Roussel F, Dalion J, Benozio M. The risk of tumoral seeding in needle biopsies. Acta Cytol. 1989;33(6):936–9.
117. Weiss H. Metastases caused by fine needle puncture? Ultraschall Med. 1989;10(3):147–51. https://doi.org/10.1055/s-2007-1005981.
118. Sulak LE, Brown RW, Butler DB. Parathyroid carcinoma with occult bone metastases diagnosed by fine needle aspiration cytology. Acta Cytol. 1989;33(5):645–8.
119. Harari A, Waring A, Fernandez-Ranvier G, Hwang J, Suh I, Mitmaker E, et al. Parathyroid carcinoma: a 43-year outcome and survival analysis. J Clin Endocrinol Metab. 2011;96(12):3679–86. https://doi.org/10.1210/jc.2011-1571.
120. Owen RP, Silver CE, Pellitteri PK, Shaha AR, Devaney KO, Werner JA, et al. Parathyroid carcinoma: a review. Head Neck. 2011;33(3):429–36. https://doi.org/10.1002/hed.21376.
121. Wei CH, Harari A. Parathyroid carcinoma: update and guidelines for management. Curr Treat Options in Oncol. 2012;13(1):11–23. https://doi.org/10.1007/s11864-011-0171-3.
122. Berenson JR. Treatment of hypercalcemia of malignancy with bisphosphonates. Semin Oncol. 2002;29(6 Suppl 21):12–8. https://doi.org/10.1053/sonc.2002.37417.
123. Zagzag J, Hu MI, Fisher SB, Perrier ND. Hypercalcemia and cancer: differential diagnosis and treatment. CA Cancer J Clin. 2018;68(5):377–86. https://doi.org/10.3322/caac.21489.
124. Karuppiah D, Thanabalasingham G, Shine B, Wang LM, Sadler GP, Karavitaki N, et al. Refractory hypercalcaemia secondary to parathyroid carcinoma: response to high-dose denosumab. Eur J Endocrinol. 2014;171(1):K1–5. https://doi.org/10.1530/EJE-14-0166.

125. Vellanki P, Lange K, Elaraj D, Kopp PA, El Muayed M. Denosumab for management of parathyroid carcinoma-mediated hypercalcemia. J Clin Endocrinol Metab. 2014;99(2):387–90. https://doi.org/10.1210/jc.2013-3031.
126. Collins MT, Skarulis MC, Bilezikian JP, Silverberg SJ, Spiegel AM, Marx SJ. Treatment of hypercalcemia secondary to parathyroid carcinoma with a novel calcimimetic agent. J Clin Endocrinol Metab. 1998;83(4):1083–8. https://doi.org/10.1210/jcem.83.4.4726.
127. Nemeth EF, Steffey ME, Hammerland LG, Hung BC, Van Wagenen BC, DelMar EG, et al. Calcimimetics with potent and selective activity on the parathyroid calcium receptor. Proc Natl Acad Sci U S A. 1998;95(7):4040–5. https://doi.org/10.1073/pnas.95.7.4040.
128. Silverberg SJ, Rubin MR, Faiman C, Peacock M, Shoback DM, Smallridge RC, et al. Cinacalcet hydrochloride reduces the serum calcium concentration in inoperable parathyroid carcinoma. J Clin Endocrinol Metab. 2007;92(10):3803–8. https://doi.org/10.1210/jc.2007-0585.
129. Marcocci C, Bollerslev J, Khan AA, Shoback DM. Medical management of primary hyperparathyroidism: proceedings of the fourth International Workshop on the Management of Asymptomatic Primary Hyperparathyroidism. J Clin Endocrinol Metab. 2014;99(10):3607–18. https://doi.org/10.1210/jc.2014-1417.
130. Fujimoto Y, Obara T, Ito Y, Kanazawa K, Aiyoshi Y, Nobori M. Surgical treatment of ten cases of parathyroid carcinoma: importance of an initial en bloc tumor resection. World J Surg. 1984;8(3):392–400. https://doi.org/10.1007/BF01655086.
131. Fang SH, Lal G. Parathyroid cancer. Endocr Pract. 2011;17(Suppl 1):36–43. https://doi.org/10.4158/EP10310.RA.
132. Betea D, Potorac I, Beckers A. Parathyroid carcinoma: challenges in diagnosis and treatment. Ann Endocrinol (Paris). 2015;76(2):169–77. https://doi.org/10.1016/j.ando.2015.03.003.
133. Hsu KT, Sippel RS, Chen H, Schneider DF. Is central lymph node dissection necessary for parathyroid carcinoma? Surgery. 2014;156(6):1336–41.; discussion 41. https://doi.org/10.1016/j.surg.2014.08.005.
134. Basceken SI, Genc V, Ersoz S, Sevim Y, Celik SU, Bayram IK. Is local resection sufficient for parathyroid carcinoma? Clinics (Sao Paulo). 2015;70(4):247–9. https://doi.org/10.6061/clinics/2015(04)05.
135. Randle RW, Schneider DF. Lymph node dissection versus no lymph node dissection for parathyroid cancer. In: difficult decisions in surgery: an evidence-based approach. Cham: Springer; 2018. p. 193–208. https://doi.org/10.1007/978-3-319-92860-9_17.
136. Enomoto K, Uchino S, Ito A, Watanabe S, Shibuya H, Enomoto Y, et al. The surgical strategy and the molecular analysis of patients with parathyroid cancer. World J Surg. 2010;34(11):2604–10. https://doi.org/10.1007/s00268-010-0618-x.
137. Vetto JT, Brennan MF, Woodruf J, Burt M. Parathyroid carcinoma: diagnosis and clinical history. Surgery. 1993;114(5):882–92.
138. Schulte KM, Talat N. Diagnosis and management of parathyroid cancer. Nat Rev Endocrinol. 2012;8(10):612–22. https://doi.org/10.1038/nrendo.2012.102.
139. Young S, Wu JX, Li N, Yeh MW, Livhits MJ. More extensive surgery may not improve survival over Parathyroidectomy alone in parathyroid carcinoma. Ann Surg Oncol. 2016; https://doi.org/10.1245/s10434-016-5256-6.
140. Villar-del-Moral J, Jimenez-Garcia A, Salvador-Egea P, Martos-Martinez JM, Nuno-Vazquez-Garza JM, Serradilla-Martin M, et al. Prognostic factors and staging systems in parathyroid cancer: a multicenter cohort study. Surgery. 2014;156(5):1132–44. https://doi.org/10.1016/j.surg.2014.05.014.
141. Medas F, Erdas E, Loi G, Podda F, Pisano G, Nicolosi A, et al. Controversies in the management of parathyroid carcinoma: a case

series and review of the literature. Int J Surg (London, England). 2016;28(Suppl 1):S94–8. https://doi.org/10.1016/j.ijsu.2015.12.040.
142. Salcuni AS, Cetani F, Guarnieri V, Nicastro V, Romagnoli E, de Martino D, et al. Parathyroid carcinoma. Best Pract Res Clin Endocrinol Metab. 2018;32(6):877–89. https://doi.org/10.1016/j.beem.2018.11.002.
143. Akirov A, Asa SL, Larouche V, Mete O, Sawka AM, Jang R, et al. The clinicopathological spectrum of parathyroid carcinoma. Front Endocrinol. 2019;10:731. https://doi.org/10.3389/fendo.2019.00731.
144. Rozhinskaya L, Pigarova E, Sabanova E, Mamedova E, Voronkova I, Krupinova J, et al. Diagnosis and treatment challenges of parathyroid carcinoma in a 27-year-old woman with multiple lung metastases. Endocrinol Diabetes Metab Case Rep. 2017;2017 https://doi.org/10.1530/EDM-16-0113.
145. Kutahyalioglu M, Nguyen HT, Kwatampora L, Clarke C, Silva A, Ibrahim E, et al. Genetic profiling as a clinical tool in advanced parathyroid carcinoma. J Cancer Res Clin Oncol. 2019;145(8):1977–86. https://doi.org/10.1007/s00432-019-02945-9.
146. Clarke CN, Katsonis P, Hsu TK, Koire AM, Silva-Figueroa A, Christakis I, et al. Comprehensive genomic characterization of parathyroid cancer identifies novel candidate driver mutations and core pathways. J Endocr Soc. 2019;3(3):544–59. https://doi.org/10.1210/js.2018-00043.
147. Chow E, Tsang RW, Brierley JD, Filice S. Parathyroid carcinoma–the Princess Margaret Hospital experience. Int J Radiat Oncol Biol Phys. 1998;41(3):569–72.
148. Munson ND, Foote RL, Northcutt RC, Tiegs RD, Fitzpatrick LA, Grant CS, et al. Parathyroid carcinoma: is there a role for adjuvant radiation therapy? Cancer. 2003;98(11):2378–84. https://doi.org/10.1002/cncr.11819.
149. Lumachi F, Basso SM, Basso U. Parathyroid cancer: etiology, clinical presentation and treatment. Anticancer Res. 2006;26(6C):4803–7.
150. Mittendorf EA, McHenry CR. Parathyroid carcinoma. J Surg Oncol. 2005;89(3):136–42. https://doi.org/10.1002/jso.20182.
151. Limberg J, Stefanova D, Ullmann TM, Thiesmeyer JW, Bains S, Beninato T, et al. The use and benefit of adjuvant radiotherapy in parathyroid carcinoma: a national cancer database analysis. Ann Surg Oncol. 2020; https://doi.org/10.1245/s10434-020-08825-8.
152. Wilhelm SM, Wang TS, Ruan DT, Lee JA, Asa SL, Duh QY, et al. The American Association of Endocrine Surgeons Guidelines for definitive management of primary hyperparathyroidism. JAMA Surg. 2016;151(10):959–68. https://doi.org/10.1001/jamasurg.2016.2310.
153. Ryhanen EM, Leijon H, Metso S, Eloranta E, Korsoff P, Ahtiainen P, et al. A nationwide study on parathyroid carcinoma. Acta Oncol. 2017;56(7):991–1003. https://doi.org/10.1080/0284186X.2017.1306103.
154. Asare EA, Silva-Figueroa A, Hess KR, Busaidy N, Graham PH, Grubbs EG, et al. Risk of distant metastasis in parathyroid carcinoma and its effect on survival: a retrospective review from a high-volume center. Ann Surg Oncol. 2019; https://doi.org/10.1245/s10434-019-07451-3.
155. Schulte KM, Gill AJ, Barczynski M, Karakas E, Miyauchi A, Knoefel WT, et al. Classification of parathyroid cancer. Ann Surg Oncol. 2012;19(8):2620–8. https://doi.org/10.1245/s10434-012-2306-6.
156. Zhu R, Wang Z, Hu Y. Prognostic role of parafibromin staining and CDC73 mutation in patients with parathyroid carcinoma: a systematic review and meta-analysis based on individual patient data. Clin Endocrinol. 2020;92(4):295–302. https://doi.org/10.1111/cen.14161.

Surgical Procedures. Parathyroidectomy: Indications, Operative Techniques, Management of Complications, Intraoperative PTH Monitoring, Role of Parathyroid Autofluorescence and ICG

Talia Burneikis and Allan E. Siperstein

Contents

A. L. Shifrin et al. (eds.), *Endocrine Surgery Comprehensive Board Exam Guide*,
https://doi.org/10.1007/978-3-030-84737-1_16

Case Presentation

A 64-year-old woman is referred for hypercalcemia with calcium levels greater than 10.5 mg/dL on multiple occasions, most recently her level was 10.9 mg/dL (normal range 8.8–10.5 mg/dL). Parathyroid hormone (PTH) was 64 pg/mL (normal 15–65 pg/mL). She has no history of kidney stones, or her renal function is normal with a glomerular filtration rate (GFR) of 75 mL/min (normal >60 mL/min). She has no significant cardiac or pulmonary comorbidities. Dual-energy x-ray absorptiometry (DEXA) scan showed osteoporosis at the distal one-third radius with a T-score of −2.1. On further inquiry, she describes symptoms of constipation, fatigue, depression, and mental fogging.

❓ Questions

1. Your patient is hesitant about surgery for primary hyperparathyroidism and wants to know the long-term benefit. You counsel her. Which of the following statements regarding parathyroidectomy for hyperparathyroidism is true?
   (a) Parathyroidectomy can slow the progression of osteoporosis but has not been associated with reversing the disease progression.
   (b) Bone mineral density significantly improves after parathyroidectomy for primary hyperparathyroidism.
   (c) Medical management has as good of outcomes as parathyroidectomy in the management of skeletal disease.
   (d) Medical management is more cost-effective than parathyroidectomy in the management of osteoporosis.
2. Preoperative imaging studies including sestamibi-SPECT CT and neck ultrasound fail to localize a parathyroid adenoma. How should you proceed based on the intraoperative findings?
   (a) Biopsy the glands as they are identified. Remove the glands that have confirmed hyperplasia. Drawing intraoperative PTH (IOPTH) levels 10 minutes after removal of each gland. Stop when the IOPTH level has dropped by at least 50% even if not all four glands have been identified.
   (b) Perform a four-gland exploration identifying all four glands before removing any abnormal appearing glands. Remove only the adenomatous appearing glands and stop when IOPTH has dropped by at least 50% and into the normal range.
   (c) The patient has four-gland hyperplasia. Perform a subtotal, three-and-a-half gland parathyroidectomy,

regardless of the appearance of the parathyroid glands leaving a normal sized superior remnant, marked with a clip, and perform cryopreservation.
   (d) The patient has four-gland hyperplasia. Use indocyanine green (ICG) intraoperatively given that preoperative imaging failed to localize any abnormal glands. ICG has been shown to aid in the identification of any parathyroid adenomas.
3. During parathyroidectomy for primary hyperparathyroidism, you identify and excise a left upper parathyroid adenoma consistent with preoperative localizing imaging studies. However, the intraoperative PTH drops from 168 preoperatively to 130 pg/mL at 10 minutes after excision. How do you proceed?
   (a) Complete the operation without any further exploration because you excised the only suspicious gland identified on preoperative imaging.
   (b) Wait 5 more minutes and recheck PTH. If the PTH level has dropped by 50% at 15 minutes, close.
   (c) Perform a subtotal three-and-a-half gland parathyroidectomy.
   (d) Perform a comprehensive parathyroidectomy, identifying all four glands and excising any abnormal appearing parathyroid glands, and recheck intraoperative PTH to confirm a PTH drop of >50% from preoperative levels.
4. During four-gland parathyroid exploration for parathyroid hyperplasia you cannot locate the left inferior parathyroid gland. What additional intraoperative maneuver should be performed next?
   (a) Perform a left thyroid lobectomy.
   (b) Perform a median sternotomy in order to find the last gland.
   (c) Perform a cervical thymectomy.
   (d) Complete the surgery, and close and monitor calcium levels postoperatively.

5. Which of the following scenarios would be an indication for bilateral exploration as the primary surgery for a patient with primary hyperparathyroidism?
   (a) A personal history of nephrolithiasis, osteoporosis, and age <45 years.
   (b) A personal history of radiation exposure.
   (c) A family history of hyperparathyroidism, pituitary adenoma, and pancreatic neuroendocrine tumor.
   (d) A drop in PTH from 160 preoperatively to 40 pg/mL 10 min post-excision after removal of a suspected right upper adenoma based on preoperative ultrasound.
6. A middle-aged woman is referred by her Primary Care Physician to your clinic for the evaluation of hyperparathyroidism as detected on routine labs. Which

of the following would be an indication for parathyroidectomy?
   (a) Calcium of 10.8 mg/dL (normal 8.5–10.5 mg/dL), PTH of 110 pg/mL (normal 10–65 pg/mL), age 45, otherwise asymptomatic.
   (b) Calcium of 10.1 mg/dL (normal 8.5–10.5 mg/dL), PTH of 50 pg/mL (normal 10–65 pg/mL), age 52, osteopenia.
   (c) Calcium of 10.6 mg/dL (normal 8.5–10.5 mg/dL), PTH of 80 pg/dL (normal 10–65 pg/mL), age 55, history of kidney stones.
   (d) A, B, and C.
   (e) A and C only.
7. Your patient undergoes preoperative neck ultrasound and sestamibi scan. Both demonstrate a right lower parathyroid adenoma. Which of the following surgical strategies would be appropriate?
   (a) Four-gland exploration with excision of the right lower gland and any additional abnormal parathyroid glands found intraoperatively with intraoperative parathyroid hormone measurement.
   (b) Right-sided neck exploration only. Intraoperative PTH is not needed because two preoperative imaging studies are concordant with a right lower gland.
   (c) Right-sided neck exploration only, with intraoperative PTH to confirm successful excision of a single adenoma.
   (d) All of the above.
   (e) A and C only.
8. A 60-year-old African American male presents with weakness, confusion, and hypertension. Physical exam is significant for a palpable left-sided neck mass. Workup reveals a calcium level of 15.9 mg/dL. A parathyroid hormone level is sent and is 520 pg/mL (10–65 pg/mL). Which of the following is the next best step in management?
   (a) Perform a sestamibi for localization, followed by focused exploration with intraoperative parathyroid hormone assay monitoring.
   (b) Four-gland exploration and three-and-a-half gland parathyroidectomy.
   (c) En bloc resection of abnormal parathyroid gland, hemithyroidectomy, and left-sided lymph node dissection.
   (d) Intravenous hydration for a goal urine output of 100–150 mL/hour.
   (e) Administration of furosemide, calcitonin, and a bisphosphonate.
9. During parathyroidectomy which of the following is true.
   (a) Dissection should be carried intimately along the thyroid to displace the parathyroid glands laterally and minimizing risk to their vascular pedicles.

   (b) The middle thyroid vein can be isolated, ligated, and divided to provide more exposure with no significant consequences.
   (c) When preoperative imaging is suggestive of a single adenoma, the suspect adenoma should be removed first before identifying any other parathyroid glands.
   (d) The middle thyroid vein courses parallel to the inferior thyroid artery, and both travel deep and posteriorly to the carotid artery.

10. During bilateral neck exploration for primary hyperparathyroidism you identify three normal-appearing glands. Which of the following is true regarding the location of missing parathyroid glands?
   (a) The most likely heterotopic location for a missing inferior parathyroid gland is the ipsilateral carotid sheath.
   (b) The most likely heterotopic location for a missing inferior parathyroid gland is undescended near the angle of the jaw.
   (c) The most likely heterotopic location for a missing superior parathyroid gland is the cervical thymus.
   (d) The most likely heterotopic location for a missing superior parathyroid gland is tracheoesophageal groove.

16.1 Introduction

Historically underrecognized and undertreated, primary hyperparathyroidism (PHPT) is the most common cause of hypercalcemia. Most cases of PHPT are diagnosed after hypercalcemia is diagnosed on routine laboratory evaluation but may also be diagnosed in patients undergoing evaluation for nephrolithiasis or symptomatic skeletal disease. After diagnosis, patients are often found to have non-specific symptoms such as mental fatigue, depression, and sleep disturbances. PHPT is more common in postmenopausal women, blacks more than whites, with an incidence of 66 per 100,000 person years in women, and 25 per 100,000 person years in men [1]. PHPT is most commonly due to single parathyroid adenomas, accounting for 80–85% of cases. However, multigland disease including double adenomas occurs in 3–5% of cases and four-gland hyperplasia in the remaining 10–15%. Surgical excision reduces nephrolithiasis and improves symptomatic osteoporosis. Surgical approach varies among practices. Some providers advocate for a routine bilateral exploration examining all four glands given the risk of multigland disease. With the improvement of preoperative localization studies and the advent of IOPTH monitoring, other providers opt for focused parathyroidectomy where only one side is explored as guided by preoperative imaging. If IOPTH drops appropriately then the contralateral side is not explored. The argued advantage of a focused approach is avoiding the potential morbidity of a bilateral exploration. However, studies have shown that even with a drop in IOPTH of at least 50% after excision of a parathyroid adenoma, there is still risk of missing an additional pathologic gland [2, 3]. This chapter aims to review the indications for parathyroidectomy and discuss the different approaches and available adjuvants to the procedure.

16.2 Indications for Surgery

Parathyroidectomy offers a surgical cure for hyperparathyroidism. All patients with symptomatic PHPT associated with hypercalcemia and elevated PTH should undergo parathyroidectomy. The latest guidelines from the American Association of Endocrine Surgeons (AAES) recommend parathyroidectomy for the following indications:

- All patients with symptomatic PHPT.
- Serum calcium level is greater than 1 mg/dL above normal reference range regardless of whether objective symptoms are present or absent.
- Objective evidence of renal involvement such as nephrocalcinosis, silent nephrolithiasis, hypercalciuria (24-hour urine calcium level >400 mg/dL), and impaired renal function (GFR <60 mL/min).
- Evidence of osteoporosis, fragility fracture, or vertebral compression fractures.
- Diagnosis of PHPT at age 50 years or younger regardless of whether objective or subjective features are present or absent.
- When clinical or biochemical evidence is consistent with parathyroid carcinoma.
- Patients unable or unwilling to comply with observation protocols.
- Presence of neurocognitive and/or neuropsychiatric symptoms that are attributable to PHPT.
- In patients with cardiovascular disease who might benefit from potential mitigation of cardiovascular sequelae other than hypertension.
- Presence of nontraditional symptoms of muscle weakness, functional capacity, abnormal sleep, gastroesophageal reflux, and fibromyalgia symptoms should be considered for parathyroidectomy [4, 5].

Studies have shown that compared to medical observation, parathyroidectomy improves fracture free survival (10-year fracture-free survival after parathyroidectomy was 94% vs. 81% in observed patients). Patients with osteoporosis demonstrated the largest impact from parathyroidectomy [6].

Additionally, the misnomer of "asymptomatic" hyperparathyroidism is increasingly recognized for neurocognitive symptoms that influence quality of life [7]. Parathyroidectomy for these patients results in objective symptom improvement based on responses to patient reported outcome measures [8–10]. Furthermore, parathyroidectomy has been shown to be more cost-effective for asymptomatic PHPT than observation and medical pharmacologic therapy [11].

When considering bilateral versus focused parathyroidectomy as the initial surgery for PHPT, the surgeon should consider the concordance of preoperative imaging, and specific patient considerations. Indications for bilateral parathyroidectomy as the initial surgery for PHPT include: known or suspected multiple endocrine neoplasia (MEN), failure of the intraoperative PTH to drop after resection of a suspected single adenoma, preoperative imaging sites suggestive of multiple disease sites, coexisting thyroid cancer, or bilateral goiter. Bilateral parathyroidectomy should be strongly considered when preoperative location studies are discordant, if IOPTH monitoring is not available, in cases of lithium-induced PHPT, other cases of familial hyperparathyroidism, or surgeon preference [4]. Focused parathyroidectomy can be considered when preoperative imaging studies suggest single gland disease. IOPTH is used by many surgeons to guide the extent of surgery.

16.3 Preoperative Evaluation

Preoperative evaluation to determine localization of parathyroid pathology is advised. Ideally, the surgeon should have concordant imaging on cervical ultrasonography (US) and ^{99}Tmc-sestamibi scan with or without four-dimensional single photon emission computed tomography (SPECT). Imaging choice is at the discretion of the surgeon, as there is variability in availability at different institutions and accuracy of localization. Cervical ultrasonography is an inexpensive, widely available tool that additionally permits evaluation for concomitant thyroid pathology, and avoids ionizing radiation [12, 13]. In experienced hands, the sensitivity of US for parathyroid is reported to be 76–79% with a specificity of 96%. These numbers decrease with multigland disease. Parathyroid adenomas will appear either hypoechoic or anechoic near the thyroid gland with an extrathyroidal feeding vessel (see ◘ Fig. 16.1). US is limited in its evaluation of retroesophageal and mediastinal glands due to overlying structures such as the esophagus and trachea and may be limited due to patient body habitus. Sestamibi sensitivity varies by institution, ranging from 45 to 92%, and is attributed to variability in institutional protocols. Similar to US, sestamibi sensitivity decreases with multiglandular disease [14–16] (see ◘ Fig. 16.2). 4D-CT is a multiphase

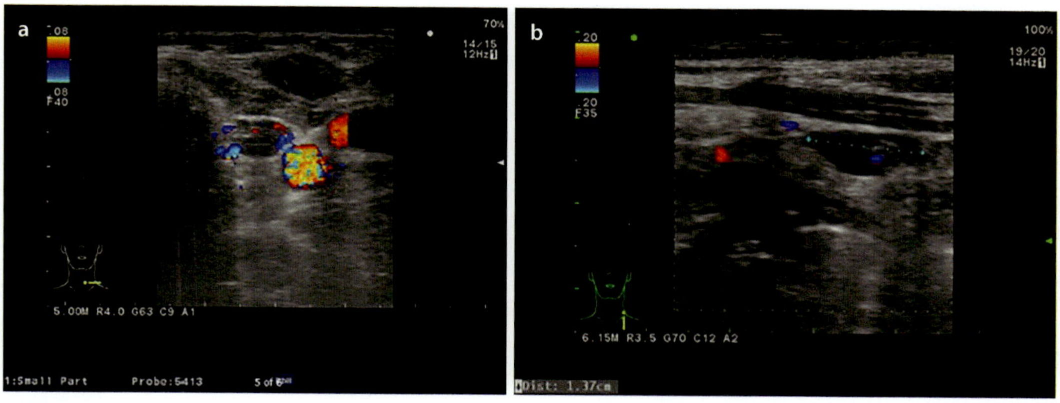

Fig. 16.1 Ultrasound imaging of classic parathyroid adenoma. Ultrasound imaging of a classic left lower parathyroid adenoma lying posterior to the inferior pole of the thyroid. Increased vascularity can be seen in the transverse **a** and sagittal **b** planes

CT technique that uses thin slices (1–3 mm) and offers a fourth dimension of assessing parathyroid gland perfusion changes with contrast attenuation over time. Rapid contrast uptake and washout is characteristic of parathyroid adenomas [17, 18] (see Fig. 16.3). In select cases, such as persistent or recurrent disease, differential jugular venous sampling can be performed for localization, with the side of pathology having at least a 10% greater PTH level than the opposite side.

Overall, preoperative imaging assists in localization and operative planning, though which modality of choice is surgeon and institution specific.

16.4 Operative Techniques

Parathyroidectomy can be performed in either a bilateral or focused approach. In contrast, focused parathyroidectomy, also described as "minimally invasive" parathyroidectomy, is often performed when adequate localization of abnormal glands is suggested by preoperative imaging. Although practices vary, intraoperative conversion from a focused parathyroidectomy to a bilateral approach may be performed if intraoperative PTH monitoring fails to confirm unilateral pathology.

16.4.1 Bilateral Exploration Parathyroidectomy

Bilateral neck exploration should be performed for patients who have non-localizing or discordant preoperative imaging studies. Some surgeons routinely use bilateral exploration as the initial approach due to the risk of missing an abnormal gland intraoperatively despite preoperative imaging. Comprehensive parathyroidectomy can be accomplished with

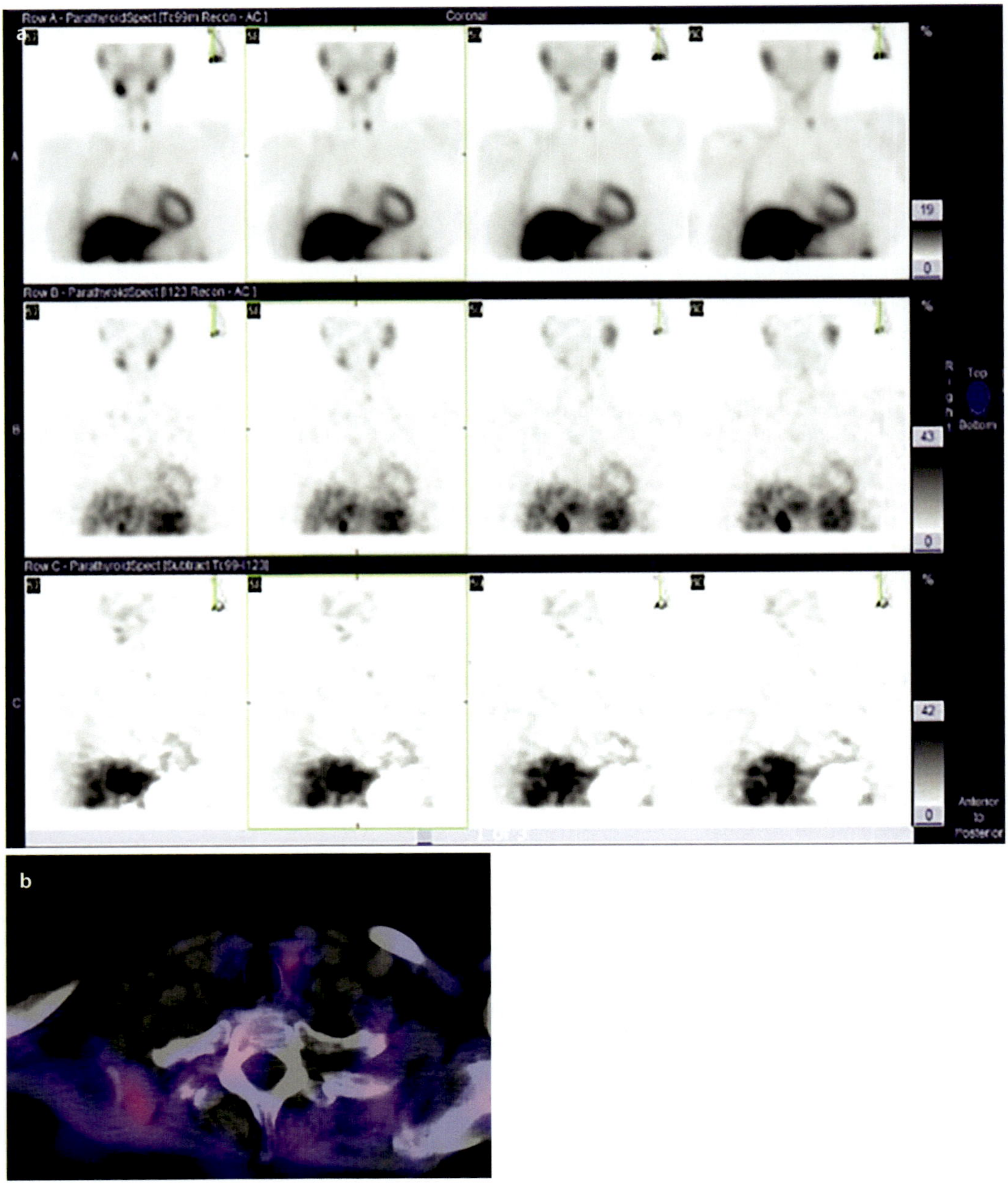

Fig. 16.2 Sestamibi subtraction images

a few essential instruments, including appendiceal retractor (lighted if available), spring retractor, peanut on a Kelly clamp, bovie, fine tipped hemostat, and Debakey forceps (see Fig. 16.4). Parathyroidectomy is most commonly performed under general anesthesia with the addition of local anesthetics, though there are variable practices using deep cervical nerve block and sedation. Antibiotics are typically not needed and sequential compression stockings are sufficient for deep vein thrombosis prophylaxis. The use of intraoperative US is a gen-

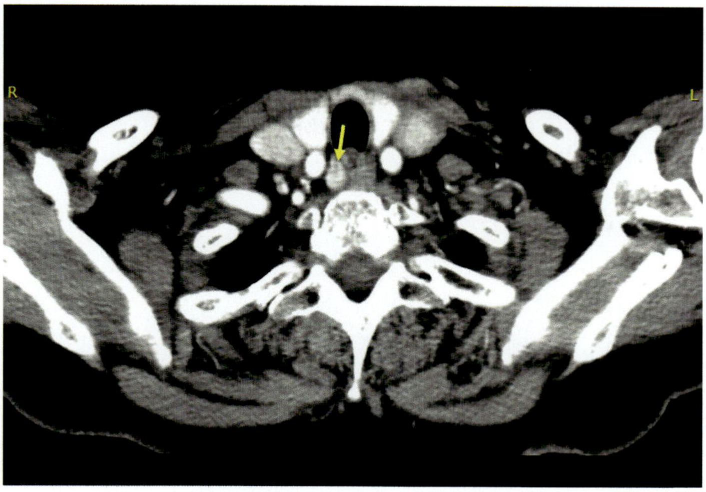

Fig. 16.3 4D CT of parathyroid adenoma. Arterial phase-contrasted CT imaging demonstrates an enhancing soft tissue lesion between the right internal carotid artery and esophagus suspicious for a parathyroid adenoma (arrow)

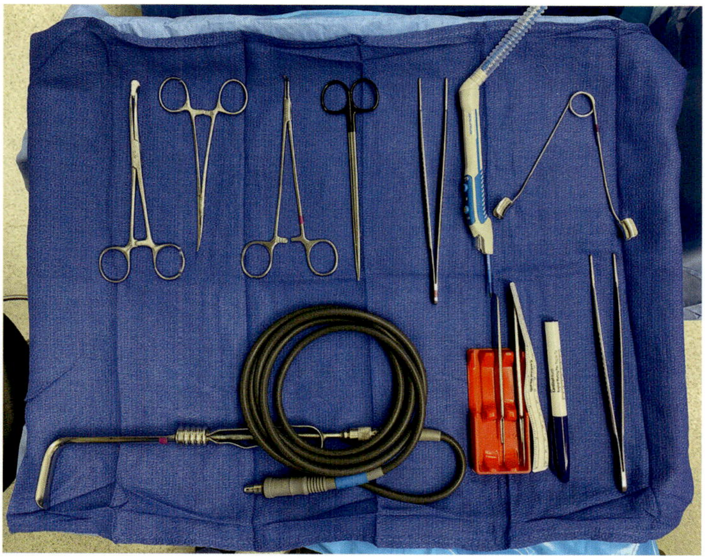

Fig. 16.4 Surgical instruments for parathyroidectomy

eral practice of the authors which allows for incision planning, and quick repeat evaluation of the neck anatomy including concomitant thyroid disease, and adenoma localization. Frozen section histology is most commonly used to confirm parathyroid pathology intraoperatively, but importantly cannot distinguish between adenoma, hyperplasia, or other parathyroid disease states.

The patient is positioned supine with arms tucked at the side, head slightly hyperextended with a roll, bean bag, or gel cushion between the scapulae. The chin and sternal notch are

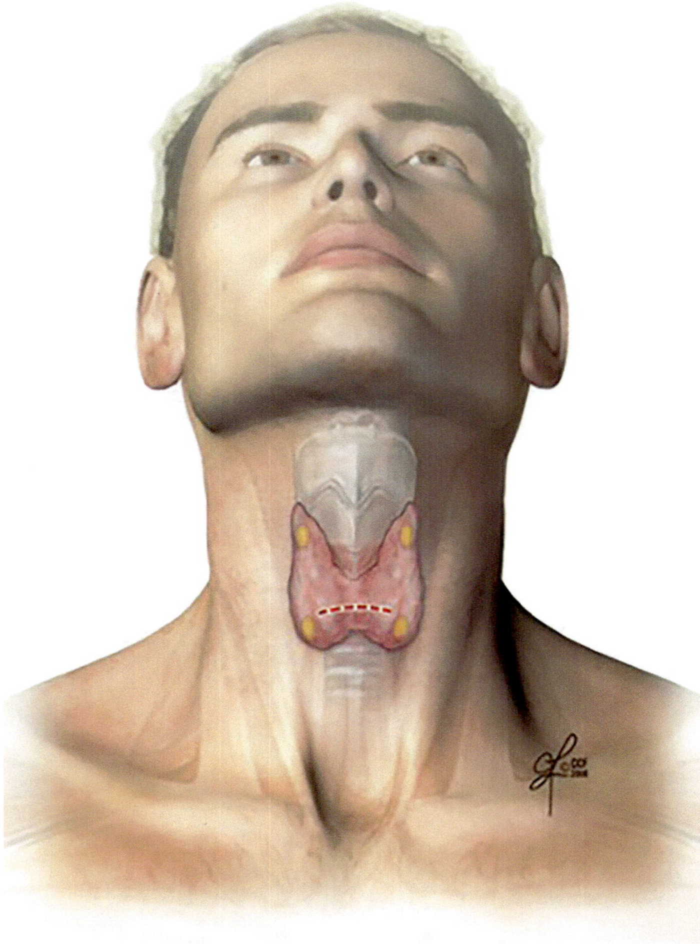

■ Fig. 16.5 Cervical incision for parathyroidectomy

positioned to provide symmetrical alignment. Potential incision sites can be marked while the patient is awake and able to flex their head to allow for cosmetic scarring at natural skin creases and is aided with the use of intraoperative ultrasound. Non-flammable chlorhexidine prep avoids skin staining and fire risk. A 4–6 cm transverse incision is made at the optimal site, usually 1.5–2 fingerbreadths above the sternal notch (see ■ Fig. 16.5). The incision is deepened using electrocautery through the platysma. Subplatysmal flaps are dissected until the thyroid cartilage is palpated superiorly and extended to the sternal notch inferiorly. This is an avascular plane superficial to the anterior jugular veins and can be accomplished using a combination of blunt dissection and electrocautery. The anterior jugular veins should be carefully preserved and can be used for IOPTH measurement (see ■ Fig. 16.6).

A self-retaining retractor is placed. The strap muscles are separated along the midline raphe exposing the thyroid. The

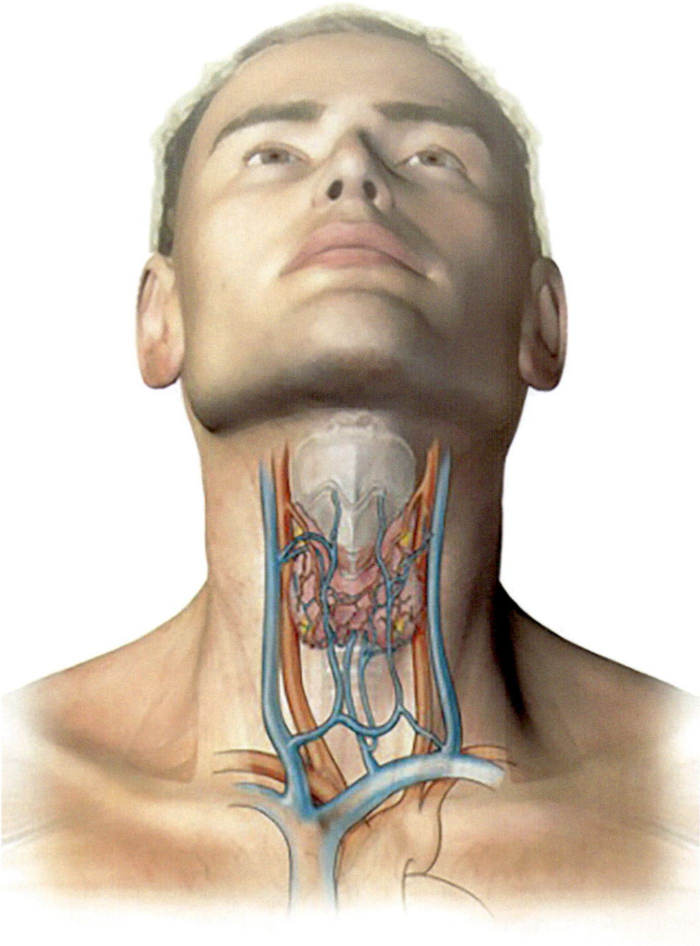

Fig. 16.6 Vascular anatomy of the neck

sternothyroid and sternohyoid muscles can be bluntly separated from each other for a short distance to further facilitate exposure. An avascular plane of loose areolar tissue between the sternothyroid muscle and thyroid gland can be separated. In order to avoid displacing parathyroid glands laterally it is important to dissect intimately along the sternothyroid muscle. The thyroid can be medially rotated and elevated using a peanut or 4x4 sponge thereby exposing the lateral and posterior thyroid surface (see Fig. 16.7). The middle thyroid vein will course medial to lateral, similar and often parallel to the inferior thyroid artery. The vein will be above the carotid artery. The inferior thyroid artery will always be situated deep to the carotid artery in its course from the thyrocervical trunk. The middle thyroid vein can be isolated, ligated, and divided to provide more exposure.

Initial dissection should be directed toward any abnormal parathyroid glands suggested by preoperative imaging. Blood

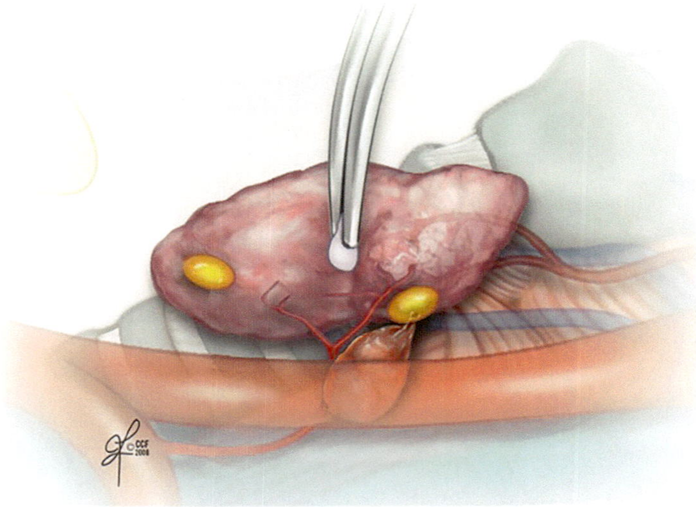

Fig. 16.7 Medial rotation of the thyroid during parathyroidectomy

staining during parathyroidectomy discolors the tissue and can make identifying parathyroid glands more difficult. If preoperative imaging is negative, the lower gland can be exposed first as it is more accessible. Purposeful observation for fatty-appearing tissue along the edges of the thyroid or adjacent to the branches of the inferior and superior thyroid artery entering the thyroid gland should be taken. Staying close to the thyroid during this dissection minimizes the risk of recurrent laryngeal nerve injury. The nerve does not need to be routinely exposed, but the direction of its course should be noted and aids in the identification of glands. When a candidate area suspicious for harboring a parathyroid gland is seen, a fine-curved hemostat is used to carefully separate the overlying fatty tissue. Parathyroid tissue appears subtly darker orange to brown in color compared to surrounding tissue. Normal parathyroid glands appear flat with a leaf-like vascular pattern. Abnormal or enlarged glands appear as a bulging mass beneath the surface (see Fig. 16.8). They will appear to slide beneath an overlying layer of tissue, this is known as the "float-sign" (see Fig. 16.9). The gland can be gently coaxed away from surrounding fat and areolar tissues to determine the true size of the gland and be sure an abnormal adenoma is not being hidden under a cap of normal parathyroid gland (see Fig. 16.10). Care should be taken not to disrupt the vascular pedicle arising medially along the thyroid. "Primary parathyroid survey" is performed by assessing the usual anatomic locations for all four glands. Our group advocates a systematic order of exploration until all four glands have been identified, usually working to identify the abnormal gland first, followed by the remaining ipsilateral gland, before exploring the contralateral side.

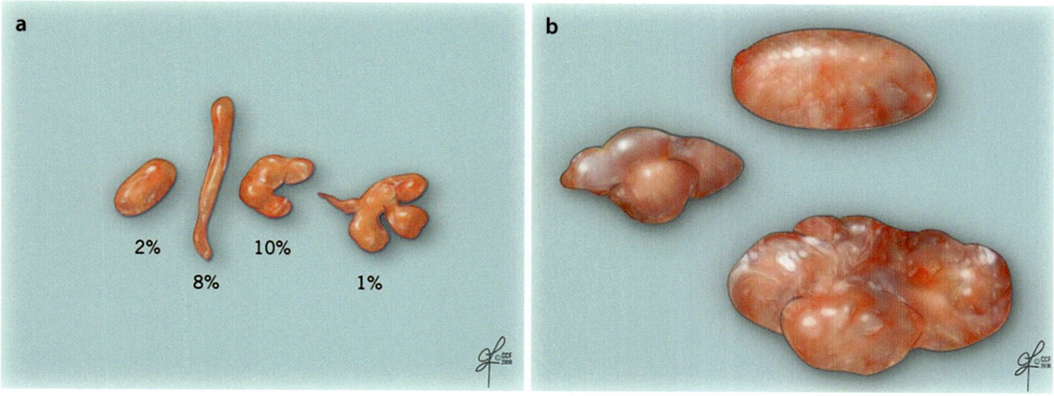

Fig. 16.8 Appearance of normal and abnormal parathyroid Glands

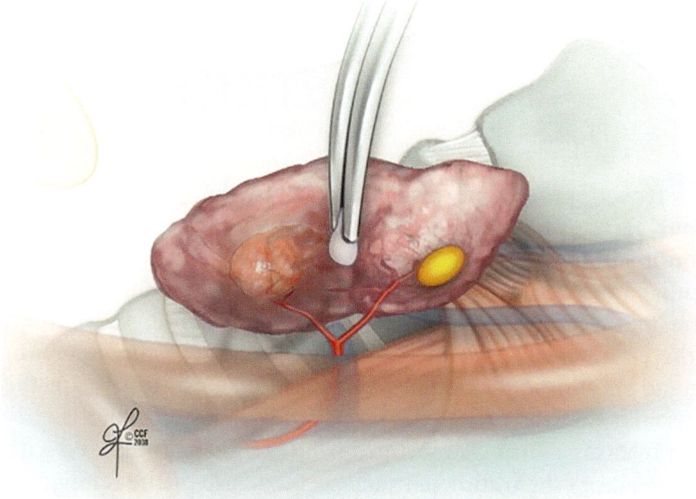

Fig. 16.9 Inferior parathyroid adenoma

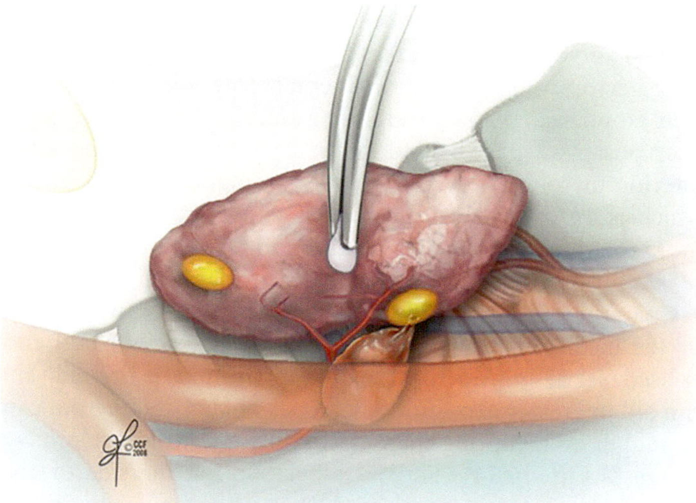

Fig. 16.10 Adenoma with cap of normal parathyroid

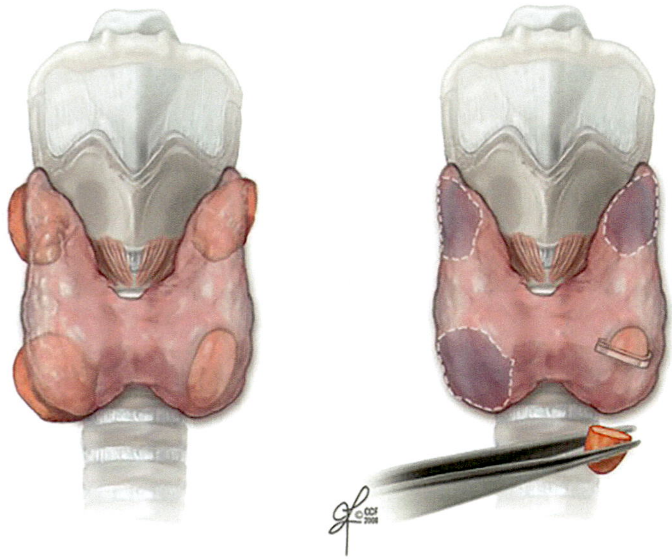

Fig. 16.11 Three-and-a-half-gland parathyroidectomy

How to proceed next is determined by the appearance of all four glands. Single or double adenomas are excised, whereas multigland hyperplasia requires subtotal parathyroidectomy and parathyroid cryopreservation. Normal remaining glands are marked with a nearby clip. When performing a subtotal (three-and-a-half gland) parathyroidectomy, the remnant gland should be fashioned first taking care not to disrupt the vascular pedicle. Usually, a more anterior lower gland is chosen in case of future reoperation. The remnant is marked with a clip across the transected surface. Goal size of the remnant is the size of a normal gland, or 6 × 4 mm, and approximately 25 mg (see Fig. 16.11).

A "secondary parathyroid survey" is performed when all four glands are not readily identified during the "primary parathyroid survey" and thus takes into consideration the possibility of ectopic glands. The most commonly missed gland is a retroesophageal parathyroid. Lying anterior to the spine in the deep posterior space behind the tracheoesophageal groove the inferior thyroid artery often courses anterior to this gland, which is an embryologically upper gland, though it appears more inferior to the actual lower gland (see Fig. 16.12). A search for missing glands is also performed during the secondary parathyroid survey. The thymus can be gently retracted out of the mediastinum without tearing the gland, palpated and excised (see Fig. 16.13). Ligation of the middle thyroid vein can aid in greater exposure. The upper pole of the thyroid can be mobilized as during thyroidectomy without devacularizing it (see Fig. 16.14). Thyroid lobectomy on the side of the missing gland may be considered when no palpable abnormality exists but can be avoided in the absence of any thyroid

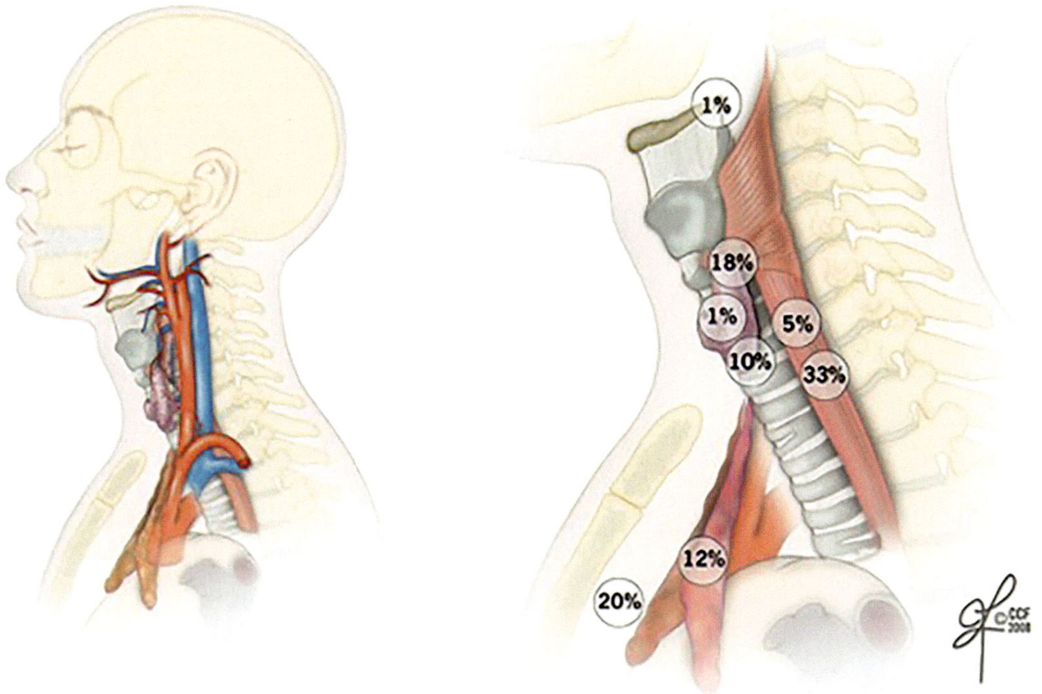

Fig. 16.12 Most common locations for ectopic parathyroid glands

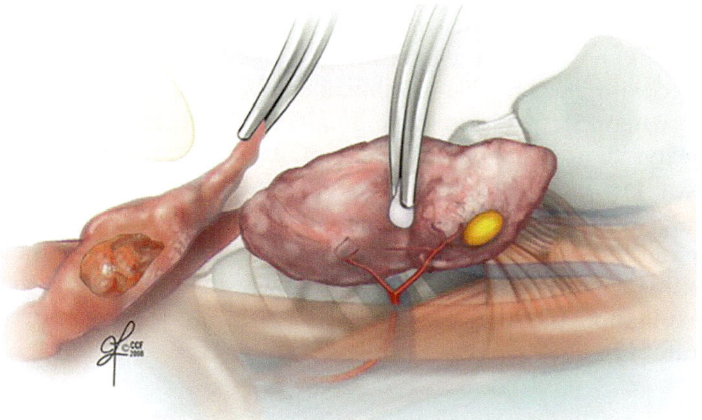

Fig. 16.13 Thymectomy for intrathymic parathyroid adenoma

nodules on preoperative ultrasound. Missing glands can also be found along the path of the carotid artery and jugular vein. Parathyroid gland locations are often symmetric on the contralateral side. A gland located in the posterior midpoint of the thyroid can be either a high-riding lower parathyroid gland or a descended superior gland. Both possibilities should be considered when encountered.

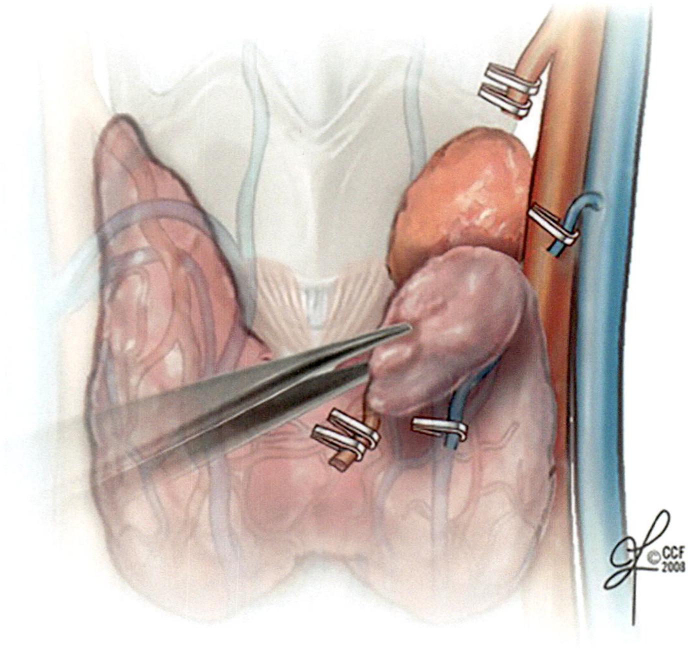

Fig. 16.14 Ligation of the middle thyroid vein

After exploration and resection are complete the neck is irrigated with sterile water, which lyses red blood cells and provides a clearer view than saline in assessing for hemostasis. Each gland is reevaluated for viability. Mild bruising is generally ok; however if the parathyroid tissue has been devascularized with questionable viability, it can be reimplanted into the ipsilateral sternocleidomastoid muscle. The strap muscles and platysma are re-approximated with absorbable suture and the skin incision closed. Our preferred method of closure, which affords an exceptional cosmetic appearance, is to run a 3–0 prolene subcuticular stitch without knots, leaving long tails on either end. Surgical glue is applied on top of the closure. After extubation, the stitch can be pulled out leaving a sutureless closure [19].

16.4.2 Focused Parathyroidectomy

Focused parathyroidectomy is performed at the discretion of the surgeon and can be considered in cases where parathyroid pathology is well localized on preoperative imaging studies. The positioning, preoperative ultrasound, and initial surgical access to the neck are as described for comprehensive parathyroidectomy above. A preoperative PTH level is obtained prior to intubation to avoid a PTH spike related to intubation or surgical manipulation prior to excision. The dissection is carried out on the side of anticipated pathology, guided by preoperative imaging. Once the abnormal gland is identified and excised, it should be confirmed to be parathyroid tissue by visual inspection, and IOPTH levels should be sent at 0, 5, and 10 minutes after excision. Conversion to a bilateral exploration is recommended if the IOPTH level fails to drop appropriately, if multigland disease is encountered, or if an abnormal parathyroid gland cannot be found. Adequate hemostasis and closure can be performed as described previously [19].

16.5 Intraoperative PTH Monitoring and Gamma-Probe Localization

The Miami criterion was first described in the early 1990s by Dr. George Irvin [20–22]. The use of IOPTH monitoring introduced the prospect of performing a focused parathyroid exploration. PTH has a short half-life on the order of 2–4 minutes [23]. Factors that influence lab results include the use of propofol, peripheral sample, dilution, and hemolysis. Using the Miami criterion, successful excision of parathyroid pathology is confirmed by at least a 50% drop in PTH from the highest preoperative or preexcision levels at 10 minutes after excision. Thus, the added potential morbidity of a bilateral exploration could be avoided. However, since its inception, the optimal algorithm for its use has been extensively studied, as there is a possibility of missing multigland disease (only 90% sensitive) [24]. Many surgeons proceed with bilateral exploration in all cases at the initial surgery, citing that parathyroid gland size does not correlate with hypersecretion, and hypercellular pathology can be seen on biopsy of normal appearing glands [25]. *Dual criteria* includes the added criteria that the PTH drop by both 50% and into the normal range and is associated with improved cure rates (97–99%) and sensitivity for multigland disease (97%) [26].

Intraoperative gamma probe comparison of in vivo and ex vivo specimen radiotracer counts has also been described. Technetium 99-m is injected 1–2 hours preoperatively and a handheld gamma probe is used to guide dissection and compare the specimen pre- and post-excision. A 20% drop in gamma emission from the surgical bed is consistent with resection of an abnormal gland. Use of gamma-probe is limited in multigland disease because the probe detects sestamibi uptake as a marker for hyperfunctioning parathyroid tissue. Additionally, thyroid nodules can retain isotope leading to false-positive results [27].

16.6 Indocyanine Green and Autofluorescence

Intraoperative identification of parathyroid glands, both normal and abnormal, has classically been credited, according to the old adage, to the experienced endocrine surgeon [28]. However, indocyanine green fluorescence (ICG) and parathyroid autofluorescence (AF) represent two novel techniques to identify parathyroid glands intraoperatively [29]. Use of these adjuncts decreases the risk of injuring the parathyroid glands and their blood supply, as well as the risk of inadvertently removing normal glands. ICG is an amphiphilic tricarbocyanine dye with near-infrared fluorescent properties at around 820-nm wavelength. ICG is administered intravenously, and fluorescence is detected using near-infrared cameras. Notably, ICG parathyroid fluorescence is limited in part due to interference from background thyroid fluorescence [30] (see ◘ Fig. 16.15).

Parathyroid tissues possess a natural fluorophore excited by 785-nm infrared light which in turn emit light at 822-nm [31]. In contrast to ICG, PAF does not require intravenous injection of fluorescent dye, can be detected using a spectrometer or modified near-infrared imaging camera, and persists regardless of gland viability. Thus, PAF can be detected after gland excision to assess for unintended parathyroidectomy. The European trial PARAFLUO showed that the use of PAF during thyroidectomy resulted in decreased postoperative hypocalcemia, parathyroid autotransplantation, and inadvertent parathyroid

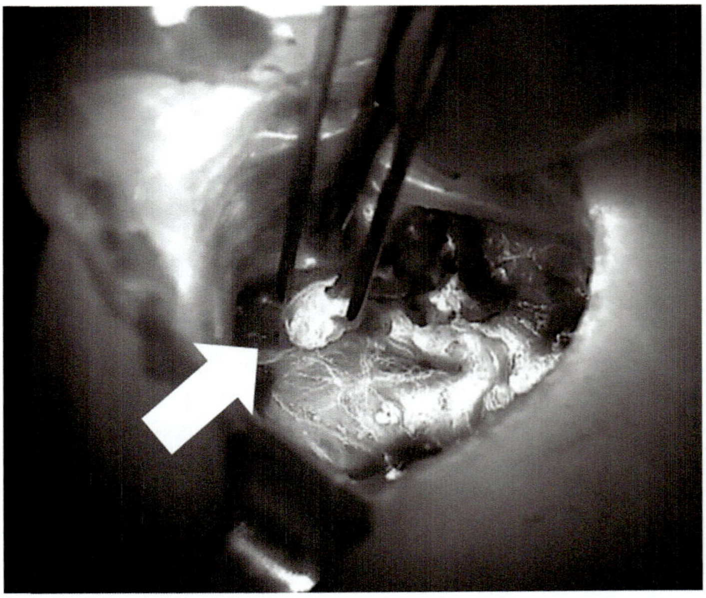

◘ **Fig. 16.15** Parathyroid ICG angiography. Image of parathyroid ICG angiography (right superior parathyroid gland after thyroidectomy) showing a well-vascularized parathyroid gland between the forceps (arrows). (Image courtesy of Demarchi et al. [30])

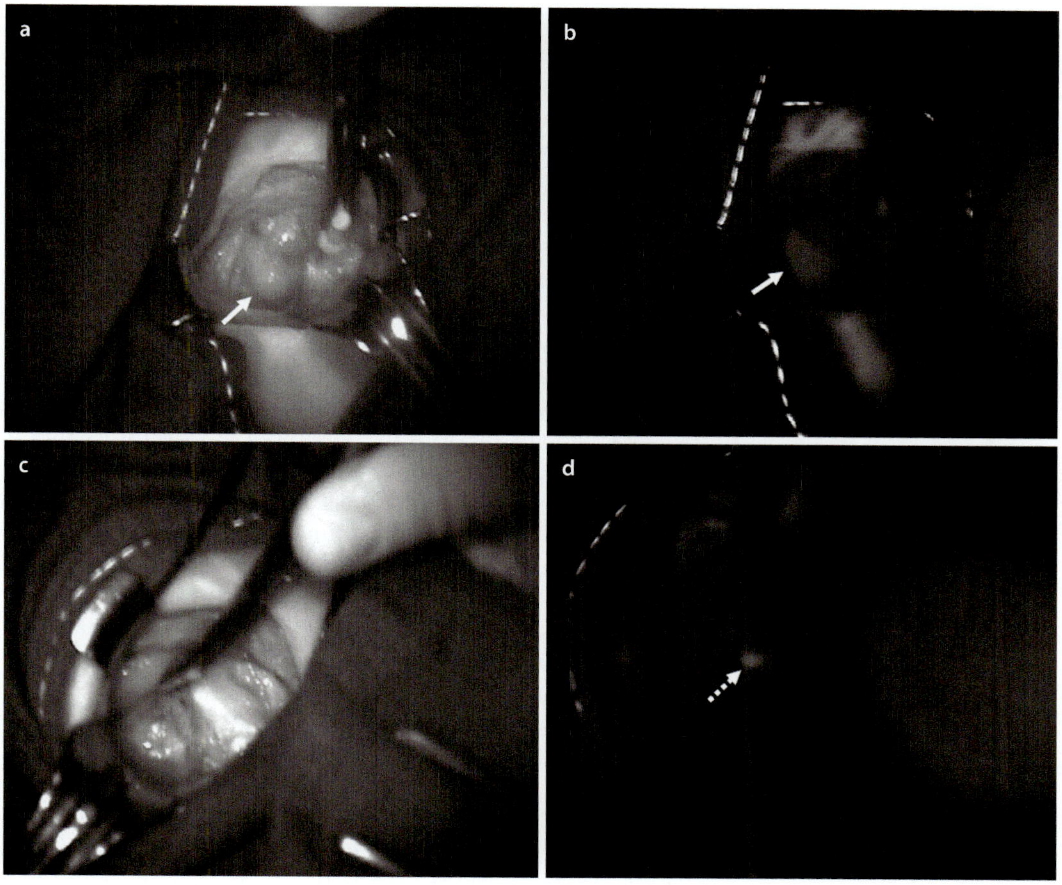

Fig. 16.16 Parathyroid autofluorescence. Four-gland parathyroid exploration demonstrating a left inferior parathyroid adenoma **a**, arrow with intraoperative autofluorescence with near infrared imaging **b**, arrow. Normal right inferior parathyroid not seen on initial visual inspection **c** detected with autofluorescence **d**, dashed arrow. (Images courtesy of Kose et al. [35])

resection [32]. Studies comparing ICG and PAF demonstrate that PAF and ICG had similar detection rates for parathyroid glands [98% (61 of 62) for PAF and 95% (60 of 63) for ICG $P = 0.31$]. When compared to naked eye identification, parathyroid glands are more frequently identified by PAF than ICG. The location of parathyroid glands was suggested before detection by the naked eye more frequently by PAF than ICG [52% (32 of 62) vs. 6% (4 of 63) of PGs; $P < 0.001$] [33–35] (see Fig. 16.16). Identification of incidentally resected parathyroid glands by autofluorescence has led to their subsequent reimplantation.

16.7 Cryopreservation and Autotransplantation

Parathyroid autotransplantation offers rescue from the devastating complication of permanent postoperative hypoparathyroidism. Parathyroid autotransplantation was first described and performed in humans during a thyroidectomy by Lahey in 1926 [36]. The procedure was largely forgotten for 50 years until Wells et al. reported the first patient series that confirmed functional autografts from the clinical, physiological, and histological perspective [37].

Immediate autotransplantation can be performed if intraoperatively there is concern that no functional parathyroid tissue remains, as may be the devastating case after performing a subtotal parathyroidectomy for hyperplasia with undue trauma to the remnant, or during total thyroidectomy with inadvertent parathyroidectomy. Delayed parathyroid autotransplantation with cryopreservation can be used in patients who develop permanent postoperative hypoparathyroidism. Identification of high-risk patients preoperatively allows the surgeon to anticipate the need for cryopreservation and tissue storage at the time of surgery. Further, it allows assessment of the outcome of the primary surgery prior to transplantation.

Immediate autotransplantation as initially described by Lahey involves the intraoperative transfer of fresh autogenous parathyroid tissue to an alternative site, most commonly the sternocleidomastoid (SCM), pectoralis, or muscle belly of the brachioradialis [36]. Immediate autotransplantation has an 85–99% success rate. The parathyroid gland is minced into 1 mm pieces which can be directly transplanted or aspirated into a syringe of balanced salt solution and then injected into the muscle belly of the SCM, pectoralis, or brachioradialis. Multiple wells within the same muscle can be created for transplantation to minimize the risk that a single site of transplanted tissue fails to take. The implantation sites are marked with either clips or non-absorbable suture [38]. Immediate autotransplantation is associated with a risk of persistent hyperparathyroidism, especially in patients with familial or renal disease who also have an inherently high risk of supernumerary or ectopic glands.

Delayed autotransplantation refers to the transplantation of previously cryopreserved autologous parathyroid tissue. Cryopreservation is done for patients who are high risk for postoperative hypoparathyroidism, including patients undergoing three-and-a-half gland parathyroidectomy for hyperplasia, total thyroidectomy with extensive lymph node dissection, or those undergoing reoperative neck surgery for persistent or recurrent disease [39]. In cases of parathyroid hyperplasia, the least abnormal hyperplastic gland should be used for cryopreservation [40]. Preserving cell viability and tissue integrity is paramount. Intraoperatively, working with chilled reagents and on ice, the harvested tissue is defatted, minced into small (1 × 1 × 1 mm) pieces, and ultimately stored in a cryopreservation medium. At our institution, parathyroid tissue is suspended in saline in the operating room and 15–20 pieces of fragmented

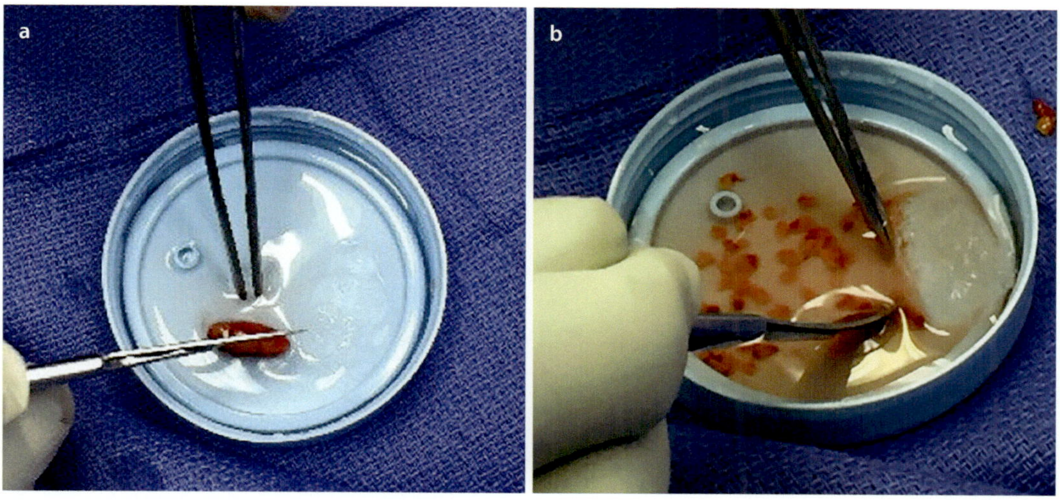

Fig. 16.17 **a** Fragmentation of parathyroid tissue for cryopreservation. **b** Parathyroid tissue is trimmed of fat and minced into 1–2 mm pieces

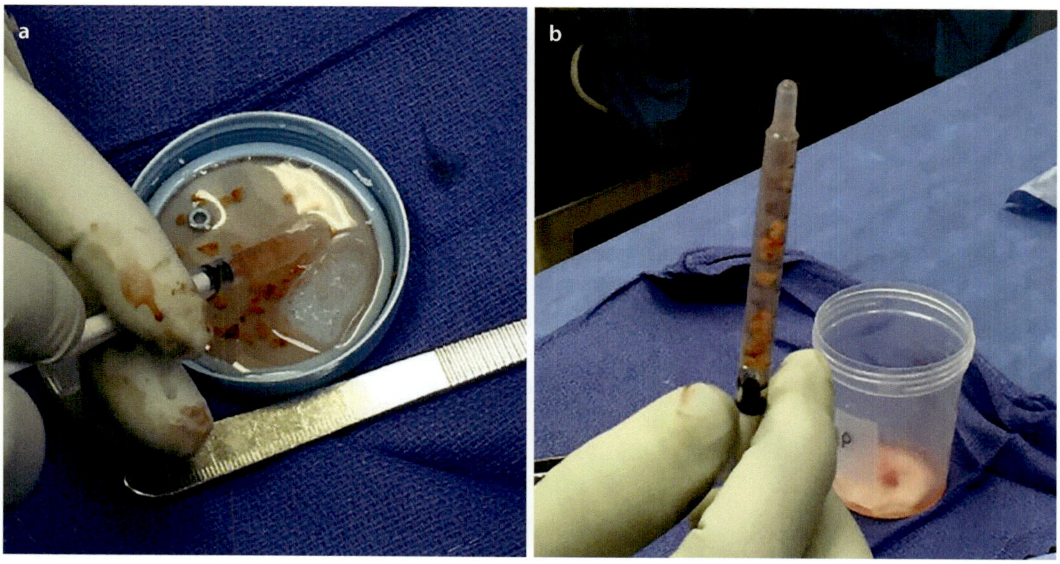

Fig. 16.18 **a** Parathyroid tissue fragments are aspirated into a tuberculin syringe. **b** Approximately 15–20 pieces per syringe suspended in injectable saline

parathyroid tissue are aspirated into 1 mL tuberculin syringes (see Figs. 16.17, 16.18, and 16.19). A venous blood sample (10–15 mL) is collected in non-additive red top vacutainers and sent to the laboratory with the parathyroid tissue for cryopreservation. Laboratory processing includes decanting the supernatant and transferring approximately ten fragments of tissue into separate sterile cryovials with cryopreservation medium. Cryopreservation medium includes Roswell Park Memorial Institute (RPMI) 1640 solution, a cytoplasmic stabilizer (dimethyl sulfoxide), and autologous serum. Specific

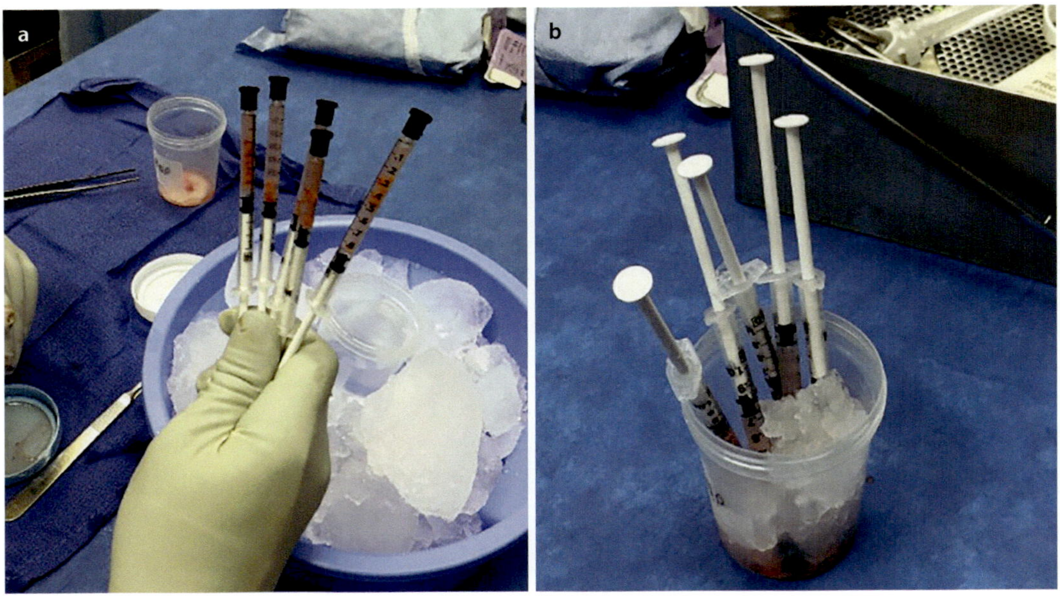

Fig. 16.19 **a** Aspirated parathyroid fragments are collected in one or more syringe per parathyroid gland. **b** Syringes are maintained on ice and transported immediately for cryopreservation (Images courtesy of Moore et al. [42])

proportions for cryopreservation medium ingredients vary by institution [41–43]. The freezing process should be gradual in order to best preserve cellular function, and long-term storage occurs at – 196 deg. C. At the time of reimplantation, 20–40 fragments, or the equivalent of two normal parathyroid glands, are transplanted into the non-dominant forearm under local anesthetic (2–3 fragments per pocket), each marked with a clip or non-absorbable suture.

Viability of cryopreserved parathyroid tissue persists up to 2 years (71% <24 months, vs. 1% >24 months) [44, 45]. Routine preservation of parathyroid tissue for all comers is not necessary. We recommend routine cryopreservation generally in patients undergoing reoperative surgery whether for thyroid or parathyroid disease or for patients with a history of other non-endocrine neck surgery. Storage of cryopreserved tissue occurs in approximately 20% of cases, but utilization of stored tissues remains low at only 1–4% [46, 47]. The majority of patients requiring autotransplantation of parathyroid tissue require transplantation within 24 months [47].

Regulatory requirements for cryopreservation or parathyroid tissue are determined by the Food and Drug Administration (FDA) and the Joint Commission on the Accreditation of Healthcare Organizations (JCAHO). Parathyroid cryopreservation, processing, storage, and recall should be performed by an experienced center specializing in long-term tissue storage such as a given hospital's blood bank, sperm bank, or andrology laboratory.

16.8 Management of Complications

Complications from parathyroidectomy are rare with an overall complication rate of approximately 4% for bilateral neck exploration. Immediate perioperative complications associated with parathyroidectomy include injury to the recurrent laryngeal nerve, hematoma, hypocalcemia, and wound infection. If injury to the recurrent laryngeal nerve, including transection, is identified at the time of surgery, repair should be attempted in order to minimize the risk of vocal cord paralysis. Direct end-to-end neurorrhaphy should be performed using fine non-absorbable suture. Bilateral recurrent laryngeal nerve injury may require reintubation and possible tracheostomy if the patient is unable to be intubated. Symptomatic postoperative hematoma may cause pain, fullness, dysphagia, or respiratory distress. Life-threatening airway compromise is best treated in the operating room for hematoma evacuation if recognized early. Wound infection after parathyroidectomy is exceedingly rare due to the hypervascular surgical bed, and prophylactic antibiotics are generally not warranted unless performing a reoperative surgery.

Postoperative hypocalcemia can be due to temporary hypoparathyroidism or rarely permanent hypoparathyroidism. Temporary hypoparathyroidism is attributed to suppression of the remaining normal parathyroid glands and resolves within a few days. Permanent hypoparathyroidism occurs when no viable parathyroid tissue remains, which can occur after subtotal parathyroidectomy where the remnant or its blood supply is compromised, or if autotransplantation fails. Permanent hypoparathyroidism is defined as persistent (>6 months) hypocalcemia, secondary to low levels of parathyroid hormone requiring calcium and vitamin D replacement without any period of normal biochemistry [48]. Permanent hypoparathyroidism has been reported to be as high as 30% after reoperative cases [49]. Assessment for postoperative hypocalcemia includes evaluation of parathyroid hormone and calcium levels on postoperative day one. Patients should be counseled to monitor for signs of hypocalcemia, including perioral or acral paresthesias, anxiety, as well as the risk of tetany, seizure, and papilledema. Routine calcium and vitamin D supplementation should be prescribed, especially if not corrected preoperatively. Though practices vary, the authors recommend 500 mg of calcium carbonate three times daily along with at least 1000 IU daily vitamin D depending on the preoperative level. Repeat serum PTH and calcium levels should be assessed at 1 to 2 weeks after surgery, and supplemental calcium may be weaned as indicated.

Hungry bone syndrome occurs when postoperative hypocalcemia is severe and prolonged despite normal or even elevated levels of PTH. It occurs in patients who have bone disease due to chronic bone resorption preoperatively [50]. Relatively decreased levels of PTH postop cause decreased bone resorption, increased bone formation, increased influx of calcium into bone, increased calcium excretion, and decreased intestinal calcium absorption.

Surgical cure after parathyroidectomy is defined as having normal calcium homeostasis 6 months after parathyroidectomy. Blood testing should be repeated at 6 months after surgery, then annually. Long-term follow-up is recommended, and cure should not be assumed based on a single set of normal postop lab values. Recurrent hyperparathyroidism after initially curative surgery occurs in approximately 2% of patients. Prior to embarking on reoperative surgery, prior operative reports should be carefully reviewed, new imaging obtained ideally demonstrating co-localization of residual disease, and direct laryngoscopy to evaluate recurrent laryngeal nerve function performed [4, 51].

16.9 Outcomes and Prognosis

Surgical cure after parathyroidectomy for primary hyperparathyroidism is greater than 95% [52–54]. Recurrent hyperparathyroidism after initially curative surgery is rare, occurring in less than 2% of patients [55]. With respect to osteoporosis, markers of bone resorption normalize rapidly after surgery, and objective improvements in bone mineral density of the lumbar spine, hip, and distal radius are observed as early as 6 months postoperatively [56]. Additionally, parathyroidectomy has been shown to be associated with a 64% reduction in the absolute risk of hip fractures [57, 58]. When compared to long-term observation or pharmacologic therapy, operative management of hyperparathyroidism is more cost-effective [4, 11]. With regard to the renal effects of hyperparathyroidism, the risk of nephrolithiasis decreases following parathyroidectomy; however renal function has not be shown to improve [59, 60]. Additionally, parathyroidectomy is associated with less well proven long-term effects on cardiovascular system including improvement of left ventricular mass index and electrocardiographic abnormalities in patients with PHPT [61, 62].

Patient quality of life improves significantly after parathyroidectomy. Objective improvement in the traditionally mislabeled "asymptomatic" neurocognitive features of PHPT has been demonstrated in numerous studies evaluating patient responses to both general and disease-specific patient reported outcomes measures including the PAS (parathyroid assessment of symptoms), SF-36 quality of life scale, and PROMPT

(Patient-Reported Outcome Measure for Parathyroid and Thyroid Disease). These improvements in depression, fatigue, thirst, and forgetfulness have stable improvement at 10 years after surgery [8–10].

Answers to the Questions

1. (b); 2. (b); 3. (d); 4. (c); 5. (c); 6. (e); 7. (e); 8. (d); 9. (b); 10. (d)

References

1. Yeh MW, Ituarte PHG, Zhou HC, Nishimoto S, Liu I-LA, Harari A, et al. Incidence and prevalence of primary hyperparathyroidism in a racially mixed population. J Clin Endocrinol Metab. 2013;98(3): 1122–9.
2. Siperstein A, Berber E, Barbosa GF, Tsinberg M, Greene AB, Mitchell J, et al. Predicting the success of limited exploration for primary hyperparathyroidism using ultrasound, sestamibi, and intraoperative parathyroid hormone: analysis of 1158 cases. Ann Surg. 2008;248(3):420–6.
3. Norman J, Lopez J, Politz D. Abandoning unilateral parathyroidectomy: why we reversed our position after 15,000 parathyroid operations. J Am Coll Surg [Internet]. 2012;214(3):260–9. Available from: https://doi.org/10.1016/j.jamcollsurg.2011.12.007
4. Wilhelm SM, Wang TS, Ruan DT, Lee JA, Asa SL, Duh QY, et al. The American association of endocrine surgeons guidelines for definitive management of primary hyperparathyroidism. JAMA Surg. 2016;151(10):959–68.
5. Bilezikian JP, Brandi ML, Eastell R, Silverberg SJ, Udelsman R, Marcocci C, et al. Guidelines for the management of asymptomatic primary hyperparathyroidism: summary statement from the fourth international workshop. J Clin Endocrinol Metab. 2014;99(10):3561–9.
6. VanderWalde LH, Liu ILA, Haigh PI. Effect of bone mineral density and parathyroidectomy on fracture risk in primary hyperparathyroidism. World J Surg. 2009;33(3):406–11.
7. Udelsman R, Åkerström G, Biagini C, Duh QY, Miccoli P, Niederle B, et al. The surgical management of asymptomatic primary hyperparathyroidism: proceedings of the Fourth International Workshop. J Clin Endocrinol Metab. 2014;99(10):3595–606.
8. Pasieka JL, Parsons L, Jones J. The long-term benefit of parathyroidectomy in primary hyperparathyroidism: a 10-year prospective surgical outcome study. Surgery [Internet]. 2009;146(6):1006–13. Available from: https://doi.org/10.1016/j.surg.2009.10.021
9. Burneikis T, Colvin J, Jin J, Berber E, Krishnamurthy VD, Shin J, et al. Validation of a novel patient-reported outcome measure for parathyroid and thyroid disease (PROMPT). Surg (United States) [Internet]. 2019;165(1):232–9. Available from: https://doi.org/10.1016/j.surg.2018.04.091.
10. Ejlsmark-Svensson H, Sikjaer T, Webb SM, Rejnmark L, Rolighed L. Health-related quality of life improves 1 year after parathyroidectomy in primary hyperparathyroidism: a prospective cohort study. Clin Endocrinol. 2019;90(1):184–91.
11. Zanocco K, Angelos P, Sturgeon C. Cost-effectiveness analysis of parathyroidectomy for asymptomatic primary hyperparathyroidism. Surgery. 2006;140(6):874–82.
12. Solorzano CC, Carneiro-Pla D. Minimizing cost and maximizing success in the preoperative localization strategy for primary hyperparathyroidism. Surg Clin North Am [Internet]. 2014;94(3):587–605. Available from: https://doi.org/10.1016/j.suc.2014.02.006

13. Arora S, Balash PR, Yoo J, Smith GS, Prinz RA. Benefits of surgeon-performed ultrasound for primary hyperparathyroidism. Langenbeck's Arch Surg. 2009;394(5):861–7.
14. Thier M, Daudi S, Bergenfelz A, Almquist M. Predictors of multiglandular disease in primary hyperparathyroidism. Langenbeck's Arch Surg. 2018;403(1):103–9.
15. Wang TS, Cheung K, Farrokhyar F, Roman SA, Sosa JA. Would scan, but which scan? A cost-utility analysis to optimize preoperative imaging for primary hyperparathyroidism. Surgery [Internet]. 2011;150(6):1286–94. Available from: https://doi.org/10.1016/j.surg.2011.09.016
16. Harari A, Mitmaker E, Grogan RH, Lee J, Shen W, Gosnell J, et al. Primary hyperparathyroidism patients with positive preoperative sestamibi scan and negative ultrasound are more likely to have posteriorly located upper gland adenomas (PLUGs). Ann Surg Oncol. 2011;18(6):1717–22.
17. Lubitz CC, Hunter GJ, Hamberg LM, Parangi S, Ruan D, Gawande A, et al. Accuracy of 4-dimensional computed tomography in poorly localized patients with primary hyperparathyroidism. Surgery [Internet]. 2010;148(6):1129–38. Available from: https://doi.org/10.1016/j.surg.2010.09.002
18. Abbott DE, Cantor SB, Grubbs EG, Santora R, Gomez HF, Evans DB, et al. Outcomes and economic analysis of routine preoperative 4-dimensional ct for surgical intervention in de novo primary hyperparathyroidism: does clinical benefit justify the cost? J Am Coll Surg. 2012;214(4):629–37.
19. Siperstein A, Milas M. Comprehensive Parathyroidectomy for the treatment of PHPT. In: Fischer J, editor. Fischer's mastery of surgery. 6th ed. Philadelphia: Lippincott Williams & Wilkins; 2012. p. 486–96.
20. Irvin GL, Dembrow VD, Prudhomme DL. Operative monitoring of parathyroid gland hyperfunction. Am J Surg. 1991;162(4):299–302.
21. Irvin G 3rd, Dembrow V, Prudhomme D. Clinical usefulness of an intraoperative "quick parathyroid hormone" assay. Surgery. 1993;114(6):1019–22.
22. Irvin GL, Prudhomme DL, Deriso GT, Sfakianakis G, Chandarlapaty SKC. A new approach to parathyroidectomy. Ann Surg. 1994;219(5):574–81.
23. Maier GW, Kreis ME, Renn W, Pereira PL, Häring HU, Becker HD. Parathyroid hormone after adenectomy for primary hyperparathyroidism. A study of peptide hormone elimination kinetics in humans. J Clin Endocrinol Metab. 1998;83(11):3852–6.
24. Lew JI, Irvin GL. Focused parathyroidectomy guided by intra-operative parathormone monitoring does not miss multiglandular disease in patients with sporadic primary hyperparathyroidism: a 10-year outcome. Surgery. 2009 Dec;146(6):1021–7.
25. Irvin GL, Carneiro DM, Solorzano CC, Leight GS, Perrier N, Nelson WR, et al. Progress in the operative management of sporadic primary hyperparathyroidism over 34 years. Ann Surg. 2004;239(5):704–11.
26. Richards ML, Thompson GB, Farley DR, Grant CS. An optimal algorithm for intraoperative parathyroid hormone monitoring. Arch Surg. 2011;146(3):280–5.
27. Chen H, Mack E, Starling JR, Irvin GL, Clark OH, Prinz RA, et al. A comprehensive evaluation of perioperative adjuncts during minimally invasive parathyroidectomy: which is most reliable? Ann Surg. 2005;242(3):375–83.
28. Doppman JL, Miller DL. Localization of parathyroid tumors in patients with asymptomatic hyperparathyroidism and no previous surgery. J Bone Min Res. 1991;Suppl 2:S153–8; discussion S159.
29. Baj J, Sitarz R, Łokaj M, Forma A, Czeczelewski M, Maani A, et al. Preoperative and intraoperative methods of parathyroid gland localization and the diagnosis of parathyroid adenomas. Molecules. 2020;25(7):1–22.

30. Demarchi MS, Karenovics W, Bédat B, Triponez F. Intraoperative autofluorescence and Indocyanine green angiography for the detection and preservation of parathyroid glands. J Clin Med. 2020;9(3):830.
31. Paras C, Keller M, White L, Phay J, Mahadevan-Jansen A. Near-infrared autofluorescence for the detection of parathyroid glands. J Biomed Opt. 2011;16(6):067012.
32. Benmiloud F, Godiris-Petit G, Gras R, Gillot JC, Turrin N, Penaranda G, et al. Association of autofluorescence-based detection of the parathyroid glands during total thyroidectomy with postoperative hypocalcemia risk: results of the PARAFLUO multicenter randomized clinical trial. JAMA Surg. 2020;155(2):106–12.
33. Kahramangil B, Berber E. The use of near-infrared fluorescence imaging in endocrine surgical procedures. J Surg Oncol. 2017;115(7):848–55.
34. Kahramangil B, Berber E. Comparison of indocyanine green fluorescence and parathyroid autofluorescence imaging in the identification of parathyroid glands during thyroidectomy. Gland Surg. 2017;6(6):644–8.
35. Kose E, Rudin AV, Kahramangil B, Moore E, Aydin H, Donmez M, Krishnamurthy V, Siperstein A, Berber E. Autofluorescence imaging of parathyroid glands: An assessment of potential indications. Surgery. 2020;167(1):173–79. https://doi.org/10.1016/j.surg.2019.04.072. Epub 2019 Sep 13. PMID: 31526579.
36. Lahey F. The transplantation of parathyroids in partial thyroidectomy. Surg Gynecol Obs. 1926;62:508–9.
37. Wells S Jr, Christiansen C. The transplanted parathyroid gland: evaluation of cryopreservation and other environmental factors which affect its function. Surgery. 1974;75(1):49–55.
38. Saxe A, Gibson G. Cryopreservation of parathyroid tissue. In: Clark O, Duh Q, Kebebew E, editors. Textbook of endocrine surgery. Philadelphia: Elsevier Saunders; 2005. p. 530–5.
39. Moffett JM, Suliburk J. Parathyroid autotransplantation. Endocr Pract. 2011;17(Suppl 1):83–9.
40. Sancho J, Sitges-Serra A. Surgical approach to secondary hyperparathyroidism. In: Clark O, Duh Q, Kebebew E, editors. Textbook of endocrine surgery, vol. 1. Philadelphia: Elsevier Saunders; 2005. p. 510–7.
41. Stotler BA, Reich-Slotky R, Schwartz J, Inabnet WB, Lee J, Wu F, et al. Quality monitoring of microbial contamination of cryopreserved parathyroid tissue. Cell Tissue Bank. 2011;12(2):111–6.
42. Moore EC, Siperstein A, Gupta S. Cryopreservation of parathyroid tissue: a white paper on establishing a local service. Endocr Pract. 2019;25:605–11.
43. Agarwal A, Waghray A, Gupta S, Sharma R, Milas M. Cryopreservation of parathyroid tissue: an illustrated technique using the Cleveland clinic protocol. J Am Coll Surg [Internet]. 2013;216(1):e1–9. Available from: https://doi.org/10.1016/j.jamcollsurg.2012.09.021
44. Guerrero MA, Evans DB, Lee JE, Bao R, Bereket A, Gantela S, et al. Viability of cryopreserved parathyroid tissue: when is continued storage versus disposal indicated? World J Surg. 2008;32(5):836–9.
45. Herrera M, Grant C, van Heerden J, Fitzpatrick L. Parathyroid autotransplantation. Arch Surg. 1992;127(7):825–9.
46. Shepet K, Alhefdhi A, Usedom R, Sippel R, Chen H. Parathyroid cryopreservation after parathyroidectomy: a worthwhile practice? Ann Surg Oncol. 2013;20(7):2256–60.
47. Borot S, Lapierre V, Carnaille B, Goudet P, Penfornis A. Results of cryopreserved parathyroid autografts: a retrospective multicenter study. Surgery. 2010;147(4):529–35.
48. Shoback D. Clinical practice. Hypoparathyroidism. N Engl J Med. 2008;359(4):391–403. https://doi.org/10.1056/NEJMcp0803050. PMID: 18650515.

49. Rothmund M, Wagner PK. Reoperations for persistent and recurrent secondary hyperparathyroidism. Ann Surg. 1988;207(3):310–4.
50. Ho LY, Wong PN, Sin HK, Wong YY, Lo KC, Chan SF, et al. Risk factors and clinical course of hungry bone syndrome after total parathyroidectomy in dialysis patients with secondary hyperparathyroidism. BMC Nephrol. 2017;18(1):1–10.
51. Shin JJ, Milas M, Mitchell J, Berber E, Ross L, Siperstein A. Impact of localization studies and clinical scenario in patients with hyperparathyroidism being evaluated for reoperative neck surgery. Arch Surg. 2011;146(12):1397–403.
52. Udelsman R. Six hundred fifty-six consecutive explorations for primary hyperparathyroidism. Ann Surg. 2002;235(5):665–72.
53. Westerdahl J, Bergenfelz A. Unilateral versus bilateral neck exploration for primary hyperparathyroidism: five-year follow-up of a randomized controlled trial. Ann Surg. 2007;246(6):976–80.
54. Powell AC, Alexander HR, Chang R, Marx SJ, Skarulis M, Pingpank JF, et al. Reoperation for parathyroid adenoma: a contemporary experience. Surgery [Internet]. 2009;146(6):1144–55. Available from: https://doi.org/10.1016/j.surg.2009.09.015.
55. Weber C, Sewell C, McGarity W. Persistent and recurrent sporadic primary hyperparathyroidism: histopathology, complications, and results of reoperation. Surgery. 1994;116(6):991–8.
56. Silverberg SJ, Clarke BL, Peacock M, Bandeira F, Boutroy S, Cusano NE, et al. Current issues in the presentation of asymptomatic primary hyperparathyroidism: proceedings of the fourth international workshop. J Clin Endocrinol Metab. 2014;99(10):3580–94.
57. Lee D, Walker MD, Chen HY, Chabot JA, Lee JA, Kuo JH. Bone mineral density changes after parathyroidectomy are dependent on biochemical profile. Surg (United States) [Internet]. 2019;165(1):107–13. Available from: https://doi.org/10.1016/j.surg.2018.04.065.
58. Cusano NE, Rubin MR, Silva BC, Tay YKD, Williams JM, Agarwal S, et al. Skeletal microstructure and estimated bone strength improve following parathyroidectomy in primary hyperparathyroidism. J Clin Endocrinol Metab. 2018;103(1):196–205.
59. Walker MD, Silverberg SJ. Primary hyperparathyroidism. Nat Rev Endocrinol [Internet]. 2018;14(2):115–25. Available from: https://doi.org/10.1038/nrendo.2017.104
60. Khan AA, Hanley DA, Rizzoli R, Bollerslev J, Young JEM, Rejnmark L, et al. Primary hyperparathyroidism: review and recommendations on evaluation, diagnosis, and management. A Canadian and international consensus. Osteoporos Int [Internet]. 2017;28(1):1–19. Available from: https://doi.org/10.1007/s00198-016-3716-2.
61. Pepe J, Cipriani C, Sonato C, Raimo O, Biamonte F, Minisola S. Cardiovascular manifestations of primary hyperparathyroidism: a narrative review. Eur J Endocrinol. 2017;177(6):R297–308.
62. Vázquez-Díaz O, Castillo-Martínez L, Orea-Tejeda A, Orozco-Gutiérrez JJ, Asensio-Lafuente E, Reza-Albarrán A, et al. Reversible changes of electrocardiographic abnormalities after parathyroidectomy in patients with primary hyperparathyroidism. Cardiol J. 2009;16(3):241–5.

Adrenals

Contents

Adrenal Glands: Anatomy, Physiology, and Pathophysiology

Sam Van Slycke, Klaas Van Den Heede, and Elisabeth-Ann Vandenwyngaerden

Contents

A. L. Shifrin et al. (eds.), *Endocrine Surgery Comprehensive Board Exam Guide*,
https://doi.org/10.1007/978-3-030-84737-1_17

Questions

1. Is an adrenal nodule always secreting?
2. If you suspect a Cushing, which hormone do you ask to dose in the first place?
3. What should always be questioned if you have a young woman without any symptoms of Cushing and a significantly elevated blood cortisol level?
4. Which lab result should you make think of a Conn in a patient with hypertension?
5. What is compatible with Conn: elevated aldosterone level–low renin level or elevated aldosterone level–elevated renin level or low aldosterone level–elevated renin level?
6. For the diagnosis of a pheochromocytoma, the dosage of epinephrine and norepinephrine is more accurate than the dosage of metanephrine and normetanephrine?
7. Performing a FNAC in an adrenal nodule is safe and recommended in the diagnostic work-out of an adrenal nodule?
8. Adrenocortical cancer has the same good prognosis as most endocrine tumors?
9. Elevated levels of cortisol and/or androgen or estrogen hypersecretion are highly suggestive for a benign adrenal nodule?
10. Elevated salivary cortisol levels is highly suggestive for Conn?
11. Hypertension is a rare phenomenon is secreting adrenal nodules?

17.1 Anatomy

The adrenal glands, also known as suprarenal glands, are endocrine organs found immediately superior to the upper pole of each kidney. They both comprise an outer cortex and an inner medulla, which are functionally and structurally distinct [1].

17.1.1 Embryology

Initially, formation of the adrenal glands is closely tied to that of the gonads as they both originate from a common region of mesoderm lying next the developing kidney. Segregation occurs, and by the ninth week, the adrenal primordia are fully enclosed by a capsule [2].

Within the adrenal glands, the cortex and medulla can be seen as two different organs with distinct embryonic origin, functions, and morphologic characteristics that unite during embryonic development [3]. First, the cortex develops in the fifth week and originates from the mesoderm. The coelomic epithelium that lies next to the developing gonadal ridge proliferates, and a subset of cells delaminates and enters the

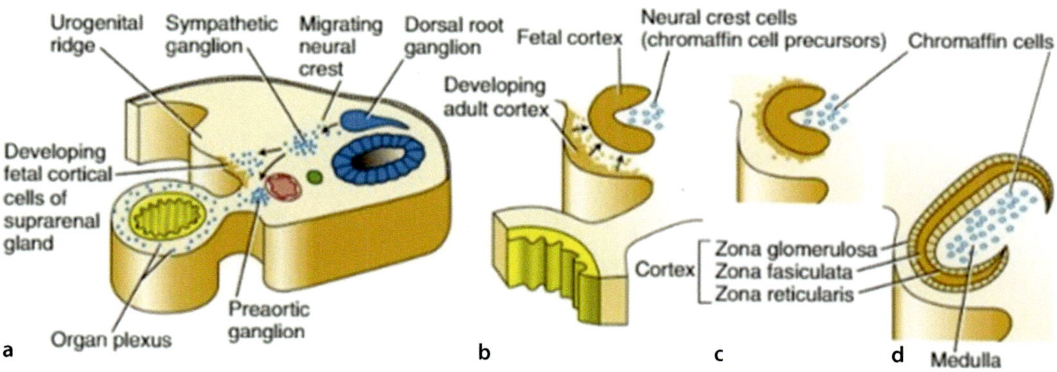

Fig. 17.1 Adrenal gland development. In the fifth week, the cortex develops and originates from the mesoderm. The coelomic epithelium that lies next to the developing gonadal ridge proliferates, and a subset of cells delaminates and enters the underlying mesoderm. They differentiate into the fetal adrenal cortical cells **a**. Next, a second group of delaminating cells migrates to surround the fetal cortex. They form a thinner definitive cortex **b**, **c**. By the second postnatal month, the fetal cortex regresses rapidly and the remaining definitive cortical cells organize into the layers known in the adult adrenal gland: the zona glomerulosa, zona fasciculata, and zona reticularis **d**. The medulla is derived from the neuroectoderm. Neural crest cells migrate into the adrenal medullary region adjoining the developing fetal cortex, where they differentiate into chromaffin cells **b**–**d**. (Reproduced from Schoenwolf et al. [2])

underlying mesoderm. They differentiate into the fetal adrenal cortical cells (Fig. 17.1a). Next, a second group of delaminating cells migrates to surround the fetal cortex. They form a thinner definitive cortex (Fig. 17.1b, c). Both cortical layers show characteristics of steroid-producing cells. During the second trimester, the fetal layer expands rapidly and produces dehydroepiandrosterone (DHEA) in the fetus, which is the substrate for placental estrogen and essential for maintaining pregnancy. Moreover, the products of the fetal cortex also influence the maturation of lungs, liver, and digestive tract, and it may contribute to regulating partition [2]. At birth, the adrenal glands are approximately one-third the size of its respective kidney [1], but the fetal cortex regresses rapidly by the second postnatal month, and the remaining definitive cortical cells organize into the layers known in the adult adrenal gland: the zona glomerulosa, zona fasciculata, and zona reticularis (Fig. 17.1d) [2].

Unlike the adrenal cortex, the medulla is derived from the neuroectoderm [4]. Neural crest cells migrate into the adrenal medullary region adjoining the developing fetal cortex, where they differentiate into chromaffin cells (Fig. 17.1b–d). These cells are specialized postganglionic sympathetic neurons innervated by preganglionic sympathetic fibers. Upon stimulation, they release epinephrine and norepinephrine [2].

17.1.2 Macroscopic Aspect

The adrenal glands are golden yellow in color [1] and have a fine granular surface [4]. The glands differ in shape: the right gland is pyramidal with two lower projections or limbs, whereas

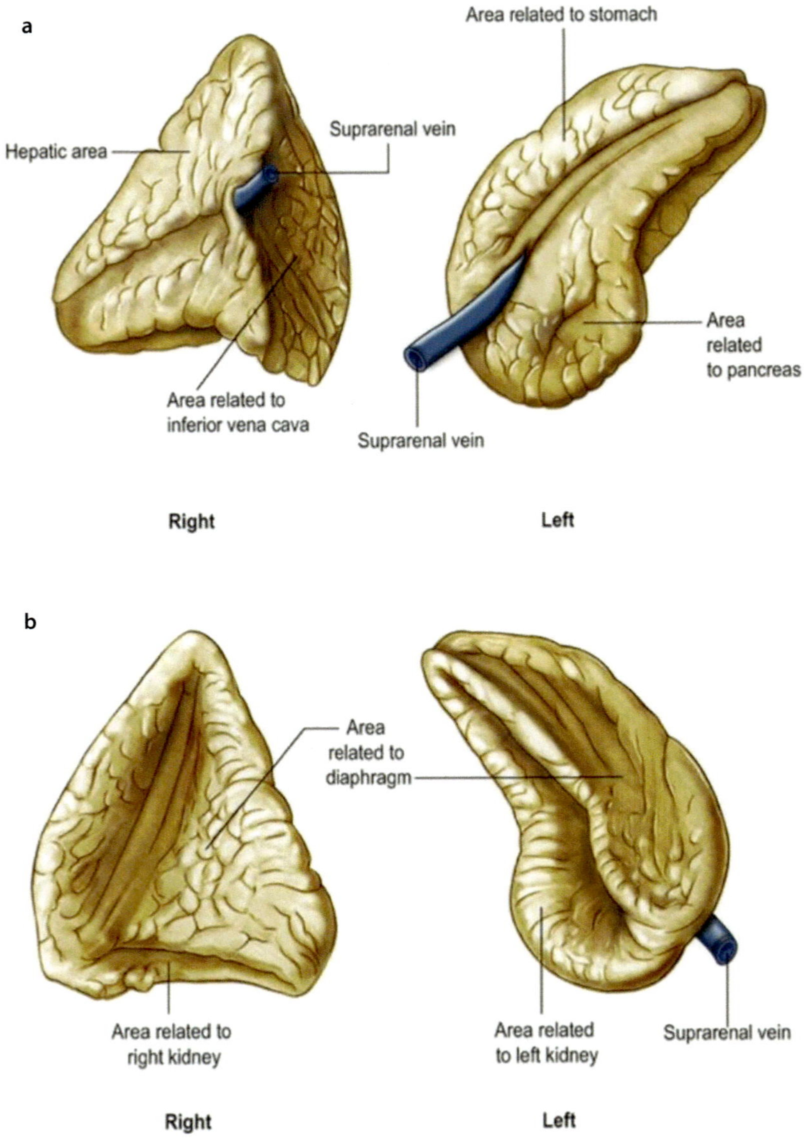

Fig. 17.2 The adrenal glands. The macroscopic anterior aspect **a** and posterior aspect **b**. (Reproduced from Standring [1])

the left gland is crescentic [1] (Fig. 17.2). The average measurements obtained from computed tomography are 0.61 cm (right) and 0.79 cm (left) for the maximum width of the body of the gland in adults. The mean width of the limbs, medial and lateral, measure approximately 0.30 cm [5]. In transverse section a suprarenal limb should not measure more than 5 mm. Each gland normally weighs approximately 5 g [1].

Small accessory adrenal nodules may be found in the areolar tissue; they are mainly composed of cortical tissue and are also known as "adrenal rests" [1].

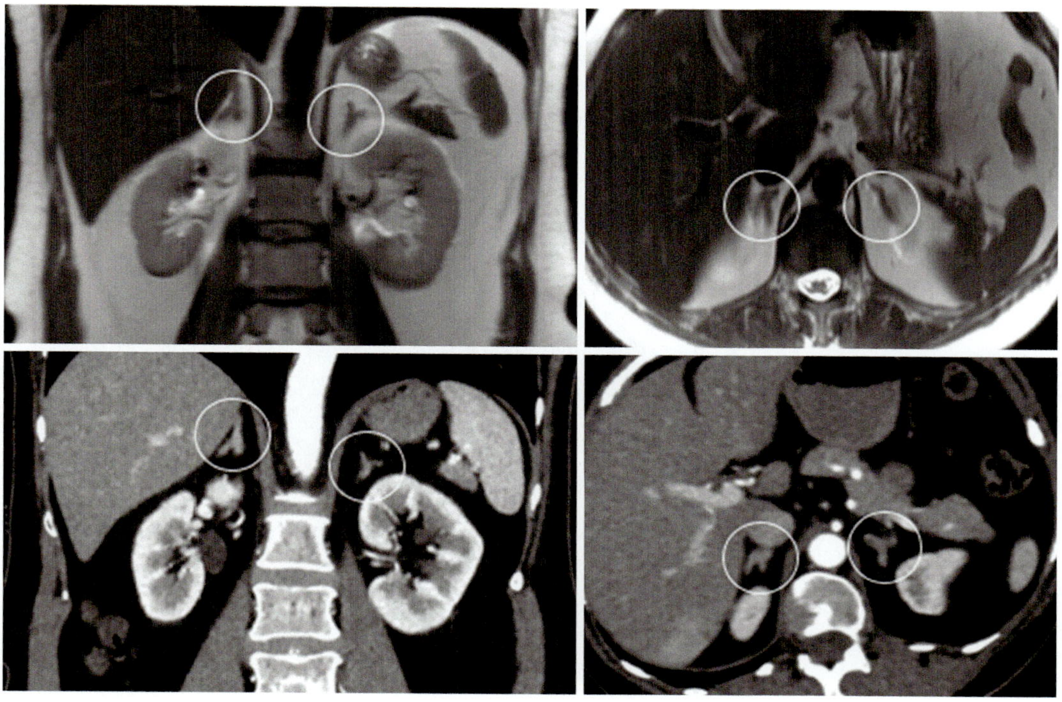

■ **Fig. 17.3** Normal adrenal glands. Triangular adrenal glands in a healthy individual on CT (above) and MR (below) images

17.1.2.1 Relationship to Surrounding Structures

The adrenal glands rest anterior of both crura of the diaphragm (■ Fig. 17.3). They lie in perinephric fat and are enclosed within the renal fascia. A limited amount of fibrous tissue separates the glands from its kidneys [1].

The majority of the right adrenal gland lies on the apex of the right kidney, slightly higher than the left gland which lies on the anteromedial part of the upper pole of the left kidney. The right adrenal gland lies posterior to right lobe of the liver, and the anterior surface lies posterior to the inferior vena cava with its medial facet (■ Fig. 17.3). The lateral facet is in contact with the bare area of the liver. Anteriorly, the left adrenal is anteriorly largely covered by peritoneum of the lesser sac, which separates the gland from the cardia of the stomach. A small part that is not covered lies closely to the pancreatic tail [1].

17.1.3 Arterial Supply

Three suprarenal arteries supply each adrenal gland with one of the highest arterial flow rates per gram of tissue [6]. The one or two inferior suprarenal arteries usually derive from the renal artery and the middle suprarenal artery arises from the abdominal aorta. The superior suprarenal artery emerges from the ipsilateral inferior phrenic artery before passing to the gland as four to five small branches (■ Fig. 17.4).

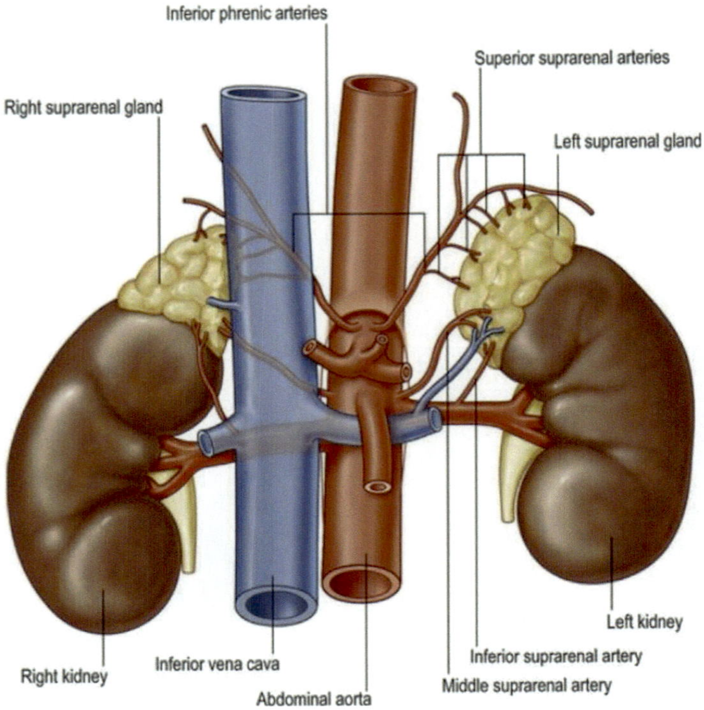

Fig. 17.4 The arterial supply and venous drainage of the suprarenal glands. (Reproduced from Drake et al. [20])

There may be multiple main branches of the suprarenal arteries, and they ramify before penetrating the gland, forming a subcapsular arterial plexus. Subsequently, sinusoids originate and pass around clusters of glomerulosa cells and between the zona fasciculata columns to form a deep plexus in the zona reticularis. Venules from this plexus pass to medullary veins [1].

17.1.4 Venous Drainage

Medullary veins arise from the hilum, usually forming a single suprarenal vein. The right vein is short and runs horizontally into the right vena cava. Occasionally, an accessory right suprarenal vein is present, running superior and medially from the hilum. The left suprarenal vein is longer and descends medially, draining into the left renal vein [1] (Fig. 17.4).

17.1.5 Lymphatic Drainage

In the adrenal capsule, lymphatic channels communicate with subserous lymphatics. These drain medially to para-aortic and paracaval nodes [7]. A few capsular channels communicate with lymph vessels passing through the diaphragm [1].

17.1.6 Nerve Supply

The adrenal gland has the largest autonomic supply of all organs, relative to its size. The nerves exist throughout the gland. A suprarenal plexus lies between the medial side of each gland and the coeliac and aorticorenal ganglia. It exists mostly of preganglionic sympathetic fibers originating from the lower thoracic spinal fragments, reaching the plexus through the splanchnic nerves. They synapse in clusters of medullary chromaffin cells, where they provoke the release of catecholamines. Other types of nerve fibers are found in the cortex, which may modulate the secretion of steroid hormones [8]. Postganglionic sympathetic nerve fibers innervate cortical blood vessels, regulating the blood flow.

17.1.7 Histology

The general histologic appearance of the adrenal gland is typical of an endocrine gland in which cells of both cortex and medulla are grouped into cords alongside wide capillaries [3].

The yellowish adrenal cortex consists out of three different zones below the capsule (■ Fig. 17.5). They are arranged concentrically. These zones differ in arrangement, quantity of lipid droplets, and the accumulation of pigment. However, they also have features in common characteristic for their function as steroid-secreting cells: acidophilic cytoplasm rich in lipid droplets, with central nuclei. Immediately inside the capsule lies the zona glomerulosa which comprises approximately 15% of the cortex. It consists out of closely packed cords of columnar or pyramidal cells with many capillaries. In the middle, 65–80% of the cortex is occupied by the zona fasciculata, in which long cords of large polyhedral cells, often one cell thick, are found. They are separated by fenestrated sinusoidal capillaries. The

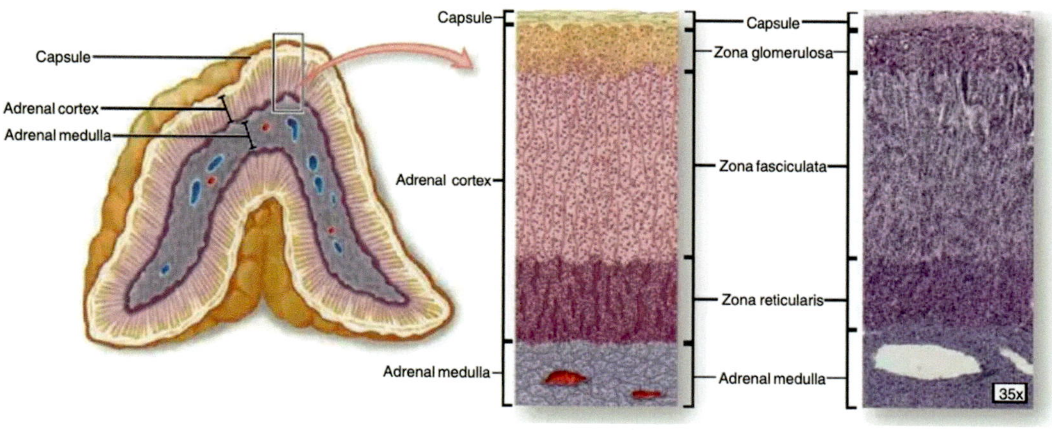

■ **Fig. 17.5** Section through an adrenal gland showing the medulla and cortex, as well as the different layers within the cortex. A hematoxylin- and eosin-stained image shows the corresponding zones. (Reproduced from Mescher [3])

innermost zona reticularis consists out of irregular cords, forming a network with smaller cells and wide capillaries in between [3].

The reddish adrenal medulla consists out of cords and clumps of large, pale-staining polyhedral cells (◘ Fig. 17.5). They are supported by a reticular fiber network. Many sinusoidal capillaries intervene between the cords. The medullary parenchymal cells are known as chromaffin cells. They contain many granules for storage and secretion of catecholamines. There is a distinction between norepinephrine-secreting cells and epinephrine-secreting cells [3].

17.2 Physiology

The adrenal glands synthetize different hormones in their different layers (◘ Table 17.1).

17.2.1 The Adrenocortical Hormones

In adrenal tissue, many steroids have been isolated. However, the adrenal cortex only hosts the synthesis and release of mineralocorticoids, glucocorticoids, and androgens in a physiologically significant amount. The mineralocorticoid aldosterone is synthetized in the outer layer, the zona glomerulosa. The glucocorticoids cortisol and corticosterone and the androgens dehydroepiandrosterone (DHEA) and androstenedione, both originate from the zona fasciculata and zona reticularis (◘ Table 17.1). From DHEA, the sex hormones can be synthetized. Deoxycorticosterone is normally secreted in approxi-

◘ **Table 17.1** Overview of the adrenocortical and adrenomedullary hormone secretion

	Adrenal layer	Hormones	Example
Adrenal cortex	Zona glomerulosa	Mineralocorticoids	Aldosterone
	Zona fasciculata	Glucocorticoids and androgens	Cortisol, corticosterone Dehydroepiandrosterone
	–		
	Zona reticularis		
Adrenal medulla	–	Catecholamines	Epinephrine Norepinephrine Dopamine

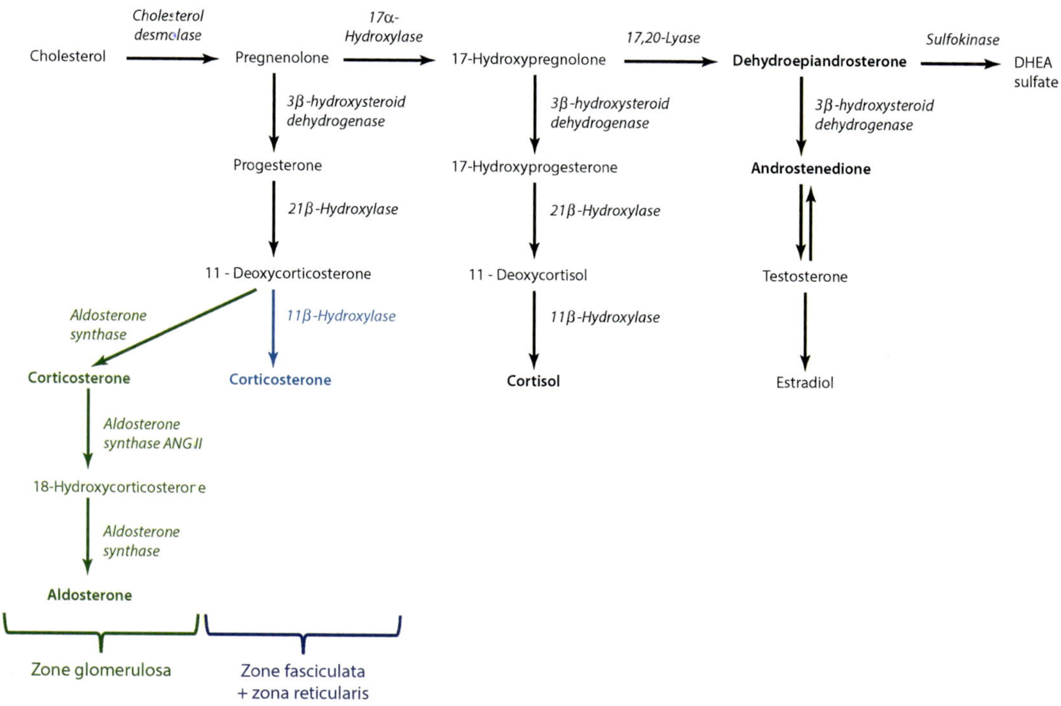

Fig. 17.6 Overview of hormone synthesis in the adrenal cortex. The major hormones are in bold. The enzymes for the reactions are indicated in italics. In the zona glomerulosa (shown in green), there is no 11 β-hydroxylase as is the case in the zona fasciculata and zona reticularis (shown in blue). However, it contains aldosterone synthase, enabling the conversion from corticosterone to aldosterone in the zona glomerulosa. DHEA: dehydroepiandrosterone; ANG II: angiotensin II

mately the same amount as aldosterone, but its effect on the metabolism is negligible. However, it is worth mentioning because its effect can be important in diseases where its secretion increases [9].

The adrenocortical hormones are all derivatives of the precursor cholesterol, containing a cyclopentanoperhydrophenanthrene nucleus. Mineralocorticoids and glucocorticoids are C_{21} steroids (with a two-carbon side chain at position 17), while androgens are of the C_{19} type (with a keto or hydroxyl group at position 17) [9]. The hormone synthesis of the adrenocortical steroids is summarized in Fig. 17.6.

17.2.1.1 Glucocorticoids: Corticosterone and Cortisol

Corticosterone and cortisol are the main human glucocorticoids. In circulation, cortisol is mainly bound to the corticosteroid-binding globulin (CBG) and in a lesser extent to albumin. Corticosterone is similarly bound, but in a lesser degree. The half-life of cortisol is therefore longer (approximately 60–90 minutes) than that of corticosterone (50 minutes). Bound steroids are biologically inactive. Changes in the CBG concentration result in changes of the bound proportion and thus also of the free cortisol level. However, at normal levels of cortisol (13,5 μg/dL), very little free cortisol is circulating. CBG is synthetized in the liver, and its production is increased by estrogen [9].

Glucocorticoids are metabolized in the liver either by a reduction reaction with the formation of first dihydrocortisol and then tetrahydrocortisol or by oxidation with the formation of cortisone. This is a very active glucocorticoid on its own, because it is converted to cortisol. Excretion occurs rapidly and mainly by the kidneys. Excretion through the liver is also possible for about 10% of the secreted cortisol, in which the metabolites enter an enterohepatic cycle and are excreted in the stool [9].

Effects of Glucocorticoids

Glucocorticoids bind to a cytoplasmatic glucocorticoid receptor that, after activation, migrates to the nucleus where transactivation causes the expression of new genes. In physiologic concentrations, glucocorticoids have impact on the intermediary metabolism of carbohydrates, protein, and fat. They increase protein catabolism, hepatic glycogenesis, and gluconeogenesis. They have an anti-insulin effect which potentially worsens diabetes. The glucocorticoids not trigger a reaction of their own but do have a permissive action effect. They must be present for certain other metabolic reactions to happen, such as the calorigenic, lipolytic, and vasopressor effects of catecholamines. Furthermore, glucocorticoids have the quality to be able to restore vascular reactivity and have an effect on the nervous system. They are also the only hormones to repair the deficit of adrenal insufficiency in cases where there is an inability to excrete water. They reduce plasma vasopressin levels and raise the glomerular filtration rate significantly. Lastly, glucocorticoids lower the concentration of circulating lymphocytes, basophils, and eosinophils and increase the number of neutrophils, platelets, and red blood cells. They decrease the size of the lymphatic organs and reduce the secretion of cytokines [9].

Regulation of Glucocorticoid Release

Secretion of glucocorticoids, both basal as stress-provoked, is regulated by ACTH. This polypeptide is released by the anterior pituitary gland. Stimulation of glucocorticoid release is acquired a few minutes after ACTH release [9].

The basal secretion of ACTH happens in irregular bursts following a circadian rhythm. The release and consecutive plasma glucocorticoids level are at its highest in the morning (approximately 25 pg/mL). The release of ACTH is regulated through the hypothalamo-hypophyseal axis depending on the secretion of corticotropin-releasing hormone (CRH) of the hypothalamus. The circadian rhythm is controlled in the suprachiasmatic nuclei of the hypothalamus. Stressor stimuli such as trauma or emotion result in an increased CRH release. Via ACTH, the glucocorticoids are mobilized as well [9].

CRH, ACTH, and the glucocorticoids are part of a feedback control loop: an increase of the plasma glucocorticoid level inhibits the release on both pituitary and hypothalamic level of respectively ACTH and CRH. The feedback control tries to keep the circulating glucocorticoids at level: decreased concentrations activate CRH and ACTH, while increased free concentrations inhibit both of their release. The feedback control is possible due to changing gene expression, which causes a certain delay of multiple hours before there is a response by activation of CRH and ACTH [9].

17.2.1.2 Mineralocorticoids: Aldosterone

Aldosterone is synthetized in the zona glomerulosa from 11-deoxycorticosterone, where no 11β-hydroxylase is present as is the case in the zona fasciculata and zona reticularis. However, it contains aldosterone synthase that shows great similarities with 11β-hydroxylase but also contains activity that enables the conversion of corticosterone to aldosterone. 11-Deoxycorticosterone itself has a limited mineralocorticoid effect.

Aldosterone in circulation is bound to protein, but less than glucocorticoids. Therefore, it has a shorter half-life (about 20 minutes). The secreted amount is in normal circumstances only about 0,006 μg/dL. Most of the aldosterone is metabolized in the liver, but some is converted into a glucuronide which is converted to free aldosterone, often called "acid-labile conjugate" because it is formed by hydrolysis at pH 1.0 (5%). Less than 1% of the secreted aldosterone is found freely in the urine [9].

Effects of Mineralocorticoids

The most important effect of mineralocorticoids is to maintain the extracellular fluid volume and normal Na + and K+ concentrations [4]. Aldosterone causes Na + retention in the extracellular fluid by reabsorption of Na + in urine, sweat, saliva, and contents of the colon. At the level of the kidneys, mineralocorticoids act on the principal cells to increase urine acidity by exchanging more Na + for K+/H+ and producing a K+ diuresis. These hormones accomplish their effect by binding to a cytoplasmic receptor, which will move to the nucleus where it alters the gene transcription [9].

Regulation of Mineralocorticoid Release

Stress-related conditions defined as conditions in which the existing optimal steady-state changes are stimuli for aldosterone secretion. Examples are surgery, anxiety, physical trauma, etc. The primary regulating and stimulating factors are ACTH, renin from the kidney (via ATII: angiotensin II), and a direct stimulatory effect of a rise in K+ concentration. Renin is released when a decrease of the intravascular volume is registered in the renal juxtaglomerular cells [4]. The secretion is regulated via a feedback loop concerning the renin-angiotensin system [9].

17.2.1.3 Adrenal Androgens

The major adrenal androgen is the 17-ketosteroid DHEA, although androstenedione is secreted as well. DHEA is primarily released by the zona reticularis [4] and appears in circulation conjugated with sulfate (DHEAS: DHEA Sulfate) for about 97.7%. Androstenedione reaches the peripheral organs through the circulation, where it converts to testosterone in the testes and to estrogens in the adipocytes of adipose tissue [9].

The daily 17-ketosteroid excretion is 15 mg (in men) or 10 mg (in women), resulting in the fact that two-thirds of the urinary ketosteroids in men are of adrenal origin. Etiocholanolone is one of the metabolites and can cause fever when unconjugated [9].

Effects of Adrenal Androgens and Estrogens

Adrenal androgens have a very weak masculinizing effect in physiological concentrations, compared to testosterone from the testes (less than 20% of the activity). They also promote protein anabolism and growth. DHEA is the basis for the synthesis of the sex hormones testosterone and estradiol [9].

The conversion of androstenedione to estrogens in fat creates an important role of estrogens in men and postmenopausal women [9].

Regulation of Adrenal Androgen Release

The release of adrenal androgens is controlled by ACTH, and not by gonadotropins. The DHEAS concentrations are higher in young people with a peak in the early 20s around 225 mg/dL. With age, these concentrations decrease. This cannot be explained by changes in ACTH secretion, but is most likely an effect of a gradual fall in lyase activity of 17α-hydroxylase [9].

17.2.2 The Adrenomedullary Hormones

The adrenal medulla synthesizes catecholamines, released into the circulation through the sinusoid capillaries. The catecholamine output is mostly epinephrine, some norepinephrine, and small amount of dopamine. The plasma level of norepinephrine is higher because it also enters the circulation from noradrenergic nerve endings. About 70% of the norepinephrine and epinephrine and 95% of the dopamine in plasma are conjugated to sulfate. Only non-conjugated catecholamines are biologically active. Catecholamines have a half-life of about 2 minutes in circulation. They are excreted through the kidney as metabolites: 50% free or conjugated metanephrine and normetanephrine, 35% vanillylmandelic acid (VMA), and small amounts of free epinephrine and norepinephrine [9].

Other substances than catecholamines are also secreted by the adrenal medulla, which are stored in the same granules. ATP, chromogranin A, peptides, and proteins are consequently released in the blood together with catecholamines [9].

17.2.2.1 Effects of Epinephrine and Norepinephrine

Catecholamines have a spectrum of effects: on the heart, vessels, brain, and metabolism. For epinephrine, effects are mostly the consequence of the free concentration. For norepinephrine, effects are mostly realized by the local release from the noradrenergic nerve endings, given that the circulating norepinephrine is too low in concentration to have effects [9].

At the level of the heart, epinephrine and norepinephrine increase the force and rate of contraction (mediated by β_1-adrenergic receptors) and stimulate myocardial excitability. At the level of the blood vessels, norepinephrine causes vasoconstriction in almost all organs via α_1-adrenergic receptors. This is in contradiction to epinephrine, which induces vasodilatation in skeletal muscles and liver via β_2-receptors. Usually, the latter predominates the vasoconstrictive effect and the total peripheral resistance drops. At the level of the brain, epinephrine and norepinephrine equally increase alertness. Furthermore, catecholamines affect blood glucose levels through several mechanisms. Epinephrine and norepinephrine both stimulate glycogenolysis, through a β_2-receptor mediated activation of phosphorylase and via α-adrenergic receptors that increase intracellular Ca^{2+}. They also stimulate insulin and glucagon secretion via β-adrenergic pathways and inhibit the secretion via α-adrenergic mechanisms. At the level of metabolism, norepinephrine and epinephrine induce a sudden rise in the metabolic rate as well as a delayed rise. The initiate increase is independent of the liver and may be due to cutaneous vasoconstriction (which decreases heat loss), the second increase is likely due to oxidation of lactate in the liver [9].

17.2.2.2 Effects of Dopamine

The physiologic functions of dopamine in the circulation are unknown, but when injected, it produces vasodilatation in the kidney and mesentery. Elsewhere, it causes vasoconstriction and increases contractibility of the heart via β_1-adrenergic receptors. This may be explained by a release of norepinephrine. The total effect of moderate doses of dopamine is an increase in systolic blood pressure and no change in diastolic pressure [9].

17.2.2.3 Regulation of Adrenal Medullary Secretion

The release of catecholamines from the adrenal gland is regulated by several factors. The most important are a lower secretion during sleep and a stimulation of secretion by arising from recumbent to standing position, during exercise, in emergency situations (followed by the flight or fight response) and when hypoglycemia, ketoacidosis, or a myocardial infarction occurs [9].

17.3 Pathophysiology

17.3.1 Introduction

Knowing normal adrenal physiology will help to understand symptoms linked to overproduction of certain adrenal hormones. In the work-up of an adrenal incidentaloma, functional studies should be carried out first before any invasive procedure. The following chapter explains basic pathophysiology of the most frequent adrenal disorders.

17.3.2 Cushing's Syndrome

Cushing's syndrome is a rare clinical entity resulting from excessive production of glucocorticoids by the adrenal cortex. As mentioned before, the zona fasciculata of the adrenal cortex secretes cortisol in a circadian rhythm [10]. Regulation is controlled through the hypothalamic-pituitary-adrenal (HPA) axis [11]. Understanding its neuroendocrine negative feedback system is essential for successfully managing a patient with Cushing's syndrome. Given the sophisticated regulation, hypercortisolism can result from a number of different pathologies that result in excessive secretion of cortisol. Causes of Cushing's syndrome are divided into three main groups [10]:

(1) *Exogenous hypercortisolism* is the result of iatrogenic glucocorticoid administration. Cushing syndrome can result even from the administration of low doses of exogenous steroids administered orally, topically, or by inhaled preparations.
(2) *Endogenous ACTH-dependent hypercortisolism* results from an elevated serum corticotropin level due to pathology extrinsic to the adrenal gland. ACTH-producing pituitary adenomas and ectopic ACTH-secreting tumors fall within this category.
(3) *Endogenous ACTH-independent hypercortisolism* results from unregulated overproduction of glucocorticoids by the adrenal(s) itself, most often by cortisol-secreting adenomas, rarely by hyperplastic glands. Autonomous overproduction of cortisol results suppression of ACTH secretion by pituitary corticotroph cells.

Loss of its diurnal secretion pattern is a cardinal feature of Cushing's syndrome. It forms the basis for screening tests aimed at differentiating pathologic hypercortisolism from other conditions with overlapping clinical findings. Non-pathologic increases in total cortisol are found in conditions affecting the level of cortisol-binding globulin (CBG) (such as pregnancy and oral contraceptive use), an important consideration in laboratory testing. Elevated plasma cortisol levels (>20 mcg/dL) will saturate CBG, resulting in elevated salivary and urinary levels [10, 12].

Effects of hypercortisolemia are mediated by the affinity of cortisol for both glucocorticoid and mineralocorticoid receptors, which are widely expressed throughout the body. Hypercortisolemia causes insulin resistance (often resulting in hyperglycemia), dyslipidemia and hypertension contributing to an elevated cardiac risk profile. Proximal muscle weakness and weight gain are caused by catabolism of skeletal muscle proteins to support increased gluconeogenesis by the liver. Changes in immune response result from deficiencies in neutrophil and macrophage function and downregulation of inflammatory cytokines. Increase in procoagulant factors and decrease in fibrinolysis lead to a prothrombotic state [12]. Hypercortisolemia also predisposes to osteoporosis by inhibiting osteoblast activity. Hypercortisolism of any etiology may result in suppression of thyroid-stimulating hormone (TSH) and gonadotropins, leading to reversible hypothyroidism and hypogonadotropic hypogonadism [10].

Diagnosis and treatment of Cushing's syndrome are multifaceted, often requiring the cooperation of internists, endocrinologists, neurosurgeons, and endocrine surgeons. Therefore, symptoms, diagnosis, and treatment will be discussed in a separate chapter.

17.3.3 Conn's Syndrome

Conn's syndrome is a rare clinical entity resulting from primary aldosteronism. Primary aldosteronism can be defined as a group of disorders with excess aldosterone production, autonomous from the renin-angiotensin system [13]. As mentioned before, the zona glomerulosa of the adrenal cortex secretes aldosterone, and regulation is controlled through a feedback loop concerning the renin-angiotensin system. Understanding this feedback system is important to manage a patient with Conn's syndrome [14].

Primary hyperaldosteronism is caused by aldosterone-producing adenomas, bilateral idiopathic adrenal hyperplasia, aldosterone-producing adrenal carcinoma, or familial aldosteronism [13, 14].

Causes of primary aldosteronism can also be divided into two main groups:

1. Unilateral disease, which can be treated and cured surgically.
2. Bilateral disease, which is treated medically in most of cases.

As explained earlier, the increased amount of aldosterone stimulates renal sodium reabsorption and water retention and potassium excretion by changing activity of basolateral membrane sodium-potassium ATPase and apical epithelial sodium channels as well as potassium channels in the tubular cells of the distal nephron. Since more sodium is reabsorbed than potassium secreted, the lumen becomes more electrically negative, causing chloride to follow sodium. H_2O follows by osmosis. In Conn's syndrome, these actions result in sodium retention, hypokalemia and metabolic alkalosis [13, 14]. The increased sodium reabsorption by the kidneys results in plasma volume expansion which is the primary initiating mechanism for hypertension. Hypokalemia causes impairment in glucose tolerance which is due to the inhibitory effects of hypokalemia on insulin secretion.

The expanded plasma volume may induce tissue inflammation and heightened sympathetic drive, with subsequent development of fibrosis in vital organs, such as heart, kidneys, and vasculature. As a result, this may lead to the development of chronic kidney disease, atrial fibrillation, stroke, ischemic heart disease, and congestive heart failure [13].

The increased blood pressure, the subsequent increased glomerular filtration rate, and subsequent decrease in renin release normally result in decreased aldosterone levels. If there is primary hyperaldosteronism, the decreased renin (and subsequent decreased angiotensin II) will not lead to a decrease in aldosterone levels. This is a helpful clinical tool in diagnosis of primary hyperaldosteronism [9, 13].

Diagnosis and treatment of Conn's syndrome are multifaceted, often requiring the cooperation of internists, endocrinologists, and endocrine surgeons. Therefore, symptoms, diagnosis, and treatment will be discussed in a separate chapter.

17.3.4 Pheochromocytoma

A pheochromocytoma is a rare clinical entity resulting from a tumor that produces catecholamines in excessive amounts and arises from the chromaffin cells of the adrenal medulla or from extra-adrenal sympathetic ganglia cells. A pheochromocytoma secretes predominantly norepinephrine. High levels of epinephrine are suggestive of an adrenal origin, since the phenylethanolamine N-methyltransferase enzyme, converting norepinephrine to epinephrine, is mainly present in the adrenal medulla and organ of Zuckerkandl (chromaffin cells at the bifurcation of the aorta) [15]. Rarely, a pheochromocytoma secretes other neurohormones such as dopamine, VIP, adrenocorticotrophic hormones, beta-endorphins, and a variety of other substances that can complicate the clinical manifestations and the differential diagnosis [15, 16].

The most common sign of a pheochromocytoma is hypertension, found in approximately 95% of patients and related to catecholamine excess. Additional symptoms seen in pheochromocytoma patients include headache, palpitations, anxiety, and sweating [17].

In addition to being a great mimicker, pheochromocytomas represent a true clinical challenge, where symptoms and signs can significantly vary in seemingly comparable clinical settings [15].

Clinical phenotype of hypertensive syndrome depends on multiple factors including the amount of catecholamine production, their intracellular processing, and the pattern of their secretion. Most patients with pheochromocytoma have significantly increased plasma catecholamine levels, with norepinephrine and epinephrine levels reaching 5 to 10 times the upper reference limit. While the cellular content can be enormous, intracellular processing can divert significant amounts into metabolites, resulting in normal or near normal plasma catecholamine levels and significantly elevated levels of (nor-)metanephrines [16, 17].

Diagnosis and treatment of a phaeochromocytoma are multifaceted, often requiring the cooperation of internists, endocrinologists, and endocrine surgeons. Therefore, symptoms, diagnosis, and treatment will be discussed in a separate chapter.

17.3.5 Adrenocortical Carcinoma

An adrenocortical carcinoma (ACC) is a very rare tumor associated with poor survival. Radical surgical excision remains the only potentially curative treatment [18]. Two-thirds of patients present with symptoms or signs of excessive hormone secretion. One-third of patients have large non-secreting tumors and present with symptoms related to its size [19].

Symptoms leading to the diagnosis can be due to hormone hypersecretion and/or tumor mass and metastasis. When careful hormonal investigations are performed, it turns out that the majority of ACC are secreting tumors, even when this is not clinically apparent. In contrast to benign adrenocortical tumors, ACC can co-secrete various types of steroids. Co-secretion of androgens and cortisol is the most frequent and highly suggestive of a malignant adrenocortical tumor [19]. Pathophysiology of cortisol and aldosterone has been discussed prior in this chapter. Androgen hypersecretion may induce various manifestations in women: hirsutism, menstrual abnormalities, infertility, and eventually frank virilization (alopecia, deepening of the voice, clitoris hypertrophy). ACC can also secrete mineralocorticoids and steroid precursors. Hypersecretion of estrogens can be observed in rare cases. Estrogen excess is responsible for gynecomastia in males.

Hormonal investigations therefore aim to characterize the steroid secretory profile [18, 19].

Diagnosis and treatment of adrenocortical cancer are multifaceted, often requiring the cooperation of internists, endocrinologists, and endocrine surgeons. Therefore, symptoms, diagnosis, genetics, classification, and treatment will be discussed in a separate chapter.

Answers to the Questions

1. No.
2. ACTH.
3. Medical oral contraceptive treatment.
4. Hypokalemia.
5. Elevated aldosterone level–low renin level.
6. No.
7. No! A phaeochromocytoma or an adrenocortical carcinoma should be ruled out first.
8. No.
9. No, this is highly suggestive for a malignant adrenocortical cancer.
10. No, it is for Cushing.
11. No.

References

1. Standring S. Chapter 71: Suprarenal (adrenal) gland. In: Standring S, editor. Gray's anatomy. 41st ed. Elsevier; London UK. 2016.
2. Schoenwolf GC, Bleyl SB, Brauer PR, Francis-West PH. Chapter 15: Development of the urogenital system. In: Larsen's human embryology. 4th ed. Churchill Livingstone Elsevier; Philadelphia, PA. 2009. p. 499–500.
3. Mescher AL. Chapter 20: Endocrine glands. In: Junqueira's basic histology. 13th ed. McGraw-Hill Education; OH, United States. 2013. p. 404–28.
4. Mihai R, Frandon JR. Chapter 64: Surgical embryology and anatomy of the adrenal glands. In: Textbook of endocrine surgery. 2nd ed. Elsevier; Philadelphia, PA. 2005. p. 557–75.
5. Vincent JM, Morrison ID, Armstrong P, Reznek RH. The size of normal adrenal glands on computed tomography. Clin Radiol. 1994;49(7):453–5.
6. Williams LR, Leggett RW. Reference values for resting blood flow to organs of man. Clin Phys Physiol Meas. 1989;10(3):187–217.
7. Merklin RJ. Suprarenal gland lymphatic drainage. Am J Anat. 1966;119(3):359–74.
8. Tóth IE, Vizi ES, Hinson JP, Vinson GP. Innervation of the adrenal cortex, its physiological relevance, with primary focus on the noradrenergic transmission. Microsc Res Tech. 1997;36(6):534–45.
9. Barrett KE, Barman SM, Boitano S, Brooks HL. Chapter 20: The adrenal medulla & adrenal cortex. In: Ganong's review of medical physiology. 24th ed. McGraw-Hill Education; United States. 2012. p. 353–76.
10. Lirov R, Gauger PG. Chapter 26: Cushing's syndrome. Evidence-based endocrine surgery. Springer; Singapore. 2018. p. 335–66.
11. Jacobson L. Hypothalamic–pituitary–adrenocortical axis regulation. Endocrinol Metab Clin N Am. 2005;34:271–92.

12. Barbot M, Ceccato F, Scaroni C. The pathophysiology and treatment of hypertension in patients with Cushing's syndrome. Front Endocrinol (Lausanne). 2019;10:321. Published 2019 May 21. https://doi.org/10.3389/fendo.2019.00321.
13. Soh LM. Chapter 27: Conn's syndrome. In: Evidence-based endocrine surgery. Springer; Singapore. 2018. p. 367–76.
14. Parmar MS, Singh S. Conn syndrome. [Updated 2020 Jun 25]. In: StatPearls [Internet]. Treasure Island (FL): StatPearls Publishing; 2020 Jan. Available from: https://www.ncbi.nlm.nih.gov/books/NBK459197/.
15. Mishra AK, Singh K, Ramakant P, Agarwal A. Phaeochromocytoma. In: Evidence-based endocrine surgery. Springer; Singapore. 2018. p. 377–88.
16. Lenders JW, Eisenhofer G, Mannelli M, Pacak K. Phaeochromocytoma. Lancet. 2005;366:665–75.
17. Zuber SM, Kantorovich V, Pacak K. Hypertension in pheochromocytoma: characteristics and treatment. Endocrinol Metab Clin N Am. 2011;40(2):295–vii. https://doi.org/10.1016/j.ecl.2011.02.002.
18. Mihai R. Surgery for adrenocortical cancer: evidence-based recommendations. In: Evidence-based endocrine surgery. Springer; Singapore. 2018. p. 389–400.
19. Libè R, Fratticci A, Bertherat J. Adrenocortical cancer: pathophysiology and clinical management. Endocr Relat Cancer. 2007;14(1):13–28. https://doi.org/10.1677/erc.1.01130.
20. Drake RL, Vogl AW, Mitchell A. Gray's anatomy for students. 2nd ed. Churchill Livingstone: Elsevier; Philadelphia, PA. 2010.

Adrenal Incidentaloma

Johnathan G. Hubbard and Frederic Sebag

Contents

A. L. Shifrin et al. (eds.), *Endocrine Surgery Comprehensive Board Exam Guide*,
https://doi.org/10.1007/978-3-030-84737-1_18

Case Presentation

A 51-year-old female was referred to clinic with an incidental finding of a left adrenal mass. The patient had undergone an enhanced CT scan 2 years previously as part of a diabetes work up. The CT report describes a round-shaped left 2 cm adrenal mass (◘ Fig. 18.1).

Medical History:
- Familial: No specific element
- Personal: Type II diabetes, HBP, hypothyroidism, bipolar troubles
- Clinical examination: 1.65 m, 61 kg
- No specific sign (skin, hair, fat repartition)
- BP: 141/84

Treatment:
- L-Thyroxine: 75 μg/d
- Metformin: 700 mg × 2/d
- Amlodipine: 10 mg/d
- Lithium carbonate: 600 mg/d

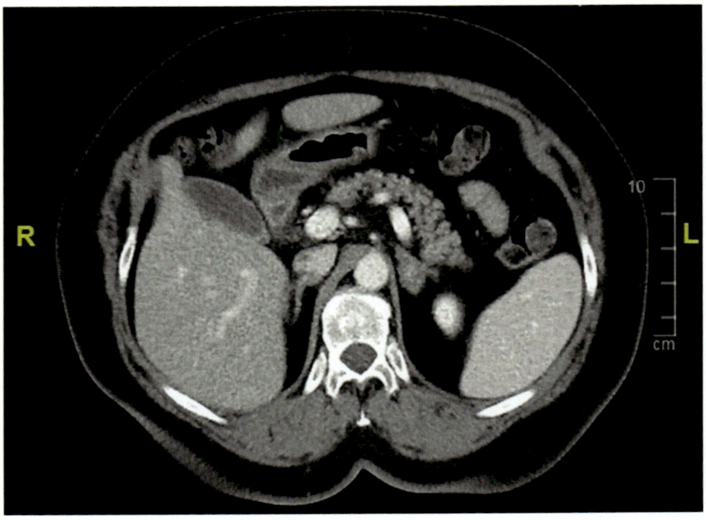

◘ **Fig. 18.1** Contrast CT showing 10 mm left adrenal nodule

Questions: (More Than One Option May Have to Be Chosen)

1. What is the most appropriate management for this patient?
    1. As no advert event happened during the last 2 years, clinical follow-up once a year is enough.
    2. Regarding the clinical presentation, there is strong evidence for a secreting adrenal tumor; surgery is mandatory.

   3. The patient requires an appropriate imaging work up.
   4. The patient requires an appropriate biochemical work up.
   5. The patient needs to be referred to a genetic counselling for advice.
2. Choose the right propositions.
   1. This case typically fits with the definition of incidentaloma.
   2. Regarding symptoms, it's a typical presentation for a secreting adrenal tumor.
   3. MRI as a first-line imaging is mandatory.
   4. Dedicated, initially unenhanced, adrenal CT scan would be the optimal approach.
   5. Regarding small size (<4 cm), no biological work up is needed.

As there were difficulties communicating with the patient, and concerns about the medical history, the GP was contacted. The GP provided further information that she had a suspicion of primary hyperaldosteronism and difficulties in managing diabetes. One plasma aldosterone assay was clearly high: 950 pmol/l.

Further information:

Blood cell count: Normal

Na^+: 142 mmol/l

K^+: 4.3 mmol/l

Normal renal function

TSH 0.83

3. What do you consider should be the next steps? (Select the right propositions)
   1. This work up is enough! Leave this patient alone!
   2. First priority: Measure sex hormones, precursors, and 17HO progesterone.
   3. Evaluate the metanephrines (plasma or urine)
   4. Cortisol secretion should be evaluated with a 1 mg overnight dexamethasone suppression test.
   5. Measure the aldosterone/renin ratio.

A dedicated CT scan was done. A 24 mm round-shaped left adrenal mass was described on the medial branch. Unenhanced density is <10 HU (◘ Fig. 18.2), after enhancement wash out is above 40%. A second mass is described on the external adrenal branch, 14 mm, with the same density and behavior. Right adrenal is considered normal.

4. What are your considerations following these results? (Select the best propositions.)
   1. To strongly consider surgery.
   2. Definitely MRI is needed.
   3. No hurry, in this case, surgical indication would rely on hormonal status
   4. Increasing should lead to FDG PET scanning.
   5. Genetic counselling is needed.

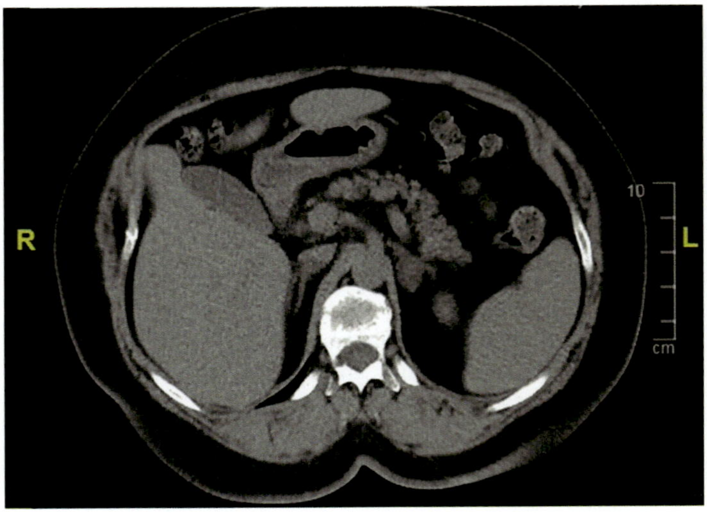

Fig. 18.2 Pre-contrast scan showing 10 mm Left adrenal nodule <10 HU

This lab work up is addressed to you:
K+: 4.1 mmol/l
TSH 1.01, calcitonin 21 pg/ml, calcium 2.52 mmol/l
Metanephrines: below the normal range, chromogranin A: 79 (N < 100)
Dexamethasone suppression test: cortisol 43 mmol/l, ACTH 0,66 pg/ml
Urinary-free cortisol (UFC): 124 nmol/24 h (30–197) 2000 cc
Ratio aldosterone/renin(rest) = 26,5
Ratio aldosterone/renin(activity) = 41,27
Urine aldosterone: 15 µg/24 h (0,58 to 26 µg/24 h)

5. These results suggest: (Select the correct propositions.)
    1. Subclinical Cushing syndrome cannot be eliminated.
    2. Evaluation of primary hyperaldosteronism should be more extensive
    3. Regarding imaging and biological results, there is no suspicion of pheochromocytoma.
    4. After this work up, the tumors should be considered as not secreting.
    5. To definitely confirm the secretion status, Norcholesterol scintigraphy is needed.

Regarding the patient's medical history, and all the information available, which other endocrine aspects do you want to explore?

6. Choose the right propositions.
    1. Let's go back to thorough interview, exploring past medical history, habits, toxics (alcohol, tobacco, etc), medication, etc.
    2. All the pituitary axis should be explored.
    3. Calcium metabolism and parathyroid function should be evaluated.

   4. More detailed and repeated thyroid test should be done.
   5. Please stop spending money!

Lab tests:

TSH 1.02, thyroid AB negative, calcitonin 18 pg/ml

Ca 2.48 mmol/l, PTH 48 pg/ml (13–65)

Interview: Patient reported smoking (20 cig/d) since age 17. She takes PPI for GORD for about 2 years. Lithium was introduced 2 months ago.

7. Choose the right propositions.
   1. Mild hypercalcitoninemia is related to lithium therapy.
   2. Mild hypercalcitoninemia could be related to smoking.
   3. Mild hypercalcitoninemia cannot be related to PPI prescription.
   4. Short-term lithium therapy can induce hyperparathyroidism.
   5. Neck US could be done, at least as referral landmark if follow up needed.
8. Regarding adrenal incidentaloma, choose the right propositions.
   1. One should first eliminate differential diagnosis and ascertain the adrenal origin.
   2. The incidence on CT scan is around 20%.
   3. The rate decreases with age.
   4. Regarding diagnosis, the case mix could significantly change because of institution recruitment bias.
   5. Diagnosing pheochromocytoma in this group of patients is almost nil.
9. Regarding work up, choose the right propositions.
   1. In a vast majority of cases, an unenhanced CT scan should be enough, avoiding further imaging studies.
   2. MRI has to be considered, at least for its safety.
   3. There is a strong correlation between FDG PET ratio (SUVmax T/SUVmax Liver) and malignancy in cortical adrenal tumor.
   4. There is a strong correlation between FDG PET ratio (SUVmax T/SUVmax Liver) and malignancy in medulla adrenal tumor.
   5. After appropriate work, a majority of patients cannot be classified (benign/malignant, secreting/non-secreting, diagnosis).
10. Regarding the management of incidentaloma, choose the right propositions.
   1. After appropriate work up, most patients will not undergo surgery.
   2. Follow-up is never required.
   3. MDT discussion is recommended to review and validate decisions.

4. In incidentaloma, as diagnosis is not assessed, open abdominal surgery is recommended.
5. Surgical excision for diagnostic purposes should be chosen selectively.

18.1 Introduction

An adrenal incidentaloma is defined as an initially considered asymptomatic adrenal mass detected on imaging not performed for suspected adrenal disease. Autopsy studies have found adrenal adenomas in around 6% [1], and on CT imaging, adrenal lesions are found in around 4%. The incidence increases with age with 10% of those >70 years having an adrenal mass [2–4]. Adrenal nodules in younger adults and in children are rare but the risk of malignancy is increased. With improved and wider use of imaging the finding of an "incidentaloma" is an increasingly common scenario. Lesions may be bilateral and each lesion should be assessed individually. The majority of lesions are benign (usually cortical adenoma) and non-functional but require evaluation to exclude malignancy and functionality. Regarding morbidity and mortality attached to such adrenal tumors, it is mandatory that the appropriate therapeutic management should not be missed. Lesions less than 1 cm in size are considered not to require further evaluation unless patients have symptoms and signs suggestive of hormonal excess [4]. The evidence base for management recommendations of adrenal lesions is generally considered to be low and recommendations are the product of evidence reviews, clinical experience, and panel discussion. Management of patients with adrenal incidentaloma should include discussion in a multidisciplinary team (MDT) meeting with a dedicated endocrine/adrenal surgeon. Work up of adrenal incidentalomas includes [4]:
1. Assessment for malignancy
2. Assessment of hormonal function
3. Indications for surgery and surgical approach
4. Follow-up of non-operated patients

Clinical assessment should be extensive, although in incidentaloma situations clinical symptoms are usually absent or mild. One should systematically look for signs of that could be related to excess cortisol secretion. Raised blood Pressure may be absent or variably present in pheochromocytoma. Patient's interview must thoroughly explore personal and familial history. If this has been done correctly before referral, the most relevant diagnostic information is provided by imaging and biological work up.
1. Assessment for Malignancy: Imaging

In incidentaloma, the assessment of malignancy or suspicious tumor will mainly rely on anatomical and functional imaging.

Dedicated adrenal imaging will usually be required as initial scan detecting the incidentaloma will be unsuitable for lesion characterization (typically an enhanced CT scan). CT and MRI are generally used to exclude malignancy (most incidentaloma are benign cortical adenoma, which have specific CT and MRI signature), while FDG PET CT is mainly used to detect/rule out malignancy/suspicious tumor. Nevertheless, functional benign tumors may demonstrate increased uptake.

18.2 Anatomical Imaging

18.2.1 CT

(i) Adrenal non-contrast CT is considered the first line assessment of adrenal incidentalomas. Homogeneous and lipid-rich lesions have Hounsfield units of <10 which is indicative of a lipid-rich benign adenoma. In patients with no known extra adrenal malignancy, these values represent a benign lesion (adenoma, myeloplipoma, cysts, ganglioneuroma) [5]. Where there is a known history of malignancy, 7% of cases with HU <10 are malignant [4].

(ii) 30% of benign adenomas have HU >10 and may represent lipid-poor adenomas. HU >10 are also found with pheochromocytoma and malignant lesions, although these lesions are typically heterogeneous in appearance.

(iii) CT contrast washout values can be informative in characterization. Relative contrast washout of >40% and absolute washout >60% indicates a benign adenoma.

(iv) After a proper evaluation and with an unenhanced dedicated adrenal CT scan, over 50–60% of adrenal incidentaloma could be classified as benign adenoma. No other imaging studies should be necessary although most of them will not require surgery.

18.2.2 MRI

MRI avoids the use ionizing radiation. Lipid-rich adrenal lesions lose signal intensity on out of phase images compared to in phase images. Malignant lesions, pheochromocytomas, and lipid-poor adenomas are all relatively lacking in intracellular fat and remain unchanged. Visual assessment of signal intensity loss is diagnostic in most situations. There is less standardization in interpreting MRI signal values compared to CT, and MRI interpretation may be more dependent on experience of radiologist than in CT. There is a clear role of MRI in the evaluation of adrenal lesions in pregnancy, children, and those under 40 when there is a desire to minimize radiation exposure [4]. Some will advocate that MRI is provides additional information to CT scan conclusions in cases of atypical imaging. If imaging follow-up is needed, repeated MRI will avoid additional radiation.

One should notice that whatever are the imaging features, tumor size remains a very strong predictive factor of malignancy (◘ Fig. 18.2).

18.3 Functional Imaging

18.3.1 FDG PET CT

PET has a role in characterizing adrenal lesions in patients. It is widely accepted in patients with a known history of extra adrenal malignancy. One should be aware that false-negative results are possible in adrenal metastasis. PET has a key role in patients whose imaging suggests potential malignant adrenal lesion. There is little evidence to support a systematic role in the general evaluation of incidentalomas [4].

Increased 18F FDG uptake represents increased glucose metabolism found in the majority of cancers and some benign lesions [6, 7]. Uptake is expressed quantitatively as the Standard Uptake Value (SUV), comparing the adrenal lesion to the average body uptake. A dedicated team showed that PET ratio (SUV max tumour/SUV max liver) is accurate to predict malignancy (ratio >1.5) or to rule out it (ratio ≤ 1) [8]. PET is combined with CT to provide better anatomical location. Mixing PET metabolic information with simple anatomical features (size) helps building predictive algorithm [9].

▪ Additional Functional Imaging Studies

The role of dedicated cortical or medulla tracers and imaging, as norcholesterol scintigraphy, MIBG scintigraphy, or F DOPA PET CT, is rarely considered in first-line management of incidentaloma.

2. Assessment of Hormonal Function

Clinical Assessment of Hormonal Excess should be performed in all patients and includes the taking of a history and examining the patient. Most patients will not have evidence of a functional syndrome. Should evidence of Cushing's syndrome, pheochromocytoma, or Conn's Syndrome be present, patients should be managed as per the relevant conditions. Autonomous cortisol secretion, previously known as subclinical Cushing's syndrome should be excluded. While less than 1% with autonomous cortisol secretion progress to overt Cushing's syndrome, there is an association of cortisol excess with cardiovascular risk factors and patients may benefit from surgical excision [4]. The management of autonomous cortisol secretion requires an individualized patient approach. The age of the patient and presence of cortisol-related comorbidities such as hypertension, Type II Diabetes, obesity, osteoporosis, vertebral fractures, and dyslipidemia will influence clinical management and require MDT discussion.

(i) Exclude cortisol excess: 1 mg overnight dexamethasone suppression test

Post dexamethasone cortisol NIH and Endocrine Society criteria:

<50 nmol/L – No excess

51–138 nmol/L – Possible excess

>138 nmol/L – Autonomous cortisol excess: additional confirmatory tests required

Low early morning ACTH confirms ACTH independence

One should know that other scientific societies (French and Italian) advocate for lower cutoff values.

(ii) Exclude pheochromocytoma: plasma-free metanephrines or urinary fractionated metanephrines.
   Plasma-free metanephrines is usually considered more sensitive and less specific than urine metanephrines. Normal level (repeated samples) should exclude pheochromocytoma. Levels above 4 times the normal range should confirm diagnosis. Chromogranin A evaluation is not systematically recommended.

(iii) Exclude primary hyperaldosteronism when hypertension or hypokalemia present: Measure the aldosterone/renin ratio
   Ratio evaluation should be done after correction of hypokalemia, under normal salted regimen, and after checking possible medication interferences.

(iv) Lesions suspicious for adrenocortical cancer should additionally have sex hormones, precursors, and urine steroid profile assessed and be managed according to ACC guidelines.

(v) In bilateral lesions consider additional assessment of 17-hydroxyprogesterone in conjunction with a non-suppressed ACTH to exclude congenital adrenal hyperplasia.

(vi) Consider adrenal insufficiency in patients with bilateral infiltrative lesions or evidence of bilateral hemorrhage. Morning cortisol will be low and ACTH elevated. Synacthen testing may be indicated.

3. Indications for Surgery
   Surgery should be tailored to the clinical scenario, imaging and hormonal results. Indications should be discussed in an MDT. All suspicious tumors after work up should be considered for surgery. Some consider that tumor size >6 cm or size pro-

gression are suspicious features that should lead to surgery. For tumors between 4 and 6 cm, surgical indication relying only on size is debatable. Surgical indications in subclinical Cushing syndrome remain a matter of debate.

   (i) Unilateral adrenalectomy is recommended in the presence of clinically significant hormonal excess.
   (ii) Asymptomatic, non-functioning, radiologically benign lesions generally do not require surgery.
   (iii) Open adrenalectomy is recommended for lesions with evidence of malignancy and local invasion on imaging.
   (iv) Laparoscopic adrenalectomy is a reasonable approach for suspicious lesions without evidence of local invasion and <6 cm size.
   (v) Adrenal biopsy is not recommended unless there is a history of extra adrenal malignancy, and the result will influence management. Pheochromocytoma should always be excluded initially.
   (vi) Peri- and post-operative glucocorticoid cover at stress doses should be used where there is evidence of "possible autonomous cortisol secretion."

4. Follow-up for patients not undergoing surgery
   (i) Clear benign lessons on imaging, <4 cm size and non-functional *may* not require further follow-up or imaging. This remains debatable and tailored to the patient characteristics.
   (ii) Indeterminate lesions not undergoing surgery should be reconsidered for surgery if the lesion enlarges on follow-up imaging at 3, 6, or 12 months. Use of RECIST Criteria [10] has been recommended [4] to determine significance of growth – 20% increase in volume and at least a 5 mm increase in maximum diameter.
   (iii) Repeated hormonal evaluation for hormone negative patients is not recommended unless the clinical scenario or comorbidities such as hypertension and diabetes worsen.
   (iv) Deterioration or the development of cortisol related comorbidities should be assessed in patients with autonomous cortisol secretion during follow up and risk benefit of surgical intervention reconsidered.

18.4 Conclusions

The vast majority of adrenal Incidentaloma are benign (cortical adenoma) non-secreting tumors. Most will not require surgery or follow-up. Unenhanced CT scan alone will characterize most lesions without the need for additional imaging. Simple ambulatory hormonal evaluation is adequate in most cases to exclude over secretion.

Regarding the potential morbidity and mortality of malignant and/or secreting adrenal tumors, these diagnoses should not be missed. Patients should be referred to dedicated management and surgery teams if needed. MDT is mandatory to plan the optimal work up and management for these patients.

Answers to the Questions

1. 3 and 4 are correct
2. 1 and 4 are correct
3. 3, 4 and 5 are correct
4. 3 is correct
5. 3 and 4 are correct
6. 1, 3 and 4 are correct
7. 2 and 5 are correct
8. 1 and 4 are correct
9. 1, 2 and 3 are correct
10. 1, 3 and 5 are correct

References

1. Young WF. Management approaches to adrenal incidentalomas. A view from Rochester, Minnesota. Endocrinol Metab Clin N Am. 2000;29:159–85.
2. Bovio S, Cataldi A, Reimondo G, et al. Prevelance of adrenal incidentaloma in a contemorary computerised tomography series. J Endocrinol Investig. 2006;29:298–302.
3. Mansmann G, Lau J, Balk E, et al. The clinically inapparent adrenal mass: update in diagnosis and management. Endocr Rev. 2004;25:309–40.
4. Fassnacht M, Wiebke A, Bancos I, et al. Management of adrenal incidentalomas: European Society of Endocrinology Clinical Practice Guideline in collaboration with the European Network for the study of Adrenal Tumors. Eur J Endocrinol. 2016;175:G1–34.
5. Dinnes J, Bancos I, Ferranti di Ruffiano L, et al. Management of endocrine disease: imaging for the diagnosis of malignancy in incidentally discovered adrenal masses: a systematic review and meta analysis. Eur J Endocrinol. 2016;175:R51–64.
6. Ansquer C, Scigliano S, Mirallie E, et al. 18F-FDG PET/CT in the characterisation and surgical decision concerning adrenal masses: a prospective multicentre evaluation. Eur J Nucl Med Mol Imaging. 2010;37:1669–78.
7. Timmers HJ, Chen CC, Carrasquillo JA, et al. Comparison of 18F-Flouro -L-DOPA, 18F-fluoro-deoxyglucose, and 18F-fluorodopamine PET and 123I-MIBG scintigraphy in the localisation of pheochromocytoma and pasraganglioma. J Clin Endocrinol Metab. 2009;94:4757–67.
8. Guerin C, Pattou F, Brunaud L, et al. Performance of 18F-FDG PET/CT in the characterization of adrenal masses in noncancer patients: a prospective study. J Clin Endocrinol Metab. 2017;102:2465–72.

9. Amodru V, Taieb D, Guerin C, et al. Large adrenal incidentalomas require a dedicated diagnostic procedure. Endocr Pract. 2019;25: 669–77.
10. Eisenhauer EA, Therasse P, Bogaerts J, et al. New response evaluation criteria in solid tumours:revised RECIST guideline (version 1.1). Eur J Cancer. 2009;45:228–47.

Cushing's Syndrome

Maurizio Iacobone and Francesca Torresan

Contents

A. L. Shifrin et al. (eds.), *Endocrine Surgery Comprehensive Board Exam Guide*,
https://doi.org/10.1007/978-3-030-84737-1_19

Case Presentation

A 44-year-old female patient presented with complains on progressive weight gain with increasing waist circumference and rounding of her face. She was evaluated for Cushing's syndrome. Past medical history was significant for hypercholesterolemia, arterial hypertension, polycystic ovary syndrome, and depression. She mentioned that she was treated for acne in her early teenage years and for a previous episode of deep vein thrombosis. No family history of endocrine diseases. Medications included calcium antagonist, statin, and benzodiazepine.

On physical examination, she showed high blood pressure (160/95 mmHg), facial plethora, supraclavicular fat pads, and abdominal purple striae. She presented with laboratory data that revealed a morning cortisol level of 17.6 nmol/L (normal 3–21 nmol/L), serum ACTH level <0.05 ng/L (reference range 10–50 ng/L), and urinary free cortisol level of 463 nmol/24 h (reference range 16–168 nmol/24 h). Other investigations revealed a plasma cortisol level of 375 nmol/L after 1 mg overnight dexamethasone suppression test and a disappeared circadian rhythm of cortisol (evening salivary cortisol level of 25.8 nmol/L, normal 0.5–2.6 nmol/L). An abdominal ultrasonography was performed, and a right retroperitoneal suprarenal mass (3 cm of diameter) was detected.

? Questions

1. With regard to the clinical case described above, which imaging techniques should be primarily considered for further investigation of the adrenal mass?
   1. CT or MRI
   2. 18F-FDG PET-CT
   3. Radiocholesterol scintigraphy
   4. Selective adrenal venous sampling
      - (a) Only (1) and (4) are correct.
      - (b) Only (1) is correct.
      - (c) Only (4) is correct.
      - (d) Only (2) and (4) are correct.
      - (e) All are correct.
2. With regard to the clinical case described above, is fine-needle aspiration biopsy (FNAB) of the mass indicated?
   1. Yes: all adrenal masses found in patients with Cushing's syndrome should undergo histological examination.
   2. Only adrenal masses >6 cm should undergo FNAB examination.
   3. In case of severe Cushing's syndrome.
   4. No.
      - (a) Only (1) is correct.
      - (b) Only (1) and (3) are correct.
      - (c) Only (4) is correct.
      - (d) Only (2) is correct.
      - (e) Only (3) is correct.
3. With regard to the clinical case described above, in case of imaging techniques suggesting the presence of an adrenal adenoma, which surgical solution would be the best option?

1. Unilateral adrenalectomy, preferably by minimal invasive approach.
2. Surgical resection of the mass and surrounding tissues via open surgery in any case, as adrenal adenomas correlated to Cushing's Syndrome have a high recurrence rate.
3. Surgical resection of the mass only after mitotane administration is started.
4. Surgery is never a first-line option.
   - (a) Only (1) is correct.
   - (b) Only (1) and (3) are correct.
   - (c) Only (4) is correct.
   - (d) Only (2) is correct.
   - (e) None is correct.

4. With regard to the clinical case described above, which medical therapy should be administered after adrenalectomy?
   1. Glucocorticoids should be administered until the normal hypothalamic–pituitary–adrenal axis is restored.
   2. No medical therapy should be given, as patients are not at risk of developing Addison's disease.
   3. No medical therapy should be administered, since the contralateral adrenal gland compensates cortisol production soon after surgery.
   4. ACTH analogues should be given to stimulate the contralateral adrenal gland.
      - (a) Only (3) is correct.
      - (b) Only (2) and (3) are correct.
      - (c) Only (1) is correct.
      - (d) Only (4) is correct.
      - (e) None is correct.
5. Which are the criteria to establish the diagnosis of Cushing's syndrome?
   1. Findings of an adrenal nodule on CT scan.
   2. History of osteoporosis and findings of an adrenal nodule at CT scan.
   3. Findings of normal cortisol levels after 1 mg dexamethasone overnight suppression test and high morning cortisol level.
   4. Elevated 24-h urine cortisol levels.
   5. Findings of normal ACTH levels and an adrenal nodule at abdominal ultrasound.
      - (a) Only (1) and (2) and (3) are correct.
      - (b) Only (3) and (5) are correct.
      - (c) Only (4) is correct.
      - (d) Only (2) and (4) and (5) are correct.
      - (e) All are correct.
6. The diagnosis of ACTH-dependent Cushing's syndrome is established in case of:

1. Elevation of both ACTH and serum morning cortisol levels
2. Elevation of ACTH but normal serum morning cortisol levels
3. Low levels of serum ACTH but high 24 h-urinary cortisol levels
4. Elevation of serum ACTH, serum morning cortisol, and 24 h-urinary cortisol levels
   (a) Only (1) and (2) and (3) are correct.
   (b) Only (1) and (2) and (4) are correct.
   (c) Only (1) and (3) and (4) are correct.
   (d) Only (1) and (4) are correct.
   (e) All are correct.

7. The diagnosis of ACTH-independent Cushing's syndrome is established in case of:
   1. Elevation of both ACTH and serum cortisol levels
   2. Low levels of ACTH and high serum cortisol and 24 h-urinary cortisol levels
   3. Elevation of ACTH and normal serum cortisol levels
   4. Normal levels of serum cortisol after 1 mg dexamethasone overnight suppression test
      (a) Only (1) and (2) and (3) are correct.
      (b) Only (1) and (2) and (4) are correct.
      (c) Only (2) is correct.
      (d) Only (2) and (4) are correct.
      (e) All are correct.
8. The diagnosis of ectopic ACTH-dependent Cushing's syndrome is established in case of:
   1. Elevation of both ACTH and serum cortisol levels, with increased ACTH levels after CRH test
   2. Elevation of serum ACTH but normal 24 h-urinary cortisol levels
   3. Elevation of serum ACTH but normal morning serum cortisol levels
   4. Elevation of serum ACTH, morning serum cortisol and 24 h-urinary cortisol levels, with unchanged ACTH levels after CRH test
      (a) Only (1) and (2) and (3) are correct.
      (b) Only (1) and (2) and (4) are correct.
      (c) Only (2) and (4) are correct.
      (d) Only (4) is correct.
      (e) All are correct.
9. What is the suggested surgical approach in case of invasive adrenocortical carcinoma associated with Cushing's syndrome?
   1. Open surgical approach with wide resections of the adrenal mass with infiltrated adjacent organs
   2. Radiotherapy alone
   3. Chemotherapy as first-line therapy to reduce the volume of the mass

4. Laparoscopic resection of the adrenal mass preserving the infiltrated adjacent organs to prevent major complications
   - (a) Only (1) and (4) are correct.
   - (b) Only (1) is correct.
   - (c) Only (2) and (4) are correct.
   - (d) Only (2) and (3) are correct.
   - (e) All are correct.

10. Which of the following genetic syndromes might be associated with Cushing's syndrome?
    1. Li-Fraumeni syndrome
    2. Turner syndrome
    3. Pheochromocytoma and paraganglioma syndrome
    4. MEN 2B
       - (a) Only (1) and (2) and (3) are correct.
       - (b) Only (2) and (3) and (4) are correct.
       - (c) Only (3) and (4) are correct.
       - (d) Only (1) is correct.
       - (e) All are correct.

11. What is the preferred technique to localize a pituitary ACTH-producing adenoma?
    1. Ultrasonography
    2. MRI imaging
    3. Bilateral inferior petrosal sinus sampling
    4. Endoscopic
       - (a) Only (1) and (4) are correct.
       - (b) Only (1) and (3) are correct.
       - (c) Only (2) and (4) are correct.
       - (d) Only (2) is correct.
       - (e) All are correct.

12. When is bilateral adrenalectomy indicated in Cushing's Syndrome?
    1. After unilateral adrenalectomy for Primary Bilateral Macronodular Adrenal Hyperplasia (PBMAH), in case of persistent hypercortisolism
    2. In case of severe occult ectopic ACTH-dependent Cushing's syndrome
    3. In emergency cases of severe not controlled ACTH-dependent hypercortisolism
    4. After reiterative pituitary surgery, in case of persistent hypercortisolism
       - (a) Only (2) and (3) and (4) are correct.
       - (b) Only (2) and (3) are correct.
       - (c) Only (1) and (3) and (4) are correct.
       - (d) Only (2) and (3) and (4) are correct.
       - (e) All are correct.

13. What is the suggested surgical approach for Primary Pigmented Nodular Adrenocortical Disease (PPNAD)?
    1. Bilateral adrenalectomy
    2. Unilateral adrenalectomy based on CT/MRI imaging results

3. Unilateral adrenalectomy based on norcholesterol scintigraphy results
4. Unilateral adrenalectomy based on adrenal vein sampling results
   (a) Only (1) and (2) and (3) are correct.
   (b) Only (2) and (3) and (4) are correct.
   (c) Only (1) and (3) and (4) are correct.
   (d) Only (1) is correct.
   (e) None of the previous is correct.

14. Which drug/combination of drugs should be used after surgical resection of adrenocortical carcinoma causing Cushing's syndrome?
    1. Mitotane as monotherapy
    2. Glucocorticoids as monotherapy
    3. Mitotane + glucocorticoids
    4. Mifepristone as monotherapy
       (a) Only (3) is correct.
       (b) Only (1) and (4) are correct.
       (c) Only (1) is correct.
       (d) Only (2) and (3) are correct.
       (e) All are correct.
15. What are possible indications for surgical treatment of subclinical or mild ACTH-independent Cushing's syndrome?
    1. Metabolic comorbidities
    2. Arterial hypertension
    3. Only for adrenal masses smaller than 6 cm
    4. Alopecia
       (a) Only (1) and (2) and (3) are correct.
       (b) Only (1) and (2) are correct.
       (c) Only (1) and (3) and (4) are correct.
       (d) Only (2) and (4) are correct.
       (e) All are correct.
16. Which of the following features may be present in Cushing's syndrome?
    1. Glucose impairment
    2. Deep vein thrombosis
    3. Diabetes mellitus
    4. Visceral obesity
       (a) Only (1) and (2) and (3) are correct.
       (b) Only (1) and (2) and (4) are correct.
       (c) Only (1) and (3) and (4) are correct.
       (d) Only (2) and (3) and (4) are correct.
       (e) All are correct.
17. Which of the following statements are correct:
    1. Carney complex usually presents with pigmented lesions of the skin.
    2. In patients affected by McCune-Albright syndrome, neonatal hypercortisolism can be detected.
    3. Li-Fraumeni syndrome is usually related to a family history of early-onset cancers.

4. Li-Fraumeni syndrome is usually related to a family history of late-onset cancers.
   (a) Only (1) and (2) and (3) are correct.
   (b) Only (1) and (2) and (4) are correct.
   (c) Only (1) and (3) and (4) are correct.
   (d) Only (2) and (3) and (4) are correct.
   (e) All are correct.

19.1 Introduction

Cushing's syndrome (CS) is a rare disease due to a wide spectrum of endogenous and exogenous conditions resulting in chronic glucocorticoid excess.

Exogenous CS (caused by excess glucocorticoid intake for chronic diseases such as asthma, obstructive pulmonary disease, rheumatologic conditions, and immunologic treatments) is the most common cause of CS and should be first excluded. Endogenous CS is a rare condition defined as adrenocorticotropic hormone (ACTH)-dependent (arising from a hypothalamic-pituitary or ectopic tumors, 80% of cases) or ACTH-independent (from adrenal origin, 20% of cases) [1] (◘ Table 19.1).

ACTH-dependent CS due to pituitary adenoma is the cause of about 70% of all cases of endogenous CS and was termed Cushing's disease (CD), since it was first described by Harvey Cushing, a neurosurgeon who found the association between the presence of a basophilic pituitary tumor and the typical clinical features of hypercortisolism. It affects prevalently women (female/male ratio of 3–4:1), usually in their fertile age, with a peak of incidence in the 3rd–4th decade of life. In most cases, it is caused by pituitary microadenoma (less than 10 mm), very rarely by pituitary carcinoma. In about 10% of ACTH-

◘ Table 19.1 Causes of endogenous hypercortisolism

ACTH-dependent hypercortisolism	ACTH-independent hypercortisolism
Pituitary tumors (Cushing disease)	Adrenal adenoma
Ectopic tumors (neuroendocrine lung tumors, thymic carcinoma, thyroid and pancreatic neuroendocrine tumors)	Adrenal carcinoma
	Primary Bilateral Macronodular (>1 cm) Adrenal Hyperplasia (PBMAH)
	Primary Pigmented Nodular (<1 cm) Adrenocortical Disease (PPNAD)

dependent CS, the source of ACTH is ectopic, mainly produced by neuroendocrine tumors of the lung or more rarely of thyroid, thymus, and pancreas with increased prevalence in male at 4th–5th decade [1, 2].

Adrenal ACTH-independent CS is less common and usually unilateral, due to an adenoma or, even more rarely, a carcinoma. A bilateral adrenal involvement is the rarest form of CS, and it is caused by primary bilateral macronodular adrenal hyperplasia (PBMAH), affecting both genders with a peak in the 5th–6-sixth decades or Primary Pigmented Nodular Adrenocortical Disease (PPNAD) and its non-pigmented variants [3, 4]. PBMAH is characterized by large asymmetric hyperplastic nodules (>1 cm) with or without internodular atrophy (type 1 or 2, respectively); it may be caused by autocrine/paracrine adrenal ACTH hypersecretion or by the presence of ectopic/aberrant receptors in adrenocortical cells and their ligands (vasopressin, serotonin, GIP, luteinizing hormone, catecholamines); in this context, hypercortisolism occurs as cyclic disease. PBMAH may present as sporadic or familial disease (associated with *ARMC5, MEN1, FH, or APC* gene mutations). PPNAD is characterized by small bilateral and symmetric micronodules (<1 cm); it may be associated to *PRKAR1A* germline mutations and may occur either as isolated disease or as part of Carney Complex (in association to cardiac myxomas, various pigmented skin lesions typically observed before puberty and with a typical distribution on the face, lips, genital area, and mucosa; somatotroph-secreting pituitary adenomas; other endocrine hyperactive tumors; testicular benign tumors and melanocytic schwannomas). The full spectrum of the disease usually develops through many years [5].

CS usually develops in adults, but cases of CS in childhood and adolescence have been also described. As in adult, CS in pediatric age occurs more commonly as ACTH-dependent pituitary hypercortisolism. Moreover, pediatric CS should lead to accurate genetic assessment aimed to assess eventual underlying genetic conditions, such as the *McCune Albright* or ***McCune-Albright syndrome*** includes a wide spectrum of diseases related to post-zygotic somatic gain-of-function mutations of the *GNAS* gene. Clinical features may include neonatal hypercortisolism (in the first year of life), leading to recurrent infantile illnesses and poor linear growth with excessive weight gain; skeletal lesions; skin hyperpigmentation; and other hyper-functioning endocrinopathies, mostly gonadotropin-independent sex steroid production and consequent precocious puberty [6]. ***Li-Fraumeni syndrome*** is an autosomal-dominant syndrome due to germline mutations resulting in loss-of-function of the tumor-suppressor *TP53 gene*, predisposing to the development of different types of cancers. This condition may lead to CS in children caused by adrenocortical carcinomas (3–4 cases per million children in Brazilian population) [7]. Moreover, these patients have a very high lifetime cumulative risk of developing other multiple and early-onset malignancies (soft tissues and osteosarcomas, premenopausal breast cancer, and brain tumors) [8, 9].

19.2 Clinical Presentation

The clinical features of CS vary in relation to the extent and duration of hormonal excess, and the variable receptor sensitivity of target organ to glucocorticoids; for these reasons, the phenotype in CS may vary from subclinical, mild to overt variants. Moreover, CS may occur as cyclic disease (in case of PBMAH due to the expression of aberrant receptors).

The clinical impact of CS is typically systemic. An excess in cortisol production induces catabolic effects on protidosynthesis in connective tissues, skeletal muscles, and skin; it induces an increased rate of gluconeogenesis, glycogenolysis, and insulin resistance; it directly affects the transcription and translation of enzyme proteins involved in the metabolism of fats. Moreover, hypercortisolism causes immune-system alterations leading to a decrease in lymphocyte levels and an increase of neutrophils. Cortisol excess influences also arterial blood pressure through its binding to mineralocorticoid receptors.

The most typical and specific signs of overt cortisol excess are facial plethora with "moon face" (◘ Fig. 19.1), violaceous cutaneous striae wider than 1 cm (striae rubrae) (◘ Fig. 19.2), fragile, and anelastic skin determining easy bruising even after only minimal injuries and proximal muscle weakness [1]. However, all these characteristics are not commonly present at diagnosis, and not all signs and symptoms are found in every patient. In fact, the clinical manifestations of CS usually begin gradually with less specific signs and symptoms that are also common in the general population: sudden weight gain with excessive abdominal centripetal adiposity and thinned limbs; metabolic syndrome with glucose intolerance or diabetes mellitus, hyperlipidemia, and arterial hypertension; acne; hirsutism; signs of protein catabolism such as osteopenia or osteoporosis and osteoporotic fractures; depression and/or psychosis; decreased libido or impotence; and recurrent infections sustained by bacterial or opportunistic microorganisms. Moreover, oligomenorrhea is common in premenopausal women and may occur before any other sign or symptoms [10]; in case of adrenocortical carcinoma, signs of virilization may be prevalent (◘ Table 19.2). For these reasons, most of the times patients are referred to different specialists depending on the dominant symptoms (i.e., gynecological, dermatological, cardiovascular, psychiatric) before a final diagnosis is established.

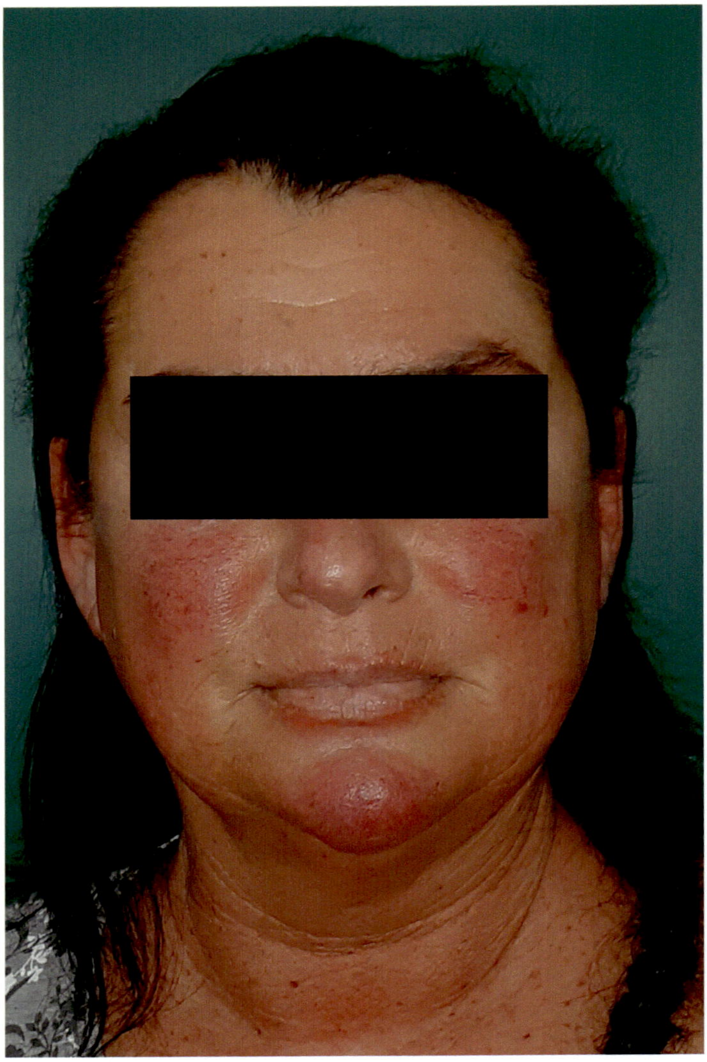

Fig. 19.1 Facial plethora with moon face in a female Cushing's syndrome patient

Nowadays, thanks to the more precise diagnostic tools and the increased awareness of physicians, CS is diagnosed earlier, when only mild or subclinical cortisol excess is detected [11].

Subclinical CS is a preclinical condition of hypercortisolism characterized by abnormal cortisol production in patients without overt clinical signs and symptoms of cortisol excess, often diagnosed during biochemical screening for hypertension, diabetes, osteoporosis, obesity, and neuropsychological impairment [1] or during the secretory work up of adrenal incidentalomas [12].

"Pseudo-Cushing's syndrome" (or "non-neoplastic hypercortisolism") refers to different pathological conditions responsible for mild-to-moderate ACTH-dependent hypercortisolism. It is probably the result of increased hypothalamic corticotro-

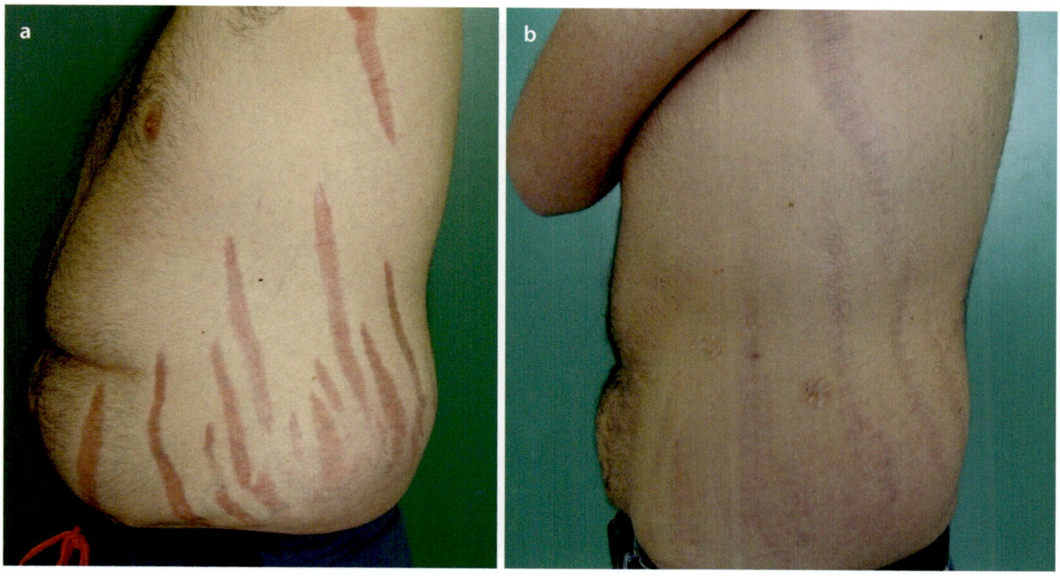

Fig. 19.2 Abdominal cutaneous striae, skin bruising, and central obesity in a Cushing's syndrome male patient before **a** and after adrenalectomy **b**

pin-releasing hormone (CRH) secretion in the context of a normal function of the hypothalamic-pituitary-adrenal axis and generally occurs in patients displaying excess central adiposity and heterogeneous group of disorders, including alcoholism and depression [13, 14].

19.3 Natural History

CS is a severe disease that significantly compromises the quality of life. High mortality rates have been reported in cases of overt untreated disease. In fact, CS patients have a significantly increased risk of morbidity and mortality due to cardiovascular and metabolic impairment. Arterial hypertension, with consequent left ventricular hypertrophy, is one of the most prevalent features and represents an independent predictor of mortality. A combination of multiple drugs, usually angiotensin converting enzyme inhibitors, sartans, or spironolactone, is often necessary to control blood pressure and eventual hypokalemia. Moreover, myocardial fibrosis and vascular atherosclerosis with coronary plaques are direct consequences of cortisol excess, leading to an increased risk of myocardial infarction and heart failure. Visceral abdominal obesity, insulin resistance, infections (caused by lymphopenia and immunodeficiency), and venous thromboembolism (caused by increased Factors VIII, IX, X, XI and von Willebrand production and polycythemia) are other common complications resulting in higher mortality rates. Bone impairment may be severe and occur early, especially in women; CS-related osteoporosis may

Table 19.2 Clinical symptoms and signs of Cushing's syndrome

Cutaneous	**Easy bruising**[a] **Facial plethora**[a] **Striae** (especially if reddish purple and 1 cm wide)[a] Thin skin Acne Poor skin healing Hirsutism or female balding
Metabolic	Facial fullness Dorsocervical fat pad (buffalo hump) Weight gain Obesity Supraclavicular fullness Polycystic ovary syndrome Changes in appetite Glucose impairment Type 2 diabetes
Cardiovascular	Hypertension Peripheral edema
Neuropsychiatric	Depression Irritability Impaired memory (especially short term) Insomnia
Musculoskeletal	**Proximal myopathy (or proximal muscle weakness)**[a] Vertebral osteoporosis Back pain
Electrolyte disturbances	Hypokalemia
In children	**Weight gain with decreasing growth velocity**[a] Short stature Abnormal genital virilization Pseudoprecocious puberty or delayed puberty
Others	Unusual infections Fatigue Decreased libido Menstrual abnormalities Kidney stones

[a]Easy bruising, facial plethora, striae rubrae, proximal myopathy/weakness, and also weight gain with decreasing growth velocity in children are the most distinctive features in Cushing's syndrome, even if most of them do not have a high sensitivity

cause multiple bone fractures and vertebral collapse with neurologic damage.

In case of subclinical CS, the natural history is uncertain. This condition may remain stable for several years, but in some cases an evolution to overt CS may occur. Therefore, in case of conservative management, a long-term monitoring is recommended. However, some studies have reported increased morbidity and mortality rate due to systemic and metabolic complication even in subclinical CS. Therefore, a surgical approach also for subclinical CS is often suggested [15].

19.4 Diagnosis

The diagnosis of CS may be challenging due to the variable clinical presentation, in particular in subclinical and mild hypercortisolism. The diagnosis of CS should begin with a detailed medical history and physical examination. Exogenous CS should be ruled out first excluding glucocorticoids intake by any route (oral, parenteral, inhaled, or topical).

As recommended by the Endocrine Society Guidelines [1], first-line biochemical screening tests to confirm endogenous CS include (1) 24-h urinary free cortisol excretion (UFC) measurement (at least two measurements); (2) overnight 1 mg dexamethasone suppression test; and (3) late-night salivary cortisol measurements (◘ Fig. 19.3). At least two of these tests are needed to confirm the diagnosis of CS. When these tests are negative, the diagnosis of CS may be formally excluded.

UFC measures the unbound cortisol filtered by renal system, and, in contrast to plasma cortisol levels, it is not influenced by corticosteroid-binding globulin whose levels may be increased in certain conditions or under some medications (oral estrogens). Normal UFC levels exclude CS and UFC values fourfold greater than the upper normal limit can be considered highly diagnostic for CS [16]. However, false-positive results should be taken into account, depending on the assay method used or on other concomitant medical conditions that could raise ACTH and cortisol in absence of an ACTH-secreting tumor (pseudo-cushing's syndrome) [1, 17]. The antibody-based immunoassays, such as RIA and ELISA, can be affected by cross-reactivity with cortisol metabolites and synthetic glucocorticoids, while some drugs such as fenofibrate and carbamazepine may interfere with UFC measurements by liquid chromatography. Therefore, normal UFC ranges vary substantially depending on the method used. False-negative UFC results may also occur in presence of renal failure or in patients with subclinical CS [17].

The 1 mg-dexamethasone overnight suppression test (Nugent test) consists in the oral intake of 1 mg of dexamethasone at 11 PM, followed by measurement of plasma cortisol in the morning of the following day. Another way to conduct the test is the 48 h-2 mg dexamethasone test that requires oral intake of 0.5 mg dexamethasone every 6 h for 2 days and measurement of plasma cortisol in the morning after the last dose of dexamethasone. The cutoff levels after dexamethasone administration for confirming the diagnosis of CS are variable: values >140 mmol/L (5 mcg/dl) are usually considered more

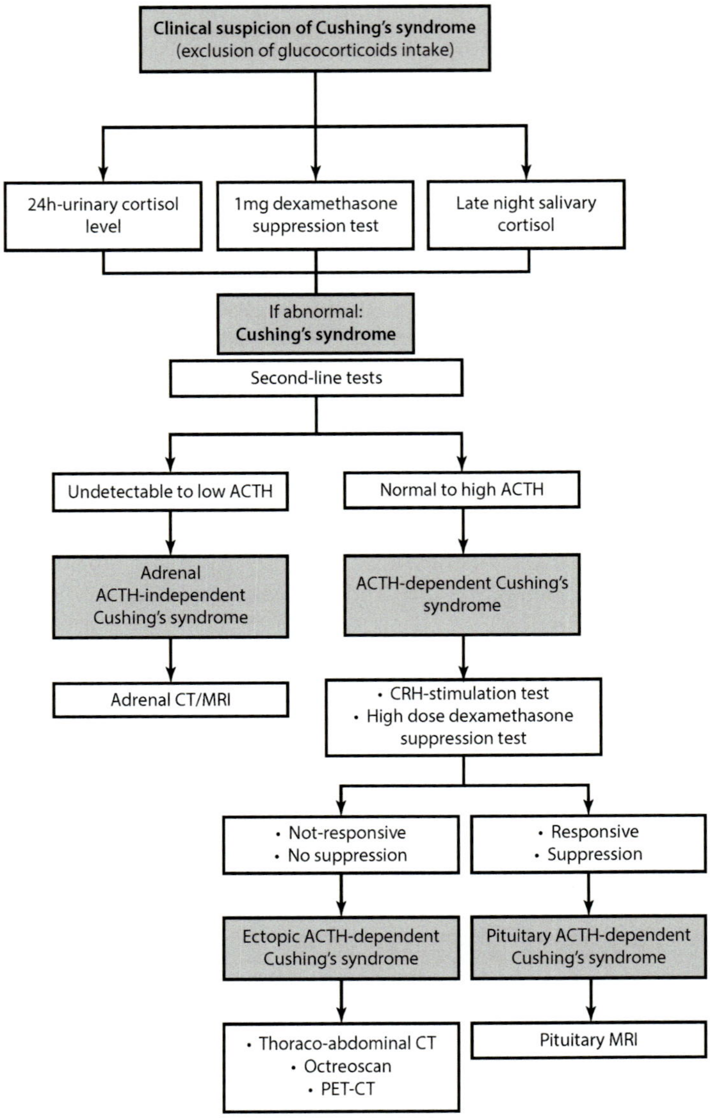

Fig. 19.3 Algorithm for the evaluation of a patient with suspected Cushing's syndrome. ACTH adrenocorticotropin hormone, CRH corticotropin-releasing hormone, CT computed tomography, MRI magnetic resonance imaging, PET-CT positron emission tomography-computed tomography

specific; the cutoff of 50 mmol/L (1.8 mcg/dl) is more sensitive [1, 11]. Certain drugs such as phenytoin, rifampicin, and alcohol induce hepatic enzymatic clearance of dexamethasone, thereby reducing the plasma dexamethasone concentrations. Moreover, dexamethasone clearance may be reduced in patients with liver and/or renal failure. Finally, dexamethasone levels are variable even in healthy individuals without medications. For this reason, measurements of both plasma cortisol and dexamethasone may be useful to ensure an adequate plasma dexamethasone concentration after suppression tests [1, 11, 17].

After the initial biochemical screening, other second-line tests and laboratory parameters could be assessed to diagnose the source of hypercortisolism.

To establish whether the CS is ACTH-dependent or ACTH-independent, the measurement of morning plasma ACTH levels should be first performed. Plasma ACTH levels higher than 20 pg/ml are indicative of ACTH-dependent CS, while lower than 10 pg/ml of ACTH-independent CS. ACTH-releasing hormone (CRH) stimulation test is particularly useful in border-line cases that present basal ACTH levels between 10 and 20 pg/ml and to discriminate pituitary from ectopic ACTH-dependent CS; only patients with pituitary-dependent CS are CRH test responsive, with an >50% increasing plasma cortisol levels [18]. Moreover, high-dose (8 mg) dexamethasone suppression test is useful to discriminate the cause of hypercortisolism; in fact, after high dose dexamethasone test, patients with pituitary CS suppress cortisol to <10% of baseline, whereas those with cortisol-secreting adrenocortical tumors or ectopic corticotropin production do not [19].

Thus, in pituitary CD, plasma basal ACTH levels are slightly increased or even normal and are frequently suppressed by high-dose dexamethasone suppression test. In Ectopic CS, plasma basal ACTH levels are markedly increased and are not suppressed by high-dose dexamethasone suppression test. In case of discordant results of the above mentioned tests, bilateral selective venous catheterization of the inferior petrosal veins after CRH stimulation is required for a conclusive diagnosis: patients with pituitary CS have an increase in corticotropin versus peripheral or prestimulation levels >50% [11].

In adrenal ACTH-independent CS, the hypothalamic-pituitary axis is suppressed; plasma ACTH levels are low or undetectable and obviously there is no suppression by dexamethasone test. Moreover, in this setting, a low level of adrenal androgen dehydroepiandrosterone sulfated form (DHEAS), due to suppression of ACTH production, has been considered a possible marker to detect an autonomous adrenal production of cortisol, especially in patients with incidentally detected adrenal incidentalomas or subclinical forms of CS.

CS may occur as cyclic disease, as in case of PBMAH with the presence of aberrant receptors. In these cases, the functional abnormalities of pituitary adrenal axis are due to other hormones and may vary overtime; thus, specific tests (standard mixed meal test; posture and other dynamic tests) are needed, sometimes repeated and should be carefully interpreted. Sexual hormones measurements may be useful in some case of malignant adrenal tumors with ACTH-independent CS, since a mixed secretion of cortisol and sexual hormones metabolites may occur.

Finally, CS may be associated with some hereditary diseases; genetic counseling (including *ARMC5, PRKAR1A, TP53* germ-line mutation analysis) may be useful in case of

PBMAH, PPNAD, and adrenocortical carcinoma in children, even in absence of familial history.

Following the biochemical diagnosis of CS, the origin of the disease must be assessed by localizing procedures. If ACTH-dependent CS is established, magnetic resonance imaging (MRI) is preferable to computed tomography (CT) scanning for identifying pituitary adenomas. In case of ectopic CS, MRI, CT scan, or Octreoscan may be useful to localize the source of ACTH hypersecretion. For ACTH-independent CS, adrenal imaging techniques required to localize the tumor and define the nature and its connections with the surrounding structures are CT and MRI scanning. Benign and malignant adrenal tumors may be potentially differentiated according to the intracellular lipid content and vascular pattern, since adenomas usually have an increased lipid content that cause a low attenuation mean value at unenhanced CT (with <10 Hounsfield Unit (HU) as suggested cutoff), high absolute and relative wash-out percentage at contrast-enhanced CT (>60% and >40%, respectively), and signal drop off in MRI at in phase and opposition phase sequences [20–22] (◘ Figs. 19.4, 19.5, and 19.6). Moreover, malignant adrenal lesions present increased metabolic activity that may be revealed by increased uptake at 18F-FDG PET-CT [23] (◘ Fig. 19.7).

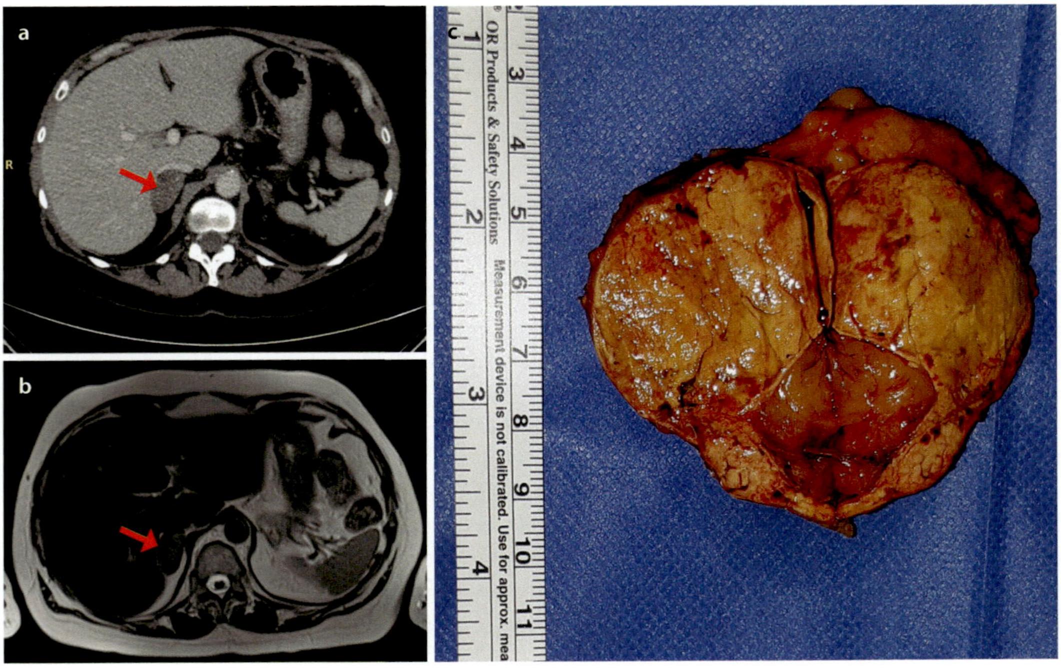

◘ **Fig. 19.4** Right adrenal adenoma at computed tomography **a**, magnetic resonance imaging **b**, and after unilateral adrenalectomy (**c**, sectioned) in a Cushing's syndrome female patient

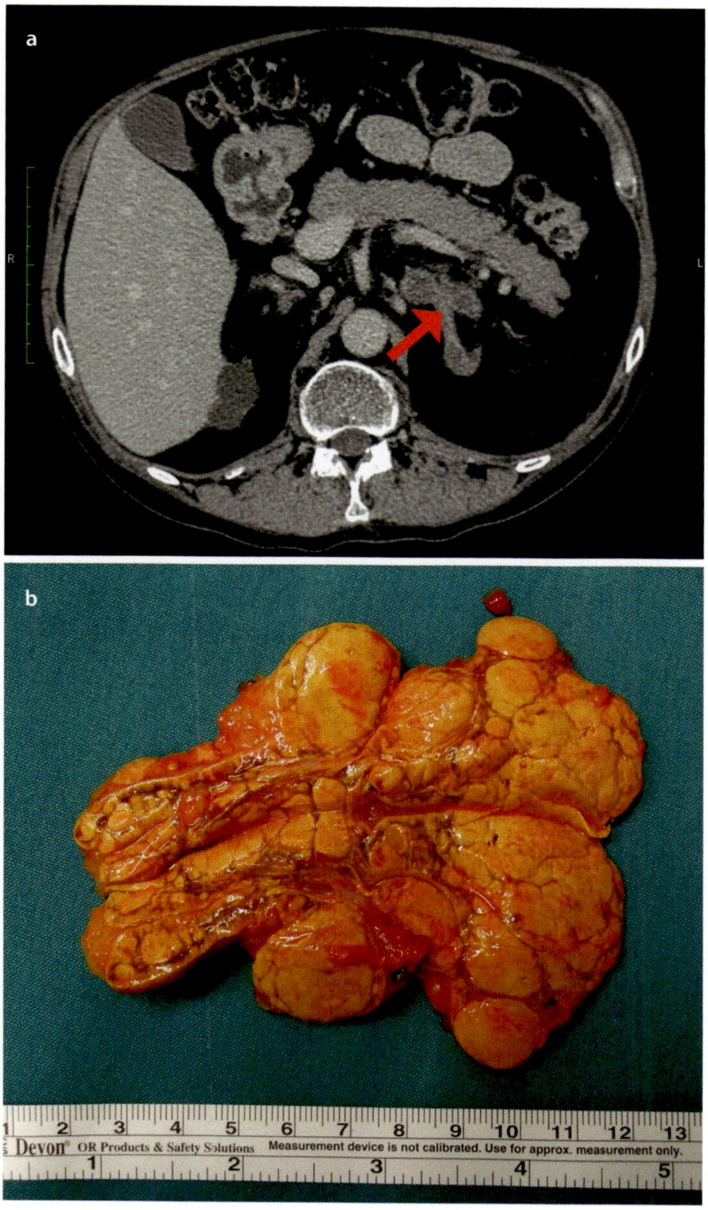

Fig. 19.5 Primary bilateral macronodular adrenal hyperplasia with prevalent left adrenal involvement (arrow, **a**), and after left unilateral adrenalectomy (sectioned, **b**) in a Cushing's syndrome patient

Radiocholesterol scintigraphy has been used as a functional examination; it may be useful in case of bilateral adrenal hyperplasia to guide the surgical resection. In these cases, however, also selective adrenal venous sampling can be helpful in determining the side of glucocorticoid overproduction; in these conditions, cortisol levels might be normalized to catecholamine or plasmatic metanephrine levels.

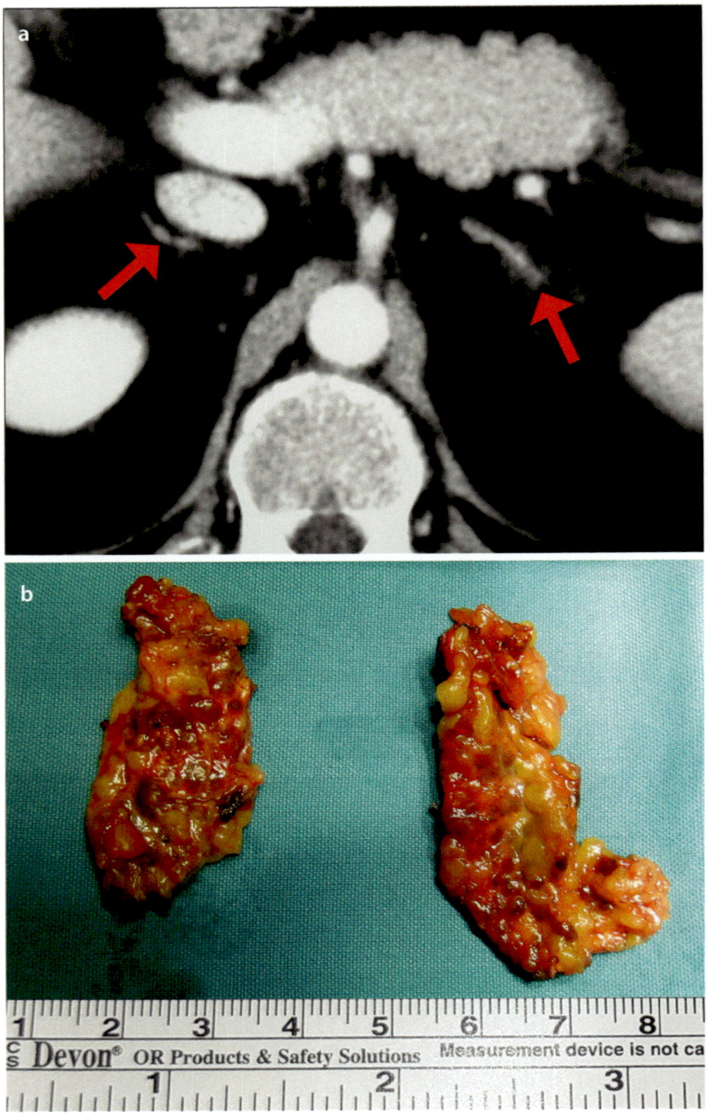

Fig. 19.6 Primary pigmented micronodular adrenal hyperplasia at computed tomography (**a**, arrows) and after bilateral adrenalectomy **b** in a Cushing's syndrome patient with Carney-complex syndrome

19.5 Treatment of CS and Indications for Surgery

The goal of treating CS is to eliminate its primary cause reducing the cortisol secretion to normal levels and to achieve definitive remission, consequently eliminating the associated signs, symptoms, and complications. Surgery, if feasible, is the recommended first-line treatment in every form of hypercortisolism [24] and should be primarily directed to pituitary in CD,

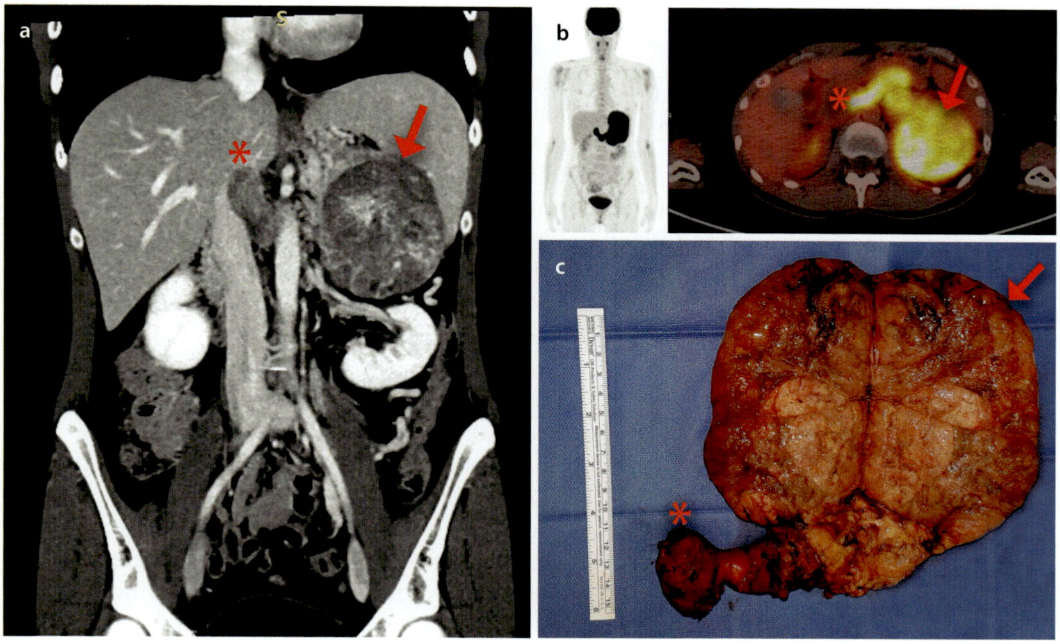

Fig. 19.7 Large left adrenocortical carcinoma (arrow) with neoplastic intracaval thrombus (*) in a 28-year-old woman with Cushing's syndrome. Coronal plane imaging at computed tomography showing the left adrenal mass and the neoplastic thrombus **a**, 18FDG-PET/CT hyperfixation **b**, surgical specimen (**c**, sectioned)

to the primary ACTH secreting tumor in vase of ectopic CS, and to adrenal(s) in ACTH-independent CS.

Medical treatments of hypercortisolism are usually considered a second-line option after failed surgery in patients with persistent CD or a primary option in those with occult or metastatic ectopic CS (in alternative to bilateral adrenalectomy) or as a complementary treatment in case of ACC [24] or before delayed surgical treatment in order to obtain a provisional decrease of hypercortisolism.

In patients with adrenal incidentaloma and subclinical ACTH-independent CS, especially with mild cortisol overproduction (values <1.5-fold upper reference range) and in absence of associated comorbidities, the benefit of the surgical treatment has not been well established; for this reason, every single patient should be evaluated independently, and managed with a tailored strategy. However, a significant benefit of adrenalectomy compared to intensive medical treatment of comorbidities in case of subclinical ACTH-independent CS with cardiovascular or metabolic impairment has been reported from some large retrospective studies [8, 9, 17].

A specific preoperative medical treatment aimed to restrict cortisol secretion and to correct its metabolic effects should be undertaken to decrease intra e postoperative morbidity, whenever possible. Hypertension and diabetes mellitus should be treated, and coagulation studies done.

In fact, CS patients are exposed to increased risk of local infections and sepsis (so that antibiotic prophylaxis and aseptic techniques should be put into practice); hemorrhage (because of the vascular fragility) and thromboembolism (because of the hypercoagulative condition) at the same time (requiring careful tissue dissection and pre and postoperative low molecular weight heparin prophylaxis, respectively); and wound healing delay (with risk of incisional hernias in case of adrenal surgery). Since the risk of deep venous thrombosis and sepsis is high in CS patients, preoperative thromboembolic and antibiotics prophylaxis is recommended. Moreover, the use of postoperative anticoagulant prophylaxis with low molecular weight heparin has demonstrated a significant reduction in the number of thromboembolic events and related mortality rate.

Operatory positioning should be carefully accomplished in consideration of osteoporosis and bone fragility; aggressive taping should also be avoided because of easy bruising; early patient mobilization should be obtained to decrease all morbidity risk. For these reasons, adrenal surgery with minimally invasive laparoscopic approaches (both transperitoneal or retroperitoneoscopic adrenalectomy) represents a safe and effective procedure and are considered the gold standard treatment, because of the decreased postoperative morbidity and shorter hospitalization [25].

19.6 ACTH-Dependent Hypercortisolism

19.6.1 Pituitary-Dependent CD

The optimal treatment for pituitary ACTH-producing tumor is surgical resection by transsphenoidal approach [24]. ACTH-producing tumors are usually microadenomas (<1 cm), evident at radiological imaging only in about 60% of patients [26]. The best results in terms of cure are obtained when micro- or macro-adenomas are visualized at preoperative imaging (CT or MRI) or during surgery, with a remission rate of 76% and 43%, respectively [27]. If the tumor is not clearly identified at radiological imaging, inferior petrosal sinus sampling for lateralization of the source of hypercortisolism and subsequent hemihypophysectomy should be performed. However, in this setting the cure rate is about 50% [28]. Morbidity related to transsphenoidal microsurgery (hemorrhage, meningitis, and oculomotor dysfunction) are uncommon (<1%). However, a transient deficit of ACTH, thyroid-stimulating hormone, prolactin, and gonadotropin occurs in most of the patients; diabetes insipidus due to the lack of adequate ADH secretion is common but usually transient [29]. Recurrence rate is high in patients with CD, ranging from 15% to 66% within 5–10 years after initial surgery [30]. When chosen, repeated surgery should be performed in a short window of time after prior surgery, usually within 2 months, to minimize additional trauma before the formation of a distorting scar tissue. Repeated surgery is associated to lower success rates and higher risk of hypopituitarism, especially in case of more aggressive surgical approaches [31]. Radiation therapy (RT) and radiosurgery are usually considered second-line option treatment for CD, often when surgical resection fails; less frequently, they can be used as first-line treatment especially in presence of macroadenomas invading the surrounding structures and/or causing mass effects, as RT seems to better control tumor size than cortisol excess [32]. Different types of radiation techniques are possible. Fractionated photon beam RT ("conventional" radiation therapy), consisting in delivering a total radiotherapic dose through small, daily doses over some weeks, allows remission in up to 83% of adults and about 78% of children, with maximum results usually achieved within 2 years [33]. Stereotactic radiotherapy and radiosurgery guarantee a specifically oriented radiation combining MRI imaging and CT-assisted planning, to minimize surrounding tissues damages. Radiosurgery aims to damage the pituitary gland or the pituitary stalk; it seems to provide a more rapid biochemical control if compared to other methods and also a more reliable preservation of the brain structures nearby, but indications for its use remain controversial.

The most common adverse effects in radiated patients (two thirds of subjects) are hypopituitarism [34], neurocognitive (particularly in children) and cerebrovascular complications, secondary tumors in the radiation field (meningiomas, gliomas and astrocytomas), and cranial neuropathies of the II, III, IV, V, and VI cranial nerves [32].

Medical therapy should be considered: (1) before surgery, especially in case of severe disease; (2) after surgery for treatment of persistent or recurrent disease; (3) before, after, or in combination with RT; (4) as first-line treatment in patients not amenable to surgery, refusing it, or without a clear surgical indication. Steroidogenesis inhibitors (ketoconazole, metyrapone, and mitotane) are the most commonly used drugs, inhibiting cortisol production via blockade of the enzymes involved in steroidogenesis. Ketoconazole (used in the past as an antifungal agent), administered orally twice or thrice daily, inhibits the cytochrome P-450 enzymes; however, its therapeutic effects tend to decrease with time, and transient hepatotoxicity may be observed [35]. Mitotane (o,p'-DDD) is an highly effective oral drug but requires several weeks to decrease the cortisol production. It causes selective destruction of the fasciculata and reticularis zones of the adrenal cortex and subsequently inhibits its adrenal steroidogenesis. Unfortunately, severe side effects (nausea, vomiting, diarrhea, skin rash) and toxic effects may occur in the majority of patients, and therefore it is used almost exclusively for treating adrenal carcinoma. Metyrapone, an

11b-hydroxylase inhibitor, may be effective for reducing cortisol secretion very quickly. However, it often results in adverse general effects (dizziness, nausea) and increases both corticotropin and androgen levels, resulting in unbearable worsening of hirsutism in women [36, 37]. Pituitary-directed drugs (neuromodulatory drugs, serotonin antagonists, GABA agonists, dopamine agonists, somatostatin analogs, or nuclear receptor ligands, PPAR-gamma agonists), inhibiting the ACTH production, represent the most physiological option in case of CD, directly targeting the source of the disease, especially in case of resistant or not operable CD.

Bilateral adrenalectomy should be considered in emergency cases that cannot be controlled by other treatments. It is effective, but it requires lifelong replacement hormonal therapy. It may be indicated after unsuccessful pituitary treatment or when transsphenoidal surgery is technically difficult, dangerous, or impossible or in patients with rapidly progressive and severe hypercortisolism. If bilateral adrenalectomy is performed and the ACTH-producing tumor remains in situ because of failed pituitary surgery, a significant risk of tumor enlargement (with headache, visual field defects, and hypopituitarism resulting from the aggressive expanding intrasellar neoplasm) and cutaneous hyperpigmentation causing the so-called Nelson's syndrome may occur in 10–30% of cases [38].

After bilateral adrenalectomy, steroid replacement therapy with glucocorticoids (hydrocortisone or cortisone acetate) must be given, and mineralocorticoids (fluorhydrocortisone acetate) are also often required. Glucocorticoid replacement must begin during surgery, immediately after adrenals ablation. Most of the symptoms of hypercortisolism recover after bilateral adrenalectomy for pituitary-dependent CD. Some patients remain hypertensive (30%) with diabetes (20%) and obesity (20%). These patients may have a reduced working capacity and quality of life, but their survival may be similar to that seen in the general population. However, life-threatening Addisonian crisis may occur; for these reasons, all patients after bilateral adrenalectomy must undergo periodic check-ups and strict follow-up; additional and supplemental corticosteroid replacement must be taken at times of stress.

19.6.2 Ectopic ACTH-Dependent CS

The low frequency of presentation of ectopic hypercortisolism makes it difficult to acquire experience in its management and thus to establish clear guidelines; generally, for localized ectopic ACTH-producing tumors, the goal of treatment is surgical resection of the primary tumor with lymph node dissection. In this setting, in absence of overt metastatic disease, cure is obtained in about 76% of patients [24]. In case of a non-localized ACTH production (metastatic or occult ectopic CS, as in small carcinoid tumors), bilateral adrenalectomy might be necessary as the most definitive solution if cortisol excess can't be controlled by medical treatments [39, 40]. In fact, in these cases, morbidity and mortality is related more strictly to the complications of hypercortisolism than to the spreading of primary neoplasm.

If surgery is not possible or advisable, a tailor-made pharmacotherapy is an option: in these cases, a combination therapy with ketoconazole and metyrapone is considered as primary treatment [41, 42]. Equally to adrenocortical carcinoma-related CS, ectopic CS confers the highest morbidity and mortality risk among CS's etiologies: for this reason, prompt treatment of this condition is essential [43].

19.7 ACTH-Independent Hypercortisolism

19.7.1 Adrenal Adenoma

Adrenal adenoma is the most common cause of ACTH-independent CS. Unilateral laparoscopic (transperitoneal or retroperitoneal) adrenalectomy is considered the gold standard treatment in unilateral benign adrenal tumors. Retroperitoneoscopic adrenalectomy might be more challenging because of the increased quantity of fat in retroperitoneum. In any case, adrenalectomy should be performed by skilled teams to avoid complications such as capsular disruption, which may lead to adrenal tissue spreading and recurrences. In the past, the morbidity rate after unilateral adrenalectomy for CS was 30%, with appreciable (1–5%) mortality, but in recent years, the morbidity rate has been reduced to less than 10%. The preoperative treatment is the same as previously described.

After surgery, as removing the cause of hypercortisolism could lead to adrenal insufficiency because of the suppression of ACTH, postoperative replacement therapy with hydrocortisone or cortisone acetate has to be administered until the contralateral gland secretion finally normalizes; however, the pituitary-adrenal axis may need several months (and sometimes years) to completely recover. The first clinical and metabolic signs of improvement start to be visible in approximately 4 or 6 weeks, while cutaneous alterations and fat redistribution regress slowly, with a complete recovery of physical appearance of these patients requiring up to 12 months [44]. Long-term cure is achieved in nearly 100% of adults and children, potentially leaving the normal hypothalamic-pituitary adrenal axis intact, and mortality in cured patients seems to be equal to that of general population [43].

19.7.2 Adrenal Carcinoma

Surgery, when feasible, is the standard of treatment for patients with adrenocortical carcinoma (ACC). Malignancies should be suspected in case of large (>6 cm) and heterogeneous masses at imaging, with a rapid onset of symptoms related to hypercortisolism and associated to a mixed hormonal secretion; in fact, in these patients' typical features of CS are often accompanied by signs of virilization due to androgen hypersecretion. In this setting, open adrenalectomy is still the gold standard surgical treatment [45].

Transperitoneal laparoscopic adrenalectomy can be considered in selected cases without evident signs of extraadrenal invasion, but most experienced endocrine surgeons believe that only open procedures can achieve en bloc resection and avoid disease recurrences; for these reasons, the role of minimally invasive surgery in the management of ACC is still controversial. As hypercortisolism seems to be negatively correlated to survival rates in these patients, cortisol levels should be lowered as much as possible administering surgery and medical compounds synchronously. Adjuvant treatments may include cytotoxic chemotherapy, radiotherapy, or combined medical approaches.

19.7.3 Primary Adrenal Hyperplasia

Primary adrenal hyperplasia is a rare cause of ACTH-independent CS. The most frequent variants of adrenal hyperplasia are PBMAH (also known as adrenocorticotropin independent macronodular adrenal hyperplasia, AIMAH) and PPNAD.

In PBMAH, adrenal glands are often widely enlarged with a massive, asymmetric macronodular pattern, but cortisol overproduction is generally mild, due to altered steroidogenic enzymatic pathways resulting in a non-effective hormone production; thus, subclinical or mild hypercortisolism may occur. In patients with overt CS, bilateral adrenalectomy might be proposed together with or alternatively to the administration of drugs aiming to block aberrant hormone receptors; if one gland is largely prevalent compared with the other, unilateral adrenalectomy should be also considered, to avoid life-long hormone replacement therapy [46]. Unilateral total adrenalectomy of the prevalent adrenal gland and subtotal contralateral adrenalectomy is another option that may represent an acceptable compromise between postoperative definitive hypocortisolism and recurrent CS.

PPNAD is characterized by small- or normal-sized adrenal glands containing multiple, small (<1 cm), pigmented cortical nodules; the adrenal involvement is typically symmetric, and

CS may be severe. In this setting, a bilateral minimally invasive adrenalectomy is the preferred option, with postoperative life-long replacement therapy.

Patients with suspected PPNAD should be periodically screened for other features of Carney complex, particularly for atrial myxoma.

Answers to the Questions

1. (b); 2. (c); 3. (a); 4. (c); 5. (c); 6. (d); 7. (c); 8. (d); 9. (b); 10. (d); 11. (d); 12. (e); 13. (d); 14. (a); 15. (b); 16. (e); 17. (a)

References

1. Nieman LK, Biller BMK, Findling JW, Newell-Price J, Savage MO, Stewart PM, Montori VM, Edwards H. The diagnosis of Cushing's syndrome: an endocrine society clinical practice guideline. J Clin Endocrinol Metab. 2008;93:1526–40.
2. Ragnarsson O, Olsson DS, Chantzichristos D, Papakokkinou E, Dahlqvist P, Segerstedt E, Olsson T, Petersson M, Berinder K, Bensing S, Höybye C, Edén Engström B, Burman P, Bonelli L, Follin C, Petranek D, Erfurth EM, Wahlberg J, Ekman B, et al. The incidence of Cushing's disease: a nationwide Swedish study. Pituitary. 2019;22:179–86.
3. Albiger NM, Regazzo D, Rubin B, Ferrara AM, Rizzati S, Taschin E, Ceccato F, Arnaldi G, Pecori Giraldi F, Stigliano A, Cerquetti L, Grimaldi F, De Menis E, Boscaro M, Iacobone M, Occhi G, Scaroni C. A multicenter experience on the prevalence of ARMC5 mutations in patients with primary bilateral macronodular adrenal hyperplasia: from genetic characterization to clinical phenotype. Endocrine. 2017;55:959–68.
4. Albiger NM, Ceccato F, Zilio M, Barbot M, Occhi G, Rizzati S, Fassina A, Mantero F, Boscaro M, Iacobone M, Scaroni C. An analysis of different therapeutic options in patients with Cushing's syndrome due to bilateral macronodular adrenal hyperplasia: a single-centre experience. Clin Endocrinol. 2015;82:808–15.
5. Correa R, Salpea P, Stratakis CA. Carney complex: an update. Eur J Endocrinol. 2015;173:M85–97.
6. Javaid MK, Boyce A, Appelman-Dijkstra N, Ong J, Defabianis P, Offiah A, Arunde P, Shaw N, Pos VD, Underhil A, Portero D, Heral L, Heegaard AM, Masi L, Monsell F, Stanton R, Dijkstra PDS, Brandi ML, Chapurlat R, et al. Best practice management guidelines for fibrous dysplasia/McCune-Albright syndrome: a consensus statement from the FD/MAS international consortium. Orphanet J Rare Dis. 2019;14:139.
7. Monteiro NML, De Sá Rodrigues KE, Vidigal PVT, De Oliveira BM. Adrenal carcinoma in children: longitudinal study in Minas Gerais, Brazil. Rev Paul Pediatr. 2019;37:20–6.
8. Correa H. Li-Fraumeni syndrome. J Pediatr Genet. 2016;5:84–8.
9. Ferreira AM, Brondani VB, Helena VP, Charchar HLS, Zerbini MCN, Leite LAS, Hoff AO, Latronico AC, Mendonca BB, Diz MDPE, de Almeida MQ, Fragoso MCBV. Clinical spectrum of Li-Fraumeni syndrome/Li-Fraumeni-like syndrome in Brazilian individuals with the TP53 p.R337H mutation. J Steroid Biochem Mol Biol. 2019;190:250–5.
10. Boscaro M, Arnaldi G. Approach to the patient with possible Cushing's syndrome. J Clin Endocrinol Metab. 2009;94:3121–31.
11. Barbot M, Zilio M, Scaroni C. Cushing's syndrome: overview of clinical presentation, diagnostic tools and complications. Best Pract Res Clin Endocrinol Metab. 2020;34:101380.

12. Fassnacht M, Arlt W, Bancos I, Dralle H, Newell-Price J, Sahdev A, Tabarin A, Terzolo M, Tsagarakis S, Dekkers OM. Management of adrenal incidentalomas: European Society of Endocrinology Clinical Practice Guideline in collaboration with the European Network for the Study of Adrenal Tumors. Eur J Endocrinol. 2016;175:G1–34.
13. Chabre O. The difficulties of pseudo-Cushing's syndrome (or "non-neoplastic hypercortisolism"). Ann Endocrinol (Paris). 2018;79: 138–45.
14. Ceroni L, Cota D, Pasquali R. Pseudo-Cushing syndrome. Physiopathologic aspects and differential diagnosis. Minerva Endocrinol. 2000;25:47–54.
15. Iacobone M, Citton M, Viel G, Boetto R, Bonadio I, Mondi I, Tropea S, Nitti D, Favia G. Adrenalectomy may improve cardiovascular and metabolic impairment and ameliorate quality of life in patients with adrenal incidentalomas and subclinical Cushing's syndrome. Surgery. 2012;152:991–7.
16. Raff H, Auchus RJ, Findling JW, Nieman LK. Urine free cortisol in the diagnosis of Cushing's syndrome: is it worth doing and, if so, how? J Clin Endocrinol Metab. 2015;100:395–7.
17. Braun LT, Riester A, Oßwald-Kopp A, Fazel J, Rubinstein G, Bidlingmaier M, Beuschlein F, Reincke M. Toward a diagnostic score in Cushing's syndrome. Front Endocrinol. 2019;10:766.
18. Lacroix A, Feelders RA, Stratakis CA, Nieman LK. Cushing's syndrome. Lancet. 2015;386:913–27.
19. Isidori AM, Kaltsas GA, Mohammed S, Morris DG, Jenkins P, Chew SL, Monson JP, Besser GM, Grossman AB. Discriminatory value of the low-dose dexamethasone suppression test in establishing the diagnosis and differential diagnosis of Cushing's syndrome. J Clin Endocrinol Metab. 2003;88:5299–306.
20. Blake MA, Kalra MK, Sweeney AT, Lucey BC, Maher MM, Sahani DV, Halpern EF, Mueller PR, Hahn PF, Boland GW. Distinguishing benign from malignant adrenal masses: multi-detector row CT protocol with 10-minute delay. Radiology. 2006;238:578–85.
21. Terzolo M, Stigliano A, Chiodini I, Loli P, Furlani L, Arnaldi G, Reimondo G, Pia A, Toscano V, Zini M, Borretta G, Papini E, Garofalo P, Allolio B, Dupas B, Mantero F, Tabarin A. AME position statement on adrenal incidentaloma. Eur J Endocrinol. 2011;164:851–70.
22. Seo JM, Park BK, Park SY, Kim CK. Characterization of lipid-poor adrenal adenoma: chemical-shift MRI and washout CT. Am J Roentgenol. 2014;202:1043–50.
23. Guerin C, Pattou F, Brunaud L, Lifante JC, Mirallié E, Haissaguerre M, Huglo D, Olivier P, Houzard C, Ansquer C, Hindié E, Loundou A, Archange C, Tabarin A, Sebag F, Baumstarck K, Täeb D. Performance of 18F-FDG PET/CT in the characterization of adrenal masses in noncancer patients: a prospective study. J Clin Endocrinol Metab. 2017;102:2465–72.
24. Nieman LK, Biller BMK, Findling JW, Murad MH, Newell-Price J, Savage MO, Tabarin A. Treatment of cushing's syndrome: an endocrine society clinical practice guideline. J Clin Endocrinol Metab. 2015;100:2807–31.
25. Vella A, Thompson GB, Grant CS, Van Heerden JA, Farley DR, Young WF. Laparoscopic adrenalectomy for adrenocorticotropin-dependent Cushing's syndrome. J Clin Endocrinol Metab. 2001;86:1596–9.
26. Storr HL, Alexandraki KI, Martin L, Isidori AM, Kaltsas GA, Monson JP, Besser GM, Matson M, Evanson J, Afshar F, Sabin I, Savage MO, Grossman AB. Comparisons in the epidemiology, diagnostic features and cure rate by transsphenoidal surgery between paediatric and adult-onset Cushing's disease. Eur J Endocrinol. 2011;164:667–74.
27. Yamada S, Fukuhara N, Nishioka H, Takeshita A, Inoshita N, Ito J, Takeuchi Y. Surgical management and outcomes in patients with

Cushing disease with negative pituitary magnetic resonance imaging. World Neurosurg. 2012;77:525–32.
28. Wind JJ, Lonser RR, Nieman LK, DeVroom HL, Chang R, Oldfield EH. The lateralization accuracy of inferior petrosal sinus sampling in 501 patients with Cushing's disease. J Clin Endocrinol Metab. 2013;98:2285–93.
29. Olson BR, Rubino D, Gumowski J, Oldfield EH. Isolated hyponatremia after transsphenoidal pituitary surgery. J Clin Endocrinol Metab. 1995;80:85–91.
30. Aranda G, Enseñat J, Mora M, Puig-Domingo M, Martínez de Osaba MJ, Casals G, Verger E, Ribalta MT, Hanzu FA, Halperin I. Long-term remission and recurrence rate in a cohort of Cushing's disease: the need for long-term follow-up. Pituitary. 2015;82:260–6.
31. Friedman RB, Oldfield EH, Nieman LK, Chrousos GP, Doppman JL, Cutler GB, Loriaux DL. Repeat transsphenoidal surgery for Cushing's disease. J Neurosurg. 1989;71:520–7.
32. Loeffler JS, Shih HA. Radiation therapy in the management of pituitary adenomas. J Clin Endocrinol Metab. 2011;96:1992–2003.
33. Acharya SV, Gopal RA, Goerge J, Menon PS, Bandgar TR, Shah NS. Radiotherapy in paediatric Cushing's disease: efficacy and long term follow up of pituitary function. Pituitary. 2010;13:293–7.
34. Hughes NR, Lissett CA, Shalet SM. Growth hormone status following treatment for Cushing's syndrome. Clin Endocrinol. 1999;51:61–6.
35. Castinetti F, Guignat L, Giraud P, Muller M, Kamenicky P, Drui D, Caron P, Luca F, Donadille B, Vantyghem MC, Bihan H, Delemer B, Raverot G, Motte E, Philippon M, Morange I, Conte-Devolx B, Quinquis L, Martinie M, et al. Ketoconazole in Cushing's disease: is it worth a try. J Clin Endocrinol Metab. 2014;99:1623–30.
36. Verhelst JA, Trainer PJ, Howlett TA, Perry L, Rees LH, Grossman AB, Wass JAH, Sesser GM. Short and long-term responses to metyrapone in the medical management of 91 patients with Cushing's syndrome. Clin Endocrinol. 1991;35:169–78.
37. Besser GM, Tomlin S, Edwards CRW. Metyrapone in long-term management of Cushing's disease. Br Med J. 1977;2:215–7.
38. Sonino N, Zielezny M, Fava GA, Fallo F, Boscaro M. Risk factors and long-term outcome in pituitary-dependent Cushing's disease. J Clin Endocrinol Metab. 1996;81:2647–52.
39. Pivonello R, De Leo M, Cozzolino A, Colao A. The treatment of Cushing's disease. Endocr Rev. 2015;36:385–486.
40. Pivonello R, Isidori AM, De Martino MC, Newell-Price J, Biller BMK, Colao A. Complications of Cushing's syndrome: state of the art. Lancet Diabetes Endocrinol. 2016;4:611–29.
41. Feelders RA, Newell-Price J, Pivonello R, Nieman LK, Hofland LJ, Lacroix A. Advances in the medical treatment of Cushing's syndrome. Lancet Diabetes Endocrinol. 2019;7:300–12.
42. Kamenický P, Droumaguet C, Salenave S, Blanchard A, Jublanc C, Gautier JF, Brailly-Tabard S, Leboulleux S, Schlumberger M, Baudin E, Chanson P, Young J. Mitotane, metyrapone, and ketoconazole combination therapy as an alternative to rescue adrenalectomy for severe ACTH-dependent Cushing's syndrome. J Clin Endocrinol Metab. 2011;96:2796–804.
43. Javanmard P, Duan D, Geer EB. Mortality in patients with endogenous Cushing's syndrome. Endocrinol Metab Clin N Am. 2018;47:313–33.
44. Berr CM, Di Dalmazi G, Osswald A, Ritzel K, Bidlingmaier M, Geyer LL, Treitl M, Hallfeldt K, Rachinger W, Reisch N, Blaser R, Schopohl J, Beuschlein F, Reincke M. Time to recovery of adrenal function after curative surgery for Cushing's syndrome depends on etiology. J Clin Endocrinol Metab. 2015;108:1085–90.
45. Gaujoux S, Mihai R, Carnaille B, Dousset B, Fiori C, Porpiglia F, Hellman P, Iacobone M, Kraimps JL, Donatini G, Langenhuijsen J,

Lorenz K, Mathonnet M, Mirallié E, Blanchard C, van Dijkum EN, Raffaelli M, Rayes N, Sébag F, et al. European Society of Endocrine Surgeons (ESES) and European Network for the Study of Adrenal Tumours (ENSAT) recommendations for the surgical management of adrenocortical carcinoma. Br J Surg. 2017;104:358–76.

46. Iacobone M, Albiger N, Scaroni C, Mantero F, Fassina A, Viel G, Frego M, Favia G. The role of unilateral adrenalectomy in ACTH-independent macronodular adrenal hyperplasia (AIMAH). World J Surg. 2008;32:882–9.

Primary Aldosteronism

Per Hellman and William F. Young Jr.

Contents

A. L. Shifrin et al. (eds.), *Endocrine Surgery Comprehensive Board Exam Guide*,
https://doi.org/10.1007/978-3-030-84737-1_20

Case Presentation

A 63-year-old man had a 10-year history of hypertension, which accelerated over the past 1 year. He had resistant hypertension with poor BP control on amlodipine 10 mg daily, lisinopril 40 mg daily, metoprolol 100 mg daily, and hydrochlorothiazide 25 mg daily. Serum potassium concentrations were low–normal (e.g., 3.5 mEq/L). PAC was 22 ng/dL (610 pmol/L) with concomitant PRA of 0.6 ng/mL/h. The 24-h urinary aldosterone excretion was 48 mcg (133 nmol) with a sodium excretion of 194 mEq. Abdominal CT scan showed bilateral adrenal nodules (see ◘ Fig. 20.1). Concomitant glucocorticoid secretory autonomy was excluded with a normal baseline serum dehydroepiandrosterone sulfate (DHEA-S) concentration of 97 mcg/dL (normal, 12–227) and normal cortisol suppression with an overnight 8-mg dexamethasone suppression test (serum cortisol concentration <1.0 mcg/dL). Adrenal venous sampling localized the aldosterone hypersecretion to the right adrenal gland (see ◘ Table 20.1). The patient underwent laparoscopic right adrenalectomy. The right adrenal gland weighed 12.5 gm (normal 4–5 gm) and contained five yellow nodules, which measured 0.8 × 0.5 × 0.5 cm; 0.8 × 0.4 × 0.4 cm; 1.3 × 0.8 × 0.7 cm; 1.1 × 0.4 × 0.4 cm; and 2.4 × 1.5 × 1.3 cm. The pathology findings were consistent with nodular hyperplasia. The serum aldosterone concentration the day after surgery was <4 ng/dL (<111 pmol/L). On hospital dismissal, his dosages of lisinopril and amlodipine were decreased by 50%, and the patient was followed with daily BP measurements and weekly serum potassium checks for 4 weeks. His weekly serum potassium checks were normal (4.3, 4.4, 4.0, and 4.1 mEq/L). His BP slowly decreased to 118/72 mm Hg at 4 weeks postoperatively at which time the amlodipine was discontinued. The plans for long-term follow-up included a return visit in 1 year for adrenal CT, baseline DHEA-S, and an 8-mg overnight dexamethasone suppression test.

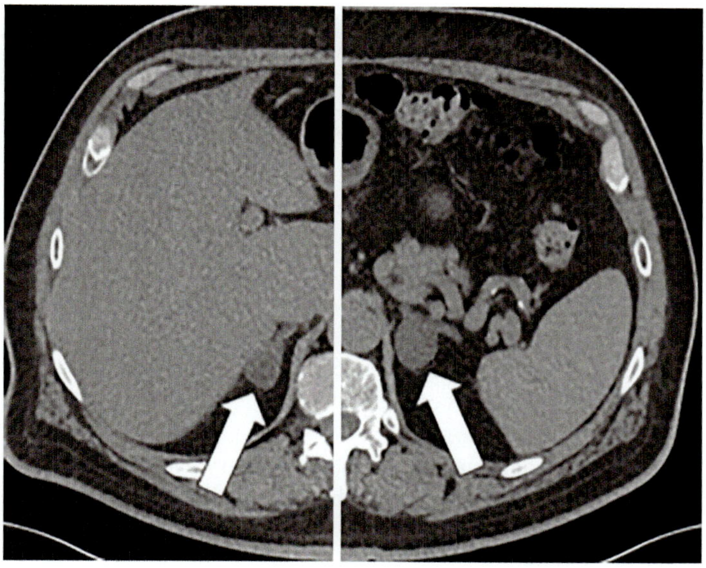

Fig. 20.1 Unenhanced axial abdominal CT images showed bilateral adrenal nodules. Two nodules were seen in the right adrenal gland. The largest right adrenal nodule measured 1.9 × 1.5 cm (arrow) had low attenuation on precontrast imaging (−3 HU) and washout characteristics indicative of a lipid-rich adenoma (venous attenuation 65 HU, delayed attenuation 9 HU). A second smaller nodule was in the inferior lateral limb measuring 1 cm in diameter—this nodule had low attenuation on precontrast imaging (5 HU) and washout characteristics indicative of a lipid rich adenoma (venous attenuation 97 HU, delayed attenuation 25 HU). The left adrenal gland contained a single nodule that measured 3.0 × 2.5 cm (arrow). This nodule also had low attenuation on precontrast imaging (4 HU) and washout characteristics also indicative of a lipid rich adenoma (venous attenuation 78 HU, delayed attenuation 18 HU)

Table 20.1 Adrenal Vein Sampling (AVS)[a]

	Right AV	IVC	Left AV
Aldosterone, ng/dL	3665	30	367
Cortisol, mcg/dL	506	29	577
A/C ratio[b]	7.24	1.0	0.64
Aldosterone lateralization ratio	11.3-to-1		
Contralateral suppression index			0.64

Abbreviations used: A aldosterone, *AV* adrenal vein, *C* cortisol, *LT* left, *RT* right, *IVC* inferior vena cava

[a]Sequential AVS completed under continuous cosyntropin infusion 50 mcg/h

[b]Each adrenal aldosterone concentration is divided by the respective cortisol concentration for the A/C ratio. The A/C ratio from the dominant adrenal is divided by the A/C ratio from the nondominant adrenal for the aldosterone lateralization ratio. In this case, 7.24 on the right is divided by 0.64 on the left yielding an aldosterone lateralization ratio of 11.3 to 1 (right-to-left). When the aldosterone lateralization ratio is >4 to 1, unilateral adrenalectomy will be curative. An additional predictor of unilateral disease is when the nondominant adrenal vein A/C ratio is less than that in the IVC, and this is termed the contralateral suppression index

Questions

1. Patients with primary aldosteronism who have an adrenal nodule >1.5 cm on CT scan should be screened for concomitant glucocorticoid secretory autonomy with which of the following:
   1. 24-h urinary-free cortisol
   2. Midnight salivary cortisol
   3. DHEA-S
   4. Overnight dexamethasone suppression test
      (a) Only (1) and (2) and (3) are correct.
      (b) Only (2) and (3) and (4) are correct.
      (c) Only (3) and (4) are correct.
      (d) Only (4) is correct.
      (e) All are correct.
2. Formal confirmatory testing for primary aldosteronism is not needed when a patient has the combination of which of the following?
   1. Spontaneous hypokalemia
   2. Plasma aldosterone concentration >20 ng/dL (>555 pmol/L)
   3. Suppressed renin (PRA <1 ng/mL/h or DRC <8 mU/L)
   4. Resistant hypertension
      (a) Only (1) and (2) and (3) are correct.
      (b) Only (2) and (3) and (4) are correct.
      (c) Only (3) and (4) are correct.
      (d) Only (4) is correct.
      (e) All are correct.
3. With regard to quality of life (QoL) in patients with primary aldosteronism, which statements are correct?
   1. QoL outcomes in patients with primary aldosteronism are superior with partial unilateral adrenalectomy vs. complete unilateral adrenalectomy.
   2. Baseline QoL metrics are equivalent between patients with essential hypertension and primary aldosteronism.
   3. QoL outcomes in patients with primary aldosteronism correlate with the size of the aldosterone-producing adenoma.
   4. QoL outcomes are superior for patients with primary aldosteronism managed surgically compared to those managed medically.
      (a) Only (1) and (2) and (3) are correct.
      (b) Only (2) and (3) and (4) are correct.
      (c) Only (3) and (4) are correct.
      (d) Only (4) is correct.
      (e) All are correct.
4. When compared to patients with bilateral idiopathic hyperplasia, most patients with aldosterone-producing adenomas have which of the following characteristics?
   1. Higher plasma aldosterone concentrations
   2. More frequent hypokalemia
   3. More difficult to control hypertension

4. Male sex predominance
   (a) Only (1) and (2) and (3) are correct.
   (b) Only (2) and (3) and (4) are correct.
   (c) Only (3) and (4) are correct.
   (d) Only (4) is correct.
   (e) All are correct.
5. Which of the following statements is correct?
   1. Hypokalemia is found in approximately 28% of people with primary aldosteronism.
   2. The prevalence of cardiac and renal target-organ damage is increased in patients with PA compared to those with essential hypertension.
   3. Somatic driver mutations account for most aldosterone-producing adenomas
   4. False-positive case detection testing may be caused by mineralocorticoid receptor antagonists (e.g., spironolactone, eplerenone)
   (a) Only (1) and (2) and (3) are correct.
   (b) Only (2) and (3) and (4) are correct.
   (c) Only (3) and (4) are correct.
   (d) Only (4) is correct.
   (e) All are correct.
6. Which of the following statements is correct?
   1. Most aldosterone-producing adenomas are >1.5 cm in diameter.
   2. Normalization of BP is the primary goal in the treatment of primary aldosteronism.
   3. Following surgery for an aldosterone-producing adenoma, mineralocorticoid receptor antagonists (e.g., spironolactone, eplerenone) and potassium supplements should be discontinued.
   4. Unilateral adrenalectomy for aldosterone-producing adenoma is cost-effective
   (a) Only (1) and (2) and (3) are correct.
   (b) Only (2) and (3) and (4) are correct.
   (c) Only (3) and (4) are correct.
   (d) Only (4) is correct.
   (e) All are correct.

20.1 Introduction

Hypertension, increased adrenal aldosterone secretion, and suppressed renin characterize the syndrome of primary aldosteronism (PA), which was first described in 1955 [1]. Although estimates vary [2, 3], the prevalence of PA is 5–20% in people with stages 1 and 2 hypertension [3, 4] and up to 20–50% in patients with treatment-resistant hypertension [3, 5, 6]. The early diagnosis of PA leads to either the cure of hypertension or to targeted pharmacotherapy in order to prevent end stage PA, which includes progressive degrees of chronic kidney disease and cardiovascular damage [7].

20.2 Clinical Presentation

Hypertension in patients with PA is usually moderate to severe and may be resistant to usual pharmacologic treatments [3, 8, 9]. In general, patients with PA caused by unilateral aldosterone-producing adenoma (APA) have higher aldosterone levels and more marked hypertension than what is found in patients with bilateral idiopathic hyperplasia (IHA). Hypokalemia is found in only 28% of people with PA [10, 11]. Thus, all patients with hypertension are candidates for PA.

The prevalence of cardiac and renal target-organ damage is increased in patients with PA compared to those with essential hypertension [12–17]. The cardiovascular and nephrotoxicity in PA is an aldosterone-specific effect and, in part, independent of hypertension.

Several studies have documented the negative impact of PA on health-related quality of life (QoL) [18–23]. A prospective QoL study compared patients with PA who were managed surgically (n = 92) versus those managed medically (n = 92) [24]. QoL was assessed with 2 validated questionnaires at baseline, 6 months, and 1 year after surgery or initiation of medical therapy. QoL at baseline was statistically significantly lower in patients with PA compared with the general population, especially in women. After 1 year, almost all QoL measures had normalized for surgically managed patients, whereas, for patients on medical treatment, most QoL measures improved but not to the level of the general population [24].

20.3 Natural History

After Conn's initial description, PA was thought by most experts to be a rare cause of hypertension [25–31]. However, over time it has been shown that most patients with PA are not hypokalemic [8, 10, 32, 33] and that case detection testing can be completed without stopping antihypertensive medications [34]. Unlike other adrenal disorders (e.g., Cushing syndrome), there is no typical PA phenotype to guide the clinician for when to suspect PA.

The two most common subtypes of PA are unilateral APA and bilateral IHA (▶ Box 20.1) [7, 33]. A less common form of PA is unilateral hyperplasia, which is caused by micronodular or macronodular hyperplasia of the zona glomerulosa of predominantly one adrenal gland. Familial hyperaldosteronism (FH) is rare, and germline pathogenic variants in four different genes have been described [7].

A major advance in the past decade has been the discovery of the underlying pathophysiology of APAs [35, 36]. Somatic driver mutations likely account for nearly all APAs and include pathogenic variants in genes encoding components of

Box 20.1 Types of Primary Aldosteronism

Aldosterone-producing adenoma (APA)—30% of cases
Bilateral idiopathic hyperplasia (IHA)—60% of cases
Primary (unilateral) adrenal hyperplasia—2% of cases
Aldosterone-producing adrenocortical carcinoma—<1% of cases
Familial hyperaldosteronism (FH)
- FH type I (glucocorticoid-remediable aldosteronism caused by germline pathogenic variants of *CYP11B2*)—<1% of cases
- FH type II (germline *CLCN2* pathogenic variants)—<6% of cases
- FH type III (germline *KCNJ5* pathogenic variants)—<1% of cases
- FH type IV (germline *CACNA1H* pathogenic variants)—<0.1% of cases

Ectopic aldosterone-producing adenoma or adrenal carcinoma—<0.1% of cases

the Kir 3.4 (GIRK4) potassium channel (KCNJ5) [37]; the sodium/potassium and calcium ATPases (ATP1A1 and ATP2B3) [38]; and a voltage-dependent C-type calcium channel (CACNA1D) [39].

20.4 Diagnosis

The three diagnostic steps for PA include case detection testing; confirmatory testing; and subtype testing. Due to the high prevalence of PA, all people with hypertension are candidates for case detection testing [7].

Case Detection Testing Case detection testing is performed with a morning venipuncture for the measurement of plasma aldosterone concentration (PAC) and renin [7, 33, 34]. Renin can be measured with either plasma renin activity (PRA) with units of measurement in ng/mL/h or direct renin concentration (DRC) with units of measurement in mU/L. The conversion rate between PRA and DRC is approximately 1 ng/mL/h to 8.2 mU/L, respectively. A positive case detection test result is a PAC >10 ng/dL (>277 pmol/L) and PRA <1 ng/mL/h or DRC <8 mU/L. False-positive case detection testing is not a problem if a cutoff for PAC is used (e.g., >10 ng/dL, >277 pmol/L). Mineralocorticoid receptor antagonists (MRAs), angiotensin-converting enzyme (ACE) inhibitors, angiotensin receptor blockers (ARBs), and diuretics have the potential to elevate renin in patients with mild PA. Thus, the finding of PRA ≥1.0 ng/mL/h or DRC >8 mU/L in a patient treated with a MRA, ACE-inhibitor, ARB, or a diuretic does not exclude the diagnosis of PA. However, when renin is below those cutoffs in a patient treated with those four classes of antihypertensive drugs, it is diagnostic of low renin hypertension and possible PA. MRAs (e.g., spironolactone and eplerenone) prevent aldosterone from activating the receptor, resulting sequentially in sodium loss, a decrease in plasma volume, and an elevation in renin. If renin is not suppressed in a patient treated with a MRA, then no further PA-related testing can be performed and the MRA should be discontinued for 6 weeks before re-testing, whereas if renin is suppressed in a patient treated with a MRA, clinicians can proceed with case detection testing, confirmatory testing, and subtype testing with adrenal vein sampling (AVS) [40–42].

Confirmatory Testing The combination of a PAC >10 ng/dL (>277 pmol/L) and low renin is not diagnostic, and PA must be confirmed by demonstration of inappropriate aldosterone secretion [7, 33]. The exception to this rule is the clinical setting of spontaneous hypokalemia, PAC >20 ng/dL (>555 pmol/L), and suppressed renin—this presentation is diagnostic of PA [33]. All other patients should have PA confirmed by demonstration of aldosterone secretory autonomy with aldosterone suppression testing, which can be performed with orally administered sodium chloride and measurement of urinary aldosterone excretion or with intravenous sodium chloride loading and measurement of PAC [7, 8, 43].

Subtype Testing The final step in the diagnosis of PA is subtype testing, which determines whether the source of aldosterone excess is from the right, left, or both adrenal glands. When localized to one adrenal gland, unilateral adrenalectomy results in (a) normalization of hypokalemia in all patients; and (b) hypertension is improved in all patients and is cured in 30–60% [44–49]. In patients with bilateral adrenal aldosterone hypersecretion (IHA and most patients with familial forms of PA), unilateral adrenalectomy debulks the disease, but does not cure the excess aldosterone secretion [9]. Thus, most patients with IHA and those with familial forms of PA should be treated medically. When PA is caused by an aldosterone-producing adrenal carcinoma, it is usually characterized by severe hypokalemia, marked hypertension, and a unilateral adrenal mass larger than 4 cm in diameter with an unenhanced CT attenuation >20 Hounsfield units (HU) [50].

In order to exclude adrenal cancer, adrenal-directed CT scan should be the first test in the subtype evaluation of PA. However, because of the age-related prevalence of nonfunctioning adrenocortical nodules [51], the reliability of CT in localizing APAs declines with patient age (e.g., >35 years of age). If the patient wants to pursue the surgical option, a subtype test more accurate than adrenal CT is required. APAs are usually small adrenal nodules (mean diameter 1.6 cm and <1.0 cm in 16.5% of patients) [49] with low unenhanced CT attenuation (<10 HU). The adrenal glands in patients with IHA may be normal on CT, may show thickening or nodular changes, or may show incidental nonfunctioning adrenal cortical nodules. Thus, adrenal CT is not accurate in distinguishing between APA and IHA [45, 49, 52, 53]. In patients seeking a surgical cure of PA, adrenal venous sampling (AVS) is an essential step.

AVS is the criterion standard test to distinguish unilateral from bilateral disease in patients with PA [32, 33, 45, 49, 52–54]. AVS is a technically demanding procedure because the right adrenal vein is small and may be difficult to locate and cannulate; the success rate depends on the expertise and degree of engagement of the interventional radiologist [55, 56]. The 5 keys to a successful AVS program include (1) appropriate patient selection; (2) careful patient preparation; (3) focused technical expertise; (4) a defined written protocol; and (5) accurate data interpretation [55]. The cortisol concentrations from the adrenal veins and inferior vena cava (IVC) are used to confirm successful catheterization. With cosyntropin-stimulated AVS, a minimal adrenal vein-to-IVC cortisol gradient is ≥5:1. The details on interpretation of AVS data can be found elsewhere [45, 49, 57–61]. As of this writing, there are no reliable noninvasive alternatives to AVS.

APAs can co-secrete cortisol that may be clinically important for perioperative management [62, 63]. Clinically important cortisol secretion from an adrenal adenoma is correlated with tumor size. Unlike aldosterone secretion from an adenoma, clinically important cortisol secretion requires a "large factory"—typically with adenoma diameters >2 cm [63]. Thus, it is reasonable to test patients with PA for cortisol co-secretion when the adrenal adenoma is >1.5 cm in diameter. Such testing includes baseline measurement of serum dehydroepiandrosterone sulfate and an overnight 1-mg dexamethasone suppression test [64]. Other tests that are used for case detection of clinical Cushing syndrome (e.g., 24-h urinary-free cortisol and midnight salivary cortisol) are not good screening tests for subclinical glucocorticoid secretory autonomy. When glucocorticoid secretory autonomy is documented in a patient with PA who has a single cortical adenoma >1.5 cm in diameter, one can argue that AVS is not needed. Clinicians do not have a good long-term medical management option for Cushing syndrome, whereas PA can be treated effectively with MRAs.

20.5 Treatment

The cause of PA directs the treatment plan. Normalization of blood pressure (BP) is not the only goal. Excessive autonomous secretion of aldosterone is associated with an increased risk of cardiovascular disease and morbidity. Thus, either curative surgery or effective MR blockade should be part of the management plan for all patients with PA. As noted above, the beneficial effects of surgical treatment are greater than for treatment with MRAs [24]. Thus, surgical management is the optimal treatment approach for those patients with unilateral adrenal disease, whereas, in patients with PA caused by bilateral adrenal disease, bilateral adrenalectomy is not a good treatment option due to the resultant primary adrenal insufficiency and need for lifelong glucocorticoid and mineralocorticoid replacement. Unilateral adrenalectomy for APA is cost-effective [65] and is significantly less expensive than long-term medical therapy [66].

20.5.1 Pharmacologic Treatment

Medical management with MRAs is the treatment of choice for patients with bilateral adrenal disease. When a longitudinal study assessing 602 patients with PA treated with MRAs were matched with 41,853 pts with essential hypertension—both with comparable cardiovascular risk profiles and BP control—the incidence of cardiovascular events was higher in patients with PA treated with MRAs than in patients with essential hypertension [15]. The excess risk for cardiovascular events and mortality was limited to patients with PA who had suppressed PRA on medical treatment—suggesting inadequate dosing of MRAs [15]. Thus, if medical management is to be pursued, it is key that the MRA dosage is adequate to fully block the toxic effects of hyperaldosteronism. Due to concomitant low renin essential hypertension in some patients with PA, measurement of renin may not be optimal to guide management; but rather, a more practical treatment target to document effective MRA dosages is a high-normal serum potassium (e.g., ≈4.5 mEq/L) without the aid of oral potassium supplements.

20.6 Indications for Surgery and Surgical Details

The common surgical treatment for PA is unilateral adrenalectomy. Which adrenal to be removed is usually guided by AVS. The histopathological reason behind the lateralization may be an adenoma but also as asymmetrical hyperplasia indicating excess aldosterone secretion on one side [67]. Very rarely, bilateral adrenalectomy may be indicated, usually in familial cases.

Preoperative management includes maintaining normokalemia to avoid perioperative morbidity. Since the affected adrenal to be removed usually is small, laparoscopic or retroperitoneoscopic approaches are the methods of choice. Open adrenalectomy is no longer used for PA, unless there are very special circumstances such as previous surgery in the area or an associated other surgical procedure to be performed simultaneously [68, 69]. Of course, in the rare event of an aldosterone-producing presumed adrenocortical cancer, an open procedure should be considered [70]. The advantages for laparoscopic (or retroperitoneoscopic) adrenalectomy include less blood loss, shorter operating time, less need of analgesics, earlier recovery, and, of course, smaller wound with less hernia complications. There seems to be a slight advantage for retroperitoneal adrenalectomy, at least for the smallest tumors, but in reality it is more up to the surgeon's own preferences [71]. Both approaches can be performed as a normal endoscopic procedure or using a robot [72]. Some authors suggest that in certain cases, partial adrenalectomy may be as successful as total adrenalectomy, although long-term follow-up studies are needed [73].

20.6.1 Adrenalectomy by the Laparoscopic Transabdominal Approach

The anatomy in this approach is familiar to general surgeons who are used to intraabdominal explorations (Fig. 20.2). The patient is placed in the lateral decubitus position, which provides the best exposure to the adrenal glands since gravity helps retraction of the liver on the right and the spleen on the left. Usually three trocars are inserted below the rib margin with enough distance apart in order to get good access from a wide angle (Fig. 20.3). A fourth trocar may be inserted for an additional grasper. CO_2 is added to a pressure of 12 mmHg, and the 30 degree camera is usually inserted in the middle tro-

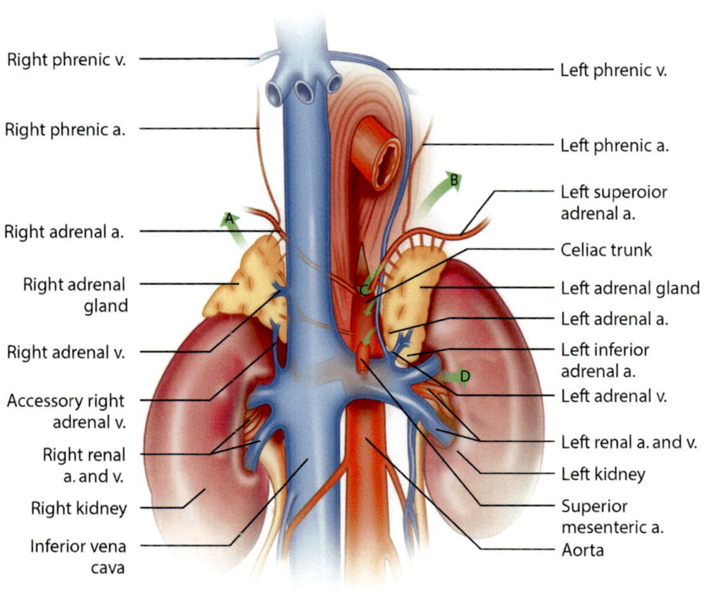

Fig. 20.2 Anatomic relationships of the adrenal glands

a

b

c

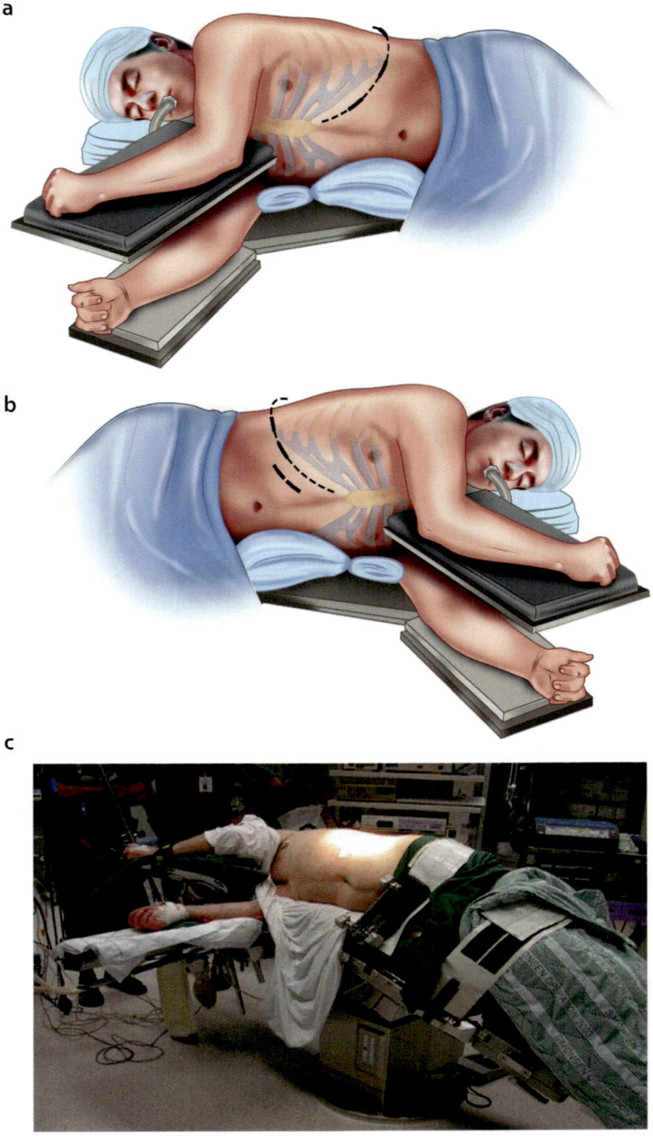

Fig. 20.3 Panel **a** and **b**, Demonstration of the lateral decubitus positioning for laparoscopic let (**a**) and right (**b**) adrenalectomy. Panel **c**, Photograph from the operating room showing the patient in lateral decubitus position in preparation for laparoscopic left adrenalectomy

car, but should of course be switched to another site if the visualization is not optimal.

For laparoscopic right adrenalectomy, the procedure continues by opening the peritoneum on the lateral and inferior side, just below the liver margin which may have to be somewhat mobilized and lifted, up to the inferior vena cava (IVC). The liver helps with its weight to open up the space where the adrenal lies. After opening the posterior peritoneum, dissection of the inferior border of the adrenal follows, separating it from the perirenal fascia. One should be cautions to avoid injury to a sometimes present arterial branch to the upper renal pole, which if accidentally injured may bleed and after securing it cause an upper pole renal infarction. Sometimes the right renal vein is also lying close in this field and should be identified and avoided. The adrenal vein and possible accessory veins drain into the IVC and can be cautiously dealt with using any of the ligating instruments such as the Ligasure or Harmonic scalpel. Ideally the device is inserted in the median trocar, since this enables the device to be inserted strictly parallel to IVC. Normally, there are no clips needed to secure the vein, unless an unusually large adrenal vein appears. The upper pole of the adrenal may be troublesome since it may proceed behind the IVC from this angle, but cautious and meticulous dissection usually mobilizes this part. Dissection is preferably performed with one of the ligating devices, also securing small arterial branches (usually many and very small). The adrenal gland is placed in a bag and extracted through one of the ports.

On the left, three trocars are inserted as on the right side, and the dissection is initially performed between the spleen and the kidney, where the posterior peritoneum is opened. The two organs separate from each other and an "open book" is created, where gravity retracts the spleen with associated pancreatic tail medially. The adrenal gland is then always found on the renal side in this cleft and can be dissected from the renal fat. On the left side, the adrenal vein drains into the renal vein and can be dealt with in a similar fashion as on the right side. The adrenal vein is much longer on the left side compared to the right and rarely misinterpreted as the left renal vein. However, if the apparent adrenal vein seems unusually large, further dissection to identify the renal vein should be performed. It may be wise not to detach the adrenal gland fully from the renal fat before securing the vein, since the gland may fall into the cleft making the dissection of the vein more troublesome. On the left side, an inferior phrenic vein can be seen medial to the adrenal and may be sharing the same drainage as the adrenal vein. This vein can be safely divided if necessary. Also here, caution should be taken to not divide any suprarenal artery, which may lead to devascularization of the upper pole of the kidney.

20.6.2 Adrenalectomy with the Retroperitoneoscopic Approach

The technique, initially described in 1995 and later refined, has probably become more popular nowadays than the laparoscopic approach [74–76]. The patient is placed in a prone, jackknife position with as close to a 90° angle as possible at the hip joints and the knees. This opens up the space between the infe-

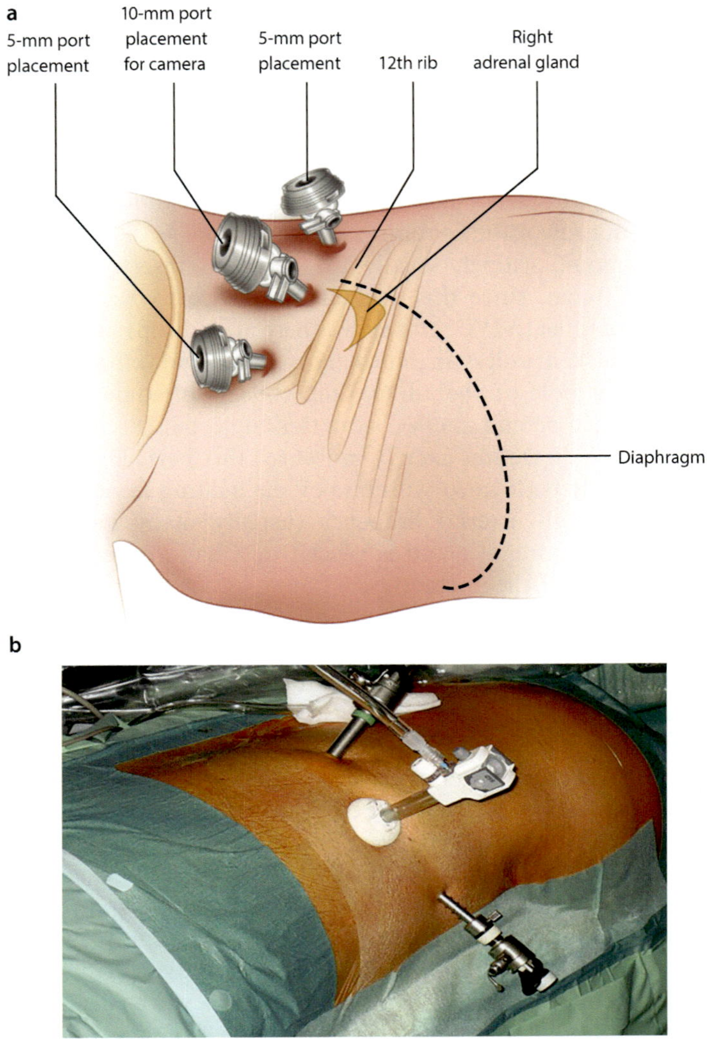

Fig. 20.4 *Panel* ***a*** depicts trocar placement for the retroperitoneoscopic approach to right adrenalectomy. *Panel* ***b***, intraoperative photograph showing trocar placement for the retroperitoneoscopic approach

rior costal margin/12th rib and the iliac crest. In short patients and in the case of high BMI, this is crucial, to really separate these bony parts from each other in order to get enough access. Three trocars are inserted (Fig. 20.4). Usually the middle one is inserted first, slightly below the 12th rib, which should be palpated and indicated with black ink. The intercostal vessels and nerve run below the 12th rib and to avoid damage to these it is suggested to go close to the rib upon insertion of the trocar. Nevertheless, some patients complain of symptoms related to nerve injury afterwards (see below). The distance from the skin to the retroperitoneal space is rather long at this position. There is a distinct "loss-of-resistance" feeling while perforating the retroperitoneal fascia and entering the proper space. This is done with a pair of Mayo scissors, followed by blunt dissection

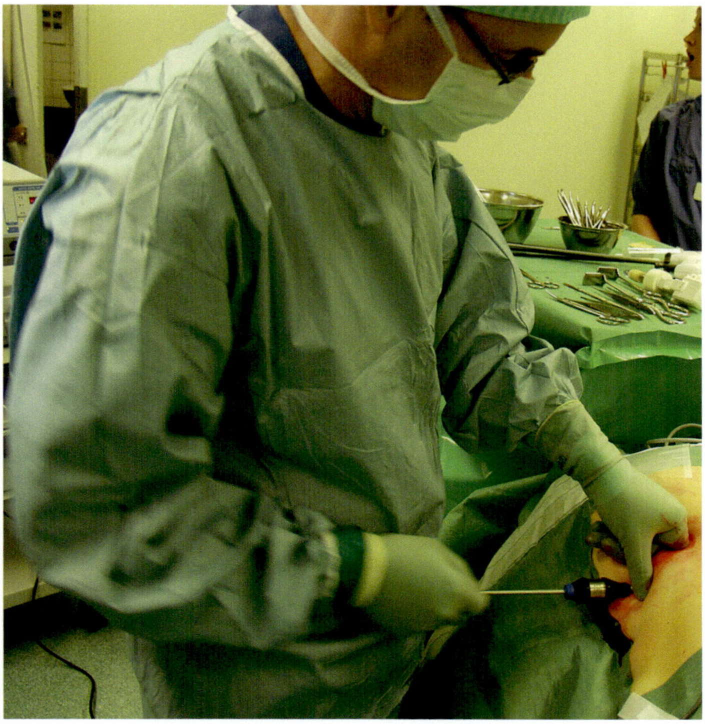

Fig. 20.5 Intraoperative photograph demonstrating lateral trocar insertion during the retroperitoneoscopic approach to adrenalectomy

of the retroperitoneal fat by the tip of the index finger, creating a small space. With a finger in this space the other two trocars are inserted, one medially and one laterally (see Fig. 20.4, Panel b). It is important to get an enough spread between these to enable easy dissection later. The lateral one can preferably be inserted rather low on the side of the patient. It is important to insert this bimanually with the index finger in space in order to direct the trocar into the created space, not to injure the lateral large bowel and to not enter into another retroperitoneal plane (Fig. 20.5). After insertion of the three trocars, high CO_2 pressure is added, up to 25 mmHg, and blunt dissection using a dissector performed in the initially small retroperitoneal space, which now opens up.

Identification of the kidney surface and the paraspinous muscles follows, which is important for anatomical orientation (Fig. 20.6). On the right side the posterior surface of the liver is visible through the peritoneum at the top of the space. The retroperitoneal fat is mobilized downward, and the angle where the right adrenal lies appears below the liver surface and medially. Traction of the upper pole of the kidney will visualize the IVC, and a following careful dissection along it will expose the adrenal vein. One may, before this part of the dissection, remove the adrenal gland from its attachments laterally and towards the retroperitoneum overlying the liver, but it is wise to leave some

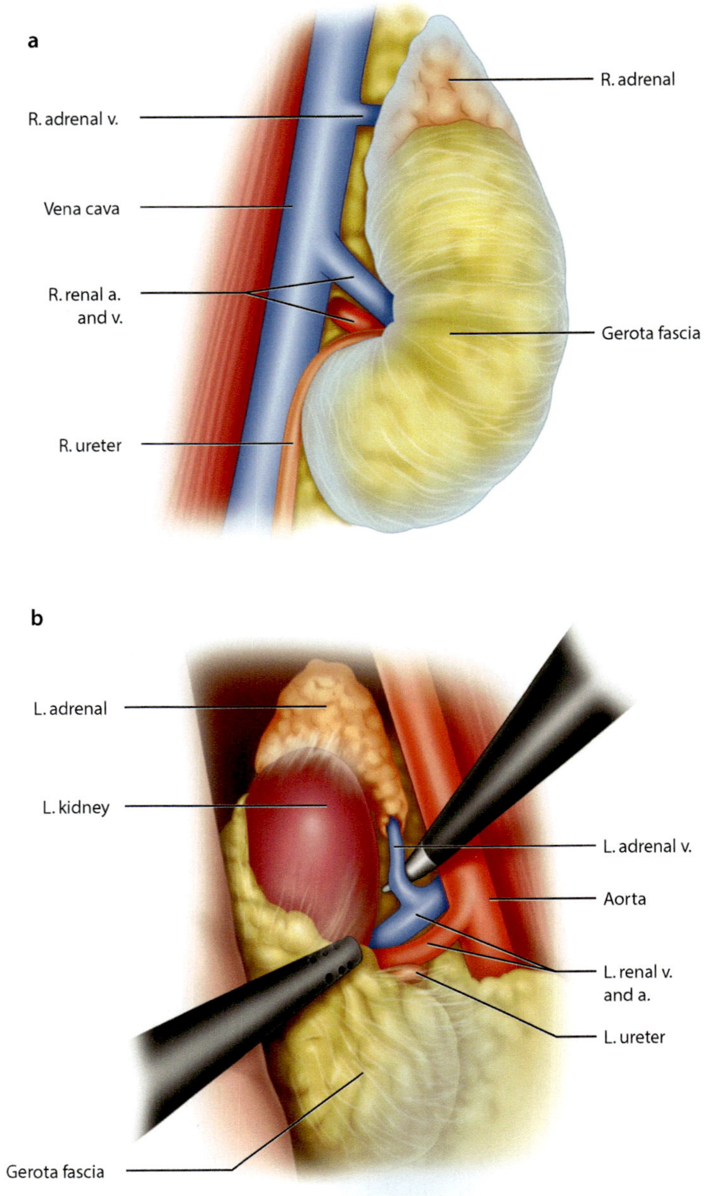

Fig. 20.6 (**a**) Right kidney and adrenal gland from a posterior view. The right adrenal vein branches directly from the inferior caval vein. (**b**) Left kidney from a posterior view. The left adrenal vein branches off the left renal vein

attachments here in order to not allow the adrenal to fall down into the operating field, making dissection of the adrenal vein more complicated. The adrenal vein is divided as in the laparoscopic approach with a device, and rarely a clip is needed.

On the left side, the procedure continues by mobilizing some of the retroperitoneal fat downwards, but leaving the most medial attachments. Downward and lateral traction of the upper pole of the kidney opens up the space where the adrenal vein is situated. This vein can on the left side usually be found rather early in the dissection, and very often in association with the phrenic vein. Renal upper pole arterial branches may be seen on both sides, but the left side is more easily injured. Sometimes one shank of the left adrenal gland lies anteriorly, just superior to the renal vessels, which may be somewhat difficult to mobilize.

Advantages with the retroperitoneal approach over the laparoscopic include less postoperative pain, no bowel paralysis, and avoidance of adhesions from previous abdominal surgery. Disadvantages of this approach may be the limitations in creating enough space in morbidly obese patients (BMI >45 kg/m^2) and CO_2 retention in patients with severe chronic obstructive pulmonary disease (COPD) [71, 72].

All the above described methods may be performed using a robot, but it is still debated whether there is any cost-benefit when compared to regular minimally invasive procedures.

20.6.3 Complications

Complications are uncommon and occur in less than 1% of patients. With the laparoscopic approach, they include intra- or postoperative bleeding, port-site infection, and incisional hernia. On the right side, injury to the IVC may occur but can usually be dealt with by suturing the defect laparoscopically after adding clamps on either side of the defect. On the left side, there may be splenic injury and bleeding, usually managed conservatively with compression. Rarely, injury to the pancreatic tail occurs on the left side, but reports of development of pancreatitis or pancreatic cysts are extremely rare.

With the retroperitoneoscopic approach, an injury to the IVC may be more complicated, due to the smaller space of the operating field. Also, conversion to an open procedure is difficult and will not gain much more exposure to the area. However, the high CO_2 pressure may keep the IVC blood in situ, and the defect may be sutured or compressed with additional glue. Generally, retroperitoneoscopic surgery bleeds less due to the up to 25 mmHg CO_2. Therefore, it is important before finishing the procedure to turn off the insufflation while removing the gland, followed by a final visualization of possible bleeding that may appear by lowering the pressure.

Injury to the 12th intercostal artery or vein may be obvious after retraction of the trocars or during the postoperative care period. Rarely, in an arterial injury, this may be handled by embolization, although most of the time the bleeding is self-limited due to achieved counter-pressure.

Pneumothorax may rarely occur due to perforation of the pleura during the dissection in the retroperitoneal space. The high CO_2 pressure will push gas into this space, which postoperatively may be seen as subcutaneous emphysema. The anesthesiology staff may comment during the surgical procedure due to lowered return amounts of CO_2, thus indicating CO_2 retention during dissection [77]. This is most often handled by increasing the ventilation, but very rarely the surgeon will have to stop, desufflate the retroperitoneal space and wait for a short while before continuing the operation. In patients with COPD, this may be especially evident. Most of the time, this is not due to iatrogenic pneumothorax.

Approximately 8% of patients will experience hypoesthesia and/or abdominal wall laxity, after a retroperitoneoscopic procedure. However, these may be temporary findings.

There seems to be similar complication rates between robotic and regular minimally invasive adrenalectomies [78].

20.6.4 Postoperative Care (Correction of Potassium and Antihypertensive Medications)

The postoperative care routinely involves proper pain control, early ambulation, and early onset of general diet. Patients undergoing the posterior approach may generally be discharged earlier than patients undergoing the lateral approach. At some centers, day surgery (23 h) is performed.

Spironolactone and eplerenone should be discontinued and potassium levels checked the morning after surgery. PAC may be measured the morning after the operation to confirm a biochemical cure [49]. Following surgery, for most patients, potassium supplements should be discontinued. In general, the number and dosages of antihypertensive medications can be reduced by 50% postoperatively. Any medications that may contribute to hyperkalemia (e.g., ACE-I, ARBs) should be discontinued. The proportion of hypertension that was associated with aldosterone excess resolves in 1–3 months after the surgery. Postoperatively, there is a risk of short-term hypoaldosteronism leading to clinically important hyperkalemia [79–81]. In a multicenter study of 142 surgically treated patients, the prevalence of postoperative hyperkalemia was 9.9%; the hyperkalemic patients were older and had worse renal function than the non-hyperkalemic patient group [82]. In a study of 192 patients with PA who were treated surgically, 12 (6.3%) developed postoperative hyperkalemia (median serum potassium 5.5 mmol/L, range 5.2–6.2 mmol/L); median time to onset was 13.5 days (range, 7–55 days) [81]. Thus, it is reasonable to monitor serum potassium weekly for 4 weeks after surgery, and a generous sodium diet should be followed to avoid the hyperkalemia of hypoaldosteronism. Short-term fludrocortisone supplementation may be required if the serum potassium concentration rises above 5.2 mEq/L. In some exceptional cases, long-term mineralocorticoid replacement may be needed.

20.7 Outcomes and Prognosis

20.7.1 Histopathology

Although an adenoma is anticipated while performing surgery, it is not unusual that the histopathological report states presence of hyperplasia, together with nodules – sometimes referred to as nodular hyperplasia. Whether this is a sign of one small APA developing in such an environment, presence of multiple aldosterone-producing small nodules or a more diffuse hyperplasia in a gland with visible nodules (non-aldosterone-producing) may be debated [83, 84]. The follow-up will reveal if the remaining adrenal gland has excess aldosterone production [84–86]. Indeed, recent findings, for instance, the aldosterone-producing cell clusters, may clarify the underlying disorder [87].

In the series by Weisbrod et al. [83], 95 patients underwent adrenalectomy for lateralized aldosterone secretion based on AVS. Of these, 66 patients had an aldosterone-producing cortical adenoma, and 14 patients demonstrated an aldosterone-producing adenoma with diffuse adrenal hyperplasia. Histopathology of the remaining 15 patients showed diffuse cortical hyperplasia without evidence of a cortical adenoma. For these 15 patients, the diagnosis manifested as multinodular hyperplasia in 10 patients and non-nodular hyperplasia in 5 patients. Interestingly, there was no significant difference between these groups in terms of age at diagnosis, gender distribution, BMI, duration of hypertension, number of preoperative antihypertensive medications, or levels of preoperative aldosterone or renin. Additionally, there was no significant difference in the clinical and laboratory features associated with patient outcome by histologic groups. These results shed light on the discussion of indication for surgery in PA.

20.7.2 Potassium and Hypertension

In general, the outcomes for hypertension, polypharmacy, and hypokalemia are excellent following adrenalectomy [88]. Normalization of potassium levels is achieved in close to 100% of patients [84–86, 88]. There is some evidence for contralateral suppression in a fraction of PA patients, and some authors propose an ACTH-stimulation test after unilateral adrenalectomy [89, 90].

Hypertension may be cured in between 30% and 60% of cases as reported by different authors [84–86]. A large proportion of patients show improved control of hypertension, but still need of antihypertensive medication to achieve normotension [84–86, 91]. Adrenalectomy has positive effects on carotid intima-media thickness and arterial stiffness in one study [92]. A small proportion of patients do not achieve any hypertensive control at all, indicating an incorrect diagnosis, failed lateralization of the AVS, or the effect of long-standing hypertension leading to advanced atherosclerosis which is not reversible by adrenalectomy. Indeed, factors associated with postoperative hypertension are age, family history, and high serum creatinine levels [44, 93, 94]. High aldosterone level itself has a vascular remodeling effect independent of hypertension and may impair both cardiac and renal functions. Adrenalectomy may reduce left ventricular hypertrophy [91]. When investigating a Norwegian population, tumors with *KCNJ5* pathogenic variants were correlated with better postoperative BP control [95].

20.7.3 Long-Term Prognosis of Cardiovascular Disease and Mortality

The effect in the long term is obvious in cases where cure is achieved—mostly in the younger patients and in those with short preoperative duration of hypertension. The longer exposure to high aldosterone levels, the more risk of secondary adverse effects in other organs. Thus, aldosterone has been found to have profound effects not only on hypertension but also directly causing vascular damage, myocardial dysfunction also in the absence of PA, but possibly being aggravated by the presence of PA. Blocking aldosterone has been suggested as one method of reducing the risk of cardiovascular disease, and the common medical (spironolactone and eplerenone) and surgical methods are presumably effective in decreasing the risk of cardiovascular disease on a long-term basis. Cardiovascular mortality is the main cause of death in PA (50% versus 34% in hypertensive controls) [96]. Another study demonstrated a significantly higher incidence of cerebral hemorrhage in patients with APA compared to patients with essential hypertension [97]. A number of other studies support these findings. Treatment of PA has been found to improve the cardiovascular outcome [98]. Some studies have noted a reduced left ventricular mass index especially after adrenalectomy [99, 100]. The risk for stroke is lower after adrenalectomy in patients with PA [101].

However, much is still unknown regarding long-term prognosis. At least a partial reversible risk for cardiovascular disease in PA seems to be clear, but whether adrenalectomy or MR blockade are equal in all situations may be debated. One meta-analysis stated that MR blockade and adrenalectomy were similar regarding reduction of left ventricular mass [102].

In a recent meta-analysis, 3039 patients with PA were compared to 45,495 patients with essential hypertension and found a higher risk for death after 3 years of observation for PA patients (RR 1.97;1.33–2.91, $P = 0.0007$); but the situation reversed after 3 years and up to 10 years—an observation interpreted as showing that following treatment for PA there is more morbidity than that found in patients with essential hypertension [103].

20.7.4 Renal Function After Surgery

Most patients with long-standing PA have some degree of renal insufficiency that is masked by the glomerular hyperfiltration associated with aldosterone excess and hypertension [104–106]. Approximately 40% of patients with PA show a clinically important decrease in renal function after surgery [107]. Glomerular hyperfiltration preoperatively masks mild to moderate underlying renal failure. In one study, the average decrease in estimated glomerular filtration rate (eGFR) was 19.7% [108]. Effective treatment of PA with either surgery or a MRA will unmask the underlying chronic kidney disease.

In conclusion, AVS-lateralized hyperaldosteronism offers patients a significant chance of cure or at least better BP control by having an adrenalectomy performed on the lateralized side. This should be done by either a laparoscopic or a retroperitoneal approach, based on the surgeon's experience and preference. The outcomes are excellent with potassium supplementation discontinued in nearly 100%, improved BP in 50–70%, and fully cured in 30–50% of patients. The probability of hypertension cure is better the younger the patient and the shorter duration of hypertension at the time of surgery. On the basis of available data, partial adrenalectomy is not recommended for APAs since there is often a background of nodular or diffuse hyperplasia on closer examination. Long-term effects after treatment of PA are positive regarding cardiovascular events and morbidity.

Key Points

- Except in the young patient (<35 yrs) with a unilateral macroadenoma (>1 cm), the findings on abdominal CT scan cannot be trusted to determine laterality of hyperaldosteronism.
- Many patients with PA have more than one nodule in the resected adrenal gland, and it is not possible to intraoperatively determine which nodule is hypersecreting aldosterone. Total adrenalectomy should be used to treat PA.

Answers to the Questions

1. (c); 2. (a); 3. (d); 4. (a); 5. (a); 6. (c)

References

1. Conn JW. Presidential address. I. Painting background. II. Primary aldosteronism, a new clinical syndrome. J Lab Clin Med. 1955;45(1): 3–17.
2. Kayser SC, Dekkers T, Groenewoud HJ, van der Wilt GJ, Carel Bakx J, van der Wel MC, et al. Study heterogeneity and estimation of prevalence of primary aldosteronism: a systematic review and meta-regression analysis. J Clin Endocrinol Metab. 2016;101(7):2826–35.
3. Brown JM, Siddiqui M, Calhoun DA, Carey RM, Hopkins PN, Williams GH, et al. The unrecognized prevalence of primary aldosteronism: a cross-sectional study. Ann Intern Med. 2020;173(1):10–20.
4. Hannemann A, Wallaschofski H. Prevalence of primary aldosteronism in patient's cohorts and in population-based studies–a review of the current literature. Horm Metab Res. 2012;44(3):157–62.
5. Douma S, Petidis K, Doumas M, Papaefthimiou P, Triantafyllou A, Kartali N, et al. Prevalence of primary hyperaldosteronism in resistant hypertension: a retrospective observational study. Lancet. 2008;371(9628):1921–6.
6. Calhoun DA, Nishizaka MK, Zaman MA, Thakkar RB, Weissmann P. Hyperaldosteronism among black and white subjects with resistant hypertension. Hypertension. 2002;40(6):892–6.
7. Young WF Jr. Diagnosis and treatment of primary aldosteronism: practical clinical perspectives. J Intern Med. 2019;285(2):126–48.
8. Young WF. Primary aldosteronism: renaissance of a syndrome. Clin Endocrinol. 2007;66(5):607–18.
9. Young WF Jr, Klee GG. Primary aldosteronism. Diagnostic evaluation. Endocrinol Metab Clin N Am. 1988;17(2):367–95.
10. Mulatero P, Stowasser M, Loh KC, Fardella CE, Gordon RD, Mosso L, et al. Increased diagnosis of primary aldosteronism, including surgically correctable forms, in centers from five continents. J Clin Endocrinol Metab. 2004;89(3):1045–50.
11. Monticone S, Burrello J, Tizzani D, Bertello C, Viola A, Buffolo F, et al. Prevalence and clinical manifestations of primary aldosteronism encountered in primary care practice. J Am Coll Cardiol. 2017;69(14):1811–20.
12. Stowasser M, Sharman J, Leano R, Gordon RD, Ward G, Cowley D, et al. Evidence for abnormal left ventricular structure and function in normotensive individuals with familial hyperaldosteronism type I. J Clin Endocrinol Metab. 2005;90(9):5070–6.
13. Milliez P, Girerd X, Plouin PF, Blacher J, Safar ME, Mourad JJ. Evidence for an increased rate of cardiovascular events in patients with primary aldosteronism. J Am Coll Cardiol. 2005;45(8):1243–8.
14. Monticone S, D'Ascenzo F, Moretti C, Williams TA, Veglio F, Gaita F, et al. Cardiovascular events and target organ damage in primary aldosteronism compared with essential hypertension: a systematic review and meta-analysis. Lancet Diabetes Endocrinol. 2018;6(1):41–50.
15. Hundemer GL, Curhan GC, Yozamp N, Wang M, Vaidya A. Cardiometabolic outcomes and mortality in medically treated primary aldosteronism: a retrospective cohort study. Lancet Diabetes Endocrinol. 2018;6(1):51–9.
16. Hundemer GL, Curhan GC, Yozamp N, Wang M, Vaidya A. Renal outcomes in medically and surgically treated primary aldosteronism. Hypertension. 2018;72(3):658–66.

17. Iwakura Y, Morimoto R, Kudo M, Ono Y, Takase K, Seiji K, et al. Predictors of decreasing glomerular filtration rate and prevalence of chronic kidney disease after treatment of primary aldosteronism: renal outcome of 213 cases. J Clin Endocrinol Metab. 2014;99(5):1593–8.
18. Sukor N, Kogovsek C, Gordon RD, Robson D, Stowasser M. Improved quality of life, blood pressure, and biochemical status following laparoscopic adrenalectomy for unilateral primary aldosteronism. J Clin Endocrinol Metab. 2010;95(3):1360–4.
19. Sonino N, Fallo F, Fava GA. Psychological aspects of primary aldosteronism. Psychother Psychosom. 2006;75(5):327–30.
20. Sonino N, Tomba E, Genesia ML, Bertello C, Mulatero P, Veglio F, et al. Psychological assessment of primary aldosteronism: a controlled study. J Clin Endocrinol Metab. 2011;96(6):E878–83.
21. Apostolopoulou K, Kunzel HE, Gerum S, Merkle K, Schulz S, Fischer E, et al. Gender differences in anxiety and depressive symptoms in patients with primary hyperaldosteronism: a cross-sectional study. World J Biol Psychiatry. 2014;15(1):26–35.
22. Kunzel HE, Apostolopoulou K, Pallauf A, Gerum S, Merkle K, Schulz S, et al. Quality of life in patients with primary aldosteronism: gender differences in untreated and long-term treated patients and associations with treatment and aldosterone. J Psychiatr Res. 2012;46(12):1650–4.
23. Velema MS, de Nooijer AH, Burgers VWG, Hermus A, Timmers H, Lenders JWM, et al. Health-related quality of life and mental health in primary aldosteronism: a systematic review. Horm Metab Res. 2017;49(12):943–50.
24. Velema M, Dekkers T, Hermus A, Timmers H, Lenders J, Groenewoud H, et al. Quality of life in primary aldosteronism: a comparative effectiveness study of adrenalectomy and medical treatment. J Clin Endocrinol Metab. 2018;103(1):16–24.
25. Fishman LM, Kuchel O, Liddle GW, Michelakis AM, Gordon RD, Chick WT. Incidence of primary aldosteronism uncomplicated "essential" hypertension. A prospective study with elevated aldosterone secretion and suppressed plasma renin activity used as diagnostic criteria. JAMA. 1968;205(7):497–502.
26. Kaplan NM. Hypokalemia in the hypertensive patient, with observations on the incidence of primary aldosteronism. Ann Intern Med. 1967;66(6):1079–90.
27. Andersen GS, Toftdahl DB, Lund JO, Strandgaard S, Nielsen PE. The incidence rate of phaeochromocytoma and Conn's syndrome in Denmark, 1977–1981. J Hum Hypertens. 1988;2(3):187–9.
28. Berglund G, Andersson O, Wilhelmsen L. Prevalence of primary and secondary hypertension: studies in a random population sample. Br Med J. 1976;2(6035):554–6.
29. Streeten DH, Tomycz N, Anderson GH. Reliability of screening methods for the diagnosis of primary aldosteronism. Am J Med. 1979;67(3):403–13.
30. Tucker RM, Labarthe DR. Frequency of surgical treatment for hypertension in adults at the Mayo Clinic from 1973 through 1975. Mayo Clin Proc. 1977;52(9):549–5.
31. Sinclair AM, Isles CG, Brown I, Cameron H, Murray GD, Robertson JW. Secondary hypertension in a blood pressure clinic. Arch Intern Med. 1987;147(7):1289–93.
32. Stowasser M. Update in primary aldosteronism. J Clin Endocrinol Metab. 2015;100(1):1–10.
33. Funder JW, Carey RM, Mantero F, Murad MH, Reincke M, Shibata H, et al. The management of primary aldosteronism: case detection, diagnosis, and treatment: an endocrine society clinical practice guideline. J Clin Endocrinol Metab. 2016;93(9):jc20154061.
34. Hiramatsu K, Yamada T, Yukimura Y, Komiya I, Ichikawa K, Ishihara M, et al. A screening test to identify aldosterone-producing adenoma by

measuring plasma renin activity. Results in hypertensive patients. Arch Intern Med. 1981;141(12):1589–93.
35. Funder JW. Genetics of primary aldosteronism. Front Horm Res. 2014;43:70–8.
36. Akerstrom T, Carling T, Beuschlein F, Hellman P. Genetics of adrenocortical tumours. J Intern Med. 2016;280(6):540–50.
37. Scholl UI, Nelson-Williams C, Yue P, Grekin R, Wyatt RJ, Dillon MJ, et al. Hypertension with or without adrenal hyperplasia due to different inherited mutations in the potassium channel KCNJ5. Proc Natl Acad Sci U S A. 2012;109(7):2533–8.
38. Beuschlein F, Boulkroun S, Osswald A, Wieland T, Nielsen HN, Lichtenauer UD, et al. Somatic mutations in ATP1A1 and ATP2B3 lead to aldosterone-producing adenomas and secondary hypertension. Nat Genet. 2013;45(4):440–4, 4e1–2.
39. Scholl UI, Goh G, Stolting G, de Oliveira RC, Choi M, Overton JD, et al. Somatic and germline CACNA1D calcium channel mutations in aldosterone-producing adenomas and primary aldosteronism. Nat Genet. 2013;45(9):1050–4.
40. Haase M, Riester A, Kropil P, Hahner S, Degenhart C, Willenberg HS, et al. Outcome of adrenal vein sampling performed during concurrent mineralocorticoid receptor antagonist therapy. J Clin Endocrinol Metab. 2014;99(12):4397–402.
41. Nanba AT, Wannachalee T, Shields JJ, Byrd JB, Rainey WE, Auchus RJ, et al. Adrenal vein sampling lateralization despite mineralocorticoid receptor antagonists exposure in primary aldosteronism. J Clin Endocrinol Metab. 2019;104(2):487–92.
42. Nagasawa M, Yamamoto K, Rakugi H, Takeda M, Akasaka H, Umakoshi H, et al. Influence of antihypertensive drugs in the subtype diagnosis of primary aldosteronism by adrenal venous sampling. J Hypertens. 2019;37(7):1493–9.
43. Funder JW, Carey RM, Fardella C, Gomez-Sanchez CE, Mantero F, Stowasser M, et al. Case detection, diagnosis, and treatment of patients with primary aldosteronism: an endocrine society clinical practice guideline. J Clin Endocrinol Metab. 2008;93(9):3266–81.
44. Sawka AM, Young WF, Thompson GB, Grant CS, Farley DR, Leibson C, et al. Primary aldosteronism: factors associated with normalization of blood pressure after surgery. Ann Intern Med. 2001;135(4):258–61.
45. Young WF, Stanson AW, Thompson GB, Grant CS, Farley DR, van Heerden JA. Role for adrenal venous sampling in primary aldosteronism. Surgery. 2004;136(6):1227–35.
46. Citton M, Viel G, Rossi GP, Mantero F, Nitti D, Iacobone M. Outcome of surgical treatment of primary aldosteronism. Langenbeck's Arch Surg. 2015;400(3):325–31.
47. Wachtel H, Cerullo I, Bartlett EK, Kelz RR, Cohen DL, Karakousis GC, et al. Long-term blood pressure control in patients undergoing adrenalectomy for primary hyperaldosteronism. Surgery. 2014;156(6):1394–403.
48. Williams TA, Lenders JWM, Mulatero P, Burrello J, Rottenkolber M, Adolf C, et al. Outcomes after adrenalectomy for unilateral primary aldosteronism: an international consensus on outcome measures and analysis of remission rates in an international cohort. Lancet Diabetes Endocrinol. 2017;5(9):689–99.
49. Lim V, Guo Q, Grant CS, Thompson GB, Richards ML, Farley DR, et al. Accuracy of adrenal imaging and adrenal venous sampling in predicting surgical cure of primary aldosteronism. J Clin Endocrinol Metab. 2014;99(8):2712–9.
50. Kendrick ML, Curlee K, Lloyd R, Farley DR, Grant CS, Thompson GB, et al. Aldosterone-secreting adrenocortical carcinomas are associated with unique operative risks and outcomes. Surgery. 2002;132(6):1008–11. discussion 12

51. Kloos RT, Gross MD, Francis IR, Korobkin M, Shapiro B. Incidentally discovered adrenal masses. Endocr Rev. 1995;16(4):460–84.
52. Kempers MJ, Lenders JW, van Outheusden L, van der Wilt GJ, Schultze Kool LJ, Hermus AR, et al. Systematic review: diagnostic procedures to differentiate unilateral from bilateral adrenal abnormality in primary aldosteronism. Ann Intern Med. 2009;151(5):329–37.
53. Nanba AT, Nanba K, Byrd JB, Shields JJ, Giordano TJ, Miller BS, et al. Discordance between imaging and immunohistochemistry in unilateral primary aldosteronism. Clin Endocrinol. 2017;87(6):665–72.
54. Ladurner R, Sommerey S, Buechner S, Dietz A, Degenhart C, Hallfeldt K, et al. Accuracy of adrenal imaging and adrenal venous sampling in diagnosing unilateral primary aldosteronism. Eur J Clin Investig. 2017;47(5):372–7.
55. Young WF, Stanson AW. What are the keys to successful adrenal venous sampling (AVS) in patients with primary aldosteronism? Clin Endocrinol. 2009;70(1):14–7.
56. Jakobsson H, Farmaki K, Sakinis A, Ehn O, Johannsson G, Ragnarsson O. Adrenal venous sampling: the learning curve of a single interventionalist with 282 consecutive procedures. Diagn Interv Radiol. 2018;24(2):89–93.
57. Monticone S, Satoh F, Viola A, Fischer E, Vonend O, Bernini G, et al. 9b.01: clinical significance of contralateral adrenal suppression during adrenal vein sampling in primary aldosteronism. J Hypertens. 2015;33(Suppl 1):e120.
58. Tagawa M, Ghosn M, Wachtel H, Fraker D, Townsend RR, Trerotola S, et al. Lateralization index but not contralateral suppression at adrenal vein sampling predicts improvement in blood pressure after adrenalectomy for primary aldosteronism. J Hum Hypertens. 2017;31(7):444–9.
59. Umakoshi H, Tanase-Nakao K, Wada N, Ichijo T, Sone M, Inagaki N, et al. Importance of contralateral aldosterone suppression during adrenal vein sampling in the subtype evaluation of primary aldosteronism. Clin Endocrinol. 2015;83(4):462–7.
60. Strajina V, Al-Hilli Z, Andrews JC, Bancos I, Thompson GB, Farley DR, et al. Primary aldosteronism: making sense of partial data sets from failed adrenal venous sampling-suppression of adrenal aldosterone production can be used in clinical decision making. Surgery. 2018;163(4):801–6.
61. Daunt N. Adrenal vein sampling: how to make it quick, easy, and successful. Radiographics. 2005;25(Suppl 1):S143–58.
62. Fujimoto K, Honjo S, Tatsuoka H, Hamamoto Y, Kawasaki Y, Matsuoka A, et al. Primary aldosteronism associated with subclinical Cushing syndrome. J Endocrinol Investig. 2013;36(8):564–7.
63. Tang L, Li X, Wang B, Ma X, Li H, Gao Y, et al. Clinical characteristics of aldosterone- and cortisol-coproducing adrenal adenoma in primary aldosteronism. Int J Endocrinol. 2018;2018:4920841.
64. Dennedy MC, Annamalai AK, Prankerd-Smith O, Freeman N, Vengopal K, Graggaber J, et al. Low DHEAS: a sensitive and specific test for the detection of subclinical hypercortisolism in adrenal incidentalomas. J Clin Endocrinol Metab. 2017;102(3):786–92.
65. Christakis I, Livesey JA, Sadler GP, Mihai R. Laparoscopic adrenalectomy for Conn's syndrome is beneficial to patients and is cost effective in England. J Investig Surg. 2017;31(4):300–6.
66. Sywak M, Pasieka JL. Long-term follow-up and cost benefit of adrenalectomy in patients with primary hyperaldosteronism. Br J Surg. 2002;89(12):1587–93.
67. Walz MK, Gwosdz R, Levin SL, Alesina PF, Suttorp AC, Metz KA, et al. Retroperitoneoscopic adrenalectomy in Conn's syndrome caused by adrenal adenomas or nodular hyperplasia. World J Surg. 2008;32(5):847–53.
68. Duncan JL 3rd, Fuhrman GM, Bolton JS, Bowen JD, Richardson WS. Laparoscopic adrenalectomy is superior to an open approach to

treat primary hyperaldosteronism. Am Surg. 2000;66(10):932–5. discussion 5-6
69. Hazzan D, Shiloni E, Golijanin D, Jurim O, Gross D, Reissman P. Laparoscopic vs open adrenalectomy for benign adrenal neoplasm. Surg Endosc. 2001;15(11):1356–8.
70. Porpiglia F, Miller BS, Manfredi M, Fiori C, Doherty GM. A debate on laparoscopic versus open adrenalectomy for adrenocortical carcinoma. Horm Cancer. 2011;2(6):372–7.
71. Gavriilidis P, Camenzuli C, Paspala A, Di Marco AN, Palazzo FF. Posterior retroperitoneoscopic versus laparoscopic transperitoneal adrenalectomy: a systematic review by an updated meta-analysis. World J Surg. 2020;45(1):168–79.
72. Ji C, Lu Q, Chen W, Zhang F, Ji H, Zhang S, et al. Retrospective comparison of three minimally invasive approaches for adrenal tumors: perioperative outcomes of transperitoneal laparoscopic, retroperitoneal laparoscopic and robot-assisted laparoscopic adrenalectomy. BMC Urol. 2020;20(1):66.
73. Anceschi U, Tuderti G, Fiori C, Zappala O, Ferriero MC, Brassetti A, et al. Minimally invasive partial versus total adrenalectomy for the treatment of primary aldosteronism: results of a multicenter series according to the PASO criteria. Eur Urol Focus. 2020;S2405-4569(20):30189.
74. Mercan S, Seven R, Ozarmagan S, Tezelman S. Endoscopic retroperitoneal adrenalectomy. Surgery. 1995;118(6):1071–5. discussion 5-6
75. Walz MK, Peitgen K, Hoermann R, Giebler RM, Mann K, Eigler FW. Posterior retroperitoneoscopy as a new minimally invasive approach for adrenalectomy: results of 30 adrenalectomies in 27 patients. World J Surg. 1996;20(7):769–74.
76. Walz MK, Alesina PF, Wenger FA, Deligiannis A, Szuczik E, Petersenn S, et al. Posterior retroperitoneoscopic adrenalectomy--results of 560 procedures in 520 patients. Surgery. 2006;140(6):943–8. discussion 8-50
77. Giebler RM, Walz MK, Peitgen K, Scherer RU. Hemodynamic changes after retroperitoneal CO2 insufflation for posterior retroperitoneoscopic adrenalectomy. Anesth Analg. 1996;82(4):827–31.
78. Inversini D, Manfredini L, Galli F, Zhang D, Dionigi G, Rausei S. Risk factors for complications after robotic adrenalectomy: a review. Gland Surg. 2020;9(3):826–30.
79. Chiang WF, Cheng CJ, Wu ST, Sun GH, Lin MY, Sung CC, et al. Incidence and factors of post-adrenalectomy hyperkalemia in patients with aldosterone producing adenoma. Clin Chim Acta. 2013;424:114–8.
80. Tahir A, McLaughlin K, Kline G. Severe hyperkalemia following adrenalectomy for aldosteronoma: prediction, pathogenesis and approach to clinical management- a case series. BMC Endocr Disord. 2016;16(1):43.
81. Shariq OA, Bancos I, Cronin PA, Farley DR, Richards ML, Thompson GB, et al. Contralateral suppression of aldosterone at adrenal venous sampling predicts hyperkalemia following adrenalectomy for primary aldosteronism. Surgery. 2018;163(1):183–90.
82. Wada N, Shibayama Y, Umakoshi H, Ichijo T, Fujii Y, Kamemura K, et al. Hyperkalemia in both surgically and medically treated patients with primary aldosteronism. J Hum Hypertens. 2017;31(10):627–32.
83. Weisbrod AB, Webb RC, Mathur A, Barak S, Abraham SB, Nilubol N, et al. Adrenal histologic findings show no difference in clinical presentation and outcome in primary hyperaldosteronism. Ann Surg Oncol. 2013;20(3):753–8.
84. Hennings J, Andreasson S, Botling J, Hagg A, Sundin A, Hellman P. Long-term effects of surgical correction of adrenal hyperplasia and adenoma causing primary aldosteronism. Langenbeck's Arch Surg. 2010;395(2):133–7.
85. Gockel I, Heintz A, Polta M, Junginger T. Long-term results of endoscopic adrenalectomy for Conn's syndrome. Am Surg. 2007;73(2):174–80.

86. Pang TC, Bambach C, Monaghan JC, Sidhu SB, Bune A, Delbridge LW, et al. Outcomes of laparoscopic adrenalectomy for hyperaldosteronism. ANZ J Surg. 2007;77(9):768–73.
87. Omata K, Anand SK, Hovelson DH, Liu CJ, Yamazaki Y, Nakamura Y, et al. Aldosterone-producing cell clusters frequently harbor somatic mutations and accumulate with age in normal adrenals. J Endocr Soc. 2017;1(7):787–99.
88. Hannon MJ, Sze WC, Carpenter R, Parvanta L, Matson M, Sahdev A, et al. Clinical outcomes following unilateral adrenalectomy in patients with primary aldosteronism. QJM. 2017;110(5):277–81.
89. Desrochers MJ, St-Jean M, El Ghorayeb N, Bourdeau I, So B, Therasse E, et al. Basal contralateral aldosterone suppression is rare in lateralized primary aldosteronism. Eur J Endocrinol. 2020;183(4):399–409.
90. Heinrich DA, Adolf C, Holler F, Lechner B, Schneider H, Riester A, et al. Adrenal insufficiency after unilateral adrenalectomy in primary aldosteronism: long-term outcome and clinical impact. J Clin Endocrinol Metab. 2019;104(11):5658–64.
91. Rossi GP, Cesari M, Cuspidi C, Maiolino G, Cicala MV, Bisogni V, et al. Long-term control of arterial hypertension and regression of left ventricular hypertrophy with treatment of primary aldosteronism. Hypertension. 2013;62(1):62–9.
92. Lin YH, Lin LY, Chen A, Wu XM, Lee JK, Su TC, et al. Adrenalectomy improves increased carotid intima-media thickness and arterial stiffness in patients with aldosterone producing adenoma. Atherosclerosis. 2012;221(1):154–9.
93. Goh BK, Tan YH, Yip SK, Eng PH, Cheng CW. Outcome of patients undergoing laparoscopic adrenalectomy for primary hyperaldosteronism. JSLS. 2004;8(4):320–5.
94. Fukudome Y, Fujii K, Arima H, Ohya Y, Tsuchihashi T, Abe I, et al. Discriminating factors for recurrent hypertension in patients with primary aldosteronism after adrenalectomy. Hypertens Res. 2002;25(1):11–8.
95. Arnesen T, Glomnes N, Stromsoy S, Knappskog S, Heie A, Akslen LA, et al. Outcome after surgery for primary hyperaldosteronism may depend on KCNJ5 tumor mutation status: a population-based study from Western Norway. Langenbeck's Arch Surg. 2013;398(6):869–74.
96. Reincke M, Fischer E, Gerum S, Merkle K, Schulz S, Pallauf A, et al. Observational study mortality in treated primary aldosteronism: the German Conn's registry. Hypertension. 2012;60(3):618–24.
97. Takeda R, Matsubara T, Miyamori I, Hatakeyama H, Morise T. Vascular complications in patients with aldosterone producing adenoma in Japan: comparative study with essential hypertension. The Research Committee of Disorders of Adrenal Hormones in Japan. J Endocrinol Investig. 1995;18(5):370–3.
98. Catena C, Colussi G, Nadalini E, Chiuch A, Baroselli S, Lapenna R, et al. Cardiovascular outcomes in patients with primary aldosteronism after treatment. Arch Intern Med. 2008;168(1):80–5.
99. Rossi GP, Sacchetto A, Visentin P, Canali C, Graniero GR, Palatini P, et al. Changes in left ventricular anatomy and function in hypertension and primary aldosteronism. Hypertension. 1996;27(5):1039–45.
100. Lin YH, Wu XM, Lee HH, Lee JK, Liu YC, Chang HW, et al. Adrenalectomy reverses myocardial fibrosis in patients with primary aldosteronism. J Hypertens. 2012;30(8):1606–13.
101. Chang YH, Chung SD, Wu CH, Chueh JS, Chen L, Lin PC, et al. Surgery decreases the long-term incident stroke risk in patients with primary aldosteronism. Surgery. 2020;167(2):367–77.
102. Marzano L, Colussi G, Sechi LA, Catena C. Adrenalectomy is comparable with medical treatment for reduction of left ventricular mass in primary aldosteronism: meta-analysis of long-term studies. Am J Hypertens. 2015;28(3):312–8.

103. Meng Z, Dai Z, Huang K, Xu C, Zhang YG, Zheng H, et al. Long-term mortality for patients of primary aldosteronism compared with essential hypertension: a systematic review and meta-analysis. Front Endocrinol. 2020;11:121.
104. Sechi LA, Di Fabio A, Bazzocchi M, Uzzau A, Catena C. Intrarenal hemodynamics in primary aldosteronism before and after treatment. J Clin Endocrinol Metab. 2009;94(4):1191–7.
105. Reincke M, Rump LC, Quinkler M, Hahner S, Diederich S, Lorenz R, et al. Risk factors associated with a low glomerular filtration rate in primary aldosteronism. J Clin Endocrinol Metab. 2009;94(3):869–75.
106. Kramers BJ, Kramers C, Lenders JW, Deinum J. Effects of treating primary aldosteronism on renal function. J Clin Hypertens (Greenwich). 2017;19(3):290–5.
107. Kim DH, Kwon HJ, Ji SA, Jang HR, Jung SH, Kim JH, et al. Risk factors for renal impairment revealed after unilateral adrenalectomy in patients with primary aldosteronism. Medicine (Baltimore). 2016;95(27):e3930.
108. Utsumi T, Kamiya N, Kaga M, Endo T, Yano M, Kamijima S, et al. Development of novel nomograms to predict renal functional outcomes after laparoscopic adrenalectomy in patients with primary aldosteronism. World J Urol. 2017;35(10):1577–83.

Pheochromocytoma and Paraganglioma

Quan-Yang Duh and William F. Young Jr.

Contents

A. L. Shifrin et al. (eds.), *Endocrine Surgery Comprehensive Board Exam Guide*,
https://doi.org/10.1007/978-3-030-84737-1_21

Case Presentation

A 53-year-old man was incidentally discovered to have a right adrenal mass on a chest CT scan that was obtained to evaluate chest pain. The subsequent CT scan of the abdomen and pelvis demonstrated a 2.4 × 3.1 cm lipid poor (35 Hounsfield units) right adrenal mass and a 2.0 × 2.8 cm retroperitoneal left para-aortic nodule (see ◘ Fig. 21.1). He was normotensive and had no symptoms referable to adrenocortical or adrenomedullary dysfunction. There was no family history of PHEO or PGL. On physical exam, BMI = 26.2 kg/m^2, blood pressure was 130/63 mmHg, and heart rate 78 beats per minute. Examination of the heart and lungs was normal. He had a firm mass in his left neck with ill-defined borders. Laboratory studies documented elevated levels of normetanephrine in the blood and urine that were diagnostic of noradrenergic PPGL (see ▶ Box 21.1). In view of the apparent abdominal PGL and left neck mass, a Ga-68 DOTATATE PET CT scan was obtained, which confirmed right adrenal PHEO, left peri-aortic retroperitoneal PGL, and three left neck PGLs. The patient was prepared for surgery with alpha-adrenergic blockade followed by beta-adrenergic blockade with titration for target systolic blood pressure of 110 mmHg and heart rate of 80 beats per minute. At open laparotomy, a 19 g right adrenal gland was resected that contained a 3.3 × 3.1 × 2.8 cm pheochromocytoma. The left para-aortic mass was resected (3.1 × 2.9 × 2.2 cm) and proved to be a PGL. When assessed 2 months after surgery, plasma fractionated metanephrines were normal with metanephrine <0.2 nmol/L (normal <0.5) and normetanephrine 0.4 nmol/L (normal <0.9). Germline genetic testing detected a pathogenic variant in *SDHD* (c.325C>T; p. Q109*). Subsequent family testing demonstrated the same *SDHD* pathogenic variant in his father and sister. Surgical management of the left neck paragangliomas is planned. The patient will be followed with plasma fractionated metanephrines measured annually, MRI of the abdomen and pelvis 1 year after surgery and then every 2–3 years, periodic MRI of the skull base and neck (frequency dependent on surgical outcome), MRI of the chest every 5 years, and Ga-68 DOTATATE PET CT every 5 years (typically 2–3 years after last chest MRI scan).

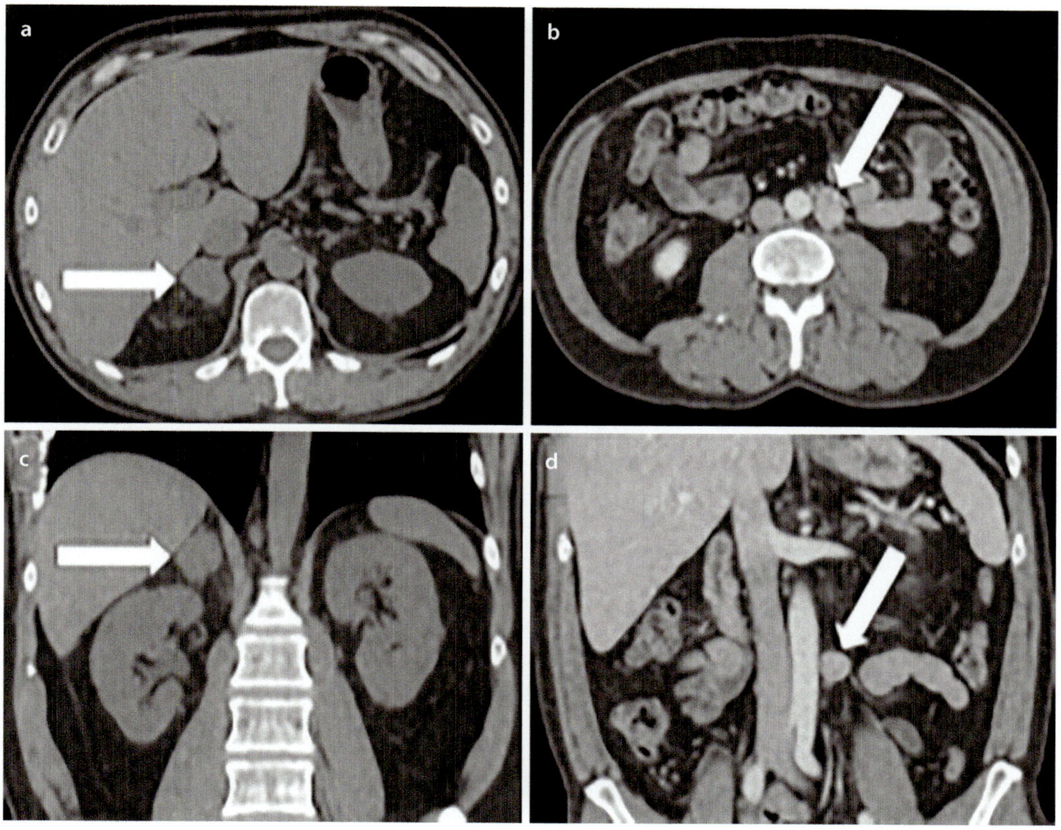

Fig. 21.1 CT scan images from a 53-year-old man with right adrenal pheochromocytoma and multiple paragangliomas. Panels **a** and **b** unenhanced axial (above) and coronal (below) images show a lipid poor (35 Hounsfield units) 2.4 × 3.1 cm right adrenal mass (arrows). With contrast administration the absolute and relative contrast washout values at 15 minutes were 50% and 27%, respectively. Panels **c** and **d** contrast-enhanced axial (above) and coronal (below) images show a 2.0 × 2.8 cm left para-aortic retroperitoneal mass (arrows)

Box 21.1 Laboratory Tests

Biochemical testing

Test	Result	Reference range
Sodium, mmol/L	141	135–145
Potassium, mmol/L	4.1	3.6–5.2
Creatinine, mg/dL	0.87	0.8–1.3
Plasma metanephrine, nmol/L	<0.2	<0.5
Plasma normetanephrine, nmol/L	3.7	<0.9
24-h urine		
Metanephrine, mcg	136	<400
Normetanephrine, mcg	1602	<900
Norepinephrine, mcg	356	<80
Epinephrine, mcg	6.7	<20
Dopamine, mcg	176	<400

Questions

1. The distinction between pheochromocytoma and paraganglioma is important for which of the following reasons:
   1. Determine risk for pancreatic neuroendocrine tumors
   2. Predict tumor size
   3. Implications for associated neoplasms and syndromes
   4. Risk for metastatic disease
      (a) Only (1) and (2) and (3) are correct.
      (b) Only (2) and (3) and (4) are correct.
      (c) Only (3) and (4) are correct.
      (d) Only (4) is correct.
      (e) All are correct.
2. Which of the following signs or symptoms would be *atypical* in a patient with a symptomatic catecholamine-secreting tumor?
   1. Forceful heartbeat
   2. Tremor
   3. Headache
   4. Flushing
      (a) Only (1) and (2) and (3) are correct.
      (b) Only (2) and (3) and (4) are correct.
      (c) Only (3) and (4) are correct.
      (d) Only (4) is correct.
      (e) All are correct.
3. A pheochromocytoma paroxysm may be precipitated by which of the following medications?
   1. Metoprolol
   2. Metoclopramide
   3. High-dose dexamethasone
   4. Doxazosin
      (a) Only (1) and (2) and (3) are correct.
      (b) Only (2) and (3) and (4) are correct.
      (c) Only (3) and (4) are correct.
      (d) Only (4) is correct.
      (e) All are correct.
4. Which of the following physical examination findings are seen in patients with neurofibromatosis type 1?
   1. Iris hamartomas
   2. Café au lait spots
   3. Axillary freckling
   4. Marfanoid body habitus
      (a) Only (1) and (2) and (3) are correct.
      (b) Only (2) and (3) and (4) are correct.
      (c) Only (3) and (4) are correct.
      (d) Only (4) is correct.
      (e) All are correct.
5. Adrenergic catecholamine-secreting tumors are typically found in which of the following genetic syndromes?
   1. Familial paraganglioma due to *SDHD* pathogenic variant
   2. Von Hippel-Lindau disease

3. Multiple endocrine neoplasia type 2
4. Neurofibromatosis type 1
   (a) Only (1) and (2) and (3) are correct.
   (b) Only (2) and (3) and (4) are correct.
   (c) Only (3) and (4) are correct.
   (d) Only (4) is correct.
   (e) All are correct.

6. Pathogenic variants in which of the following genes are associated with maternal imprinting?
   1. SDHB
   2. SDHC
   3. SDHD
   4. SDHAF2
      (a) Only (1) and (2) and (3) are correct.
      (b) Only (2) and (3) and (4) are correct.
      (c) Only (3) and (4) are correct.
      (d) Only (4) is correct.
      (e) All are correct.
7. Pheochromocytoma can be resected surgically by:
   1. Laparoscopic transperitoneal adrenalectomy
   2. Retroperitoneal endoscopic adrenalectomy
   3. Hand-assisted laparoscopic adrenalectomy
   4. Robot-assisted adrenalectomy
      (a) Only (1) and (2) and (3) are correct.
      (b) Only (2) and (3) and (4) are correct.
      (c) Only (3) and (4) are correct.
      (d) Only (4) is correct.
      (e) All are correct.
8. Complication(s) associated with unilateral adrenalectomy for pheochromocytoma are:
   1. Bleeding
   2. Fracturing of tumor
   3. Hypoglycemia
   4. Addisonian crisis
      (a) Only (1) and (2) and (3) are correct.
      (b) Only (2) and (3) and (4) are correct.
      (c) Only (3) and (4) are correct.
      (d) Only (4) is correct.
      (e) All are correct.
9. Initial treatment of a patient in pheochromocytoma crisis usually involves:
   1. Beta-adrenergic blockade
   2. ECMO (extracorporeal membrane oxygenation)
   3. Emergency adrenalectomy
   4. Alpha-adrenergic blockade
      (a) Only (1) and (2) and (3) are correct.
      (b) Only (2) and (3) and (4) are correct.
      (c) Only (3) and (4) are correct.
      (d) Only (4) is correct.
      (e) All are correct.

10. Subtotal adrenalectomy can be a good option for a:
    1. 3 cm para-aortic PGL in a patient with known *SDHB* mutation
    2. 8 cm right adrenal PHEO in a patient with MEN2B
    3. 3 cm left adrenal PHEO in a patient with VHL
    4. 3 cm right adrenal PHEO in a patient with MEN2A who already had a left adrenalectomy
       (a) Only (1) and (2) and (3) are correct.
       (b) Only (2) and (3) and (4) are correct.
       (c) Only (3) and (4) are correct.
       (d) Only (4) is correct.
       (e) All are correct.
11. Intraoperative hemodynamic instability:
    1. Can usually be treated with blood transfusion
    2. Can be reduced by preoperative preparation with alpha-adrenergic blockade and volume expansion
    3. Can be treated with vasopressors and vasodilators by experienced anesthesiologists
    4. Can be best anticipated and managed by an experienced multidisciplinary team
       (a) Only (1) and (2) and (3) are correct.
       (b) Only (2) and (3) and (4) are correct.
       (c) Only (3) and (4) are correct.
       (d) Only (4) is correct.
       (e) All are correct.
12. After an apparently successful resection of a PHEO, recurrences can be caused by:
    1. Incomplete resection of the PHEO
    2. Growth of tumor cells seeded from fracturing the PHEO during initial operation
    3. Development of a PHEO in the contralateral adrenal gland
    4. Growth of metastases to the liver or bones
       (a) Only (1) and (2) and (3) are correct.
       (b) Only (2) and (3) and (4) are correct.
       (c) Only (3) and (4) are correct.
       (d) Only (4) is correct.
       (e) All are correct.

21.1 Introduction

Catecholamine-secreting tumors that arise from the chromaffin cells in the adrenal medulla and the sympathetic ganglia are referred to as *pheochromocytoma* (PHEO) and *catecholamine-secreting paraganglioma* (PGL), respectively [1]. Because the tumors have similar clinical presentations and are treated with similar approaches, many clinicians use the term *pheochromocytoma* to refer to both adrenal PHEO and extra-adrenal catecholamine-secreting PGLs. However, the distinction between PHEO and PGL (PPGL) is important because of the implications for associated neoplasms and syndromes are different and the risk for metastatic disease is higher in patients with PGL. Catecholamine-secreting PPGLs are rare, with an annual incidence of 2–8 cases per 1 million people [2]. However, it is important to suspect, confirm, localize, and resect these tumors because (a) the associated hypertension is curable with surgical resection, (b) a catecholamine crisis may result in multiorgan failure and death, and (c) at least 10% of PPGLs will prove to be metastatic and an early resection may prevent this outcome (◘ Fig. 21.2).

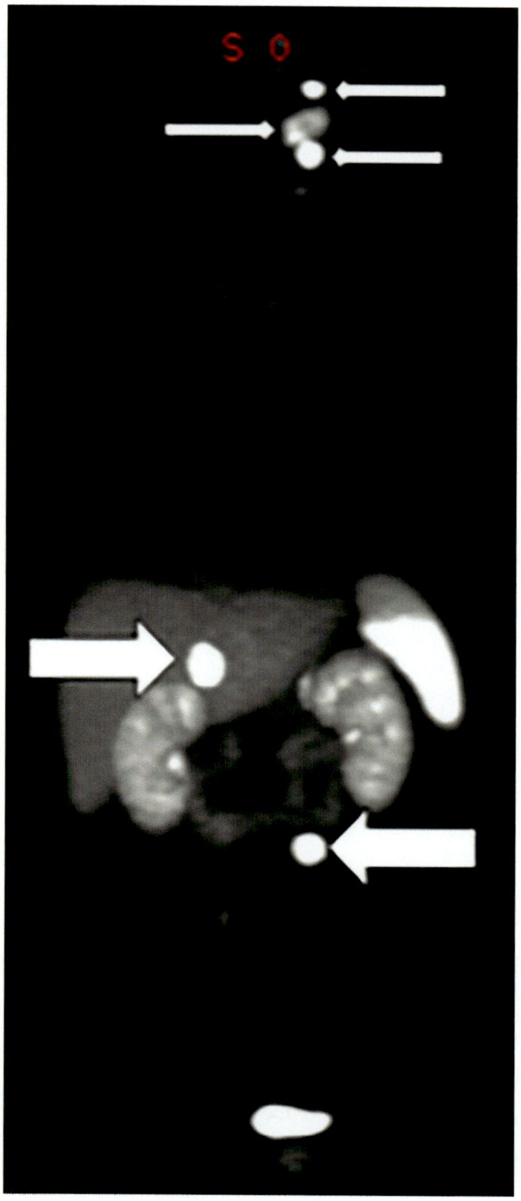

◘ **Fig. 21.2** Coronal image from Ga-68 DOTATATE PET-CT shows that the right adrenal mass and left para-aortic nodule were intensely tracer avid (large arrows). In addition, there were 3 sites of intense tracer uptake in the left neck—in the left carotid space, the left jugular foramen, and inferiorly along the left carotid vessels (small arrows)

21.2 Clinical Presentation

PPGLs occur with equal frequency in men and women, primarily in the third, fourth, and fifth decades. These tumors are rare in children, and when discovered, they may be multifocal and associated with a hereditary syndrome. The symptoms, listed in ▶ Box 21.2, are caused by the pharmacologic effects of excess concentrations of circulating catecholamines [3].

Box 21.2 Signs and Symptoms Associated with Catecholamine-Secreting Tumors

Paroxysm-related signs and symptoms

Anxiety and fear of impending death
Diaphoresis
Dyspnea
Epigastric and chest pain
Headache
Hypertension
Nausea and vomiting
Pallor
Palpitation (forceful heartbeat)
Tremor

Chronic signs and symptoms

Cold hands and feet
Congestive heart failure—dilated or hypertrophic cardiomyopathy
Constipation
Diaphoresis
Dyspnea
Ectopic hormone secretion–dependent symptoms (e.g., CRH/ACTH, GHRH, PTHrP, VIP)
Epigastric and chest pain
Fatigue
Fever
General increase in sweating
Grade II to IV hypertensive retinopathy
Headache
Hyperglycemia
Hypertension
Nausea and vomiting
Orthostatic hypotension
Painless hematuria (associated with urinary bladder paraganglioma)
Pallor
Palpitation (forceful heartbeat)
Tremor
Weight loss

Not typical of pheochromocytoma

Flushing

ACTH corticotropin, *CRH* corticotropin–releasing hormone, *GHRH* growth hormone-releasing hormone, *PTHrP* parathyroid hormone-related peptide, *VIP* vasoactive intestinal polypeptide
Adapted from Young [3]

When present, the associated hypertension may be sustained or paroxysmal. However, when a PPGL is diagnosed in the presymptomatic stage, it is common for these patients to have normal blood pressure [4].

Episodic symptoms may occur in spells, or paroxysms, that can be extremely variable in presentation but typically include forceful heartbeat, pallor, tremor, headache, and diaphoresis [5, 6]. The spell may start with a sensation of a "rush" in the chest and a sense of shortness of breath, followed by a forceful heartbeat and a throbbing headache [5]. Peripheral vasoconstriction associated with a spell results in cool or cold hands and feet and facial pallor. Spells may appear to be either spontaneous or precipitated by postural change, anxiety, medications (e.g., beta-adrenergic blockers, metoclopramide, anesthetic agents, and high-dose corticosteroids), exercise, or maneuvers that increase intra-abdominal pressure (e.g., change in position, lifting, defecation, exercise, colonoscopy, pregnancy, and trauma). However, the clinician should be aware that most patients with spells do not have a catecholamine-secreting PPGL [5].

Additional clinical signs of catecholamine-secreting PPGL include hypertensive retinopathy, orthostatic hypotension, angina, nausea, constipation (megacolon may be the presenting symptom), hyperglycemia, diabetes mellitus, hypercalcemia, Raynaud phenomenon, livedo reticularis, erythrocytosis, and mass effects from the tumor. Although hypercalcemia may be a sign of primary hyperparathyroidism in patients with multiple endocrine neoplasia type 2 (MEN2), in most patients with PPGL, the hypercalcemia is an isolated finding and resolves with resection of the catecholamine-secreting neoplasm. Fasting hyperglycemia and diabetes mellitus are caused in part by the alpha-adrenergic inhibition of insulin release. Painless hematuria and paroxysmal attacks induced by micturition and defecation are associated with urinary bladder PPGLs.

The clinical presentations of PPGL that are frequently missed as signs of underlying PPGL are cardiomyopathy, congestive heart failure, myocarditis, and myocardial infarction with normal coronary arteries. The cardiomyopathy, whether dilated or hypertrophic, may be totally reversible with tumor resection [7]. In addition, Takotsubo cardiomyopathy with ventricular apical ballooning can also be a presentation of catecholamine-secreting PPGL. Many physical examination findings can be associated with genetic syndromes that predispose to catecholamine-secreting PPGL—these findings include retinal angiomas (von Hippel Lindau [VHL] disease); iris hamartomas (neurofibromatosis type 1 [NF1]); Marfanoid body habitus (MEN2B); café au lait spots (NF1); axillary freckling (NF1); subcutaneous neurofibromas (NF1); thyroid nodule or goiter related to medullary thyroid carcinoma (MEN2A and 2B); and, mucosal neuromas on the eyelids and tongue (MEN2B). Clinicians may be confused when a patient with PPGL is asymptomatic despite high circulating levels of catecholamines; this presentation most likely reflects adrenergic receptor desensitization related to chronic stimulation.

21.3 Natural History

Because of the increased and widespread use of computed tomography (CT) and magnetic resonance imaging (MRI) in patients with abdominal symptoms, PPGLs may be detected as an incidental adrenal mass or retroperitoneal mass in many patients before any symptoms develop. Approximately 60% of patients with adrenal PHEO have their tumors discovered incidentally on imaging performed for other reasons [4, 8–10]. Although usually these incidentally discovered tumors in asymptomatic patients are small (e.g., <3 cm), they may be up to 10 cm in diameter.

At the time of symptom-based detection, PHEOs have an average diameter of 4.5 cm [11]. PGLs are found where there is chromaffin tissue: along the para-aortic sympathetic chain, within the organ of Zuckerkandl (at the origin of the inferior mesenteric artery), in the wall of the urinary bladder, and along the sympathetic chain in the neck or mediastinum [12]. During early postnatal life, the extra-adrenal sympathetic paraganglionic tissues are prominent; later they degenerate, leaving residual foci associated with the vagus nerves, carotid vessels, aortic arch, pulmonary vessels, and mesenteric arteries. Odd locations for PGLs include the intra-atrial cardiac septum, spermatic cord, vagina, scrotum, and sacrococcygeal region. PGLs in the skull base and neck region (e.g., carotid body tumors, glomus tumors, and chemodectomas) usually arise from parasympathetic tissue and typically do not hypersecrete catecholamines and metanephrines. PGLs in the lower mediastinum, abdomen, and pelvis usually arise from sympathetic chromaffin tissue and usually do hypersecrete catecholamines and metanephrines.

21.3.1 Genetic Forms of Pheochromocytoma and Paraganglioma

Pathogenic variants in PPGL susceptibility genes have three general transcription signatures: (a) cluster 1, genes encoding proteins that function in the cellular response to hypoxia; (b) cluster 2, genes encoding proteins that activate kinase signaling; and (c) cluster 3, Wnt signaling pathway genes (see Table 21.1). Cluster 1 tumors are mostly extra-adrenal PGLs (except in VHL, in which most tumors are localized to the adrenal gland), and nearly all have a noradrenergic biochemical phenotype (the predominant catecholamine is norepinephrine and the predominant metabolite is normetanephrine) [13].

Table 21.1 Pheochromocytoma and paraganglioma susceptibility genes

Syndrome/name	Gene	Typical tumor location and other associations
Hypoxic pathway: Cluster 1[a]		
SDHD pathogenic variant	*SDHD*	Primarily skull base and neck; occasionally adrenal medulla, mediastinum, abdomen, pelvis; GIST; possible pituitary adenoma
SDHAF2 pathogenic variant[b]	*SDHAF2*	Primarily skull base and neck; occasionally abdomen and pelvis
SDHC pathogenic variant	*SDHC*	Primarily skull base and neck; occasionally abdomen, pelvis, or chest; GIST; possible pituitary adenoma
SDHB pathogenic variant	*SDHB*	Abdomen, pelvis, and mediastinum; rarely adrenal medulla, skull base, and neck; GIST; renal cell carcinoma; possible pituitary adenoma
SDHA pathogenic variant	*SDHA*	Primarily skull base and neck; occasionally abdomen and pelvis; GIST; possible pituitary adenoma
von Hippel-Lindau (VHL) disease	*VHL*	Adrenal medulla, frequently bilateral; occasionally paraganglioma that may be localized from skull base to pelvis; VHL-associated findings—including: retinal angiomas, cerebellar hemangioblastomas, spinal hemangioblastomas, renal cell carcinoma, pancreatic neuroendocrine tumors, and endolymphatic sac tumor
Hereditary leiomyomatosis and renal cell carcinoma (Reed syndrome)—fumarate hydratase mutation	*FH*	Multifocal and metastatic paraganglioma; associated with hereditary leiomyomatosis, uterine fibroids, and renal cell carcinoma
Endothelial PAS	*EPAS1*	Paraganglioma, polycythemia, and rarely somatostatinomas

(continued)

Table 21.1 (continued)

Syndrome/name	Gene	Typical tumor location and other associations
Familial erythrocytosis associated with pathogenic variant in prolyl hydroxylase isoform 1 (*PDH1*)	*EGLN2* (Egl-9 Family)	Polycythemia associated with pheochromocytoma and paraganglioma
Familial erythrocytosis associated with pathogenic variant in prolyl hydroxylase isoform 2 (*PDH2*)	*EGLN1* (Egl-9 Family)	Polycythemia associated with pheochromocytoma and paraganglioma
Kinesin family member 1B	*KIF1B*	Paraganglioma, ganglioneuroma, leiomyosarcoma, lung adenocarcinoma, neuroblastoma, ganglioneuroma
Malate dehydrogenase 2	*MDH2*	Pheochromocytoma and paraganglioma—penetrance and associated conditions not yet characterized
Solute carrier family 25 member 11	*SLC25A11*	Pheochromocytoma and paraganglioma—penetrance and associated conditions not yet characterized
DNA methyltransferase 3 alpha	*DNMT3A*	Pheochromocytoma and paraganglioma—penetrance unknown; acute myeloid leukemia
Isocitrate dehydrogenase (NADP(+)) 1	*IDH1*	Pheochromocytoma and paraganglioma—penetrance and associated conditions not yet characterized
Dihydrolipoamide S-succinyltransferase	*DLST*	Pheochromocytoma and paraganglioma—penetrance and associated conditions not yet characterized
Glutamic-oxaloacetic Transaminase 2	*GOT2*	Pheochromocytoma and paraganglioma—penetrance and associated conditions not yet characterized
Kinase signaling pathway: Cluster 2[c]		
MEN2A	*RET*	Pheochromocytoma in 50% (frequently bilateral); medullary thyroid carcinoma in 100%, primary hyperparathyroidism in 20%, and cutaneous lichen amyloidosis in 5%

(continued)

Table 21.1 (continued)

Syndrome/name	Gene	Typical tumor location and other associations
MEN2B	*RET*	Pheochromocytoma in 50% (frequently bilateral); medullary thyroid carcinoma in 100%; mucocutaneous neuromas in most (typically involving the tongue, lips, and eyelids); skeletal deformities (kyphoscoliosis or lordosis) in most; joint laxity in most; myelinated corneal nerves in many; and, intestinal ganglio-neuromas (Hirschsprung disease) in most
Neurofibromatosis type 1 (NF1)	*NF1*	Pheochromocytoma or periadrenal paraganglioma in 3%; cafe au lait spots; subcutaneous or plexiform neurofibromas; axillary or inguinal freckling; optic glioma; iris hamartomas (Lisch nodules); and osseous lesions (e.g., sphenoid dysplasia),
MYC associated factor X[b]	*MAX*	Adrenal medulla
Transmembrane protein 127	*TMEM127*	Adrenal medulla; possible renal cell carcinoma
Wnt signaling pathway: Cluster 3[d]		
Cold shock domain containing E1	*CSDE1*	Pheochromocytoma and paraganglioma—penetrance and associated conditions not yet characterized
Mastermind like transcriptional coactivator 3	*MAML3*	Pheochromocytoma and paraganglioma—penetrance and associated conditions not yet characterized

Abbreviations used: GIST gastrointestinal stromal tumor, *MEN* multiple endocrine neoplasia, *SDH* succinate dehydrogenase

[a]Cluster 1 tumors are mostly extra-adrenal paragangliomas (except in VHL where most tumors are localized to the adrenal) and nearly all have a noradrenergic biochemical phenotype

[b]Associated with maternal imprinting—see text

[c]Cluster 2 tumors are usually adrenal pheochromocytomas with an adrenergic biochemical phenotype

[d]Cluster 3 tumors are adrenal or extra-adrenal in location with variable biochemical phenotype

Cluster 2 tumors are usually adrenal PHEOs with an adrenergic biochemical phenotype (the predominant catecholamine is epinephrine and the predominant metabolite is metanephrine). Cluster 3 tumors are adrenal and extra-adrenal in location and the biochemical phenotype is adrenergic or noradrenergic, respectively (see ◘ Table 21.1). Since 1990, 23 germline PPGL susceptibility genes have been reported: *RET, NF-1, MAX, TMEM127, SDHA, SDHAF2, SDHB, SDHC, SDHD, VHL, FH, EGLN1 (PHD2), EGLN2 (PDH1), KIF1B, IDH1, MDH2, EPAS* [1, 2], *SLC25A11, DNMT3A, DLST, GOT2, CSDE1,* and *MAML3* [1, 14, 15].

Most cases of familial PGLs are caused by mutations in the succinate dehydrogenase (SDH) (succinate: ubiquinone oxidoreductase) subunit genes (*SDHB*, *SDHC*, *SDHD*, *SHDA*, and *SDHAF2*), which make up portions of mitochondrial complex II. In patients with *SDHD* or *SDHAF2* mutations, penetrance depends on the mutation's parent of origin—with rare exceptions, the disease is not manifested when the mutation is inherited from the mother but is approximately 44% penetrant when inherited from the father [1, 16]. This phenomenon is known as *maternal imprinting* [17]. *SDHB* pathogenic variants have lower penetrance (≈22%), but are associated with a higher risk of metastatic disease [1, 18].

21.4 Diagnosis

21.4.1 Differential Diagnosis

Numerous disorders can cause signs and symptoms that may prompt the clinician to test for catecholamine-secreting PPGL. The disorders span much of medicine and include psychological disorders (e.g., panic disorder), endocrine disorders (e.g., primary hypogonadism), cardiovascular disorders (e.g., idiopathic orthostatic hypotension), pharmacologic causes (e.g., withdrawal from an adrenergic inhibitor), neurologic disorders (e.g., postural orthostatic tachycardia syndrome), and miscellaneous disorders (e.g., mast cell disease) [5]. Indeed, most patients tested for catecholamine-secreting PPGL do not have it. In addition, levels of fractionated catecholamines and metanephrines may be elevated in several clinical scenarios, including any acute illness (e.g., subarachnoid hemorrhage, migraine headache, preeclampsia), withdrawal from medications or drugs (e.g., clonidine, alcohol), and administration of many drugs and medications (► Box 21.3) [6].

Box 21.3 Medications that May Increase Measured Levels of Fractionated Catecholamines and Metanephrines

Tricyclic antidepressants (including cyclobenzaprine)—up to tenfold elevations in NE and Normet
Levodopa—up to 20-fold elevations in DA and 4-fold in NE and Normet
Antipsychotic agents and buspirone—up to tenfold elevations in NE and Normet
Serotonin-norepinephrine reuptake inhibitor—up to fivefold elevations in NE and Normet
Selective serotonin reuptake inhibitors—up to twofold elevations in NE and Normet
Prochlorperazine—up to fivefold elevations in NE and Normet
Reserpine—up to tenfold elevations in NE and Normet
Drugs containing adrenergic receptor agonists (e.g., decongestants)—up to fivefold elevations in NE and Normet
Amphetamines—up to tenfold elevations in NE and Normet
Withdrawal from clonidine and other drugs—up to tenfold elevations in NE and Normet
Illicit drugs (e.g., cocaine, heroin)—up to 10-fold elevations in NE and Normet
Ethanol—up to fivefold elevations in NE and Normet

Abbreviations used: *DA* dopamine, *NE* norepinephrine, *Normet* normetanephrine

21.4.2 When to Do Case Detection Testing

Catecholamine-secreting PPGL should be suspected in patients who have one or more of the following: an incidentally discovered adrenal mass with imaging characteristics consistent with PHEO; a familial syndrome that predisposes to catecholamine-secreting PPGLs (e.g., MEN2, NF1, VHL); a family history of PPGL; pressor response during anesthesia, surgery, or angiography; hyperadrenergic spells (e.g., self-limited episodes of nonexertional forceful palpitations, diaphoresis, headache, tremor, or pallor); treatment-resistant hypertension; onset of hypertension at a young age (e.g., <20 years); and, idiopathic dilated cardiomyopathy.

21.4.3 Measurement of Fractionated Metanephrines and Catecholamines in Urine and Plasma

The diagnosis must be confirmed biochemically by the presence of increased concentrations of fractionated metanephrines and catecholamines in urine or plasma [6]. The metabolism of catecholamines is primarily intratumoral, with formation of metanephrine from epinephrine and normetanephrine from norepinephrine. Most laboratories measure fractionated catecholamines (dopamine, norepinephrine, and epinephrine) and fractionated metanephrines (metanephrine and normetanephrine) by high-performance liquid chromatography with electrochemical detection or tandem mass spectrometry.

Although it is preferred that patients not receive any medication during the diagnostic evaluation, treatment with most medications may be continued. Tricyclic antidepressants are the drug class that interferes most frequently with the interpretation of fractionated metanephrines and catecholamines. To effectively screen for catecholamine-secreting tumors, treatment with tricyclic antidepressants and other psychoactive agents listed in ► Box 21.3 should be tapered and discontinued at least 2 weeks before any hormonal assessments. In some clinical situations, it is contraindicated to discontinue certain medications (e.g., antipsychotics), and if case-detection testing is positive, then CT or MRI of the abdomen and pelvis would be needed to exclude a catecholamine-secreting tumor. Measurements of urinary catecholamines and metabolites may be invalid if the patient has advanced renal failure [19]. Concentrations of plasma fractionated metanephrines are falsely elevated in patients with end-stage renal disease and are not useful in this setting [20]. In patients without PPGL who are receiving hemodialysis, plasma norepinephrine and dopamine concentrations are increased threefold and twofold above the upper limit of normal, respectively [21]. However, standard normal ranges can be used for interpreting plasma epinephrine concentrations [19, 22]. Therefore, when patients with renal failure have plasma norepinephrine concentrations more than three times above the upper normal limit or epinephrine concentrations greater than the upper normal limit, PPGL should be suspected.

21.4.4 Genetic Testing

Genetic testing should be considered in all patients with PPGL. The probability of finding a pathogenic variant in a PPGL susceptibility gene is inversely correlated with age—germline pathogenic variants are found in approximately 85% of those with a PPGL detected in the first decade of life and 25% when PPGL is diagnosed in the 6th decade of life [1]. An asymptomatic person at risk for disease on the basis of family history of PPGL should have genetic testing only if an affected family member has a known mutation. Genetic testing can be complex and testing of one family member has implications for related individuals. Genetic counseling is recommended to help families understand the implications of genetic test results, to coordinate testing of at-risk individuals, and to help families work through the psychosocial issues that may arise before, during, or after the testing process.

21.4.5 Localization

Localization studies should not be initiated until biochemical studies have confirmed the diagnosis of a catecholamine-secreting tumor. CT or MRI of the abdomen and pelvis should be the first localization test (sensitivity, >95%; specificity, >65%) [6]. Approximately 85% of these tumors are found in the adrenal glands, and 95% are found in the abdomen and pelvis. The most common locations of catecholamine-secreting PGLs include superior abdominal para-aortic region, 46%; inferior abdominal para-aortic region, 29%; urinary bladder, 10%; mediastinum, 10%; head and neck, 3%; and pelvis, 2% [12].

When the results of abdominal and pelvic imaging are negative in patients with biochemically confirmed catecholamine-secreting PPGL, additional localization imaging is indicated with either gallium 68 (68-Ga) 1,4,7,10-tetraazacyclododecane-1,4,7,10-tetraacetic acid (DOTA)-octreotate (DOTATATE) positron emission tomography (PET) (^{68}Ga-DOTATATE PET) or scintigraphy with iodine 123 (^{123}I) metaiodobenzylguanidine (^{123}I-MIBG). These agents accumulate preferentially in PPGLs. ^{123}I-MIBG scintigraphy is not as sensitive as was initially hoped (sensitivity, 80%; specificity, 99%) [23]. If a typical (<10 cm) unilateral adrenal PHEO is found on CT or MRI, ^{123}I-MIBG scintigraphy is superfluous, and the results may even confuse the clinician [24, 25]. On the other hand, if the adrenal PHEO is more than 10 cm in diameter or if a PGL is identified on CT or MRI, then ^{68}Ga-DOTATATE PET-CT or ^{123}I-MIBG scintigraphy is indicated, because the patient has increased risk of metastatic disease and additional PGLs. ^{68}Ga-DOTATATE PET-CT is proving to be more sensitive in some patients than ^{123}I-MIBG, CT/MRI, or ^{18}F-fluorodeoxyglucose (FDG) PET-CT for detection of metastatic disease [26].

21.5 Treatment

The treatment of choice for PHEO is complete surgical resection. The most common complications are intra-operative blood pressure lability and postoperative hypotension. Careful preoperative pharmacologic preparation is crucial for successful treatment [6, 27]. Most catecholamine-secreting tumors are benign and can be totally excised.

21.5.1 Preoperative Management

Some form of preoperative pharmacologic preparation is indicated for all patients with catecholamine-secreting neoplasms, including those who are asymptomatic and normotensive [6, 27]. However, no randomized controlled trials have compared the different approaches. Combined alpha- and beta-adrenergic blockade is one approach to control blood pressure and prevent intraoperative hypertensive crises. Alpha-adrenergic blockade with either doxazosin or phenoxybenzamine should be started at least 7–10 days preoperatively to normalize blood pressure and expand the contracted blood volume. When compared to doxazosin, use of phenoxybenzamine is more effective in preventing intraoperative hemodynamic instability [28]. A longer duration of preoperative alpha-adrenergic blockade is indicated for patients with recent myocardial infarction, catecholamine cardiomyopathy, or catecholamine-induced vasculitis. Blood pressure should be monitored with the patient in the seated and standing positions twice daily. Target blood pressure is low-normal blood pressure for age (e.g., <120/80 mm Hg in the seated position), with systolic blood pressure greater than 90 mm Hg (standing); both targets should be modified on the basis of the patient's age and comorbid disease. Orthostasis is not a goal of treatment but rather a side effect. Therefore, on the second or third day of alpha-adrenergic blockade, patients are encouraged to start a diet high in sodium content (>5000 mg/day) because of the catecholamine-induced volume contraction and the orthostasis associated with alpha-adrenergic blockade. This degree of volume expansion may be contraindicated in patients with congestive heart failure or renal insufficiency. After adequate alpha-adrenergic blockade has been achieved, beta-adrenergic blockade (e.g., extended release metoprolol) is initiated, typically 2–3 days preoperatively.

21.5.2 Acute Hypertensive Crises

Acute hypertensive crises may occur before or during an operation, and they should be treated with intravenously administered sodium nitroprusside, phentolamine, or nicardipine. Sodium nitroprusside is an ideal vasodilator for intraoperative management of hypertensive episodes because of its rapid onset of action and short duration of effect. Phentolamine is a short-acting, nonselective alpha-adrenergic blocker that is available in lyophilized form in 5-mg vials.

21.6 Indications for Surgery and Details

21.6.1 Adrenalectomy for Pheochromocytoma: Surgical Approach

The definitive treatment of PHEO is surgical resection [6]. Most (90%) PHEOs can be removed by laparoscopic adrenalectomy using either the transperitoneal approach [29] or the retroperitoneal approach [30, 31]. Very large tumors (>6–8 cm on the right or >8–10 cm on the left) may require hand-assisted or open resection. Invasive tumors require open adrenalectomy. Robot-assisted laparoscopic adrenalectomy may help in resecting large adrenal tumors but adds significant time and expense [32, 33]. In general, the choice of surgical approach depends on available local surgical expertise; posterior approach can save operating time for bilateral operation and transabdominal approach is favored for larger tumors or those at risk for conversion to open resection [34, 35].

The standard adrenalectomy for PHEO is complete removal of the tumor and the whole adrenal gland en bloc with periadrenal tissue. All PHEOs should be treated as potentially malignant. Breaching the tumor capsule or fracturing the tumor will lead to tumor cell seeding of the resection bed and cause pheochormocytomatosis and recurrent PHEO [36].

Adrenal Veins The right adrenal vein is short and drains anteriomedially into the inferior vena cava (IVC). The left adrenal vein drains inferiorly, usually joined by the left inferior phrenic vein, then drains into the left renal vein. Understanding the venous anatomy and the variations are crucial to prevent bleeding complications [37]. Life-threatening hemorrhage is usually caused by injury to the IVC on the right or injury to the inferior phrenic vein or splenic vein on the left. Anomalous drainage and/or supernumerary veins also increase the risk of bleeding during dissection. PHEOs, especially larger tumors, are more likely to have multiple or anomalous adrenal veins. Old textbook suggestion of "ligating the adrenal vein first" is rarely practical nor necessary. The tissue attachments around the adrenal vein need to be carefully dissected to free the vein for ligation. This may be easier and safer after some feeding adrenal arteries have already been taken to open the space around the adrenal vein. Once the adrenal vein is ligated and transected, the tumor can become engorged and further dissection bloodier. A vessel sealing device or metal clips are usually used to ligate the main adrenal veins. Very large adrenal veins can be transected with a vascular-load GIA stapler, but only after the length of vein is dissected free enough to safely accommodate the relatively wide tip of the stapler. When using metal clips or staples, careful tactical planning is necessary, because vessel sealer device is ineffective if metal is caught between the jaws.

21.6.2 Perioperative Concerns

Collaboration by an experienced multidisciplinary team of endocrinologists, anesthesiologists and surgeons ensure good perioperative care of patients with PHEO. Preoperative preparation with alpha-adrenergic blockade and volume repletion lessens intraoperative and postoperative hemodynamic instability [6]. Experienced anesthesia team can manage the intraoperative hemodynamic changes with antihypertensive drugs or vasopressors. An arterial line and large bore intravenous lines are usually necessary. Prophylactic antibiotic and stress dose glucocorticoid are not needed routinely. Rarely (<5%) blood transfusion may be required, especially for very large tumors or if large vessels such as the IVC is injured. The blood bank should be prepared and type, and cross of blood products should be considered.

In patients who have been appropriately prepared with alpha-adrenergic or other blockade, hemodynamic fluctuation during the operation can be easily treated by an experienced anesthesiologist. Communication between the surgeon and the anesthesiologist is paramount, especially when the tumor is manipulated and when the adrenal vein is ligated. Vasopressin should be considered for blood pressure support when usual catecholamine type pressors may be less effective.

Immediate postoperative hypoglycemia can occur in 5–10% of patients. It needs to be anticipated and treated. Hypoglycemia is more common in children because of lower glycogen reserve in liver and muscles. Until the patient is fully awake from anesthesia, blood glucose needs to be monitored. Because catecholamine excess worsens diabetes, removing the PHEO usually improve long-term glycemic control. Patients with diabetes mellitus usually will need to lower the dosage of insulin or other anti-glycemic drugs [38].

With appropriate preoperative blockade and operative treatment, most patients can be monitored and treated on the ward after a period of observation in the recovery room. Care in the intensive care unit is needed in about 5–10% of patients whose hemodynamic instability requires continuous monitoring.

21.6.3 Special Cases

Pheochromocytoma Crisis Some patients present with PHEO crisis with multisystem failure. Emergency adrenalectomy is rarely indicated. Urgent or semi-elective adrenalectomy after resuscitation and medical treatment with alpha-adrenergic blockade is associated with lower mortality and morbidity than emergency resection [39].

Pregnancy PHEO during pregnancy is associated with high morbidity and mortality for the mother and fetus, especially if unrecognized [40]. PHEO diagnosed during pregnancy can usually be treated medically with alpha-adrenergic blockade. Alpha-blockade can be continued through pregnancy, and the baby can be delivered at or near term, usually by Cesarean section. Adrenalectomy can be planed a few weeks postpartum with the usual surgical approach. If resection is necessary during pregnancy, adrenalectomy can be performed safely during the second trimester.

21.6.4 Abdominal Paraganglioma

PGLs usually do not have a single main draining vein and usually have multiple feeding arteries from neighboring aorta, renal arteries, or mesentery arteries. Although some PGLs can be safely removed via laparoscopy by experienced surgeons, most will require open resection. The risk of malignancy and recurrence for PGL is higher than for adrenal PHEO. The risk of bleeding is higher because of extensive vascular supply. The risk of compromising the vascular supply to the kidney or the small bowel needs to be considered during resection of PGL.

21.6.5 Subtotal (Partial, Cortex-Sparing) Adrenalectomy

Subtotal adrenalectomy can be considered for some patients with genetic causes of PHEO. The risk of adrenal cortical insufficiency needs to be balanced with the risk of recurrent PHEO and the need for reoperation on the remnant adrenal gland [41, 42]. Patients with von Hippel-Lindau or MEN2A syndromes are potential candidates for subtotal resection, especially if the PHEO is small and located peripherally [43, 44]. About one third to one half of an adrenal gland remnant is usually enough to avoid long-term adrenal cortical insufficiency. Vessel sealing devices are usually used to transect the adrenal gland, to lessen bleeding from the cut edges and lessen shedding of medullary tissue which can be nidus of recurrence. The location of the remnant adrenal gland should be planned to facilitate potential future reoperation for recurrence.

21.7 Outcomes and Recurrences

Overall, the long-term results of laparoscopic adrenalectomy for PHEO are excellent [45–47]. There are several causes of recurrent PHEO. Incomplete resection will cause recurrent tumor in the resection bed. Fracturing the tumor will cause pheochromocytomatosis that can be both in the resection bed and with intraperitoneal dissemination [48]. PHEO cancer can metastasize, most commonly to the liver. Patient can also develop additional primary tumor because of genetic predisposition, usually in the contralateral adrenal gland or in a remnant gland after a subtotal resection.

Because of the risk of recurrence, all patients with PPGL should have at least a yearly follow up, with measurement of tumor markers associated with the originally resected PPGL, such as plasma-free fractionated metanephrines. If there is evidence of recurrence by tumor markers or symptoms, imaging studies should follow. Genetic screening, if not already done, facilitates the most appropriate follow-up.

In addition to CT scan and MRI, I-123 MIBG, F18-FDG PET-CT, or Ga68 DOTATATE PET-CT scans can be used to localize recurrences. If a recurrence is resectable, surgery is preferred. Debulking surgery, if able to remove more than 90% of tumor mass, should be considered. The role of other local ablative treatments, such as radiofrequency ablation, is being investigated [49, 50]. For non-resectable PHEO, systemic treatment options may include high-dose I-131 MIBG [51] or lutetium Lu 177 DOTATATE [52].

Key Points

- The clinical presentation of approximately 60% of all patients with adrenal PHEO is that of an adrenal incidentaloma.
- Many patients with catecholamine-secreting PPGL are asymptomatic.
- When a patient has a PGL, total body imaging with either Ga-68 DOTATATE PET-CT or 123-I-MIBG is indicated to screen for additional PGLs or metastatic disease.
- When a patient has more than one PHEO or PGL, the probability of a germline pathogenic variant in a PPGL susceptibility gene is 100%.
- Following surgical resection, all patients with PPGL should be followed with annual biochemical testing for life because all PPGLs have malignant potential.
- In patients with pathogenic variants in SDHx, periodic imaging from skull base to pelvis is indicated to detect nonfunctioning PGLs.

Answers to the Questions

1. (c); 2. (d); 3. (a); 4. (a); 5. (c); 6. (c); 7. (e); 8. (a); 9. (d); 10. (c); 11. (b); 12. (e)

References

1. Neumann HPH, Young WF Jr, Eng C. Pheochromocytoma and paraganglioma. N Engl J Med. 2019;381(6):552–65.
2. Stenstrom G, Svardsudd K. Pheochromocytoma in Sweden 1958–1981. An analysis of the National Cancer Registry Data. Acta Med Scand. 1986;220(3):225–32.
3. Young WF Jr. Pheochromocytoma: 1926-1993. Trends Endocrinol Metab. 1993;4(4):122–7.

4. Gruber L, Young WF, Bancos I. Pheochromocytoma characteristics and behavior differ depending on method of discovery. J Clin Endocrinol Metab. 2019;104(5):1386–93.
5. Young WF Jr, Maddox DE. Spells: in search of a cause. Mayo Clin Proc. 1995;70(8):757–65.
6. Lenders JW, Duh QY, Eisenhofer G, Gimenez-Roqueplo AP, Grebe SK, Murad MH, et al. Pheochromocytoma and paraganglioma: an endocrine society clinical practice guideline. J Clin Endocrinol Metab. 2014;99(6):1915–42.
7. Giavarini A, Chedid A, Bobrie G, Plouin PF, Hagege A, Amar L. Acute catecholamine cardiomyopathy in patients with phaeochromocytoma or functional paraganglioma. Heart. 2013;99(19):1438–44.
8. Oshmyansky AR, Mahammedi A, Dackiw A, Ball DW, Schulick RD, Zeiger MA, et al. Serendipity in the diagnosis of pheochromocytoma. J Comput Assist Tomogr. 2013;37(5):820–3.
9. Motta-Ramirez GA, Remer EM, Herts BR, Gill IS, Hamrahian AH. Comparison of CT findings in symptomatic and incidentally discovered pheochromocytomas. AJR Am J Roentgenol. 2005;185(3):684–8.
10. Wachtel H, Cerullo I, Bartlett EK, Roses RE, Cohen DL, Kelz RR, et al. Clinicopathologic characteristics of incidentally identified pheochromocytoma. Ann Surg Oncol. 2015;22(1):132–8.
11. Kinney MA, Warner ME, van Heerden JA, Horlocker TT, Young WF, Schroeder DR, et al. Perianesthetic risks and outcomes of pheochromocytoma and paraganglioma resection. Anesth Analg. 2000;91(5):1118–23.
12. Erickson D, Kudva YC, Ebersold MJ, Thompson GB, Grant CS, van Heerden JA, et al. Benign paragangliomas: clinical presentation and treatment outcomes in 236 patients. J Clin Endocrinol Metab. 2001;86(11):5210–6.
13. Yan Q, Bancos I, Gruber LM, Bancos C, McKenzie TJ, Babovic-Vuksanovic D, et al. When biochemical phenotype predicts genotype: pheochromocytoma and paraganglioma. Am J Med. 2018;131(5):506–9.
14. Neumann HP, Young WF Jr, Krauss T, Bayley JP, Schiavi F, Opocher G, et al. 65 years of the double helix: genetics informs precision practice in the diagnosis and management of pheochromocytoma. Endocr Relat Cancer. 2018;25(8):T201–T19.
15. Yamazaki Y, Gao X, Pecori A, Nakamura Y, Tezuka Y, Omata K, et al. Recent advances in histopathological and molecular diagnosis in pheochromocytoma and paraganglioma: challenges for predicting metastasis in individual patients. Front Endocrinol. 2020;11:587769.
16. Astuti D, Douglas F, Lennard TW, Aligianis IA, Woodward ER, Evans DG, et al. Germline SDHD mutation in familial phaeochromocytoma. Lancet. 2001;357(9263):1181–2.
17. Baysal BE. Mitochondrial complex II and genomic imprinting in inheritance of paraganglioma tumors. Biochim Biophys Acta. 2013;1827(5):573–7.
18. Young AL, Baysal BE, Deb A, Young WF Jr. Familial malignant catecholamine-secreting paraganglioma with prolonged survival associated with mutation in the succinate dehydrogenase B gene. J Clin Endocrinol Metab. 2002;87(9):4101–5.
19. Godfrey JA, Rickman OB, Williams AW, Thompson GB, Young WF Jr. Pheochromocytoma in a patient with end-stage renal disease. Mayo Clin Proc. 2001;76(9):953–7.
20. Marini M, Fathi M, Vallotton M. Determination of serum metanephrines in the diagnosis of pheochromocytoma. Ann Endocrinol (Paris). 1994;54(5):337–42.

21. Stumvoll M, Radjaipour M, Seif F. Diagnostic considerations in pheochromocytoma and chronic hemodialysis: case report and review of the literature. Am J Nephrol. 1995;15(2):147–51.
22. Morioka M, Yuihama S, Nakajima T, Kobayashi T, Sone A, Furukawa Y, et al. Incidentally discovered pheochromocytoma in long-term hemodialysis patients. Int J Urol. 2002;9(12):700–3.
23. Wiseman GA, Pacak K, O'Dorisio MS, Neumann DR, Waxman AD, Mankoff DA, et al. Usefulness of 123I-MIBG scintigraphy in the evaluation of patients with known or suspected primary or metastatic pheochromocytoma or paraganglioma: results from a prospective multicenter trial. J Nucl Med. 2009;50(9):1448–54.
24. Miskulin J, Shulkin BL, Doherty GM, Sisson JC, Burney RE, Gauger PG. Is preoperative iodine 123 meta-iodobenzylguanidine scintigraphy routinely necessary before initial adrenalectomy for pheochromocytoma? Surgery. 2003;134(6):918–22. discussion 22-3
25. van Berkel A, Pacak K, Lenders JW. Should every patient diagnosed with a phaeochromocytoma have a (1)(2)(3) I-MIBG scintigraphy? Clin Endocrinol. 2014;81(3):329–33.
26. Janssen I, Blanchet EM, Adams K, Chen CC, Millo CM, Herscovitch P, et al. Superiority of [68Ga]-DOTATATE PET/CT to other functional imaging modalities in the localization of SDHB-associated metastatic pheochromocytoma and paraganglioma. Clin Cancer Res. 2015;21(17):3888–95.
27. Weingarten TN, Welch TL, Moore TL, Walters GF, Whipple JL, Cavalcante A, et al. Preoperative levels of catecholamines and metanephrines and intraoperative hemodynamics of patients undergoing pheochromocytoma and paraganglioma resection. Urology. 2017;100:131–8.
28. Buitenwerf E, Osinga TE, Timmers H, Lenders JWM, Feelders RA, Eekhoff EMW, et al. Efficacy of alpha-blockers on hemodynamic control during pheochromocytoma resection: a randomized controlled trial. J Clin Endocrinol Metab. 2020;105(7):2381–91.
29. Gagner M, Lacroix A, Bolte E. Laparoscopic adrenalectomy in Cushing's syndrome and pheochromocytoma. N Engl J Med. 1992;327(14):1033.
30. Mercan S, Seven R, Ozarmagan S, Tezelman S. Endoscopic retroperitoneal adrenalectomy. Surgery. 1995;118(6):1071–5. discussion 5-6
31. Walz MK, Peitgen K, Hoermann R, Giebler RM, Mann K, Eigler FW. Posterior retroperitoneoscopy as a new minimally invasive approach for adrenalectomy: results of 30 adrenalectomies in 27 patients. World J Surg. 1996;20(7):769–74.
32. Brunaud L, Ayav A, Zarnegar R, Rouers A, Klein M, Boissel P, et al. Prospective evaluation of 100 robotic-assisted unilateral adrenalectomies. Surgery. 2008;144(6):995–1001; discussion
33. Greilsamer T, Nomine-Criqui C, Thy M, Ullmann T, Zarnegar R, Bresler L, et al. Robotic-assisted unilateral adrenalectomy: risk factors for perioperative complications in 303 consecutive patients. Surg Endosc. 2019;33(3):802–10.
34. Barczynski M, Konturek A, Nowak W. Randomized clinical trial of posterior retroperitoneoscopic adrenalectomy versus lateral transperitoneal laparoscopic adrenalectomy with a 5-year follow-up. Ann Surg. 2014;260(5):740–7. discussion 7-8
35. Marrero AP, Kazaure HS, Thomas SM, Stang MT, Scheri RP. Patient selection and outcomes of laparoscopic transabdominal versus posterior retroperitoneal adrenalectomy among surgeons in the Collaborative Endocrine Surgery Quality Improvement Program (CESQIP). Surgery. 2020;167(1):250–6.

36. Li ML, Fitzgerald PA, Price DC, Norton JA. Iatrogenic pheochromocytomatosis: a previously unreported result of laparoscopic adrenalectomy. Surgery. 2001;130(6):1072–7.
37. Scholten A, Cisco RM, Vriens MR, Shen WT, Duh QY. Variant adrenal venous anatomy in 546 laparoscopic adrenalectomies. JAMA Surg. 2013;148(4):378–83.
38. Beninato T, Kluijfhout WP, Drake FT, Lim J, Kwon JS, Xiong M, et al. Resection of pheochromocytoma improves diabetes mellitus in the majority of patients. Ann Surg Oncol. 2017;24(5):1208–13.
39. Scholten A, Cisco RM, Vriens MR, Cohen JK, Mitmaker EJ, Liu C, et al. Pheochromocytoma crisis is not a surgical emergency. J Clin Endocrinol Metab. 2013;98(2):581–91.
40. Bancos I, Atkinson E, Eng C, Young WF Jr, Neumann HPH, et al. Maternal and fetal outcomes in phaeochromocytoma and pregnancy: a multicentre retrospective cohort study and systematic review of literature. Lancet Diabetes Endocrinol. 2021;9(1):13–21.
41. Hahner S, Spinnler C, Fassnacht M, Burger-Stritt S, Lang K, Milovanovic D, et al. High incidence of adrenal crisis in educated patients with chronic adrenal insufficiency: a prospective study. J Clin Endocrinol Metab. 2015;100(2):407–16.
42. Neumann HPH, Tsoy U, Bancos I, Amodru V, Walz MK, Tirosh A, et al. Comparison of pheochromocytoma-specific morbidity and mortality among adults with bilateral pheochromocytomas undergoing total adrenalectomy vs cortical-sparing adrenalectomy. JAMA Netw Open. 2019;2(8):e198898.
43. Benhammou JN, Boris RS, Pacak K, Pinto PA, Linehan WM, Bratslavsky G. Functional and oncologic outcomes of partial adrenalectomy for pheochromocytoma in patients with von Hippel-Lindau syndrome after at least 5 years of followup. J Urol. 2010;184(5):1855–9.
44. Castinetti F, Qi XP, Walz MK, Maia AL, Sanso G, Peczkowska M, et al. Outcomes of adrenal-sparing surgery or total adrenalectomy in phaeochromocytoma associated with multiple endocrine neoplasia type 2: an international retrospective population-based study. Lancet Oncol. 2014;15(6):648–55.
45. Walz MK, Alesina PF, Wenger FA, Koch JA, Neumann HP, Petersenn S, et al. Laparoscopic and retroperitoneoscopic treatment of pheochromocytomas and retroperitoneal paragangliomas: results of 161 tumors in 126 patients. World J Surg. 2006;30(5):899–908.
46. Shen WT, Grogan R, Vriens M, Clark OH, Duh QY. One hundred two patients with pheochromocytoma treated at a single institution since the introduction of laparoscopic adrenalectomy. Arch Surg. 2010;145(9):893–7.
47. Chen Y, Scholten A, Chomsky-Higgins K, Nwaogu I, Gosnell JE, Seib C, et al. Risk factors associated with perioperative complications and prolonged length of stay after laparoscopic adrenalectomy. JAMA Surg. 2018;153(11):1036–41.
48. Rafat C, Zinzindohoue F, Hernigou A, Hignette C, Favier J, Tenenbaum F, et al. Peritoneal implantation of pheochromocytoma following tumor capsule rupture during surgery. J Clin Endocrinol Metab. 2014;99(12):E2681–5.
49. Deljou A, Kohlenberg JD, Weingarten TN, Bancos I, Young WF Jr, Schroeder DR, et al. Hemodynamic instability during percutaneous ablation of extra-adrenal metastases of pheochromocytoma and paragangliomas: a case series. BMC Anesthesiol. 2018;18(1):158.
50. Kohlenberg J, Welch B, Hamidi O, Callstrom M, Morris J, Sprung J, et al. Efficacy and safety of ablative therapy in the treatment of patients with metastatic pheochromocytoma and paraganglioma. Cancers (Basel). 2019;11(2):195.

51. Pryma DA, Chin BB, Noto RB, Dillon JS, Perkins S, Solnes L, et al. Efficacy and safety of high-specific-activity (131)I-MIBG therapy in patients with advanced pheochromocytoma or paraganglioma. J Nucl Med. 2019;60(5):623–30.
52. Kong G, Grozinsky-Glasberg S, Hofman MS, Callahan J, Meirovitz A, Maimon O, et al. Efficacy of peptide receptor radionuclide therapy for functional metastatic paraganglioma and pheochromocytoma. J Clin Endocrinol Metab. 2017;102(9):3278–87.

Adrenocortical Carcinoma, Adrenal Lymphoma and Metastases to Adrenal Gland

Mechteld C. de Jong, Shahab Khan, and Radu Mihai

Contents

A. L. Shifrin et al. (eds.), *Endocrine Surgery Comprehensive Board Exam Guide*,
https://doi.org/10.1007/978-3-030-84737-1_22

Case Presentation

The patient is a 50-year-old female who was presented with left flank pain for 3 months associated with nausea, significant weight loss and reduced appetite. She also had an episode of haematuria. Past medical history was significant for anxiety and depression, with the former increasing over recent months as well. There is no significant comorbidity. Medication includes quetiapine, sertraline and propranolol. On physical examination, her vital signs are within normal range, and her abdomen is soft with some mild tenderness in the left upper quadrant with a palpable fullness over this area.

A CT of the abdomen and pelvis with contrast was performed, showing a large heterogeneous high-attenuation mass originating from the left adrenal gland. The mass measured approximately 14 cm in the greatest dimension. The mass was pushing the left kidney inferiorly and the small and large bowel loops anteriorly. The left renal vein appeared to be thrombosed. Minor clot burden was also noted at the confluence of the left renal vein and the inferior vena cava (IVC).

A subsequent whole-body PET/CT scan showed the large necrotic left adrenal mass to be markedly FDG-avid (SUVmax = 16.5). The tumour was invading the left renal vein with tumour thrombus extending into the IVC. There was a concern for invasion into the upper pole of the left kidney. There was no evidence of distant disease.

Urine metanephrines were all within normal ranges: 3-methoxytyramine = 50 nmol/mmol (normal, 0–220 nmol/mmol), metadrenaline = 60 nmol/mmol (normal, 0–150 nmol/mmol) and normetadrenalin = 360 nmol/mmol (normal, 0–450 nmol/mmol). In addition, her laboratory data show increased levels of androstenedione = 25.9 nmol/L (normal, 3–8 nmol/L), dehydroepiandrosterone sulphate = 62.1 umol/L (normal, 0.0–10.4) and testosterone = 7.2 nmol/L (normal, 0.5–2.6 nmol/L). Her urine steroid profile showed high concentrations of dehydroepiandrosterone = 115,210 μg/L (normal $\mu = 327 \pm 244$) and androstenedione = 44,955 μg/L (normal $\mu = 770 \pm 420$).

Questions

1. A 36-year-old patient presents at the emergency room with severe hypertension (210/110 mmHg) and right upper quadrant pain. He is very anxious and sweaty. His routine bloods are normal. A CT scan identifies a 10 cm right adrenal mass. The next step should be:
   1. Measure plasma metanephrines' level.
   2. Cancel the previously planned biopsy of this mass.
   3. Measure the blood response to a 40 mg propranolol dose.
   4. Check full blood count and blood film for possible lymphoma.

   (a) Only (1) and (2) and (3) are correct.
   (b) Only (1) and (2) and (4) are correct.
   (c) Only (3) is correct.
   (d) Only (1) and (2) are correct.
   (e) All are correct.
2. A 56-year-old patient presents with abdominal pain and microscopic blood in urine. A computed tomography of kidneys, ureters and bladder is performed to look for renal stones. An 8 cm left suprarenal mass is seen consistent with adrenal origin. The next steps should be:

1. Arrange PET/CT (depending on the biochemical work-up).
2. Check urine/plasma metanephrines.
3. Refer to appropriate MDT.
4. Arrange biopsy of mass.
   (a) Only (1) and (2) and (3) are correct.
   (b) Only (1) and (2) and (4) are correct.
   (c) Only (3) is correct.
   (d) Only (1) and (2) are correct.
   (e) All are correct.

3. An 88-year-old male with heart failure and dementia is referred from nursing home with abdominal pains. CT scan reveals a 12 cm right adrenal mass with suspicion of invasion into the IVC and liver. The next appropriate steps would be:
   1. Refer to MDT.
   2. Palliative care.
   3. PET/CT.
   4. Check urine steroid profile.
      (a) Only (1) and (2) and (3) are correct.
      (b) Only (1) and (2) and (4) are correct.
      (c) Only (3) is correct.
      (d) Only (1) and (2) are correct.
      (e) All are correct.
4. A 45-year-old female attends with suspected gallstones and has an MRCP. This reveals gallstones and an incidental 10 cm right adrenal mass with tumour extension into the IVC. The next steps should be:
   1. PET/CT.
   2. Urine metanephrines and steroid profile.
   3. Refer to MDT with plan for mitotane chemotherapy.
   4. Refer to MDT with plan for surgical excision.
      (a) Only (1) and (2) and (3) are correct.
      (b) Only (1) and (2) and (4) are correct.
      (c) Only (3) is correct.
      (d) Only (1) and (2) are correct.
      (e) All are correct.
5. An 80-year-old fit and healthy patient with a previous history of surgically excised sigmoid cancer 6 years ago is referred with an enlarging PET-avid right adrenal mass measuring 22 mm. It is suspected to be a metastasis. This is the sole site of recurrence. The next steps should include:
   1. Refer to MDT.
   2. Biopsy of the lesion.
   3. Check renin/angiotensin levels.
   4. Check urine steroid profile.
      (a) Only (1) and (2) and (3) are correct.
      (b) Only (1) and (2) and (4) are correct.
      (c) Only (3) is correct.
      (d) Only (1) and (2) are correct.
      (e) All are correct.

6. The correct treatment for a 22 mm isolated left adrenal metastasis could include:
   1. Laparoscopic resection
   2. Retroperitoneoscopic resection
   3. Open surgery
   4. Radiotherapy
      (a) Only (1) and (2) and (3) are correct.
      (b) Only (1) and (2) and (4) are correct.
      (c) Only (3) is correct.
      (d) Only (1) and (2) are correct.
      (e) All are correct.
7. A 70-year-old male presents with marked weight loss, nausea, anorexia, orthostatic dizziness and joint pain. On clinical suspicion, a paired morning cortisol and ACTH are taken, revealing a decreased cortisol with a raised ACTH. A contrast-enhanced CT revealed bilateral adrenal masses. It is suspected to be bilateral lymphoma with adrenal insufficiency. The next steps should include:
   1. Refer to MDT.
   2. Biopsy of the lesion.
   3. Check urine metanephrines.
   4. Check urine steroid profile.
      (a) Only (1) and (2) and (3) are correct.
      (b) Only (1) and (2) and (4) are correct.
      (c) Only (3) is correct.
      (d) Only (1) and (2) are correct.
      (e) All are correct.
8. An 85-year-old patient presenting with intentional weight loss undergoes a CT scan which reveals bilateral adrenal masses, measuring 3.4 × 3.2 cm lesion on the right side and a 3.1 × 2.2 cm lesion on the left side. A subsequent biopsy shows diffuse large B-cell lymphoma.

The next steps should include:
   1. Refer to MDT.
   2. Check urine metanephrines and urine steroid profile.
   3. Check paired morning cortisol and ACTH.
   4. Laparoscopic removal of the largest tumour.
      (a) Only (1) and (2) and (3) are correct.
      (b) Only (1) and (2) and (4) are correct.
      (c) Only (4) is correct.
      (d) Only (1) and (3) are correct.
      (e) All are correct.

22.1 Introduction

The adrenal glands are frequently affected by a wide variety of growths that either cause symptoms or are found incidentally on cross-sectional imaging performed for not related issues. Their overall incidence is about 3–10% for the whole population and is increasing with the age [1]. The majority of these tumours are small, benign and non-functioning adenomas. This chapter will focus on three rare entities: adrenocortical carcinoma (ACC), primary adrenal lymphoma (PAL) and metastases to adrenal gland from other primary tumour sites.

22.2 Adrenocortical Carcinoma

22.2.1 Clinical Presentation

Adrenocortical carcinoma (ACC) is a rare tumour with an incidence of one to two/million population/year. It often presents at an advanced stage, and the median age at the time of diagnosis is in the fifth or sixth decade of life [2].

About two-thirds of patients present with signs of increased hormone secretion (i.e. Cushing's syndrome, virilization in females, feminization in males) [3]. Although cortisol overproduction is the most common (~40%), in the majority of patients, the tumour produces a range of hormones including both glucocorticoids and sex hormones [3, 4]. The overproduction of aldosterone is very rare [4].

Another one-third of patients present with symptoms related to the size and mass effect of their (large) tumour (i.e. pain, abdominal distension, early satiety, nausea/vomiting, weight loss, leg oedema) [3, 5]. The average diameter of palpable ACCs is about 12–15 cm, with a weight of >500 g [6].

More recently, an increasing number of ACCs are discovered as incidentalomas on cross-sectional imaging done for other indications [6, 7].

A minority of patients can be identified during screening of families with genetic mutations known to be associated with increased risk of ACC (e.g. Li-Fraumeni, multiple endocrine neoplasia type 1, Lynch syndrome, familial adenomatous polyposis, Gardner syndrome and Beckwith-Wiedemann syndrome) [5, 8].

22.2.2 Natural History

ACC has a dismal prognosis with an overall 5-year survival of <30%. This is partly due to the nature of the tumour and partly due to the often late presentation. In an analysis including 320 patients with stage III and IV disease [9], the outcomes for patients who did not undergo surgery were very poor, with a 1-year survival of ~15%.

Sites of metastatic disease include regional lymph nodes (25–46%), lungs (45–97%), the liver (48–96%) and bones (11–33%) [10].

22.2.3 Diagnosis

(i) *Clinical suspicion*

Both the presentation with symptoms of newly onset and rapid progression of hypersecretion of adrenal hormones and a palpable abdominal tumour are highly suspicious for a malignancy.

(ii) *Biochemical assessment*

As for all adrenal tumours, initial biochemical assessment should include:

- Plasma-free levels of metanephrines (to exclude phaeochromocytoma).
- Measurements of urinary free cortisol levels and overnight 1 mg dexamethasone suppression test (formal assessment of glucocorticoid axis).
- Measurements of DHEAS (dehydroepiandrosterone sulphate) and androstenedione for assessment of androgen secretion.
- Determination of plasma renin activity and aldosterone concentration is reserved for those individuals with hypertension (though aldosterone is seldom secreted by ACC).
- A urine steroid profiling can be undertaken [11]. This is a highly sensitive and specific biomarker tool for malignant adrenal lesions, as a pattern of predominantly immature, early-stage steroidogenesis can be seen in the urine of patients with ACC [11–13].
- Measurement of serum electrolytes should be done in all patients, as adrenal steroids can induce severe hypokalaemia needing preoperative correction.

(iii) *Cross-sectional imaging*

Most ACCs are large at presentation, with a diameter of >6 cm in over 90% of cases [14, 15], and there is an increasing risk of malignancy for larger tumours.

While the risk of malignancy is thought to be already considerably high at ~20% for tumours >6 cm, this increases to ~50% for those larger than 8 cm [16]. The risk of a tumour smaller than 4 cm being malignant was found to be considerably lower, hence the recommendation of adrenalectomy for non-functional incidentalomas measuring larger than 4 cm.

Other characteristics of ACC on computed tomography (CT) scan, besides a relatively large tumour size, include a well-defined margin with a thin enhancing rim, a central area of low attenuation and a tendency for extension into the inferior vena cava [15]. Relatively high unenhanced CT scan attenuation values (>10 Hounsfield units (HU)) on non-contrast CT scan have a high sensitivity for diagnosing ACC but a rather low specificity [14, 15, 17].

On magnetic resonance imaging (MRI scan), ACC appears iso- or hypo-intense compared to the liver on T1-weighted images, while their appearance is hyper-intense on T2-weighted images [14, 18]. The chemical shifting that is usually seen in benign lipid-rich adenomas is virtually absent in the contrast-enhanced MR images of patients with ACC.

(iv) *Functional molecular imaging*

The majority of ACCs are avid on positron emission tomography/computed tomography (PET/CT) labelled with fluorine-18 fluorodeoxyglucose (FDG). The sensitivity and specificity for the diagnosis of ACC on FDG-PET/CT are high, at around 95% for both [19–21]. However, as metastatic lesions in the adrenal gland give a similar appearance, the FDG-PET/CT should not be used as a standalone diagnostic modality.

Imaging with ^{123}I-iodometomidate (i.e. radioactive iodine-labelled metomidate) is another promising imaging modality. Metomidate has a high affinity for 11β-hydroxylase, which is an enzyme located in the cortex of the adrenal gland that is essential in the synthesis of the hormones aldosterone and cortisol [21, 22]. In a study of 430 lesions, metomidate PET had 100% specificity, but a many lesions failed to show uptake leading to a low sensitivity of 38% [22].

(v) *Biopsy is not indicated*

Biopsy is not indicated in the work-up of possible ACC in order to avoid rupture of the capsule and spilling of tumour cells [6]. In general, adrenal biopsy should only be considered when primary adrenal lymphoma (PAL) is suspected or when trying to demonstrate adrenal metastases, as discussed later in this chapter.

(vi) *Histological assessment*

The difference between ACC and a benign adrenal tumour can be challenging. Some of the histological features associated with malignancy (capsular invasion or vascular invasion) can also be encountered in benign adrenal adenomas.

The *Weiss scoring system* remains the standard for the diagnosis of ACC. This score is based on the assessment of nine morphological parameters at light microscopy: nuclear grade, mitotic rate >5 per 50 HPFs, atypical mitotic figures, diffuse architecture, necrosis, venous invasion, and invasion of tumour capsule. A score <3 defines benign adenomas, a score >6 is associated with ACC, and a score of 3–6 raises suspicion of malignancy.

The proliferation marker Ki67 is considered an important prognostic marker for recurrence-free survival and overall survival. For example, in a study of over 300 patients, the clinical outcome differed significantly between patients with Ki67 <10%, 10–19% and >20% (median overall survival, 180 versus 113 versus 42 months) [23].

22.2.4 Treatment

Surgery is considered the only curative treatment. Patients with locally advanced disease treated without surgery have poor survival [9]. This will later be discussed in more details.

Adrenolytic chemotherapy with mitotane can be given either as adjuvant or palliative therapy. Mitotane is an isomer of dichlorodiphenyltrichloroethane (DDT) that is directly cytotoxic to adrenal tissue [24]. In the palliative setting, the aim of mitotane treatment is both the control of tumour growth progression and the reduction of hormone secretion. It has severe side effects (e.g. anorexia, nausea and vomiting but also adrenal insufficiency and crisis in some patients); moreover, the target therapeutic level and toxic range are narrowly together (14–20 ng/dL). While mitotane is frequently used as a monotherapy, for more aggressive tumours, it can be combined with chemotherapy treatment [25]. Based on the results of an international randomized trial (FIRM-ACT trial), mitotane plus etoposide, doxorubicin and cisplatin is now the established first-line cytotoxic therapy owing to a higher response rate and longer median progression-free survival than achieved with streptozocin-mitotane.

Retrospective studies on the use of adjuvant mitotane in ACC have shown mixed results [24]. A prospective randomized trial (ADIUVO) is currently recruiting patients, and possibly its results will impact on future protocols for ACC.

Although there are no guidelines that currently advise neoadjuvant medical treatment for ACC, clinicians at MD Anderson [26] described preoperative systemic treatment for patients with *borderline resectable tumours*, in order to achieve reduction of tumour burden. They reported a prolonged disease-free survival for those who underwent surgery after downstaging neoadjuvant systemic therapy.

Radiotherapy for ACC is limited because of technical difficulties to limit the irradiation field of the adrenal bed without affecting surrounding viscera. In a study of 78 patients treated at the University of Michigan, USA, the 3-year overall survival estimate for patients improved from 48.6% for patients without RT to 77.7% with RT (HR, 3.59) [27]. In addition, a systematic review of 362 citations showed that adjuvant RT dramatically reduces the local recurrence of ACC after surgery and that the treatment has a low acute and late toxicity, resulting in a high therapeutic index [28].

22.2.4.1 Indications for Surgery and Surgical Details

Complete surgical resection of the ACC is the backbone of treatment for localized disease.

For tumours not invading surrounding organs, guidelines advise to remove the adrenal gland and the surrounding fat and lymph node tissue. There is little data supporting a benefit of a more extensive lymph node dissection [6, 29]. Although lymph node dissection obviously does aid in the correct tumour staging, its influence on overall and disease-free survival remains controversial [30].

A topic of debate is the type of surgical approach that should be employed for these patients, i.e. an open resection or a minimally invasive approach. In general, the main objective is to obtain a complete R0 excision without tumour spill, including at least a nodal dissection of the renal pedicle. While open resection in the hands of an experienced adrenal surgeon currently is the gold standard for operative management of this disease [7], there are some studies supporting the performance of a laparoscopic resection, at least for a selected set of patients with small tumours.

Available data show that, as for other diseases, a laparoscopic approach is associated with a shorter length of stay, at least for tumours measuring ≤10 cm [31]. Moreover, a recent review of non-randomized controlled trials [32] reported that for patients with localized/locally advanced primary ACC, a laparoscopic approach seems to be comparable to a laparotomy not only in terms of obtaining negative surgical margins but also when addressing overall recurrence, disease-free survival and overall survival.

In order to achieve R0 resection margins, wide en bloc resection is necessary for many large tumours. As the cranial border of the perirenal space is not covered by Gerota's fascia, invasion of the liver and/or diaphragm (right-sided tumour) or spleen, pancreas and/or diaphragm (left-sided tumour) might occur and can sometimes only be appreciated during the surgical procedure [6, 10]. For these patients, an en bloc resection that includes not only the tumour but also the kidney, the adjacent invaded organs and the entire continuity of peri-adrenal and perirenal fat might be indicated in order to achieve negative margins [6]. Although only limited data exists to provide precise guidance, it is generally considered that the threshold for en bloc resection of adjacent organs should be low, mainly if there is macroscopic suspicion of invasion [8]. For such cases, an open adrenalectomy is the preferred approach.

An important subgroup of patients is those in whom the inferior vena cava is involved by tumour. In general, this involvement consists more often of a caval tumour thrombus than of actual direct tumour extension into the venous wall [6, 33, 34]. For these patients, a formal thrombectomy should be undertaken. When there is frank invasion of the wall of the vena cava, this is usually only over a limited tract and is therefore amenable for partial caval resection with direct closure or by a patch. It has been shown that large vessel extension of the ACC is associated with poorer overall and recurrence-free survival [35].

Data on surgical debulking for ACC are scarce, but in general, several studies have shown that progression-free survival is similar in patients who undergo debulking (i.e. R2 resections) and for those treated non-surgically [36, 37]. Therefore, current guidelines state that only in selected cases (e.g. patients with severe hormone excess or serious symptoms from the tumour's mass effect such as vena cava compression), debulking surgery might be an option. It is generally advised that surgery should be considered if >80% of the tumour burden can be removed [38].

There is an ongoing effort to identify methods to centralize surgery for ACC, as the current service provision is unsatisfactory. The European Society of Endocrine Surgeons reviewed the evidence for a volume-outcome correlation in adrenal surgery and made the recommendations that adrenal surgery should continue only in centres performing at least 6 cases per year and that surgery for adrenocortical cancer should be restricted to centres performing at least 12 adrenal operations per year. Moreover, an integrated multidisciplinary team should be established in all such centres [39]. How this should be achieved will vary in each country. It is, however, the duty of every clinician to provide patients with the correct advice before reaching an informed decision about referral to a regional centre where appropriate expertise exists for the care of patients with such an aggressive malignancy.

22.2.5 Outcomes or Prognosis

ACC remains a disease with a dismal prognosis, with a reported overall 5-year survival rate between 16% and 47% [25, 40]. For the very few patients with stage I disease (i.e. tumours <5 cm with no signs of lymph node or distant metastases), median survival could be in excess of 10 years, but those with stage IV disease (distant metastases) are unlikely to survive more than 1 year after initial diagnosis [41]. Overall, ACC is a diverse cancer, and outcomes may therefore vary even among patients within the same tumour stage, due to the largely still unknown impact of different clinical, pathological and molecular factors [42].

22.3 Metastases to the Adrenal Gland

22.3.1 Clinical Presentation

The adrenal glands can be infiltrated with metastases from a variety of oncological diseases [43]. Moreover, metastatic tumours are the most common lesions of the adrenal gland at post-mortem examinations [44]. Adrenal metastases most commonly occur in patients with lung cancer, breast cancer, melanoma, renal cancer and gastrointestinal carcinomas [45, 46].

The typical route of spread is generally understood to be haematogenous, with the tumour cells nesting in the adrenal gland while travelling through its sinusoid-like blood vessel network. However, for lung cancer, there might be lymphatic spread instead [47].

Clinical presentation is usually silent, as metastatic lesions fail to destruct enough adrenal tissue to produce clinical signs or symptoms of insufficiency, although there are case reports of Addison's crisis due to bilateral adrenal metastases [48–55]. Consequently, most adrenal metastases are picked up on follow-up imaging.

As the cancer-related mortality for most malignancies has decreased over the past decades and patients therefore have a longer survival, the incidence of adrenal metastases diagnosed during oncological follow-up has gone up. Moreover, with the concomitant increased use of more protocolized follow-up regimens, these metastases are detected at an earlier stage.

22.3.2 Natural History

As adrenal metastases are always a sign of spreading of the primary malignant disease, not treating these lesions will result in a shorter survival. In a review of seven studies discussing the non-surgical treatment of adrenal metastases from different primary tumours, there were large variances per primary tumour site, and the median overall survival was poor (3–15 months) [43].

22.3.3 Diagnosis

As stated earlier, most metastatic adrenal lesions are silent in their presentation, and the diagnosis is therefore usually made on imaging scans which are part of the work-up for patients' initial disease.

Specific characteristics of adrenal metastases on computed tomography (CT) scan include their irregular shape and inhomogeneous nature, their tendency to be bilateral, their high unenhanced CT scan attenuation values (>20 Hounsfield units

(HU)) and their enhancement with intravenous contrast on CT scan [56]. Moreover, there is a distinct delay in contrast medium washout (an absolute contrast medium washout of less than 50% at 10 minutes post administration of contrast). This latter is mainly due to the increased microvascular density, which causes a slower flow of contrast fluid exiting the tumour, and to a high endothelial permeability resulting in accumulation of contrast fluid within the tumour [57]. Furthermore, some authors suggest that every isolated adrenal mass 'inciden-taloma' measuring more than 3 cm in diameter in patients with a known history of cancer should be interpreted as suspicious for metastasis [58].

On magnetic resonance imaging (MRI scan), metastatic adrenal lesions generally are isointense or slightly less intense than the liver on T1-weighted images and have a high to intermediate signal intensity on T2-weighted MRI [59].

Due to their increased glucose metabolism, most adrenal metastases are avid on positron emission tomography/computed tomography (PET/CT) labelled with fluorine-18 fluorodeoxyglucose (FDG) [60, 61]. Several authors have reported a sensitivity of over 90% with a specificity close to 100% for FDG-PET/CT to differentiate benign from malignant adrenal lesions [62, 63].

The role of biopsy for adrenal lesions has been somewhat controversial. While open biopsy of the adrenal gland has now been abandoned in the work-up, most authors agree that CT- or US-guided fine-needle aspiration (FNA) cytology can be considered the procedure of choice in the diagnostic evaluation of adrenal nodules in patients with known malignant neoplasms [64–66]. Other techniques to obtain tissue for biopsy can be via *endoscopic ultrasound* (*EUS*)-guided *FNA* [67, 68]. While performing an image-guided FNA may be indicated in patients with known malignant disease and a newly discovered adrenal mass with suspicious characteristics on imaging, it is important to exclude increased metanephrine production (i.e. phaeochromocytoma) before proceeding with such a biopsy. Moreover, adrenal biopsy might not be indicated in patients with already known widespread metastatic disease. Risks of FNA biopsy of the adrenal gland include haematoma of the adrenal gland or liver, pancreatitis, pneumothorax, formation of an adrenal abscess and tumour seeding along the needle track; however, overall this is considered a safe procedure with complication rates reported as low as 2.8% [69, 70].

A rare scenario involves patients presenting with an adrenal incidentaloma but no previous history of malignancy. If the incidentaloma is enlarging on serial scans or if the initial tumour dimeter is over 4 cm, such patients are offered laparoscopic adrenalectomy for the potential risk of malignancy (i.e. ACC), and occasionally the final histological diagnosis could be of a metastatic lesion from a clinically silent primary tumour.

22.3.4 Treatment

To establish a tailor-made treatment, all patients with adrenal metastases require multidisciplinary evaluation to determine the appropriateness of surgical intervention [71]. Such decisions are likely to be different based on the primary site of malignancy and the suspicion/evidence for any additional metastatic disease.

Overall, the only curative option for patients with metastatic disease to their adrenal gland is complete (R0) resection of all known disease. Several studies have underlined the more favourable outcomes for patient after resection of disease compared with non-operative management [43, 71–73]. Therefore, as a general principle, resection of a single-site adrenal metastatic disease should be attempted, considering that the operation is feasible with minimal morbidity.

For synchronous metastases, the treatment for the adrenal metastasis should be offered after completion of curative treatment for the primary tumour (e.g. lung resection followed by laparoscopic adrenalectomy).

For metachronous metastases, the decision to operate for the adrenal metastasis would be influenced by the time to recurrence (better outcomes when metastasis was diagnosed some 6–12 months after the initial treatment for primary malignancy).

For patients with metastases in multiple sites or extensive tumour burden, treatment with systemic chemotherapy or palliative-supportive care should be undertaken [71]. Alternatively, recent reports on stereotactic body radiation therapy (SBRT) for adrenal metastasis show that this treatment has the possibility to provide good short-term local control with an excellent safety profile [74, 75].

For non-surgical candidates, percutaneous image-guided ablation therapy, such as chemical ablation, radiofrequency ablation, cryoablation and microwave ablation, has been shown of clinical value [76–80]. Overall, adrenal ablation is well-tolerated by patients and has the advantage that it can be performed under sedation or general anaesthesia. Although several studies have shown this technique to be feasible and that there does seem to be some survival benefit from this therapy, clear data on oncological outcomes is not yet available.

22.3.4.1 Indications for Surgery and Surgical Details

Before surgery is contemplated, assessment of plasma-free levels of metanephrines is mandatory to rule out phaeochromocytoma. In general, a complete endocrine assessment should also include measurements of urinary free cortisol levels and overnight 1 mg dexamethasone suppression test.

Adrenal metastasis is often confined within the gland itself, providing a good opportunity for achieving en bloc removal. The main features of a successful adrenalectomy are a wide resection with negative margins (i.e. a R0 surgical resection) and the absence of tumour spill during the procedure.

As for most adrenal tumours, traditionally, open surgery was the preferred operation for patients with adrenal metastasis. The first report of laparoscopic adrenalectomy for malignancy was published in 1999 [81]. Although it has taken nearly two decades to do so, laparoscopic adrenalectomy is currently the standard treatment for metastatic disease to the adrenal glands. The non-oncological benefits of minimally invasive surgery have long been established also for other indications, i.e. shorter postoperative hospitalization, less intra- and postoperative complications as well a greater patient compliance [82, 83]. Furthermore, several large studies showed that the survival for patients undergoing a laparoscopic adrenalectomy for metastasis is similar to the open approach [83, 84].

More recently, posterior retroperitoneoscopic adrenalectomy has been utilized in the resection of adrenal metastasis [85]. Similar as for the anterior laparoscopic approach, several studies have shown this to be a safe and feasible technique [85–87]. An added benefit of the retroperitoneoscopic approach is that it avoids the need for mobilization of adjacent intra-abdominal organs and that there is no impact of adhesions from possible previous abdominal surgeries. The main limitation is that the technique is more difficult to be mastered in centres with low-volume practice and that the small operative space creates additional challenges for an oncological resection (i.e. no tumour breaching/fragmentation during the dissection).

For cases in which wide surgical margins with en bloc excision of peri-adrenal fat cannot be achieved through a laparoscopic or retroperitoneoscopic approach, open adrenalectomy remains the gold standard technique. For those patients in whom local invasion is suspected on preoperative imaging, whose tumour is large, when there is significant lymphadenopathy or tumour thrombus in the vena cava, open adrenalectomy also remains the technique of choice. Several authors also suggested relative contraindications for a laparoscopic approach, such as morbid obesity, cardiovascular comorbidity or adhesions due to multiple prior abdominal surgeries [43, 71, 88].

A specific subgroup of patients who should be considered candidates for adrenalectomy are those in whom one or more other sites of metastatic disease are responding to systemic therapy, but there is a non-response deposit in one of the adrenal glands. This situation has been described as *sanctuary metastases*, and cases involving primary tumours as melanoma and the uterus have been published [89, 90]. Overall advice from available literature is to perform early adrenal surgery in these patients.

22.3.5 Outcomes or Prognosis

Overall oncological outcomes for adrenalectomy for metastases are not easily assessed, as it comprises a heterogeneous group of patients with various primary tumour sites. Although there have not been any randomized studies performed to assess this and while there is a presumed bias in the patient selection for surgery, most studies report favourable outcomes after adrenalectomy for metastases. In a large multicentre European study of a total of 317 patients with histologically confirmed adrenal metastatic disease who underwent laparoscopic (n = 146) or open (n = 171) adrenalectomy, the median overall survival was 24 months for open adrenalectomy and 45 for laparoscopic adrenalectomy. Survival rates at 1 and 5 years were 68% and 29% for open surgery versus 88% and 46% for laparoscopy, respectively. Patients who underwent laparoscopic adrenalectomy showed a longer survival than open adrenalectomy individuals, although minimally invasive approach was attempted more commonly in less advanced disease which led to higher number of R0 resections [82].

22.4 Adrenal Lymphoma

22.4.1 Clinical Presentation

While series on autopsies have reported adrenal gland involvement in up to 25% of lymphoma patients (mainly non-Hodgkin's lymphoma) [91], actual primary adrenal lymphoma (PAL) is a very rare clinical entity. The majority of PAL (~70%) are diffuse large B-cell lymphoma subtype [92].

In a review of about 100 cases of PAL available in literature [92], a large portion of patients presented with symptoms common in lymphoma, including abdominal or lumbar back pain, fever of unknown origin, anorexia, weight loss and malaise. However, interestingly, as more than two-thirds of all patients had bilateral enlargement of the adrenal glands, these authors reported that a significant percentage of patients presented with signs of adrenal insufficiency. Moreover, PAL can also rarely manifest as frank Addison's disease [93]. Furthermore, the majority of cases on PAL available in literature included older males, with a mean age at presentation of 65 years and a male-to-female ratio of 2:1 [91, 92, 94].

22.4.2 Natural History

Overall, this disease has a very poor prognosis – even when treatment is provided. Available data shows that patients given only palliative treatment succumbed at a rapid rate [92]. However, due to the paucity of available data, how PAL compares with other types of lymphoma with similar histology is not known; therefore, no reliable statements regarding its natural history can be made [95].

22.4.3 Diagnosis

As PAL is a very rare disease, limited reports on the preferred diagnostic pathway are available [96]. Most diagnoses are made after performance of cross-sectional imaging scans. On imaging, PAL can easily be confused with an adrenal metastatic lesion.

On computed tomography (CT) scan, necrosis, haemorrhage and calcifications within the adrenal lesion are frequently seen [97, 98].

On magnetic resonance imaging (MRI scan), PAL tends to be hypo-intense on T1-weighted images, while it tends to be hyper-intense on T2-weighted images [94].

Positron emission tomography/computed tomography (PET/CT) labelled with fluorine-18 fluorodeoxyglucose (FDG) seems to be useful in demonstrating extra-adrenal locations of PAL, with one study reporting incidence of extra-adrenal locations in 70% of patients [94].

For the definite histological diagnosis, a biopsy is required. This can be obtained by a CT-guided needle biopsy or as a surgical biopsy [97, 98].

22.4.4 Treatment

Currently, no empirical protocols specifically for the treatment of PAL are available. Most authors describe local regimens consisting of multimodality treatment including chemotherapy or radiotherapy, while data supporting the preferred treatment options are not existing.

Chemotherapy is the most commonly used regimen. In a SEER-based analysis, receipt of chemotherapy was an independent factor for prolonged overall survival [95].

Traditionally, CHOP regimens were most frequently administered. This combination therapy consists of cyclophosphamide and hydroxydaunorubicin with oncovin and prednisone. Unfortunately, the outcomes were generally poor with overall reported survival rates from 20 to 50% [96]. More recently, regimens containing rituximab combined with CNS prophylaxis have been proposed as alternate and, possibly, more promising treatment options for the treatment of PAL [99]. A complete remission rate of 55% and an overall response rate of 87% were reported in 31 patients who received R-CHOP (i.e. with rituximab) regimens [100].

The role of surgery in this disease has been controversial. While case reports on patients who underwent unilateral or even bilateral adrenalectomy for PAL are available [92, 101], the largest cohorts on surgical treatment for this disease reported no survival benefit for those who underwent surgery compared to those who were treated with medical treatment only [94, 100].

22.4.5 Indications for Surgery and Surgical Details

Although most data on the indications for adrenalectomy for patients with PAL are anecdotal, there are some case reports addressing this subject. It is therefore questionable if reliable statements regarding the benefit or indications of surgical treatment for this disease can be made [92].

The largest series addressing the surgical treatment for PAL included 28 patients of whom 4 underwent surgery, and it was found that adrenalectomy brought no survival benefit [94].

Similarly, there was no survival benefit for surgery in a group of 31 patients treated with an R-CHOP regimen, of whom 7 underwent adrenalectomy [100].

22.4.6 Outcomes or Prognosis

As mentioned before, the outcomes for patients presenting with PAL are poor. Less than 50% of patients who were treated with curative intent achieve a complete remission, while many of these develop relapse of their disease during the first months of follow-up as about a third of patients survived disease-free for at least 6 months [92]. Similarly, a report of 136 patients identified on the Surveillance, Epidemiology, and End Results (SEER) program (1983–2015) showed that the majority of patients presented with advanced-stage disease and reported an overall survival at 5 and 10 years of 19% and 3%, respectively. Independent prognostic factors correlated with adverse overall survival were age over 70 years and bilateral lesions [95].

Answers to the Questions

1. (d); 2. (a); 3. (d); 4. (b); 5. (d); 6. (a); 7. (a); 8. (a)

References

1. Mansmann G, Lau J, Balk E, Rothberg M, Miyachi Y, Bornstein SR. The clinically inapparent adrenal mass: update in diagnosis and management. Endocr Rev. 2004;25(2):309–40.
2. Fassnacht M, Allolio B. Clinical management of adrenocortical carcinoma. Best Pract Res Clin Endocrinol Metab. 2009;23(2):273–89.
3. Nakamura Y, Yamazaki Y, Felizola SJ, Ise K, Morimoto R, Satoh F, Arai Y, Sasano H. Adrenocortical carcinoma: review of the pathologic features, production of adrenal steroids, and molecular pathogenesis. Endocrinol Metab Clin N Am. 2015;44(2):399–410.
4. Ng L, Libertino JM. Adrenocortical carcinoma: diagnosis, evaluation and treatment. J Urol. 2003;169(1):5–11.
5. Else T, Kim AC, Sabolch A, Raymond VM, Kandathil A, Caoili EM, Jolly S, Miller BS, Giordano TJ, Hammer GD. Adrenocortical carcinoma. Endocr Rev. 2014;35(2):282–326.
6. Gaujoux S, Weinandt M, Bonnet S, Reslinger V, Bertherat J, Dousset B. Surgical treatment of adrenal carcinoma. J Visc Surg. 2017;154(5):335–43.
7. Dickson PV, Kim L, Yen TWF, Yang A, Grubbs EG, Patel D, Solorzano CC. Evaluation, staging, and surgical management for adrenocortical carcinoma: an update from the SSO endocrine and head and neck disease site working group. Ann Surg Oncol. 2018;25(12):3460–8.
8. Gaujoux S, Mihai R, joint working group of ESES and ENSAT. European Society of Endocrine Surgeons (ESES) and European Network for the Study of Adrenal Tumours (ENSAT) recommendations for the surgical management of adrenocortical carcinoma. Br J Surg. 2017;104(4):358–76.
9. Tran TB, Liou D, Menon VG, Nissen NN. Surgical management of advanced adrenocortical carcinoma: a 21-year population-based analysis. Am Surg. 2013;79(10):1115–8.
10. Libe R, Fratticci A, Bertherat J. Adrenocortical cancer: pathophysiology and clinical management. Endocr Relat Cancer. 2007;14(1):13–28.
11. Arlt W, Biehl M, Taylor AE, Hahner S, Libe R, Hughes BA, Schneider P, Smith DJ, Stiekema H, Krone N, et al. Urine steroid metabolomics as a biomarker tool for detecting malignancy in adrenal tumors. J Clin Endocrinol Metab. 2011;96(12):3775–84.
12. Velikanova LI, Shafigullina ZR, Lisitsin AA, Vorokhobina NV, Grigoryan K, Kukhianidze EA, Strelnikova EG, Krivokhizhina NS, Krasnov LM, Fedorov EA, et al. Different types of urinary steroid profiling obtained by high-performance liquid chromatography and gas chromatography-mass spectrometry in patients with adrenocortical carcinoma. Horm Cancer. 2016;7(5–6):327–35.
13. Hines JM, Bancos I, Bancos C, Singh RD, Avula AV, Young WF, Grebe SK, Singh RJ. High-resolution, accurate-mass (HRAM) mass spectrometry urine steroid profiling in the diagnosis of adrenal disorders. Clin Chem. 2017;63(12):1824–35.
14. Zini L, Porpiglia F, Fassnacht M. Contemporary management of adrenocortical carcinoma. Eur Urol. 2011;60(5):1055–65.
15. Zhang HM, Perrier ND, Grubbs EG, Sircar K, Ye ZX, Lee JE, Ng CS. CT features and quantification of the characteristics of adrenocortical carcinomas on unenhanced and contrast-enhanced studies. Clin Radiol. 2012;67(1):38–46.

16. Sturgeon C, Shen WT, Clark OH, Duh QY, Kebebew E. Risk assessment in 457 adrenal cortical carcinomas: how much does tumor size predict the likelihood of malignancy? J Am Coll Surg. 2006;202(3):423–30.
17. Petersenn S, Richter PA, Broemel T, Ritter CO, Deutschbein T, Beil FU, Allolio B, Fassnacht M, German ACCSG. Computed tomography criteria for discrimination of adrenal adenomas and adrenocortical carcinomas: analysis of the German ACC registry. Eur J Endocrinol. 2015;172(4):415–22.
18. Ilias I, Sahdev A, Reznek RH, Grossman AB, Pacak K. The optimal imaging of adrenal tumours: a comparison of different methods. Endocr Relat Cancer. 2007;14(3):587–99.
19. Gust L, Taieb D, Beliard A, Barlier A, Morange I, de Micco C, Henry JF, Sebag F. Preoperative 18F-FDG uptake is strongly correlated with malignancy, Weiss score, and molecular markers of aggressiveness in adrenal cortical tumors. World J Surg. 2012;36(6):1406–10.
20. Nunes ML, Rault A, Teynie J, Valli N, Guyot M, Gaye D, Belleannee G, Tabarin A. 18F-FDG PET for the identification of adrenocortical carcinomas among indeterminate adrenal tumors at computed tomography scanning. World J Surg. 2010;34(7):1506–10.
21. McDuffie LA, Aufforth RD. Adrenocortical carcinoma: modern management and evolving treatment strategies. Int J Endocr Oncol. 2016;3(2):161–74.
22. Kreissl MC, Schirbel A, Fassnacht M, Haenscheid H, Verburg FA, Bock S, Saeger W, Knoedler P, Reiners C, Buck AK, et al. [(1)(2)(3)I] Iodometomidate imaging in adrenocortical carcinoma. J Clin Endocrinol Metab. 2013;98(7):2755–64.
23. Beuschlein F, Weigel J, Saeger W, Kroiss M, Wild V, Daffara F, Libe R, Ardito A, Al Ghuzlan A, Quinkler M, et al. Major prognostic role of Ki67 in localized adrenocortical carcinoma after complete resection. J Clin Endocrinol Metab. 2015;100(3):841–9.
24. Bedrose S, Daher M, Altameemi L, Habra MA. Adjuvant therapy in adrenocortical carcinoma: reflections and future directions. Cancers (Basel). 2020;12(2):508.
25. Puglisi S, Calabrese A, Basile V, Pia A, Reimondo G, Perotti P, Terzolo M. New perspectives for mitotane treatment of adrenocortical carcinoma. Best Pract Res Clin Endocrinol Metab. 2020;34(3):101415.
26. Bednarski BK, Habra MA, Phan A, Milton DR, Wood C, Vauthey N, Evans DB, Katz MH, Ng CS, Perrier ND, et al. Borderline resectable adrenal cortical carcinoma: a potential role for preoperative chemotherapy. World J Surg. 2014;38(6):1318–27.
27. Gharzai LA, Green MD, Griffith KA, Else T, Mayo CS, Hesseltine E, Spratt DE, Ben-Josef E, Sabolch A, Miller BS, et al. Adjuvant radiation improves recurrence-free survival and overall survival in adrenocortical carcinoma. J Clin Endocrinol Metab. 2019;104(9):3743–50.
28. Viani GA, Viana BS. Adjuvant radiotherapy after surgical resection for adrenocortical carcinoma: a systematic review of observational studies and meta-analysis. J Cancer Res Ther. 2019;15(Supplement):S20–6.
29. Reibetanz J, Jurowich C, Erdogan I, Nies C, Rayes N, Dralle H, Behrend M, Allolio B, Fassnacht M, German ACC study group. Impact of lymphadenectomy on the oncologic outcome of patients with adrenocortical carcinoma. Ann Surg. 2012;255(2):363–9.
30. Saade N, Sadler C, Goldfarb M. Impact of regional lymph node dissection on disease specific survival in adrenal cortical carcinoma. Horm Metab Res. 2015;47(11):820–5.
31. Donatini G, Caiazzo R, Do Cao C, Aubert S, Zerrweck C, El-Kathib Z, Gauthier T, Leteurtre E, Wemeau JL, Vantyghem MC, et al. Long-term survival after adrenalectomy for stage I/II adrenocortical carcinoma (ACC): a retrospective comparative cohort study of laparoscopic versus open approach. Ann Surg Oncol. 2014;21(1):284–91.
32. Mpaili E, Moris D, Tsilimigras DI, Oikonomou D, Pawlik TM, Schizas D, Papalampros A, Felekouras E, Dimitroulis D. Laparoscopic versus

open adrenalectomy for localized/locally advanced primary adrenocortical carcinoma (ENSAT I-III) in adults: is margin-free resection the key surgical factor that dictates outcome? A review of the literature. J Laparoendosc Adv Surg Tech A. 2018;28(4):408–14.
33. Chiche L, Dousset B, Kieffer E, Chapuis Y. Adrenocortical carcinoma extending into the inferior vena cava: presentation of a 15-patient series and review of the literature. Surgery. 2006;139(1):15–27.
34. Mihai R, Iacobone M, Makay O, Moreno P, Frilling A, Kraimps JL, Soriano A, et al. Outcome of operation in patients with adrenocortical cancer invading the inferior vena cava–a European Society of Endocrine Surgeons (ESES) survey. Langenbeck's Arch Surg. 2012;397(2):225–31.
35. Turbendian HK, Strong VE, Hsu M, Ghossein RA, Fahey TJ 3rd. Adrenocortical carcinoma: the influence of large vessel extension. Surgery. 2010;148(6):1057–64. discussion 1064
36. Schimmack S, Strobel O. Resection strategies for adrenocortical carcinoma. Chirurg. 2019;90(1):9–14.
37. Bilimoria KY, Shen WT, Elaraj D, Bentrem DJ, Winchester DJ, Kebebew E, Sturgeon C. Adrenocortical carcinoma in the United States: treatment utilization and prognostic factors. Cancer. 2008;113(11):3130–6.
38. Fassnacht M, Dekkers OM, Else T, Baudin E, Berruti A, de Krijger R, Haak HR, Mihai R, Assie G, Terzolo M. European Society of Endocrinology Clinical Practice Guidelines on the management of adrenocortical carcinoma in adults, in collaboration with the European Network for the Study of Adrenal Tumors. Eur J Endocrinol. 2018;179(4):G1–G46.
39. Mihai R, Donatini G, Vidal O, Brunaud L. Volume-outcome correlation in adrenal surgery-an ESES consensus statement. Langenbeck's Arch Surg. 2019;404(7):795–806.
40. Fassnacht M, Libe R, Kroiss M, Allolio B. Adrenocortical carcinoma: a clinician's update. Nat Rev Endocrinol. 2011;7(6):323–35.
41. Mihai R. Diagnosis, treatment and outcome of adrenocortical cancer. Br J Surg. 2015;102(4):291–306.
42. Terzolo M, Daffara F, Ardito A, Zaggia B, Basile V, Ferrari L, Berruti A. Management of adrenal cancer: a 2013 update. J Endocrinol Investig. 2014;37(3):207–17.
43. Spartalis E, Drikos I, Ioannidis A, Chrysikos D, Athanasiadis DI, Spartalis M, Avgerinos D. Metastatic carcinomas of the adrenal glands: from diagnosis to treatment. Anticancer Res. 2019;39(6):2699–710.
44. Lam KY, Fu KH, Wong MP, Wang EP. Significant changes in the distribution of histologic types of lung cancer in Hong Kong. Pathology. 1993;25(2):103–5.
45. Lam KY, Lo CY. Metastatic tumours of the adrenal glands: a 30-year experience in a teaching hospital. Clin Endocrinol. 2002;56(1):95–101.
46. Angelousi A, Alexandraki KI, Kyriakopoulos G, Tsoli M, Thomas D, Kaltsas G, Grossman A. Neoplastic metastases to the endocrine glands. Endocr Relat Cancer. 2020;27(1):R1–R20.
47. Onuigbo WI. Lymphangiogenesis may explain adrenal selectivity in lung cancer metastases. Med Hypotheses. 2010;75(2):185–6.
48. Vieweg WV, Reitz RE, Weinstein RL. Addison's disease secondary to metastatic carcinoma: an example of adrenocortical and adrenomedullary insufficiency. Cancer. 1973;31(5):1240–3.
49. Akcay MN, Tekin SB, Akcay G. Addisonian crisis due to adrenal gland metastasis in Hodgkin's disease. Int J Clin Pract. 2003;57(9):840–1.
50. Munoz A, Onate J, Mane JM, Rubio I, Fernandez R, Barcelo JR, Lopez Vivanco G. Addisonian crisis as first manifestation of adrenal gland insufficiency in patient diagnosed with lung cancer. An Med Interna. 2001;18(1):35–7.
51. Miyamura T, Obama K, Takahira H, Uike N, Kozuru M. A case of primary non-Hodgkin lymphoma of the adrenal gland presenting with Addison's disease. Rinsho Ketsueki. 1993;34(7):882–4.

52. Kennedy RL, Ball RY, Dixon AK, ApSimon AT. Metastatic transitional cell carcinoma of the bladder causing Addison's disease. J Urol. 1987;137(5):986–8.
53. Herndon J, Nadeau AM, Davidge-Pitts CJ, Young WF, Bancos I. Primary adrenal insufficiency due to bilateral infiltrative disease. Endocrine. 2018;62(3):721–8.
54. Iqbal MS, Hardman J. Addisonian crisis secondary to bilateral adrenal metastases in rectal carcinoma: report of a rare case and literature review. J Gastrointest Cancer. 2013;44(2):225–7.
55. Hernandez IR, Hernandez Lavado R, Ortega PR, Carmona CG, Perez de Madrid JD. Primary adrenal insufficiency due to bilateral adrenal lymphoma. Endocrinol Nutr. 2011;58(2):96–7.
56. Dunnick NR, Korobkin M, Francis I. Adrenal radiology: distinguishing benign from malignant adrenal masses. AJR Am J Roentgenol. 1996;167(4):861–7.
57. Blake MA, Cronin CG, Boland GW. Adrenal imaging. AJR Am J Roentgenol. 2010;194(6):1450–60.
58. Sandler MA, Pearlberg JL, Madrazo BL, Gitschlag KF, Gross SC. Computed tomographic evaluation of the adrenal gland in the preoperative assessment of bronchogenic carcinoma. Radiology. 1982;145(3):733–6.
59. Platzek I, Sieron D, Plodeck V, Borkowetz A, Laniado M, Hoffmann RT. Chemical shift imaging for evaluation of adrenal masses: a systematic review and meta-analysis. Eur Radiol. 2019;29(2):806–17.
60. Brady MJ, Thomas J, Wong TZ, Franklin KM, Ho LM, Paulson EK. Adrenal nodules at FDG PET/CT in patients known to have or suspected of having lung cancer: a proposal for an efficient diagnostic algorithm. Radiology. 2009;250(2):523–30.
61. Stone WZ, Wymer DC, Canales BK. Fluorodeoxyglucose-positron-emission tomography/computed tomography imaging for adrenal masses in patients with lung cancer: review and diagnostic algorithm. J Endourol. 2014;28(1):104–11.
62. Metser U, Miller E, Lerman H, Lievshitz G, Avital S, Even-Sapir E. 18F-FDG PET/CT in the evaluation of adrenal masses. J Nucl Med. 2006;47(1):32–7.
63. Elaini AB, Shetty SK, Chapman VM, Sahani DV, Boland GW, Sweeney AT, Maher MM, Slattery JT, Mueller PR, Blake MA. Improved detection and characterization of adrenal disease with PET-CT. Radiographics. 2007;27(3):755–67.
64. Ettinghausen SE, Burt ME. Prospective evaluation of unilateral adrenal masses in patients with operable non-small-cell lung cancer. J Clin Oncol. 1991;9(8):1462–6.
65. de Agustin P, Lopez-Rios F, Alberti N, Perez-Barrios A. Fine-needle aspiration biopsy of the adrenal glands: a ten-year experience. Diagn Cytopathol. 1999;21(2):92–7.
66. Zhang CD, Delivanis DA, Eiken PW, Atwell TD, Bancos I. Adrenal biopsy: performance and use. Minerva Endocrinol. 2019;44(3):288–300.
67. Zhang CD, Erickson D, Levy MJ, Gleeson FC, Salomao DR, Delivanis DA, Bancos I. Endoscopic ultrasound-guided fine-needle aspiration in the diagnosis of adrenal metastasis in a high-risk population. Endocr Pract. 2017;23(12):1402–7.
68. Eloubeidi MA, Black KR, Tamhane A, Eltoum IA, Bryant A, Cerfolio RJ. A large single-center experience of EUS-guided FNA of the left and right adrenal glands: diagnostic utility and impact on patient management. Gastrointest Endosc. 2010;71(4):745–53.
69. Welch TJ, Sheedy PF 2nd, Stephens DH, Johnson CM, Swensen SJ. Percutaneous adrenal biopsy: review of a 10-year experience. Radiology. 1994;193(2):341–4.
70. Arellano RS, Harisinghani MG, Gervais DA, Hahn PF, Mueller PR. Image-guided percutaneous biopsy of the adrenal gland: review of

indications, technique, and complications. Curr Probl Diagn Radiol. 2003;32(1):3–10.
71. Sancho JJ, Triponez F, Montet X, Sitges-Serra A. Surgical management of adrenal metastases. Langenbeck's Arch Surg. 2012;397(2):179–94.
72. Luketich JD, Burt ME. Does resection of adrenal metastases from non-small cell lung cancer improve survival? Ann Thorac Surg. 1996;62(6):1614–6.
73. Sarela AI, Murphy I, Coit DG, Conlon KC. Metastasis to the adrenal gland: the emerging role of laparoscopic surgery. Ann Surg Oncol. 2003;10(10):1191–6.
74. Chen WC, Baal JD, Baal U, Pai J, Gottschalk A, Boreta L, Braunstein SE, Raleigh DR. Stereotactic body radiation therapy of adrenal metastases: a pooled meta-analysis and systematic review of 39 studies with 1006 patients. Int J Radiat Oncol Biol Phys. 2020;107(1):48–61.
75. Torok J, Wegner RE, Burton SA, Heron DE. Stereotactic body radiation therapy for adrenal metastases: a retrospective review of a noninvasive therapeutic strategy. Future Oncol. 2011;7(1):145–51.
76. Yamakado K. Image-guided ablation of adrenal lesions. Semin Intervent Radiol. 2014;31(2):149–56.
77. Zhou K, Pan J, Yang N, Shi HF, Cao J, Li YM, Zhang HZ, Wang KF, Chen SH. Effectiveness and safety of CT-guided percutaneous radiofrequency ablation of adrenal metastases. Br J Radiol. 2018;91(1085):20170607.
78. Wolf FJ, Dupuy DE, Machan JT, Mayo-Smith WW. Adrenal neoplasms: effectiveness and safety of CT-guided ablation of 23 tumors in 22 patients. Eur J Radiol. 2012;81(8):1717–23.
79. Hasegawa T, Yamakado K, Nakatsuka A, Uraki J, Yamanaka T, Fujimori M, Miki M, Sasaki T, Sakuma H, Sugimura Y. Unresectable adrenal metastases: clinical outcomes of radiofrequency ablation. Radiology. 2015;277(2):584–93.
80. Botsa EI, Thanou IL, Papatheodoropoulou AT, Thanos LI. Thermal ablation in the management of adrenal metastasis originating from non-small cell lung cancer: a 5-year single-center experience. Chin Med J. 2017;130(17):2027–32.
81. Heniford BT, Arca MJ, Walsh RM, Gill IS. Laparoscopic adrenalectomy for cancer. Semin Surg Oncol. 1999;16(4):293–306.
82. Moreno P, de la Quintana Basarrate A, Musholt TJ, Paunovic I, Puccini M, Vidal O, Ortega J, Kraimps JL, European Study Group for Metastatic Adrenalectomy. Laparoscopy versus open adrenalectomy in patients with solid tumor metastases: results of a multicenter European study. Gland Surg. 2020;9(Suppl 2):S159–65.
83. Frattolillo G, Paradiso G, Scarano Catanazaro V, Giordano L, Avantifiori R, D'Ermo G, Letizia C, De Toma G. The role of laparoscopic surgery in isolated adrenal metastasis: our personal experience. G Chir. 2020;41(1):46–490.
84. Edmonds BT, Koenig E. Transmembrane cytoskeletal modulation in preterminal growing axons: I. Arrest of bulk and organelle transport in goldfish retinal ganglion cell axons regenerating in vitro by lectins binding to sialoglycoconjugates. Cell Motil Cytoskeleton. 1990;17(2):106–17.
85. Kaneko G, Katsui M, Orikasa H, Hattori S, Hara S. Retroperitoneoscopic partial adrenalectomy for metachronous renal cell carcinoma metastasis to solitary adrenal gland. Int Cancer Conf J. 2020;9(1):1–4.
86. Glenn JA, Kiernan CM, Yen TW, Solorzano CC, Carr AA, Evans DB, Wang TS. Management of suspected adrenal metastases at 2 academic medical centers. Am J Surg. 2016;211(4):664–70.
87. Perrier ND, Kennamer DL, Bao R, Jimenez C, Grubbs EG, Lee JE, Evans DB. Posterior retroperitoneoscopic adrenalectomy: preferred technique for removal of benign tumors and isolated metastases. Ann Surg. 2008;248(4):666–74.

88. Uberoi J, Munver R. Surgical management of metastases to the adrenal gland: open, laparoscopic, and ablative approaches. Curr Urol Rep. 2009;10(1):67–72.
89. Zippel D, Yalon T, Nevo Y, Markel G, Asher N, Schachter J, Goitein D, Segal TA, Nissan A, Hazzan D. The non-responding adrenal metastasis in melanoma: the case for minimally invasive adrenalectomy in the age of modern therapies. Am J Surg. 2020;20(2):349–53.
90. Nguyen MC, Shah MH, Liebner DA, Backes FJ, Phay J, Shirley LA. The adrenal gland as a sanctuary site of metastases after pembrolizumab treatment: a case series. J Natl Compr Cancer Netw. 2018;16(11): 1279–83.
91. Kita M, Mandala E, Saratzis A, Ventzi L, Venizelos I, Kteryttopoulos P, Efstathiadou Z, Garyfallos A, Avramides A. Primary adrenal lymphoma presenting as Addison's disease. Case report and review of the literature. Exp Clin Endocrinol Diabetes. 2008;116(6):363–5.
92. Mantzios G, Tsirigotis P, Veliou F, Boutsikakis I, Petraki L, Kolovos J, Papageorgiou S, Robos Y. Primary adrenal lymphoma presenting as Addison's disease: case report and review of the literature. Ann Hematol. 2004;83(7):460–3.
93. Oelkers W. Adrenal insufficiency. N Engl J Med. 1996;335(16):1206–12.
94. Laurent C, Casasnovas O, Martin L, Chauchet A, Ghesquieres H, Aussedat G, Fornecker LM, Bologna S, Borot S, Laurent K, et al. Adrenal lymphoma: presentation, management and prognosis. QJM. 2017;110(2):103–9.
95. Li S, Wang Z, Wu Z, Zhuang H, Xu Y. Clinical characteristics and outcomes of primary adrenal diffuse large B cell lymphoma in a large contemporary cohort: a SEER-based analysis. Ann Hematol. 2019;98(9):2111–9.
96. Grigg AP, Connors JM. Primary adrenal lymphoma. Clin Lymphoma. 2003;4(3):154–60.
97. Falchook FS, Allard JC. CT of primary adrenal lymphoma. J Comput Assist Tomogr. 1991;15(6):1048–50.
98. Alvarez-Castells A, Pedraza S, Tallada N, Castella E, Gifre L, Torrents C. CT of primary bilateral adrenal lymphoma. J Comput Assist Tomogr. 1993;17(3):408–9.
99. Ichikawa S, Fukuhara N, Inoue A, Katsushima H, Ohba R, Katsuoka Y, Onishi Y, Yamamoto J, Sasaki O, Nomura J, et al. Clinicopathological analysis of primary adrenal diffuse large B-cell lymphoma: effectiveness of rituximab-containing chemotherapy including central nervous system prophylaxis. Exp Hematol Oncol. 2013;2(1):19.
100. Kim YR, Kim JS, Min YH, Hyunyoon D, Shin HJ, Mun YC, Park Y, Do YR, Jeong SH, Park JS, et al. Prognostic factors in primary diffuse large B-cell lymphoma of adrenal gland treated with rituximab-CHOP chemotherapy from the Consortium for Improving Survival of Lymphoma (CISL). J Hematol Oncol. 2012;5:49.
101. Ram N, Rashid O, Farooq S, Ulhaq I, Islam N. Primary adrenal non-Hodgkin lymphoma: a case report and review of the literature. J Med Case Rep. 2017;11(1):108.

Surgical Procedure: Adrenalectomy – Indications, Operative Techniques and Management of Complications

Rocco Bellantone and Carmela De Crea

Contents

A. L. Shifrin et al. (eds.), *Endocrine Surgery Comprehensive Board Exam Guide*,
https://doi.org/10.1007/978-3-030-84737-1_23

Case Presentation

A 55-year-old male was referred in September 2020 for a 24-mm right adrenal mass, increased in size during 6-month follow-up. The adrenal mass was homogeneous without any suspicious features at the contrast computed tomography (CT) scan.

The patient reported no significant complaints. No adrenal hypersecretion was discovered at hormonal evaluation. The patient's BMI was 31 Kg/m^2. Past medical history was significant for previous history of kidney clear cell carcinoma (pT3a pN0 pMx, grade 2 Fuhrman, grade 2 WHO/ISUP 2016) treated with open (median laparotomy) radical left nephrectomy plus left adrenalectomy plus regional lymphadenectomy in September 2018, complicated by postoperative fluid collection.

Questions

1. What is the next step in diagnosis?
   1. If an 18F-FDG PET/CT is performed, we should consider the possibility of an inconclusive result since metastasis from kidney carcinoma might be FDG negative.
   2. Adrenal biopsy should be considered.
   3. A magnetic resonance imaging (MRI) can be done in order to definitively rule out whether the adrenal mass is benign or malignant.
   4. No further studies are needed.
      - (a) Only (1) is correct.
      - (b) Only (1) and (2) are correct.
      - (c) Only (2) is correct.
      - (d) Only (3) and (4) are correct.
2. Adrenal biopsy should be performed:
   1. In the diagnostic work-up of all patients with adrenal masses when the radiological imaging is inconclusive
   2. Only in selected cases of patients with adrenal masses and history of extra-adrenal malignancy
   3. If the lesion is hormonally inactive (in particular, a phaeochromocytoma needs to be excluded)
   4. If the subsequent management would be altered by knowing the histology
      - (a) Only (1) is correct.
      - (b) Only (2) and (3) are correct.
      - (c) Only (3) and (4) are correct.
      - (d) Only (2) and (3) and (4) are correct.

3. The adrenal lesion resulted in site of exclusive uptake at 68Ga-DOTATOC PET/CT. How should you proceed based on the clinical data?
   1. The patient should be directly referred to surgery.
   2. Surgery is not an option since the patient already underwent left adrenalectomy, and therefore, the resection of the remaining right adrenal gland would expose the patients to adrenal insufficiency with the necessity of lifelong steroid replacement.
   3. A strict follow-up should be planned in order to figure out a potential further increase in size of the adrenal lesion.
   4. The case requires a consultation with a multidisciplinary expert board.
      (a) Only (1) is correct.
      (b) Only (2) is correct.
      (c) Only (4) is correct.
      (d) Only (3) is correct.
4. The patient's relatively young age and the fact that the adrenal mass was the only metastatic site led the multidisciplinary board to conclude that the surgical resection was reasonable from an oncological point of view. Which approach of adrenalectomy would be more appropriate in this case?
   1. Open adrenalectomy would be the best choice, given the suspicious for malignancy of the adrenal lesion.
   2. Posterior retroperitoneoscopic adrenalectomy would be ideal in this case since the history of previous surgery.
   3. Lateral transabdominal adrenalectomy can be performed even if potentially more challenging because of the history of previous surgery.
   4. Robot-assisted adrenalectomy is indicated because of the suspicious for malignancy.
      (a) Only (2) and (3) are correct.
      (b) Only (1) is correct.
      (c) Only (2) is correct.
      (d) Only (2), (3) and (4) are correct.
5. In the posterior retroperitoneoscopic adrenalectomy:
   1. The kidney is the main landmark.
   2. The working space is relatively limited, and therefore, lesions ranging in size within 6 cm represent the ideal indication for this approach.
   3. The prone position exposes both adrenals at the same time, without the need to reposition the patient in bilateral diseases.
   4. Extreme obesity (body mass index >40) does not represent a concern since the route is extra-peritoneal thus avoiding the abdominal fat.
      (a) Only (1) is correct.
      (b) Only (3) is correct.

   (c) Only (4) is correct.
   (d) Only (1), (2) and (3) are correct.

6. What surgical steps can be undertaken to successfully perform a posterior retroperitoneoscopic adrenalectomy?
   1. The dissection should start from the cranial aspect of the adrenal gland in order to create an adequate working space.
   2. The dissection should follow an upward direction, leaving the mobilization of the cranial aspect of the adrenal gland as the last step.
   3. Dissection of the upper kidney pole should be as complete as possible, in order to allow an adequate exposure of the inferior aspect of the adrenal.
   4. The adrenal gland should be removed en bloc with the peri-adrenal fat.
      (a) Only (1) and (4) are correct.
      (b) Only (2), (3) and (4) are correct.
      (c) Only (2) is correct.
      (d) Only (4) is correct.
7. During right lateral transabdominal adrenalectomy, which of the following is true?
   1. The key factor for exposure of the right adrenal gland is a wide dissection of the right triangular ligament of the liver and of the posterior peritoneum.
   2. The main landmark for the right adrenalectomy is the inferior vena cava.
   3. The adrenal gland should be removed en bloc with the peri-adrenal fat.
   4. Thanks to the gravity-facilitated exposure of the adrenal glands, no mobilization at all of the structures overlying the adrenals is required.
      (a) Only (2) and (4) are correct.
      (b) Only (4) is correct.
      (c) Only (2) is correct.
      (d) Only (1), (2) and (3) are correct.
8. During left lateral transabdominal adrenalectomy, which of the following is true?
   1. Thanks to the gravity-facilitated exposure of the adrenal glands, no mobilization at all of the structures overlying the adrenals is required.
   2. The first step in left adrenalectomy is the dissection of the left colic flexure.
   3. The spleno-parietal ligament should be dissected far enough to visualize the fundus of the stomach and the left crus of the diaphragm.
   4. A complete mobilization of the spleno-pancreatic bloc is required.
      (a) Only (2), (3) and (4) are correct.
      (b) Only (2) and (4) are correct.
      (c) Only (4) is correct.
      (d) Only (1) is correct.

9. Which are the advantages of robot-assisted adrenalectomy over its conventional laparoscopic counterpart?
   1. A significant decrease of complication rates
   2. A significant decrease of operative time in all cases of adrenalectomy
   3. Improved ergonomics, stereoscopic vision, tremor filtration and greater range of motion within the operative field
   4. A significant decrease of overall costs
      (a) Only (2) and (4) are correct.
      (b) Only (4) is correct.
      (c) Only (1) is correct.
      (d) Only (3) is correct.
10. Specific indications for open adrenalectomy include:
   1. Adrenal mass with evidence of local invasion or suspected metastatic lymph nodes (ENSAT stage III).
   2. Conversion to open approach is required whenever, during laparoscopic adrenalectomy, the dissection is challenging and potentially prevents a complete and oncologically correct adrenal removal.
   3. Recurrent malignant phaeochromocytoma or adrenocortical carcinoma.
   4. All cases of adrenal metastases.
      (a) Only (1), (2) and (3) are correct.
      (b) All the answers are correct.
      (c) Only (3) and (4) are correct.
      (d) Only (3) is correct.

23.1 Introduction

Adrenal tumours are a common disease, with a prevalence rate higher than 4% in the adult population, as reported by systematic analyses of abdominal/thoracic computed tomography investigations [1, 2]. In contrast, adrenalectomy is a quite uncommon procedure [3, 4].

Adrenal pathologies exhibit heterogeneous patterns of presentation, depending on their hormonal status and oncologic potential, based on which adrenalectomy is indicated. Evaluation of the patient with adrenal disease requires a thorough understanding of physiology and proper application of biochemical testing and conventional and nuclear medicine imaging in order to guide the suitable therapeutic approach.

In general, adrenalectomy is indicated in case of hormone hypersecretion, suspected or proven malignancy and lesion size >4 cm (4–6 cm in diameter is the agreed threshold above which adrenalectomy is indicated because of the increased risk for non-secreting adrenocortical carcinoma) [5, 6].

Adrenalectomy is a technically demanding procedure, which requires careful and meticulous dissection around major vessels and organs in a relatively narrow space as retroperitoneum is. The peculiar retroperitoneal location of the adrenal glands explains the early development of several surgical accesses for adrenalectomy [7–10]. Indeed, open adrenalectomy has typically been described and performed through anterior, flank or posterior approaches [7–10]. Thornton first performed the transperitoneal approach in 1889 to remove a huge (20 kilograms) adrenal tumour en bloc with the left kidney in a 36-year-old woman [7]. Charles Mayo described the flank approach in 1927 when he successfully removed a phaeochromocytoma [8]. Young from Johns Hopkins first realized the adrenalectomy with the posterior approach in 1936 [9].

Similar to what happened in open adrenalectomy after its first description, different approaches have been described also for endoscopic adrenalectomy [10, 11]. These include laparoscopic approaches with the patient in a supine (anterior approach) or lateral (lateral approach) position and retroperitoneoscopic approaches with the patient in a lateral (lateral approach) or prone (posterior approach) position [10, 11]. The anterior transperitoneal approach with the patient in supine position allows the exploration of the entire abdominal cavity and the removal of both adrenal glands without the need for patient repositioning. However, few surgeons favoured the routine use of the anterior approach that requires a challenging dissection to guarantee an adequate exposition of the adrenal region [10, 11]. Retroperitoneoscopic adrenalectomy has been described either through the posterior and lateral routes, respectively, implying the jackknife or the lateral decubitus position. The lateral retroperitoneoscopic approach is a unilateral access, requiring patient repositioning for bilateral adrenalectomy. Some surgeons favour the lateral decubitus position for the easier conversion to an open extra-peritoneal or transabdominal procedure if needed [10, 11]. However, the most widespread endoscopic accesses to adrenalectomy are the lateral transabdominal and the posterior retroperitoneoscopic ones [10, 11], which will be treated in detail in the present chapter.

Each technique of adrenalectomy has theoretic advantages relating to adrenal gland exposure and dissection. Several advantages concern the definition of the most direct route of access to the adrenal glands, thereby avoiding excessive dissection and manipulation of surrounding structures.

Selecting the optimal approach for surgical resection of an adrenal mass requires consideration of multiple factors, including tumour size and the suspicion for malignancy [6, 11–16]. Other factors influencing the therapeutic approach include laterality of the disease [17], presence of multiple or extra-adrenal tumours, additional intra-abdominal disease, distant metastases, history of prior abdominal surgery, patient's body habitus and surgeon's experience [10, 11, 18].

Regardless of the technical approach, a thorough understanding of endocrine pathophysiology, adrenal anatomy, proper positioning and the advantages and disadvantages of the various approaches are the key to a successful adrenalectomy.

23.2 Minimally Invasive Adrenalectomy

23.2.1 Laparoscopic Lateral Transabdominal Adrenalectomy

Gagner et al. first described laparoscopic transabdominal adrenalectomy with the flank approach in the lateral decubitus position in 1992 [19]. Soon after the initial description and standardization of laparoscopic lateral transabdominal adrenalectomy (LTA) [20, 21], its application has expanded significantly and quickly became the gold standard treatment for most adrenal surgical disorders [10, 22, 23].

The success of LTA is mainly due to some key factors: the laparoscopic approach allows an optimal exposure of the adrenal area; the magnification provided by the endoscope is particularly helpful during dissection of an anatomically complex and dangerous region as retroperitoneum is; from an anatomical point of view, the adrenal vascular supply is well defined; and the adrenalectomy is an ablative procedure, thus particularly suitable for a laparoscopic approach [10, 22, 23].

Although no randomized controlled studies have been conducted to compare the laparoscopic and open approaches for adrenalectomy, the current literature shows that laparoscopic adrenalectomy is associated with the expected benefits of minimally invasive surgery such as less postoperative pain, shorter hospital stay and recovery time and lower perioperative morbidity [24–31].

LTA is currently one of the most widely used approach, since it allows an optimal and comprehensive view of the adrenal glands and surrounding structures, and it provides a working space adequate for the dissection. An additional advantage of the transabdominal approach is the possibility to explore the abdominal cavity allowing the simultaneous treatment of potentially associated diseases [18]. Moreover, this approach allows a quick conversion to hand-assisted or open surgery in the case of troublesome dissection or intraoperative, otherwise untreatable, bleeding, without the need to reposition the patient.

▪▪ Indications

Laparoscopic adrenalectomy is the recommended approach for the treatment of small- to medium-sized (≤6 cm) adrenal tumours [6, 10, 15, 22, 23].

There is general agreement in the literature concerning the indication of LTA for all conditions of hypersecreting glands and tumours, such as primary hyperaldosteronism, phaeochromocytoma, and hypercortisolism with benign imaging features [6, 10, 22, 23].

The suitability of the laparoscopic approach for the treatment of large and potentially malignant adrenal tumours remains a controversial topic [12, 13, 15, 16, 32–35].

The 2002 NIH statement addressed that the prevalence of primary adrenocortical carcinoma (ACC) is clearly related to the size of the tumour, accounting for 2% of tumours ≤4 cm, 6% of tumours between 4.1 and 6 cm and 25% of tumours >6 cm [5]. However, tumour size alone as a limiting factor for the choice of the surgical approach for adrenalectomy has been considered relatively insensitive and nonspecific, since about 75% of adrenal tumours >6 cm will be benign at the final pathological report [12, 13, 35, 36]. Thus, if a tumour size >6 cm is recognized as a contraindication to laparoscopic adrenalectomy, the advantages of minimally invasive approach will be denied to patients having a most likely benign disease [12, 35, 36]. Indeed, the early experience with laparoscopic adrenalectomy from referral centres reported the safety of endoscopic approach for the removal of large adrenal lesions (up to 10 cm in maximum diameter), in absence of suspicious imaging features [12, 22, 23].

In the case of adrenal lesions with radiological evidence of local extension (invasion of surrounding structures, lymph node or distant metastases, intravenous thrombus), laparoscopic adrenalectomy is contraindicated [6, 15, 32, 35–40].

However, in the absence of radiological suspicious findings, it may be difficult to predict pre- and even intraoperatively the oncologic potential of an adrenal incidentaloma.

Indeed, the increased rate of adrenal incidentalomas referred to surgery with the widespread diffusion of minimally invasive adrenalectomy [41] led to a rise in the number of unexpected and "incidentally" pathological diagnosis of ACC after endoscopic adrenalectomy, up to 10% in some series [42].

Therefore, the surgical technique plays a key role in the treatment of adrenal tumours and should involve in all the cases a meticulous procedural approach that follows the oncological principles of dissection as adequate resection margin and en bloc removal of the adrenal with the peri-adrenal fat and intact tumour capsule, in order to prevent the risk of cell dissemination. In this context, it is significant to emphasize the importance of the rule of conversion to open approach whenever the dissection is challenging and potentially prevents a complete and oncologically correct adrenal removal.

Indeed, it is well known that a complete surgical resection is the mainstay treatment for localized ACC [43], since a R0 resection is the only means to achieve long-term disease control in ACC patients [38, 44].

Several reports found an increased risk for R1-R2 resection or tumour spill [16], peritoneal carcinomatosis [34, 45] and earlier recurrence [16] in patients undergoing endoscopic adrenalectomy for localized ACC. Therefore, based on these findings, an international consensus conference on ACC strongly discouraged endoscopic adrenalectomy for the treatment of known or suspicious ACC [33].

On the other hand, recently published comparative studies based on single-centre [46] or multi-institutional series [47] demonstrated that the oncologic outcomes of localized ACC following endoscopic adrenalectomy could be similar to that of open adrenalectomy.

The debate on this topic has been increasingly supported in the last years, due to the report of several series from the USA that further discouraged the laparoscopic approach in case of unknown/localized ACC [48–50], while some multi-institutional European comparative studies demonstrated that endoscopic adrenalectomy does not compromise the oncologic outcome of selected cases of ACC with respect to their open counterpart [51, 52].

More recently, it has been demonstrated that in referral high-volume centres, the oncologic outcome of unknown/localized ACC treated with endoscopic approach is not inferior to that achieved with open adrenalectomy, if strict selection criteria and the rule of conversion to open approach in case of challenging dissection are followed [4, 15, 40, 53].

The importance of the volume-outcome correlation in this specific field has been further underlined, in recent statements [4], recommendations [15] and guidelines [40] from European scientific societies, where the role of high-volume centres is addressed, together with the importance of a multi-disciplinary approach for ACC, both being achievable only in dedicated referral centres.

However, if an endoscopic approach is considered for an adrenal tumour at increased risk for malignancy (a mass with radiological intra-tumoural signs of suspicion and without clear loco-regional involvement), the transabdominal lateral adrenalectomy might be the preferred approach since it might allow intraoperative evaluation of the presence of distant metastasis and larger en bloc resection of the tumour [15].

General contraindications for LTA include patient comorbidities such as unacceptable cardiopulmonary risk and untreated or uncorrectable coagulopathy [10, 22, 23].

Relative contraindications may include large size, prior extensive abdominal or adrenal surgery and trauma in the vicinity and are mostly dependent on the surgeon's experience [54]. The history of abdominal surgery, especially previous upper mesocolic or retroperitoneal surgery, has been reported to increase the risk of intra- and postoperative complications as well as the risk of conversion [55].

Operative Technique

One of the main advantages of the transabdominal lateral approach is to allow the gravity-facilitated exposure of the adrenal glands. Indeed, after the mobilization of the structures overlying the adrenals, the liver on the right and the spleen and tail of the pancreas on the left, there is no need to manipulate further these structures during the following steps of the procedure.

From a technical point of view, essential requirements for a successful laparoscopic adrenalectomy are an appropriate knowledge of retroperitoneal anatomy, a gentle tissue manipulation and a precise haemostasis technique in order to adequately identify the structures of interest and avoid the troublesome oozing that could make the surgical procedure challenging.

Patient and trocars' position. The LTA requires a general anaesthesia, with muscle relaxation and controlled ventilation. The patient should be initially placed in a supine position for induction anaesthesia. An orogastric tube for gastric decompression (mainly helpful in left-sided adrenalectomy) and a Foley catheter are usually positioned. The current guidelines for antibiotic prophylaxis [56] and for prevention of venous thromboembolism [57] are applicable to most of adrenal pathologies, whereas some diseases (e.g. Cushing) are associated with a higher operative and perioperative risk [58].

The patient is then turned in a full lateral left decubitus position for the right and in a full lateral right decubitus position for the left adrenalectomy, respectively, with the 10th rib positioned over the breakpoint in the operating table. A cushion is placed under the opposite flank with respect to the side of adrenalectomy. The table is flexed in order to maximize the exposure of the space between the costal margin and the iliac crest. The right/left arm is elevated and secured on an elevated arm board. The patient's legs are flexed to avoid stretching of the crural nerve. The area from the umbilicus to the spine and from the nipple down to the superior anterior iliac crest should be exposed. Adequate patient positioning is essential for technical success in laparoscopic adrenalectomy. The surgeons stand on the abdominal side of the patient, facing the monitor at the head of the patient.

Atraumatic graspers, scissor, hook and clip applier are common to many laparoscopic procedures. More specific for adrenalectomy are small swabs, allowing atraumatic retraction of the gland. A right-angled grasper, a vascular clamp and a needle holder must be available on the operative table. An atraumatic grasper is useful for the mobilization of the adrenal gland in order to avoid bleeding during the manipulation of the periadrenal fat. Safe dissection requires a high-quality CCD camera. The operation is performed using a 30-degree 5/10-mm endoscope.

Initial peritoneal access is achieved about 2 cm inferior to the right/left costal margin in the midclavicular line, with either the blind (Veress needle) access, with the open (Hasson) access and with the optical access trocar. We use the optical access trocars that allow inserting the endoscope directly inside the clear trocar tip, enabling the surgeon to visualize all the abdominal layers during port placement. A pressure of 12–14 mmHg is generally used for CO2 insufflation.

For the right adrenalectomy, four trocars are used. A 5- or 12-mm trocar for the endoscope is placed in the subcostal area in the midclavicular line. A diagnostic laparoscopy is then performed. The ascending colon, the liver, the right kidney, the diaphragm and the duodenum are inspected. If there are signs suggestive of adrenal malignancies (e.g. local invasion), conversion is mandatory. Under direct vision, the second 12-mm trocar is placed in the subcostal area about 4 cm medially to the first. It receives graspers for exposure of the operative field, hook, scissors, retractors, instruments with peanut swabs and energy devices or clip applier to achieve adequate haemostasis. The third trocar (5 mm) is inserted in the epigastric area, receiving a smooth retractor in order to retract the liver during the whole procedure. The fourth trocar (5 mm) is inserted at the subcostal angle (◘ Fig. 23.1).

Left adrenalectomy, generally, may be performed with three trocars. The first one, a 5- or 12-mm trocar, is positioned in the subcostal space at the anterior axillary line for the endoscope. Diagnostic laparoscopy is then performed. The ligament of the colonic splenic flexure and the descending colon are inspected. The spleen, the lateral segments of the left liver, the diaphragm and the greater curvature of the stomach are inspected. If there are signs suggestive of adrenal malignancies (e.g. local inva-

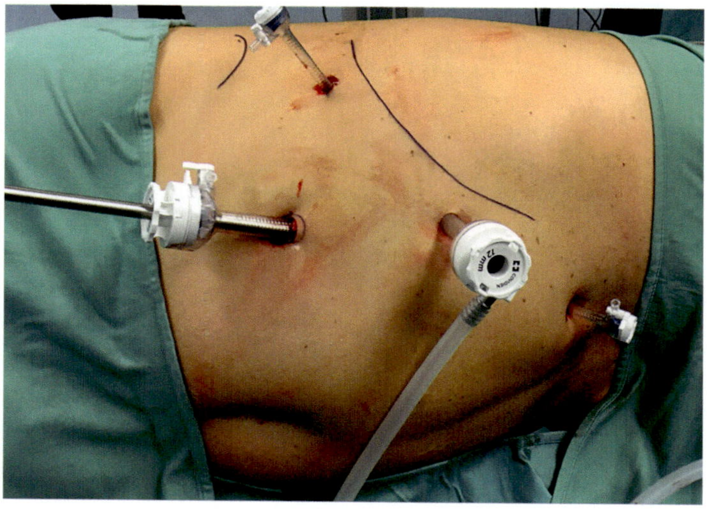

◘ **Fig. 23.1** Trocars' position for right laparoscopic lateral transabdominal adrenalectomy (LTA)

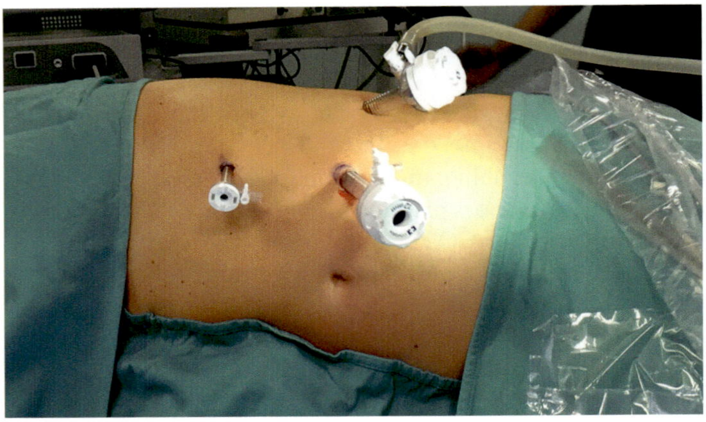

Fig. 23.2 Trocars' position for left LTA

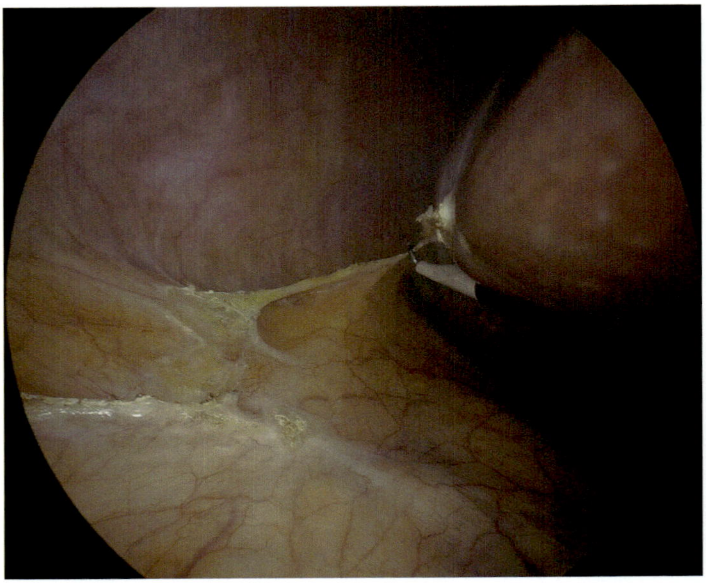

Fig. 23.3 Dissection of the right triangular ligament of the liver during right LTA

sion), conversion is mandatory. If the inspection is satisfactory, two other 5- or 10-mm trocars are placed under direct vision about 7 cm on each side of the first trocar below the costal margin (Fig. 23.2). As in the right side, they will take graspers for exposure of the operative field, hook, scissors, retractors, instruments with peanut swabs, clip applier and energy devices to achieve adequate haemostasis.

23.2.1.1 Right Adrenalectomy

Exposure. The key factor for exposure of the right adrenal region is a wide dissection of the right triangular ligament of the liver (Fig. 23.3) and of the posterior peritoneum (Fig. 23.4), allowing to achieve a complete mobilization of

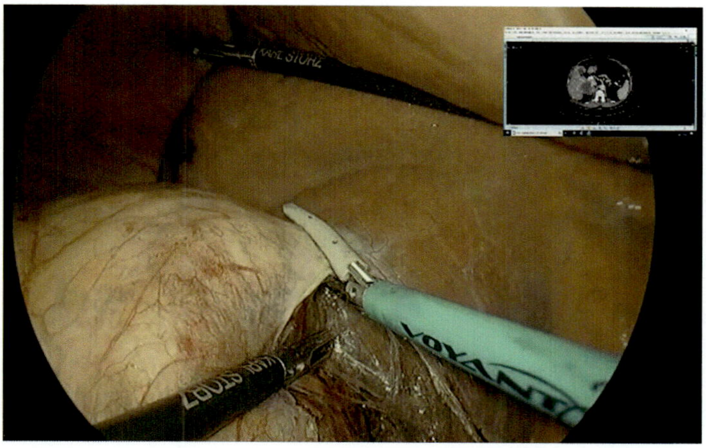

Fig. 23.4 Dissection of the posterior peritoneum (hepatoparietal ligament) during right LTA

the liver. The effective liver mobilization enables its cranial and medial retraction, opening the space between the liver and kidney and thus exposing the adrenal gland and the inferior vena cava (IVC).

Dissection of the main right adrenal vein. The main landmark for the right adrenalectomy is the IVC. Once the IVC has been identified, the procedure continues with the dissection of the plane between the adrenal gland and the IVC. The dissection of the lateral edge of the IVC should be accomplished starting from the right renal vein and proceeding superiorly. The medial edge of the adrenal gland is thus identified, and the plane between the IVC and the gland is opened, allowing the lateral retraction of the adrenal and exposing the area where the main adrenal vein runs. The right adrenal vein is generally short and wide. Once the main adrenal vein is identified (Fig. 23.5) and dissected with a right angle, it is doubly clipped and divided, completing the most difficult step of the dissection. The precocious dissection of the adrenal vein can be more demanding in the case of large adrenal lesions. Indeed, in this case, it can be suitable to start the dissection from the lateral and superior aspect of the lesion and then moving inferiorly along the IVC. In about 20% of cases, an accessory adrenal vein is encountered 2–3 cm above the main adrenal vein and when present should be dissected, clipped and divided.

End dissection/extraction. The adrenalectomy then proceeds with the dissection of the inferior aspect of the adrenal gland en bloc with the peri-adrenal fat. Once the posterior muscle plane is gained, the adrenal gland is lifted up, and the dissection is continued at the posterior and lateral aspect of the gland and finally superiorly. During these last steps of the dissection, the three main adrenal arteries and the accessory veins are identified and divided. The adrenal gland is then placed inside a retrieval bag and removed through a 10–12-mm trocar. The

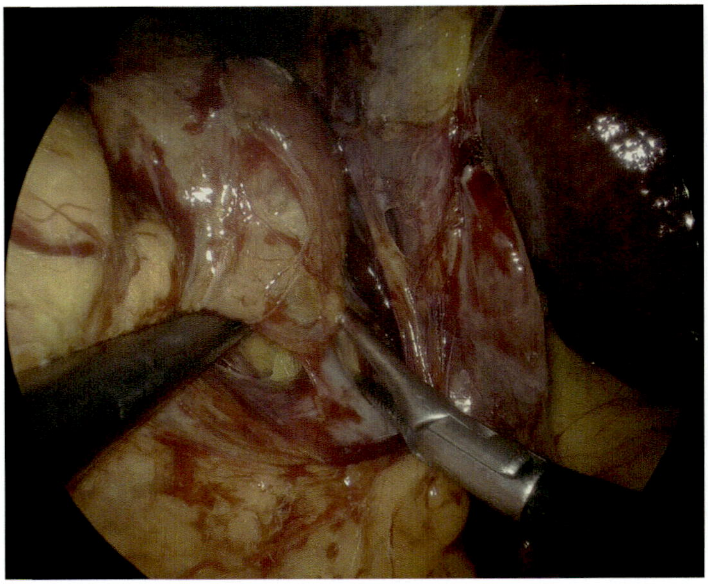

Fig. 23.5 Identification of the right main adrenal vein

placement of a drain in the adrenal region is optional but generally advisable. Careful port site closure is recommended in order to prevent incisional hernias.

23.2.1.2 Left Adrenalectomy

Several factors, such as the lack of major anatomic landmarks (e.g. the inferior IVC in the right side), the relative small size of the left adrenal gland, the location of main adrenal vein within the retroperitoneal fat and the close proximity of the pancreatic tail, may render left adrenalectomy a challenging procedure.

The prerequisite in order to achieve an adequate exposure of the left adrenal gland is a complete mobilization of the spleno-pancreatic bloc. Indeed, an effective dissection of the spleen along with the tail of the pancreas allows taking advantage of the gravity-facilitated exposure of the left adrenal gland, since the spleen will fall away from the operative field.

Exposure. The first step of left adrenalectomy is the dissection of the left colic flexure (Fig. 23.6).

Afterwards, the next step of the procedures is the mobilization of the spleen, accomplished by dissecting the spleno-parietal ligament easily exposed thanks to the lateral decubitus position (Fig. 23.7). The dissection of the spleno-parietal ligament is started at the posterior and inferior edge of the spleen, taking care to leave a margin of about 2 cm of peritoneum for an effective retraction of the spleen, allowing the exposure of its posterior aspect. The spleno-parietal ligament dissection is continued until the diaphragm, far enough to visualize the fundus of the stomach and the left crus of the diaphragm.

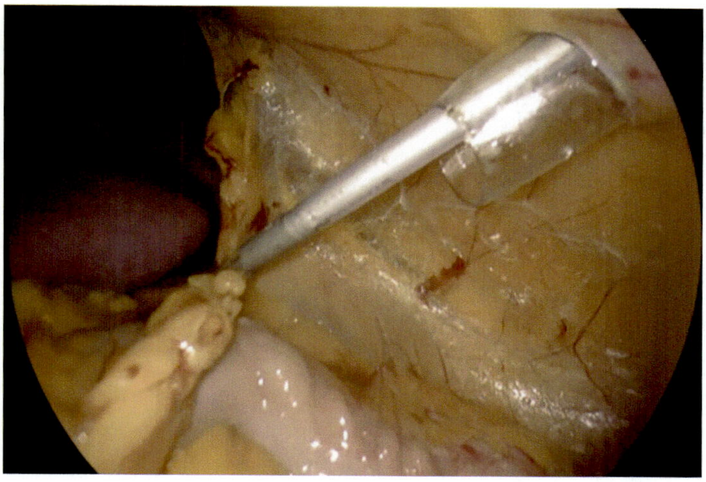

Fig. 23.6 Dissection of the left colonic flexure during left LTA

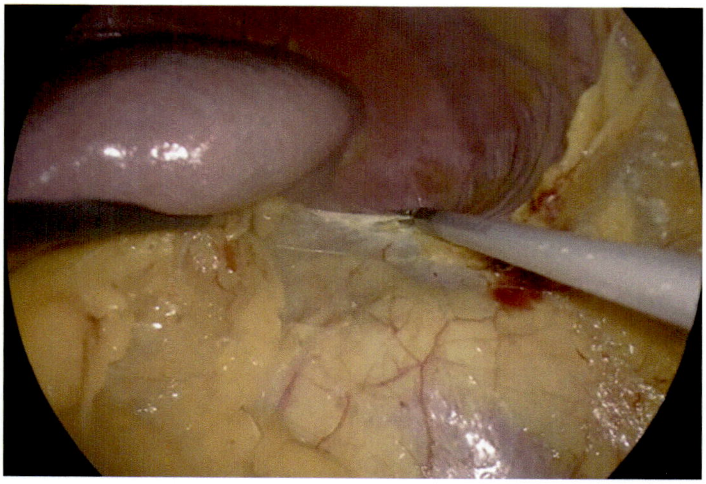

Fig. 23.7 Dissection of the spleno-parietal ligament during left LTA

The full dissection of the spleno-parietal ligament allows a complete mobilization of the spleen.

Then, the dissection proceeds with the division of the spleno-renal ligament, starting from the posterior aspect of the spleen and continuing with the tail of the pancreas. The medial and anterior retraction of the spleno-renal ligament allows its dissection in a superficial plane (Fig. 23.8), preventing opening of the renal fascia and avoiding the deep dissection in the peri-renal fat. At this point, the spleno-pancreatic bloc is displaced medially, out of the operative field, with gravity playing a major role, and the renal upper pole and adrenal area are exposed.

Dissection of the main left adrenal vein. The dissection of the left adrenal gland should start on the medial aspect of the gland, proceeding from upper to lower adrenal pole, keeping

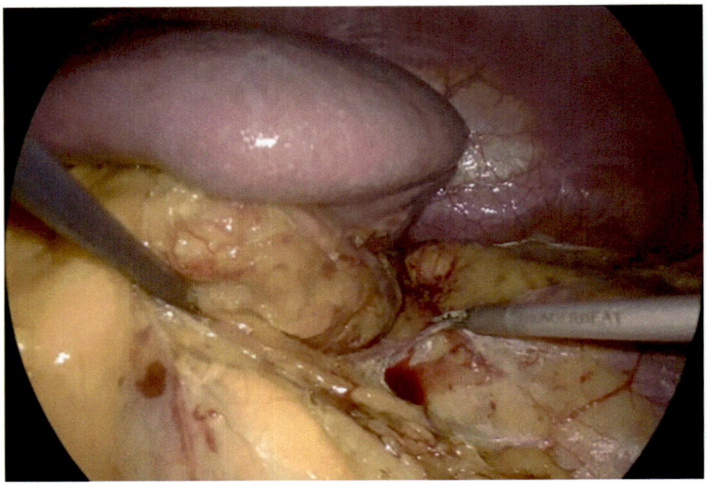

Fig. 23.8 Dissection of the spleno-renal ligament in the left LTA

close to the posterior muscular plane. This manoeuvre allows the lateral rotation of the adrenal and exposes the space where the left adrenal vein runs. Dissection of the lateral aspect of the gland should be avoided, since the adrenal gland would fall medially, preventing the access to its medial and inferior edge. During dissection of the medial aspect of the adrenal gland, the diaphragmatic vein is often encountered: it represents an important landmark for the identification of the main left adrenal vein. The main adrenal vein is identified at its entry in the left renal vein; it is isolated, often using a right-angle dissector, doubly clipped (Fig. 23.9) and divided.

End dissection/extraction. After dissection of the main adrenal vein, the adrenal is lifted en bloc with the peri-adrenal fat, and the dissection continues at the posterior and lateral aspects of the gland. The adrenal upper pole is dissected lastly (hanging technique). Dissection can be performed using a hook, coagulating scissors or energy devices. The adrenal within the retrieval bag is removed through a 10–12-mm trocar. The placement of a drain in the adrenal lodge is optional but generally advisable. Careful port site closure is recommended in order to prevent incisional hernias.

23.2.1.3 Pitfalls and Management of Complications

During each step of adrenalectomy, special attention must be paid in the dissection of the adrenal gland in order to avoid any tissue fragmentation and/or capsular breach. The surgical removal of the adrenal en bloc with the peri-adrenal fat helps to maximize the concept of oncological dissection.

Besides the general pitfalls related to the laparoscopic approach (bowel and vascular injuries, gas embolism, operative difficulties linked to adhesions, obesity, etc.), in the right adrenalectomy, there are some specific side-related problems, such

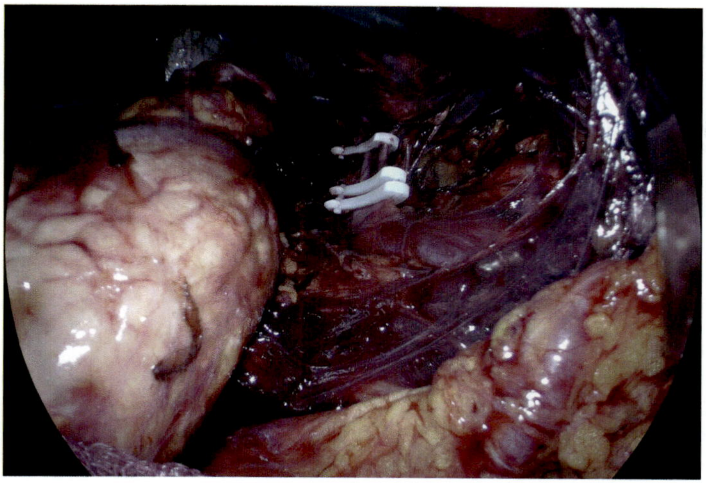

■ **Fig. 23.9** Identification of the left main adrenal vein at its entry in the left renal vein: it is isolated and doubly clipped

as liver injury, duodenum injury, IVC injury, division of a polar renal artery and injury of the diaphragm.

Specific side-related problems that can be observed for a left adrenalectomy are splenic injury and pancreatic injury. In the left-sided lesion, moreover, uncertainty can occur between the main adrenal vein and the renal vein especially in the case of large adrenal tumours that can displace the generally oblique left adrenal vein in a horizontal fashion. As in the right, also in the left adrenalectomy, inadvertent division of an unrecognized polar renal artery and diaphragmatic injury can occur.

Evidence of local invasion or difficulty in dissection that may prevent an adequate oncological resection or may portend capsular breach implies prompt conversion to an open approach for definitive en bloc resection.

Most of the bleeding encountered during laparoscopic adrenalectomy can be successfully treated laparoscopically in expert hands. However, in the case of uncontrolled bleeding presaging major lesion of the IVC or of the renal vessels, conversion to open approach is advisable for haemostasis. One of the advantages of LTA is that the lateral position allows a fast and easy conversion without the need to reposition the patient.

23.2.2 Posterior Retroperitoneoscopic Adrenalectomy

In 1992, Gaur published for the first time the technique of retroperitoneoscopy using a dissecting balloon to develop acceptable exposure for endoscopic exploration [59]. Soon after, in 1995, Mercan et al. reported their experience with posterior endoscopic approach in 11 adrenalectomies [60]. However, the technique failed to reach a wide diffusion probably for the inability to gain adequate exposure in the retroperitoneal space with standard insufflation pressure. Higher insufflation pressure was considered prohibitive at that time for the potential obstructive effect on the IVC and the consequent detrimental effect on the cardiac filling. Giebler et al. observed that patients who underwent posterior retroperitoneoscopic adrenalectomy (PRA) in the prone position had normal filling pressures and no evidence of decreased cardiac output despite the use of high insufflation pressure (20 mmHg) [61], demonstrating that retropneumoperitoneum at high pressure with the patient in prone position did not alter the cardiovascular haemodynamics and it is well-tolerated [61].

Indeed, thanks to these observations and after the standardization by Walz et al. [62, 63], the retroperitoneal approach was widely adopted, with minimal modifications, worldwide [11, 64, 65].

Subsequently, several large experiences demonstrated that PRA is safe and associated with decreased operative time and fast patient recovery [11, 63–65].

The posterior retroperitoneoscopic approach provides a direct access to the adrenal gland, without requiring the dissection of adjacent structures (the liver on the right and splenopancreatic bloc on the left), implying a theoretically decrease of the operative time.

However, the paucity of conventional landmarks and the difficult orientation, as well as the relatively small working space, are addressed by some surgeons as the major criticisms of this approach [23].

▪▪ Indications

Indications for PRA involve benign adrenal tumours, both functional and non-functional, isolated adrenal metastases in patients with known history of prior malignancy and bilateral benign adrenal disease.

Being an extra-peritoneal approach, PRA represents a valid alternative route of access to LTA in cases of extensive previous abdominal surgery, where the transabdominal access may be more challenging.

The posterior retroperitoneoscopic approach is particularly suitable in cases of bilateral adrenalectomy, since the prone position exposes both adrenals at the same time, without the need to reposition the patient in bilateral diseases. This could imply a potential decrease in the operative time, particularly relevant in the case of patients with Cushing's syndrome requiring bilateral adrenalectomy, for the potential impact on the surgical stress and thus on the postoperative morbidity. Simultaneous bilateral PRA is performed with two different surgical teams operating at the same time, one per side [66]. Indeed, recently, in a multicentre study comparing laparoscopic versus posterior retroperitoneoscopic versus robotic approach for synchronous bilateral adrenalectomy for Cushing's syndrome, Raffaelli et al. [67] reported a significantly shorter operative time in the group of patients who underwent posterior retroperitoneoscopic adrenalectomy.

The main disadvantage of PRA is perhaps the small working space, which limits the size of the lesions suitable for this approach to diameters ≤7 cm in very expert hands [68]. However, in most of the experience [11, 64, 65], benign lesions ranging in sizes within 6 cm represent the ideal indication for this approach.

Extreme obesity (body mass index >40) makes PRA more difficult but does not represent a contraindication in expert hands [63].

Absolute contraindication for PRA is suspected or known primary adrenal malignancy. Relative contraindications are lesion size greater than 4–6 cm and limited distance between the ribs and iliac crest, both of which make the procedure more technically challenging.

Although it has been hypothesized that the PRA is preferable to the LTA in the treatment of benign small- and medium-sized adrenal lesions, because of the theoretical advantages in terms of reduced operating time, lower rates of conversion and minimal dissection of the peri-adrenal structures [63], to date there are no definitive data in the literature which incontrovertibly demonstrate the superiority of an endoscopic approach over the other [11, 65]. Therefore, the choice of the best endoscopic approach still depends on surgeon experience rather than on objectively measurable arguments.

The ability to perform both LTA and PRA offers the possibility to choose the most appropriate approach tailored on the specific patients and tumour characteristics [11].

▪▪ Operative Technique

The patient is in prone position with the chest and the abdomen supported by the Wilson frame. The table is flexed in jackknife position with the back level, opening the space between the posterior costal margin and the posterior iliac crest (◘ Fig. 23.10).

The surgical team (surgeon, one assistant and one nurse) and equipment (insufflator, camera, surgical instrumentation) are assembled on the same side of the adrenal lesion. The monitor is positioned in front of to the surgical team.

Patient and trocars' position. A 1.5-cm transverse incision is performed just below the tip of the 12th rib. The retroperitoneal space is reached by blunt and sharp dissection of the abdominal wall. With this technique, a small cavity is prepared for the insertion of two standard trocars (5–10 mm), introduced with internal finger guidance 4–5 cm laterally (midaxillary line) and medially (erector spinae muscle) to the initial incision site (◘ Fig. 23.11). During the insertion of the medial trocar, particular attention must be paid in order to avoid the

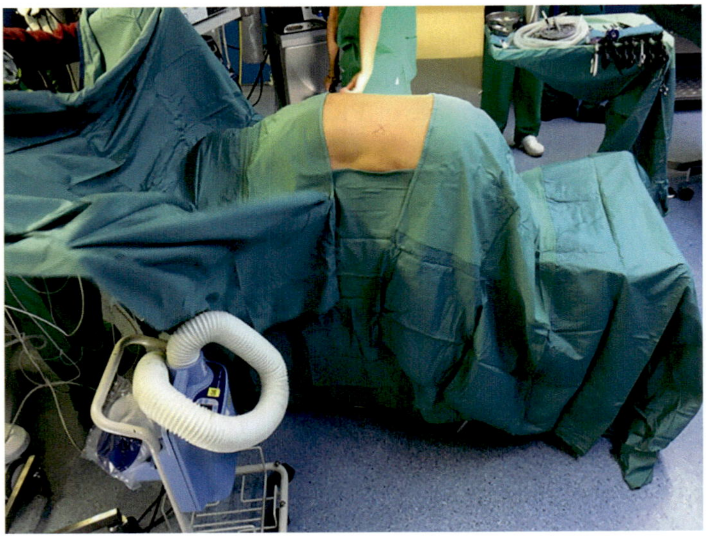

Fig. 23.10 Patient's position in posterior retroperitoneoscopic adrenalectomy (PRA)

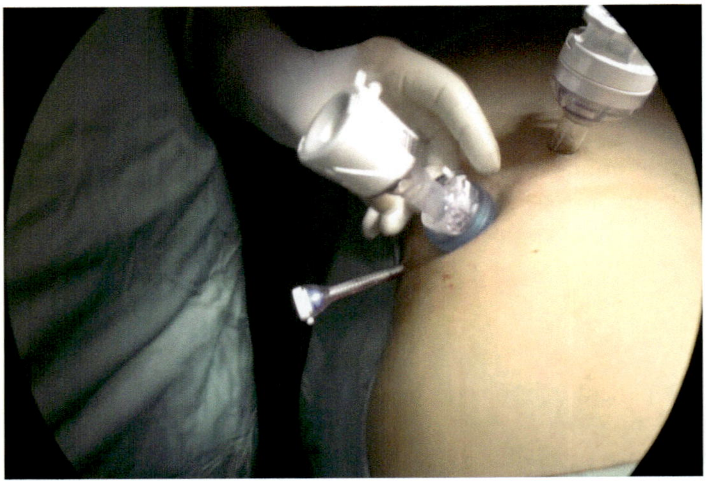

Fig. 23.11 Trocars' position in PRA

subcostal nerve. A blunt trocar with an inflatable balloon and an adjustable sleeve is introduced into the initial incision site and blocked. The retropneumoperitoneum is created by maintaining a CO2 pressure of 20 mmHg. Retroperitoneoscopy is usually performed with a 5–10-mm 30° endoscope, which is introduced into the first trocar.

Retroperitoneal dissection. Zuckerkandl's fascia (Fig. 23.12) is opened under direct vision by blunt and sharp dissection: the dissection should be as wide and far as possible, in order to allow an adequate access to the retroperitoneum. After the Zuckerkandl's fascia is opened, the retroperitoneal fat must be dissected downwards to expose the paravertebral muscles medially, diaphragm cranially and peritoneum later-

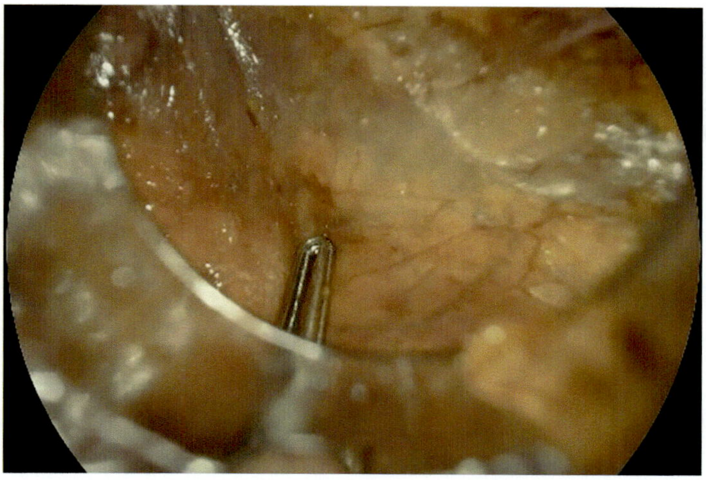

Fig. 23.12 Zuckerkandl's fascia

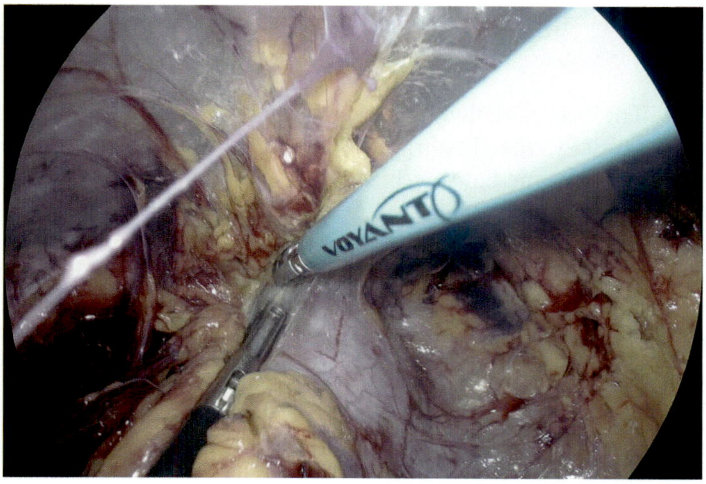

Fig. 23.13 Identification and dissection of the kidney upper pole in PRA

ally (with the liver and the spleen on the right and left side, respectively). This step is critical for the creation of an adequate working space. If the peritoneum is inadvertently opened at this time, the procedures could be continued, even if the pneumoperitoneum may reduce the working space.

Kidney upper pole dissection. Following the creation of the retroperitoneal space, the kidney upper pole should be exposed and dissected (Fig. 23.13). The kidney represents the most important landmark in the retroperitoneoscopic approach, crucial for the subsequent dissection of the adrenal gland. The dissection of the renal upper pole can be achieved by blunt and sharp dissection (monopolar coagulation and/or ultrasonic or radiofrequency activated shears). The dissection of the upper pole of the kidney should be as complete as possible, in order to allow an adequate exposure of the inferior aspect of the adrenal, essential for a safe identification of the main adrenal

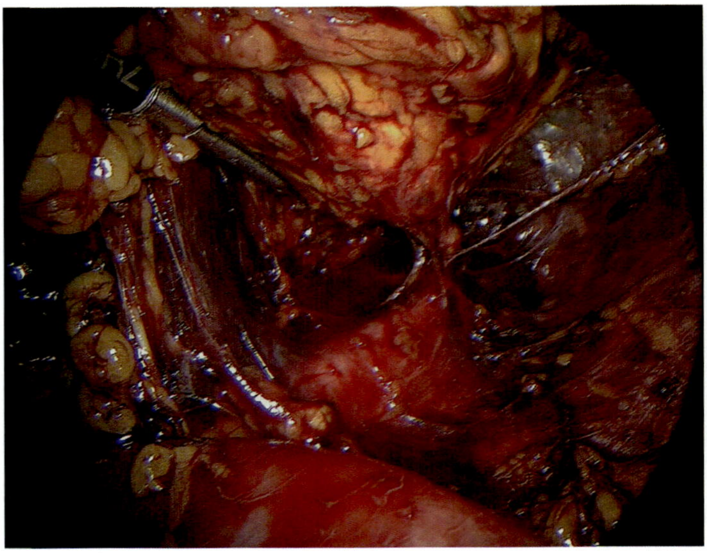

■ **Fig. 23.14** Inferior vena cava (IVC) in its retroperitoneal cranial aspect during PRA

vein. The operative field is now delimited by the kidney upper pole caudally, the diaphragm cranially, the spine and paraspinal muscles medially and the peritoneum laterally. The muscles of the posterior abdominal wall are the top of the space of dissection.

Adrenal gland and main adrenal vein dissection. The dissection of the adrenal gland begins caudally. All adrenal gland manipulations must be performed carefully using blunt palpation probes in order to avoid any capsular disruption and/or adrenal tissue fragmentation. Dissection is continued medially. In this area, on the *right side*, the adrenal gland arteries cross the vena cava posteriorly. These vessels are divided by means of activated shears or clips. After dissecting the right adrenal caudally and medially, the gland can be lifted up in order to expose the vena cava in its retroperitoneal cranial aspect (■ Fig. 23.14). The short right adrenal vein becomes then clearly visible running in a posterolateral direction. The right main adrenal vein is prepared for a length of about 1 cm and then dissected with a right angle and divided between clips (■ Fig. 23.15).

On the *left side*, the main adrenal vein must be prepared in the space between the adrenal gland and the diaphragmatic branch medial to the upper pole of the kidney. In this space, it is possible to identify the diaphragmatic vein joining the main adrenal vein: this represents an important landmark for identifying the left main adrenal vein. Once identified and adequately prepared with a right angle, the left adrenal vein is sectioned between clips (■ Fig. 23.16).

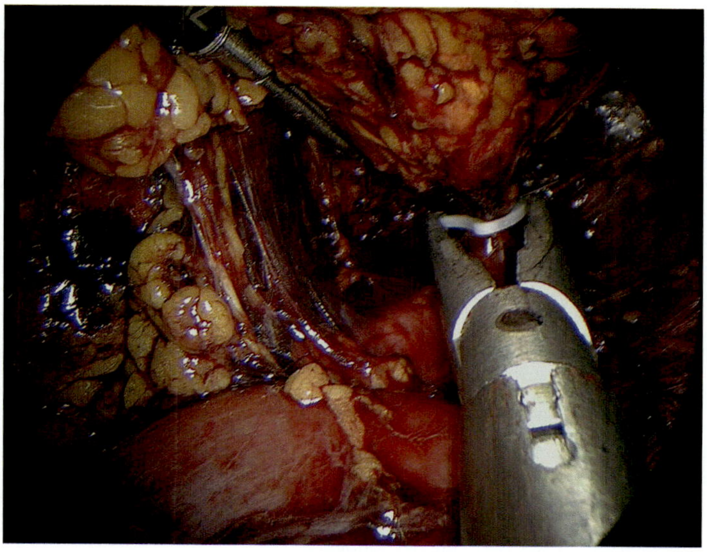

Fig. 23.15 The right main adrenal vein during PRA

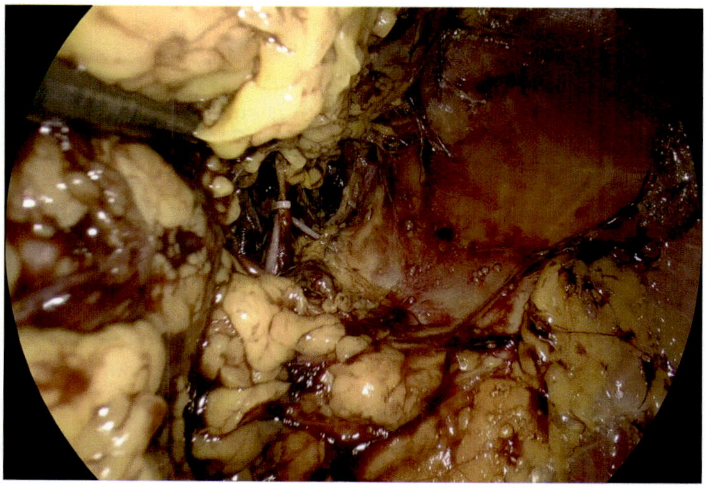

Fig. 23.16 Left adrenal vein in its junction with diaphragmatic vein during PRA

End dissection/extraction. The adrenal gland is then laterally and cranially dissected. The dissection of the cranial aspect of the adrenal gland as the last step of the procedure is of the utmost importance since it prevents falling of the gland in the operative field, thus reducing the need for its retraction (hanging technique) (Fig. 23.17). The resected adrenal gland is extracted within an endoscopic specimen bag through the central trocar port. The retroperitoneal space is then inspected for haemostasis. Insufflation is gradually decreased to a pressure of 12 mmHg, in order to identify eventual venous bleeding, hidden by the high insufflation pressure. The insertion of a suction drain is optional but advisable.

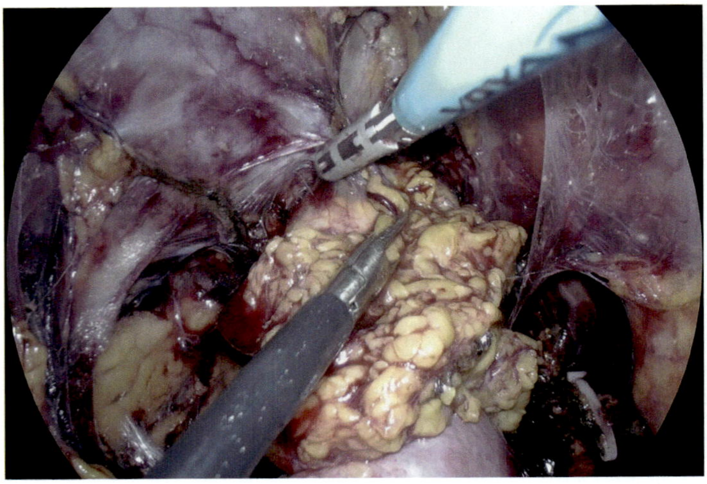

Fig. 23.17 The dissection of the cranial aspect of the adrenal gland is the last step of the PRA (hanging technique)

23.2.2.1 Pitfalls and Management of Complications

All manoeuvres on the adrenal gland should be carried out using atraumatic instruments, in order to prevent capsular disruption. In addition, also in PRA, it is suitable to remove the adrenal en bloc with the peri-adrenal fatty tissue.

Small inadvertent breach of the peritoneum can limit the working space but rarely prevents successful completion of the procedure.

A complication characteristic of PRA is a neuralgia caused by damage to the intercostal nerve at the level of the 12th rib during the trocar insertion. Injury to this nerve can determine hypoesthesia of the ipsilateral abdominal wall and can be associated with transversis abdominis relaxation. These injuries can be transient or permanent depending on the type of lesion of the nerve. They are reported in about 2–3% of the cases [63, 65].

In the case of troublesome intraoperative oozing, a slight increase of the CO2 pressure highly assists in the bleeding control.

In PRA, the upward direction of the dissection, both in the right and in the left side, guarantees an anatomical fixed hanging of the gland at its upper pole, reducing the need of adrenal manipulation and retraction.

In the case of failure to progress during a PRA, conversion to LTA should be considered.

As for LTA, also in PRA, most of intraoperative bleeding can be successfully treated; however, for uncontrolled bleeding, conversion to a transabdominal approach is indicated. Conversion to an open posterior approach may be an option.

23.2.3 Robot-Assisted Adrenalectomy

In 1999, Piazza et al. [69] and Hubens et al. [70] reported the first cases of robot-assisted adrenalectomy (RAA) using the ZEUS-AESOP (Computer Motion, Inc., Santa Barbara, CA). After the introduction of the da Vinci system (Intuitive Surgical, Sunnyvale, CA, USA), several series of robotic surgical procedures have been reported.

The widespread diffusion of robotic technology has led to the development and standardization of robot-assisted approach to adrenalectomy [71]. RAA has been proved to be feasible and safe in several centres [71–79]. The perceived advantages of RAA can be considered the improved ergonomics, the stereoscopic vision, the tremor filtration and greater range of motion within the operative field [80], potentially resulting in an ameliorated surgical dexterity and, theoretically, maximization of the surgical efficiency of conventional laparoscopic adrenalectomy. Indeed, it has been reported that RAA may improve the performance of surgeons without extensive laparoscopic experience who wish to perform minimally invasive adrenalectomy [81].

▪▪ Indications

Several variables, such as BMI [72, 75], previous abdominal surgery and tumour size [82], have been evaluated in different clinical settings, in order to figure out whether the RAA approach is preferable to the conventional laparoscopic approach in selected complex patients and/or in selected complex adrenal masses.

It has been observed that the effects of obesity (BMI ≥30) on laparoscopic adrenalectomy are a risk factor for complication [83] or significantly increase the operative time [54, 84].

It seems reasonable that the application of robotic technology in the case of adrenalectomy for obese patients can lead to some advantages over the conventional laparoscopic approach. Despite the relative scarcity of available data regarding this topic, it has been demonstrated that RAA in obese patients is able to overcome the technical difficulties in terms of exposure and dissection encountered in conventional laparoscopic adrenalectomy, reducing the need for conversion [75] and decreasing the mean operative time [78], without additional detrimental effects in terms of complication rate and length of hospital stay.

Large tumour size is generally associated with difficult dissection during conventional laparoscopic adrenalectomy, potentially leading to the risk of capsular breach and eventually impairment of oncologic outcome in the case of unknown malignant lesions [12, 14]. Currently, different threshold sizes have been considered to be large ranging from 5 to 10 cm with a general consensus of 6 cm [5, 12, 14, 35].

Several studies showed that adrenalectomy is feasible with both laparoscopic [12, 22, 23] and robotic [80] approaches in patients with large adrenal tumours. From a theoretical point of view, if the interposition of the surgeon-computer interface can maximize the efficiency of surgical procedure, RAA would be more suitable in this situation. Besides the inhomogeneous available data on this very controversial topic, it seems that RAA, in expert hands, can significantly reduce the operative time when dealing with large and challenging adrenal lesion [78, 85].

Partial adrenalectomy is considered as an option to spare adrenal parenchyma in selected patients with familial predisposition as an alternative to total adrenalectomy, in order to avoid the lifelong risk of morbidity and death related to adrenocortical insufficiency or long-term glucocorticoid replacement therapy. After laparoscopic partial adrenalectomy, it is considered that about 9% of patients developed local recurrence over time and 86% of them do not require routine steroid supplementation [80, 86]. Unfortunately, macroscopic intraoperative distinction between the cortex and the medulla can be very difficult, even with laparoscopic magnification [86]. In this context, the use of indocyanine green fluorescence imaging represents an emerging technology that facilitates the assessment of tissue vascularity, tissue distinction and tumour localization during surgery [87] (◘ Fig. 23.18). The application of robotic technology can be promising in this particular subset of patients, since the three-dimensional view can help in the definition of the adrenal parenchyma. Although the available literature on this topic refers to case series of few patients, the

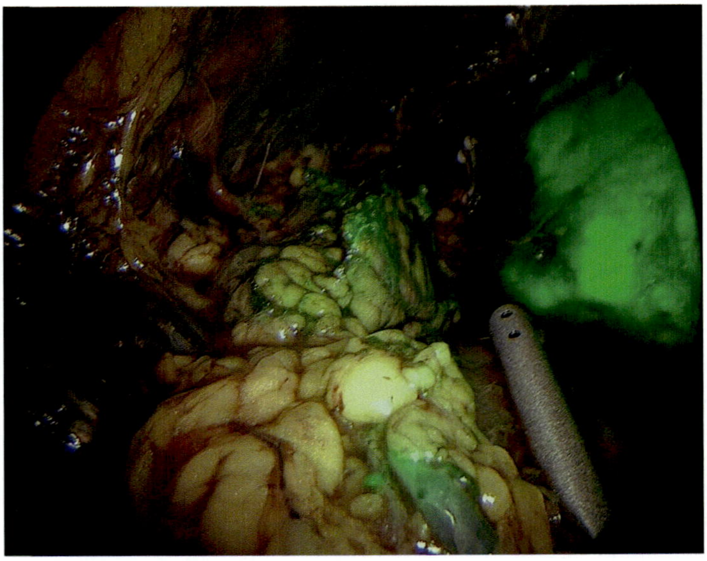

◘ **Fig. 23.18** Posterior retroperitoneoscopic bilateral partial adrenalectomy with indocyanine green fluorescence: assessment of tissue vascularity of the right adrenal remnant

preliminary reports appear encouraging in terms of functional and oncologic outcome [80].

However, to date, no clear benefit from the use of the RAA approach has been found [79], and cost increase still represents a major drawback correlated to RAA [4, 79, 82]. Moreover, in the healthcare system of several European countries such as France and Italy, the reimbursement recognized to robotic procedure is the same of laparoscopic ones (flat reimbursement). However, the increasing of the surgical load, the decreasing of the operative time and the efficacious employment of the operating room and its resources can allow to reach a positive cost margin, even when the robot-assisted approach for adrenalectomy is used [88].

23.2.4 Operative Technique

▪▪ Lateral Transabdominal Robot-Assisted Adrenalectomy

The da Vinci Robotic Surgical System (Intuitive Surgical, Sunnyvale, CA) includes a robotic engineering with three or four arms depending on the robot version (the central arm holds the camera, and the two or three other arms hold the surgical instruments) and a remote console from where the first operator performs the procedure. Once the pneumoperitoneum is created (15 mmHg), trocars are placed, and the right and left robot arms are connected. The docking step can be challenging at the beginning of the experience, but it can be reduced to 5–10 min after having acquired adequate expertise with the procedure [82, 88]. Usually, a 30° endoscope is used.

For the right lateral transabdominal RAA, the patient is in the left lateral decubitus position. The first port, a 12-mm camera port, is placed along the line between the umbilicus and the right costal margin. Two 8-mm robotic trocars are then inserted medially and laterally to the first camera trocar (these are the operative trocars for the first operator) at about 2–3 cm from the costal margin. A 5-mm trocar is positioned in the epigastrium to hold the liver retractor. A 10-mm accessory trocar (fifth trocar) is placed between the camera trocar and the medial operative robotic trocar to hold the clip applier for the assistant at the operating table (◘ Figs. 23.19 and 23.20). By the means of the accessory trocar (the fifth port), the assistant at the operating table clips and divides the adrenal vein and can use the suction if necessary. The surgical step of right transabdominal RAA reproduces the same step of LTA (see the specific section in the chapter).

Left transabdominal RAA is performed with the patient in the right lateral decubitus position. Trocar position includes the placement of the 12-mm camera port in the midway between the umbilicus and the left subcostal angle. The two

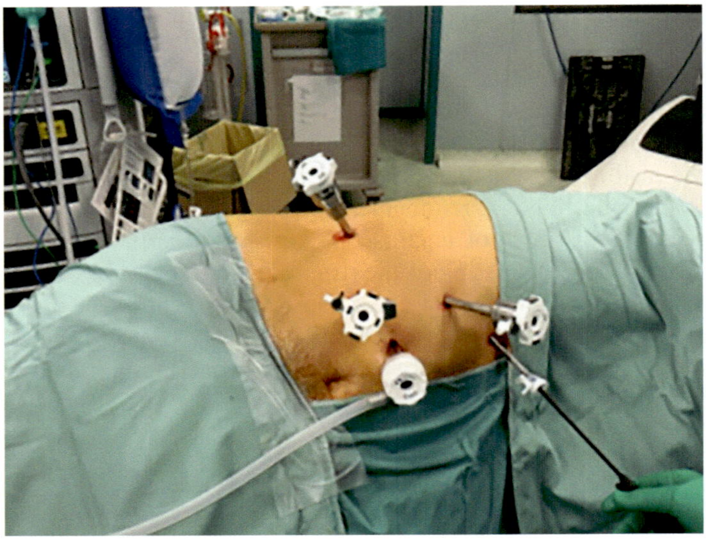

Fig. 23.19 Trocar position in the right lateral transabdominal robot-assisted adrenalectomy (RAA)

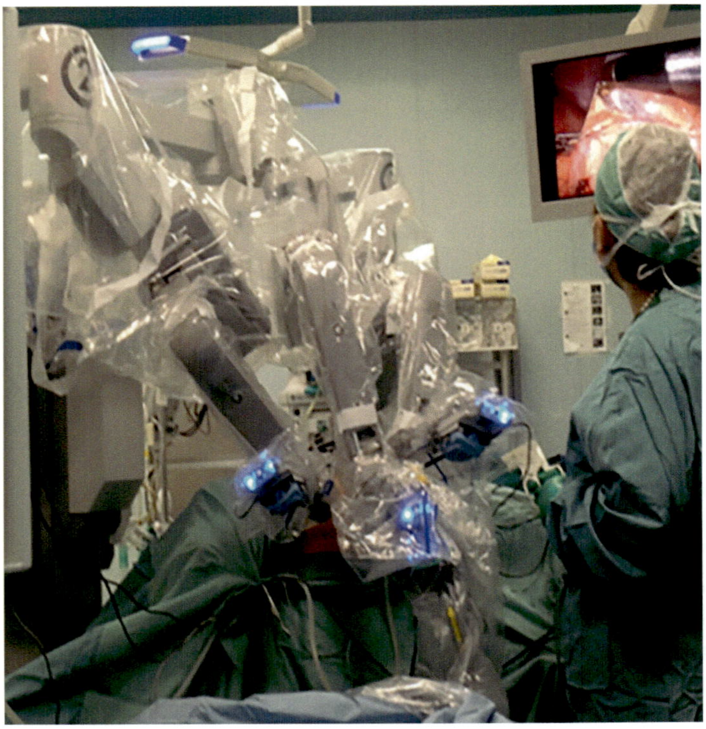

Fig. 23.20 Robotic arms' connection in the right lateral transabdominal RAA

8-mm robotic trocars are then inserted medially and laterally to the camera port and will hold the robotic instrument for the first operator at the console.

A 12-mm accessory trocar (the fourth port) is placed in between the camera port and the lateral robotic port to receive the clip applier for the assistant at the operating table.

Similarly to right transabdominal RAA, also the surgical step of left transabdominal RAA reproduces those of the left LTA (see the specific section in the chapter).

▪▪ Posterior Retroperitoneoscopic Robot-Assisted Adrenalectomy

Despite the direct access to the adrenal, the PRA implies several technical difficulties mainly related to the small working space and to the proximity of the trocar that can limit the triangulation of the rigid laparoscopic armamentarium. The robotic surgical technology has been applied to posterior adrenalectomy in order to overcome the limitation of conventional endoscopic approach. Although the reported series are small, and the diffusion of the technique is still limited to the proponent centres [89–91], the posterior robotic approach has demonstrated to be feasible and safe [89–91].

The patient and trocar position are the same to that described for conventional PRA. After conventional positioning of the three ports, the robot is docked, brought in front the head of the table, between the patient's shoulders. The 8-mm robotic ports are those medial and lateral to the camera port and are used by the first operator from the console. Thus, the adrenal vein is generally dissected with the vessel sealer or other energy devices. The use of a clip applier or of the suction implies the removal of one of the robotic instruments. The remaining steps of the procedure are similar to those of conventional PRA (see the specific section in the chapter).

23.3 Open Approaches for Adrenalectomy

Despite, today, most of adrenalectomies are approached with laparoscopic technique, open approach to adrenalectomy still plays a key role in the management of selected adrenal diseases. Several open approaches have been used for adrenalectomy [7–10]. The posterior open approach, being the most direct access to the adrenal gland, results in low postoperative morbidity. However, the small working space restricts the application of this approach to the treatment of adrenal lesions of limited size (generally <5 cm). The flank approach offers a quite good access to the adrenal region and to the relative major vascular structures, but it can be troublesome in the treatment of large adrenal lesion or in the case of tumours with local invasion requiring en bloc resection. The thoracoabdominal approach allows a wide exposure with the cost of a potential high postoperative morbidity. The anterior approach allows optimal access and exposure of adrenal regions with the morbidity of a major laparotomy.

Indications

Specific indications for an open adrenalectomy include adrenal masses with preoperative finding of invasion of surrounding structures and extension of the tumour into the renal vein or inferior vena cava (IVC) [15]. Indeed, the European Society of Endocrine Surgeons (ESES) and European Network for the Study of Adrenal Tumours (ENSAT) recommendations for the surgical management of adrenocortical carcinoma recently do not recommend "the laparoscopic approach for an adrenal mass with evidence of local invasion or suspected metastatic lymph nodes (ENSAT stage III)" [15]. To date, the most powerful prognostic factor for ACC remains the completeness of initial operative resection [92–94]. Therefore, the capability to extend the local resection, thanks to the improvement of operative management [95], could decrease the high local recurrence rate [92]. An open approach may be the preferred choice in the case of recurrent malignant phaeochromocytoma or ACC.

23.3.1 Operative Technique

Anterior approach. The anterior approach is the most commonly used for an open adrenalectomy. The anterior approach can be performed through a bilateral/chevron, unilateral subcostal or midline incision. The bilateral subcostal/chevron incision offers an optimal exposure of the peritoneal cavity and of both adrenal glands. A unilateral subcostal incision may be adequate for unilateral adrenalectomy (Fig. 23.21). The advantage of anterior access is the excellent control of the abdominal cavity allowing for a safe resection of the adrenal en bloc with any adjacent structure potentially involved by malignant invasion.

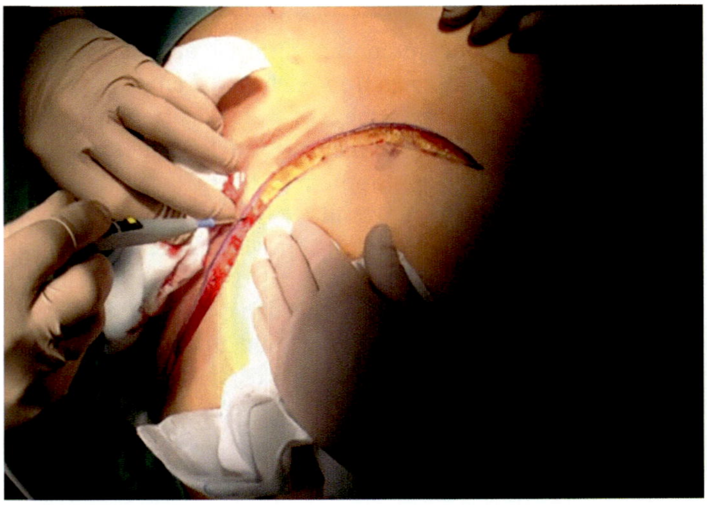

Fig. 23.21 Unilateral subcostal incision for open anterior right adrenalectomy

After opening the abdomen for an adrenalectomy, a careful inspection of the liver and peritoneum is mandatory to figure out the presence of metastatic disease. The first step of the surgical procedure is the dissection of the hepatic flexure of the colon. A subsequent ample Kocher manoeuvre allows to expose the IVC, the right adrenal gland and the upper pole of the right kidney.

In the right adrenalectomy, a wide dissection of the lateral and triangular ligament of the right lobe of the liver allows an adequate liver mobilization. For huge adrenal masses extending beyond the Morrison's pouch, a full mobilization of the right hepatic lobe may be requested. This implies the dissection of the falciform ligament up to the point of conjunction with the right triangular ligament. During the dissection of the lateral and triangular hepatic ligaments, attention should be paid in order to avoid unintentional injury respectively to the inferior diaphragmatic and middle hepatic veins. The liver mobilization with its superior and medial retraction provides wide access to the adrenal region. At this point, the dissection is continued exposing the lateral aspect of the IVC starting from the junction of the right renal vein and proceeding cephalad (◘ Fig. 23.22): the short right adrenal vein is then encountered

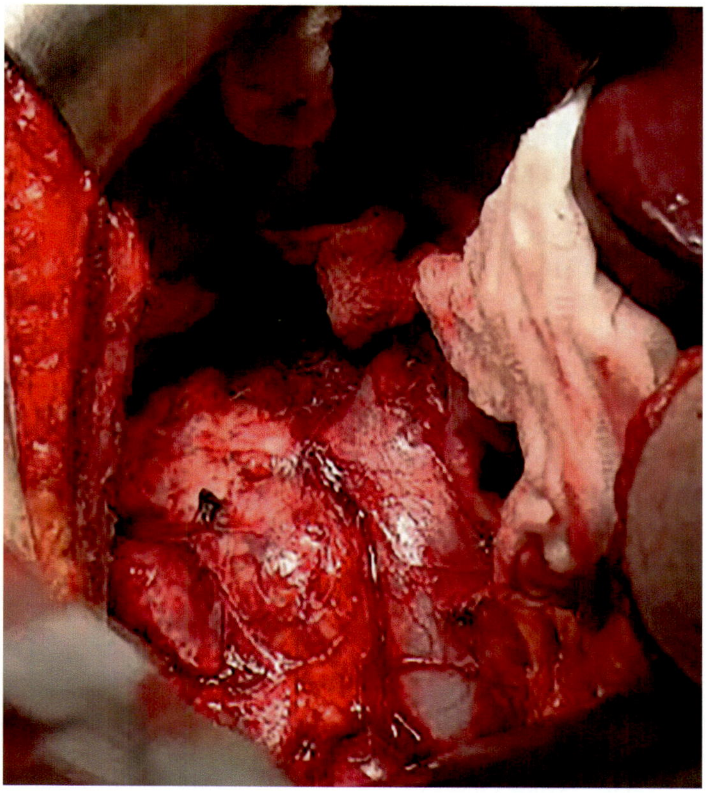

◘ **Fig. 23.22** Exposition of IVC during open anterior adrenalectomy: the dissection of the lateral aspect of the IVC is started from the junction of the right renal vein and proceeds cephalad

running from the anterior surface of the adrenal to the posterior face of the IVC.

In the case in which a right kidney en bloc resection is planned, it is advisable to expose and recount the left renal vein at its conjunction with the IVC. The right adrenal vein can be clipped, ligated or sutured according to the vein size. In the case of phaeochromocytoma, a precocious vascular control is advisable in order to avoid catecholamine release during the tumour manipulation.

The dissection is then continued along the superior, lateral and inferior aspect of the adrenal gland. The accessory adrenal veins and the arterial adrenal pedicles can be ligated, clipped or dissected by means of activated shears, according to the surgeon preference. Involvement of the IVC with tumour thrombus is considered loco-regional disease and does not preclude resection of the adrenal tumour (stage III ACC – ENSAT) [43, 95]. Anterior approach provides optimal exposure in treating extension of tumour thrombus into the IVC: a small venotomy allows extracting the tumour thrombus that, typically, is not adherent to the wall of the IVC. Proximal and distal control of the IVC is essential to prevent tumour embolus.

In left adrenalectomy, a wide dissection of the left colic flexure extended downwards along the paracolic gutter and medially along the gastrocolic ligaments far enough to expose the inferior mesenteric vein allows inferior retraction of transverse and left colon, and it represents the first step of the surgical procedure. Then the lateral attachment of the spleen is dissected until the left diaphragm crus and the gastric fundus are exposed. During this step, special care should be taken in order to avoid excessive traction on the spleen causing troublesome capsular rupture.

Then, a Mattox manoeuvre or, more properly, a Jinnai variant of Mattox manoeuvre is performed in order to medialize the spleno-pancreatic bloc. The peritoneal layer of descending mesocolon is detached by incising the white line of Toldt. This line is a lateral avascular reflection of the visceral peritoneum covering the colon and its mesentery over the lateral abdominal wall to become the parietal peritoneum. This opens the plane of dissection in the retroperitoneal space.

If tumour invasion prevents the mobilization of the spleno-pancreatic bloc, the access to the adrenal can be gained by opening the lesser sac dissecting the gastrocolic ligament. The correct oncological approach to large malignant tumours implies en bloc resection of the pancreas, spleen and/or kidney, if indicated.

At this point, the incision of the renal fascia exposes the adrenal gland and allows access to adrenal vein that runs from the infero-medial aspect of the adrenal draining into the renal vein. The dissection should start from the infero-lateral border of the adrenal gland in order to identify the adrenal vein. Then the left adrenal is dissected by means of ligatures or clips or activated shears. Once the adrenal vein is ligated, it is advisable to not complete the dissection of the inferior aspect of the adrenal gland, to prevent the cranial retraction of the adrenal vein. Indeed, different from the laparoscopic approach, the dissection is continued with the mobilization of the adrenal upper pole allowing downward retraction of the gland. In the case of tumour thrombus involving the adrenal vein and usually extending also in renal vein, besides nephrectomy, other possibilities include thrombus extraction as previously described for right adrenalectomy.

Thoracoabdominal/Lateral Transthoracic Approach. This approach finds its application in the treatment of widely invasive malignant adrenal tumours with major vascular involvement. It provides adequate access to the supradiaphragmatic vena cava, in cases of wide vena cava tumour involvement, requiring proper control of the thoracic vena cava.

The patient position implies a full lateral or semi-lateral (45°) position with the operating table flexed at the level of the 11th rib in order to open the space between the thorax and the iliac crest.

The incision for a right adrenalectomy should follow the superior aspect of the 10th rib directing inferiorly and medially with oblique direction towards the rectus muscle. The 10th rib is resected with partial excision of costal cartilage. The diaphragm is dissected along the lateral abdominal wall avoiding damage to the phrenic nerve. The full mobilization of the liver allows its supero-medial retraction and provides wide access to adrenal region with optimal exposition of infra- and suprahepatic vena cava. Then, the careful dissection of Gerota's fascia allows to expose and mobilize the right kidney. Subsequently, the surgical steps are similar to those of the anterior approach.

On the left side, since the left adrenal gland takes place slightly lower than the right, the incision can follow the 11th rib, thus possibly avoiding to entering in the pleural cavity.

Posterior approach. Today, with widespread diffusion of laparoscopic adrenalectomy, which shares the same indication with this approach, the application of open posterior approach is very limited and perhaps restricted to those cases of conversion of PRA to open approach. Like its endoscopic counterpart, the open posterior approach is a direct access to adrenals that eludes entering the peritoneal cavity. The small working space limited this approach to adrenal lesion up to 5 cm in size. The patient's position is the same of retroperitoneoscopic adrenalectomy. According to the Young technique [10], the incision follows the 10th rib, starting about 5 cm laterally to the spine and directing inferiorly and laterally towards the iliac crest. However, an oblique incision following the course of the 12th rib can also be used.

Then the exposition of the 12th rib is achieved by means of dissection of latissimus dorsi and erector spinae muscles. The lumbodorsal fascia is then dissected and the retroperitoneum entered. The subsequent dissection, dissimilar to endoscopic approach that implies the hanging technique, will start superiorly and will proceed downwards.

Flank approach. The flank approach is a posterolateral extra-peritoneal access to the adrenal, providing a quite larger working space than posterior approach. The indications to flank approach are similar to those of posterior ones. Being extra-peritoneal, the flank approach can be proposed in the case of previous abdominal surgery. However, the exposure of adrenal region is limited, mainly in the right side. The patient is positioned in a full lateral position. The incision is made at the tip of the 11th rib on the right and of the 12th rib on the left at the level of the midaxillary line, and it is prolonged along the costal margin posteriorly. It is a unilateral access, requiring the reposition of the patient in the case of bilateral adrenalectomy.

23.3.1.1 Pitfalls and Management of Complications

Complications risks of the open approach are intrinsic to the chosen approach. Iatrogenic injury to any of the surrounding organs is possible, resulting in haemorrhage, enteric fistulae, pancreatic leak or splenic injury.

During the liver mobilization in the right open adrenalectomy, attention should be paid in order to avoid injury to hepatic veins, which run in the medial posterior attachments of the liver.

In the left adrenalectomy, injury to the pancreatic parenchyma can lead to postoperative pseudocysts or pancreatic fistula. These injuries should be repaired with either ligation, parenchymal transection or proper and adequate drainage.

The left adrenal gland extends infero-medially almost to the renal hilum, placing the renal vessels at risk of injury especially in the case of large size lesion. Moreover, a superior renal pole artery may be present in up to 15% of patients and should be searched either in the preoperative imaging studies or intraoperatively.

It is known that compared to the minimally invasive counterpart, the open approach is associated with a longer operative time, longer hospital stay, increased intraoperative blood loss and more intraoperative complications [96, 97]. However, the greater risk of morbidity of open adrenalectomy is also affected by a selection bias, since open surgery is primarily chosen for larger adrenal mass and malignant and/or invasive adrenal tumours.

Answers to the Questions

1. (b); 2. (d); 3. (c); 4. (a); 5. (d); 6. (b); 7. (d); 8. (a); 9. (d); 10. (a)

References

1. Young WF Jr. Clinical practice. The incidentally discovered adrenal mass. N Engl J Med. 2007;356(6):601–10.
2. Davenport C, Liew A, Doherty B, Win HHN, Misran H, Hanna S, Kealy D, Al-Nooh F, Agha A, Thompson CJ, Lee M, Smith D. The prevalence of adrenal incidentaloma in routine clinical practice. Endocrine. 2011;40:80–3.
3. Gimm O, Duh QY. Challenges of training in adrenal surgery. Gland Surg. 2019;8(Suppl 1):S3–9.
4. Mihai R, Donatini G, Vidal O, Brunaud L. Volume-outcome correlation in adrenal surgery-an ESES consensus statement. Langenbeck's Arch Surg. 2019;404:795–806.
5. NIH state-of-the-science statement on management of the clinically inapparent adrenal mass ("incidentaloma"). NIH Consens State Sci Statements. 2002;19(2):1–25.
6. Fassnacht M, Arlt W, Bancos I, Dralle H, Newell-Price J, Sahdev A, Tabarin A, Terzolo M, Tsagarakis S, Dekkers OM. Management of adrenal incidentalomas: European Society of Endocrinology Clinical Practice Guideline in collaboration with the European Network for the Study of Adrenal Tumors. Eur J Endocrinol. 2016;175:G1–34.
7. Thornton JK. Abdominal nephrectomy for large sarcoma of the left suprarenal capsule: recovery. Trans Clin Soc Lond. 1890;23:150.
8. Mayo CH. Paroxysmal hypertension with tumor of retroperitoneal nerve. JAMA. 1927;89:1047.
9. Young HH. A technique for simultaneous exposure and operation on the adrenals. Surgery. 1936;63:179.
10. Smith CD, Weber CJ, Amerson JR. Laparoscopic adrenalectomy: new gold standard. World J Surg. 1999;23:389–96.
11. Lombardi CP, Raffaelli M, De Crea C, Sollazzi L, Perilli V, Cazzato MT, Bellantone R. Endoscopic adrenalectomy: is there an optimal operative approach? Results of a single-center case-control study. Surgery. 2008;144(6):1008–14.
12. Henry JF, Sebag F, Iacobone M, Mirallie E. Results of laparoscopic adrenalectomy for large and potentially malignant tumors. World J Surg. 2002;26(8):1043–7.
13. Lombardi CP, Raffaelli M, De Crea C, Bellantone R. Role of laparoscopy in the management of adrenal malignancies. J Surg Oncol. 2006;94:128–31.
14. Bellantone R, Lombardi CP, Raffaelli M. What is the appropriate role of minimally invasive vs. open surgery for small adrenocortical cancers? Curr Opin Oncol. 2015 Jan;27(1):44–9.
15. Gaujoux S, Mihai R. Joint working group of ESES and ENSAT. European Society of Endocrine Surgeons (ESES) and European Network for the Study of Adrenal Tumours (ENSAT) recommendations for the surgical management of adrenocortical carcinoma. Br J Surg. 2017;104(4):358–76.
16. Miller BS, Ammori JB, Gauger PG, Broome JT, Hammer GD, Doherty GM. Laparoscopic resection is inappropriate in patients with known or suspected adrenocortical carcinoma. World J Surg. 2010;34:1380–5.
17. Gaujoux S, Bonnet S, Leconte M, Zohar S, Bertherat J, Bertagna X, Dousset B. Risk factors for conversion and complications after unilateral laparoscopic adrenalectomy. Br J Surg. 2011;98(10):1392–9.
18. Raffaelli M, De Crea C, Bellantone R. Laparoscopic adrenalectomy. Gland Surg. 2019;8(Suppl 1):S41–52.

19. Gagner M, Lacroix A, Boltè E. Laparoscopic adrenalectomy in Cushing's syndrome and pheochromocytoma. N Engl J Med. 1992;327:1033.
20. Gagner M, Lacroix A, Bolte E, Pomp A. Laparoscopic adrenalectomy. The importance of a flank approach in the lateral decubitus position. Surg Endos. 1994;8:135–8.
21. Marescaux J, Mutter D, Wheeler MH. Laparoscopic right and left adrenalectomies. Surgical procedures. Surg Endosc. 1996;10(9):912–5.
22. Assalia A, Gagner M. Laparoscopic adrenalectomy. Br J Surg. 2004;91(10):1259–74.
23. Henry JF. Minimally invasive adrenal surgery. Best Pract Res Clin Endocrinol Metab. 2001;15(2):149–60.
24. Prinz RA. A comparison of laparoscopic and open adrenalectomies. Arch Surg. 1995;130:489–92.
25. Brunt LM, Doherty GM, Norton JA, Soper NJ, Quasebarth MA, Moley JF. Laparoscopic adrenalectomy compared to open adrenalectomy for benign adrenal neoplasms. J Am Coll Surg. 2001;183:1–10.
26. Thompson GB, Grant CS, van Heerden JA, Schlinkert RT, Young WF Jr, Farley DR, Ilstrup DM. Laparoscopic versus open posterior adrenalectomy: a case-control study of 100 patients. Surgery. 1997;122:1132–6.
27. Dudley NE, Harrison BJ. Comparison of open posterior versus transperitoneal laparoscopic adrenalectomy. Br J Surg. 1999;86:656–60.
28. Imai T, Kikumori T, Ohiwa M, Mase T, Funahashi H. A case-controlled study of laparoscopic compared with open lateral adrenalectomy. Am J Surg. 1999;178:50–3.
29. Lee J, El-Tamer M, Schifftner T, Turrentine FE, Henderson WG, Khuri S, Hanks JB, Inabnet WB 3rd. Open and laparoscopic adrenalectomy: analysis of the National Surgical Quality Improvement Program. J Am Coll Surg. 2008;206(5):953–9.
30. Elfenbein DM, Scarborough JE, Speicher PJ, Scheri RP. Comparison of laparoscopic versus open adrenalectomy: results from American College of Surgeons-National Surgery Quality Improvement Project. J Surg Res. 2013;184(1):216–20.
31. Eichhorn-Wharry LI, Talpos GB, Rubinfeld I. Laparoscopic versus open adrenalectomy: another look at outcome using the Clavien classification system. Surgery. 2012;152(6):1090–5.
32. Miller BS, Doherty GM. Surgical management of adrenocortical tumours. Nat Rev Endocrinol. 2014;10:282–92.
33. Schteingart DE, Doherty GM, Gauger PG, Giordano TJ, Hammer GD, Korobkin M, Worden FP. Management of patients with adrenal cancer: recommendations of an international consensus conference. Endocr Relat Cancer. 2005;12(3):667–80.
34. Gonzalez RJ, Shapiro S, Sarlis N, Vassilopoulou-Sellin R, Perrier ND, Evans DB, Lee JE. Laparoscopic resection of adrenal cortical carcinoma: a cautionary note. Surgery. 2005;138:1078–85.
35. Carnaille B. Adrenocortical carcinoma: which surgical approach? Langenbeck's Arch Surg. 2012;397:195–9.
36. MacGillivray DC, Whalen GF, Malchoff CD, Oppenheim DS, Shichmann SJ. Laparoscopic resection of large adrenal tumors. Ann Surg Oncol. 2002;9(5):480–5.
37. Fassnacht M, Kroiss M, Allolio B. Update in adrenocortical carcinoma. J Clin Endocrinol Metab. 2013;98:4551–64.
38. Else T, Kim AC, Sabolch A, Raymond VM, Kandathil A, Caoili EM, Jolly S, Miller BS, Giordano TJ, Hammer GD. Adrenocortical carcinoma. Endocr Rev. 2014;35:282–326.
39. Ronchi CL, Kroiss M, Sbiera S, Deutschbein T, Fassnacht M. Current and evolving treatment options in adrenocortical carcinoma: where do we stand and where do we want to go? Eur J Endocrinol. 2014;171:R1–R11.

40. Fassnacht M, Dekkers O, Else T, Baudin E, Berruti A, de Krijger R, Haak H, Mihai R, Assie G, Terzolo M. European Society of Endocrinology Clinical Practice Guidelines on the management of adrenocortical carcinoma in adults, in collaboration with the European Network for the Study of Adrenal Tumors. Eur J Endocrinol. 2018;179(4):G1–G46.
41. Miccoli P, Raffaelli M, Berti P, Materazzi G, Massi M, Bernini G. Adrenal surgery before and after the introduction of laparoscopic adrenalectomy. Br J Surg. 2002;89:779–82.
42. O'Neill CJ, Spence A, Logan B, Suliburk JW, Soon PS, Learoyd DL, Sidhu SB, Sywak MS. Adrenal incidentalomas: risk of adrenocortical carcinoma and clinical outcomes. J Surg Oncol. 2010;102:450–3.
43. Fassnacht M, Johanssen S, Quinkler M, Bucsky P, Willenberg HS, Beuschlein F, Terzolo M, Mueller HH, Hahner S, Allolio B, German Adrenocortical Carcinoma Registry Group; European Network for the Study of Adrenal Tumors. Limited prognostic value of the 2004 international union against cancer staging classification for adrenocortical carcinoma: proposal for a Revised TNM classification. Cancer. 2009;115:243–50.
44. Grubbs EG, Callender GG, Xing Y, Perrier ND, Evans DB, Phan AT, Lee JE. Recurrence of adrenal cortical carcinoma following resection: surgery alone can achieve results equal to surgery plus mitotane. Ann Surg Oncol. 2010;17:263–70.
45. Leboulleux S, Deandreis D, Al Ghuzlan A, Aupérin A, Goéré D, Dromain C, Elias D, Caillou B, Travagli JP, De Baere T, Lumbroso J, Young J, Schlumberger M, Baudin E. Adrenocortical carcinoma: is the surgical approach a risk factor of peritoneal carcinomatosis? Eur J Endocrinol. 2010;162:1147–53.
46. Porpiglia F, Fiori C, Daffara F, Zaggia B, Bollito E, Volante M, Berruti A, Terzolo M. Retrospective evaluation of the outcome of open versus laparoscopic adrenalectomy for stage I and II adrenocortical cancer. Eur Urol. 2010;57:873–8.
47. Brix D, Allolio B, Fenske W, Agha A, Dralle H, Jurowich C, Langer P, Mussack T, Nies C, Riedmiller H, Spahn M, Weismann D, Hahner S, Fassnacht M, German Adrenocortical Carcinoma Registry Group. Laparoscopic versus open adrenalectomy for adrenocortical carcinoma: surgical and oncologic outcome in 152 patients. Eur Urol. 2010;58:609–15.
48. Miller BS, Gauger PG, Hammer GD, Doherty GM. Resection of adrenocortical carcinoma is less complete and local recurrence occurs sooner and more often after laparoscopic adrenalectomy than after open adrenalectomy. Surgery. 2012;152:1150–7.
49. Cooper AB, Habra MA, Grubbs EG, Bednarski BK, Ying AK, Perrier ND, Lee JE, Aloia TA. Does laparoscopic adrenalectomy jeopardize oncologic outcomes for patients with adrenocortical carcinoma? Surg Endosc. 2013;27:4026–32.
50. Mir MC, Klink JC, Guillotreau J, Long JA, Miocinovic R, Kaouk JH, Simmons MN, Klein E, Krishnamurthi V, Campbell SC, Fergany AF, Reynolds J, Stephenson AJ, Haber GP. Comparative outcomes of laparoscopic and open adrenalectomy for adrenocortical carcinoma: single, high-volume center experience. Ann Surg Oncol. 2013;20:1456–61.
51. Lombardi CP, Raffaelli M, De Crea C, Boniardi M, De Toma G, Marzano LA, Miccoli P, Minni F, Morino M, Pelizzo MR, Pietrabissa A, Renda A, Valeri A, Bellantone R. Open vs endoscopic adrenalectomy in the treatment of localized (stage I/II) adrenocortical carcinoma: results of a multiinstitutional Italian survey. Surgery. 2012;152:1158–64.
52. Donatini G, Caiazzo R, Do Cao C, Aubert S, Zerrweck C, El-Kathib Z, Gauthier T, Leteurtre E, Wemeau JL, Vantyghem MC, Carnaille B, Pattou F. Long-term survival after adrenalectomy for stage I/II adreno-

cortical carcinoma (ACC): a retrospective comparative cohort study of laparoscopic versus open approach. Ann Surg Oncol. 2014;21:284–91.
53. Lombardi CP, Raffaelli M, Boniardi M, De Toma G, Marzano LA, Miccoli P, Minni F, Morino M, Pelizzo MR, Pietrabissa A, Renda A, Valeri A, De Crea C, Bellantone R. Adrenocortical carcinoma: effect of hospital volume on patient outcome. Langenbeck's Arch Surg. 2012;397(2):201–7.
54. Economopoulos KP, Phitayakorn R, Lubitz CC, Sadow PM, Parangi S, Stephen AE, Hodin RA. Should specific patient clinical characteristics discourage adrenal surgeons from performing laparoscopic transperitoneal adrenalectomy? Surgery. 2016;159(1):240–8.
55. Coste T, Caiazzo R, Torres F, Vantyghem MC, Carnaille B, Do Cao C, Douillard C, Pattou F. Laparoscopic adrenalectomy by transabdominal lateral approach: 20 years of experience. Surg Endosc. 2017;31(7):2743–51.
56. Berríos-Torres SI, Umscheid CA, Bratzler DW, Leas B, Stone EC, Kelz RR, Reinke CE, Morgan S, Solomkin JS, Mazuski JE, Patchen Dellinger E, Itani KMF, Berbari EF, Segreti J, Parvizi J, Blanchard J, Allen G, Kluytmans JAJW, Donlan R, Schecter WP, Healthcare Infection Control Practices Advisory Committee. Centers for disease control and prevention guideline for the prevention of surgical site infection, 2017. JAMA Surg. 2017;152(8):784–91.
57. Bates SM, Greer IA, Middeldorp S, Veenstra DL, Prabulos AM, Vandvik PO. VTE, thrombophilia, antithrombotic therapy, and pregnancy: antithrombotic therapy and prevention of thrombosis, 9th ed: American College of Chest Physicians Evidence-Based Clinical Practice Guidelines. Chest. 2012 Feb;141(2 Suppl):e691S–736S.
58. Babic B, De Roulet A, Volpe A, Nilubol N. Is VTE prophylaxis necessary on discharge for patients undergoing adrenalectomy for Cushing syndrome? J Endocr Soc. 2018;3(2):304–13.
59. Gaur DD. Laparoscopic operative retroperitoneoscopy: use of a new device. J Urol. 1993;149:973–6.
60. Mercan S, Seven R, Ozarmagan S, Tezelman S. Endoscopic retroperitoneal adrenalectomy. Surgery. 1995;118:1071–107.
61. Giebler RM, Walz MK, Peitgen K, Scherer RU. Hemodynamic changes after retroperitoneal CO2 insufflation for posterior retroperitoneoscopic adrenalectomy. Anesth Analg. 1996;82:827–31.
62. Walz MK, Peitgen K, Hoermann R, Giebler RM, Mann K, Eigler FW. Posterior retroperitoneoscopy as a new minimally invasive approach for adrenalectomy: results of 30 adrenalectomies in 27 patients. World J Surg. 1996;20:769–74.
63. Walz MK, Alesina PF, Wenger FA, Deligiannis A, Szuczik E, Petersenn S, Ommer A, Groeben H, Peitgen K, Janssen OE, Philipp T, Neumann HPH, Schmid KW, Mann K. Posterior retroperitoneoscopic adrenalectomy-results of 560 procedures in 520 patients. Surgery. 2006;140:943–50.
64. Dickson PV, Jimenez C, Chisholm GB, Kennamer DL, Ng C, Grubbs EC, Evans DB, Lee JE, Perrier ND. Posterior retroperitoneoscopic adrenalectomy: a contemporary American experience. J Am Coll Surg. 2011;212(4):659–65.
65. Gavriilidis P, Camenzuli C, Paspala A, Di Marco AN, Palazzo FF. Posterior retroperitoneoscopic versus laparoscopic transperitoneal adrenalectomy: a systematic review by an updated meta-analysis. World J Surg. 2020;45(1):168–79. https://doi.org/10.1007/s00268-020-05759-w.
66. Lombardi CP, Raffaelli M, De Crea C, Bellantone R, Fusco A, Bianchi A, Pontecorvi A, De Marinis L. ACTH-dependent Cushing's syndrome: the potential benefits of simultaneous bilateral posterior retroperitoneoscopic adrenalectomy. Surgery. 2011;149(2):299–300.
67. Raffaelli M, Brunaud L, De Crea C, Hoche G, Oragano L, Bresler L, Bellantone R, Lombardi CP. Synchronous bilateral adrenalectomy for

Cushing's syndrome: laparoscopic versus posterior retroperitoneoscopic versus robotic approach. World J Surg. 2014;38:709–15.
68. Walz MK, Petersen S, Koch JA, Mann K, Neumann HPH, Schmid KW. Endoscopic treatment of large primary adrenal tumours. Br J Surg. 2005;92:719–23.
69. Piazza L, Caragliano P, Scardilli M, Sgroi AV, Marino G, Giannone G. Laparoscopic robot-assisted right adrenalectomy and left ovariectomy (case reports). Chir Ital. 1999;51:465–6.
70. Hubens G, Ysebaert D, Vaneerdeweg W, Chapelle T, Eyskens E. Laparoscopic adrenalectomy with the aid of the AESOP 2000 robot. Acta Chir Belg. 1999;99:125–7.
71. Desai MM, Gill IS, Kaouk JH, Matin SF, Sung GT, Bravo EL. Robotic-assisted laparoscopic adrenalectomy. Urology. 2002;60:1104–7.
72. Brunaud L, Bresler L, Ayav A, Zarnegar R, Raphoz AL, Levan T, Weryha G, Boissel P. Robotic-assisted adrenalectomy: what advantages compared to lateral transperitoneal laparoscopic adrenalectomy? Am J Surg. 2008;195:433–8.
73. Brunaud L, Ayav A, Zarnegar R, Rouers A, Klein M, Boissel P, Bresler L. Prospective evaluation of 100 robotic-assisted unilateral adrenalectomies. Surgery. 2008;144:995–1001.
74. Giulianotti PC, Buchs NC, Addeo P, Bianco FM, Ayloo SM, Caravaglios G, Coratti A. Robot-assisted adrenalectomy: a technical option for the surgeon? Int J Med Robot. 2011;7:27–32.
75. Aksoy E, Taskin HE, Aliyev S, Mitchell J, Siperstein A, Berber E. Robotic versus laparoscopic adrenalectomy in obese patients. Surg Endosc. 2013;27:1233–6.
76. Brandao LF, Autorino R, Laydner H, Haber GP, Ouzaid I, De Sio M, Perdonà S, Stein RJ, Porpiglia F, Kaouk JH. Robotic versus laparoscopic adrenalectomy: a systematic review and meta-analysis. Eur Urol. 2014;65:1154–61.
77. Tang K, Li H, Xia D, Yu G, Guo X, Guan W, Xu H, Ye Z. Robot-assisted versus laparoscopic adrenalectomy: a systematic review and meta-analysis. Surg Laparosc Endosc Percutan Tech. 2015;25:187–95.
78. Morelli L, Tartaglia D, Bronzoni J, Palmeri M, Guadagni S, Di Franco G, Gennai A, Bianchini M, Bastiani L, Moglia A, Ferrari V, Fommei E, Pietrabissa A, Di Candio G, Mosca F. Robotic assisted versus pure laparoscopic surgery of the adrenal glands: a case-control study comparing surgical techniques. Langenbeck's Arch Surg. 2016;401:999–1006.
79. Economopoulos KP, Mylonas K, Stamou AA, Theocharidis V, Sergentanis TN, Psaltopoulou T, Richards ML. Laparoscopic versus robotic adrenalectomy: a comprehensive metaanalysis. Int J Surg. 2017;38:95–104.
80. Nomine-Criqui C, Germain A, Ayav A, Bresler L, Brunaud L. Robot-assisted adrenalectomy: indications and drawbacks. Updat Surg. 2017;69:127–33.
81. Talamini MA, Chapman S, Horgan S, Melvin WS, Academic Robotics Group. A prospective analysis of 211 robotic assisted surgical procedures. Surg Endosc. 2003;17:1521–4.
82. Greilsamer T, Nomine-Criqui C, Thy M, Ullmann T, Zarnegar R, Bresler L, Brunaud L. Robotic-assisted unilateral adrenalectomy: risk factors for perioperative complications in 303 consecutive patients. Surg Endosc. 2018;33:802–10.
83. Kazaure HS, Roman SA, Sosa JA. Obesity is a predictor of morbidity in 1,629 patients who underwent adrenalectomy. World J Surg. 2011;35(6):1287–95.
84. Chen Y, Scholten A, Chomsky-Higgins K, Nwaogu I, Gosnell JE, Seib C, Shen WT, Suh I, Duh QY. Risk factors associated with perioperative complications and prolonged length of stay after laparoscopic adrenalectomy. JAMA Surg. 2018;153(11):1036–41.

85. Thompson LH, Nordenström E, Almquist M, Jacobsson H, Bergenfelz A. Risk factors for complications after adrenalectomy: results from a comprehensive national database. Langenbeck's Arch Surg. 2017;402(2):315–22.
86. Rossitti HM, Söderkvist P, Gimm O. Extent of surgery for phaeochromocytomas in the genomic era. Br J Surg. 2018;105:e84–98.
87. Moore EC, Berber E. Fluorescence techniques in adrenal surgery. Gland Surg. 2019;8(Suppl 1):S22–7.
88. De Crea C, Arcuri G, Pennestrì F, Paolantonio C, Bellantone R, Raffaelli M. Robotic adrenalectomy: evaluation of cost-effectiveness. Gland Surg. 2020;9(3):831–9.
89. Dickson PV, Alex GC, Grubbs EG, Jimenez C, Lee JE, Perrier ND. Robotic-assisted retroperitoneoscopic adrenalectomy: making a good procedure even better. Am Surg. 2013;79(1):84–9.
90. Kahramangil B, Berber E. Comparison of posterior retroperitoneal and transabdominal lateral approaches in robotic adrenalectomy: an analysis of 200 cases. Surg Endos. 2018;32(4):1984–9.
91. Kim WW, Lee YM, Chung KW, Hong SJ, Sung TY. Comparison of robotic posterior retroperitoneal adrenalectomy over laparoscopic posterior retroperitoneal adrenalectomy: a single tertiary center experience. Int J Endocrinol. 2019;2019:9012910.
92. Pommier RF, Brennan MF. An eleven-year experience with adrenocortical carcinoma. Surgery. 1992;112:963–70.
93. Bellantone R, Ferrante A, Boscherini M, Lombardi CP, Crucitti P, Crucitti F, Favia G, Borrelli D, Boffi L, Capussotti L, Carbone G, Casaccia M, Cavallaro A, Del Gaudio A, Dettori G, Di Giovanni V, Mazziotti A, Marrano D, Masenti E, Miccoli P, Mosca F, Mussa A, Petronio R, Piat G, Marazano L, et al. Role of reoperation in recurrence of adrenal cortical carcinoma: results from 188 cases collected in the Italian National Registry for Adrenal Cortical Carcinoma. Surgery. 1997;122:1212–8.
94. Gaujoux S, Brennan MF. Recommendation for standardized surgical management of primary adrenocortical carcinoma. Surgery. 2012;152:123–32.
95. Mihai R, Iacobone M, Makay O, Moreno P, Frilling A, Kraimps JL, Soriano A, del Moral JV, Barczynski M, Durán MC, Sadler GP, Niederle B, Dralle H, Harrison B, Carnaille B. Outcome of operation in patients with adrenocortical cancer invading the inferior vena cava – a European Society of Endocrine Surgeons (ESES) survey. Langenbeck's Arch Surg. 2012;397:225–31.
96. Bittner JG 4th, Gershuni VM, Matthews BD, Moley JF, Brunt LM. Risk factors affecting operative approach, conversion, and morbidity for adrenalectomy: a single-institution series of 402 patients. Surg Endosc. 2013;27:2342–50.
97. Heger P, Probst P, Hüttner FJ, Gooßen K, Proctor T, Müller-Stich BP, Strobel O, Büchler MW, Diener MK. Evaluation of open and minimally invasive adrenalectomy: a systematic review and network meta-analysis. World J Surg. 2017;41(11):2746–57.

Neuroendocrine Tumors (Thymic and Gastroentero-pancreatic)

Contents

Neuroendocrine Tumors (Thymic and Gastroenteropancreatic): Anatomy, Endocrine Physiology, and Pathophysiology

Michael J. Stechman and Robert Bränström

Contents

A. L. Shifrin et al. (eds.), *Endocrine Surgery Comprehensive Board Exam Guide*,
https://doi.org/10.1007/978-3-030-84737-1_24

Case Presentation

A previously healthy 63-year-old male presents to the emergency room with a history of 3 days of abdominal pain, which has become increasingly severe over the last 24 hours and associated with profuse vomiting. He has no medical history apart from appendicectomy during adolescence. On clinical examination, he is dehydrated with a distended abdomen and generalized tenderness on palpation but no peritonitis. An emergency CT scan with oral and intravenous contrast clearly shows small bowel obstruction secondary to a tumor mass in the mesentery and multiple liver metastases. A more detailed patient history reveals weight loss, intermittent abdominal pain during the past 6 months, and a change in bowel habit to diarrhea but no family history.

Questions

Q1. What is the annual incidence of NET in the population (all variants included)?
1. 1/100,000
2. 5/100,000
3. 50/100,000
4. 100/100,000.

Q2. What is the most likely reason for the increasing prevalence of NET in the population?
1. The prevalence has not increased in society.
2. Better diagnostic methods and improved knowledge about NET.
3. Survival improved in the last decades.
4. 2 + 3.

Q3. What are the classical symptoms in carcinoid syndrome?
1. Diarrhea.
2. Flushing attacks.
3. Bronchospasm.
4. Heart valve stenosis.
5. All of the above.

Q4. Pathologists can usually diagnose NET in H&E sections, but the diagnosis can be additionally verified with immunohistochemistry. Which marker(s) has high specificity for NET?
1. Human epidermal growth factor receptor 2 (HER2).
2. Chromogranin A.
3. Synaptophysin.
4. Carcinoembryonic antigen (CEA).
5. 2 + 3, but not 1 + 4
6. All of the above (1 + 2 + 3 + 4).

Q5. Grading of NET is crucial for the choice of treatment. A cornerstone of the grading is Ki67. What does Ki67 measure?
1. Number of lymph nodes in surgical specimens with tumor growth.
2. A blood test for NET.
3. Cellular marker for proliferation.
4. The degree of surgical margin.

Q6. ^{68}Ga-DOTATOC-PET/CT scan is a modern method for visualizing NET. The method is based on NET cells expressing a certain receptor, which one?
1. Somatostatin receptor.
2. Calcitonin receptor.
3. Insulin receptor.
4. Glucagon receptor.
5. Serotonin receptor.
6. All of the above.

Q7. Chromogranin A can be measured in blood and is a relatively good marker for NET. However, there are several pitfalls, and some are mentioned below.
1. Proton pump inhibitors.
2. Certain foods like walnuts, pineapple, avocado, soy sauce, tomatoes, and more.
3. Prostate and urothelial cancer.
4. Chronic atrophic gastritis.
5. 1 + 2 + 3
6. 1 + 3 + 4
7. All of the above (1 + 2 + 3 + 4).

Q8. 5-HIAA, or 5-hydroxyindoleacetic acid, can now days not only be measured in urine, but some laboratories can also measure this in blood samples. 5-HIAA is a metabolite from a signaling substance that is rapidly metabolized when released, which is?
1. Somatostatin.
2. Catecholamines like adrenaline/epinephrine and noradrenaline/norepinephrine.
3. Chromogranin A.
4. Serotonin.
5. 1 + 4
6. 1 + 2 + 4
7. All of the above (1 + 2 + 3 + 4).

Q9. Appendix NETs are often diagnosed after appendectomy. How high is the incidence among appendectomies?
1. 1/10
2. 1/100
3. 1/300
4. 1/5000
5. 1/10,000.

Q10. A pathology report shows an appendix NET of 1.5 cm in diameter, with Ki67 of 10% but radically excised with clear margins (R0). There are no other abnormal findings in the pathology report. Does this patient require any additional investigation and treatment?
1. The tumor is radically excised, so no additional treatment or follow-up is needed.
2. Additional investigation with chromogranin A and PET/CT scan. If positive, re-operation with right hemicolectomy.
3. Upfront right hemicolectomy. No additional preoperative investigation is needed.

Q11. Liver metastases are common in small intestinal NET. What treatment options are available?
1. Somatostatin analogs.
2. Liver embolization.
3. Liver resection.
4. SIRT (selective internal radiation therapy).
5. ^{177}Lu-DOTATATE.
6. Liver transplantation.
7. All of the above are possible treatments.

Q12. The diagnosis gastrinoma is set by elevated levels of gastrin and chromogranin A, in combination with high acid production and low pH in the stomach. Where is the most common site of gastrinoma?
1. Pancreas.
2. Liver.
3. Small intestine.
4. Duodenum.
5. Stomach.
6. None of the above.

Q13. The gastrinoma diagnosis is set via blood samples, and the patient suffers from recurrent severe ulcer problems. Investigation using ^{68}Ga-DOTATOC-PET/CT scan and MRI does not show any tumor in the pancreas, duodenum, or other locations. Gastroscopy and EUS show no abnormality. You have tried medical treatments with little or no effect. What is the next step?
1. Capsule endoscopy.
2. Cholecystectomy.
3. Laparotomy and manual palpation of the duodenum.
4. Colonoscopy.

Q14. A patient with acute bowel obstruction is taken to the OR. During laparotomy, a tumor burden is found that binds the small intestine in a hard knot, and multiple liver metastases are seen. At the same time, the anesthesiologist complains of low swinging blood pressure and that the patient shows a mysterious redness in the skin. No major bleeding can be observed. What is your immediate action?
1. Ask anesthesiologist to administer more i.v. fluid.
2. End the operation as soon as possible.
3. Resect liver metastases and small intestinal tumor.
4. Ask anesthesiologist to administer i.v. somatostatin.
5. All of the above.

Q15. Continuing from question 14 (Q14), what is the most likely cause of the low blood pressure?
1. The tumor burden causes compression of the *inferior vena cava*.
2. Stenosis of heart valves.
3. Release of serotonin and other vasoactive peptides from primarily the liver metastases.
4. Decreased perfusion of the pulmonary circulation.

Q16. Continuing from questions 14 and 15 (Q14 + Q15), after solving the issue with low blood pressure, you have decided to proceed with surgery. One of the first steps is to palpate through the small intestine. Why?
1. Trigger and stimulate additional hypotension.
2. NET can be multiple.
3. Check for pancreatic tumors.
4. Make sure there are no other adherents.
5. 1 + 2 + 3.
6. 2 + 4.
7. All of the above (1 + 2 + 3 + 4).

Q17. Nowadays, somatostatin can be administered as an injection in a depot preparation. What is the recommended starting interval with the standard dose?
1. Once a week.
2. Every 4 weeks.
3. Twice a week.
4. Every other month.
5. When the patient has symptoms.

Q18. NET can be associated with certain types of hereditary syndromes. Which is?
1. Multiple endocrine neoplasia type 1 (MEN1).
2. Von Hippel-Lindau (VHL) syndrome.
3. Neurofibromatosis type 1 (von Recklinghausen's disease).
4. Tuberous sclerosis.
5. 1 + 3 + 4, but not 2
6. 3 + 4, but not 1 and 2
7. All of the above (1 + 2 + 3 + 4).

Q19. And speaking of heredity diseases, many hereditary conditions are inherited autosomal dominantly. What is the risk for first-degree relatives to carry the condition?
   1. 10%
   2. 25%
   3. 50%
   4. 75%
   5. 100%
   6. Needs to be calculated individually.

Q20. Low differentiated NETs with high proliferation and high Ki67 (>20%) are referred to as NEC (neuroendocrine cancer). What is the preferred method of visualizing tumor status in these cases?
   1. ^{18}FDG-PET/CT scan
   2. MRI.
   3. Regular CT scan.
   4. ^{68}Ga-DOTATOC-PET/CT scan.

Q21. Continuing from question 20 (Q20), what is the most common first line of treatment in NEC?
   1. Surgery.
   2. Somatostatin analogs.
   3. Chemotherapy.
   4. ^{177}Lu-DOTATATE
   5. SIRT (selective internal radiation therapy).

Q22. Multidisciplinary conferences are strongly encouraged in patients with NETs. Why?
   1. Excellent teaching opportunity.
   2. Treatment of NET is multimodal.
   3. The treatment involves several different specialties.
   4. These patients live a long time and will need several additional requirements during their lifetime.
   5. Equal patient care.
   6. All of the above.

Q23. The pancreatic NET can be both functional and non-functional, reflecting the tumor's ability to release hormones. What is the ratio between functional and non-functional pancreatic NETs?
   1. 20% functional/80% non-functional
   2. 40% functional/60% non-functional
   3. 60% functional/40% non-functional
   4. 80% functional/20% non-functional.

Q24. The diagnosis of insulinoma is biochemical. After prolonged 72-hour fasting, which laboratory findings are diagnostic of insulinoma?
   1. Elevated insulin levels of 60 pmol/L or more (normal <36 pmol/L).
   2. Glucose levels of less than 2.2 mmol/L (less than 40 mg/dL).
   3. C-peptide levels exceeding 6.25 nmol/L (normal <5 nmol/L).
   4. 1 + 2, but not 3

5. 2 + 3, but not 1
6. All of the above (1 + 2 + 3).

Q25. In European and American guidelines, the gold standard for surgical strategy in small intestinal NET is open laparotomy. What is the main reason for this?
1. Tumors release greater amounts of hormones during laparoscopy and abdominal inflation with CO_2.
2. NETs are indolent tumors and are often multiple. Careful palpation and inspection of the entire small intestine are necessary.
3. If multiple liver metastases are present, these must be resected at the same operation.

24.1 Introduction

The discovery of neuroendocrine tumors (hereon referred to as NET) of the gastrointestinal tract and pancreas began in the late eighteenth century when the German physiologist Rudolf Peter Heidenhain in 1870 described neuroendocrine cells from which these tumors arise. Later Siegfried Oberndorfer introduced the term carcinoid in 1907, where he characterized a tumor that was different from classic epithelial cancer but still possessed malignant features – a "cancer-like" tumor. The name carcinoid has been used ever since and can still be seen in some literature. Over time, nomenclature has changed with the addition of the terms foregut, midgut, and hindgut carcinoid to describe the embryonic location of the tumor. The pancreatic islet cells were first described in 1869 by Paul Langerhans, and in 1924, Seale Harris was the first to describe insulinoma. This was followed by the discovery of other tumors from neuroendocrine cells, such as gastrinoma (Robert Zollinger and Edwin Ellison in 1955) and VIPoma (John Verner and Ashton Morrison in 1958) [1]. The state of NET knowledge is continuously advancing, and the area is extremely broad in scope. The aim of this chapter is to provide a summary of NET, with a particular focus on surgical intervention and treatment strategies. For comprehensive, detailed knowledge, reference is made to dedicated literature and clinical guidelines. The most recent WHO classification for gastrointestinal neuroendocrine tumors dates from 2017 [2].

24.1.1 Incidence and Prevalence

NETs are relatively uncommon, and their incidence varies by tumor site between 0.1 and 1 per 100,000/year [3]; however, their prevalence is much higher because of prolonged patient survival due to their indolent nature. According to international data collection from US National Cancer Institute Surveillance Epidemiology and End Results (US NCI SEER), the overall annual incidence of NETs in 2004 was 5.25 per 100,000 inhabitants [4]. Increasing incidence and prevalence are probably due to improved diagnostics and increased knowledge in the field [5, 6]. NETs are equally common in men and women, and the median age at diagnosis is approximately 60 years, although they can occur at any age. Tumors may rise in most organs, but common sites are the gastrointestinal tract, pancreas, and lungs, followed by less common locations such as ovaries, kidneys, and testicles. Within the group of gastroenteropancreatic tumors (GEP-NETs), the origin of the tumor is distributed in the following manner: small intestine (35%), rectum (20%), appendix (15%), pancreas (10%), ventricle (10%), and colon (10%). NETs are usually malignant, but the majority are slow growing and may not give specific symptoms until significant local and distant spread has occurred. For these reasons, it is not uncommon for the diagnosis to be delayed for several years. Altered bowel habit, weight loss, bleeding, and abdominal pain are most commonly associated with advanced disease. At diagnosis, approximately 50% of the tumors are localized, 25% of the patients have locoregional spread, and about 25% of patients have distant metastases. NETs may also be classified according to whether they are functional (a syndrome attributed to hormone(s) or pre-hormone(s) secreted by the tumor is present) or non-functional tumors (no syndrome present). Around 60% are non-functioning, and this is because the hormones and pre-hormones produced may have no biological significance, such as chromogranin A, or are secreted at sub-physiological levels (see ▶ Sect. 24.5).

24.1.2 Heredity in NET

Most NETs are sporadic without known cause. Familial forms occur in multiple neuroendocrine neoplasia types 1 and 4 (MEN1 and MEN4), von Hippel-Lindau syndrome, neurofibromatosis type 1 (von Recklinghausen's disease), polycythemia-paraganglioma syndrome, and tuberous sclerosis. Individuals with these syndromes often have multiple tumors in several neuroendocrine organs simultaneously. These syndromes are generally inherited in an autosomal dominant fashion, which means that one of the index patient's parents will have the disorder and their siblings and children have a 50% risk of inheriting the disease.

24.2 Clinical Presentation

24.2.1 Gastric NET

Most NETs in the stomach are detected during gastroscopy and rarely cause symptoms. They are divided into three types where type 1 is the most common. These tumors are often referred to as ECLomas, that is, they originate from the mucosal enterochromaffin-like (ECL) cells. Occasional patients with ECLoma type 1, 2, or 3 tumors may exhibit atypical carcinoid syndrome with attacks of mucosal edema, usually in the respiratory tract, urticaria, and asthma-like symptoms caused by histamine secretion. The rarer ECLoma type 3 and neuroendocrine cancers (NECs) in the stomach can cause hematemesis/anemia or, in more advanced tumor disease, symptoms analogous to other malignant tumors of the stomach.

24.2.2 Endocrine Pancreas

Pancreatic NETs occur with an annual incidence of 0.5–1 per 100,000 of population. The vast majority are sporadic tumors, but pancreatic NET may occur with hereditary tumor syndromes such as MEN1, von Hippel-Lindau disease, tuberous sclerosis, and neurofibromatosis type 1. They are commonly detected either because the patient is being investigated for specific hormone-related symptoms that can be attributed to an endocrine tumor of the pancreas (see below), in the course of investigations for upper abdominal symptoms or pain, or as a side effect of a computer tomography (CT) scan examination performed for any other reasons (incidentalomas in the pancreas). There are both functional (40%) and non-functional (60%) pancreatic NETs.

24.2.3 Duodenal NET

Like other NETs, duodenal NETs can also be functional or non-functional. The average age for onset is approximately 65 years, and the tumors are slightly more common in men. They are extremely rare, making up about 1–3% of all NETs and similarly 1–3% of all duodenal tumors. The most common are gastrinomas, and in 90% of cases, they occur in the first part of the duodenum, while most of the remaining tumors are periampullary. Duodenal NETs are small, >75% are less than 2 centimeters, and they are usually submucosal. Spread to regional lymph nodes occurs in about 50% of cases, while liver metastases are uncommon. If multiple tumors are detected, MEN1 should be suspected, which is present in 6–10% of all cases of duodenal NET. In Zollinger-Ellison syndrome, the risk of MEN1 is up to 30%.

24.2.4 Small Intestinal NET

NETs of the small intestine (in older literature described as small bowel carcinoid) make up about a third of all GEP-NETs and just under half of all malignant small bowel tumors. Other small bowel tumors consist largely of GIST (gastrointestinal stromal cell tumors). The annual incidence is 1–2/100,000 of population, and the median age at diagnosis is between 60 and 70 years without a major gender difference. They are almost always sporadic, but in rare cases, a familial association is seen.

24.2.5 Appendix NET

NET of the appendix occurs in approximately 0.3–0.9% of appendectomies [7] and represents half of all appendix tumors. Most originate from enterochromaffin cells and are found in the appendix tip. Typically, they behave in a clinical fashion, stain positively for chromogranin A and serotonin, and are found by coincidence in connection with surgery.

24.2.6 NETs of the Colon and Rectum

Colonic NETs are very rare, and the average age of onset is about 60 years. Nearly half arise in the cecum (high proportion of enterochromaffin cells) and should be considered and treated as NETs of the small intestine. Spread to regional lymph nodes is seen in up to 45%, and distant metastases occur in approximately 40% of all colonic NET patients. Colonic NETs distal to the cecum, however, do not usually arise from enterochromaffin cells and should be considered as a separate entity. The 5-year survival for NETs of the colon is generally about 60%, but this falls to about 30% in the presence of metastatic disease. Rectal NETs are more common and make up about 20% of all NETs. The average age for onset is about 55 years. Most rectal NETs occur in the mid-rectum (5–10 cm from the dentate line) and are less than 1 cm. Lymph node metastases and distant metastases are seen in <10% of all patients with rectal NETs.

24.2.7 Neuroendocrine Cancer (NEC)

NEC is highly proliferative with Ki67 index >20%, and these tumors may occur anywhere in the gastrointestinal tract. NECs are predominantly seen in the esophagus and colon, with a median age at diagnosis of 60 years. In the latest WHO classification [2], the concept of pancreatic NET grade 3 (G3 NET) was introduced, which comprises highly differentiated pancreatic NETs with a proliferation >20% but usually <55%. These tumors were previously classified as pancreatic NEC but reclassified due to enhanced survival and requirement for less aggressive treatment.

24.2.8 Thymic NET

Primary NETs of the thymus are rare and highly aggressive tumors. They are usually located in the anterior mediastinal space and rarely in the middle or posterior mediastinum. They exhibit a male preponderance and slightly younger mean age at diagnosis of ~50 years [8]. In approximately half of the cases, thymic NETs are associated with other endocrinopathies like MEN1, Cushing's syndrome, and acromegaly. In MEN1 patients, these tumors represent the major cause of death [9].

24.3 Natural History

The natural history of NETs may exist on a spectrum from a very benign process with a long survival lasting several decades at one end to a very aggressive process where expected average survival is counted in months, at the other. It is therefore difficult to generalize since tumor behavior is largely dependent on the origin of the NET, its grade, whether it is functional or non-functional, and in particular whether it is surgically resectable at presentation.

24.4 Diagnosis and Common Syndromes

Since NETs are derived from cells that secrete hormones, amines, and peptides, they can give rise to a series of typical clinical symptoms, which are classically described as syndromes that are linked to the respective tumor type. Common medical conditions can often explain individual symptoms in a previously healthy patient. However, a specific combination of symptoms and clinical findings should raise the suspicion of a NET, followed by prompt in-depth history, examination, and investigation. Below is a review of the most common signs and symptoms, along with which conditions should be considered.

24.4.1 Classic Carcinoid Syndrome

Carcinoid syndrome is usually due to NET of the small bowel (embryonic midgut) and is derived from enterochromaffin cells that primarily produce serotonin and other vasoactive peptides. To cause hormonal symptoms, a certain tumor burden is usually required, usually the presence of liver metastases or retroperitoneal or ovarian metastases, which are not drained via the portal vein. The carcinoid syndrome is thus a late manifestation of the disease. Another common symptom of small intestinal NET is severe colicky abdominal pain due to obstruction.

The classical symptoms in carcinoid syndrome are:

- Diarrhea.
- Flushing attacks (reddening of the skin).
- Bronchospasm.
- Tricuspid valve stenosis ("carcinoid heart disease").

The diarrhea is sometimes profuse and watery (secretory) and in some cases very frequent. The flush comes in attacks, has a bluish red color, and usually affects the upper part of the torso and face. It is often provoked by food and alcohol intake or catecholamine release during stress or pain and may be associated with a significant drop in blood pressure. In carcinoid heart disease, the most common lesions are tricuspid insufficiency and pulmonary stenosis, which leads to right-sided cardiac failure in pronounced cases. The symptoms of failure can be triggered by anesthesia with positive pressure ventilation. A small proportion of patients with classic carcinoid syndrome may be affected by bronchospasm. This may be exacerbated by asthma treatment with sympathomimetics.

24.4.2 Atypical Carcinoid Syndrome

In rare cases, NETs of the stomach, duodenum, and bronchi can cause overproduction of histamine and vasoactive peptides, causing the so-called atypical carcinoid syndrome. In addition to diarrhea, the patient may suffer from anaphylactoid symptoms, skin rash, mucosal swelling, bronchospasm, and urticaria. The condition can imitate severe types of allergic reactions.

24.4.3 Diarrhea

Diarrhea is part of both the classic and atypical carcinoid syndrome. In small intestinal NETs, the cause is multifactorial. NETs derived from pancreatic islet cells may secrete VIP (vasoactive intestinal peptide) which leads to frequent, watery diarrhea. Effects of the peptide and the subsequent disorders in the electrolyte and fluid balance are often summarized as WDHA syndrome ("watery diarrhea, hypokalemia, and achlorhydria") or Verner-Morrison syndrome. Gastrin-producing tumors from G cells in the pancreas or duodenum can increase hydrochloric acid production, leading to diarrhea, which is a partial manifestation of Zollinger-Ellison syndrome. Somatostatin-producing tumors from delta cells in the pancreas can cause steatorrhea due to impaired fat absorption. NETs of the colon and rectum are rarely functional but can cause diarrhea (sometimes bloody) due to local tumor reaction. Glucagon-producing tumors in the pancreas (glucagonomas) also have diarrhea as a partial manifestation.

24.4.4 Small Bowel Obstruction

Small intestinal NETs commonly present with bowel obstruction, and many patients have repeatedly sought medical attention symptoms before the diagnosis is made and classic hormone-related symptoms occur. The obstruction can be due to the tumor itself and fibrosis around the primary tumor or mesenteric lymph node metastases. Bowel obstruction can also become acute and require emergency surgery (see Section "Indications for Surgery and Surgical Strategy").

24.4.5 Gastrointestinal Bleeding

Gastrointestinal NET can in rare cases lead to hematemesis or rectal bleeding. Bleeding ulcers arising from gastrin overproduction in gastrinoma can cause acute or chronic upper gastrointestinal bleeding, which is sometimes life-threatening.

24.4.6 Epigastric Pain and Dyspepsia

Increased hydrochloric acid production in gastrinoma causes acid-related symptoms with recurrent ulcers in the duodenum (Zollinger-Ellison syndrome) [10]. Other NETs, like other abdominal tumors, can cause nonspecific abdominal problems of varying intensity.

24.4.7 Flushing

Inflammatory flushing arises primarily from the amine-producing NET in the small intestine or (more uncommonly) in the bronchi or stomach (see above). Flushing can also be seen in VIPoma and gastrinoma patients. "Weathered appearance" in the form of telangiectasias and chronic blue-red discoloration of the face often becomes the result of long-term exposure to vasoactive hormones and is seen mainly in patients with small intestinal NET.

24.4.8 Jaundice

NET in the pancreas or duodenum can cause biliary or pancreatic obstruction and cause jaundice, steatorrhea, or pancreatitis. The same can be seen in widespread lymph node metastases of small intestine NET. Pronounced liver metastasis can, in rare cases, cause liver failure with jaundice.

24.4.9 Effects on Blood Pressure

Intermittent and sometimes dramatic hypotension is often seen combined with flushing in gastrointestinal NET and VIPomas. Pronounced peripheral vasodilation in severe and prolonged flushing can cause severe hypotension leading to shock. In rare cases, paradoxical hypertension may be seen in patients with small bowel NET.

24.4.10 Heart Failure

Heart failure due to advanced NET usually involving the right-side heart valves leading to right heart failure [11].

24.4.11 Pulmonary Obstructive Disorders

NET in the bronchi and upper gastrointestinal tract sometimes produces histamine which can give pronounced bronchospasm and anaphylactoid symptoms. The small intestinal NET can in rare cases give rise to obstructive disorders in classical carcinoid syndrome.

24.4.12 Abdominal Angina

Vascular effects of metastases or surrounding fibrosis in small intestinal NETs may result in mesenteric angina and eventual acute intestinal ischemia.

24.4.13 Pallor

Hypoglycemia attacks in insulinoma may cause catecholamine secretion, leading to the patient becoming pale and cold sweaty. Severe pallor, tremor, and sweating and tachycardia are also classical symptoms of pheochromocytoma (see Chap. 21 in this book).

24.4.14 Hypoglycemia

Hypoglycemia is the main symptom of insulinoma and causes tachycardia, tremor, sweating, and anxiety (as a result of hypoglycemia-triggered catecholamine secretion), which may result in disturbances of consciousness and seizures in severe hypoglycemia. Patients can often describe recurring problems during fasting or demanding physical activity, and over time, they may describe significant weight gain due to overeating as a method of avoiding attacks.

24.4.15 Hyperglycemia

In glucagonoma, hyperglycemia is the classical finding and can give rise to diabetes mellitus. Similarly, VIPoma, somatostatinomas, and ACTH-producing tumors (hypercortisolism) can occur in the pancreas and give rise to hyperglycemia.

24.4.16 Tachycardia

Insulinoma may cause tachycardia in hypoglycemic attacks (see above). Tachycardia can also occur in association with hypotension in severe flushing attacks in patients with small bowel NET.

24.4.17 Necrolytic Migratory Exanthema

A classical symptom of glucagon is migratory spots with redness of the skin, blisters, sores, and crusting that is primarily seen on the legs and around the mouth but also in the gluteal region, the groin, and the perineum.

24.5 Diagnostics

The diagnosis of NETs usually requires the use, in combination, of biochemical, radiological, nuclear medicine, and histopathology investigations. Biochemical diagnosis involves the measurement of general and specific hormonal markers. Radiological diagnostics are usually based on a CT scanning or magnetic resonance imaging (MRI) examination, and nuclear medicine investigation relies primarily on the expression of somatostatin receptors by tumor cells. Latterly, the combination of functional and cross-sectional imaging has been advanced by the introduction of Gallium-68 (^{68}Ga)-DOTATATE and ^{68}Ga-DOTATOC positron emission tomography (PET) scanning.

24.5.1 Biochemical Markers

Biochemical testing to establish the presence of elevated levels of hormones in plasma or urine is a key step in determining if:

1. The patient has a NET.
2. It is hormonally active.
3. The tumor responds to a given treatment.

Plasma concentrations are usually determined after a night of fasting and are often measured by the concentration of hormones or their metabolites in daily urine [12]. Hormones can be divided into general and specific, where chromogranin A is a general tumor marker for NET. This means that chromogranin A is expressed in all neuroendocrine cells with hormone-containing granules, and thus high levels are frequently present in patients with different types of NET. Specific hormones are usually expressed only in one cell type, for example, serotonin expressed predominantly in the small intestinal enterochromaffin cells, insulin expressed in the pancreatic β-cell islets, and glucagon expressed in the pancreatic α-cells.

24.5.1.1 Chromogranin A

Plasma chromogranin A (CgA) is one of the most widely used biochemical markers for NET, although it is not completely specific to this tumor group. The hormone is produced in all neuroendocrine cells and stored in secretory granules. There is continued speculation about its function, but there is no conclusive evidence for any functional role to date. In the individual patient, the plasma concentration of CgA correlates well with tumor burden when the patient is untreated. CgA is also a sensitive marker for detecting a small tumor burden, for example, to diagnose relapse early after radical surgery. In a treated patient, CgA reflects changes in tumor burden and can evaluate the treatment effect. Treatment with somatostatin analogs usually leads to a fall in CgA levels, without affecting the tumor burden. To evaluate CgA, one must be aware that several other conditions also result in an elevated serum CgA level. These include chronic atrophic gastritis (which can generate very high serum levels) and treatment with proton pump inhibitors. In both cases, the elevated CgA values are caused by a lack of acid production in the stomach, which leads to compensatory increased gastrin production. Elevated CgA can also be seen in prostate cancer and other tumors. Other non-tumor-related causes include renal impairment, liver failure, heart failure, stress, and inflammatory bowel disease. At the population level, the majority of people with elevated CgA will not be found to have a NET. Neuron-specific enolase (NSE) is another general biomarker for NETs but has its greatest significance in neuroblastoma, and there is currently no reason to measure NSE at adult patients with NET diagnosis.

24.5.1.2 Serotonin and 5-Hydroxyindoleacetic Acid (5-HIAA)

5-Hydroxyindoleacetic acid is a metabolite of serotonin and one of the diagnostic cornerstones for diagnosis and monitoring of NETs of the small intestine. Measurement is by 24-hour urine collection. In difficult cases, two collections may be necessary and then an average value calculated. Although morning urine tests have replaced daily measurements in some centers, more recently, serum 5-HIAA assays have become available, and this method is now recommended as it is easier for the patient and reduces errors due to the patient failing to collect a full 24-hour urine sample. Errors in 5-HIAA may also arise from intake of serotonin-containing foods (see below). Therefore, patient should be instructed to maintain certain dietary restrictions during the collection period and avoid certain foods (banana, pineapple, walnut, tomato, red wine, blue cheese, avocado, kiwi, plum, chocolate, and eggplant), nicotine, and alcohol.

24.5.1.3 Gastrin

The diagnosis of gastrinoma is biochemical and is made by measuring elevated levels of serum gastrin and CgA, in combination with high acid production in the stomach and low pH (<2). Note that the majority of patients with elevated levels of gastrin and CgA do not have gastrinoma. More commonly, the cause is either treatment with proton inhibitors or atrophic gastritis. The proton inhibitors should therefore be discontinued at least 2 weeks before sampling. If necessary, the patient uses antacids as an alternative, which do not affect gastrin levels. However, it is essential to remember that discontinuing proton inhibitors in a patient with gastrinoma can cause potentially life-threatening bleeding from gastrointestinal ulceration.

24.5.1.4 Insulin, C-Peptide, and Pro-insulin

Insulin, C-peptide, and pro-insulin are analyzed when insulinoma is suspected, partly as a screening test and in connection with 72-h fasting. Sampling for glucose, C-peptide, and insulin is performed every 3 h and monitored for symptoms of hypoglycemia. It is crucial to secure blood samples before the patient's hypoglycemia is treated to evaluate the test. Symptoms of hypoglycemia usually appears when glucose is less than 2.5 mmol/L (45 mg/dl). The insulin/glucose ratio should exceed 5 for the diagnosis of insulinoma to be secure. Individual patients have pro-insulin production instead of insulin, which should be measured at the start and end of fasting. It is essential to measure C-peptide to rule out that hypoglycemia can be caused by self-medicated insulin and/or oral hypoglycemic drugs.

24.5.1.5 Glucagon, Vasoactive Intestinal Peptide (VIP), Pancreatic Polypeptide (PP), and Others

Glucagon is analyzed on suspicion of glucagonoma (hyperglycemia and skin lesions compatible with *necrolytic migratory exanthema*). High levels of VIP are seen in VIPomas, and such tumors are also located in the pancreas or duodenum. Elevated levels of PP are seen in some pancreatic NETs, but these tumors frequently produce other peptides as well. It has been suggested that PP is one of the many satiety hormones and leads to decreased appetite at high levels and may also contribute to watery diarrhea at VIPomas. In experimental settings, several "non-functional" pancreatic NETs have been found to secrete PP [13]. ACTH is analyzed when ectopic ACTH-producing NET is suspected as the cause of Cushing's syndrome. Hyperglycemia in former non-diabetics may be a symptom of this. Calcitonin is produced by C-cells in the thyroid and is an excellent biomarker in medullary thyroid cancer. Calcitonin can, in rare cases, also be seen in pancreatic NET.

24.5.2 Endoscopy

Endocrine tumors of the stomach and duodenum are usually diagnosed during gastroscopy, often for dyspepsia symptoms. When examining the pancreatic NET, EUS (endoscopic ultrasound) has a higher sensitivity than radiology and is therefore recommended, especially in difficult-to-locate tumors. The role of endoscopy in the diagnosis of small intestinal NET is unclear, even though small intestinal NET can be diagnosed via colonoscopy if the tumor is located near the ileocecal valve. Push enteroscopy, or per-operative endoscopy, is rarely performed, and only anecdotes are described. Capsule endoscopy can sometimes be a useful tool for finding NETs in the small intestine if there are particular reasons to locate the primary tumor preoperatively, but the risk of the capsule lodging in a stenotic segment of small bowel must be taken into account. In the investigation of colorectal NETs, colonoscopy and proctoscopy have an important role as does endorectal ultrasound.

24.5.3 Radiological Diagnostics

CT scanning is the primary method for tumor staging, evaluating treatment, and determining the presence of relapse [14]. Mesenteric fibrosis, or desmoplastic reaction, surrounding a mesenteric mass is a pathognomonic feature of small intestinal NETs (◘ Fig. 24.1). The liver and pancreas should be evaluated before (native) and during intravenous contrast enhancement in the arterial phase (portal vein inflow phase) and the entire abdomen in the venous phase three-phase examination. Thoracic CT scan is always included initially in case of spread to the thorax. NET metastases in the liver and NET in the pancreas can show different contrast charging patterns and can sometimes only be seen in one phase and, therefore, missed if the examination is performed incorrectly.

MRI of the abdomen, including dynamic contrast-enhanced examination of the liver-pancreas and diffusion-weighted sequences, generally offers better diagnostics than CT scanning alone. This also applies to the detection of skeletal metastases for which CT scan lacks sensitivity. However, if MRI capacity

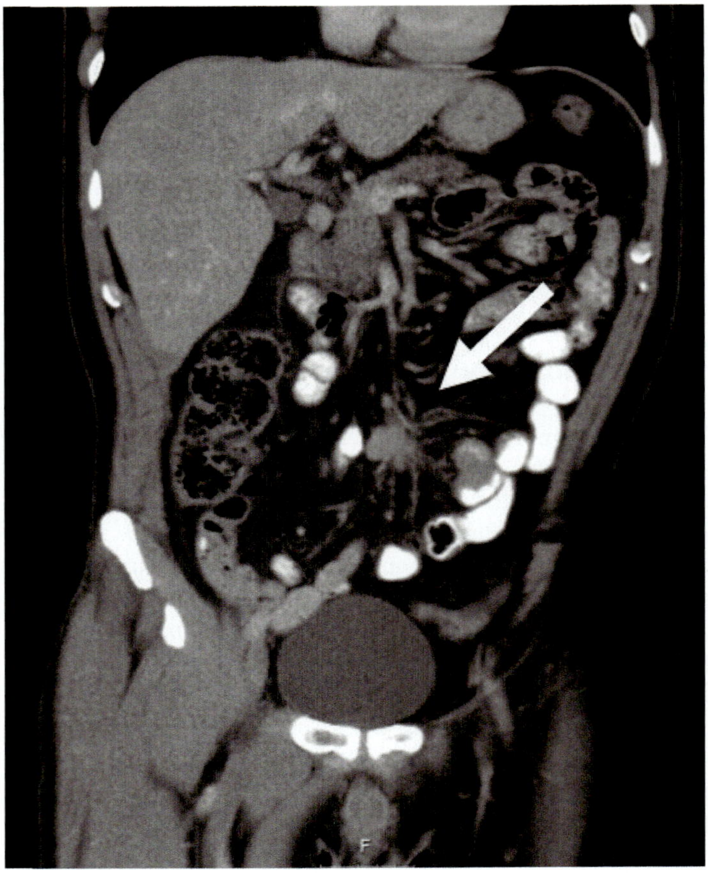

Fig. 24.1 Coronal sections from regular CT scan with oral and intravenous contrast enhancement, showing a small intestinal NET and a desmoplastic reaction in the mesentery (arrow)

is limited, it may be limited to cases where tumor detection, delimitation, and characterization are uncertain with CT scan. MRI may be an alternative in young patients with predicted long-term survival should not be exposed to the radiation dose from repeated CT scans checks should be examined with MRI, including those being screening for genetic NETs. However, small lung metastases can be missed with MRI due to the lower resolution compared with CT of the thorax. The latter should therefore be selected and performed with low radiation dose. Intravenous contrast-enhanced MRI is also better than CT scan for the diagnosis of brain metastases. Lastly, contrast-enhanced ultrasound has proven to be very useful for visualizing liver metastases, characterization of unclear CT scan findings, and the guidance of biopsies and ablation of liver metastases.

EUS has a high sensitivity for detecting pancreatic tumors as well as tumors localized in the esophagus, stomach, and duodenum. EUS should be performed in gastric and rectal

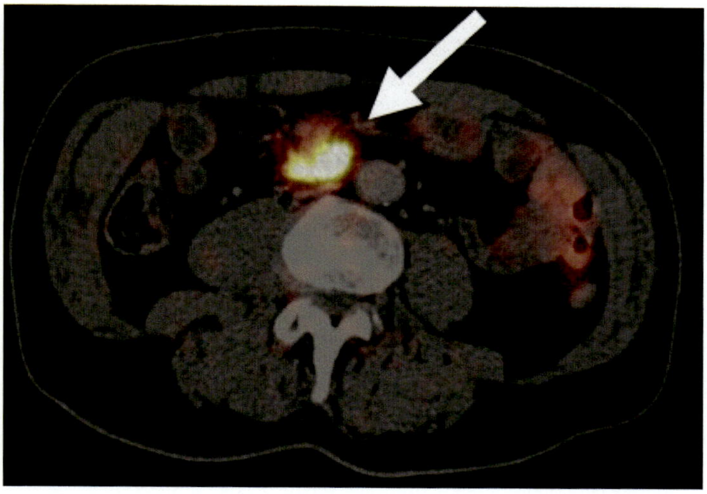

Fig. 24.2 ^{68}Ga-DOTATOC-PET/CT scan, transverse section, on the same patient as in Fig. 24.1. Apparent tracer uptake in a mesenteric metastasis of small intestinal NET (arrow)

NET ≥1 cm to assess invasion depth. Per-operative ultrasound examination is used in liver and pancreatic surgery (mandatory in MEN1), and to locate small duodenal NETs, and to guide ablation of liver metastases.

24.5.3.1 Nuclear Medicine Diagnostics

In recent years, PET/CT scan with ^{68}Ga-labeled somatostatin analogs has in high degree replaced somatostatin receptor scintigraphy for molecular imaging of low-grade NETs (Fig. 24.2). The most used preparations are ^{68}Ga-DOTATOC and ^{68}Ga-DOTATATE, which allow PET/CT scan 0.5–1 hour after injection, giving very high-resolution image contrast. For NETs with a Ki67 > 15% (see below) and NEC, which usually expresses little or no somatostatin receptors, metabolic ^{18}FDG-PET/CT scan is often a better choice [15].

24.5.3.2 Pathology

NETs consist of tumor cells that have similarities to the neuroendocrine cells and express genes central to the specific common functions such as synthesis, storage, and exocytosis of hormones. Well-established markers for NET are CgA and synaptophysin (Fig. 24.3), as well as specific hormone products. In routine hematoxylin-eosin sections, NETs can usually be identified by a typical pathological characteristic, but the diagnosis is confirmed by immunohistochemical staining for CgA and synaptophysin. Histopathological diagnosis of NETs in the gastrointestinal tract should confirm to the current WHO classification (2019) [16]. For NETs in the pancreas, classification is described in WHO 2017 classification [2]. The

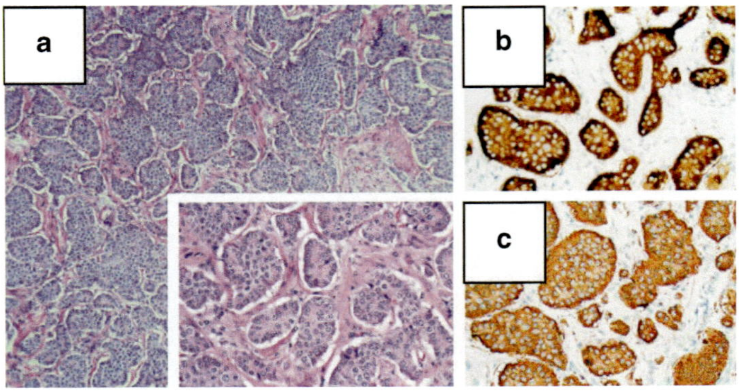

Fig. 24.3 H&E section **a** from a small intestinal NET at 100× and 400× (inset) magnification and immunohistochemistry section stained for synaptophysin **b** and CgA **c**. Both **b** and **c** are 400×. Courtesy of Dr. Christofer Juhlin, Endocrine pathologist at Karolinska University Hospital, Stockholm, Sweden

WHO criteria make the general assumption that all NETs are potentially malignant. The malignancy potential is reflected by the tumor grading from 1 to 3 (referred to as G1, G2, and G3), which in turn is determined by the proportion of tumor cells undergoing proliferation. The fraction of proliferating tumor cells is estimated by analysis of Ki67 index and mitotic count; G1 NETs possess a Ki67 ≤ 2%, G2 a Ki67 of 3–20%, and G3 a Ki67 > 20% (NEC). G1 and G2 NETs often have a characteristic pattern of minimal cellular atypia, while NEC (and G3) usually has a solid pattern with widespread tumor cell necrosis and a high degree of cellular atypia.

A pathology report for NET should contain:

- The anatomical location and multifocality if present.
- Tumor size (largest diameter in mm).
- Morphological description of the tumor and its spread and relation to resection surfaces.
- If the tumor has been radically resected.
- Immunohistochemical results for general neuroendocrine markers (CgA, synaptophysin) and specific cell type markers (amines, peptides).
- Ki67 index and mitotic count.
- WHO classification [2].
- TNM classification, version 8 [17], including the number of positive lymph nodes/total number of lymph nodes, size of greatest metastasis, and presence of lymphovascular and perineural invasion.

24.5.3.3 TNM Staging

Currently, no one staging system covers all NETs. Well-differentiated lesions (G1 and G2) generally have their own staging system based on tumor location, whereas poorly differentiated (G3 and NEC) and mixed lesions are staged as carcinomas. Details of staging for NET are outside the scope of this chapter, and reference is made to specialist literature in the field [2, 17].

24.5.3.4 Multidisciplinary Conference

The management of NET patients is often complex, owing to their heterogeneric nature, clinical presentation, frequent diagnosis with advanced disease, and a wide range of treatment options. Despite these issues, even patients with advanced disease can have long-term survival. Surgery is only one of the several treatment modalities. The patient will likely need other specialists and other modes of treatment, and so all patients diagnosed with a NET should be discussed at a multidisciplinary conference, particularly in connection with diagnosis, tumor progression, and/or change of therapy. The conference will generally comprise visceral surgeons, endocrinologists, pathologists, radiologists, and oncologist.

24.6 Treatment

24.6.1 Surgery

Surgery is the primary treatment for G1 and G2 tumors and the only modality that can offer potential cure. Some types of NET rarely have metastases at diagnosis, while others usually do. Compared to gastrointestinal adenocarcinoma, active surgery is also indicated in certain patients with disseminated NET [18]. Details of indications for surgical treatment and surgical strategy are summarized below.

24.6.2 Oncological and Medical Treatment

The choice of oncological and medical treatment will depend on the type of tumor the patient has as well as tumor spread and tumor biological factors. The treatment recommended for specific tumors may vary according to whether a patient has stable or progressive disease. Available options include:

Somatostatin Analogs A randomized, placebo-controlled study has demonstrated extended progression-free survival in patients with metastatic small intestinal NET treated with octreotide LAR (Sandostatin LAR) [19]. The result for small intestinal NET has also been confirmed in one randomized, placebo-controlled study with Somatuline Autogel (Lanreotide Autogel) in which the progression-free survival was prolonged in the treatment arm for both small intestinal NET and non-functional pancreatic NET [20]. There are currently two different preparations available: Sandostatin LAR (octreotide LAR) and Somatuline Autogel (Lanreotide Autogel). There is no documented difference in effect between the two preparations. What sets them apart is that Somatuline Autogel is given deeply subcutaneously, allowing some patients to administer it themselves. Sandostatin LAR is given through injection intramuscularly and must therefore be administered by medical staff. Somatostatin analog therapy is recommended for patients with G1–G2 tumor hormonally triggered symptoms, where several studies have shown a very good effect on both symptoms and quality of life. Sometimes patients with G3 NETs have endocrine symptoms, and these may be alleviated with a somatostatin analog therapy. Both preparations have been shown to have anti-proliferation effect in grade 1–2 tumors and can, therefore, also be given as antitumor treatment. A normal starting dose for a patient with hormone-induced symptoms is Sandostatin LAR 30 mg every 4 weeks or Somatuline Autogel 120 mg every 4 weeks, but the dose intervals can be reduced. For individual patients, extradoses of short-acting octreotide may be necessary in addition to the long-acting octreotide somatostatin analog to control symptoms.

Patients with metastatic non-functional pancreatic NET with a Ki67 < 10% may be treated with a somatostatin analog, and there are also other possible options for such patient in this category, which makes the place of somatostatin analogs unclear. Many patients need treatment with pancreatic enzymes because the use of somatostatin analog inhibits pancreatic secretions leading to fat malabsorption with concomitant diarrhea. In some patients, this arises in the course of treatment, and it is essential to distinguish this deficiency of pancreatic enzyme as a cause of diarrhea from diarrhea caused by the disease itself.

Peptide Receptor Radionuclide Therapy (PRRT) Radiolabeled somatostatin analogs are a treatment option for patients with non-resectable or metastatic NETs with high somatostatin receptor expression. In studies, up to 60% of patients demonstrated reduced tumor size, and additional patients had symptom relief while on treatment [21]. In Europe, treatment is mostly performed with ^{177}Lu-DOTATATE, which is a molecule consisting of one radioactive isotope (lutetium-177) coupled to a somatostatin analog (octreotate “TATE”). There are also examples where yttrium-90 is used, but this isotope has been shown to increase the risk of nephrotoxicity [22]. The treatment is aimed at somatostatin receptor subtypes 2 and 5, which are often strongly expressed on these tumors and can be described as an internal target radiation therapy, where the target is the somatostatin receptor and the radiation treatment the β-radiation emitted by the radioisotope. The treatment with ^{177}Lu-DOTATATE is usually given on four separate occasions. The number of treatments with 7.4 GBq has been determined based on renal dosimetry, possible side effects (especially hematological), and treatment responses [23]. Dose-limiting organs are often the kidneys and bone marrow. There is no indication for ^{177}Lu-DOTATATE on NEC.

Immunotherapy α-Interferon has been used to treat several different malignancies since the 1980s and has also been involved in the treatment of hepatitis C. α-Interferon is mainly used to treat low-proliferative G1 and G2 tumors and usually to treat small intestinal NET [24].

Chemotherapy Cytostatics are predominantly used to treat pancreatic NETs, whereas small intestinal NETs do not generally respond to chemotherapy. In treating pancreatic NETs, streptozocin and 5-fluorouracil have long been the first choice if the Ki67 index is <20%. At higher Ki67 (>20%), the first choice has traditionally been cisplatin, carboplatin, and etoposide. In recent years, temozolomide either alone or combined with capecitabine has become a treatment option for patients with a highly differentiated G3 NET of the pancreas and patients with NEC that exhibits intermediate proliferation (Ki67 10–55%). There are no comparative studies between these different treatment options.

24.7 Indications for Surgery and Surgical Strategy

24.7.1 Pancreatic NET

Resection of the primary tumor should be considered whenever possible, especially if an R0 resection can be achieved. Open, laparoscopic, and robot-assisted pancreatectomies are all feasible methods, and tumor stage and local expertise will primarily guide the choice. Tumors of the pancreatic tail will usually mandate distal pancreatectomy, whereas tumors of the pancreatic head may be treated by enucleation if small or Whipple's operation if >1 cm or multiple. Surgery for metastatic disease should be considered if appropriate in the context of the patient's presentation and performance status. Unlike other NETs, pancreatic NETs that are judged to be primarily irresectable may be suitable for neoadjuvant treatment with chemotherapy to facilitate future surgery.

24.7.2 Gastric NET

ECLoma types 1 and 2 less than 5 mm (T1) usually only require local excision. Tumors 0.5–1 cm are often resectable with polypectomy/excision via gastroscopy. For tumor sizes 1–2 cm (T2), without invasion into the *muscularis propria* (evaluated via EUS), polypectomy or endoscopic mucosal resection (EMR) or endoscopic submucosal dissection (ESD) is recommended. For tumor with invasion into the *muscularis propria* (T2–T3), radical tumor excision is performed. For ECLoma type 3 (T3 or higher), curative surgery with total or partial gastrectomy with lymph node dissection should be considered as for other malignant tumors in the stomach. In the case of functional or histamine-secreting (type 3) tumors, somatostatin analogs are indicated. H2 blockade may be indicated in histamine production. For type 1 tumors, iron supplements and vitamin B12 are given according to pernicious anemia treatment protocols. In gastric NET type 3, especially at high proliferation, chemotherapy is considered for patients with metastatic disease. NEC in the stomach is in a similar fashion to other NECs.

24.7.3 Duodenal NET

Tumor less than 1 cm (T1, N0, M0) should preferably be resected endoscopically via polypectomy or endoscopic mucosal resection (EMR). For tumors ≥1 cm or with invasion into the *muscularis propria* (T2–T3, N0, M0), resection of the primary tumor is the goal. Different methods exist, for example, transduodenal excision at laparotomy, Whipple's procedure, or pancreatic duodenectomy. Periampullary tumors are a particular difficulty due to their proximity to the bile duct. More advanced disease with metastatic tumor (stages III–IV) may, in special cases, also undergo surgery, especially in limited metastasis. Resection of liver metastases may be considered.

24.7.4 Small Intestinal NET

Surgery is the primary oncological treatment for G1–G2 small intestinal NETs and can potentially cure the patient. The gold standard is exploratory laparotomy [25, 26] with careful palpation of the entire jejunum-ileum to identify small and/or multifocal NETs. The most common site for small intestinal NET is the distal ileum, and the most common bowel resection is small bowel resection, including right hemicolectomy. R0 resection is feasible in only 20% of small intestinal NET due to advanced stage at diagnosis [27]. It should be emphasized that surgery of small intestinal NET requires significant expertise since all types of bowel surgery may be required. Compared with gastrointestinal adenocarcinoma, active surgery is meaningful even in disseminated disease [18]. In the case of symptoms, tumor debulking surgery should always be considered, which often provides adequate symptom relief. However, it is doubtful whether active surgery of the primary tumor in disseminated and advanced disease prolongs survival [28]. North American and European guidelines do not consider laparoscopic surgery or minimally invasive surgery ideal for managing small intestinal NET because of their small size and multifocal nature [29, 30]. NEC is usually treated with chemotherapy and is rarely accessible for radical surgery [31]. Palliative surgery may also be necessary to prevent, for example, bowel obstruction or ischemia (see "Emergency Surgery in NET"). The incidence of metastases and the metastasis location vary with the different NET subtypes and are low for the stomach, duodenum, appendix, and rectum, while they are high for the pancreas, small intestine, and colon. Metastases can be found in the peritoneum, lymph nodes, and liver and more rarely in the skeleton, brain, and lungs.

Lymph Node Dissection Radical excision of locoregional lymph node metastases is recommended. Also, other abdominal lymph node metastases, e.g., para-aortic, may be considered for excision. Even in the presence of liver metastases, resection of lymph node metastases should be considered as the alternative treatment options for these are limited, while there are several effective locoregional treatment methods for liver metastases.

Liver Metastasis Liver metastases are common in several NET types, and it is not uncommon for these to be diagnosed before the primary tumor. As a result, the most significant tumor burden is often found in the liver, which is often the source of primary hormone secretion. In many cases, therefore, treatment of liver metastasis is crucial for symptom control and prognosis. Liver metastases in NET are usually multiple, and limited residual extrahepatic metastasis is not a contraindication for liver surgery. Liver surgery should not be performed on NEC other than in very selected cases. Curative liver surgery is rarely possible, while tumor reduction surgery can be performed in those cases. For a select few patients, liver transplantation may be considered [32]. It can be considered for young patients (<50 years) who have no metastatic site other than the liver and where other treatment has failed. NETs are one of the very few diagnoses where liver transplantation can be considered in liver metastases, due to their slow growth. Ki67 > 10% is a contraindication.

Peritoneal Metastasis Metastasis in the peritoneum is only amenable to radical excision in exceptional cases, and so systemic therapy becomes more relevant instead. Peritonectomy +/– chemotherapy (HIPEC) has not been established in NET. Ovarian metastases are often associated with peritoneal metastasis and should be resected.

Remote metastases are usually treated with systemic treatment. One should, however, always consider palliative radiation therapy for brain metastases or symptomatic skeletal metastases. In rare and selected cases, such as an isolated or occasional remote metastasis with other metastases well under control, it may be feasible to attempt local curative treatment, such as surgery or radiation. Bone resorption inhibitors in skeletal metastasis may also be considered.

Cholecystectomy As long-term treatment with somatostatin analogs increases the risk of gallstone disease, cholecystectomy should be considered during all primary surgery.

24.7.5 Appendix NET

Most appendix NETs are diagnosed by coincidence after appendicectomy. Classic appendiceal NETs are rarely the cause of appendicitis. Carcinoid syndrome occurs very rarely, and in such cases, the diagnosis of small intestinal NET should be considered. Risk factors for metastasis or residual tumor are tumor size >2 cm, narrow or non-radical surgical margin, G2, lymphovascular invasion, invasion of the subserosa or mesoappendix ≥3 mm, and tumor growth through the peritoneum or into surrounding organs.

■ **Surgical Treatment Strategy**

- Appendix NET ≤2 cm without risk factors that are radically operated or appendix NET <1 cm with only one risk factor that is radically operated: appendectomy is sufficient.
- Appendix NET that is >2 cm, or with involved or doubtful margins after surgery, should be offered reoperation with right hemicolectomy and lymph node dissection, preceded by basal examination (biochemistry and somatostatin receptor PET/CT scan).
- Patients with radically operated appendix NET 1–2 cm who have only one risk factor should be examined with basal examination (the same as above); if this is positive, right hemicolectomy with lymph node dissection is offered, and if the investigation is negative, the patient can instead be offered follow-up for 10 years with annual biochemistry and somatostatin receptor PET/CT scan after 5 and 10 years.
- Patients with two or more risk factors should be offered right hemicolectomy with lymph node dissection, preceded by basal examination (the same as above).

Locally advanced unresectable or metastatic appendix NET is treated as small intestinal NET.

24.7.6 Thymic NET

Surgery is the primary treatment with a complete resection through a median sternotomy. Downstaging treatment with chemotherapy ± radiotherapy is usually required since many tumors often present with an invasion of the surrounding structures. The long-term outcome is poor, even in completely resected tumors, due to the high risk of recurrence and distant metastases. Prognosis mainly depends on tumor stage, invasiveness, completeness of resection, associated endocrinopathies, and development of recurrence or distant metastases.

24.7.7 Other NETs

Colonic NETs have similar properties to small intestinal NETs and should therefore be treated in a similar fashion with segmental colectomy. NETs in the testis, ovaries, and other locations are very rare, and as a general rule, these should be surgically removed, if feasible, and treated as small intestinal NET.

24.7.8 Emergency Surgery in NET

Emergency surgery in NETs is almost exclusively in the context of small intestinal disease with either obstruction or ischemic bowel due to compromise of the mesenteric vessels by nodal disease. Although several studies have not shown any difference in long-term survival when comparing elective and emergency surgery [33], in the emergency situation, extensive surgery should be avoided, and a damage control approach should be employed.

24.8 Prognosis

24.8.1 Follow-Up

Patients with NET usually have a very long life expectancy. Late relapses after radical surgery are the rule rather than the exception; however, the tumor is often slow growing. Follow-up protocols are dictated by origin of the NET and treatment modalities employed.

Answers to the Questions

Q1. 2
Q2. 2
Q3. 5
Q4. 5
Q5. 3
Q6. 1
Q7. 6
Q8. 4
Q9. 3
Q10. 2
Q11. 7

Q12. 4
Q13. 3
Q14. 4
Q15. 3
Q16. 2 and possibly 6 can be accepted
Q17. 2
Q18. 7
Q19. 3
Q20. 1
Q21. 3
Q22. 6
Q23. 2
Q24. 6
Q25. 2

References

1. Verner JV, Morrison AB. Islet cell tumor and a syndrome of refractory watery diarrhea and hypokalemia. Am J Med. 1958;25(3):374–80.
2. Lloyd RV, Osamura R, Klöppel G, Rosai J. WHO Classification of Tumours of Endocrine Organs. WHO; IARC Publications. 2017. ISBN 978-92-832-4493-6
3. Fraenkel M, Kim M, Faggiano A, de Herder WW, Valk GD. Incidence of gastroenteropancreatic neuroendocrine tumours: a systematic review of the literature. Endocr Relat Cancer. 2014;21(3):R153–63.
4. Yao JC, Hassan M, Phan A, Dagohoy C, Leary C, Mares JE, et al. One hundred years after "carcinoid": epidemiology of and prognostic factors for neuroendocrine tumors in 35,825 cases in the United States. J Clin Oncol. 2008;26(18):3063–72.
5. Modlin IM, Oberg K, Chung DC, Jensen RT, de Herder WW, Thakker RV, et al. Gastroenteropancreatic neuroendocrine tumours. Lancet Oncol. 2008;9(1):61–72.
6. Huguet I, Grossman AB, O'Toole D. Changes in the epidemiology of neuroendocrine tumours. Neuroendocrinology. 2017;104(2):105–11.
7. Connor SJ, Hanna GB, Frizelle FA. Appendiceal tumors: retrospective clinicopathologic analysis of appendiceal tumors from 7,970 appendectomies. Dis Colon Rectum. 1998;41(1):75–80.
8. Dusmet ME, McKneally MF. Pulmonary and thymic carcinoid tumors. World J Surg. 1996;20(2):189–95.
9. Phan AT, Oberg K, Choi J, Harrison LH Jr, Hassan MM, Strosberg JR, et al. NANETS consensus guideline for the diagnosis and management of neuroendocrine tumors: well-differentiated neuroendocrine tumors of the thorax (includes lung and thymus). Pancreas. 2010;39(6): 784–98.
10. Ito T, Cadiot G, Jensen RT. Diagnosis of Zollinger-Ellison syndrome: increasingly difficult. World J Gastroenterol. 2012;18(39):5495–503.
11. Ram P, Penalver JL, Lo KBU, Rangaswami J, Pressman GS. Carcinoid heart disease: review of current knowledge. Tex Heart Inst J. 2019;46(1):21–7.
12. Oberg K, Couvelard A, Delle Fave G, Gross D, Grossman A, Jensen RT, et al. ENETS consensus guidelines for standard of care in neuroendocrine tumours: biochemical markers. Neuroendocrinology. 2017;105(3):201–11.
13. Rindi G, Grant SG, Yiangou Y, Ghatei MA, Bloom SR, Bautch VL, et al. Development of neuroendocrine tumors in the gastrointestinal

tract of transgenic mice. Heterogeneity of hormone expression. Am J Pathol. 1990;136(6):1349–63.
14. Sundin A, Arnold R, Baudin E, Cwikla JB, Eriksson B, Fanti S, et al. ENETS consensus guidelines for the standards of care in neuroendocrine tumors: radiological, nuclear medicine & hybrid imaging. Neuroendocrinology. 2017;105(3):212–44.
15. Nilica B, Waitz D, Stevanovic V, Uprimny C, Kendler D, Buxbaum S, et al. Direct comparison of (68)Ga-DOTA-TOC and (18)F-FDG PET/CT in the follow-up of patients with neuroendocrine tumour treated with the first full peptide receptor radionuclide therapy cycle. Eur J Nucl Med Mol Imaging. 2016;43(9):1585–92.
16. Nagtegaal ID, Odze RD, Klimstra D, Paradis V, Rugge M, Schirmacher P, et al. The 2019 WHO classification of tumours of the digestive system. Histopathology. 2020;76(2):182–8.
17. O'Sullivan B, Brierley J, Byrd D, Bosman F, Kehoe S, Kossary C, et al. The TNM classification of malignant tumours-towards common understanding and reasonable expectations. Lancet Oncol. 2017;18(7):849–51.
18. Partelli S, Bartsch DK, Capdevila J, Chen J, Knigge U, Niederle B, et al. ENETS consensus guidelines for standard of care in neuroendocrine tumours: surgery for small intestinal and pancreatic neuroendocrine tumours. Neuroendocrinology. 2017;105(3):255–65.
19. Rinke A, Müller HH, Schade-Brittinger C, Klose KJ, Barth P, Wied M, et al. Placebo-controlled, double-blind, prospective, randomized study on the effect of octreotide LAR in the control of tumor growth in patients with metastatic neuroendocrine midgut tumors: a report from the PROMID Study Group. J Clin Oncol. 2009;27(28):4656–63.
20. Caplin ME, Pavel M, Ćwikła JB, Phan AT, Raderer M, Sedláčková E, et al. Lanreotide in metastatic enteropancreatic neuroendocrine tumors. N Engl J Med. 2014;371(3):224–33.
21. Kwekkeboom DJ, de Herder WW, Kam BL, van Eijck CH, van Essen M, Kooij PP, et al. Treatment with the radiolabeled somatostatin analog [177 Lu-DOTA 0,Tyr3]octreotate: toxicity, efficacy, and survival. J Clin Oncol. 2008;26(13):2124–30.
22. Lambert B, Cybulla M, Weiner SM, Van De Wiele C, Ham H, Dierckx RA, et al. Renal toxicity after radionuclide therapy. Radiat Res. 2004;161(5):607–11.
23. Garske-Román U, Sandström M, Fröss Baron K, Lundin L, Hellman P, Welin S, et al. Prospective observational study of (177)Lu-DOTA-octreotate therapy in 200 patients with advanced metastasized neuroendocrine tumours (NETs): feasibility and impact of a dosimetry-guided study protocol on outcome and toxicity. Eur J Nucl Med Mol Imaging. 2018;45(6):970–88.
24. Oberg K, Funa K, Alm G. Effects of leukocyte interferon on clinical symptoms and hormone levels in patients with mid-gut carcinoid tumors and carcinoid syndrome. N Engl J Med. 1983;309(3):129–33.
25. Deguelte S, Perrier M, Hammoutene C, Cadiot G, Kianmanesh R. Surgery and perioperative management in small intestinal neuroendocrine tumors. J Clin Med. 2020;9(7):2319.
26. Howe JR, Cardona K, Fraker DL, Kebebew E, Untch BR, Wang YZ, et al. The surgical management of small bowel neuroendocrine tumors: consensus guidelines of the North American Neuroendocrine Tumor Society. Pancreas. 2017;46(6):715–31.
27. Moris D, Ntanasis-Stathopoulos I, Tsilimigras DI, Vagios S, Karamitros A, Karaoanis G, et al. Update on surgical management of small bowel neuroendocrine tumors. Anticancer Res. 2018;38(3):1267–78.
28. Daskalakis K, Karakatsanis A, Hessman O, Stuart HC, Welin S, Tiensuu Janson E, et al. Association of a prophylactic surgical approach to stage IV small intestinal neuroendocrine tumors with survival. JAMA Oncol. 2018;4(2):183–9.

29. Boudreaux JP, Klimstra DS, Hassan MM, Woltering EA, Jensen RT, Goldsmith SJ, et al. The NANETS consensus guideline for the diagnosis and management of neuroendocrine tumors: well-differentiated neuroendocrine tumors of the jejunum, ileum, appendix, and cecum. Pancreas. 2010;39(6):753–66.
30. Niederle B, Pape UF, Costa F, Gross D, Kelestimur F, Knigge U, et al. ENETS consensus guidelines update for neuroendocrine neoplasms of the jejunum and ileum. Neuroendocrinology. 2016;103(2):125–38.
31. Haugvik SP, Janson ET, Österlund P, Langer SW, Falk RS, Labori KJ, et al. Surgical treatment as a principle for patients with high-grade pancreatic neuroendocrine carcinoma: a Nordic Multicenter Comparative Study. Ann Surg Oncol. 2016;23(5):1721–8.
32. Olausson M, Friman S, Cahlin C, Nilsson O, Jansson S, Wängberg B, et al. Indications and results of liver transplantation in patients with neuroendocrine tumors. World J Surg. 2002;26(8):998–1004.
33. Manguso N, Gangi A, Nissen N, Harit A, Siegel E, Hendifar A, et al. Long-term outcomes after elective versus emergency surgery for small bowel neuroendocrine tumors. Am Surg. 2018;84(10):1570–4.

Neuroendocrine Tumors of the Thymus

Benoît Bédat and Frédéric Triponez

Contents

A. L. Shifrin et al. (eds.), *Endocrine Surgery Comprehensive Board Exam Guide*,
https://doi.org/10.1007/978-3-030-84737-1_25

25

Case Presentation

A 25-year-old man with a history of asthma and Poland syndrome underwent chest CT in 2016 owing to chest pain, dyspnea on exertion, and headache. An anterior mediastinal mass measuring 15 cm was discovered, associated with incomplete obstruction of the superior vena cava (◘ Fig. 25.1). A transthoracic needle biopsy of the mass was performed. The cytological description of the mass was consistent with the presence of trabecular growth pattern and rosette formation. Immunohistochemical staining was positive for synaptophysin, chromogranin A, CD56, and NSE, with a Ki-67 index of 5%, consistent with the diagnosis of atypical carcinoid tumor of the thymus. A 6-fluoro-(^{18}F)-L-3,4-dihydroxyphenylalanine (18*F-DOPA*) positron emission tomography (PET)/CT showed no extrathymic metastases. Complete thymectomy was then performed by hemiclamshell thoracotomy with resection of the right phrenic nerve. A large, well-circumscribed tumor was found without any invasion into the adjacent structure. Final pathology revealed an atypical carcinoid tumor with Ki-67 index between 10% and 20%. This tumor was classified as stage IIB based on TNM classification (7th edition) and Masaoka classification, due to infiltration of the perithymic fat, and pT2R0. Surgical treatment was complemented by adjuvant radiotherapy (50 Gy). However, there was a recurrence 3 years later with cervical and mediastinal lymph node metastases, which was confirmed with needle biopsy vand Ga-68-labeled dodecanetetraacetic acid-tyrosine-3-octreotate (DOTATATE) PET/CT. Complete left lateral neck dissection (by cervicotomy) with left mediastinal lymph node dissection (by VATS) was then performed. Thirteen of 41 lymph nodes were positive for metastatic disease. Immunohistochemistry showed absence of SSTR2 and PDL1 expression. Whole-genome sequencing showed the presence of MEN1 mutation. Ten months later, the patient presented with new lymph node, as well as lung, and bone metastases (◘ Fig. 25.2). Systemic treatment with lutetium (177Lu) oxodotreotide was initiated which stabilized the patient's condition.

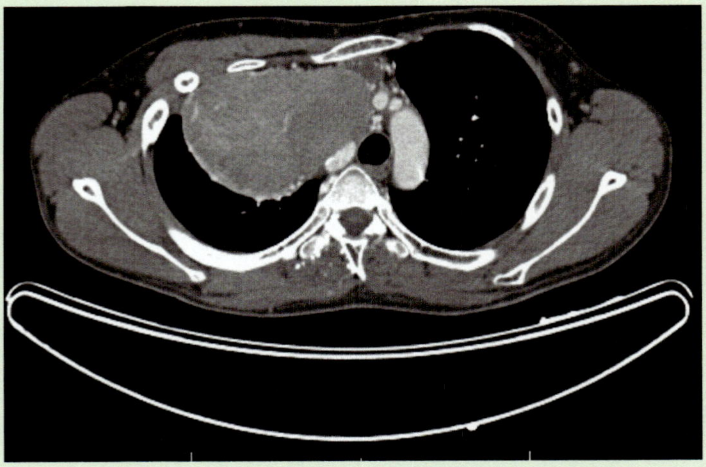

◘ **Fig. 25.1** Chest computed tomography shows anterior mediastinal mass with partial obstruction of the superior vena cava

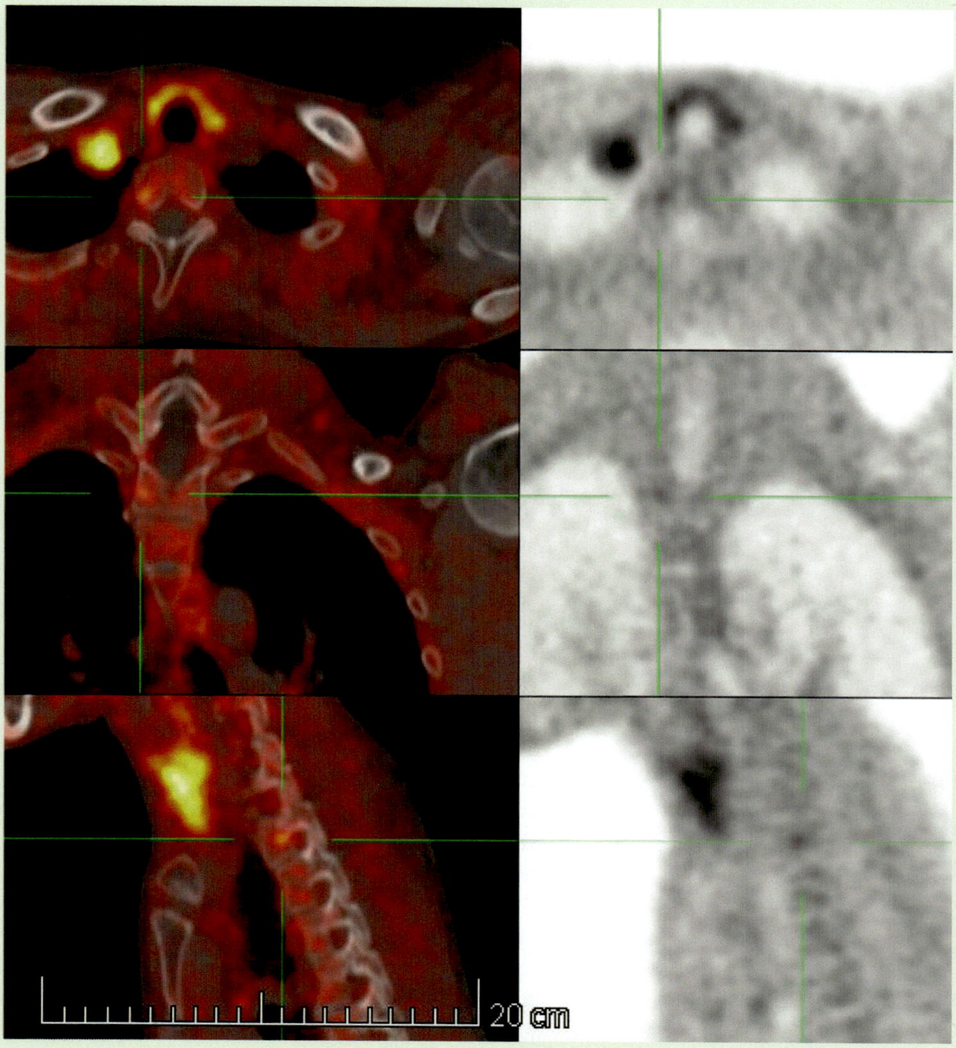

Fig. 25.2 A Ga-68 dodecanetetraacetic acid-tyrosine-3-octreotate (DOTATATE) PET/CT showed mediastinal and cervical lymph node and bone metastases

Questions

1. What are the epidemiological characteristics of TNET?
   1. TNET is a rare tumor in patients with the MEN1 syndrome but is a common tumor of the thymus.
   2. TNET is predominant in males and in patients with smoking history.
   3. Phenotype-genotype correlation in patients with MEN1 mutations is low.
   4. Twenty-five percent of thymic carcinoids are associated with the MEN1 syndrome.
      - (a) Only 1) and 4) are correct.
      - (b) Only 1) and 2) are correct.
      - (c) Only 2), 3), and 4) are correct.
      - (d) Only 2) is correct.
      - (e) All are correct.
2. Which imaging test(s) or serum marker(s) is/are used when thymic NET is suspected?
   1. Serum chromogranin A
   2. Chest MRI
   3. Presence of *MEN1* mutations
   4. Ga-18 DOTATATE PET/CT
      - (a) Only 1) is correct.
      - (b) Only 2) and 4) are correct.
      - (c) Only 3) is correct.
      - (d) Only 4) is correct.
      - (e) All are incorrect.
3. Which of the following clinical presentation(s) is/are most commonly seen in patients with thymic NET?
   1. Skin flushing
   2. Chest pain
   3. Diarrhea
   4. Moon face
   5. Absence of symptoms
      - (a) Only 1), 2), and 3) are correct.
      - (b) Only 2) and 5) are correct.
      - (c) Only 2) is correct.
      - (d) Only 5) is correct.
      - (e) All are correct.
4. Which of the following factors negatively influence the survival of patients with thymic NET?
   1. The histological grade
   2. Incomplete radical surgical resection
   3. Thymectomy by video-assisted thoracic surgery
   4. Thymectomy by sternotomy
      - (a) Only 1) is correct.
      - (b) Only 4) is correct.
      - (c) Only 1), 2), and 3) are correct.
      - (d) Only 1) and 2) are correct.
      - (e) All are correct.

5. Which statement(s) regarding the management of thymic NET is/are correct?
   1. Active surveillance with MRI every 3 months is recommended for early-stage tumors.
   2. Multidisciplinary management of thymic tumors is recommended.
   3. Centers with expertise in thoracic and cardiovascular surgery are recommended for management of patients with thymic NET.
   4. Complete and radical resection of the tumor is recommended if the tumor is resectable.
      (a) Only 1) is correct.
      (b) Only 2) is correct.
      (c) Only 2) and 4) are correct.
      (d) Only 2), 3), and 4) are correct.
      (e) All are correct.
6. Which statement(s) regarding thymic surgery is/are correct?
   1. A transcervical approach should always be performed in patients with thymic NET associated with the MEN1 syndrome.
   2. Thymectomy including perithymic fat is the standard of care surgical approach for thymic tumors.
   3. Surgery by minimally invasive approach can always be performed.
   4. Thymectomy by sternotomy is an obsolete procedure.
      (a) Only 2) is correct.
      (b) Only 1) and 2) are correct.
      (c) Only 3) and 4) are correct.
      (d) All are correct.
7. The benefits of minimally invasive surgery as compared to open procedures are as follows:
   1. Reduced operative time
   2. Reduced intraoperative blood loss
   3. Shorter hospital stay
   4. Lower rate of cancer recurrence at 5 years
   5. Lower rate of postoperative pneumonia
      (a) Only 4) is correct.
      (b) Only 1) and 3) are correct.
      (c) Only 2), 3), and 5) are correct.
      (d) Only 2) and 5) are correct.
      (e) All are correct.
8. Radiotherapy is currently used as follows:
   1. In association with chemotherapy
   2. As adjuvant treatment for patients with positive margins
   3. As palliative treatment in case of vena cava syndrome
   4. In all cases with MEN1 syndrome
      (a) Only 1) is correct.
      (b) Only 2) is correct.

   (c) Only 2) and 3) are correct.
   (d) Only 4) is correct.
   (e) All are correct.
9. Which statement(s) regarding the prognosis of thymic NET is/are correct?
   1. The Masaoka staging system is specific to predict the prognosis.
   2. Reported 10-year survival rate for atypical carcinoid thymic tumors is 30%.
   3. Patients with TNET secondary to the MEN1 syndrome have better prognosis with a 10-year survival rate of 90% as compared to sporadic cases.
   4. Recurrence is frequent.
      (a) Only 1) and 4) are correct.
      (b) Only 1) is correct.
      (c) Only 2) and 4) are correct.
      (d) Only 3) is correct.
      (e) All are correct.
10. A 20-year-old patient presented with the MEN1 syndrome and primary hyperparathyroidism. Chest CT did not reveal any thymic masses. Which statement(s) is/are correct?
   1. Performing a prophylactic transcervical thymectomy during a parathyroidectomy surgery for primary hyperparathyroidism is sufficient to prevent TNET.
   2. A prophylactic transcervical thymectomy can be performed during a parathyroid surgery for primary hyperparathyroidism with routine pathological evaluation of the thymus for thymic pathology.
   3. A minimally invasive complete thymectomy could be performed during surgery for primary hyperparathyroidism to avoid the risk of TNET.
   4. Transcervical thymectomy is currently not necessary during surgery for primary hyperparathyroidism.
      (a) Only 1) is correct.
      (b) Only 2) is correct.
      (c) Only 3) is correct.
      (d) Only 4) is correct.
      (e) Only 2) and 3) are correct.

25.1 Introduction

Neuroendocrine tumors of the thymus (TNETs) are rare. They account for approximately 5% of all tumors of the mediastinum and 0.4% of all neuroendocrine tumors [1–3]. The reported incidence of TNET is 0.02/100,000 population per year and shows male predominance (male-to-female ratio of

3:1) [2]. Although most TNETs are sporadic, some are associated with multiple neuroendocrine neoplasia type 1 syndrome (TNETs-MEN1), thymoma, or thymic carcinoma [1, 4, 5]. In a prospective study of 85 patients, Gibril et al. showed that 8% of patients with the MEN1 syndrome developed TNET [6]. In the American/European series, TNET-MEN1 occurs predominantly in male patients (10:1) [7]. However, the genotype-phenotype correlations in patients with the MEN1 syndrome are reported to be lower in TNET than in pulmonary neuroendocrine tumors (PNET) [8–11]. TNET in patients with the MEN1 syndrome is associated with a higher risk of death (hazard ratio [HR] = 4.64, 95% CI = 1.73–12.41) than in patients without the MEN1 syndrome [12].

Thoracic NETs (pulmonary and thymic) are often referred to as foregut NETs. TNET and PNET are traditionally classified using the same World Health Organization (WHO) criteria into low-grade typical carcinoids (TC), intermediate-grade atypical carcinoids (ACs), and two high-grade malignancies: large cell neuroendocrine carcinoma (LCNEC) and small cell carcinoma (SCC). However, TNET and PNET have clinicopathological and genetic differences. For example, AC and LCNEC are the most frequent subtypes in the thymus, whereas TC and SCC are prevalent in the lung. The WHO classification is based on morphology. However, other classifications have been proposed based on mitotic count and Ki-67 index [13] or a morphomolecular grading system using a copy number instability (CNI) score [14].

25.2 Clinical Presentation

One-third of patients with TNET are asymptomatic, and tumors are discovered incidentally. Local symptoms, such as chest pain, cough, and respiratory distress, occur in about half of patients. Superior vena cava syndrome and hoarseness can occur depending on the extent of the tumor. Liver, bone, and lung metastases are often found. TNET can be accompanied by paraneoplastic syndromes, such as Cushing's syndrome, hypertrophic osteoarthropathy, or ectopic acromegaly. Carcinoid syndrome is rare [15].

Due to the higher risk of death associated with TNET, screening for thymic tumors is required every 1–3 years in patients with the MEN1 syndrome using thoracic (low-dose) computed tomography (CT) or magnetic resonance imaging (MRI) [16]. Since patients with foregut NET often lack aromatic amino acid decarboxylase, which is necessary to convert tryptophan to serotonin, urinary serotonin or 5-HIAA measurement is not routinely recommended for screening and/or diagnosis of TNET.

25.3 Prognosis

According to the WHO classification of TNET, the reported 5-year survival rate, 10-year survival rate, and median survival time were 100%, 60%, and 126 months, respectively, for TC, and 50%, 30%, and 52 months, respectively, for AC. The reported 5-year survival rate and median survival time was 30% and 21 months, respectively, for LCNEC, and 0% and 13.5 months, respectively, for SCC [11]. According to the Groupe d'Etude des Tumeurs Endocrines (GTE) network, the median survival time of patients with TNET-MEN1 is 9 years and 7 months, and the 10-year survival rate is 36% [12].

There is no established method for staging TNET. The most common method includes the Masaoka system, which was initially established for thymoma. However, neither the Masaoka staging nor the proposed TNM classification suggested by the International Association for the Study of Lung Cancer (IASLC)/International Thymic Malignancy Interest Group (ITMIG) seems relevant for prognosis of TNET [17, 18]. In contrast, histological grade, high proliferative rate (Ki-67 index >10%), incomplete radical surgical resection, and absence of surgical resection seem to be negative prognostic factors [2, 18, 19].

25.4 Treatment of TNET

TNET should be referred to an experienced medical team. Multidisciplinary management of thymic tumors is recommended. According to the European Society for Medical Oncology and North American Neuroendocrine Tumor Society guidelines, complete and radical resection is recommended, if the tumor is resectable [19, 20].

25.5 Surgical Details

Centers with expertise in thoracic and cardiovascular surgery are recommended to manage patients with TNET. The completeness of resection (R0) is the most important prognostic factor. Therefore, complete resection of the thymus (thymectomy) is the standard of care for thymic tumors. To evaluate the resectability of the tumor, thoracic MRI might be necessary. However, judgment during surgery is critical for determining invasion of adjacent structures and resectability. The aim of thymectomy is to remove the entire thymus without opening the tumor capsule and the perithymic fat (including cervical, mediastinal, and cardiophrenic fat) between the two phrenic nerves. Anterior lymph node dissection (N1) is also mandatory in thymic cancer [21]. Sometimes, resection of the mediastinal pleura, pericardium, adjacent lung, innominate vein, or phrenic nerve is required to achieve resection with negative margins.

To complete the resection of the thymus (R0), open mediastinal sternotomy and minimally invasive thymectomy (MIT) are usually performed. These different approaches can vary depending on the extent of the tumor, its size, and the experience of the surgeon.

Median sternotomy is the standard for thymomectomy/thymectomy and remains the preferred approach in cases of pleuropulmonary invasion of TNET. It provides excellent exposure to the neck, anterior mediastinum, and thymus. MIT is an increasingly used alternative to the traditional open approach for thymic tumors, especially for small and well-encapsulated tumors, with a similar 10-year recurrence-free survival [22]. In contrast to sternotomy, MIT demonstrates reduced intraoperative blood loss and shorter hospital stays [22, 23]. However, an appropriately designed prospective trial would be required to assess whether MIT is as safe as sternotomy. There is a wide range of MIT procedures used: robot-assisted thoracic surgery (RATS); video-assisted thoracic surgery (VATS) with a left, right, or bilateral approach; subxiphoid single-port VATS; video-assisted transcervical thymectomy; or a hybridization of these procedures [23–26]. None of these procedures showed any real benefit over the other.

25.6 Prophylactic Transcervical Thymectomy

Given the frequency of supernumerary parathyroid glands in the thymus, there is a general agreement to perform transcervical thymectomy at the time of surgery for primary hyperparathyroidism in patients with the MEN1 syndrome [27]. This procedure is advocated for resection of ectopic parathyroid glands, for reduction of the rate of persistent and recurrent hyperparathyroidism, and as prophylaxis against development of TNET. However, transcervical thymectomy only partially removes the thymus, mostly the superior thymic horns, leaving behind a significant part of the thymus. Although partial thymectomy is useful in the treatment of hyperparathyroidism, its efficacy in finding or preventing TNET and its impact on patient survival have not been demonstrated [28, 29]. Furthermore, the development of thymic carcinoids has been documented after prophylactic transcervical thymectomy [30]. Due to poor survival associated with TNET and the high risk of recurrence, complete thymectomy (preferentially minimally invasive) in addition to parathyroidectomy for treatment of primary hyperparathyroidism is currently debated. Long-term screening with thoracic imaging is therefore required in patients with the MEN1 syndrome after transcervical thymectomy.

25.7 Medical Treatment and Radiotherapy

Adjuvant radiotherapy is currently used in the treatment of incomplete resection, resection with positive margins, and unresectable cases. Systemic treatments include cytotoxic chemotherapy, somatostatin analogs, and everolimus. Systemic treatment may be administered as curative therapy for advanced TNET, as induction therapy to reduce the tumor burden before surgery, as postoperative therapy to reduce the risk of recurrence, and as palliative therapy for unresectable, metastatic, and recurrent TNET. The management of patients with TNET requires multidisciplinary expertise at every step of disease progression.

Answers

1. (c); 2. (e); 3. (b); 4. (d); 5. (d); 6. (a); 7. (c); 8. (c); 9. (c); 10. (e)

References

1. Strobel P, Marx A, Chan JK, et al. Thymic neuroendocrine tumors. In: Travis WD, Brambilla E, Burke AP, et al., editors. WHO classification of tumors of the lung, pleura, thymus, and heart. Lyon: IARC Press; 2015. p. 234–41.
2. Gaur P, Leary C, Yao JC. Thymic neuroendocrine tumors: an SEER database analysis of 160 patients. Ann Surg. 2010;251:1117–21.
3. Filosso PL, Yao X, Ahmad U, et al. Outcome of primary neuroendocrine tumors of the thymus: a joint analysis of the International Thymic Malignancy Interest Group and the European Society of Thoracic Surgeons databases. J Thorac Cardiovasc Surg. 2015;149:103 e2–109 e2.
4. Rosai J, Higa E, Davie J. Mediastinal endocrine neoplasm in patients with multiple endocrine adenomatosis: a previously unrecognized association. Cancer. 1972;29:1075–83.
5. Teh BT, Zedenius J, Kytölä S, et al. Thymic carcinoids in multiple endocrine neoplasia type 1. Ann Surg. 1998;228:99–105.
6. Gibril F, Chen YJ, Schrump DS, Vortmeyer A, Zhuang Z, Lubensky IA, Reynolds JC, Louie A, Entsuah LK, Huang K, Asgharian B, Jensen RT. Prospective study of thymic carcinoids in patients with multiple endocrine neoplasia type 1. J Clin Endocrinol Metab. 2003;88:1066–81.
7. Ye L, Wang W, Ospina NS, et al. Clinical features and prognosis of thymic neuroendocrine tumors associated with multiple endocrine neoplasia type 1: a single-center study, systematic review, and meta-analysis. Clin Endocrinol. 2017;87:706–16.
8. Teh BT, Hayward NK, Walters MK, et al. Genetic studies of thymic carcinoids in multiple endocrine neoplasia type 1. J Med Genet. 1994;31: 261–2.
9. Zhao J, de Krijger RR, Meier D, et al. Genomic alterations in well-differentiated gastrointestinal and bronchial neuroendocrine tumors (carcinoids): marked differences indicate diversity in molecular pathogenesis. Am J Pathol. 2000;157:1431–8.
10. Petzmann S, Ullmann R, Klemen H, et al. Loss of heterozygosity on chromosome arm 11q in lung carcinoids. Hum Pathol. 2001;32:333–8.
11. Strobel P, Zettl A, Shilo K, et al. Tumor genetics and survival of thymic neuroendocrine neoplasms: a multi-institutional clinicopathologic study. Genes Chromosomes Cancer. 2014;53:738–49.

12. Goudet P, Murat A, Binquet C, Cardot-Bauters C, Costa A, Ruszniewski P, et al. Risk factors and causes of death in MEN1 disease A GTE (Groupe d'Etude des Tumeurs Endocrine) cohort study among 758 patients. World J Surg. 2010;34:249–55.
13. Pelosi G, Pattini L, Morana G, et al. Grading lung neuroendocrine tumors: controversies in search of a solution. Histol Histopathol. 2017;32:223–41.
14. Dinter H, Bohnenberger H, Beck J, et al. Molecular classification of neuroendocrine tumors of the thymus. J Thorac Oncol. 2019;8: 1472–83.
15. Soga J, Yakuwa Y, Osaka M. Evaluation of 342 cases of mediastinal/ thymic carcinoids collected from literature: a comparative study between typical carcinoids and atypical varieties. Ann Thorac Cardiovasc Surg. 1999;5:285–92.
16. Thakker RV, Newey PJ, Walls GV, et al. Clinical practice guidelines for multiple endocrine neoplasia type 1 (MEN1). J Clin Endocrinol Metab. 2012;97:2990–3011.
17. Zhao Y, Shi J, Fan L, et al. Evaluation of the proposed International Association for the Study of Lung Cancer (IASLC)/International Thymic Malignancies Interest Group (ITMIG) staging revisions in thymic well-differentiated neuroendocrine carcinoma patients. Eur J Cardiothorac Surg. 2016;49:569–73.
18. Crona J, Björklund P, Welin S, Kozlovacki G, Oberg K, Granberg D. Treatment, prognostic markers and survival in thymic neuroendocrine tumors. a study from a single tertiary referral center. Lung Cancer. 2013;79:289–93.
19. Oberg K, Jelic S, ESMO Guidelines Working Group. Neuroendocrine bronchial and thymic tumors: ESMO clinical recommendation for diagnosis, treatment, and follow-up. Ann Oncol. 2009;20:147–9.
20. Phan AT, Oberg K, Choi J, et al. NANETS consensus guideline for the diagnosis and management of neuroendocrine tumors: well-differentiated neuroendocrine tumors of the thorax (includes lung and thymus). Pancreas. 2010;39:784–98.
21. Bhora FY, Chen DJ, Detterbeck FC, et al. The ITMIG/IASLC Thymic epithelial tumors staging project: a proposed lymph node map for thymic epithelial tumors in the forthcoming 8th edition of the TNM classification of malignant tumors. J Thorac Oncol. 2014;9:S88.
22. Xie A, Tjahjono R, Phan K, Yan TD. Video-assisted thoracoscopic surgery versus open thymectomy for thymoma: a systematic review. Ann Cardiothorac Surg. 2015;4:495–508.
23. O'Sullivan KE, Kreaden US, Hebert AE, Eaton D, Redmond KC. A systematic review of robotic versus open and video assisted thoracoscopic surgery (VATS) approaches for thymectomy. Ann Cardiothorac Surg. 2019;8:174–93.
24. Lemaître PH, Keshavjee S. Uniportal video-assisted transcervical thymectomy. Thorac Surg Clin. 2019;29:187–94.
25. Zieliński M, Rybak M, Wilkojc M, Fryzlewicz E, Nabialek T, Pankowski J. Subxiphoid video-assisted thoracoscopic thymectomy for thymoma. Ann Cardiothorac Surg. 2015;4:564–6.
26. Suda T. Robotic subxiphoid thymectomy. J Vis Surg. 2016;22:118.
27. Montenegro FLM, Neves MC, Lourenço DM Jr, Arap SS, Nascimento CP Jr, Toledo SPA, et al. Thymectomy in the surgical approach to hyperparathyroidism in type 1 multiple endocrine neoplasia. Rev Bras Cir Cab Pesc. 2010;39:174–8.
28. Powell AC, Alexander HR, Pingpank JF, et al. The utility of routine transcervical thymectomy for multiple endocrine neoplasia 1-related hyperparathyroidism. Surgery. 2008;144:878–83.

29. Welch K, McHenry CR. The role of transcervical thymectomy in patients with hyperparathyroidism. Am J Surg. 2012;203:292–5. discussion 295–296
30. Burgess JR, Giles N, Shepherd JJ. Malignant thymic carcinoid is not prevented by transcervical thymectomy in multiple endocrine neoplasia type 1. Clin Endocrinol. 2001;55:689–93.

Neuroendocrine Tumors: Stomach

Jiping Wang and Gerard Doherty

Contents

A. L. Shifrin et al. (eds.), *Endocrine Surgery Comprehensive Board Exam Guide*,
https://doi.org/10.1007/978-3-030-84737-1_26

Case Presentation

A 67-year-old female had history of a chronic vague right upper quadrant tenderness for a year. This led to subsequent esophagogastroduodenoscopy (EGD), which reviewed more than 12 polyps in the cardia and body of the stomach. All are less than 2 cm. The antrum is free from tumors. The tissue biopsy showed gastric neuroendocrine tumor (gNET). Ki-67 is <3%.

Questions

1. Which of the following is true?
   - A. These are well-differentiated gastric neuroendocrine tumors.
   - B. These are moderately differentiated gastric neuroendocrine tumors.
   - C. These are poorly differentiated gastric neuroendocrine tumors.
   - D. These are G1 gastric neuroendocrine tumors.
   - E. Cannot determine with the available information.
2. What is the next step for this patient's work-up?
   - A. Serum chromogranin A
   - B. Serum gastrin
   - C. *CT* scan of the abdomen and pelvis
   - D. Dotatate scan
   - E. All of the above
3. The patient's chromogranin A level is 686 pg/mL and gastrin level 3133 pg/mL. This patient likely has:
   - A. Type I gNET
   - B. Type II gNET
   - C. Type III gNET
   - D. Gastrinoma
   - E. Needs more study
4. The patient's *CT* scan showed a hyperintense lesion in the second portion of the duodenum, and *EGD* tissue biopsy showed gastrinoma. This patient has:
   - A. Type I gNET
   - B. Type II gNET
   - C. Type III gNET
   - D. Type IV gNET
   - E. Needs more study

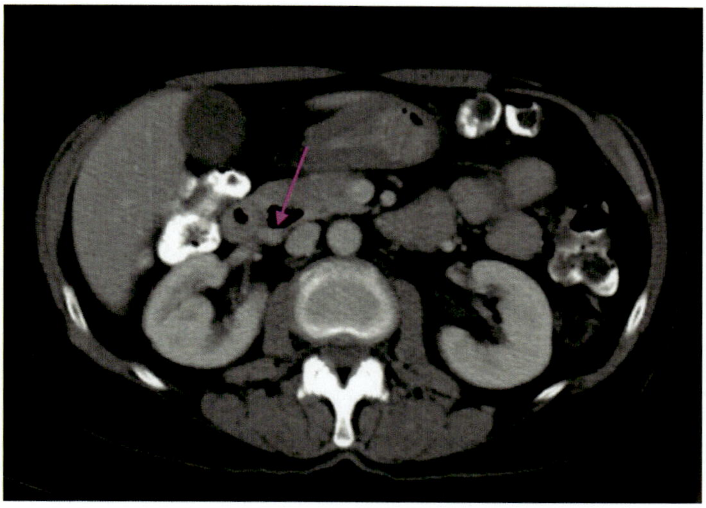

5. What is the most appropriate treatment for this patient?
   A. *ESD* for duodenal gastrinoma
   B. Duodenal wedge resection/Whipple with local lymph node dissection
   C. Antrectomy to remove G cells
   D. Total gastrectomy
   E. Long-acting somatostatin analogue
6. Which is *NOT* a major factor contributing to the recent increased incidence of gastric neuroendocrine tumor (gNET)?
   A. Readily availability of endoscopy
   B. Better pathology definition
   C. Increased awareness of neuroendocrine tumor
   D. Availability of Dotatate scan
   E. New *WHO* grading system
7. Which is the *LEAST* common site for *NETs* in the digestive system?
   A. Pancreas
   B. Stomach
   C. Small intestine
   D. Rectum
   E. Large intestine
8. The most common reason that led to the diagnosis of type I gNET is:
   A. Atrophic gastritis/pernicious anemia
   B. Abdominal pain
   C. Peptic ulcer
   D. *MEN* 1
   E. Bleeding

9. Which of the following statement regarding chromogranin A is true?
   A. Serum chromogranin A is both sensitive and specific for the diagnosis of gNET.
   B. Serum chromogranin A is specific but not sensitive for the diagnosis of gNET.
   C. Serum chromogranin A is elevated in type I and II but not type III gNET.
   D. Serum chromogranin A is elevated in type III but not in type I/II gNET.
   E. Serum chromogranin A can be used to monitor tumor response.
10. Which of the following statement is NOT true?
   A. Gastrinoma is a type of neuroendocrine tumor.
   B. Gastrinoma is associated with Zollinger-Ellison syndrome.
   C. Significant gastrin elevation is observed in all gastrinoma cases.
   D. Gastrinoma and gNET are the same disease entity.
   E. Gastrinoma usually is associated with peptic ulcer.

26.1 Introduction

Gastric neuroendocrine tumors (gNETs), also known as gastric carcinoids, originate from gastric enterochromaffin-like (ECL) cells. ECL cells locate in the gastric oxyntic mucosa and are in close contact with both chief cells and parietal cells [1]. ECL cells produce, store, and secrete histamine, which plays a critical role in gastric acid secretion. Gastrin stimulates ECL cell proliferation, hypertrophy, and hyperplasia and can eventually lead to the formation of neuroendocrine tumor [2, 3]. The incidence of gNETs has been steadily increased longitudinally (0.3/100,000 in 2000, 0.45/100,000 in 2012, and 0.61/100,000 in 2016) [4, 5]. The major contributing factors to this incidence increase include the standardization of the nomenclature and staging, the increase awareness of the disease, and the readily availability of endoscopic surveillance. The stomach is the least common site for NET in the digestive tract and only represents 5–6% of all NETs [6, 7].

26.2 Classification

The three subtypes of gNETs have been well-accepted in the endocrine tumor field after Rindi et al. published their clinicopathologic study of 55 endocrine tumor cases in 1993 [8]. Type I gNETs account for 60–80% of all gNETs. Women have a higher likelihood of suffering from this condition than men. Patients usually have no clinically significant symptom and are diagnosed by endoscopic examination. Most type I gNET cases are associated with atrophic gastritis and/or pernicious anemia. Type II gNETs are associated with multiple endocrine neoplasia type I (MEN 1) syndrome and represent 3–5% of all gNETs. It is believed to be the sequela of the prolonged exposure to hypergastrinemia from gastrinoma. Type III gNETs are also known as sporadic gNETs and represent about 17–37% of all gNETs.

26.3 Clinical and Pathological Characteristics

Table 26.1 shows the characteristics of the three subtypes of gNET [8–13].

Most type I gNETs are multiple and smaller than 1 cm [9]. Seventy-four to 90% of patients present with G1 disease [11, 13, 14]. Lymph node metastases (<7%) and distant metastases (<2%) are uncommon and are associated with larger tumors (>2 cm) and deeper invasion (beyond muscularis propria) [8–11, 13]. The majority of type I gNETs has significant elevation of serum chromogranin A (CgA) and gastrin levels (86–100%) [9, 10]. Approximately 40% of patients are diagnosed due to screening endoscopy for atrophic gastritis or pernicious anemia without significant clinical symptom [9]. The most common symptoms that lead to further investigation and the diagnosis of type I gNETs are abdominal pain and/or gastrointestinal bleeding/anemia (40%).

Type II gNETs are associated with MEN 1 or Wermer's syndrome. MEN 1 is the result of inactivation of the

Table 26.1 Subtypes of gastric neuroendocrine tumors (gNETs)

	Type I	Type II	Type III
Proportions	60–80%	3–5%	17–37%
Female/male	1.2–2.9:1	–	0.37–0.57:1
Age (median)	56–66	51–54	58–59
Associated condition	Atrophic gastritis	MEN 1	None
	Pernicious anemia		
Grade	G1/G2	G1/G2	G1/G2/G3
Serum CgA	86–100%	100%	83%+
Gastrin	86–100%	100%	22%
Tumor size	Small	Large	Large
Metastasis	<7%	50–100%	50–100%

tumor suppressor gene *MEN1*, which codes for the tumor-suppressing protein, MENIN. Zollinger-Ellison syndrome (ZES) was first described by Zollinger and Ellison in 1955 [15]. The hallmark clinical presentation of ZES is severe, recurrent, and multifocal ulcers at the proximal gastrointestinal tract associated with hypersecretion of gastric acid in response to an elevated gastrin level. Although type II gNETs are rare (3–5% of all the gNETs), it is common among patients with MEN 1/ZES. It has been reported that 22–46% of patients with ZES are associated with MEN 1 [16–18]. The remainder of ZES cases are considered sporadic. It is important to differentiate patients with ZES who have associated MEN 1 since patients with ZES/MEN 1 have a 20- to 30-fold higher chance of developing a type II gastric carcinoid than patients with sporadic ZES [19]. Both serum chromogranin A and gastrin levels are elevated in type II gNETs. Most patients' tumor size is greater than 1 cm with a high likelihood to metastases (50–100%).

Type III gNET (sporadic) is usually diagnosed in the absence of chronic gastritis or pernicious anemia. It is not associated with hypergastrinemia, ZES, or MEN 1. It happens twice as often in men than in women. The tumor usually is single and larger than 2 cm and is associated with aggressive behavior. Lymph node and distant metastases are present in about 50–100% at the time of diagnosis.

Typical carcinoid syndrome, including flushing, diarrhea, tachycardia, pellagra, and dyspnea, is rarely (0.5–11%) observed in gNET patients since most of those tumors lack DOPA decarboxylase [20]. Instead of producing serotonin (5-hydroxytryptamine), those gNETs release 5-hydroxytryptophan which can lead to atypical purple flushing in the trunk and extremities [21, 22].

26.4 Diagnosis and Staging

26.4.1 Upper Endoscopy

Esophagogastroduodenoscopy is the most common and important tool in the diagnosis of gNETs. A standardized procedure report is highly recommended since it plays an important role in the diagnosis and management. The report should include a diagram of the stomach and markings for lesion location(s). In addition, characteristics of the lesions, number, size, and companion findings such as ulcers and polyps should be reported. Endoscopic ultrasound is commonly used to evaluate the depth of tumor invasion. Tissue biopsies should be obtained whenever it is feasible.

26.4.2 Imaging Studies

There are many imaging modalities available for the staging and follow-up of gNETs. Combined multiple modalities are often used depending on the purposes and availabilities.

26.4.2.1 CT Scans

Most neuroendocrine tumors are hypervascular; therefore, contrast-enhanced CT scan is usually used for staging when primary tumor is larger than 1 cm with suspicion of lymph node or distant metastases and surveillance. This is especially useful for gNETs that are not identified with tracers targeted to somatostatin receptors.

26.4.2.2 Nuclear Medicine

The expression of somatostatin receptors on the cell surface of NET provides a unique opportunity for the development of difference nuclear imaging techniques in evaluating this type of tumors. Krenning et al. reported their initial experience using ^{123}I-labelled tyr-3-octreotide in gastrinoma localization in 1989 [23]. Since then, the tracer has been modified and optimized, and ^{111}In-labeled octreotide scan has been widely accepted in the clinical practice [24]. Although the overall resolution is low, SPECT images provided clinician a useful alternative tool for NET staging. Complementing to contrast CT or MRI, it helps to identify additional metastatic diseases. In 2000, a study found that ^{68}Ga-Dotatate has significant strong affinity to human somatostatin receptor 2 [25]. Pauwels reviewed the comparison of the sensitivity between ^{111}In-DTPA-octreotide planar and/or SPECT and ^{68}Ga-DOTA-peptide PET from 7 reports which included 443 neuroendocrine patients. ^{68}Ga-DOTA-peptide PET is 24–64% more sensitive than ^{111}In-DTPA-octreotide scan [26]. In fact, ^{68}Ga-dotatate can achieve very high diagnostic accuracy (sensitivity 81% and specificity 90%) [25, 27, 28].

26.4.2.3 Magnetic Resonance Imaging (MRI)

MRI is usually reserved for suspected gNETs with liver or retroperitoneal metastases. Gadolinium contrast is often used to enhance the performance. For NET patients with lesions suspicious for liver metastasis, the diagnostic accuracy of dynamic contrast-enhanced (DCE) MRI was compared with 18F-fluorodeoxyglucose (18F-FDG) or ^{68}Ga-Dotatate. Area under the curve (AUC) was used as the comparison for the differentiation between metastases and liver background. AUC was similar for ^{68}Ga-Dotatate (AUC = 0.966) and 18F-FDG PET/CT (AUC = 0.989) and DCE MRI (AUC of 0.949) [29]. Nevertheless, the investigators recommended that combining MRI with PET may improve the diagnostic power since they may provide complementary information [30].

26.4.3 Biochemical Tests

26.4.3.1 Gastrin

Type I and type II gNETs usually are associated with an elevated gastrin level, whereas type III gNETs rarely have abnormal gastrin elevation. Therefore, a fasting serum gastrin level can help to differentiate different types of gNETs. Nevertheless, hypergastrinemia can be observed in many non-gNET clinical settings. Chronic atrophic gastritis, gastrinoma, and antacid treatment including H2 blocker, proton pump inhibitors, or truncal vagotomy can all cause serum gastrin level elevation.

26.4.3.2 Chromogranin A (CgA)

Chromogranin A is a 49 kDa hydrophilic glycoprotein that resides in the neurosecretory vesicles of the NET cells throughout the gastrointestinal tract. Most patients with NET have elevated serum CgA levels. Peracchi et al. studied serum CgA levels in 45 healthy volunteers, 9 type I gNET patients, and 43 consecutive atrophic gastritis patients (21 without and 22 with ECL cell hyperplasia/dysplasia) [31]. The study found that the sensitivity of CgA is 100% but the specificity is only 20% because CgA can be elevated in the presence of other disorders such as chronic gastritis, inflammatory bowel disease, chronic pancreatitis, and *H. pylori* infection. The authors concluded that CgA is not useful for the diagnosis of type I gNETs. However, the high negative predictive value (100%) makes it a useful tool to rule out type I gNETs. Thus, if serum CgA is not elevated, then a patient is very unlikely to have type I gNETs [32]. In addition, changes in CgA level have been associated with disease recurrence or tumor response [33, 34]. CgA was recommended by the European Neuroendocrine Tumor Society (ENETS) for follow-up of type III gNET patients [35].

Finally, chromogranin A is heavily influenced by proton pump inhibitor (PPI) therapy. Pregun et al. studied 54 patients who took PPI and found that 5 days of PPI use can significantly increase serum CgA level [36]. After long-term use (6 months), both CgA and gastrin levels can be significantly elevated. It takes at least 5 days for both CgA and gastrin to normalize after withholding PPI therapy. Therefore, it is recommended to measure CgA and gastrin level after discontinuing PPI for at least 1 week.

26.5 Clinical and Pathologic Evaluation and Staging

The number and size of tumors, depth of invasion, tumor differentiation, mitotic counts, and Ki-67 index are all significantly associated with patient's outcome. Therefore, it is important to have accurate tumor assessment. Grading of gastric NETs has been evolving in recent years. The most recent World Health Organization (WHO) grading system from 2019 defines [37]:

- G1 – mitotic count less than 2 per 10 high-power fields (HPFs) and/or Ki-67 index 3% or less
- G2 – mitotic count 2–20 per 10 HPFs and/or Ki-67 index 3–20%
- G3 – mitotic count over 20 per 10 HPFs and/or Ki-67 index exceeding 20%

Table 26.2 shows the American Joint Committee on Cancer (AJCC) TNM 8th edition staging system. The staging system does not take the subtypes of gNET into account. In addition, the N stage only categorizes patient into node-negative and node-positive disease. Pak et al. analyzed both the National Cancer Database (NCDB) and the Surveillance, Epidemiology, and End Results (SEER) database to further explore the relationship between the number of positive lymph nodes and patients' outcome. The study identified and validated that patients who have six or fewer positive lymph nodes have significantly different survival than those who had seven or more positive lymph nodes (5-year overall survival (OS), 65% vs. 43%, respectively) [38]. When patients had tumor confined within the stomach (AJCC stage I/II, without lymph node involvement), the cancer-specific survival (CSS) remains high (95.6%) [39]. However, patient with distant metastatic disease have a 5-year CSS of 20%. There are no national or population data regarding subtype-specific prognosis for gNETs. Yang et al. analyzed 3740 gNET patients from the SEER database. The 5-year OS was 86.7± 0.7% for those who were diagnosed between 2002 and 2014. Time and age at diagnosis, gender, marital status, tumor grade, tumor size, tumor stage, and surgery were all significantly associated with patients' prognosis [39].

Figure 26.1 shows the work-up algorithm to differentiate subtypes of gNETs. Once the tissue diagnosis has been established, serum gastrin level should be measured. If the gastrin level is within normal limits, then patient likely has a type III gNET. If gastric level is elevated, 24-hour gastric pH should be measured. If the gastric pH is less than 2, then that suggests a type II gNET. If it is greater than 4, then the diagnosis of type I gNET is established.

Table 26.2 AJCC pathologic TNM staging of neuroendocrine tumors of the stomach (8th edition)

Primary tumor (pT)			
TX: Primary tumor cannot be assessed			
T0: No evidence of primary tumor			
T1: Invades the lamina propria or submucosa and is ≤1 cm in size			
T2: Invades the muscularis propria or is >1 cm in size			
T3: Invades through the muscularis propria into subserosal tissue without penetration of overlying serosa			
T4: Invades visceral peritoneum (serosa) or other organs or adjacent structures			
Regional lymph nodes (pN)			
NX: Regional lymph nodes cannot be assessed			
N0: No regional lymph node metastasis has occurred			
N1: Regional lymph node metastasis			
Distant metastasis (pM)			
M0: No distant metastasis			
M1: Distant metastasis			
M1a: Metastasis confined to the liver			
M1b: Metastasis in at least one extrahepatic site (e.g., lung, ovary, nonregional lymph node, peritoneum, bone)			
M1c: Both hepatic and extrahepatic metastases			
Stage grouping			
Stage I:	T1	N0	M0
Stage II:	T2–T3	N0	M0
Stage III:	T4	N0	M0
	Any T	N1	M0
Stage IV:	Any T	Any N	M1

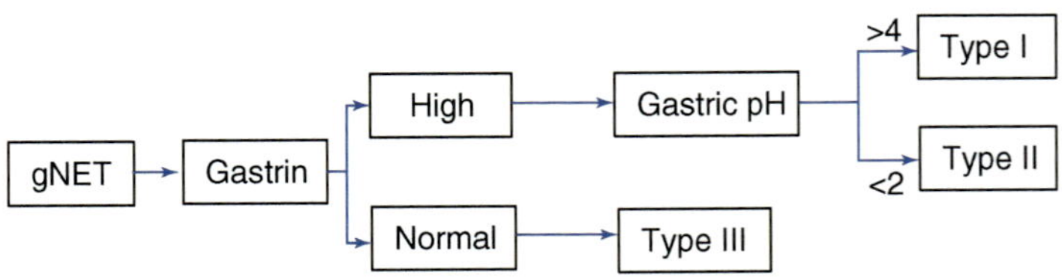

Fig. 26.1 Work-up algorithm to differentiate subtypes of gNETs

26.6 Local Treatment Modalities for gNETs

The common curative treatment modalities include both endoscopic [40] and surgical approaches.

Endoscopic mucosal resection (EMR) has been widely used for endoscopic treatment for benign or low-risk-for-metastasis gastrointestinal tumor. Its indication is generally limited to mucosal tumors less than 2 cm in size. Due to the use of snare technique after submucosal injection, it is hard to control the resection margin status both horizontally and vertically. Sometimes, it requires more than one attempt since the tumor was resected in a piecemeal fashion, which is less ideal for accurate pathological examination.

Endoscopic submucosal dissection (ESD) by submucosal injections of sodium hyaluronate or saline is used to achieve long-lasting mucosal elevation, so the ESD procedures are capable of resecting larger lesions or lesions with scarring. Facciorusso et al. performed a meta-analysis comparing EMR and ESD in treating early gastric cancer [41]. The result showed that ESD has almost 10 times higher complete tumor resection rates and significant lower local recurrence rates.

Surgical approaches include antrectomy, wedge resection, and subtotal or total gastrectomy depending on the type of gNET and the tumor location. Those procedures can be performed open, laparoscopically, or robotically. D1+ or D2 lymph node dissection should be performed if needed.

26.7 Management of gNETs

Saund et al. analyzed SEER gNET patients who underwent lymph node sampling. Of patients with tumors smaller than 2 cm but larger than 1 cm, approximately 20% had lymph node metastasis. This fraction increased to 32% for those with tumors >2 cm. If the tumor involves the muscularis propria or deeper, approximately 50% of patients had lymph node metastasis. For those with a shallower depth of invasion, <20% of patients had lymph node involvement [42]. It has been well-established that patients with small (<1 cm) type I gNET rarely develop local or distant metastasis, whereas patients with diffuse or large type III gNET had much aggressive behavior. Therefore, the management plan should be customized according to the tumor characteristics, including tumor size, differentiation, Ki-67, mitotic count, depth of invasion, and potential of lymph node metastasis and distant metastasis.

26.7.1 Management of Type I gNETs

Panzuto et al. studied 137 type I gNETs. The majority of them (82.5%) underwent endoscopic resection as the first therapy, and 34.3% experienced disease recurrence. The 5-year OS was 100%, and mortality rate was 0.7% [43]. Merola et al. reported their experience regarding the management of type I gNETs using the endoscopic approach. Among 33 patients with a follow-up of 46 months, the survival was 100%. However, 63.6% of the patients experienced disease recurrence after a median of 8 months. Felder et al. studied the treatment pattern for 86 type I gNET patients. The majority of them (78.9%) had G1 disease with smaller tumors (83.6% <2 cm). Only 11.6% of those patients underwent surgery. For all type I gNET patients, the 10-year overall survival was close to 90% [10]. Other smaller size case series supported the management principle [10, 44]. Sato et al. reported 82 type I gNET patients from multiple institutions in Japan. Patients underwent either active endoscopic surveillance (n = 25), endoscopic resection (n = 41), or surgery (n = 16). Only one patient had tumor that invaded beyond the submucosa (muscularis propria). With a median follow-up of 7 years, recurrence-free survival (RFS) was 97.6%, and disease-specific survival (DSS) was 100%. This further supports the conservative treatment strategy [45]. The surgical literature suggests that gastric antrectomy might be the most efficacious treatment for type I gNETs. Dakin reviewed 18 type I gNETs treated medically (8 patients) or surgically (10 patients) [46]. Mean gastrin levels decreased by 94% in the surgical group versus 37.2% in the medical group. The serum gastrin level can be normalized as early as within 8 hours after surgery.

26.7.1.1 Medical Treatment

Thomas et al. have reported the treatment effect of long-acting somatostatin analogues (SSAs) on type I gNETs. Among 32 patients treated with SSAs, 8 had a complete response (CR), 15 had partial response (PR), 3 patients had stable disease (SD), and 6 had progressive disease (PD) [47]. Grozinsky-Glasberg et al. studied 15 patients with type I gNETs treated with long-acting octreotide (LAR) or Lanreotide for at least 6 months [48]. With a median follow-up of 18 months, all patients had reduction in both the size and number of carcinoid tumors at 6 months' gastroscopy examination. Complete tumor regression was observed at 1-year gastroscopy in 11 (73%) of the patients.

Netazepide is a highly selective and competitive gastrin/cholecystokinin 2 (CCK2) receptor antagonist. Boyce et al. studied this in 16 type I gNET patients who were treated with netazepide 50 mg once daily for 12 weeks [49]. The number and size of the largest tumor(s) were all significantly decreased, and the serum CgA fell into the normal range. After discontinuation of the drug for 12 weeks, all the related measures rebounded although all remained better than before treatment. Thirteen of the 16 patients resumed the treatment and continued for 53 weeks. Netazepide resulted in tumor clearance in 38.5% (5/13) of the patients, and the tumor number and size of all other patients had decreased. Serum CgA remained in the normal range. This study suggested that this gastrin/CCK2 receptor antagonist is a potential alternative treatment for type I gNET.

26.7.1.2 Type I gNETs' Treatment Summary

The overall prognosis of type I gNETs is excellent even for patients with recurrent disease. Lymph node or distant metastases are rare for patients with type I gNET. Therefore, EMR and ESD are common treatments of choice upon confirming the diagnosis of type I gNETs. However, due to the persistent hypergastrinemia, tumor recurrence is also common. Patients should be informed of the high recurrence rate following endoscopic treatment and the need for close endoscopic follow-up. According to the ENETS guidelines, yearly EGD is recommended for patients after recurrence and EGD every 24 months for surveillance of patients who have not yet recurred. Surgical resection with antrectomy is indicated for patients with numerous tumors that make surveillance challenging, as well as for bleeding, noncompliance, repeated recurrence, or co-existence with another gastric malignancy. Antrectomy removes the source of gastrin production and hence prevents disease recurrence [9]. As minimally invasive approaches to antrectomy gain in application, the low morbidity and mortality have made the treatment more easily accepted by patients [50]. Although evidence suggests that medical treatment with SSA or netazepide may significantly decrease the number and size of tumors, this approach has not been adopted by professional society consensus as a definitive therapy.

26.7.2 Management of Type II gNETs

Both type II gNET and gastrinoma tumors are associated with ZES and both are neuroendocrine tumors. However, gastrinomas are of G cell origin, whereas gNETs are of ECL cell origin. Unlike type II gNETs, most gastrinomas are present in the pancreas, duodenum, or "gastrinoma triangle" – with three vertices defined by the confluence of the cystic and common bile duct, the junction between the neck and body of the pancreas, and the junction of the second and third part of the duodenum. It is a well-accepted hypothesis that persistent hypergastrinemia produced by gastrinoma leads to hyperplasia/dysplasia of ECL cells in the stomach, hence leading to the formation of type II gNETs. Therefore, the treatment principle for type II gNETs is to control the source, i.e., resection of gastrinoma. Details of gastrinoma treatment will be discussed elsewhere.

In general, type II gNETs are thought to be associated with aggressive tumor behavior. They have a high likelihood of lymph node and distant metastasis. Hence, radical gastrectomy with aggressive lymph node dissection has been recommended. However, due to the low incidence of type II gNET, there is limited evidence from the literature to support the treatment recommendations [8–11, 14]. Since gastrinomas are accountable for gNET formation, removing the gastrinoma might be the only treatment needed for some type II gNETs with indolent tumor biology. Richards et al. reported two type II gNET patients who underwent resection of gastrinomas in the pancreas/duodenum along with any gNETs >1 cm [51]. Both patients showed long-term normalization of gastrin level after radical resection of the gastrinomas and rapid regression of gNETs without recurrence. Tomassetti et al. reported their experience in treating three type II gNET patients with Lanreotide or long-acting analogue octreotide. All three patients showed a reduction in the size and number of the carcinoid tumors observed after 6 months of treatment and complete disappearance of the tumors after 1 year [52]. On the other hand, some type II gNETs can be aggressive. Among 107 MEN 1 ZES patients, Norton et al. identified 5 type II gNET patients with significant clinical symptoms (bleeding, carcinoid syndrome, weight loss and pain, and gastric outlet obstruction), which required surgical intervention [53]. Among the five patients, three had liver metastases at the time of diagnosis. Four of the five patients underwent total gastrectomy with D2 lymph node dissection, and three patients underwent concurrent partial hepatectomy. Four of the five patients had lymph node metastases. Hence, authors advocated total gastrectomy for type II gNETs due to the concern that partial gastrectomy could not remove all of the disease. During the 5± 2-year follow-up, all the five patients remain alive.

26.7.2.1 Type II gNETs' Treatment Summary

Once the diagnosis of type II gNET is established, patients should be referred for genetic testing and if tested positive for MEN 1 appropriately managed for other MEN 1-related disease. Gastrinomas should be localized and appropriately treated with surgery and lymph node dissection [12, 54]. Both the National Comprehensive Cancer Network (NCCN) and ENETS recommend local or limited excision of gNETs at that time. However, detailed indications are not provided. In our institution, we recommended concurrent surgical resection of gNETs >1 cm when performing the primary gastrinoma resection. For tumor <1 cm, endoscopic resection and observation with close endoscopic follow-up are acceptable options due to the possible spontaneous regression after effective control of hypergastrinemia. However, radical gastrectomy with appropriate lymph node dissection should be performed if clinically indicated (e.g., for a larger tumor, numerous tumors, tumor causing obstruction or bleeding, or tumors with lymph node or liver metastasis).

26.7.3 Management of Type III gNETs

Both NCCN and ENETS unanimously agree that radical resection with appropriate lymphadenectomy is the preferred treatment modality for type III gNETs due to the high risk for local, regional, and distant metastasis [12, 54]. However, recent data suggest that for low-risk patients, endoscopic resection is an acceptable alternative treatment modality. Min et al. reported their experience in treating 32 type III gNET (25 G1, 5 G2, and 2 G3) patients. Endoscopic resection was performed on 17 G1 patients (all <2 cm). One of the patients with tumor >1.5 cm developed lymph node recurrence. Wedge resection without lymph node dissection was performed on seven patients. Subtotal or total gastrectomy was performed on eight patients. The overall 5-year survival for all patients was 96% [40]. Kwon et al. studied 50 type III gNET patients who received either ESD or EMR. All patients had submucosa or shallower disease except one with a muscularis propria lesion. Complete resection was achieved in 80% of the patients. Among ten patients received incomplete endoscopic resection, three patients who had lymphovascular invasion received additional surgery. Among 45 patients with median follow-up time of 46 months, no disease recurrence was observed [55]. In fact, NCCN allowed the consideration of endoscopic or wedge resection of the stomach for patients without evidence of lymphadenopathy [54].

26.7.3.1 Type III gNETs' Treatment Summary

The standard of care for type III gNETs is radical gastrectomy with appropriate lymphadenectomy. Given the fact that gNETs have a better prognosis compared to gastric adenocarcinoma, it is reasonable to extrapolate the treatment recommendation from early gastric adenocarcinoma data [56]. Less invasive approach such as ESD or EMR may be considered for patients with T1a tumor and low-grade and smaller tumor (<2 cm).

26

Answers

1. E; 2. E; 3. E; 4. B; 5. B; 6. D; 7. B; 8. A; 9. E; 10. D

References

1. Kamoshida S, Saito E, Fukuda S, Kato K, Iwasaki A, Arakawa Y. Anatomical location of enterochromaffin-like (ECL) cells, parietal cells, and chief cells in the stomach demonstrated by immunocytochemistry and electron microscopy. J Gastroenterol. 1999;34(3):315–20.
2. Hakanson R, Chen D, Lindstrom E, Norlen P, Bjorkqvist M, Lehto-Axtelius D. Physiology of the ECL cells. Yale J Biol Med. 1998;71(3–4):163–71.
3. Zhao CM, Chen D. The ECL cell: relay station for gastric integrity. Curr Med Chem. 2012;19(1):98–108.
4. Dasari A, Shen C, Halperin D, Zhao B, Zhou S, Xu Y, et al. Trends in the incidence, prevalence, and survival outcomes in patients with neuroendocrine tumors in the United States. JAMA Oncol. 2017;3(10):1335–42.
5. Hu P, Bai J, Liu M, Xue J, Chen T, Li R, et al. Trends of incidence and prognosis of gastric neuroendocrine neoplasms: a study based on SEER and our multicenter research. Gastric Cancer. 2020;23(4):591–9.
6. Yao JC, Hassan M, Phan A, Dagohoy C, Leary C, Mares JE, et al. One hundred years after "carcinoid": epidemiology of and prognostic factors for neuroendocrine tumors in 35,825 cases in the United States. J Clin Oncol. 2008;26(18):3063–72.
7. Hallet J, Law CH, Cukier M, Saskin R, Liu N, Singh S. Exploring the rising incidence of neuroendocrine tumors: a population-based analysis of epidemiology, metastatic presentation, and outcomes. Cancer. 2015;121(4):589–97.
8. Rindi G, Luinetti O, Cornaggia M, Capella C, Solcia E. Three subtypes of gastric argyrophil carcinoid and the gastric neuroendocrine carcinoma: a clinicopathologic study. Gastroenterology. 1993;104(4):994–1006.
9. Borch K, Ahren B, Ahlman H, Falkmer S, Granerus G, Grimelius L. Gastric carcinoids: biologic behavior and prognosis after differentiated treatment in relation to type. Ann Surg. 2005;242(1):64–73.
10. Felder S, Jann H, Arsenic R, Denecke T, Prasad V, Knappe-Drzikova B, et al. Gastric neuroendocrine neoplasias: manifestations and comparative outcomes. Endocr Relat Cancer. 2019;26(9):751–63.
11. Manfredi S, Walter T, Baudin E, Coriat R, Ruszniewski P, Lecomte T, et al. Management of gastric neuro-endocrine tumours in a large French national cohort (GTE). Endocrine. 2017;57(3):504–11.
12. Delle Fave G, O'Toole D, Sundin A, Taal B, Ferolla P, Ramage JK, et al. ENETS consensus guidelines update for gastroduodenal neuroendocrine neoplasms. Neuroendocrinology. 2016;103(2):119–24.
13. Vanoli A, La Rosa S, Miceli E, Klersy C, Maragliano R, Capuano F, et al. Prognostic evaluations tailored to specific gastric neuroendocrine neoplasms: analysis of 200 cases with extended follow-up. Neuroendocrinology. 2018;107(2):114–26.
14. Chung CS, Tsai CL, Chu YY, Chen KC, Lin JC, Chen BC, et al. Clinical features and outcomes of gastric neuroendocrine tumors after endoscopic diagnosis and treatment: a Digestive Endoscopy Society of Taiwan (DEST). Medicine (Baltimore). 2018;97(38):e12101.
15. Zollinger RM, Ellison EH. Primary peptic ulcerations of the jejunum associated with islet cell tumors of the pancreas. Ann Surg. 1955;142(4):709–23; discussion 24–8.

16. Farley DR, van Heerden JA, Grant CS, Miller LJ, Ilstrup DM. The Zollinger-Ellison syndrome. A collective surgical experience. Ann Surg. 1992;215(6):561–9; discussion 9–70.
17. Roy PK, Venzon DJ, Shojamanesh H, Abou-Saif A, Peghini P, Doppman JL, et al. Zollinger-Ellison syndrome. Clinical presentation in 261 patients. Medicine (Baltimore). 2000;79(6):379–411.
18. Berna MJ, Annibale B, Marignani M, Luong TV, Corleto V, Pace A, et al. A prospective study of gastric carcinoids and enterochromaffin-like cell changes in multiple endocrine neoplasia type 1 and Zollinger-Ellison syndrome: identification of risk factors. J Clin Endocrinol Metab. 2008;93(5):1582–91.
19. Jensen RT, Fraker DL. Zollinger-Ellison syndrome. Advances in treatment of gastric hypersecretion and the gastrinoma. JAMA. 1994;271(18):1429–35.
20. Modlin IM, Gilligan CJ, Lawton GP, Tang LH, West AB, Darr U. Gastric carcinoids. The Yale experience. Arch Surg. 1995;130(3):250–5; discussion 5–6.
21. Burkitt MD, Pritchard DM. Review article: pathogenesis and management of gastric carcinoid tumours. Aliment Pharmacol Ther. 2006;24(9):1305–20.
22. Oates JA, Sjoerdsma A. A unique syndrome associated with secretion of 5-hydroxytryptophan by metastatic gastric carcinoids. Am J Med. 1962;32:333–42.
23. Krenning EP, Bakker WH, Breeman WA, Koper JW, Kooij PP, Ausema L, et al. Localisation of endocrine-related tumours with radioiodinated analogue of somatostatin. Lancet. 1989;1(8632):242–4.
24. Krenning EP, Kwekkeboom DJ, Bakker WH, Breeman WA, Kooij PP, Oei HY, et al. Somatostatin receptor scintigraphy with [111In-DTPA-D-Phe1]- and [123I-Tyr3]-octreotide: the Rotterdam experience with more than 1000 patients. Eur J Nucl Med. 1993;20(8):716–31.
25. Reubi JC, Schar JC, Waser B, Wenger S, Heppeler A, Schmitt JS, et al. Affinity profiles for human somatostatin receptor subtypes SST1-SST5 of somatostatin radiotracers selected for scintigraphic and radiotherapeutic use. Eur J Nucl Med. 2000;27(3):273–82.
26. Pauwels E, Cleeren F, Bormans G, Deroose CM. Somatostatin receptor PET ligands - the next generation for clinical practice. Am J Nucl Med Mol Imaging. 2018;8(5):311–31.
27. Haug AR, Cindea-Drimus R, Auernhammer CJ, Reincke M, Beuschlein F, Wangler B, et al. Neuroendocrine tumor recurrence: diagnosis with 68Ga-DOTATATE PET/CT. Radiology. 2014;270(2):517–25.
28. Haug AR, Cindea-Drimus R, Auernhammer CJ, Reincke M, Wangler B, Uebleis C, et al. The role of 68Ga-DOTATATE PET/CT in suspected neuroendocrine tumors. J Nucl Med. 2012;53(11):1686–92.
29. Armbruster M, Zech CJ, Sourbron S, Ceelen F, Auernhammer CJ, Rist C, et al. Diagnostic accuracy of dynamic gadoxetic-acid-enhanced MRI and PET/CT compared in patients with liver metastases from neuroendocrine neoplasms. J Magn Reson Imaging. 2014;40(2):457–66.
30. Armbruster M, Sourbron S, Haug A, Zech CJ, Ingrisch M, Auernhammer CJ, et al. Evaluation of neuroendocrine liver metastases: a comparison of dynamic contrast-enhanced magnetic resonance imaging and positron emission tomography/computed tomography. Investig Radiol. 2014;49(1):7–14.
31. Peracchi M, Gebbia C, Basilisco G, Quatrini M, Tarantino C, Vescarelli C, et al. Plasma chromogranin A in patients with autoimmune chronic atrophic gastritis, enterochromaffin-like cell lesions and gastric carcinoids. Eur J Endocrinol. 2005;152(3):443–8.
32. Bashir S, Gibril F, Ojeaburu JV, Asgharian B, Entsuah LK, Ferraro G, et al. Prospective study of the ability of histamine, serotonin or serum chromogranin A levels to identify gastric carcinoids in patients with gastrinomas. Aliment Pharmacol Ther. 2002;16(7):1367–82.

33. Yao JC, Phan AT, Chang DZ, Wolff RA, Hess K, Gupta S, et al. Efficacy of RAD001 (everolimus) and octreotide LAR in advanced low- to intermediate-grade neuroendocrine tumors: results of a phase II study. J Clin Oncol. 2008;26(26):4311–8.
34. Wang YH, Yang QC, Lin Y, Xue L, Chen MH, Chen J. Chromogranin A as a marker for diagnosis, treatment, and survival in patients with gastroenteropancreatic neuroendocrine neoplasm. Medicine (Baltimore). 2014;93(27):e247.
35. Delle Fave G, Kwekkeboom DJ, Van Cutsem E, Rindi G, Kos-Kudla B, Knigge U, et al. ENETS consensus guidelines for the management of patients with gastroduodenal neoplasms. Neuroendocrinology. 2012;95(2):74–87.
36. Pregun I, Herszenyi L, Juhasz M, Miheller P, Hritz I, Patocs A, et al. Effect of proton-pump inhibitor therapy on serum chromogranin a level. Digestion. 2011;84(1):22–8.
37. Klimstra DSKG, La Rosa S, Rindi G, the WHO Classification of Tumours Editorial Board, editors. WHO classification of neuroendocrine neoplasms of the digestive system. 5th ed. France: IRAC; 2019.
38. Pak LM, Yang T, Wang J. Further classification for node-positive gastric neuroendocrine neoplasms. J Gastrointest Surg. 2019;23(4):720–9.
39. Yang Z, Wang W, Lu J, Pan G, Pan Z, Chen Q, et al. Gastric neuroendocrine tumors (G-Nets): incidence, prognosis and recent trend toward improved survival. Cell Physiol Biochem. 2018;45(1):389–96.
40. Uygun A, Kadayifci A, Polat Z, Yilmaz K, Gunal A, Demir H, et al. Long-term results of endoscopic resection for type I gastric neuroendocrine tumors. J Surg Oncol. 2014;109(2):71–4.
41. Facciorusso A, Antonino M, Di Maso M, Muscatiello N. Endoscopic submucosal dissection vs endoscopic mucosal resection for early gastric cancer: a meta-analysis. World J Gastrointest Endosc. 2014;6(11):555–63.
42. Saund MS, Al Natour RH, Sharma AM, Huang Q, Boosalis VA, Gold JS. Tumor size and depth predict rate of lymph node metastasis and utilization of lymph node sampling in surgically managed gastric carcinoids. Ann Surg Oncol. 2011;18(10):2826–32.
43. Panzuto F, Campana D, Massironi S, Faggiano A, Rinzivillo M, Lamberti G, et al. Tumour type and size are prognostic factors in gastric neuroendocrine neoplasia: a multicentre retrospective study. Dig Liver Dis. 2019;51(10):1456–60.
44. Schindl M, Kaserer K, Niederle B. Treatment of gastric neuroendocrine tumors: the necessity of a type-adapted treatment. Arch Surg. 2001;136(1):49–54.
45. Sato Y. Endoscopic diagnosis and management of type I neuroendocrine tumors. World J Gastrointest Endosc. 2015;7(4):346–53.
46. Dakin GF, Warner RR, Pomp A, Salky B, Inabnet WB. Presentation, treatment, and outcome of type 1 gastric carcinoid tumors. J Surg Oncol. 2006;93(5):368–72.
47. Thomas D, Tsolakis AV, Grozinsky-Glasberg S, Fraenkel M, Alexandraki K, Sougioultzis S, et al. Long-term follow-up of a large series of patients with type 1 gastric carcinoid tumors: data from a multicenter study. Eur J Endocrinol. 2013;168(2):185–93.
48. Grozinsky-Glasberg S, Kaltsas G, Gur C, Gal E, Thomas D, Fichman S, et al. Long-acting somatostatin analogues are an effective treatment for type 1 gastric carcinoid tumours. Eur J Endocrinol. 2008;159(4):475–82.
49. Boyce M, Moore AR, Sagatun L, Parsons BN, Varro A, Campbell F, et al. Netazepide, a gastrin/cholecystokinin-2 receptor antagonist, can eradicate gastric neuroendocrine tumours in patients with autoimmune chronic atrophic gastritis. Br J Clin Pharmacol. 2017;83(3):466–75.

50. Hirschowitz BI, Griffith J, Pellegrin D, Cummings OW. Rapid regression of enterochromaffin-like cell gastric carcinoids in pernicious anemia after antrectomy. Gastroenterology. 1992;102(4 Pt 1):1409–18.
51. Richards ML, Gauger P, Thompson NW, Giordano TJ. Regression of type II gastric carcinoids in multiple endocrine neoplasia type 1 patients with Zollinger-Ellison syndrome after surgical excision of all gastrinomas. World J Surg. 2004;28(7):652–8.
52. Tomassetti P, Migliori M, Caletti GC, Fusaroli P, Corinaldesi R, Gullo L. Treatment of type II gastric carcinoid tumors with somatostatin analogues. N Engl J Med. 2000;343(8):551–4.
53. Norton JA, Melcher ML, Gibril F, Jensen RT. Gastric carcinoid tumors in multiple endocrine neoplasia-1 patients with Zollinger-Ellison syndrome can be symptomatic, demonstrate aggressive growth, and require surgical treatment. Surgery. 2004;136(6):1267–74.
54. (NCCN) NCCN. NCCN clinical practice guidelines in oncology: neuroendocrine tumors https://www.nccn.org: National Comprehensive Cancer Network (NCCN); 2019 [updated 3/5/2019]. Available from: https://www.nccn.org/professionals/physician_gls/default.aspx.
55. Min BH, Hong M, Lee JH, Rhee PL, Sohn TS, Kim S, et al. Clinicopathological features and outcome of type 3 gastric neuroendocrine tumours. Br J Surg. 2018;105(11):1480–6.
56. Japanese Gastric Cancer Association. Japanese gastric cancer treatment guidelines 2014 (ver. 4). Gastric Cancer. 2017;20(1):1–19.

Diagnosis and Management of Functional Pancreatic Neuroendocrine Tumors

Els J. M. Nieveen van Dijkum and Anton F. Engelsman

Contents

A. L. Shifrin et al. (eds.), *Endocrine Surgery Comprehensive Board Exam Guide*,
https://doi.org/10.1007/978-3-030-84737-1_27

27

Case Presentation (Adapted from Ref. [1])

The patient is a 50-year-old male with an insignificant medical history until age of 40, when he was diagnosed with a non-functional pNET of 11.5 cm with splenic metastasis of 1.4 cm. He underwent curative resection of the primary tumor and the metastasis. Histological examination showed a well-differentiated neuroendocrine tumor (Ki-67 index 10%, grade 2) and one positive lymph node. After 2 years of follow-up, liver metastases developed which were treated with radiofrequency ablation, and a somatostatin analogue was started. Because of disease progression, he was subsequently treated in a phase II clinical trial and later in a palliative setting with streptozocin/5-fluorouracil. A year after his last chemotherapy, 8 years after initial diagnosis, he was admitted with severe symptomatic hypercalcemia. Laboratory results showed albumin-corrected serum calcium of 3.49 mmol/l and parathyroid hormone (PTH) levels of 0.76 pmol/l, and parathyroid hormone-related peptide (PTHrP) was undetectable (<0.3 pmol/l). In contrast, levels of 1,25-dihydroxycholecalciferol (1,25(OH)2D3) were increased (342 pmol/l). The hypercalcemia was resistant to zoledronate but declined after hyperhydration and dietary calcium restriction. 68Ga-DOTATATE PET and 18F-FDG PET scans showed progression of liver metastasis and an enlarged portacaval lymph node. Due to aberrant arterial supply of the liver tumor, embolization was not possible. Instead patient underwent a palliative hepatectomy of segments 4b/5/6 and portacaval lymph node dissection to achieve tumor load reduction. Pathological examination showed a radically resected, well-differentiated NET grade 2 (Ki-67 index <20%), with areas of higher proliferation (grade 3, Ki-67 index 20–25%). Tumor genetics revealed mRNA expression of CYP27B1, which encodes 25-hydroxyvitamin D3 1-alpha-hydroxylase, the enzyme that converts 25-hydroxyvitamin D3 into the active metabolite 1,25(OH)2D3. The patient's condition improved rapidly after the operation, including normalization of calcium and 1,25(OH)2D3 levels. Unfortunately, 3 months after hepatectomy, CT imaging revealed new peritoneal and hepatic metastases, and 8 months after initiation of nivolumab, severe hypercalcemia relapsed. CT imaging showed an increase of the liver mass and significant reduction of the peritoneal metastases. Palliative hemihepatectomy was performed revealing further dedifferentiation of the pancreatic neuroendocrine tumor metastasis to grade 3 with a Ki-67 index of 40%.

Questions

1. Which criteria are required to establish the diagnosis of insulinoma?
   - I. Finding 68Ga-DOTATATE-avid tumor in the pancreas
   - II. A positive result of the 72-hour fasting test with hypoglycemia
   - III. 5 mIU/L (36 pmol/L) insulin threshold
   - IV. 0.6 ng/mL (0.2 nmol/L) C-peptide threshold
   - V. Insulin/C-peptide ratio <1.0
   - VI. 20 pmol/L proinsulin cutoff level
   - VII. Absence of sulfonylurea (metabolites) in the plasma or urine
     - (a) All of the above
     - (b) All answers except I
     - (c) Answer II only
     - (d) Answers II, III, and VI

2. Which conditions might elevate serum gastrin levels and can cause a false-positive result?
   I. PPI use
   II. Increased serum calcium levels
   III. Kidney failure
   IV. Atrophic gastritis
   V. History of smoking
      (a) II and III
      (b) IV only
      (c) I, II, III, and IV
      (d) I, III, and IV
      (e) All of the above
3. Pancreatic fistula rate is lower after enucleation of functional pNETs as compared to pancreatic resection.
   (a) Correct
   (b) Incorrect
4. Which criteria establish the diagnosis of gastrinoma?
   I. Can only be diagnosed by a pathologist with highly specific gastrin staining
   II. By clinical confirmation of the Zollinger-Ellison syndrome
   III. Confirmation of a tumor in the gastrinoma triangle on a 68Ga-DOTATATE PET/CT
      (a) Answer I only
      (b) Answer II only
      (c) All of the above
      (d) Answers II and III
      (e) Answers I and II
5. The most common location of MEN 1-related gastrinoma is:
   (a) In the pancreatic head
   (b) In the distal duodenum
   (c) In the proximal duodenum
   (d) All of the above
6. What are the criteria to establish Verner-Morrison syndrome?
   I. Elevated serum VIP levels >200 pg/ml
   II. Diarrhea
   III. Hypokalemia
   IV. Achlorhydria
   V. Flushing
      (a) All of the above
      (b) I only
      (c) I, II, III, and IV
      (d) II, III, and IV

7. How can you differentiate between an overt hypergastrinemia due to a gastrinoma and patients with other conditions causing elevated gastrin levels (PPI use, kidney failure, atrophic gastritis)?
   I. By clinical confirmation of the Zollinger-Ellison syndrome
   II. By establishing a gastric pH >7
   III. By establishing a gastric pH <2
      (a) Answer I only
      (b) Answers I and III
      (c) Answer II only
      (d) Answer III only
8. For which case(s) is/are formal resection including lymph node dissection preferred over enucleation?
   I. Gastrinoma in MEN 1 patient
   II. Sporadic gastrinoma
   III. Insulinoma
      (a) Answers I and II
      (b) Answer III
      (c) Answer II

27.1 Introduction

Functional pancreatic neuroendocrine tumors (F-pNETs) are defined as tumors located in the pancreas with hormonal overproduction which causes a specific clinical syndrome. Functional and non-functional pNETs have a distinct biological behavior as compared to pancreatic adenocarcinoma, and therefore, clinical management differs between both tumor types. Of all pNETs, 60–90% are non-functional and often asymptomatic. These are discussed in ► Chap. 28.

The most frequent F-pNETs are insulinomas which cause hypoglycemia and gastrinomas which cause gastrin overproduction (also known as the Zollinger-Ellison syndrome, ZES). Other less frequent occurring F-pNETs include glucagonomas, VIPomas, somatostatinomas, and others (see ◘ Table 27.1).

Most pNETs occur as sporadic tumors; however, a significant proportion of F-pNETs are part of an inherited syndrome. MEN 1 remains the most predominant inherited condition responsible for F-pNET, followed by Von Hippel-Lindau (VHL) disease, von Recklinghausen's syndrome (neurofibromatosis type 1, NF-1) and, in rare cases, tuberous sclerosis [2].

Diagnostic work-up and management of F-pNETs may be challenging due to the diversity in clinical presentation, confounding factors in serum hormone measurements, and localization difficulties of sometimes very small F-pNET. Determining the best treatment strategy for these rare tumors is often complex and should be decided by a multidisciplinary team in a dedicated center including endocrine, oncology, imaging, gastrointestinal, and surgical expertise.

Table 27.1 Rare functional pancreatic neuroendocrine tumors

Name	Hormone	Incidence (per 1 million person-years)	Localization	Malignant (%)	MEN 1 associated (%)	Symptoms
VIPoma, Verner-Morrison syndrome	Vasoactive intestinal peptide	0.05–0.2	Pancreas (90%), others (neuronal, adrenal, periganglionic, 10%)	40–70	6	Diarrhea (90–100%) Hypokalemia (80–100%) Dehydration (83%)
Glucagonoma	Glucagon	0.01–0.1	Pancreas (100%)	50–80	1–20	Skin rash (67–90%) Glucose intolerance (38–87%) Weight loss (66–96%)
SSoma	Somatostatin	Rare	Pancreas (55%), duodenum/jejunum (41%)	>70	45	Diabetes (63–90%) Cholelithiasis (65–90%) Diarrhea (35–90%)
GHRHoma	Growth hormone-releasing hormone	Unknown	Pancreas (30%), lung (54%), jejunum (7%), others (13%)	>60	16	Acromegaly (100%)
ACTHoma	ACTH	Rare	Pancreas (4–16% of ectopic Cushing)	>95	Rare	Cushing syndrome (100%)
pNET with carcinoid syndrome	Serotonin	Very rare	Pancreas <1% of all carcinoids	60–88	Rare	Carcinoid syndrome
pNET with hypocalcemia	PTHrp	Rare	Pancreatic location rare	84	Rare	Hypocalcemia-related symptoms
pNET with calcitonin production	Calcitonin	Rare	Pancreatic location rare	>80	16	Diarrhea (50%)
pNET with renin production	Renin	Rare	Pancreas	Unknown	Unknown	Hypertension
pNET with LH production	LH	Rare	Pancreas	Unknown	Unknown	Anovulation, virilization (female), reduced libido (male)
pNET with erythropoietin production	Erythropoietin	Rare	Pancreas	100	Unknown	Polycythemia
pNET with IGF-II production	Insulin-like growth factor II	Rare	Pancreas	Unknown	Unknown	Hypoglycemia

This chapter will discuss epidemiology, diagnosis, treatment, and outcomes of the most frequent F-pNETs.

27.2 Insulinoma

An insulinoma is a tumor of the pancreas originating from the beta cells and secretes insulin. The incidence of insulinomas is four per million person-years, and it is the most frequently occurring functioning neuroendocrine tumor of the pancreas. Data from some large series showed that the median age at the time of surgery is 50 years (range 17–86 years) and 57% of patients are female. Placzkowski et al. reported on a large cohort of 237 patients with insulinomas, of which 14 patients (6%) were MEN 1 related [3]. Data from another large cohort of 224 patients with insulinomas showed that 194 (87%) had single benign tumors, 16 (7%) had multiple benign tumors, and only 13 (6%) had malignant insulinomas, as defined as the presence of metastases [4].

27.2.1 Clinical Presentation

Patients present with symptoms of neuroglycopenia, such as confusion, visual impairment, unusual behavior, palpitations, tremors, and seizure-like presentations. Mean time from the start of symptoms to diagnosis is 18 months; however, some patients may even been misdiagnosed with neurologic or psychiatric disorders for years. Symptoms typically occur during fasting; however, 20% of patients have postprandial complaints.

27.2.2 Diagnosis

Originally the clinical diagnosis of an insulinoma depends on Whipple's triad with [5]:

1. Complaints of hunger, tremor, dizziness, and other hypoglycemic symptoms.
2. A serum glucose level <50 mg/dl or <4 pmol/l.
3. Relief of symptoms after glucose administration.

The diagnosis is established by inappropriately high insulin concentrations during a 72-hour supervised fasting period (fasting test). In case patients have postprandial symptoms, a mixed meal test can be used to confirm the diagnosis. Normal insulin levels do not exclude the presence of an insulinoma, because the absolute insulin level is not elevated in all patients with insulinoma. Proinsulin may be considered to be a more reliable marker, because the proportion of proinsulin secreted by insulinoma cells is generally higher than by normal β-cells.

An important disorder to consider which simulates insulinoma test results is self-induced hypoglycemia. Sulfonylurea-induced hypoglycemia is induced by ingestion of oral insulin secretagogue medication (gliclazide) and can be confirmed by measuring serum sulfonylurea. Factitious hypoglycemia is induced by self-injected insulin. Measuring C-peptide may help in discriminating between insulinoma and factitious hypoglycemia. C-peptide is the natural breakdown peptide of insulin and should be high in endogenous insulin overproduction due to continuous insulin release and low in case of factitious hypoglycemia.

The present consensus in diagnosis of an insulinoma includes:

1. Hypoglycemia during a 72-hour supervised fasting test
2. 5 mIU/L (36 pmol/L) insulin threshold
3. 0.6 ng/mL (0.2 nmol/L) C-peptide threshold
4. Insulin/C-peptide ratio <1.0
5. 20 pmol/L proinsulin cutoff level
6. Absence of sulfonylurea (metabolites) in the plasma or urine.

27.2.3 Localization

Adequate localization is imperative for preoperative planning and preparation of both surgeon and patient. CT scan, MRI scanning, and endoscopic ultrasonography (EUS) may be used for localization of the insulinoma [6]. Sensitivity of SSTR2 receptor-mediated imaging (68Gallium-DOTATATE PET/CT) is low (45%) as compared to other neuroendocrine tumors (80–100%) and therefore is not included in the standard work-up for localization of an insulinoma [7]. It has been shown that targeting the glucagon-like peptide-1 receptors (GLP-1R) using the specific exendin-4-based ligand is a very sensitive (≥95% sensitivity) method to localize benign and more recently also malignant insulinomas with SPECT [8]. However, this imaging technique may not be generally available.

Intraoperative ultrasonography and/or selective arterial calcium stimulation (SACS) test combined with venous sampling are available when noninvasive techniques failed to localize the insulinoma. As a last resort to localize an insulinoma, intraoperative selective arterial stimulation with calcium may be considered. Selective injection of calcium in the splenic artery, superior mesenteric artery, and gastroduodenal artery will increase insulin secretion by an insuloma located in the pancreatic tail, corpus, or head, respectively. Increased insulin secretion can be detected by sampling the hepatic vein 30–120 seconds after calcium injection [9].

27.2.4 Treatment

Since most insulinomas are benign and unifocal, enucleation is the preferred treatment strategy, especially for insulinomas located in the pancreatic head or corpus region. However, postoperative complication rates associated with enucleations from the pancreatic head region are comparable with complication rates of formal pancreatic resections. However, most importantly, the long-term effect of enucleations as compared to pancreatic resections is preservation of the exocrine function of the pancreas.

Insulinomas located in the pancreatic tail region can be treated with enucleation or pancreatic tail resection, preferably sparing the spleen. Both short-term and long-term complication rates are comparable between both techniques [10–12].

In case a patient has not been cured after insulinoma resection, medical treatment may be helpful to bridge during further reoperation planning. Patients in very poor condition can also be treated symptomatically with diazoxide, octreotide, or verapamil; however, cure can only be achieved with insulinoma resection. Some authors have started radiofrequency ablation for these benign lesions, but results from this treatment have yet to be balanced against enucleation and formal resection techniques.

27.3 Gastrinoma

A gastrinoma is a tumor derived from G-cells in the duodenum, pancreas, or less commonly stomach that secretes the peptide hormone gastrin. Gastrin-secreting neuroendocrine tumors of the pancreas or duodenum cause the clinical syndrome called Zollinger-Ellison syndrome (ZES). Although many neuroendocrine tumors stain positive for gastrin, only tumors with the overt clinical ZES are classified as gastrinoma. The annual incidence of gastrinoma is 0.5–2 per million person-years, and approximately 80% of gastrinomas are sporadic tumors [13].

Only 25% of all gastrinomas are located in the pancreas, whereas the other patients have duodenal gastrinomas, mainly located in the first part of the duodenum. MEN 1 patients have 70–100% localization of gastrinomas in the duodenal area [14].

27.3.1 Clinical Presentation

The clinical presentation in patients with ZES is related to overproduction of gastrin, causing gastric acid hypersecretion resulting in peptic ulcer disease (73–98%), abdominal pain or heart burn (50–55%), and diarrhea (60–75%) and complications of ulcerative disease including bleeding, stricture, and perforation [15]. Endoscopic features include peptic ulcers, typically smaller than 1 cm in diameter, and in 75% of cases located in the first part of the duodenum. In MEN 1 patients, ulcers are often smaller (<0.5 cm), and the gastrinomas are more often multifocal and associated with lymph node involvement (40–60%) [16].

27.3.2 Diagnosis

Fasting serum gastrin level greater than 10 times the upper limit of normal in the presence of gastric pH <2 is diagnostic for ZES. Measurement of gastric pH is important to exclude secondary hypergastrinemia due to renal failure, atrophic gastritis, or PPI use. If fasting gastrin levels are less than tenfold the upper limit of normal, a secretin stimulation test can be performed. Secretin stimulates gastrin release by the gastrinoma, whereas normal G-cells are inhibited by secretin [17].

This secretin stimulation test has a 94% sensitivity and 100% specificity for gastrinoma diagnosis. Patients with severe symptoms may not be able to pause PPI use during the diagnostic process. In these cases, high dosage of H2 receptor blockers should be administered to replace PPI use.

27.3.3 Localization

Localization studies include CT scan, MRI, and PET/CT using 68Ga-DOTATATE or 68Ga-DOTATOC. If these studies are negative, EUS can be performed, possibly with fine needle aspiration or biopsy. Preoperative imaging identifies over 90% of gastrinoma localizations. As in insulinoma patients, selective arterial secretin injection (SASI) test can be performed to localize gastrinomas in the pancreas (sensitivity 75–100%) or duodenum (sensitivity 30–63%) [17]. Intraoperative imaging with ultrasonography or duodenal transillumination may aid in localizing the gastrinoma in patients with non-localized disease on preoperative imaging, especially in MEN 1 patients.

27.3.4 Treatment

Medical management with PPIs and somatostatin analogues such as octreotide or Lanreotide aims at symptom control. H2 receptor antagonists such as cimetidine can be used additionally to PPIs.

Resection of a solitary gastrinoma is the treatment of choice and is curative in about 50% of patients (◘ Fig. 27.1). Additional lymphadenectomy has shown to improve cure rates as compared to gastrinoma resection alone [18, 19]. Since lymphadenectomy should be performed, enucleation is less

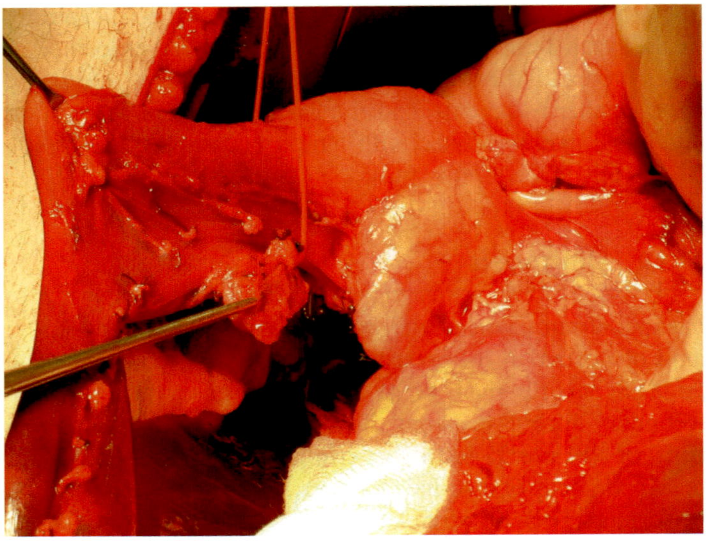

Fig. 27.1 Pancreatic head sparing duodenectomy with lymph node metastasis of gastrinoma

often indicated and should be reserved for large solitary tumors in the pancreatic head. Long-term biochemical cure is achieved in only 30% of patients, and some of these patients benefit from reoperations, especially if localization of the recurrent gastrinoma is confirmed preoperatively [20, 21].

27.4 Other F-pNETs

Among other F-pNETs, a wide variety of extremely rare tumors exist (see Table 27.1), all of which have their distinct presentation based on the hormone that is secreted. Many are related to hereditary syndromes such as MEN 1 [22].

27.4.1 Glucagonoma

Glucagonomas are F-pNETs originating from the pancreatic alpha cells that result in the overproduction of glucagon. Glucagon, a hormone produced by pancreatic islet α-cells, plays an opposite role to insulin in glycometabolism. Mostly, these tumors are large at diagnosis (>5 cm), which makes localization easier as compared to gastrinomas or insulinomas. Eighty percent of glucagonomas are located in the pancreatic head or body. Glucagonomas occurring in patients with MEN 1 syndrome have malignancy potential.

The diagnosis of glucagonoma is established by the presence of typical symptoms, the elevated levels of glucagon above 500 pg/mL, and the presence of a tumor in the pancreas [23]. Glucagonoma syndrome includes symptoms of necrotic migratory erythema, weight loss, hypoalbuminemia, and diabetes mellitus or impaired glucose tolerance. However, glucagon level, the only specific indicator, is also elevated in other conditions, such as cirrhosis, diabetes mellitus, sepsis, and burns. Therefore, hyperglucagonemia must be considered together with other typical symptoms of glucagonoma syndrome for diagnosis. A 68Ga-DOTATATE scan is highly sensitive to assess for metastases.

The treatment of glucagonoma is resection; however, metastases may exist rendering the tumor uncurable. Even after cytoreductive surgery in combination with chemotherapy, 5-year survival rates of up to 50% may be reached. If cytoreductive surgery of liver metastases is not feasible, liver embolization may be considered to provide symptom relief from the excess of hormone production. Also, octreotide is effective for symptom relief from unresectable glucagonoma.

27.4.2 VIPoma

VIPomas are characterized by overproduction of vasoactive intestinal polypeptide (VIP) hormone, which results in a characteristic clinical presentation (Verner-Morrison syndrome), involving watery diarrhea, hypokalemia, and achlorhydria.

The diagnosis of Verner-Morrison syndrome is confirmed by increased serum VIP concentration >200 pg/ml. 68Ga-DOTATATE scan is sensitive to localize the primary tumor as well as potential metastases. Most VIPomas are located in the pancreas (90%) and are generally solitary and >3 cm. Seventy-five percent of pancreatic VIPomas are located in the pancreatic tail region [24, 25]. At initial diagnosis, 50% of VIPomas are classified as malignant, of which 75% show metastases (regional lymph nodes and liver).

Due to the malignant potential, aggressive surgical approach including resection and lymph node dissection is warranted. In case of unresectable disease, octreotide may be considered for symptom relief.

27.4.3 SSomas

Somatostatin-producing NETs (SSomas) mainly originate from the pancreas, the duodenum close to the ampulla, and the peri-ampullary area. Because somatostatin inhibits the endocrine secretion and the motility of the stomach and gallbladder, somatostatin-producing NETs always cause a classical triad of syndromes: hyperglycemia, cholelithiasis, and maldigestion of food. However, recently, the actual existence of a distinct clinical somatostatinoma (SSoma) syndrome has been questioned because in one extensive review of cases, none of the 46 patients with pathologically diagnosed SSomas, nor any of 821 other pNET cases reviewed, had the full features of the proposed SSoma clinical syndrome [26]. Serum somatostatin levels can be elevated with regard to various extra-pancreatic NETs, and a prevalence of 1 in 40 million in the morbidity of pancreatic somatostatin-producing NETs makes drawing conclusions difficult based on both typical clinical symptoms and laboratory assessments.

Answers to the Questions

1. (b); 2. (c); 3. (b); 4. (b); 5. (c); 6. (c); 7. (b); 8. (c)

References

1. Van Lierop AH, Bisschop PH, Boelen A, van Eeden S, Engelsman AF, Nieveen van Dijkum EJM, Klumpen HJ. Hypercalcemia due to a calcitriol producing tumor. J Surg Case Rep. 2019;12:1–3.
2. Tirosh A, Kebebew E. Genetic and epigenetic alterations in pancreatic neuroendocrine tumors. J Gastrointest Oncol. 2020;11(3):567–77.
3. Placzkowski KA, Vella A, Thompson GB, Grant CS, Reading CC, Charboneau JW, Andrews JC, Lloyd RV, Service FJ. Secular trends in the presentation and management of functioning insulinoma at the Mayo Clinic, 1987–2007. J Clin Endocrinol Metab. 2009;94(4):1069.
4. Service FJ, McMahon MM, O'Brien PC, Ballard DJ. Functioning insulinoma--incidence, recurrence, and long-term survival of patients: a 60-year study. Mayo Clin Proc. 1991;66(7):711.
5. Cryer PE, Axelrod L, Grossman AB, Heller SR, Montori VM, Seaquist ER, Service FJ, Endocrine Society. Evaluation and management of adult hypoglycemic disorders: an Endocrine Society clinical practice guideline. J Clin Endocrinol Metab. 2009;94(3):709.
6. Rösch T, Lightdale CJ, Botet JF, Boyce GA, Sivak MV Jr, Yasuda K, Heyder N, Palazzo L, Dancygier H, Schusdziarra V. Localization of pancreatic endocrine tumors by endoscopic ultrasonography. N Engl J Med. 1992;326(26):1721.
7. Mirallié E, Pattou F, Malvaux P, Filoche B, Godchaux JM, Maunoury V, Palazzo L, Lefebvre J, Huglo D, Paris JC, Carnaille B, Proye C. Value of endoscopic ultrasonography and somatostatin receptor scintigraphy in the preoperative localization of insulinomas and gastrinomas. Experience of 54 cases. Gastroenterol Clin Biol. 2002;26(4):360.
8. Christ E, Wild D, Ederer S, Béhé M, Nicolas G, Caplin ME, Brändle M, Clerici T, Fischli S, Stettler C, Ell PJ, Seufert J, Gloor B, Perren A, Reubi JC, Forrer F. Glucagon-like peptide-1 receptor imaging for the localisation of insulinomas: a prospective multicentre imaging study. Lancet Diabetes Endocrinol. 2013;1:115–22.
9. Doppman JL, Miller DL, Chang R, Shawker TH, Gorden P, Norton JA. Insulinomas: localization with selective intraarterial injection of calcium. Radiology. 1991;178(1):237.
10. Jilesen APJ, van Eijck CHJ, Busch ORC, van Gulik TM, Gouma DJ, Nieveen van Dijkum EJM. Postoperative outcomes of enucleation and standard resections in patients with a pancreatic neuroendocrine tumor. World J Surg. 2016;40:715–28.
11. Kabir T, Tan ZZX, Syn N, Chung AYF, Ooi LPJ, Goh BKP. Minimally-invasive versus open enucleation for pancreatic tumours: a propensity-score adjusted analysis. Ann Hepatobiliary Pancreat Surg. 2019;23(3):258–64.
12. Zhou Y, Zhao M, Wu L, Ye F, Si X. Short- and long-term outcomes after enucleation of pancreatic tumors: an evidence-based assessment. Pancreatology. 2016;16(6):1092–8.

13. Berna MJ, Hoffmann KM, Serrano J, Gibril F, Jensen RT. Serum gastrin in Zollinger-Ellison syndrome: I. Prospective study of fasting serum gastrin in 309 patients from the National Institutes of Health and comparison with 2229 cases from the literature. Medicine. 2006;85(6):295.
14. Norton JA. Neuroendocrine tumors of the pancreas and duodenum. Curr Probl Surg. 1994;31(2):77–9.
15. Zollinger RM, Ellison EH. Primary peptic ulcerations of the jejunum associated with islet cell tumors of the pancreas. Ann Surg. 1955;142(4):709.
16. Norton JA, Foster DS, Ito T, Jensen RT. Gastrinomas: medical or surgical treatment. Endocrinol Metab Clin N Am. 2018;47(3):577.
17. Mendelson AH, Donowitz M. Catching the zebra: clinical pearls and pitfalls for the successful diagnosis of Zollinger-Ellison syndrome. Dig Dis Sci. 2017;62(9):2258.
18. Bartsch DK, Waldmann J, Fendrich V, Boninsegna L, Lopez CL, Partelli S, Falconi M. Impact of lymphadenectomy on survival after surgery for sporadic gastrinoma. Br J Surg. 2012;99(9):1234–40.
19. Giovinazzo F, Butturini G, Monsellato D, Malleo G, Marchegiani G, Bassi C. Lymph nodes metastasis and recurrences justify an aggressive treatment of gastrinoma. Updat Surg. 2013;65(1):19.
20. Grobmyer SR, Vogel SB, McGuigan JE, Copeland EM, Hochwald SN. Reoperative surgery in sporadic Zollinger-Ellison syndrome: long-term results. J Am Coll Surg. 2009;208(5):718.
21. Norton JA, Fraker DL, Alexander HR, Venzon DJ, Doppman JL, Serrano J, Goebel SU, Peghini PL, Roy PK, Gibril F, Jensen RT. Surgery to cure the Zollinger-Ellison syndrome. N Engl J Med. 1999;341: 635–44.
22. Jensen RT, Berna MJ, Bingham MD, et al. Inherited pancreatic endocrine tumor syndromes: advances in molecular pathogenesis, diagnosis, management and controversies. Cancer. 2008;113(7 suppl):1807–43.
23. Appetecchia M, Lauretta R, Rota F, Carlini M. Neuroendocrine tumors biomarkers. In: Massimo C, editor. Abdominal neuroendocrine tumors. Milano: Springer; 2018. p. 65–78.
24. Solcia E, Capella C, Riva C, Rindi G, Polak JM. The morphology and neuroendocrine profile of pancreatic epithelial VIPomas and extrapancreatic, VIP-producing, neurogenic tumors. Ann N Y Acad Sci. 1988;527:508–17.
25. Bloom SR. Vasoactive intestinal peptide, the major mediator of the WDHA (pancreatic cholera) syndrome: value of measurement in diagnosis and treatment. Am J Dig Dis. 1978;23:373–6.
26. Garbrecht N, Anlauf M, Schmitt A, et al. Somatostatin-producing neuroendocrine tumors of the duodenum and pancreas: incidence, types, biological behavior, association with inherited syndromes, and functional activity. Endocr Relat Cancer. 2008;15:229–41.

Non-functional Pancreatic Neuroendocrine Tumors

Reto M. Kaderli and Dietmar Simon

Contents

A. L. Shifrin et al. (eds.), *Endocrine Surgery Comprehensive Board Exam Guide*,
https://doi.org/10.1007/978-3-030-84737-1_28

Case Presentation

A 55-year-old patient presented with abdominal pain. As part of the diagnosis, an abdominal CT scan was performed. This revealed a cystic mass of approximately 2 cm in the pancreatic tail. There were no signs of compression of the pancreatic duct. The mass was assumed to have no correlation to the complained symptoms and thus assessed as an incidental finding. Comorbidities were diabetes mellitus with diabetic polyneuropathy and a hypertensive cardiac disease. Further diagnosis was performed to assess the lesion. Thin-slice CT scan showed the same lesion with some irregular border. On endoscopic ultrasound, the 2 cm mass was described as partly cystic with a well-vascularized wall which was up to 4 mm thick. A fine needle biopsy was not performed. Tumor markers (CEA, CA 19–9, chromogranin A) were in the normal range. Because of the young age of the patient, indication to operation was proposed. A laparoscopic spleen-preserving pancreatic tail resection was performed. Postoperative course was uneventful, and the patient was discharged from hospital 6 days postoperatively. Histology demonstrated a 1.8 cm highly differentiated, partly cystic neuroendocrine tumor. Proliferative index was less than 2%. The tumor was classified as pNET pT1 L0 V0 Pn0 G1 R0. Tumor aftercare was recommended by the tumor board.

Questions

1. Which of the clinical aspects of pNETs are correct?
   1. Most of the pNETs are poorly differentiated.
   2. All pNETs secrete hormones or peptides.
   3. Hormone- or peptide-secreting pNETs can be asymptomatic.
   4. Immunohistochemical positivity for hormones defines the clinical symptoms.
      (a) Only (3) is correct.
      (b) Only (1) and (2) are correct.
      (c) Only (1) and (4) are correct.
      (d) Only (1), (2), and (4) are correct.
      (e) All are correct.
2. Which answers about inherited pNETs are correct?
   1. About 10% of pNETs are caused by germline mutations.
   2. Typical inherited syndromes for pNETs are VHL and MEN 1 syndrome.
   3. pNETs in MEN 1 occur in all parts of the pancreas.
   4. The most frequent manifestation in MEN 1 is pNETs.
      (a) Only (1) is correct.
      (b) Only (1), (2), and (3) are correct.
      (c) Only (1), (3), and (4) are correct.
      (d) Only (3) and (4) are correct.
      (e) All are correct.
3. Frequent symptoms of the clinical presentation of pNETs are:
   1. Weight loss.
   2. Palpable mass.
   3. Intra-abdominal hemorrhage.
   4. Abdominal pain.

   (a) Only (2) is correct.
   (b) Only (1) and (2) are correct.
   (c) Only (1) and (4) are correct.
   (d) Only (1), (2), and (3) are correct.
   (e) Only (3) and (4) are correct.

4. The diagnostic procedure(s) for detection of NF-pNETs is/are favorably?
   1. Computed tomography (CT).
   2. Magnetic resonance imaging (MRI).
   3. PET/CT with Ga 68-DOTATATE.
   4. Transabdominal ultrasound.
      (a) Only (3) is correct.
      (b) Only (1) and (2) are correct.
      (c) Only (2) and (3) are correct.
      (d) Only (1), (2), and (3) are correct.
      (e) Only (4) is correct.
5. The following diagnostic tools are helpful in the assessment of NF-pNETs. Which of the answer(s) is/are correct?
   1. Endoscopic ultrasound is useful in the follow-up of NF-pNETs in MEN 1.
   2. Assessment of CgA (chromogranin A) may facilitate diagnosis of NF-pNETs.
   3. Germline DNA testing for MEN 1 and VHL is routinely performed in NF-pNETs.
   4. Ga 68-DOTATATE PET/CT has the highest sensitivity with about 90% for localizing NF-pNETs.
      (a) Only (1) and (2) are correct.
      (b) Only (2) and (3) are correct.
      (c) Only (1), (2), and (3) are correct.
      (d) Only (1), (2), and (4) are correct.
      (e) All are correct.
6. On which option(s) for the treatment of NF-pNETs would you decide?
   1. The first choice for treatment of NF-pNETs is the surgical resection.
   2. Some NF-pNETs can be observed and followed up.
   3. Surgery is recommended for young patients and in case of signs of invasion.
   4. Size of the tumor has no influence on the decision for treatment.
      (a) Only (1) is correct.
      (b) Only (2) is correct.
      (c) Only (4) is correct.
      (d) Only (2) and (4) are correct.
      (e) Only (1), (2), and (3) are correct.
7. Which of the following statements about small NF-pNETs would you agree on?
   1. Small NF-pNETs can be managed conservatively.
   2. Typical indication for conservative management of small NF-pNETs is old patients with necessity of major resection.

3. NF-pNETs of <2 cm size have a clear indication to operation.
4. The malignancy rate of small NF-pNETs (<2 cm) is >30%.
   (a) Only (1) is correct.
   (b) Only (3) is correct.
   (c) Only (4) is correct.
   (d) Only (3) and (4) are correct.
   (e) Only (1) and (2) are correct.

8. The following therapies are performed in advanced stage of disease in NF-pNETs:
   1. TACE (transarterial chemoembolization) and RFA (radiofrequency ablation) are treatment options for metastatic hepatic disease.
   2. Liver transplantation is indicated in patients with poorly differentiated G3 NF-pNETs.
   3. Less than 60% of NF-pNETs express somatostatin receptors making them less suitable for therapy with SSA (somatostatin analogues).
   4. PRRT (peptide receptor radiotherapy) is recommended after failure of medical therapy.
      (a) Only (1) is correct.
      (b) Only (2) is correct.
      (c) Only (2) and (3) are correct.
      (d) Only (1) and (4) are correct.
      (e) Only (1), (2), and (3) are correct.
9. Which operative strategy would you follow in the following settings?
   1. Small NF-pNETs can be enucleated.
   2. Large tumors and invasion or lymph node involvement indicate pancreatic resection.
   3. Splenectomy is mandatory for left pancreatic resection of malignant NF-pNETs with lymph node involvement.
   4. Pancreatic resection is obsolete when hepatic metastases are present.
      (a) Only (1) is correct.
      (b) Only (1) and (2) are correct.
      (c) Only (3) and (4) are correct.
      (d) Only (1), (2), and (3) are correct.
      (e) All are correct.
10. Surgical management of NF-pNETs in MEN 1 syndrome remains controversial. Which of the following statements would you agree on?
    1. NF-pNETs in MEN 1 are almost always multifocal.
    2. Prophylactic surgery may prevent development of malignant tumors and improve survival.
    3. Risk of malignancy increases with tumor size.
    4. Therapy ranges from active surveillance over enucleation up to total pancreatectomy.

(a) Only (2) is correct.
(b) Only (1) and (2) are correct.
(c) Only (2) and (3) are correct.
(d) Only (4) is correct.
(e) All are correct.

11. Prognosis of NF-pNETs depends on various aspects. Which answers are correct?
    1. NF-pNETs are slowly growing tumors with a good prognosis.
    2. Survival is mostly affected by the presence of hepatic metastases.
    3. Prognosis is independent of grading and age.
    4. The median overall survival of patients with NF-pNETs is >60 months.
    (a) Only (1) is correct.
    (b) Only (1) and (2) are correct.
    (c) Only (3) is correct.
    (d) Only (3) and (4) are correct.
    (e) Only (2), (3), and (4) are correct.
12. There are various treatment options available for therapy of advanced-stage disease of NF-pNETs. Which of the answer(s) is/are correct?
    1. The goal of systemic therapy is to improve survival and control symptoms.
    2. About 80% of NF-pNETs present somatostatin receptors making them suitable for therapy with SSA (somatostatin analogues).
    3. Systemic chemotherapy is indicated in bulky disease of G1/G2 NF-pNETs, G3 NF-pNETs, and G3 NF-pNECs, respectively.
    4. Targeted drugs (e.g., everolimus, sunitinib) can be used sequential to previous SSA therapy and/or chemotherapy.
    (a) Only (1) and (2) are correct.
    (b) Only (2) and (3) are correct.
    (c) Only (1), (3), and (4) are correct.
    (d) Only (2), (3), and (4) are correct.
    (e) All are correct.

28.1 Introduction

Non-functional pancreatic neuroendocrine tumors (NF-pNETs) exhibit a wide range of malignant potential. Most NF-pNETs are well-differentiated slow-growing and non-infiltrative tumors, whereas poorly differentiated WHO grade 3 (G3) neuroendocrine carcinomas (NECs) are uncommon [1].

pNETs are classified based on the existence or non-existence of symptoms caused by hormone hypersecretion. NF-pNETs may secrete some hormones and peptides such as chromogranin

A, pancreatic polypeptide, and others, but without a clinical syndrome due to hormone hypersecretion [2]. They may show immunohistochemical positivity for hormones which may be produced, but not secreted, which are clinically inert such as pancreatic polypeptide, and whose serum concentrations are insufficient to induce symptoms [1].

NF-pNETs account for 60–90% of all pNETs according to the Surveillance, Epidemiology, and End Results (SEER) database [3] and are usually diagnosed at a more advanced stage due to their relatively indolent nature and slow growth causing a delay in the onset of symptoms.

28.2 Hereditary Tumor Syndromes

While most NF-pNETs are sporadic, approximately 10% are inherited because of germline mutations associated with multiple endocrine neoplasia type 1 (MEN 1) or von Hippel-Lindau (VHL) disease [4].

MEN 1 is a rare autosomal dominant condition characterized by the development of well-differentiated tumors of the parathyroids, pancreas, duodenum, and pituitary. NF-pNETs are the most common pancreatic neoplasms (80–100%) in MEN 1, occurring in 19% of patients with MEN 1 [1]. Patients with MEN 1 frequently present with multiple pNETs throughout the pancreas [5].

VHL is an autosomal dominant disorder that is associated with pancreatic tumors or cysts. NF-pNETs occur in 13–17% [1].

28.3 Clinical Presentation

NF-pNETs usually become clinically apparent when they reach a size that causes compression or invasion of adjacent organs or when they metastasize [1]. Therefore, NF-pNETs are usually diagnosed late in the course of the disease. According to SEER data, localized, regional, and distant stages correspond to 14%, 23%, and 54% of cases [3]. Frequent symptoms are abdominal pain (35–78%), weight loss (20–35%), and anorexia and nausea (45%). Less frequent signs are jaundice (17–50%), intraabdominal hemorrhage (4–20%), or a palpable mass (7–40%) [1].

28.4 Diagnosis

Computed tomography (CT) and magnetic resonance imaging (MRI) constitute the basic radiological method for NET imaging because of their wide availability, standardized reproducible technique, and generally high diagnostic yield [6] (◘ Fig. 28.1).

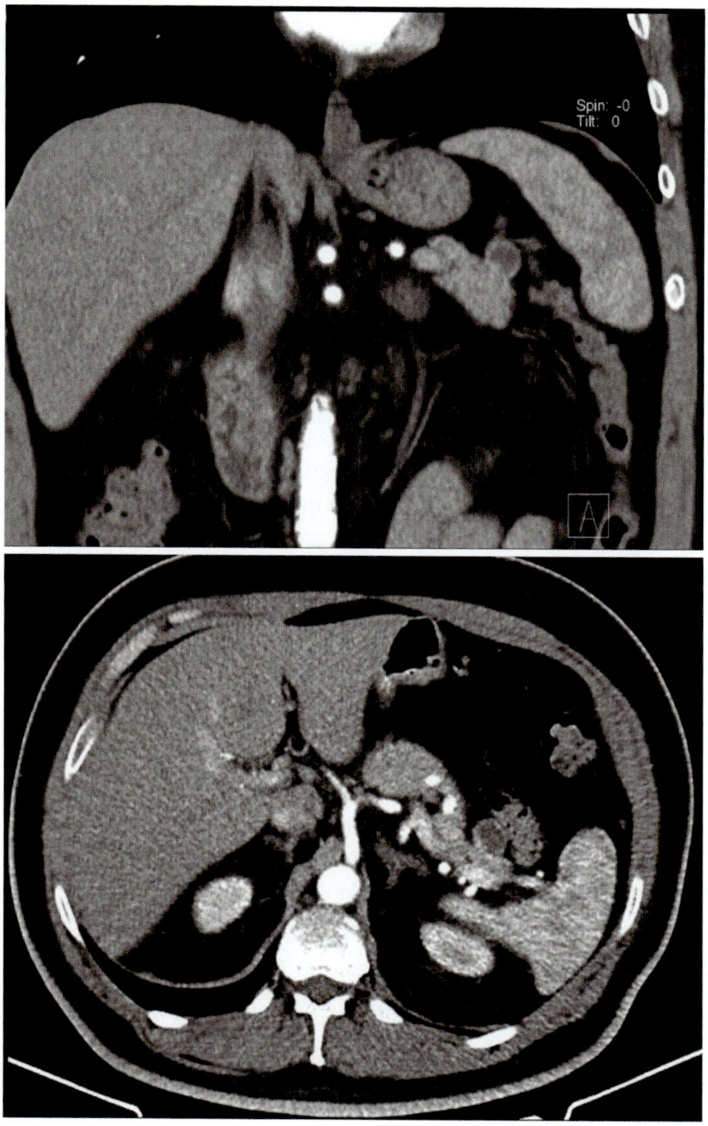

Fig. 28.1 CT scan of a patient with a small cystic NF-pNET in the pancreatic tail

Imaging with positron emission tomography and CT (PET/CT) using ^{68}Ga-labeled somatostatin has the highest sensitivity with 86–100% and also a high specificity with 79–100% for localizing NF-pNETs [7, 8]. It is therefore the first-line diagnostic method to evaluate and stage the extent of the disease [9, 10]. If the PET/CT is not available, somatostatin receptor scintigraphy is a useful single-screening method for NF-pNETs. Patients with small NF-pNETs may be assessed using endoscopic ultrasound (EUS), in particular in small lesions and multiple lesions in MEN 1 syndrome [11]. Although not recommended as a standard diagnostic procedure, EUS-guided fine needle aspiration (FNA) with immunostaining for synaptophysin and chromogranin A (CgA) is a useful method for the diagnosis of NF-pNETs [10, 12].

The assessment of CgA may facilitate the diagnosis of NF-pNETs, and, if elevated, it may be used as a tumor marker to predict disease recurrence, outcome, and efficacy of therapy [13]. The findings regarding sensitivity and specificity of meal-stimulated pancreatic polypeptide (PP) are controversial.

Germline DNA testing is only justified in clinical situations strongly suggesting MEN 1 or VHL [1].

28.5 Treatment

Surgery represents the curative treatment of choice for NF-pNETs, with improved survival especially in localized disease [14–16]. However, a non-operative management for asymptomatic, sporadic, and diagnostically proven NF-pNETs ≤2 cm is suggested in selected cases, especially in elderly patients, the presence of important comorbidities, and when a major pancreatic resection is required [17–20, 24]. Only 6% of NF-pNETs ≤2 cm are considered to be malignant [21]. At present, it is still challenging to accurately assess the tumor's natural history. Therefore, the risk of a wait-and-see policy has to be weighed against the operative morbidity and mortality of pancreatic surgery [18, 20–23]. Surgery is recommended for young patients and in cases when signs of local invasiveness (e.g., dilatation of the main pancreatic duct and/or presence of jaundice and/or suspicion of nodal involvement) are present [20]. In case of a non-operative approach, a follow-up after 6 months and thereafter every 6–12 months is recommended [9, 25]. However, the level of evidence for expectant management of small asymptomatic NF-pNETs is low. Studies with longer follow-up are needed to define patients who benefit from upfront surgery in contrast to the wait-and-see strategy. Until now, there are no clear prognostic factors that can distinguish between tumors suitable for observation and tumors with increased malignant potential and more aggressive surgery. Possible selection criteria can be tumor size and grading, intensity of uptake in functional imaging (Ga 68-DOTATATE PET/CT), stage of disease, and patient's desire [25].

28.5.1 Locoregional Ablative Therapy

Hepatic transarterial (chemo-)embolization (TA[C]E) or percutaneous/laparoscopic radiofrequency ablation (RFA) represents a valid locoregional ablative therapy or an adjunct to palliative surgery. Experience is limited; however, palliation seems possible in patients with a tumor burden of less than 75%, small metastases (<5 cm), and no extrahepatic metastases [1].

28.5.2 Liver Transplantation

Liver transplantation may be an option in patients without extrahepatic metastases, low proliferation rate (G1 and G2, Ki-67 <10%), previous removal of the primary tumor, metastatic diffusion <50% of the total liver volume, stable disease in response to therapy for at least 6 months prior to transplant consideration, and age <60 years, when all other surgical and medical therapies have failed [20, 26]. Most transplanted patients have recurrences within months to years, possibly due to postoperative immunosuppressive treatment and/or undiagnosed extrahepatic metastases prior to procedure.

28.5.3 Medical Therapy in Advanced Disease

The goal of systemic therapy is to improve survival in recurrent NF-pNETs as well as to improve quality of life by controlling symptoms. Currently, there is no evidence to support the use of various systemic modalities in an adjuvant fashion following complete surgical resection of NF-pNETs [16].

Nearly 80% of NF-pNETs express somatostatin receptors, making them a suitable target for therapy with somatostatin analogues (SSA) [16]. SSA are recommended for the prevention and inhibition of tumor growth [20, 27].

Targeted drugs, everolimus or sunitinib, may be used as first- or second-line options with respect to chemotherapy or subsequent to SSA therapy in patients with surgically non-resectable progressive G1 and G2 NF-pNETs [20, 27]. Due to their potential toxicity, they should not be used as first-line therapy. There is no robust evidence that the combination therapy of targeted drugs and SSA is superior to monotherapy [20, 27]. Furthermore, there is no evidence on the exact sequencing of different treatment options in NF-pNETs [20, 27, 28].

Systemic chemotherapy is indicated in progressive or bulky G1/G2 NF-pNETs and in G3 NF-pNETs and G3 NF-pNECs, respectively [27]. Streptozotocin (STZ) and 5-fluorouracil (5-FU) are recommended in G1/G2 NF-pNET patients with a higher tumor burden or in patients with significant tumor progression in ≤6–12 months [27]. Furthermore, the STZ/5-FU regimen is indicated in G3 NF-pNET patients. Temozolomide and capecitabine may replace the STZ/5-FU regimen in case it is not available. In G3 NF-pNECs, platinum-based chemotherapy (e.g., cisplatin and etoposide) is recommended as a first-line therapy, and second-line therapy options include FOLFOX and FOLFIRI [27].

The use of peptide receptor radionuclide therapy (PRRT) is recommended after failure of medical therapy, if a high and homogeneous expression of somatostatin receptor type

2 (sstr2) was found by somatostatin receptor imaging [9]. Radionuclide therapy with ^{177}Lu-labeled SSA is most frequently used [27].

28.6 Indications for Surgery and Surgical Details

Surgery is the treatment of choice for localized NF-pNETs >2 cm in patients without contraindications for surgery due to significant comorbidities [14, 15].

The surgical strategy depends on tumor size and site [10, 15]: For NF-pNETs >2 cm or in case of suspicion of nodal involvement, typical resections should be performed. Lesions of the pancreatic head are treated with a pancreaticoduodenectomy, while lesions of the body and tail are treated with a left pancreatectomy with or without spleen preservation, depending on the technical possibilities. Atypical resections (central pancreatectomy, enucleation) might be considered for small NF-pNETs ≤2 cm with benign or uncertain behavior, which are located more than 2–3 mm from the main pancreatic duct [29]. The main advantage is the improved endocrine and exocrine long-term function of the pancreas. On the other hand, atypical resections are associated with a higher rate of postoperative pancreatic fistula.

Nodal sampling should be performed consequently, whereas a systematic lymphadenectomy with a removal of 11–15 lymph nodes for an accurate nodal staging is only indicated in case of a formal resection.

Laparoscopic distal pancreatectomy and enucleation are safe and feasible in patients with pancreatic endocrine tumors [30].

28.6.1 Surgery in Metastatic Patients

All patients with liver metastases from NF-pNETs should be considered for surgery, since this improves progression-free survival and symptom control [31].

Surgery of the primary tumor in case of unresectable metastatic disease is handled in different ways, since this approach is only supported by retrospective data [10]. Resection of the primary tumor might allow to focus the treatment on liver metastases, avoid local complications of the tumor, and possibly improve response to PRRT.

The indication for cytoreductive surgery in metastatic disease is discussed controversially [10]: Symptom control and survival might be improved if more than 70% of liver metastases are resected. However, the rate of tumor recurrence is high. Preoperatively, the following conditions have to be assessed: (1) the absence of extra-abdominal disease, (2) the presence of low proliferation index (Ki-67) by FNA (G1 or G2), and (3) the existence of somatostatin receptors in order to deliver radiolabeled therapies as they are effective after cytoreductive surgery [32].

28.6.2 Palliative Surgery

No data support debulking surgery for unresectable, locally advanced NF-pNET, although in selected cases, surgery could alleviate mass-related symptoms by reducing tumor burden.

28.6.3 Surgery in High-Grade NF-pNET

High-grade (G3) NF-pNETs should be stratified into NF-pNECs and NF-pNETs and managed accordingly: Patients with poorly differentiated NF-pNECs should not undergo any resection due to the extremely poor prognosis [10]. In the context of a multimodal therapy, patients with G3 NF-pNETs should be evaluated for resection if localized. Cytoreduction of liver metastases may not be indicated due to high relapse rates and poor survival.

28.6.4 Surgery in MEN 1 Patients

The surgical management of MEN 1-associated NF-pNETs remains controversial since these NF-pNETs are almost always multifocal and usually distributed throughout the pancreatic parenchyma [22, 33]. Prophylactic surgery could remove these lesions before malignancy develops, which might improve survival [34]. Others suggest a more conservative approach, as their data indicate that only tumors >2 cm are associated with an increased risk of malignancy of 30% [35].

It is therefore recommended to perform surgery in MEN 1 patients in case of NF-pNETs >2 cm, in case of suspicion of nodal involvement after exclusion of distant metastases and relevant comorbidities, or in case of relatively rapid rate of growth over 6 to 12 months, whereas NF-pNETs ≤1 cm should not be resected [10, 15, 20, 22]. NF-pNETs 1–2 cm can be treated by active surveillance or surgery [10, 15, 22].

Surgery ranges from enucleation to total pancreatectomy with intraoperative US to detect multicentric lesions [5]. However, parenchyma-preserving surgery is recommended due to the high risk of developing new NF-pNETs in the remaining pancreatic tissue and the slow growth [15]. Nodal sampling should be performed consequently, whereas a systematic lymphadenectomy is not indicated [15].

28.7 Outcomes or Prognosis

NF-pNETs are usually slow-growing neoplasms with a favorable overall prognosis [18]. Due to the widespread use of cross-sectional imaging, asymptomatic and sporadic NF-pNETs are more and more frequently diagnosed at an early stage [36]. According to a population-based study, the median overall survival of patients with NF-pNETs is 38 months [3]. The survival is mostly affected by the presence of distant metastases [37]. Other influencing factors are tumor grade, age >40 years, positive surgical margins, time of diagnosis, and size and location of the tumor [37–39].

28.7.1 Follow-Up

Follow-up investigations should be adjusted to the type of tumor (G1, G2, or G3) and the stage of the disease (radically resected or advanced disease). The follow-up should include biochemical markers (CgA) and conventional imaging (CT and/or MRI) every 3–9 months in patients with G1 and G2 tumors [9]. In case of stable disease, the interval can be increased. If positive, somatostatin receptor imaging should be repeated every 2 years or earlier if progression is suspected [20]. NF-pNEC patients should be followed up every 2–3 months [20, 40].

Answers to the Questions

1. (a); 2. (b); 3. (c); 4. (d); 5. (d); 6. (e); 7. (e); 8. (d); 9. (b); 10. (e); 11. (b); 12. (e)

References

1. Falconi M, Bartsch DK, Eriksson B, Kloppel G, Lopes JM, O'Connor JM, et al. ENETS consensus guidelines for the management of patients with digestive neuroendocrine neoplasms of the digestive system: well-differentiated pancreatic non-functioning tumors. Neuroendocrinology. 2012;95(2):120–34.
2. Krampitz GW, Norton JA. Pancreatic neuroendocrine tumors. Curr Probl Surg. 2013;50(11):509–45.
3. Yao JC, Hassan M, Phan A, Dagohoy C, Leary C, Mares JE, et al. One hundred years after "carcinoid": epidemiology of and prognostic factors for neuroendocrine tumors in 35,825 cases in the United States. J Clin Oncol. 2008;26(18):3063–72.
4. Kuo JH, Lee JA, Chabot JA. Nonfunctional pancreatic neuroendocrine tumors. Surg Clin North Am. 2014;94(3):689–708.
5. Jensen RT, Berna MJ, Bingham DB, Norton JA. Inherited pancreatic endocrine tumor syndromes: advances in molecular pathogenesis, diagnosis, management, and controversies. Cancer. 2008;113(7 Suppl):1807–43.
6. Sundin A, Arnold R, Baudin E, Cwikla JB, Eriksson B, Fanti S, et al. ENETS consensus guidelines for the standards of care in neu-

roendocrine tumors: radiological, nuclear medicine & hybrid imaging. Neuroendocrinology. 2017;105(3):212–44.
7. Koukouraki S, Strauss LG, Georgoulias V, Eisenhut M, Haberkorn U, Dimitrakopoulou-Strauss A. Comparison of the pharmacokinetics of 68Ga-DOTATOC and [18F]FDG in patients with metastatic neuroendocrine tumours scheduled for 90Y-DOTATOC therapy. Eur J Nucl Med Mol Imaging. 2006;33(10):1115–22.
8. Sharma P, Arora S, Dhull VS, Naswa N, Kumar R, Ammini AC, et al. Evaluation of (68)Ga-DOTANOC PET/CT imaging in a large exclusive population of pancreatic neuroendocrine tumors. Abdom Imaging. 2015;40(2):299–309.
9. Falconi M, Eriksson B, Kaltsas G, Bartsch DK, Capdevila J, Caplin M, et al. ENETS consensus guidelines update for the management of patients with functional pancreatic neuroendocrine Tumors and non-functional pancreatic neuroendocrine tumors. Neuroendocrinology. 2016;103(2):153–71.
10. Howe JR, Merchant NB, Conrad C, Keutgen XM, Hallet J, Drebin JA, et al. The North American Neuroendocrine Tumor Society consensus paper on the surgical management of pancreatic neuroendocrine tumors. Pancreas. 2020;49(1):1–33.
11. Dumlu EG, Karakoç D, Özdemir A. Nonfunctional pancreatic neuroendocrine tumors: advances in diagnosis, management, and controversies. Int Surg. 2015;100(6):1089–97.
12. Klimstra DS, Modlin IR, Coppola D, Lloyd RV, Suster S. The pathologic classification of neuroendocrine tumors: a review of nomenclature, grading, and staging systems. Pancreas. 2010;39(6):707–12.
13. Modlin IM, Gustafsson BI, Moss SF, Pavel M, Tsolakis AV, Kidd M. Chromogranin A--biological function and clinical utility in neuro endocrine tumor disease. Ann Surg Oncol. 2010;17(9):2427–43.
14. Hill JS, McPhee JT, McDade TP, Zhou Z, Sullivan ME, Whalen GF, et al. Pancreatic neuroendocrine tumors: the impact of surgical resection on survival. Cancer. 2009;115(4):741–51.
15. Practice guideline neuroendocrine tumors – AWMF-Reg. 021-27. Z Gastroenterol. 2018;56(6):583–681.
16. Cloyd JM, Poultsides GA. Non-functional neuroendocrine tumors of the pancreas: advances in diagnosis and management. World J Gastroenterol. 2015;21(32):9512–25.
17. Crippa S, Partelli S, Zamboni G, Scarpa A, Tamburrino D, Bassi C, et al. Incidental diagnosis as prognostic factor in different tumor stages of nonfunctioning pancreatic endocrine tumors. Surgery. 2014;155(1):145–53.
18. Gaujoux S, Partelli S, Maire F, D'Onofrio M, Larroque B, Tamburrino D, et al. Observational study of natural history of small sporadic nonfunctioning pancreatic neuroendocrine tumors. J Clin Endocrinol Metab. 2013;98(12):4784–9.
19. Partelli S, Cirocchi R, Crippa S, Cardinali L, Fendrich V, Bartsch DK, et al. Systematic review of active surveillance versus surgical management of asymptomatic small non-functioning pancreatic neuroendocrine neoplasms. Br J Surg. 2017;104(1):34–41.
20. Pavel M, Öberg K, Falconi M, Krenning E, Sundin A, Perren A, et al. Gastroenteropancreatic neuroendocrine neoplasms: ESMO clinical practice guidelines for diagnosis, treatment and follow-up. Ann Oncol. 2020;31(7):844–60.
21. Bettini R, Partelli S, Boninsegna L, Capelli P, Crippa S, Pederzoli P, et al. Tumor size correlates with malignancy in nonfunctioning pancreatic endocrine tumor. Surgery. 2011;150(1):75–82.
22. Masui T, Anazawa T, Takaori K, Shinji U. The surgical management of non-functioning pancreatic neuroendocrine tumors. Pancreas (online). 2018;S(3):354–7.

23. Yang G, Ji M, Chen J, Chen R, Chen Y, Fu D, et al. Surgery management for sporadic small (≦2cm), non-functioningpancreatic neuroendocrine tumors: a consensus statement by the Chinese Study Group for Neuroendocrine Tumors (CSNET). 2016. https://doi.org/10.3892/ijo.2016.3826:567-74.
24. Sallinen V, Le Large TYS, Galeev S, Kovalenko Z, Tieftrunk E, et al. Surveillance strategy for small asymptomatic nonfunctional pancreatic neuroendocrine tumors – a systematic review and meta-analysis. 2HPB 017;19:310–20. https://doi.org/10.1016/j.hpb.2016.12.010.
25. Bar-Moshe Y, Mazeh H, Grozinsky-Glasberg S. Non-functioning pancreatic neuroendocrine tumors: surgery or observation. World J Gastrointest Endosc. 2017;9(4):153–61.
26. Pavel M, Baudin E, Couvelard A, Krenning E, Oberg K, Steinmuller T, et al. ENETS consensus guidelines for the management of patients with liver and other distant metastases from neuroendocrine neoplasms of foregut, midgut, hindgut, and unknown primary. Neuroendocrinology. 2012;95(2):157–76.
27. Pavel M, O'Toole D, Costa F, Capdevila J, Gross D, Kianmanesh R, et al. ENETS consensus guidelines update for the management of distant metastatic disease of intestinal, pancreatic, bronchial neuroendocrine neoplasms (NEN) and NEN of unknown primary site. Neuroendocrinology. 2016;103(2):172–85.
28. Kaderli RM, Spanjol M, Kollár A, Bütikofer L, Gloy V, Dumont RA, et al. Therapeutic options for neuroendocrine tumors: a systematic review and network meta-analysis. JAMA Oncol. 2019;5(4):480–9.
29. Falconi M, Zerbi A, Crippa S, Balzano G, Boninsegna L, Capitanio V, et al. Parenchyma-preserving resections for small nonfunctioning pancreatic endocrine tumors. Ann Surg Oncol. 2010;17(6):1621–7.
30. Fernández-Cruz L, Blanco L, Cosa R, Rendón H. Is laparoscopic resection adequate in patients with neuroendocrine pancreatic tumors? World J Surg. 2008;32(5):904–17.
31. Cusati D, Zhang L, Harmsen WS, Hu A, Farnell MB, Nagorney DM, et al. Metastatic nonfunctioning pancreatic neuroendocrine carcinoma to liver: surgical treatment and outcomes. J Am Coll Surg. 2012;215(1):117–24; discussion 24–5/
32. Bloomston M, Muscarella P, Shah MH, Frankel WL, Al-Saif O, Martin EW, et al. Cytoreduction results in high perioperative mortality and decreased survival in patients undergoing pancreatectomy for neuroendocrine tumors of the pancreas. J Gastrointest Surg. 2006;10(10):1361–70.
33. Anlauf M, Schlenger R, Perren A, Bauersfeld J, Koch CA, Dralle H, et al. Microadenomatosis of the endocrine pancreas in patients with and without the multiple endocrine neoplasia type 1 syndrome. Am J Surg Pathol. 2006;30(5):560–74.
34. Kouvaraki MA, Shapiro SE, Cote GJ, Lee JE, Yao JC, Waguespack SG, et al. Management of pancreatic endocrine tumors in multiple endocrine neoplasia type 1. World J Surg. 2006;30(5):643–53.
35. Triponez F, Goudet P, Dosseh D, Cougard P, Bauters C, Murat A, et al. Is surgery beneficial for MEN1 patients with small (< or = 2 cm), nonfunctioning pancreaticoduodenal endocrine tumor? An analysis of 65 patients from the GTE. World J Surg. 2006;30(5):654–62; discussion 63–4.
36. Cheema A, Weber J, Strosberg JR. Incidental detection of pancreatic neuroendocrine tumors: an analysis of incidence and outcomes. Ann Surg Oncol. 2012;19(9):2932–6.
37. Bilimoria KY, Talamonti MS, Tomlinson JS, Stewart AK, Winchester DP, Ko CY, et al. Prognostic score predicting survival after resection of pancreatic neuroendocrine tumors: analysis of 3851 patients. Ann Surg. 2008;247(3):490–500.

38. Jarufe NP, Coldham C, Orug T, Mayer AD, Mirza DF, Buckels JA, et al. Neuroendocrine tumours of the pancreas: predictors of survival after surgical treatment. Dig Surg. 2005;22(3):157–62.
39. Wu J, Sun C, Li E, Wang J, He X, Yuan R, Yi C, Liao W, Wu L. Non-functional pancreatic neuroendocrine tumours: emerging trends in incidence and mortality. BMC Cancer. 2019;19:334.
40. Garcia-Carbonero R, Sorbye H, Baudin E, Raymond E, Wiedenmann B, Niederle B, et al. ENETS consensus guidelines for high-grade gastroenteropancreatic neuroendocrine tumors and neuroendocrine carcinomas. Neuroendocrinology. 2016;103(2):186–94.

Small Intestine NETs

Andrea Goldmann and Thomas Clerici

Contents

A. L. Shifrin et al. (eds.), *Endocrine Surgery Comprehensive Board Exam Guide*,
https://doi.org/10.1007/978-3-030-84737-1_29

Case Presentation and Case-Specific Questions

A 72-year-old man presents to his general practitioner (GP) because of a loss of general well-being, general fatigue, recurrent nausea, and weight loss (3 kg in 2 months). His past medical history includes prostatic cancer (pT2 pN0 cM0) which had been treated with radical prostatectomy and adjuvant radiotherapy (66Gy) 5 years before. So far, there has been no evidence for a relapse of the disease. There are no further comorbidities and the patient is under no relevant medication.

On physical examination the GP finds some clinic findings suggesting anemia which is confirmed later (Hb 10.5 g/dl). An ultrasound of the abdomen performed by the GP does not reveal any pathology or an obvious structural alterations of the liver.

The GP orders a colonoscopy which does not show any pathology or a source of a blood loss, and therefore the patient undergoes a gastroduodenoscopy which does also show an inconspicuous finding.

Because of deteriorating symptoms including vomiting, the patient presents at the emergency room of the closest county hospital the night after the gastroduodenoscopy. An abdominal CT-scan reveals a mass in the lower right abdomen with local signs of infiltration suggestive of a malignant process of unknown origin without signs of relevant liver involvement. Under conservative treatment the bowel obstruction resolves, and the patient is referred to the tertiary center for the further workup of his condition.

There, the specific properties of the mass in the CT, classically corresponding to a desmoplastic stromal reaction of the mesentery, give rise to the suspicion of a siNET being the cause of the chronic blood loss and the transient bowel obstruction.

❓ Questions

1. What additional biochemical investigations would you recommend at this point of the workup?
    1. No further investigations are necessary; because of imminent complete bowel obstruction, the patient should be operated rather sooner than later – the presented CT scan provides all tactical information needed for the planning of the operation and tumor stage.
    2. Baseline-measurement of chromogranin A in serum as a general tumor marker for neuroendocrine tumors for the later follow-up.
    3. Measurement of 24 h urinary chromogranin A excretion as a general tumor marker for neuroendocrine tumors.
    4. Measurement of 5-HIAA as a specific test for serotonin-producing neuroendocrine tumors in the serum.
    5. Measurement of the 24 h urinary excretion of 5-HIAA excretion as a specific test for serotonin-producing neuroendocrine tumors.
        - (a) Only 1 is correct.
        - (b) Only 3 and 5 are correct.
        - (c) Only 2 and 4 are correct.
        - (d) Only 2 and 4 and 5 are correct.

2. What additional imaging studies would you recommend at this point of the workup?
   1. If the operation is performed under SSA-prophylaxis, further imaging is not likely to change the surgical strategy intraoperatively.
   2. Because of its proven benefits for adequate tumor staging in many malignancies, I would recommend ^{18}F-fluorodeoxyglucose PET/CT to look for hepatic and systemic manifestations of the suspected siNET.
   3. I would recommend an MRI investigation of the liver as cross-sectional imaging modality, since it is superior to the CT scan in detecting the extent of a hepatic spread.
   4. The actual manifestations in the CT scan suggest a slow dynamic to the disease with a low or moderate proliferation rate of the tumor (G1 or G2). In this situation I would go for a somatostatin receptor specific functional imaging modality, preferably a ^{68}Ga-SSA PET/CT (if available).
   (a) Only 2 and 3 are correct.
   (b) Only 1 is correct.
   (c) Only 1, 3, and 4 are correct.
   (d) Only 3 and 4 are correct.

MRI and ^{68}Ga-SSA PET/CT show no evidence for liver metastasis and a positivity for somatostatin-receptors in the mesenteric masses as well as a potential primary in the distal ileum (◘ Figs. 29.1 and 29.2).

Chromogranin A levels show a fivefold increase in relation to the upper norm, and 24 h urinary 5-HIAA levels are normal.

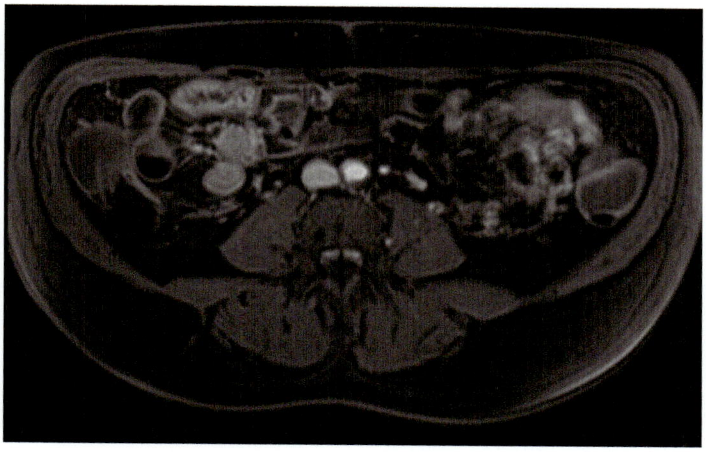

◘ **Fig. 29.1** Classical appearance of siNET lymph node metastasis with a desmoplastic stromal reaction in the mesentery of the terminal ileum

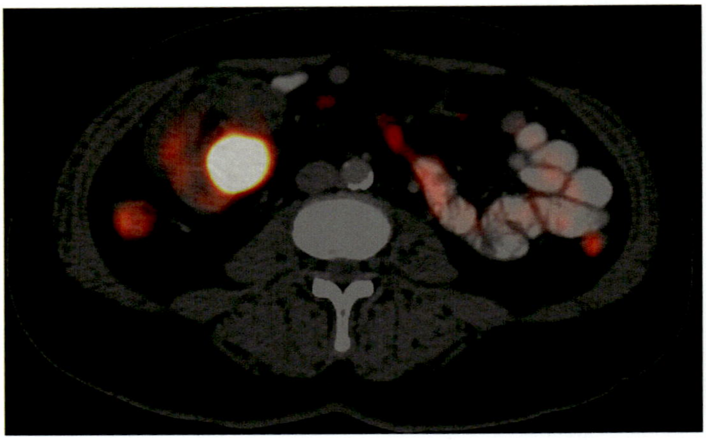

Fig. 29.2 Corresponding ^{68}Ga-SSA PET/CT image showing SSR-positivity of lymph node metastasis in the ileal mesentery

3. The patient was found to have an elevated chromogranin A value more than 5 times above the normal range. Which of the following statements regarding chromogranin A are correct?
   1. The fivefold increase of the chromogranin A value is clearly attributable to a neuroendocrine tumor and proves the siNET suspected in the CT-scans.
   2. This chromogranin A value might be influenced by a so far unknown renal insufficiency.
   3. The medication of PPIs can substantially lower chromogranin A values.
   4. In the presence of significant arterial hypertension and a chronic atrophic gastritis, chromogranin A levels can be raised.
   5. A high cholesterol level leads to an increase in the chromogranin A value.
   6. Chromogranin A is a valuable tool in the screening for neuroendocrine tumors.
   7. Chromogranin A levels are typically elevated in patients with pheochromocytomas and paragangliomas.
      (a) Only 1, 2, and 4 are correct.
      (b) Only 2 and 4 are correct.
      (c) Only 2, 4, and 6 are correct.
      (d) Only 2, 4, and 7 are correct.
      (e) Only 3, 4, and 7 are correct.
4. Which statements regarding imaging in siNETs are correct?
   1. If CT and MRI are equally available for accurate detection of liver metastasis preoperatively and for further follow-up, MRI should be the preferred option.
   2. Due to its high anatomical resolution, MRI is the imaging modality of choice to determine the extent of nodal involvement in the mesentery.

3. ^{18}F-FDG PET/CT should be considered in the workup of a neuroendocrine tumor with a proliferation rate >20%.
4. If as in the presented case the MRI would show no liver metastases and 24 h urinary 5-HIAA levels would be normal, a ^{68}Ga-SSA PET/CT would not be mandatory at this stage of the workup.
   (a) Only 1, 3, and 4 are correct.
   (b) Only 1 and 2 are correct.
   (c) Only 3 and 4 are correct.
   (d) All are correct.
   (e) Only 1 and 2 and 4 are correct.

5. What further examinations or treatments would you consider mandatory in this patient before the planned operation?
   1. The repetition of the colonoscopy to obtain a biopsy and therefore a grading of the siNET.
   2. An echocardiography and a NT-proBNP to exclude a carcinoid heart disease (CHD).
   3. In another case with a tenfold increase of chromogranin A: an adjuvant treatment with SSA in asymptomatic patients with no evidence of hepatic metastasis, since these levels of chromogranin A are biochemical evidence of a carcinoid syndrome.
   4. In another case with a pronounced carcinoid syndrome with severe diarrhea: a correctly applied perioperative prophylaxis with SSA will address the issue appropriately and reliably prevent a carcinoid crisis.
   (a) Only 1 and 2 are correct.
   (b) None is correct.
   (c) Only 1, 3, and 4 are correct.
   (d) Only 1, 2, and 4 are correct.

6. Considering a laparoscopic resection of the tumor in the presented case:
   1. There is no absolute contraindication to start the procedure video-endoscopically.
   2. A complete intraoperative assessment of the tumor and the abdominal site is achieved by inspection of the liver, the whole small intestine, the peritoneal cavity, and the ovaries.
   3. Regarding SAA-prophylaxis it does not make a difference if you operate through a conventional laparotomy or videoendoscopically.
   4. Big or very centrally located mesenteric metastasis and a pronounced desmoplastic stromal reaction in the mesentery are to be considered at least a relative contraindication to a videoendoscopic approach, since endoscopic preparation in these conditions is extremely demanding and carries an increased risk of insufficient radicality and complications.

5. Combining a cholecystectomy with the ileal resection is only recommended if gallstones have been diagnosed in the preoperative workup.
   (a) Only 1, 2, 3, and 4 are correct.
   (b) Only 1, 3, and 4 are correct.
   (c) Only 1 and 3 are correct.
   (d) Only 2 and 3 and 4 are correct.
   (e) All are correct.

Surgery is then scheduled based on the diagnosis of a locally advanced siNET without evidence of a hepatic spread, and a conventional, oncologic right hemicolectomy with extended ileal resection (◘ Fig. 29.3) is performed under perioperative prophylaxis with SSA; a prophylactic cholecystectomy is included to the procedure. The postoperative course is uneventful, and the histopathological workup confirms a siNET pT3 pN1(3/25) L1 V0 Pn0 G1 R0.

7. Which statements about the tumor stage and prognosis are correct?
   1. Due to the R0-resection, the G1-grading and the fact that only 3 out of 25 lymph nodes showed metastasis, the patient can be considered cured with an outstanding long-term prognosis and no need of a further tumor-specific follow-up.
   2. Because of the locally advanced tumor (pN1), the patient should be put under an adjuvant therapy with SSAs and followed-up at intervals of 6 months.
   3. Since the tumor has metastasized into the mesentery showing a pronounced desmoplasia, it must be considered aggressive and therefore followed-up by imaging every 3 months.

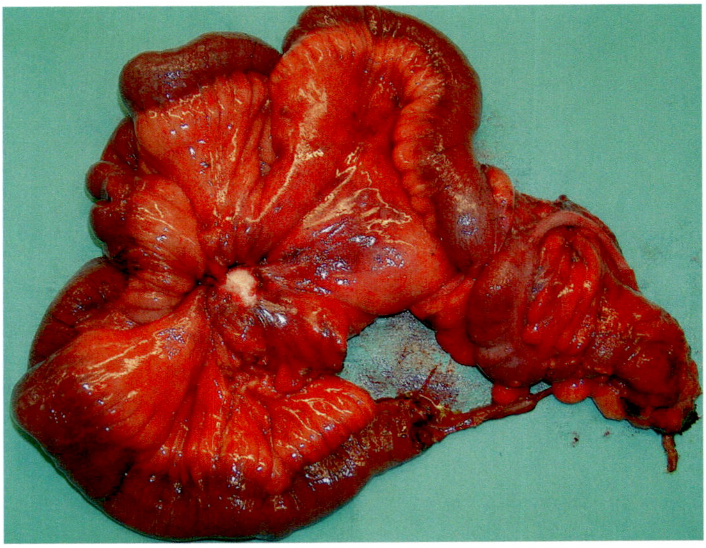

◘ **Fig. 29.3** Specimen showing lymph node metastasis in in the mesentery of the terminal ileum with serotonin-induced fibrosis and contraction

4. The patient's long-term prognosis is good. A follow-up consisting in chromogranin A measurement and cross-sectional imaging every 6 months is sufficient, and in the case of an uneventful course the tumor-specific follow-up could be eventually stopped after 10 years.
   (a) Only 1 is correct.
   (b) Only 2 is correct.
   (c) Only 3 is correct.
   (d) Only 4 is correct.
   (e) No answer is correct.

8. Generally speaking, what should a tumor-specific, long-term follow-up for siNET consist of?
   1. For cross-sectional imaging, MRI should be preferred in relation to CT to reduce long-term and cumulative exposure to radiation, especially in young patients.
   2. An ideal follow-up for G1 or G2-tumors operated on in curative intent consists of patient history, a physical examination, laboratory tests, and cross-sectional imaging every 6–12 months.
   3. If preoperative chromogranin A levels were normal, the measurement of chromogranin A levels during follow-up without evidence of a hepatic spread in cross-sectional imaging is unnecessary.
   4. Regardless of tumor stage, routine screening for CHD with echocardiography and measurement of NT-pro-BNP is important and should be performed every 2 years.
   5. Since during follow-up metastasis to the bone are predominantly detected by a ^{68}Ga-SSA PET/CT, this investigation is recommended in approximatively 5 years intervals.
   (a) Only 1 is correct.
   (b) Only 1, 2, 3, and 4 are correct.
   (c) Only 1 and 2 are correct.
   (d) Only 1, 3, and 5 are correct.
   (e) Only 1, 3, and 4 are correct.

After discharge, the patient is enrolled in a tumor-specific follow-up program including patient history, chromogranin A measurements, and cross-sectional imaging by MRI initially in 6 months, later in 12 months intervals.

In the sixth year of a so far uneventful follow-up, a single hepatic growth of 10 mm diameter in the liver segment V shows up at the MRI without any change to chromogranin A levels, which remains normal. It does not light up in the ^{68}Ga-SSA PET/CT which might be contributed to its small diameter at this point.

9. Which statements regarding the management of the newly found liver lesion are correct?
   1. As the patient had no recurrence for 6 years, chances are that the growth in the liver does originate from a different tumor than the siNET. Therefore, a wholesome checkup to locate another primary should be planned.
   2. With a newly detected spread to the liver probably originating from the siNET, it is time to check the 24 h urinary excretion of 5-HIAA excretion and have the cardiologist perform a baseline echocardiography looking for a thickening of the right heart valves as morphological evidence of CHD.
   3. The fact that the hepatic growth does not light up in the ^{68}Ga-SSA PET/CT excludes the possibility that it corresponds to a metastasis of the siNET.
   4. With evident and measurable disease to the liver with an extremely high likelihood of coming from the siNET, a therapy with SSAs is to be recommended.
   5. Since the new finding is to be followed by new investigations and probably will entail a new strategy, a presentation of the case at the interdisciplinary tumor board should be strongly recommended.
   6. If in doubt of the provenience of the hepatic growth, a percutaneous ultrasound guided FNA of biopsy could be helpful to determine its origin and determine proliferative activity of a siNET liver metastasis.
   7. Since the hepatic growth does not show up in the ^{68}Ga-SSA PET/CT, a ^{18}F-FDG PET/CT should be ordered at this stage.
      (a) Only 1, 3, and 7 are correct.
      (b) Only 1, 3, 6, and 7 are correct.
      (c) Only 2, 4, 5, and 6 are correct.
      (d) Only 1, 3, 5, 6, and 7 are correct.

   The patient is put under an anti-proliferative therapy with SSA, and an anticipated MRI is performed 6 months later. At this time, the lesion has grown in size and measures 15 mm in diameter. An ultrasound-guided core-biopsy done at its histopathological workup proves indeed a metastasis of a NET with a proliferation rate <2% and a strong positivity for somatostatin receptors 2 and 5.
10. What are your most appropriate treatment options in this situation? What would an interdisciplinary tumor conference possibly agree upon at this stage?
    1. Because of the somatostatin receptors status of siNET metastasis and its growth despite SSA therapy, peptide receptor radionuclide therapy (PRRT) is the best option at this stage of the disease.

2. Since it is still a solitary, slowly growing metastasis and there are no elevated 24 h urinary 5-HIAA levels or echocardiographic signs of CHD, a "watchful-waiting" strategy could be advised for and the SAA baseline therapy continued.
3. Addressing the metastasis surgically is not an option in the current situation.
4. Since no additional metastasis could be found 6 months after detecting the solitary metastasis, a locally ablative procedure like a percutaneous RFA would be well suited to address this solitary metastasis.
5. Because SSA therapy does not seem to be effective, the prescription of everolimus should be evaluated.
   (a) Only 1 is correct.
   (b) Only 2 is correct.
   (c) Only 3 is correct.
   (d) Only 4 is correct.
   (e) Only 2 and 4 are correct.
   (f) Only 4 and 5 are correct.

11. Generally speaking (not related to the presented case), which statements regarding surgical therapy of liver metastases are correct?
    1. Liver surgery is only to be considered for metastasis of well-differentiated G1- or G2-siNETs.
    2. Generally, absence of extra-abdominal metastasis is a precondition for liver surgery.
    3. Liver surgery should only be evaluated if a radical resection (R0) of the hepatic tumor load can be achieved.
    4. Debulking liver surgery should only be considered if at least 50% of the tumor burden can be reduced.
       (a) Only 1 and 2 and 3 are correct.
       (b) Only 1 and 2 and 4 are correct.
       (c) Only 1 and 2 are correct.
       (d) Only 2 is correct.

    Based on a decision of an interdisciplinary NET conference, a percutaneous radiofrequency ablation (RFA) of the metastasis is performed.

    For 18 months, consecutive MRI show no vital growth-remnants, but the next MRI 6 months later reveals another growth of 10 mm in segment VII. In the meanwhile, the patient has reached an age of 80 years and is enjoying an excellent health status biking, hiking, and skiing without any restrictions whenever possible.

12. What are your most appropriate treatment options now after the second recurrence in the liver 8 years after the initial therapy of the siNET? What could an interdisciplinary tumor conference probably agree on in this patient at this stage?

1. The course of the disease suggests that there might be still many, slowly growing metastasis to the liver well below the detection threshold of cross-sectional and functional imaging. Since the somatostatin receptors status of the first treated metastasis is known to be positive for somatostatin receptors 2 and 5, peptide receptor radionuclide therapy (PRRT) might reduce or even eliminate micro-metastasis at an early stage of development and therefore prevent metastasis developing into growths of a clinically relevant size for a relevant amount of time. Therefore, PRRT seems to be a valuable option at this stage of the disease.
2. Since again, the new finding represents only a solitary, slowly growing metastasis and there are no elevated 24 h urinary 5-HIAA levels or signs of CHD, a "watchful-waiting" strategy could be advised for and the SAA baseline therapy continued.
3. Since there is no additional metastasis at this moment, a locally ablative procedure like a percutaneous RFA would be well suited to address again this new solitary metastasis.
4. Because everolimus can have relevant side effects and the patient enjoys an excellent wellbeing, this therapeutic option should not yet be considered.
   (a) Only 2 and 3 are correct.
   (b) Only 2, 3, and 4 are correct.
   (c) Only 1, 3, and 4 are correct.
   (d) All answers are correct.

29.1 Introduction

Small intestine neuroendocrine tumors (siNETs) are derived from serotonin-producing enterochromaffin cells of the small intestine. The tumors may be hormonally active due to excessive serotonin release, leading to a specific clinical syndrome, or may be so-called non-functional if there is no pathological increase in hormone levels. As in other neuroendocrine tumor entities, siNETs have had a relevant increase in incidence (more than sixfold) in recent decades [1]. This is probably due to better awareness and understanding of this disease, well-defined histopathological classification, readily accessible guidelines, and improved detection rates [2]. Clinical manifestation of a siNET can be discrete or hardly noticeable for a long time, delaying diagnosis and resulting in advanced tumor stages being seen at the time of diagnosis [2]. The publication of detailed, siNET-specific guidelines by the European Neuroendocrine Tumor Society (ENETS) and North American Neuroendocrine Tumor Society (NANETS) have greatly facilitated and promoted interdisciplinary management and treatment of patients with siNETs [2–6]. No medical discipline can treat these complex patients singlehandedly – siNET treatment requires interdisciplinary teamwork at its best.

29.2 Natural History

SiNETs usually develop as small submucosal tumors, very rarely exceeding 2 cm in size, and are typically found on the antimesenteric bowel wall. Most siNETs occur in the distal ileum. A characteristic property of siNETs is their multifocality, which is observed in up to 30% of the cases [3, 5, 7]. The majority of ileal siNETs are well-differentiated and graded as G1 and G2 by biopsy or definitive histology [8, 9]. Badly differentiated G3 tumors (G3 NETs and neuroendocrine carcinomas [NECs]) are exceedingly rare [2, 8, 9].

Typically, siNETs develop lymphatic metastasis at an early stage of the disease [3, 5, 7]. Serotonin released by the primary tumor and regional lymph node metastasis can lead to pronounced fibrosis in the mesentery, causing mesenteric contraction with consecutive bowel ischemia, bowel obstruction, or intraluminal hemorrhage. These local complications and their surgical treatment may be life-threatening already at this stage of the disease [10, 11].

The liver is the most frequent site of distant metastases of siNETs (~60%) [5, 12]. Further progression of the disease with increasing liver involvement gives rise to specific, systemic, serotonin-induced symptoms (i.e., carcinoid syndrome). SiNETs may also metastasize into the peritoneal cavity in approximately 20% of cases [7]. Later in the course of the disease, patients may also develop metastasis to the lungs and bones.

Progressive, extensive liver involvement with increasing serotonin exposure to the right heart valves induces fibrotic thickening of the valves, resulting in valve insufficiency, progredient right-sided heart failure, and ultimately death [13].

29.3 Incidence

Recently, the age-adjusted incidence of siNETs in the United States (1.05 per 100'000) has narrowly overtaken the incidence rate of rectum NET (1.04 per 100,000) and is now second behind lung NETs [1]. Similar data are available for Europe [14]. SiNETs are the most common tumors of the small intestine, and are more frequent than adenocarcinomas [6]. The average age at initial diagnosis is 50–70 years [2]. Women and men have been equally affected in some studies [15–17], whereas in other publications siNETs seem to be slightly more common in men [18, 19]. African-Americans appear to be slightly more affected than Caucasians [2].

29.4 Risk Factors

Some studies have found an increased prevalence of siNETs in families of patients diagnosed with siNETs, suggesting a possible genetic predisposition to the disease [20–22]. Known risk factors for the development of siNETs are a family history of any cancer and the patient's past or present (but not specifically heavy) smoking habits [23, 24]. Gall bladder diseases and cholecystectomy are also associated with a 1.5-fold increased risk of developing siNETs [25, 26]. This seems to be due to an alteration in bile homeostasis, which modifies bile salt catabolite production and alters the intestinal microbiota, as well as the mucosal immune response [26]. These catabolites (e.g., deoxycholic acid) are known tumor promoters and are primarily absorbed in the distal ileum, exposing the neuroendocrine cells to these tumor promoters [27].

29.5 Prognosis

The median overall survival for patients with siNETs is 14 years, regardless of tumor site and stage. Survival rates vary from 70 months in advanced stages with distant metastasis to 170 months in localized disease. Patients with well-differentiated, G1 siNETs have significantly better survival of 160 months compared to patients with G3 siNETs, who have an overall survival of 30 months [1]. Multivariate analyses have shown that overall survival is dependent on age, ethnicity, differentiation, tumor stage, and site [12], with Caucasians of young age (<50 years) with a localized, well-differentiated siNET having the longest survival.

29.6 Clinical Presentation

29.6.1 Non-specific Symptoms and Intestinal Obstruction

A very typical feature of siNETs is varied clinical manifestation; 37% of patients experience discrete or non-specific symptoms, such as vague abdominal pain or weight loss. Therefore, general practitioners may initially decide to do without an extended workup, or even mis-diagnose as irritable bowel syndrome, for example. Delaying accurate diagnosis of siNETs by years is not uncommon, and tumors are often (30–80%) diagnosed in an advanced, metastasized stage [7, 28, 29]. Rarely, siNET tumors are found "incidentally" in standard cross-sectional imaging of the abdomen, functional imaging (e.g., hybrid tomographic positron emission tomography with computed tomography), or during colonoscopy.

If the primary tumor or a metastatic mesenteric mass leads to intestinal obstruction, the patient will experience the classical clinical symptoms: nausea, vomiting, abdominal colic, and stool retention. These rather distinctive symptoms are present in approximately 21.5% of all patients with siNET [2, 9] and will almost certainly lead to a speedy, specific, and accurate diagnostic path.

29.6.2 Desmoplastic Reaction

An absolute typical and unique property of siNETs is the development of a serotonin-mediated, desmoplastic stromal reaction in the mesentery of the tumor-bearing ileum or jejunum, which in time causes progressive fibrosis and subsequent contraction of the mesentery [5, 7, 30]. This contraction and fibrotic encasement of the mesenteric root and its main feeding vessels to the bowel will eventually entail small bowel ischemia with subsequent chronic or intermittent abdominal pain, luminal obstruction, and intraluminal hemorrhage [29]. If the desmoplastic reaction reaches the retroperitoneum, obstruction of the ureter with consequent hydronephrosis may occur [2].

29.6.3 Carcinoid Syndrome

Well-differentiated siNETs predominantly produce serotonin, but also other active amines and polypeptides [31, 32]. In localized disease affecting only the small bowel and its mesentery, no serotonin-induced symptoms typically occur, as these amines are metabolized and inactivated in the liver and do not reach relevant systemic levels. Serotonin-associated symptoms are usually referred to as "carcinoid syndrome," and are an expression of the relevant metastatic tumor load in the liver [29, 33]. Serotonin-producing neuroendocrine tumors and their metastases from other primary localizations that do not primarily drain via the portal vein may develop carcinoid syndrome at an earlier disease stage because the liver does not inactivate serotonin in these cases [34].

The most common symptoms of carcinoid syndrome consist of watery diarrhea (58–100%), cutaneous flushing (45–96%), and wheezing from bronchospasms (3–18%) [19, 35, 36]. The carcinoid syndrome may secondarily include dehydration, weight loss, electrolyte imbalances, and protein deficiency as symptoms due to severe diarrhea [37].

29.6.4 Carcinoid Heart Disease (Hedinger Syndrome)

Typically, systemic serotonin excess leads to a fibrotic thickening of the right heart valves (tricuspid and pulmonary), and long-term to right-sided heart failure [6, 34]. This heart condition is called carcinoid heart disease (CHD), or Hedinger syndrome. Recent studies have shown the prevalence of CHD in patients with metastatic siNET to be as high as 20% [38]. The emergence of CHD during the clinical course of the disease significantly worsens the survival of patients with siNETs [2, 13, 36].

29.6.5 Carcinoid Crisis

A life-threatening carcinoid crisis can be triggered by stimuli, including general anesthesia, invasive procedures, or surgery in patients with known carcinoid syndrome, as well as asymptomatic or oligosymptomatic patients with unknown, but already advanced, disease [2, 5, 39]. For further information on carcinoid crisis, see ► Chap. 43, which is exclusively devoted to this topic.

29.7 Diagnostic Workup

Specific, efficient, complete, and cost-effective assessment of a patient with siNET is fundamental for the development of a therapeutic concept and is ideally discussed and decided upon in an interdisciplinary tumor conference. In addition to the patient history and physical examination, a biochemical workup, cross-sectional and functional imaging studies, endoscopy, and cytology or histology of the primary tumor and, eventually, its liver metastases are necessary.

29.7.1 Biochemistry

The specific biochemistry workup for siNETs requires measurement of plasma chromogranin A and urinary 5-hydroxy indole acetic acid (5-HIAA) excretion [2].

29.7.1.1 Chromogranin A

Chromogranin A is an acidic glycoprotein secreted by a variety of different neuroendocrine tumors, including non-functional neuroendocrine tumors [40, 41]. It is by far the most important biochemical marker for neuroendocrine tumors in the primary workup and follow-up of the patient. However, chromogranin A values are susceptible to a variety of clinical conditions, which are important to know when assessing the result of a chromogranin A measurement. Proton pump inhibitors (PPIs), renal insufficiency, and hypertension may lead to sometimes impressive, but false positive, chromogranin A levels [41]. Therefore, it is crucial to take note of these conditions prior to chromogranin A measurements and to cease PPI use whenever possible at least 1 week before taking the blood sample. The level of chromogranin A usually correlates well with tumor burden and tumor-related prognosis, making it the most valuable biochemical factor in an evaluation of the mid- and long-term course of the disease [6, 29, 41, 42].

29.7.1.2 5-Hydroxy Indole Acetic Acid (5-HIAA)

Serotonin is difficult to measure, and its excretion presents with heavy daily fluctuations, but its degradation product 5-HIAA can easily be measured in a 24-h urine sample and is a reliable surrogate parameter for serotonin activity [26, 43]. 5-HIAA can now also be determined in serum, but the availability of this test is still limited [44]. When ordering a serum or urine 5-HIAA measurement, some strict dietary rules must be observed (► Box 29.1). If these requirements are met, 5-HIAA has a sensitivity of nearly 100% and specificity of 85–90% for the detection of carcinoid syndrome [33, 41]. For biochemical confirmation of the presence of a siNET, the sensitivity of 5-HIAA is 70–75% with a specificity of nearly 100% [2, 45].

Box 29.1: Foods and Medications That Could Affect the Result of 24 h Urinary 5-HIAA

Foods rich in serotonin should be avoided at least 24 h before the urine collection:

Pineapples, aubergines, avocados, bananas, capsaicin-containing foods (peppers, peperoncini, chilli, pepper, tabasco), currants, coffee, kiwi, melons, nicotine, nuts, chocolate, black tea, gooseberries, tomatoes, vanilla-containing foods, plums

The following medicines influence the level of 5-hydroxyindoleacetic acid. They should be discontinued 1 week before collection or, if withdrawal is not possible, be taken into account when interpreting the results:

Increased readings by: Acetanilide, coumarins, ephedrine, mephenesin, methamphetamine, methocarbamol, paracetamol, phenacetin, phenobarbital, phentolamine

Lowered measured values by: Antidepressants, aspirin, chlopromazine, isoniazid, levodopa, methenamine, promethazine, streptozocin, theophylline

29.7.2 Imaging

For localization of the primary tumor and accurate pre-therapeutic staging of siNETs, a combination of anatomical and functional imaging is recommended [2, 3, 5, 29].

29.7.2.1 Anatomical Cross-Sectional Imaging

Computed tomography (CT) is the most frequently used first-line imaging modality in the siNET workup. The obvious advantages of CT are its availability, its excellent anatomical resolution, and the ability to investigate the entire abdomen and thorax with a short examination time. To detect these mostly small primary tumors, multi-slice CT may be preferred. Three-phase contrast-enhanced CT will also assess the liver regarding potential metastases, which are characteristically hyper-vascular and best seen in the arterial phase. However, some metastases may be hypo-vascular and best detected in the venous phase, where they have a dark appearance [29, 46, 47].

Alternatively, magnetic resonance imaging (MRI) is more sensitive for the detection of liver metastases, but is less readily available and provides poorer anatomical resolution of nodal involvement in the mesentery [5]. SiNETs and their metastases are typically hypointense lesions in the T1-weighted sequence and hyperintense in the T2-weighted and diffusion-weighted sequence. They have similar contrast behavior in both MRI and CT [46, 48].

Ultrasound has important limitations for the localization of the primary tumor and staging in siNETs. However, it can be very useful for guiding fine needle aspiration (FNA) or biopsy of a liver metastasis, and it can be an important intraoperative adjunct to localize liver metastasis or guide intraoperatively ablative treatment modalities [29, 46, 49].

29.7.2.2 Functional Imaging

Functional imaging has become a particularly important tool for accurately assessing the degree of hepatic or systemic spread of a neuroendocrine malignancy. As 80–100% of all siNETs express a high density of somatostatin receptors on the cell surface, they constitute an ideal tumor type for imaging with radiolabeled somatostatin analogs (SSAs) [50]. The imaging modality of choice is currently hybrid tomographic positron emission tomography (PET/CT), which uses gallium-68-labeled SSAs such as DOTATOC, DOTANOC, and DOTATATE [26, 51, 52]. ^{68}Ga-SSA PET/CT has >90% sensitivity for the detection of all types of neuroendocrine neoplasms [26, 46, 53]. As well-differentiated siNETs normally do not show a relevant uptake of radiolabeled glucose, ^{18}F-fluorodeoxyglucose PET/CT (^{18}F-FDG PET/CT) has not been recommended for imaging siNETs. ^{18}F-FDG PET-CT should only be considered as an option in the workup of poorly differentiated siNETs [54].

29.7.3 Endoscopy

Preoperative colonoscopy is a mandatory diagnostic step prior to any type of operation for an siNET of the distal small bowel to exclude relevant colon pathology. In many cases, this allows for the exact localization and biopsy of siNETs in the terminal ileum [2, 3, 55]. To reach siNETs higher up in the ileum, a double-balloon technique during endoscopy may be necessary. Alternatively, capsule endoscopy could be performed, but routine use is not recommended due to a lack of supportive data in siNETs [29].

29.7.4 Biopsy and Histopathology

Biochemical results and findings in cross-sectional imaging may be extremely suggestive of the presence of a siNET, and functional imaging can definitively prove that the tumor in question is a neuroendocrine tumor, but only histopathology can deliver the key element in determining the therapeutic concept: grading. Direct biopsies of the primary tumor and core needle biopsies of liver metastasis are better suited to achieving this objective than FNA [2]. A standard histopathological workup consists of hematoxylin eosin (HE) staining in combination with immunohistochemical staining for chromogranin A and synaptophysin [2, 6, 56]. Because the proliferative rates or grading of the primary tumor and its hepatic metastasis may differ, it is often important to establish the proliferation rate of both the primary tumor and its hepatic metastasis, as the higher grading will determine the course of therapeutic action [57]. Neuroendocrine tumors of the gastrointestinal tract are graded according to the 2010 WHO classification of tumors of the digestive system [58, 59]. This grading is based on the mitotic rate or Ki-67 proliferation index. The most recent WHO classification was published in 2019 and is summarized in ▫ Table 29.1 [60]. SiNETs are also classified according to the ENETS and American Joint Committee on Cancer (AJCC)/ Union for International Cancer Control (UICC) staging system (▫ Tables 29.1 and 29.2) [60, 61].

29.7.5 Cardiac Workup

If there is evidence of carcinoid syndrome or clinically oligosymptomatic but morphologically relevant tumor load in the liver, the threshold for ordering a cardiac assessment to exclude or prove CHD should be low before embarking on any kind of therapy. For this purpose, the measurement of N-terminal pro-B-type natriuretic peptide (NT-proBNP) and echocardiography are widely accepted [13, 37, 62].

Table 29.1 2019 World Health Organization (WHO) Classification and grading criteria for neuroendocrine neoplasms of the gastrointestinal tract [60]

Classification/ grade	Ki-67 proliferative index (%)	Mitotic index (per 10 HPF)
Well-differentiated NET		
Grade 1	<3	<2
Grade 2	3–20	2–20
Grade 3	>20	>20
Poorly differentiated NEC		
Grade 3 NEC		
Small cell type	>20	>20
Large cell type	>20	>20

29

29.8 Treatment

Surgeons can come across siNETs in a variety of different situations. For example, young colleagues may unexpectedly encounter a siNET during a nightshift emergency operation for bowel obstruction, which could be associated with considerable technical difficulties in the case of massive desmoplastic stromal reaction. On the other side of the spectrum, elective operations can involve anything from a straightforward standard resection to a very demanding multi-visceral resection involving extensive liver surgery [63].

Because more than 50% of patients with siNETs have already metastasized by diagnosis, the treatment and timing of the surgical intervention should be discussed and decided upon in an interdisciplinary tumor conference [2]. Moreover, the prevention of serotonin-induced, systemic complications (see ▶ Chap. 43 on carcinoid crisis) as a special feature of siNETs should be addressed early on during this conference, prior to any interventional procedures [5].

29.8.1 Surgery for siNETs

29.8.1.1 Indication

Intestinal obstruction, imminent or established intestinal ischemia represent an acute and absolute indication for an emergency operation. Oncological, elective resection with curative or palliative intent is also a well-established indication for surgical intervention unless relevant contraindications are pres-

Table 29.2 TNM classification, staging, and grading of Si-NENs according to the AJCC UICC 8th edition [61]

Si-NENs	
T-Primary tumor	
X	Primary tumor cannot be assessed
0	No evidence of primary tumor
1	Tumor invades lamina propria or submucosa and size ≤1 cm
2	Tumor invades muscularis propria or size >1 cm
3	Tumor invades subserosa
4	Tumor invades peritoneum or other organs
N-Lymph nodes	
X	Regional lymph nodes cannot be assessed
0	No regional lymph node metastasis
1	Regional lymph node metastasis <12 nodes
2	Large mesenteric masses (>2 cm) and/or ≥12 nodes, especially those with encasement of the superior mesenteric vessels
M-Metastases	
0	No distant metastasis
1	Distant metastasis
1a	Metastasis confined to liver
1b	Metastasis in at least one extrahepatic site
1c	Both hepatic and extrahepatic metastases
Stage	
0	Tis N0 M0 (ENETS only)
I	T1, N0, M0
II	T2 or 3, N0, M0
III	T4, N0, M0 or any T, N1 or N2, M0
IV	Any T, any N, M1

ent [3, 5, 29]. In the special case of an advanced siNET, this may consist of relevant cardiac involvement in the context of CHD. In such a situation, it may be advisable to consider cardiac surgery before performing any visceral resection in a second step [13].

One of the intrinsic properties of hepatic metastasis of siNETs is that they tend to exhibit slow progression over years, or even decades, in contrast to the typical behavior of liver metastases originating from colonic carcinoma. Therefore, knowledge of the patient-specific growth dynamics of liver metastasis is an important factor when deciding on the indication and timing of resection for the primary tumor [3, 5].

29.8.1.2 Pre- and Peri-operative Care

Massive preoperative, systemic serotonin exposure, reflected by elevated 5'HIAA levels, and established CHD are significant risk factors for perioperative complications and death [64]. Due to severe watery diarrhea in the case of a clinically manifest carcinoid syndrome, patients often suffer from dehydration, electrolyte abnormalities, and hypoproteinemia [65]. These conditions should be corrected before planning major abdominal interventions. In extreme cases, parenteral feeding may even be necessary [66].

In the case of a manifest carcinoid syndrome with elevated 5'HIAA levels or morphologically proven liver metastasis, patients should receive preoperative prophylaxis with SSAs, such as octreotide, to prevent a carcinoid crisis during surgery [5, 37]. Various regimens are recommended for the perioperative administration of SSAs [5, 37, 67]. If patients have not previously received SSA treatment, ENETS guidelines [37] recommend subcutaneous administration of 100–200 μg octreotide 3 times/day 2 weeks prior to surgery. When surgery cannot be delayed this long, octreotide is given as an intravenous infusion for 1–2 days prior to surgery. Perioperative treatment with intravenous octreotide is recommended starting 12 h before anesthesia at a dose of 50–100 μg/h using dose titration until the resolution of symptoms.

Others [5, 68] recommend starting at least 1 day prior to surgery with subcutaneous or intravenous SSAs and continue a minimum 1 day after surgery. The patient should then be gradually weaned off [68]. However, perioperative prophylactic treatment with octreotide does not seem to prevent an intraoperative carcinoid crisis in all cases [69, 70], but it does lower the rate to 3.4% if administered intravenously at high doses (500 μg/h) [70]. Therefore, surgeons and anesthesiologists need to recognize that a carcinoid crisis occurs intraoperatively at a significant rate, even in asymptomatic patients or patients with established perioperative octreotide prophylaxis or therapy. In the event of a carcinoid crisis despite perioperative prophylaxis, immediate reaction and treatment is crucial to prevent serious complications or death [5].

29.8.1.3 Surgery for Locoregional Disease (Stage I– III)

In the absence of hepatic spread, the surgical standard of care for siNETs consists of resection of the primary tumor and its corresponding lymphatic drainage area with the aim of R0 resection [68, 71]. In proximal ileal siNETs, this will be achieved by segmental bowel resection with its mesentery.

However, for most distal ileal siNETs, right-sided hemicolectomy will represent the resection type of choice [2, 3].

29.8.1.4 Systematic Intraoperative Exploration and Primary Tumor Resection

While exploring a patient with siNET, the surgeon must understand that approximately 30% of the patients have multifocal primary tumors <1 cm in size. Even an optimal preoperative assessment with morphological and functional imaging techniques usually does not detect all siNETs in multifocal cases, and often underestimates the stage of the disease [68, 72]. For this reason, careful intraoperative exploration of the entire small intestine, abdominal cavity, liver, and ovaries is mandatory. This wholesome exploratory approach has been shown to be superior to all imaging techniques and should be performed systematically [3, 5, 68]. A pure inspection of the small intestine alone is not sufficient; bi-digital palpation must be performed to detect the often very small, submucosal, and multifocal siNETs [3]. Thus, an open laparotomy is generally recommended [2, 3, 5, 68]. Laparoscopic surgery should only be considered at early stages with no or limited lymph node involvement. A laparoscopic-assisted procedure would also allow an open, palpatory revision of the small intestine and combine reduced invasiveness with the possibility of bi-digital palpation of the small intestine. If the resection is performed laparoscopically, no concession should be made on oncological radicality regarding the length of bowel resection and the extent and radicality of the lymphadenectomy [3, 5].

29.8.1.5 Lymphadenectomy

One of the specific characteristics of siNETs is the development of lymph node metastases at an early stage of the disease. Almost 50% of all siNETs smaller than 1 cm already have lymph node metastases [73]. This implies that, even at early stages, tubular segmental small bowel resection is an inadequate primary resection type, and that resection of even small tumors should include resection of the corresponding mesentery.

Systematic lymphadenectomy with at least eight lymph nodes has shown significantly better survival than selective lymph node resection [74, 75] and is recommended by the ENETS guidelines [3]. The minimum number of resected lymph nodes required for sufficient lymphadenectomy is controversial due to a lack of data. In contrast to ENETS, the NANETS guidelines do not recommend a minimum number of lymph nodes to be resected [5]. The number of lymph nodes does not depend on the length of the small bowel specimen; thus, a "generous" pizza slice technique, removing an inappropriate length of small bowel cannot be recommended. Reverse lymphadenectomy with sparse small bowel resection seems to be the optimal procedure [3].

Unfortunately, mesenteric lymph node metastases are frequently associated with extensive mesenteric fibrosis due to the serotonin-induced desmoplastic stromal reaction. The specific alterations often involve the mesenteric root, and sometimes even the retroperitoneum. If the mesenteric root is fibrotic and contracted, lymphadenectomies are to be considered highly demanding and should be performed in specialized centers [3, 5]. In experienced hands, complete surgical resection of the primary tumor and its involved lymph nodes can be achieved in up to 80% of cases [74, 76, 77]. In the case of pronounced fibrosis around the central mesenteric root, removal of the lymph node metastasis may technically not be possible because the major mesenteric vessels could not possibly be preserved, and their damage will inevitably cause subtotal bowel ischemia, resulting in short bowel syndrome. However, if central mesenteric debulking succeeds, patients will be relieved from their obstructive symptoms and enjoy a far better prognosis than patients treated palliatively only [76].

29.8.1.6 Prophylactic Cholecystectomy

Treatment with SSAs decreases gallbladder function and promotes the formation of gallstones in patients undergoing long-term therapy. The prevalence of gallstones in patients on SSAs is much higher than in the general population (up to 63%) [78]. Approximately 77% of all siNET patients will require SSA therapy in the long-term [79], and simultaneous prophylactic cholecystectomy is recommended during first time surgery to avoid specific complications, such as biliary obstruction or cholecystitis. Patients with significant lymph node involvement or liver or peritoneal metastasis are most likely to be receive SSA therapy soon during follow-up [2, 5, 68].

29.8.1.7 Surgery in Metastatic Disease (Stage IV)

Unfortunately, 50–80% of patients present with metastatic spread to the liver at diagnosis and cannot be treated with curative intent [31, 68]. Nevertheless, even in this setting, surgery can reduce the tumor burden and improve the quality of life and survival of the patients who are part of a multimodal therapeutic concept [80]. In addition, 40–50% of patients will develop isolated or multiple liver metastases only during follow-up [81, 82]. There are a variety of options to address liver involvement, including surgery, locally ablative procedures, a combination of surgery and local ablation, embolization, or liver-directed systemic treatment, such as peptide receptor radionuclide therapy (PRRT) or medical treatment [83].

29.8.1.8 Surgery in Metastatic Liver Disease (M1a)

Because patients with surgically treated liver metastasis have significantly better 5-year survival than patients treated conservatively, surgical resection of liver metastases remains the first-line therapy [83, 84]. In addition to the survival benefit, with 5-year survival rates of 60–90%, complete relief, or at least improvement, of serotonin-induced symptoms can be expected in 96% of patients [49, 85, 86].

As liver metastasis can de-differentiate compared to the primary tumor and, therefore, may have a higher grading, one is well advised to determine the proliferation rate of dominant liver metastasis before deciding on the type and extent of surgical treatment of the liver. Usually, a low grading (G1 or G2) of hepatic metastasis and absence of extra-abdominal metastasis [3, 5] are considered preconditions for the indication of hepatic surgery.

The distribution and size of the liver metastasis are also decision-relevant factors. Single resectable liver metastases can be addressed surgically, whereas surgery in cases with many broadly disseminated, small metastasis is not recommended. Complex bilateral but potentially resectable liver involvement can be addressed in a two-step surgical strategy (e.g., associating liver partition and portal vein ligation for staged hepatectomy [ALPPS]) or in combination with locally ablative techniques [5, 87].

Recurrence rates after hepatic surgery, even for R0 resected patients, are exceedingly high (95%), and patients with R1 and R2 resections have comparable 5-year survival rates. Thus, the surgical strategy has recently shifted from curative intent to a more palliative attitude in the sense of debulking surgery [49, 86, 88, 89]. Healthy liver tissue must be maintained; excessive resections of liver metastasis in the presence of scarce normal liver tissue can lead to organ failure and death [5]. A careful preoperative evaluation of the prospective liver function is important; patient-related factors, such as performance status and other relevant comorbidities, must also be considered in the decision-making process for potential liver interventions [87].

As a rule, debulking surgery should only be considered if the tumor burden can be reduced at least 70%. Otherwise, other therapeutic modalities should be pursued [3, 5]. Liver transplantation for the treatment of metastatic liver disease in the context of neuroendocrine tumors is controversial. It may be an option in highly selected patients with unresectable liver metastases if strict Milan and ENETS criteria are met [3, 90].

29.8.1.9 Surgery for the Primary Tumor in Inoperable Liver Disease (M1a)

Due to the lack of prospective studies, it is not entirely clear whether resection of the primary ileal or jejunal tumor with adequate lymphadenectomy improves survival in locally asymptomatic patients with inoperable liver metastases. Nevertheless, it may be recommended in patients with very slowly advancing hepatic tumor load and general wellbeing in order to prevent local complications, such as intestinal obstruction and ischemia caused by a progressive desmoplastic stromal reaction [3, 5, 91].

29.8.1.10 Surgery in Cases with Peritoneal Spread

Peritoneal spread of the siNET occurs in approximately 20% of patients undergoing exploration [7]. Unfortunately, no validated therapeutic concepts are available for this situation, though some patients treated with cytoreductive surgery may benefit from prolonged survival [92]. Currently, there is no evidence for the additive use of hyper-thermic intraperitoneal chemotherapy (HIPEC) for the treatment of peritoneal metastases of neuroendocrine tumors in general [5].

29.8.2 Non-surgical Treatment Options

29.8.2.1 Somatostatin Analogs (SSAs)

As already mentioned, SSAs play an important role in preventing a carcinoid crisis during interventions for serotonin-excreting neuroendocrine tumors. They are also considered the first-line treatment modality after surgical R1 or R2 resection or in non-resectable metastatic disease. This is due to its proven antiproliferative and antisecretory effect [6, 82, 93–95]. At the beginning of SSA therapy, a short-acting octreotide (100–200 μg, 3 times/day) is usually applied subcutaneously to test its tolerability and possible side effects. Later, the therapy is switched to a long-acting SSA, such as octreotide long-acting repeatable (LAR) or lanreotide. These are usually administered every 4 weeks [82]. For a dose increase, the interval can be shortened to 3, or even 2, weeks. Octreotide LAR and lanreotide have been shown to be equally effective in symptom control [96, 97].

29.8.2.2 Interferon Alpha (IFN)

In Europe, interferon alpha (IFN) is approved for the treatment of neuroendocrine tumors associated with carcinoid syndrome. IFN can be used in addition to SSA therapy for refractory carcinoid syndrome or somatostatin receptor negative siNETs. IFN represents another treatment option in cases of poor SSA tolerance. Its efficacy has been comparable to SSA therapy in uncontrolled and controlled studies [98–100]. However, in the US, IFN has not been approved by the Food and Drug administration (FDA) for this indication [6].

29.8.2.3 Everolimus

Everolimus is an immune-suppressive drug belonging to the mTOR inhibitors. Its effects have been studied in patients with advanced neuroendocrine tumors associated with carcinoid syndrome and in patients with non-functional neuroendocrine tumors [101, 102]. Because of the improved median survival compared to placebo, everolimus is approved for therapy of advanced, progressive, grade 1 or grade 2 non-functioning gastro-entero-pancreatic (including siNETs) and lung neuroendocrine tumors [29, 103].

29.8.2.4 Peptide Receptor Radionuclide Therapy (PRRT)

PRRT allows for very selective, targeted application of radioactivity to a somatostatin receptor-positive tumor or metastasis using radiolabeled SSAs. The most frequently used radionuclides in therapeutic applications are yttrium-90 or lutetium-177. Due to its response rates and positive effects on overall survival, PRRT has become an important and well-established second-line therapy in the treatment of siNETs with progression under SSA therapy [6, 82, 104, 105].

29.8.2.5 Liver-Directed Therapy

As discussed earlier, metastatic liver disease should preferentially be addressed surgically because of its beneficial effect on survival [2, 6, 68]. However, if the surgical approach is not feasible, locally ablative procedures or embolization for dominant metastasis should be evaluated [6, 29].

In radiofrequency ablation (RFA) or microwave destruction, heat is applied locally via a probe inserted into the metastasis, which induces necrosis of the metastatic tissue. These methods can be used intraoperatively as an adjunct to the surgical resection, or percutaneously. Each method has certain limitations. Locally ablative procedures are not recommended for metastases larger than 5 cm. Furthermore, peripheral subcapsular localization of metastasis, and metastases located in the immediate vicinity of vital structures or vessels may limit their applicability [83].

Other therapeutic options include trans-arterial embolic procedures. These procedures take advantage of the fact that the blood flow to neuroendocrine tumor metastasis is mainly provided by the hepatic artery. Embolization can be performed in three different variations: bland embolization, chemoembolization, or radioembolization [83].

Due to the lack of prospective comparative studies for liver-directed treatment modalities, it is not known, whether relevant differences exist in regard to the response rate, complication rates, and survival [6, 29, 83]. Therefore, the chosen path for liver-targeted therapy will depend on individual patient features (e.g., size, distribution, localization and number of lesions, vascularization, and proliferative index), local availability, and local skills [106, 107].

All liver-targeted treatments should be performed under prophylactic SSA medication to prevent a carcinoid crisis.

29.8.2.6 Chemotherapy

Chemotherapy plays a minor role in the treatment of grade 1 and grade 2 siNETs [29]. Only a few retrospective studies with low case numbers have shown some beneficial effect in well-differentiated siNETs [108]. Neuroendocrine carcinomas of the small intestine are extremely rare, and their treatment is primarily chemotherapy using platinum-based chemotherapeutics (cisplatin, carboplatin) in combination with etoposide [82].

29.8.2.7 Symptomatic Therapy for Serotonin-Induced Diarrhea

SSAs are the first choice for the treatment of serotonin-induced diarrhea. If fatty stools or other signs of excretory pancreatic insufficiency occur as adverse effects of SSA therapy, pancreatic enzymes should also be administered [103]. Loperamide and other anticholinergics, ondansetron, and opium tincture can be used to address diarrhea [34]. Recently, telotristat was approved as a new drug to treat refractory serotonin-induced diarrhea [109]. Telotristat ethyl is an inhibitor of tryptophan hydroxylase, which has been shown to significantly lower serotonin levels [110, 111] and, therefore, has a beneficial effect on diarrhea in carcinoid syndrome.

29.8.2.8 Treatment of Carcinoid Heart Disease (CHD, Hedinger Syndrome)

If CHD is diagnosed, treatment with SSAs is mandatory to reduce serotonin exposure to the heart. SSAs have been shown to improve the cardiac reserve, but it does not stop progression of the cardiac condition [13]. In CHD, there is no evidence of a benefit of standard heart failure treatment [13]. If a general improvement in the patient's situation and stabilization of tumor progression can be achieved, cardiac surgery with right-sided valve replacement should be attempted in moderate or severe CHD [13, 112]. These patients have an otherwise short life expectancy [113]. Cardiac surgery is to be envisaged especially prior to major liver surgery or embolization, despite the fact that a surgical reduction of the hepatic metastatic load can also slow CHD progression [8]. For major liver surgery before correcting the heart condition, surgeons should keep in mind that, due to the venous congestion associated with increased right heart pressure, major liver surgery can cause massive blood loss. For optimal treatment of CHD, a multidisciplinary therapeutic strategy is essential and should be ensured at all stages [13].

29.9 Follow-Up

Even in patients with curatively resected siNETs, the long-term recurrence rate is approximately 50% [114, 115]. These local recurrences or distant metastases can radiologically manifest many years after initial therapy, as micro-metastasis with a low proliferation rate can take a long time to grow to a size that is captured by imaging during follow-up. Because the developing cumulative tumor load may also be small, it can take many years until the patients develop clinically detectible, serotonin-induced symptoms. Thus, specific, long-term surveillance of these patients by clinical, biochemical, and radiological means is important to timely detect and eventually treat a recurrence [6, 116].

In patients with persistent disease after initial therapy, the tumor-specific follow-up aims to capture the moment of significant tumor progression to adapt ongoing therapies or initiate the next line of treatment in order to slow the biochemical or morphological progression of the disease. Patients should be discussed regularly at interdisciplinary tumor conferences, particularly in the case of tumor progression, to decide on the next therapeutic steps [2, 3, 6].

29.9.1 Frequency and Duration of the Follow-Up

While the NANETS guidelines recommend a surveillance period of 10 years with the option of prolonging it in young patients or in the case of an increased risk of developing recurrence or metastasis (e.g., numerous affected lymph nodes) for curatively treated patients [6], the ENETS guidelines recommend lifelong follow-up [116]. The follow-up intervals depend mainly on the tumor stage and grading, as well as the completeness of the tumor resection. Curatively resected patients with G1/G2 siNETs should be followed up every 6–12 months, and patients with residual tumor or metastases in 3–6-month intervals. Patients with G3 siNETs or tumors with rapid progression should be checked at least every 3 months [116].

29.9.2 Investigations

The follow-up examinations include the patient history and a physical examination, looking specifically for symptoms associated with carcinoid syndrome or CHD. The biochemical investigation will focus on the tumor marker chromogranin A and the breakdown products of serotonin (i.e., 5-HIAA). Regarding cross-sectional imaging, one should be aware that these patients will eventually be followed up for decades. Thus, for the longitudinal observation of the liver, MRI may be preferable to CT to reduce the cumulative exposure to radiation. For the same reasons, somatostatin receptor-specific imaging should not be used as a standard imaging modality during follow-up, but should be reserved for situations in which systemic spread beyond the liver needs to be objectified, or in preparation for an eventual PRRT [116]. In the case of a relevant metastatic load to the liver with preexisting carcinoid syndrome, the follow-up should also encompass a workup of the heart condition. For this purpose, echocardiography and measurement of NT-pro-BNP are recommended [116].

Answers to the Questions

1. (d); 2. (c); 3. (d); 4. (a); 5. (b); 6. (b); 7. (d); 8. (c); 9. (c); 10. (e); 11. (c); 12. (d)

References

1. Dasari A, Shen C, Halperin D, Zhao B, Zhou S, Xu Y, et al. Trends in the incidence, prevalence, and survival outcomes in patients with neuroendocrine tumors in the United States. JAMA Oncol. 2017;3(10):1335–42.
2. Niederle B, Pape UF, Costa F, Gross D, Kelestimur F, Knigge U, et al. ENETS consensus guidelines update for neuroendocrine neoplasms of the jejunum and ileum. Neuroendocrinology. 2016;103(2):125–38.
3. Partelli S, Bartsch DK, Capdevila J, Chen J, Knigge U, Niederle B, et al. ENETS consensus guidelines for standard of care in neuroendocrine tumors: surgery for small intestinal and pancreatic neuroendocrine tumors. Neuroendocrinology. 2017;105(3):255–65.
4. Pavel M, de Herder WW. ENETS consensus guidelines for the standard of care in neuroendocrine tumors. Neuroendocrinology. 2017;105(3):193–5.
5. Howe JR, Cardona K, Fraker DL, Kebebew E, Untch BR, Wang YZ, et al. The surgical management of small bowel neuroendocrine tumors: consensus guidelines of the North American Neuroendocrine Tumor Society. Pancreas. 2017;46(6):715–31.
6. Strosberg JR, Halfdanarson TR, Bellizzi AM, Chan JA, Dillon JS, Heaney AP, et al. The North American Neuroendocrine Tumor Society consensus guidelines for surveillance and medical management of midgut neuroendocrine tumors. Pancreas. 2017;46(6):707–14.
7. Norlen O, Stalberg P, Oberg K, Eriksson J, Hedberg J, Hessman O, et al. Long-term results of surgery for small intestinal neuroendocrine tumors at a tertiary referral center. World J Surg. 2012;36(6):1419–31.
8. Niederle MB, Hackl M, Kaserer K, Niederle B. Gastroenteropancreatic neuroendocrine tumors: the current incidence and staging based on the WHO and European Neuroendocrine Tumor Society classification: an analysis based on prospectively collected parameters. Endocr Relat Cancer. 2010;17(4):909–18.
9. Niederle MB, Niederle B. Diagnosis and treatment of gastroenteropancreatic neuroendocrine tumors: current data on a prospectively collected, retrospectively analyzed clinical multicenter investigation. Oncologist. 2011;16(5):602–13.
10. Lardiere-Deguelte S, de Mestier L, Appere F, Vullierme MP, Zappa M, Hoeffel C, et al. Toward a preoperative classification of lymph node metastases in patients with small intestinal neuroendocrine tumors in the era of intestinal-sparing surgery. Neuroendocrinology. 2016;103(5):552–9.

11. Akerstrom G, Hellman P. Surgical aspects of neuroendocrine tumors. Eur J Cancer. 2009;45(Suppl 1):237–50.
12. Modlin IM, Lye KD, Kidd M. A 5-decade analysis of 13,715 carcinoid tumors. Cancer. 2003;97(4):934–59.
13. Steeds RP, Sagar V, Shetty S, Oelofse T, Singh H, Ahmad R, et al. Multidisciplinary team management of carcinoid heart disease. Endocr Connect. 2019;8(12):R184–R99.
14. Fraenkel M, Kim M, Faggiano A, de Herder WW, Valk GD, Knowledge N. Incidence of gastroenteropancreatic neuroendocrine tumors: a systematic review of the literature. Endocr Relat Cancer. 2014;21(3):R153–63.
15. Ellis L, Shale MJ, Coleman MP. Carcinoid tumors of the gastrointestinal tract: trends in incidence in England since 1971. Am J Gastroenterol. 2010;105(12):2563–9.
16. Garcia-Carbonero R, Capdevila J, Crespo-Herrero G, Diaz-Perez JA, Martinez Del Prado MP, Alonso Orduna V, et al. Incidence, patterns of care and prognostic factors for outcome of gastroenteropancreatic neuroendocrine tumors (GEP-NETs): results from the National Cancer Registry of Spain (RGETNE). Ann Oncol. 2010;21(9):1794–803.
17. Ploeckinger U, Kloeppel G, Wiedenmann B, Lohmann R, Representatives of 21 German NETC. The German NET-registry: an audit on the diagnosis and therapy of neuroendocrine tumors. Neuroendocrinology. 2009;90(4):349–63.
18. Lepage C, Bouvier AM, Manfredi S, Dancourt V, Faivre J. Incidence and management of primary malignant small bowel cancers: a well-defined French population study. Am J Gastroenterol. 2006;101(12):2826–32.
19. Bergestuen DS, Aabakken L, Holm K, Vatn M, Thiis-Evensen E. Small intestinal neuroendocrine tumors: prognostic factors and survival. Scand J Gastroenterol. 2009;44(9):1084–91.
20. Hassan MM, Phan A, Li D, Dagohoy CG, Leary C, Yao JC. Family history of cancer and associated risk of developing neuroendocrine tumors: a case-control study. Cancer Epidemiol Biomark Prev. 2008;17(4):959–65.
21. Hemminki K, Li X. Familial carcinoid tumors and subsequent cancers: a nation-wide epidemiologic study from Sweden. Int J Cancer. 2001;94(3):444–8.
22. Jarhult J, Landerholm K, Falkmer S, Nordenskjold M, Sundler F, Wierup N. First report on metastasizing small bowel carcinoids in first-degree relatives in three generations. Neuroendocrinology. 2010;91(4):318–23.
23. Leoncini E, Carioli G, La Vecchia C, Boccia S, Rindi G. Risk factors for neuroendocrine neoplasms: a systematic review and meta-analysis. Ann Oncol. 2016;27(1):68–81.
24. Rinzivillo M, Capurso G, Campana D, Fazio N, Panzuto F, Spada F, et al. Risk and protective factors for small intestine neuroendocrine tumors: a prospective case-control study. Neuroendocrinology. 2016;103(5):531–7.
25. Nogueira L, Freedman ND, Engels EA, Warren JL, Castro F, Koshiol J. Gallstones, cholecystectomy, and risk of digestive system cancers. Am J Epidemiol. 2014;179(6):731–9.
26. Clift AK, Kidd M, Bodei L, Toumpanakis C, Baum RP, Oberg K, et al. Neuroendocrine neoplasms of the small bowel and pancreas. Neuroendocrinology. 2020;110(6):444–76.
27. Schottenfeld D, Beebe-Dimmer JL, Vigneau FD. The epidemiology and pathogenesis of neoplasia in the small intestine. Ann Epidemiol. 2009;19(1):58–69.
28. Yao JC, Hassan M, Phan A, Dagohoy C, Leary C, Mares JE, et al. One hundred years after "carcinoid": epidemiology of and prognostic factors for neuroendocrine tumors in 35,825 cases in the United States. J Clin Oncol. 2008;26(18):3063–72.

29. Scott AT, Howe JR. Management of small bowel neuroendocrine tumors. J Oncol Pract. 2018;14(8):471–82.
30. Modlin IM, Shapiro MD, Kidd M. Carcinoid tumors and fibrosis: an association with no explanation. Am J Gastroenterol. 2004;99(12): 2466–78.
31. Modlin IM, Oberg K, Chung DC, Jensen RT, de Herder WW, Thakker RV, et al. Gastroenteropancreatic neuroendocrine tumors. Lancet Oncol. 2008;9(1):61–72.
32. Vinik AI, Silva MP, Woltering EA, Go VL, Warner R, Caplin M. Biochemical testing for neuroendocrine tumors. Pancreas. 2009;38(8): 876–89.
33. Vinik AI, Chaya C. Clinical presentation and diagnosis of neuroendocrine tumors. Hematol Oncol Clin North Am. 2016;30(1):21–48.
34. Naraev BG, Halland M, Halperin DM, Purvis AJ, O'Dorisio TM, Halfdanarson TR. Management of diarrhea in patients with carcinoid syndrome. Pancreas. 2019;48(8):961–72.
35. Helland SK, Prosch AM, Viste A. Carcinoid tumors in the gastrointestinal tract--a population-based study from Western Norway. Scand J Surg. 2006;95(3):158–61.
36. Pape UF, Berndt U, Muller-Nordhorn J, Bohmig M, Roll S, Koch M, et al. Prognostic factors of long-term outcome in gastroenteropancreatic neuroendocrine tumors. Endocr Relat Cancer. 2008;15(4):1083–97.
37. Kaltsas G, Caplin M, Davies P, Ferone D, Garcia-Carbonero R, Grozinsky-Glasberg S, et al. ENETS consensus guidelines for the standards of care in neuroendocrine tumors: pre- and perioperative therapy in patients with neuroendocrine tumors. Neuroendocrinology. 2017;105(3):245–54.
38. Bhattacharyya S, Raja SG, Toumpanakis C, Caplin ME, Dreyfus GD, Davar J. Outcomes, risks and complications of cardiac surgery for carcinoid heart disease. Eur J Cardiothorac Surg. 2011;40(1):168–72.
39. Castillo JG, Filsoufi F, Adams DH, Raikhelkar J, Zaku B, Fischer GW. Management of patients undergoing multivalvular surgery for carcinoid heart disease: the role of the anaesthetist. Br J Anaesth. 2008;101(5):618–26.
40. Deftos LJ. Chromogranin A: its role in endocrine function and as an endocrine and neuroendocrine tumor marker. Endocr Rev. 1991;12(2):181–7.
41. Oberg K, Couvelard A, Delle Fave G, Gross D, Grossman A, Jensen RT, et al. ENETS consensus guidelines for standard of care in neuroendocrine tumors: biochemical markers. Neuroendocrinology. 2017;105(3):201–11.
42. Yang X, Yang Y, Li Z, Cheng C, Yang T, Wang C, et al. Diagnostic value of circulating chromogranin a for neuroendocrine tumors: a systematic review and meta-analysis. PLoS One. 2015;10(4):e0124884.
43. Feldman JM, O'Dorisio TM. Role of neuropeptides and serotonin in the diagnosis of carcinoid tumors. Am J Med. 1986;81(6B):41–8.
44. Tohmola N, Itkonen O, Sane T, Markkanen H, Joenvaara S, Renkonen R, et al. Analytical and preanalytical validation of a new mass spectrometric serum 5-hydroxyindoleacetic acid assay as neuroendocrine tumor marker. Clin Chim Acta. 2014;428:38–43.
45. Ardill JE, Erikkson B. The importance of the measurement of circulating markers in patients with neuroendocrine tumors of the pancreas and gut. Endocr Relat Cancer. 2003;10(4):459–62.
46. Sundin A, Arnold R, Baudin E, Cwikla JB, Eriksson B, Fanti S, et al. ENETS consensus guidelines for the standards of care in neuroendocrine tumors: radiological, nuclear medicine & hybrid imaging. Neuroendocrinology. 2017;105(3):212–44.
47. Ruf J, Schiefer J, Furth C, Kosiek O, Kropf S, Heuck F, et al. 68Ga-DOTATOC PET/CT of neuroendocrine tumors: spotlight on the CT phases of a triple-phase protocol. J Nucl Med. 2011;52(5):697–704.

48. Dromain C, de Baere T, Lumbroso J, Caillet H, Laplanche A, Boige V, et al. Detection of liver metastases from endocrine tumors: a prospective comparison of somatostatin receptor scintigraphy, computed tomography, and magnetic resonance imaging. J Clin Oncol. 2005;23(1): 70–8.
49. Maxwell JE, Sherman SK, O'Dorisio TM, Bellizzi AM, Howe JR. Liver-directed surgery of neuroendocrine metastases: what is the optimal strategy? Surgery. 2016;159(1):320–33.
50. Plockinger U, Rindi G, Arnold R, Eriksson B, Krenning EP, de Herder WW, et al. ENETS guidelines: guidelines for the diagnosis and treatment of neuroendocrine gastrointestinal tumors. Neuroendocrinology. 2005;80(6):394–424.
51. Deppen SA, Liu E, Blume JD, Clanton J, Shi C, Jones-Jackson LB, et al. Safety and efficacy of 68Ga-DOTATATE PET/CT for diagnosis, staging, and treatment management of neuroendocrine tumors. J Nucl Med. 2016;57(5):708–14.
52. Barrio M, Czernin J, Fanti S, Ambrosini V, Binse I, Du L, et al. The impact of Somatostatin receptor-directed PET/CT on the management of patients with neuroendocrine tumor: a systematic review and meta-analysis. J Nucl Med. 2017;58(5):756–61.
53. Sundin A, Vullierme MP, Kaltsas G, Plockinger U. ENETS consensus guidelines for the standards of care in neuroendocrine tumors: radiological examinations. Neuroendocrinology. 2009;90(2):167–83.
54. Reubi JC. Somatostatin and other peptide receptors as tools for tumor diagnosis and treatment. Neuroendocrinology. 2004;80(Suppl 1): 51–6.
55. Prommegger R, Ensinger C, Steiner P, Sauper T, Profanter C, Margreiter R. Neuroendocrine tumors and second primary malignancy--a relationship with clinical impact? Anticancer Res. 2004;24(2C):1049–51.
56. Bellizzi AM. Assigning site of origin in metastatic neuroendocrine neoplasms: a clinically significant application of diagnostic immunohistochemistry. Adv Anat Pathol. 2013;20(5):285–314.
57. Keck KJ, Choi A, Maxwell JE, Li G, O'Dorisio TM, Breheny P, et al. Increased grade in neuroendocrine tumor metastases negatively impacts survival. Ann Surg Oncol. 2017;24(8):2206–12.
58. Klimstra DS, Modlin IR, Coppola D, Lloyd RV, Suster S. The pathologic classification of neuroendocrine tumors: a review of nomenclature, grading, and staging systems. Pancreas. 2010;39(6):707–12.
59. Bosman FT, Carneiro F, Hruban R, Theise N, editors. WHO classification of tumors of the digestive system. 4th ed. Lyon: International Agency for Research on Cancer (IARC); 2010.
60. Nagtegaal ID, Odze RD, Klimstra D, Paradis V, Rugge M, Schirmacher P, et al. The 2019 WHO classification of tumors of the digestive system. Histopathology. 2020;76(2):182–8.
61. Amin MES, Greene F. AJCC cancer staging manual. 8th ed. Springer; 2017.
62. Mancuso K, Kaye AD, Boudreaux JP, Fox CJ, Lang P, Kalarickal PL, et al. Carcinoid syndrome and perioperative anesthetic considerations. J Clin Anesth. 2011;23(4):329–41.
63. Modlin IM, Moss SF, Chung DC, Jensen RT, Snyderwine E. Priorities for improving the management of gastroenteropancreatic neuroendocrine tumors. J Natl Cancer Inst. 2008;100(18):1282–9.
64. Kinney MA, Warner ME, Nagorney DM, Rubin J, Schroeder DR, Maxson PM, et al. Perianaesthetic risks and outcomes of abdominal surgery for metastatic carcinoid tumors. Br J Anaesth. 2001;87(3): 447–52.
65. Graham GW, Unger BP, Coursin DB. Perioperative management of selected endocrine disorders. Int Anesthesiol Clin. 2000;38(4):31–67.
66. O'Toole D, Salazar R, Falconi M, Kaltsas G, Couvelard A, de Herder WW, et al. ENETS guidelines: rare functioning pancreatic endocrine tumors. Neuroendocrinology. 2006;84(3):189–95.

67. Massimino K, Harrskog O, Pommier S, Pommier R. Octreotide LAR and bolus octreotide are insufficient for preventing intraoperative complications in carcinoid patients. J Surg Oncol. 2013;107(8):842–6.
68. Moris D, Ntanasis-Stathopoulos I, Tsilimigras DI, Vagios S, Karamitros A, Karaolanis G, et al. Update on surgical management of small bowel neuroendocrine tumors. Anticancer Res. 2018;38(3):1267–78.
69. Falconi M, Plockinger U, Kwekkeboom DJ, Manfredi R, Korner M, Kvols L, et al. ENETS guidelines: well-differentiated pancreatic non-functioning tumors/carcinoma. Neuroendocrinology. 2006;84(3):196–211.
70. Woltering EA, Wright AE, Stevens MA, Wang YZ, Boudreaux JP, Mamikunian G, et al. Development of effective prophylaxis against intraoperative carcinoid crisis. J Clin Anesth. 2016;32:189–93.
71. Schnirer II, Yao JC, Ajani JA. Carcinoid--a comprehensive review. Acta Oncol. 2003;42(7):672–92.
72. Clift AK, Faiz O, Al-Nahhas A, Bockisch A, Liedke MO, Schloericke E, et al. Role of staging in patients with small intestinal neuroendocrine tumors. J Gastrointest Surg. 2016;20(1):180–8; discussion 8
73. Walsh JC, Schaeffer DF, Kirsch R, Pollett A, Manzoni M, Riddell RH, et al. Ileal "carcinoid" tumors-small size belies deadly intent: high rate of nodal metastasis in tumors </=1 cm in size. Hum Pathol. 2016;56:123–7.
74. Watzka FM, Fottner C, Miederer M, Weber MM, Schad A, Lang H, et al. Surgical treatment of NEN of small bowel: a retrospective analysis. World J Surg. 2016;40(3):749–58.
75. Landry CS, Lin HY, Phan A, Charnsangavej C, Abdalla EK, Aloia T, et al. Resection of at-risk mesenteric lymph nodes is associated with improved survival in patients with small bowel neuroendocrine tumors. World J Surg. 2013;37(7):1695–700.
76. Chambers AJ, Pasieka JL, Dixon E, Rorstad O. The palliative benefit of aggressive surgical intervention for both hepatic and mesenteric metastases from neuroendocrine tumors. Surgery. 2008;144(4):645–51; discussion 51–3
77. Pasquer A, Walter T, Hervieu V, Forestier J, Scoazec JY, Lombard-Bohas C, et al. Surgical management of small bowel neuroendocrine tumors: specific requirements and their impact on staging and prognosis. Ann Surg Oncol. 2015;22(Suppl 3):S742–9.
78. Trendle MC, Moertel CG, Kvols LK. Incidence and morbidity of cholelithiasis in patients receiving chronic octreotide for metastatic carcinoid and malignant islet cell tumors. Cancer. 1997;79(4):830–4.
79. Norlen O, Hessman O, Stalberg P, Akerstrom G, Hellman P. Prophylactic cholecystectomy in midgut carcinoid patients. World J Surg. 2010;34(6):1361–7.
80. Farley HA, Pommier RF. Surgical treatment of small bowel neuroendocrine tumors. Hematol Oncol Clin North Am. 2016;30(1):49–61.
81. Frilling A, Modlin IM, Kidd M, Russell C, Breitenstein S, Salem R, et al. Recommendations for management of patients with neuroendocrine liver metastases. Lancet Oncol. 2014;15(1):e8–21.
82. Pavel M, O'Toole D, Costa F, Capdevila J, Gross D, Kianmanesh R, et al. ENETS consensus guidelines update for the management of distant metastatic disease of intestinal, pancreatic, bronchial neuroendocrine neoplasms (NEN) and NEN of unknown primary site. Neuroendocrinology. 2016;103(2):172–85.
83. Dermine S, Palmieri LJ, Lavole J, Barre A, Dohan A, Abou Ali E, et al. Non-pharmacological therapeutic options for liver metastases in advanced neuroendocrine tumors. J Clin Med. 2019;8(11):1907.
84. Kacmaz E, Heidsma CM, Besselink MGH, Dreijerink KMA, Klumpen HJ, Nieveen van Dijkum EJM, et al. Treatment of liver metastases from

midgut neuroendocrine tumors: a systematic review and meta-analysis. J Clin Med. 2019;8(3):403.
85. Sarmiento JM, Heywood G, Rubin J, Ilstrup DM, Nagorney DM, Que FG. Surgical treatment of neuroendocrine metastases to the liver: a plea for resection to increase survival. J Am Coll Surg. 2003;197(1):29–37.
86. Mayo SC, de Jong MC, Pulitano C, Clary BM, Reddy SK, Gamblin TC, et al. Surgical management of hepatic neuroendocrine tumor metastasis: results from an international multi-institutional analysis. Ann Surg Oncol. 2010;17(12):3129–36.
87. Linecker M, Kambakamba P, Raptis DA, Malago M, Ratti F, Aldrighetti L, et al. ALPPS in neuroendocrine liver metastases not amenable for conventional resection – lessons learned from an interim analysis of the International ALPPS Registry. HPB (Oxford). 2020;22(4):537–44.
88. Glazer ES, Tseng JF, Al-Refaie W, Solorzano CC, Liu P, Willborn KA, et al. Long-term survival after surgical management of neuroendocrine hepatic metastases. HPB (Oxford). 2010;12(6):427–33.
89. Graff-Baker AN, Sauer DA, Pommier SJ, Pommier RF. Expanded criteria for carcinoid liver debulking: maintaining survival and increasing the number of eligible patients. Surgery. 2014;156(6):1369–76; discussion 76–7
90. Mazzaferro V, Sposito C, Coppa J, Miceli R, Bhoori S, Bongini M, et al. The long-term benefit of liver transplantation for hepatic metastases from neuroendocrine tumors. Am J Transplant. 2016;16(10):2892–902.
91. Capurso G, Rinzivillo M, Bettini R, Boninsegna L, Delle Fave G, Falconi M. Systematic review of resection of primary midgut carcinoid tumor in patients with unresectable liver metastases. Br J Surg. 2012;99(11):1480–6.
92. Wright MF, Cates J, Gonzalez RS, Das S, Berlin JD, Shi C. Impact of peritoneal metastasis on survival of patients with small intestinal neuroendocrine tumor. Am J Surg Pathol. 2019;43(4):559–63.
93. Singh S, Asa SL, Dey C, Kennecke H, Laidley D, Law C, et al. Diagnosis and management of gastrointestinal neuroendocrine tumors: an evidence-based Canadian consensus. Cancer Treat Rev. 2016;47:32–45.
94. Caplin ME, Pavel M, Cwikla JB, Phan AT, Raderer M, Sedlackova E, et al. Lanreotide in metastatic enteropancreatic neuroendocrine tumors. N Engl J Med. 2014;371(3):224–33.
95. Rinke A, Muller HH, Schade-Brittinger C, Klose KJ, Barth P, Wied M, et al. Placebo-controlled, double-blind, prospective, randomized study on the effect of octreotide LAR in the control of tumor growth in patients with metastatic neuroendocrine midgut tumors: a report from the PROMID Study Group. J Clin Oncol. 2009;27(28):4656–63.
96. Eriksson B, Annibale B, Bajetta E, Mitry E, Pavel M, Platania M, et al. ENETS consensus guidelines for the standards of care in neuroendocrine tumors: chemotherapy in patients with neuroendocrine tumors. Neuroendocrinology. 2009;90(2):214–9.
97. Ruszniewski P, Ish-Shalom S, Wymenga M, O'Toole D, Arnold R, Tomassetti P, et al. Rapid and sustained relief from the symptoms of carcinoid syndrome: results from an open 6-month study of the 28-day prolonged-release formulation of lanreotide. Neuroendocrinology. 2004;80(4):244–51.
98. Oberg K. Interferon in the management of neuroendocrine GEP-tumors: a review. Digestion. 2000;62(Suppl 1):92–7.
99. Faiss S, Pape UF, Bohmig M, Dorffel Y, Mansmann U, Golder W, et al. Prospective, randomized, multicenter trial on the antiproliferative effect of lanreotide, interferon alfa, and their combination for therapy of metastatic neuroendocrine gastroenteropancreatic tumors--the International Lanreotide and Interferon Alfa Study Group. J Clin Oncol. 2003;21(14):2689–96.
100. Arnold R, Rinke A, Klose KJ, Muller HH, Wied M, Zamzow K, et al. Octreotide versus octreotide plus interferon-alpha in endocrine gastro-

enteropancreatic tumors: a randomized trial. Clin Gastroenterol Hepatol. 2005;3(8):761–71.
101. Pavel ME, Hainsworth JD, Baudin E, Peeters M, Horsch D, Winkler RE, et al. Everolimus plus octreotide long-acting repeatable for the treatment of advanced neuroendocrine tumors associated with carcinoid syndrome (RADIANT-2): a randomised, placebo-controlled, phase 3 study. Lancet (London, England). 2011;378(9808):2005–12.
102. Yao JC, Fazio N, Singh S, Buzzoni R, Carnaghi C, Wolin E, et al. Everolimus for the treatment of advanced, non-functional neuroendocrine tumors of the lung or gastrointestinal tract (RADIANT-4): a randomised, placebo-controlled, phase 3 study. Lancet (London, England). 2016;387(10022):968–77.
103. Pavel M, Valle JW, Eriksson B, Rinke A, Caplin M, Chen J, et al. ENETS consensus guidelines for the standards of care in neuroendocrine neoplasms: systemic therapy – biotherapy and novel targeted agents. Neuroendocrinology. 2017;105(3):266–80.
104. Hicks RJ, Kwekkeboom DJ, Krenning E, Bodei L, Grozinsky-Glasberg S, Arnold R, et al. ENETS consensus guidelines for the standards of care in neuroendocrine neoplasia: peptide receptor radionuclide therapy with radiolabeled somatostatin analogues. Neuroendocrinology. 2017;105(3):295–309.
105. Strosberg J, El-Haddad G, Wolin E, Hendifar A, Yao J, Chasen B, et al. Phase 3 trial of (177)Lu-Dotatate for midgut neuroendocrine tumors. N Engl J Med. 2017;376(2):125–35.
106. Pavel M, Baudin E, Couvelard A, Krenning E, Oberg K, Steinmuller T, et al. ENETS consensus guidelines for the management of patients with liver and other distant metastases from neuroendocrine neoplasms of foregut, midgut, hindgut, and unknown primary. Neuroendocrinology. 2012;95(2):157–76.
107. de Baere T, Deschamps F, Tselikas L, Ducreux M, Planchard D, Pearson E, et al. GEP-NETS update: interventional radiology: role in the treatment of liver metastases from GEP-NETs. Eur J Endocrinol. 2015;172(4):R151–66.
108. Kotteas EA, Syrigos KN, Saif MW. Profile of capecitabine/temozolomide combination in the treatment of well-differentiated neuroendocrine tumors. Onco Targets Ther. 2016;9:699–704.
109. Anthony L, Ervin C, Lapuerta P, Kulke MH, Kunz P, Bergsland E, et al. Understanding the patient experience with carcinoid syndrome: exit interviews from a randomized, placebo-controlled study of telotristat ethyl. Clin Ther. 2017;39(11):2158–68.
110. Kulke MH, Horsch D, Caplin ME, Anthony LB, Bergsland E, Oberg K, et al. Telotristat ethyl, a tryptophan hydroxylase inhibitor for the treatment of carcinoid syndrome. J Clin Oncol. 2017;35(1):14–23.
111. Pavel M, Gross DJ, Benavent M, Perros P, Srirajaskanthan R, Warner RRP, et al. Telotristat ethyl in carcinoid syndrome: safety and efficacy in the TELECAST phase 3 trial. Endocr Relat Cancer. 2018;25(3):309–22.
112. Garcia-Carbonero R, Sorbye H, Baudin E, Raymond E, Wiedenmann B, Niederle B, et al. ENETS consensus guidelines for high-grade gastroenteropancreatic neuroendocrine tumors and neuroendocrine carcinomas. Neuroendocrinology. 2016;103(2):186–94.
113. Luis SA, Pellikka PA. Carcinoid heart disease: diagnosis and management. Best Pract Res Clin Endocrinol Metab. 2016;30(1):149–58.
114. Le Roux C, Lombard-Bohas C, Delmas C, Dominguez-Tinajero S, Ruszniewski P, Samalin E, et al. Relapse factors for ileal neuroendocrine tumors after curative surgery: a retrospective French multicentre study. Dig Liver Dis. 2011;43(10):828–33.

115. Dieckhoff P, Runkel H, Daniel H, Wiese D, Koenig A, Fendrich V, et al. Well-differentiated neuroendocrine neoplasia: relapse-free survival and predictors of recurrence after curative intended resections. Digestion. 2014;90(2):89–97.

116. Knigge U, Capdevila J, Bartsch DK, Baudin E, Falkerby J, Kianmanesh R, et al. ENETS consensus recommendations for the standards of care in neuroendocrine neoplasms: follow-up and documentation. Neuroendocrinology. 2017;105(3):310–9.

Large Intestine NETs

Rafael H. Pérez-Soto, Alicia M. Trolle-Silva, and Miguel F. Herrera

Contents

A. L. Shifrin et al. (eds.), *Endocrine Surgery Comprehensive Board Exam Guide*,
https://doi.org/10.1007/978-3-030-84737-1_30

Case Presentation

A 56-year-old man came to the outpatient clinic complaining of constipation, change in bowel habits, night sweats, and right-upper quadrant abdominal pain for the last 3 months. His past medical history included a recent diagnosis of type-2 diabetes mellitus treated with oral hypoglycemic agents. No family history of cancer was present. Physical examination showed a pulse of 96 bpm, with the rest of vital signs within normal range. He was pale and presented painful hepatomegaly. A firm, right-sided rectal mass 5 cm from the anal verge was found at digital rectal examination, with a positive fecal occult blood test. No murmurs were identified in chest examination. Initial laboratory workup was performed with the following results: hemoglobin 9.7 g/dL (14.5–17.7 g/dL), hematocrit 29% (42.6–52.6%), mean corpuscular volume of 90.3 fL (83.5–96.5 fL), mean corpuscular hemoglobin concentration 33.4% (32.8–34.9%), white blood cells 3700 c/mm^3 (4000–12,000 c/mm^3), neutrophils 78.9% (40–85%), lymphocytes 11.7% (12–46%), glucose 102 mg/dL (70–99 mg/dL), creatinine 0.33 mg/dL (0.7–1.3 mg/dL), serum sodium 133 mEq/L (126–146 mEq/L), total bilirubin 0.76 mg/dL (0.3–1.0 mg/dL), alkaline phosphatase 258 U/L (34–104 U/L), alanine aminotransferase 56.8 U/L (7–52 U/L), aspartate aminotransferase 27 U/L (13–39 U/L), and albumin 3 g/dL (3.5–5.7 g/dL). A contrast-enhanced CT scan of the abdominopelvic cavity was performed (▣ Fig. 30.1), showing a right-sided rectal mass with extension to the perirectal fat tissue and a heterogenous large mass in the right lobe of the liver, suggestive of metastatic disease (▣ Fig. 30.2).

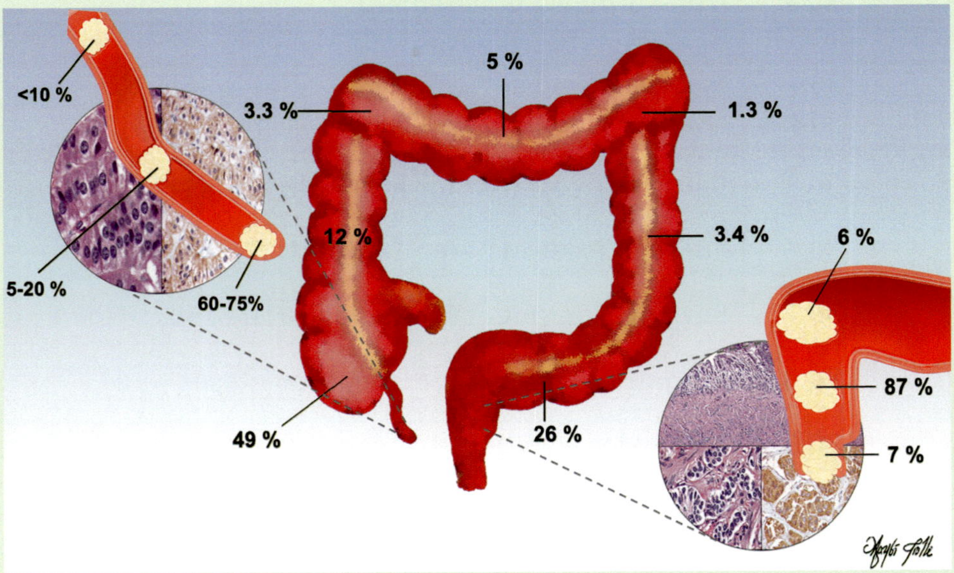

▣ **Fig. 30.1** Location distribution of large intestine neuroendocrine tumors [14, 33, 61]

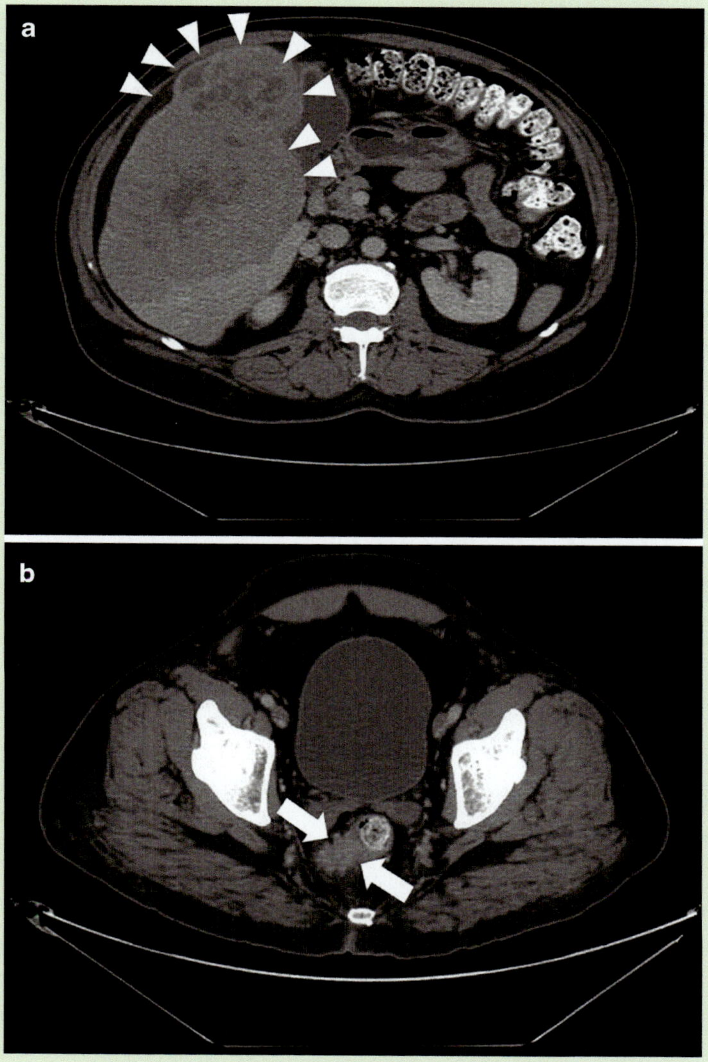

Fig. 30.2 Computed tomography axial slices of the patient. **a** Shows a mass in the right lobe of the liver suggestive of metastatic disease (white arrowheads). **b** White arrows point to a rectal mass with mesorectal and fat tissue invasion, which seems to be the primary tumor

Questions

1. Which of the following histological features of an appendix neuroendocrine tumor are considered risk factors for aggressive disease?
   1. Mesoappendix invasion
   2. Lymphovascular invasion
   3. Chromogranin A positive immunohistochemistry
   4. High Ki67 index
      - (a) Only 1) and 2) are correct
      - (b) Only 1) is correct
      - (c) Only 1) and 4) are correct
      - (d) Only 1) and 2) and 4) are correct
      - (e) All are correct
2. What is (are) the best surgical treatment for a 33-year-old male with a diagnosis of a neuroendocrine tumor of the appendix located in the base with no evidence of distant metastatic disease?
   1. Active surveillance
   2. Right hemicolectomy
   3. *En bloc* resection of appendix and mesoappendix
   4. Simple appendectomy
      - (a) Only 4) is correct
      - (b) Only 1) and 4) are correct
      - (c) Only 2) is correct
      - (d) Only 3) and 4) are correct
      - (e) All are correct
3. In which of the following patients determination of 24-hour urinary 5-HIAA is NOT indicated:
   1. 43-year-old man with a neuroendocrine tumor of the appendix, and heart failure symptoms
   2. 53-year-old woman with a rectal neuroendocrine tumor
   3. 60-year-old man with a neuroendocrine tumor of sigmoid colon and liver metastatic disease
   4. 45-year-old woman with a rectal neuroendocrine tumor and abnormally elevated serum Chromogranin A
      - (a) Only 1) and 3) are correct
      - (b) Only 2) and 3) and 4) are correct
      - (c) Only 3) and 4) are correct
      - (d) Only 1) is correct
      - (e) All are correct
4. What is the most appropriate management for a 45-year-old man surgically treated of appendectomy for acute appendicitis with a histopathological report consisting of a neuroendocrine tumor <1 cm located at the tip, with a Ki67% >3%, with no lymphovascular invasion, deep mesoappendix invasion, and positive surgical margins?
   1. Anatomical or functional imaging for staging
   2. No further evaluation
   3. Complementary right colectomy
   4. Colonoscopy

   (a) Only 2) is correct
   (b) Only 1) and 3) and 4) are correct
   (c) Only 1) and 4) are correct
   (d) Only 1) and 3) are correct
   (e) All are correct

5. Which of the following resection techniques are alternative treatments for a 45-year-old male with a 9 mm rectal neuroendocrine tumor located 5 cm from the anal verge and limited to the submucosa?
   1. Polypectomy
   2. Endoscopic mucosal resection
   3. Endoscopic submucosal resection
   4. Transanal endoscopic microsurgery
      (a) Only 4) is correct
      (b) Only 1) and 2) and 4) are correct
      (c) Only 2) and 3) are correct
      (d) Only 1) is correct
      (e) All are correct
6. In which of the following patients with an appendix neuroendocrine tumor, a right hemicolectomy is the most appropriate surgical treatment?
   1. Base located NET with mesoappendix invasion
   2. Tip located NET < 1 cm, with a G1-G2 histology
   3. Goblet cell variant NET, lesion <1 cm
   4. Body located NET with Ki67 of 10%
      (a) Only 3) and 1) are correct
      (b) Only 3) is correct
      (c) Only 1) and 3) and 4) are correct
      (d) Only 1) and 2) are correct
      (e) All are correct
7. Which of the following statements is (are) true regarding prophylactic cholecystectomy in patients with neuroendocrine tumors?
   1. Patients with prophylactic cholecystectomy have inferior rates of complications associated with gallbladder disease
   2. It is not recommended for patients who may receive liver-directed therapies due to advanced neuroendocrine tumors
   3. Performing prophylactic cholecystectomy during primary tumor resection surgical procedure increases the rate of complications and mortality
   4. Prophylactic cholecystectomy is recommended for patients who may receive long-term Telistrat treatment
      (a) Only 1) is true
      (b) Only 1) and 3) are true
      (c) Only 1) and 2) and 3) are true
      (d) Only 1) and 4) are true
      (e) All are true

8. Which of the following rectal NETs is (are) candidate (s) for endoscopic resection?
   1. Rectal NET of 1.5 cm, limited to submucosa
   2. A 2 cm rectal NET invading the *muscularis propria* with no lymphadenopathies or distant metastases
   3. NET of 1.4 cm with N1 lymphadenopathy
   4. 1.3 cm rectal NET at 3 cm from the anal verge, limited to submucosa
      (a) Only 4) is correct
      (b) Only 1) and 4) are correct
      (c) Only 1) and 2) and 4) are correct
      (d) Only 1) and 3) are correct
      (e) All are correct
9. Which of the following studies are required to properly stage a patient with a rectal neuroendocrine tumor >2 cm identified in a screening sigmoidoscopy?
   1. Complete colonoscopy
   2. Pelvic magnetic resonance imaging
   3. Endorectal ultrasound
   4. Chest/abdomen/pelvic CT scan
      (a) Only 2) and 3) are correct
      (b) Only 2) and 3) and 4) are correct
      (c) Only 1) and 3) are correct
      (d) Only 1) and 2 are correct
      (e) All are correct
10. According to the NET location within the colon, which of the following sequences (order from the highest to the lowest incidence rate) is correct?
   1. Sigmoid colon, cecum, ascending colon, transverse colon, descending colon
   2. Cecum, sigmoid colon, ascending colon, transverse colon, descending colon
   3. Cecum, ascending colon, transverse colon, descending colon, sigmoid colon
   4. Transverse colon, sigmoid colon, cecum, ascending colon, descending colon
      (a) Only 1) is correct
      (b) Only 3) is correct
      (c) Only 2) is correct
      (d) Only 4) is correct
      (e) None is correct
11. Regarding the use of Chromogranin A measurements for the diagnosis of large intestine NETs, the following sentences are true:
   1. Chromogranin A can help to distinguish between a well-differentiated appendix carcinoid tumor from a more aggressive histology
   2. Chromogranin A is a specific biochemical marker for appendix NETs

3. Chromogranin A has a direct association with tumor burden
4. Chromogranin A has no role during follow-up
   (a) Only 1) and 4) are true
   (b) Only 2) and 3) are true
   (c) Only 1) and 2) and 3) are true
   (d) Only 1) and 3) are true
   (e) All are true

30.1 Incidence and Presentation

Large intestine neuroendocrine tumors (NETs) comprehend a wide spectrum of neoplasms arising from the diffuse neuroendocrine system located in the appendix, ascending, transverse, and descending colon, as well as the rectum. As a consequence of the wide distribution of these tumors within the colon and the different embryologic origin (midgut for ascending colon and appendix neuroendocrine tumors, and hindgut for transverse, descending colon and rectum), their clinical scenario and the biochemical profile may be different depending on their location [1, 2].

The estimated incidence rate (IR) of neuroendocrine tumors in the appendix (aNETs) ranges from 0.09 to 0.4/100,000 persons, being this location one of the most frequent places for gastrointestinal neuroendocrine tumors. Female patients have an IR twice as much as males with higher incidence rates in younger ages (15–19 years for women and 20–29 years for men) [3–5]. The most common presentation of aNETs is acute appendicitis, but patients can also present with intermittent vague abdominal pain in the right lower quadrant. In 0.2% of the appendectomy specimens, aNETs are found incidentally at histology [5, 6]. Carcinoid syndrome is rare and occurs when patients develop liver metastases. Metastatic disease at diagnosis has been described in only 3% of the patients. Larger tumor size and mesoappendiceal invasion are predictive factors for liver metastases [7, 8].

The IR of NETs of the colon, from cecum to sigmoid, ranges from 0.04 to 0.15 per 100,000 persons, with a predominance on the right side. The mean age at diagnosis is 63.3 years in the USA (range from 63 to 68 years), which is higher than the age of presentation in Europe and Asia [3, 9]. The most common clinical scenarios of these NETs are gastrointestinal bleeding, change in bowel habits, non-specific abdominal pain, and weight loss. Symptomatic patients often have tumors larger than 2 cm. This late presentation is responsible for locoregional and distant metastasis at diagnosis in up to two-thirds of the patients. Patients with advanced locoregional disease may develop bowel obstruction and anemia. Carcinoid syndrome occurs in the presence of liver metastases and occurs in approximately 5% of the patients at the time of diagnosis [9, 10].

The rectum is the third most common location for gastrointestinal NETs with an estimated IR of 1.04 per 100,000 persons [11]. Mean age at diagnosis is 56 years. Although rectal bleeding, tenesmus, pain, and bowel habit changes are the most frequent symptoms, screening colonoscopy programs have increased the detection of small lesions (<1 cm) in asymptomatic patients. Early detection has increased the 5-year survival rate by 20%. Serotonin production is rare in rectal NETs; thus, the carcinoid syndrome is not a frequent clinical presentation. In advanced disease, bowel obstruction and systemic symptoms may appear [10, 12, 13]. The distribution of NETs within the large intestine is shown in ◘ Fig. 30.1.

30.2 Diagnosis

When aNETs are found incidentally after an appendectomy, the diagnostic workup is usually implemented after the initial treatment, and it is focused on staging and follow-up. Laboratory tests include Chromogranin A (CgA) as a non-specific biochemical marker for NETs, and 24-hour urinary 5-hydroxy-indol-acetic-acid (5-HIAA) when carcinoid syndrome is suspected. CgA measurement is recommended in patients with advanced or metastatic aNETs, and no role for diagnosis or follow-up has been validated. However, CgA plays an important role in differential diagnosis between aNETs and appendix goblet cell carcinoma. Imaging studies aim to detect lymph node or distant metastasis, and their use depends on the initial tumor size and risk factors for aggressive behavior. Cross-sectional imaging studies of the abdomen (CT or MRI) are recommended for patients with aNETs between 1 and 2 cm, especially if they have grade 2 histology, they are located at the base of the appendix, and there is deep mesoappendiceal infiltration or vascular/lymphatic invasion. For tumors >2 cm with deep mesoappendiceal infiltration or vascular invasion, aside from cross-sectional imaging, functional imaging (somatostatin receptor scintigraphy or PET/CT) is recommended. For patients with well-differentiated aNETs <1 cm and R0 resection, no further investigation is needed. Colonoscopy has no major role in the follow-up of aNETs [15–17].

Histopathological diagnosis of aNETs must include immunohistochemistry for CgA and synaptophysin. The mitotic count, the Ki-67 index, the evaluation of vascular/lymphatic invasion, surgical margins, histological grading, and the classification according to the WHO, ENETS, and AJCC pTNM systems must be properly reported [17, 18].

Diagnostic workup for suspected colon NETs must include measurements of CgA. It helps to establish the disease burden and the follow-up of patients with advanced or metastatic disease. Full colonoscopy to exclude synchronous tumors and a cross-sectional imaging study of the chest, abdomen, and pelvis are needed. Measurement of 5-HIAA is indicated when there are symptoms of carcinoid syndrome. Functional imaging such as Indium-111 octreotide scan and gallium-68 (Ga-68) DOTA octreotide (ate) PET have a primary role in the identification of metastatic disease. Fluorodeoxyglucose (FDG) PET is preferred over other functional imaging modalities in patients with histologically proven high-grade/poorly differentiated NETs. Abdominal ultrasound (US) can be used to assess liver metastases [9, 19, 20].

Rectal NETs are incidental findings in approximately 40% of lower gastrointestinal tract endoscopies. There are two possible scenarios: (a) the diagnosis of a NET in a specimen of polypectomy. In this case, if an R0 resection is performed, the tumor is less than 10 mm and has a low Ki67 index, no further workup is needed, and (b) the finding of a tumor in which the biopsy makes the diagnosis of a NET. This scenario allows for preoperative/pre-resection staging and planning. A full colonoscopy should be performed to identify concomitant colonic disease or synchronous tumors. Endorectal ultrasound (EUS) and pelvic MRI are useful to evaluate tumor size, depth, invasion, and lymph node disease, and additional imaging modalities such as chest/abdomen/pelvic CT scan or functional imaging studies are indicated when tumor size >2 cm or distant metastatic disease is suspected. Tattooing of the tumor site is recommended to facilitate future identification [20–22].

In terms of biochemical markers, CgA has a value in the patient's follow-up, particularly for metastatic rectal NETs. Determinations of 5-HIAA are useful when the carcinoid syndrome is present. Other serum markers, such as acid phosphatase, pancreatic polypeptide, and ß-HCG, have limited value [20, 23].

In addition, patients with carcinoid syndrome and clinical suspicion of cardiac involvement (cardiac murmurs or raised brain natriuretic peptide or pro-b-type natriuretic peptide, etc.) should undergo echocardiographic evaluation, as tricuspid valve thickening and retraction are common findings [24].

30.3 Treatment

30.3.1 Preoperative Management

General anesthesia and major surgical procedures are well-known factors for carcinoid crisis in patients with serotonin-secreting NETs. Patients may present severe hypotension, flushing, bronchospasm, and arrhythmias as a result of the rapid release of vasoactive hormones by the tumor into the bloodstream [25]. Intravenous octreotide before the induction of anesthesia may prevent the crisis [26]. Despite octreotide administration, physicians should be prepared for the use of vasopressor agents [27].

30.3.2 Prophylactic Cholecystectomy

Patients with a preoperative diagnosis of appendiceal or colorectal NETs, who require surgical treatment for advanced or metastatic disease or in whom long-term medical therapy with somatostatin analogs (SSA) is planned, might benefit from prophylactic cholecystectomy. This recommendation becomes stronger if the patient is likely to receive radiofrequency ablation or hepatic artery embolization for liver metastatic disease [28, 29]. The recommendation is supported by data from Norlén et al. that shows a 63% incidence of gallbladder stones with SSA treatment with a 15% incidence of gallbladder-related complications [30]. In addition, the risk of postoperative morbidity and mortality is not increased in patients undergoing primary tumor resection plus prophylactic cholecystectomy [31].

30.3.3 Endoscopic Management

Endoscopic resection is feasible for rectal NETs. Indications for local resection through endoscopic approach include lesions <1 cm and tumors between 1 and 2 cm with low mitotic index and without invasion to the *muscularis propria*. Endoscopic techniques for rectal NETs resection include traditional polypectomy, endoscopic mucosal resection with or without submucosal dissection, and band ligation. After endoscopic resection, assessment of risk factors and histological evaluation of the specimen are imperative for further management [21, 32, 33]. Pros and cons regarding endoscopic techniques for rectal NETs resection are displayed in ◘ Table 30.1 [34]. Endoscopic treatment is not recommended for appendiceal and colonic NETs.

30.3.4 Carcinoid Syndrome Management

Due to the fact that 80% of carcinoid tumors express somatostatin receptors, SSA are the main medical treatment for carcinoid syndrome (CS) symptoms. This group of drugs includes Octreotide, Sandostatin, and Lanreotide. In addition to the inhibitory effect of SSA on TNEs cells secretion, these medications have proven to inhibit tumor growth. Telotistrat, an oral tryptophan hydroxylase inhibitor, is another pharmacologic therapy approved by the FDA for CS treatment in

Table 30.1 Advantages and disadvantages of endoscopic techniques for rectal NETs resection

Technique	Advantages	Disadvantages
Polypectomy	Simple procedure, short procedural time, low risk for complications	High rate of incomplete resection
Endoscopic mucosal resection	Simple procedure, short procedural time, low risk for complications	Complete resection (30–70%)
Endoscopic submucosal dissection	Complete resection (80–100%)	Long procedural time, high risk for complications, increased cost, and length of stay

combination with SSA. The use of this agent has been limited for adult patients with refractory diarrhea associated with CS. Interferon has antitumor effects through induction of cell cycle arrest and inhibition of angiogenesis and has been used as an alternative option for the treatment of refractory CS. Dietary modifications avoiding simple carbohydrates, restricting fat consumption, and increasing fiber consumption, the use of Cholestyramine, Colestipol, or Colesevelam, antidiarrheal agents (loperamide, diphenoxylate), and other agents such as Ondansetron or Cyproheptadine have been useful in patients with refractory diarrhea due to CS [24, 35].

Peptide receptor radionuclide therapy (PRRT) has shown to be superior to long-acting release octreotide therapy for CS-related symptoms and should be considered as an option for refractory cases. A more aggressive treatment for refractory CS includes liver metastasis-directed therapies such as cytoreductive surgery, radiofrequency ablation, radioembolization, transarterial embolization, and transarterial chemoembolization [35].

30.4 Non-surgical Management of Metastatic Disease

30.4.1 Systemic Treatment

Numerous drugs have been proven to improve progression-free survival in patients with metastatic NETs. Therefore, these medications are commonly used for the treatment of liver-metastatic NETs patients, despite their limited impact on overall survival. A summary of these drugs, mechanism of action, and side effects are shown in Table 30.2 [36, 37].

Table 30.2 Systemic treatment drugs for neuroendocrine tumors

Group	Drugs	Mechanism	Side Effects
First-generation somatostatin receptor ligands	**Octreotide Lanreotide**	Binds to somatostatin receptors in NET cells, inhibiting secretion and growth (SSTR 2 primarily)	Nausea, abdominal discomfort, loose stools, gallstones, and gallbladder dysfunction
Mammalian target of rapamycin inhibition	**Everolimus**	Regulation of cell proliferation, metabolism and survival of cells through mTOR signaling pathway	Pneumonitis, thrombocytopenia, stomatitis, rash, diarrhea, renal failure, peripheral edema, hyperglycemia
Vascular endothelial growth factor (VEGF) receptor inhibitor	**Sunitinib**	Inhibition of multiple tyrosine kinase receptors	Diarrhea, nausea, vomiting, fatigue, and hypertension
Monoclonal antibody for VEGF	**Bevacizumab**	Inhibition of VEGF and VEGF receptor interaction	Diarrhea, nausea, vomiting, mouth sores, headache, dry mouth and eyes, hypertension
Interferon	**Interferon alpha**	Effects on cell proliferation, apoptosis, differentiation, and angiogenesis	Pyrexia, fatigues, anorexia, depression, weight loss, flu-like symptoms, myelosuppression, thyroid dysfunction, polymyalgia
Tryptophan hydroxylase inhibitors	**Telistrat**	Inhibition of serotonin synthesis through tryptophan hydroxylase inhibition	Nausea, vomiting, constipation, anorexia, elevated transaminases and gamma-glutamyltransferase, depression, pyrexia, headache, flatulence, peripheral edema
Next-generation somatostatin receptor ligands	**Pasireotide**	Binds to somatostatin receptors in NET cells, inhibiting secretion and growth (SSTR 1, 3, and 5)	Hyperglycemia
Peptide radionuclide therapy (PRRT)	^{177}**Lu-dotatate**	Directed radiation injury to NET cells	Liver toxicity, myelodysplastic syndrome, leukemia, cytopenia, infertility, acute renal injury, carcinoid syndrome crisis

30

30.4.2 Liver-Directed Therapy

Liver-directed therapy can be classified into two groups, the locally ablative techniques and the angiographic techniques. The former group includes radiofrequency, microwave, laser, and cryotherapy ablations. Radiofrequency ablation (RA) therapy is the most commonly used technique for NETs liver metastases, with proven effectiveness for rapidly improving carcinoid syndrome symptoms and survival. Microwave ablation has comparable efficacy to RA, with lesser procedural time with a 5-year survival rate of 37–57%. Patients with unresectable NET liver metastases with dominant liver lesions <5 cm are candidates for these therapies. Both are safe for palliative care, with the possibility of repeated sessions. Angiographic techniques include transarterial embolization (TAE), transarterial chemoembolization (TACE), and selective internal radiotherapy (SIRT). Their main indication is hypervascular liver metastases, and they have also shown to reduce progression and overall survival [37–39]. Regarding SIRT, multiple prospective studies have shown symptom response rates from 50 to 61% with survival rates between 15 and 29.4 months [40, 41]. Angiographic techniques are recommended for patients with well-differentiated NETs, and a better response is obtained with limited hepatic tumor burden (<50%) and no extrahepatic disease.

30.5 Surgical Treatment for Appendix NETs

For diagnosed patients with aNETs, surgical treatment extension depends on known risk factors for aggressive behavior. According to current guidelines, simple appendectomy (SA) is sufficient for aNETs with less than 1 cm. Right hemicolectomy (RH) is reserved for patients with any of the following:

(a) Appendix base located NET
(b) Incomplete surgical margins
(c) Lymphovascular or mesoappendix invasion
(d) Intermediate or high-grade tumors
(e) Goblet cell carcinoid variant

For aNETs >2 cm, RH is the standard surgical treatment. Controversy still exists in the group of patients with tumors between 1 and 2 cm. SA may be sufficient when the following criteria are absent:

(a) Base or caecum invasion
(b) Positive surgical margins
(c) Lymphovascular or mesoappendix invasion
(d) High Ki67 index (≥3%)
(e) High or intermediate-grade tumors
(f) Mixed histology (goblet cell carcinoid)

When tumor size cannot be determined, RH is advised [17, 42–44]. Patients in need of RH should receive an oncologic RH procedure, meaning *en bloc* resection with a division of supplying arteries close to the superior mesenteric artery in order to include the regional lymph nodes [45].

In most patients treated for acute appendicitis, the appendix is skeletonized during laparoscopic appendectomy, leaving the mesoappendix in situ. Some authors have advised to include the mesoappendix in the *en bloc* resection of the appendix in all patients for better staging and decision-making regarding the need for further surgery when an aNET is incidentally diagnosed in the specimen of a laparoscopic appendectomy [46].

30.6 Surgical Treatment for Colonic NETs

Colon NETs are more aggressive and have worse survival compared with appendiceal and rectal NETs. This is in part due to more advanced disease (tumor >2 cm and *muscularis propria* invasion). Surgical treatment recommendations for colonic NETs are similar to those regarding colonic adenocarcinomas. Patients with colonic NETs without evidence of distant metastasis should undergo open or laparoscopic segmental colonic resection with lymphadenectomy. In the presence of metastatic disease, palliative resection (hemicolectomy plus lymphadenectomy) or maximal cytoreduction should be offered with previous multidisciplinary evaluation. Multiple organ resections including segmental colectomy plus lymphadenectomy are advised for patients with adjacent organ invasion when an R0 resection is feasible. In patients with metastatic disease and clinical or impending bowel obstruction, surgical bowel diversion or tumor resection is recommended for palliative purposes [32, 33, 47].

Regarding endoscopic resection of colonic NETs, there is no clear recommendation. ENETS guidelines mention endoscopic polypectomy and endoscopic mucosal resection for colonic NETs <2 cm as therapy options, encouraging surgical oncological resection for grade 3 or incomplete resected tumors [20, 26, 47].

30.7 Surgical Treatment for Rectal NETs

There are many factors involved in the surgical treatment of rectal NETs. These include tumor location, size, staging, and histopathological features. The most common surgical options include transanal endoscopic microsurgery (TEM), low anterior resection (LAR), and abdominoperineal resection (APR) [33].

TEM is a minimally invasive surgical technique performed through a multi-channel transanal port using CO_2 insufflation and endosurgical instruments. The endoscopic optical equipment allows a magnified view of the surgical field. Surgical steps in the TEM resection are (a) delimitation of the area of resection, (b) full-thickness resection (down to the outer fatty tissue), and (c) rectal defect closure. Indications for TEM include tumors <1 cm, distal rectal tumors between 1 and 2 cm confined to the submucosa, and for patients with tumors invading the *muscularis propria*, but without evidence of lymph node metastasis by EUS or MRI. TEM has been also used to remove positive surgical margins after purely endoscopic resections [19, 21, 33, 48–50].

Rectal NETs >2 cm should be treated similarly as adenocarcinomas. The choice between LAR, extended low anterior resection (eLAR), and APR mainly relies on tumor location within the rectum. Lesions located in the middle or upper rectum can be treated with a LAR. LAR procedure requires sigmoid colon and rectum mobilization, ligation, and division of the inferior mesenteric vessels, followed by rectum transection 5 cm distal to the tumor and further reconstruction through a hand-sewn or circular stapling device anastomosis. Tumors located at 2 cm from the anal sphincter can be resected by eLAR, which follows the same steps of LAR but requires a more distal dissection to the level of the elevator ani muscle. The APR procedure is reserved for rectal tumors located very low. The main oncological principle of these surgical techniques is total mesorectal excision [10, 12, 51].

30.8 Surgical Treatment for Liver Metastases

Liver metastases of NETs treatment are commonly treated by nonanatomic metastasectomies, and in selected cases, liver transplantation. Criteria for resection include:

(a) Grade 1 or 2 NETs
(b) No evidence of non-resectable extrahepatic disease
(c) Possible R0 or R1 liver resection, sparing at least 30% of liver remnant
(d) No right heart failure (carcinoid heart disease)
(e) Access to an experience center

Hepatic resection is not recommended for most poorly differentiated liver metastasis from NET. In patients with a primary tumor and concomitant liver metastasis at diagnosis, a one- or two-step surgical approach is selected depending on the tumor and patient characteristics. After an R0/R1 hepatic resection, survival rates at 5 years range from 46 to 86% and 35 to 79% at 10 years [52–55].

Liver metastatic NET is one of the few indications for liver transplantation in malignant disease. Factors such as effectiveness of the therapy, shortage of donor organs, and recurrence of liver disease in the graft induce significant controversy to the indication. Several criteria have been suggested to consider patients as candidates for a liver transplant [21, 38, 52, 56]. Here are two sets of guidelines:

Milan criteria:

(a) Histological diagnosis of low-grade NET regardless of the presence or absence of syndrome
(b) Primary tumor located in the pancreas or intermediate gut (distal stomach to sigmoid colon), thereby tributary of the portal vein, already removed with a curative resection
(c) Less than 50% of liver involvement
(d) Stable disease for at least 6 months during the pre-transplantation period
(e) Age <55 years

ENETS guidelines:
(a) Well-differentiated NET with Ki67 index ≤10%
(b) Primary tumor removed at least 6 months prior to transplantation
(c) Less than 50% of liver involvement or <75% of liver involvement in patients with refractory hormonal symptoms
(d) Stable disease for at least 6 months
(e) Age <55 years
(f) Diffuse unresectable disease confined to the liver – robust extrahepatic exclusion

30.9 Follow-Up

Follow-up for >2 cm colorectal NETs is compulsory. Grade 1 or grade 2 tumors require at least a colonoscopy or an imaging study and CgA determinations within the first year and then annually; follow-up for G3 tumors is recommended every 4–6 months in the first 12 months and then annually. For tumors between 1 and 2 cm independently of histological grade and tumors <1 cm with histological grade 3, colonoscopy is advised every 12 months. In patients with tumors <1 cm without lymph node disease and no invasion of the *muscularis propria*, further follow-up after the curative treatment is not recommended [20, 32].

For aNET, follow-up is recommended if the tumor measures between 1 and 2 cm and has nodal metastases, lymphovascular or mesoappendix invasion, intermediate or high-grade histology, or an aggressive variant (goblet cell carcinoid, adenocarcinoid). Although the follow-up schedule for these patients has not been clearly described, aNETs >2 cm, tumors with distant metastasis or incomplete resections, should be initially followed 3 to 6 months after treatment, and then every 6 to 12 months. No further follow-up is needed for well-differentiated aNETs <2 cm with complete resection and the absence of negative prognostic factors [17, 42].

30.10 Prognosis

aNETs discovered after surgical treatment for acute appendicitis enjoy a very good prognosis. When a localized disease is present, 5-year overall survival ranges between 95 and 100%, decreasing to 75–100% and 25% with regional disease and distant metastases, respectively [3, 33]. Goblet cell variant tumor has a worse prognosis, and staging of these tumors is performed based on the criteria for appendiceal adenocarcinomas. Estimated overall mean survival for goblet cell tumor is

43 months, with a 10-year survival of 78%, 33%, and 4% for low-grade, intermediate grade, and high grade, respectively [57, 58].

From all NETs of the large bowel, colonic neuroendocrine tumors have the worse outcomes. Five-year survival rates for localized, regional, and metastatic disease are 76%, 72%, and 30%, respectively. Estimated median survival for regional and metastatic disease are 52 months and 7 months, respectively [33, 59].

Similar to aNETs, rectal NETs have an excellent prognosis as many are detected incidentally during screening sigmoidoscopy. In fact, rectal NETs have the best overall survival compared with the rest of the gastro-entero-pancreatic NETs. Patients with localized disease have a 5-year survival of 98–100%; for regional and metastatic disease, 5-year survival ranges from 54 to 74% and 15 to 37%, respectively [22, 60].

Answers

1. (d); 2. (c); 3. (b); 4. (d); 5. (e); 6. (c); 7. (a); 8. (b); 9. (e); 10. (c); 11. (d)

References

1. Arnold R. Introduction: definition, historical aspects, classification, staging, prognosis and therapeutic options. Best Pract Res Clin Endocrinol Metab. 2005;19:491–505.
2. Northop JA, Lee JH. Large bowel carcinoid tumors. Curr Opin Gastroenterol. 2007;23(1):74–8.
3. Fraenkel M, Kim MK, Faggiano A, Valk GD. Epidemiology of gastroenteropancreatic neuroendocrine tumours. Best Pract Res Clin Gastroenterol. 2012;26(6):691–703.
4. Amr B, Froghi EM, Haq K, Thengungal-Kochupapy R. Management and outcomes of appendicular neuroendocrine tumours: retrospective review with 5-year follow-up. Eur J Surg Oncol. 2015;41(9):1243–6.
5. Moris D, Tsilimigras DI, Vagios S, Ntanasis-Stathopoulos I, Karachaliou GS, Papalampros A, Alexandrou A, Blazer DG 3rd, Felekouras E. Neuroendocrine neoplasms of the appendix: a review of the literature. Anticancer Res. 2018;38(2):601–11.
6. Şenel F, Karaman H, Demir H. Neuroendocrine tumors detected in appendectomy specimens: ten-year single-center experience. Turk J Med Sci. 2018;48(1):68–73.
7. Riihimaki M, Hemminki A, Sundquist K, Sundquist J, Hemminki K. The epidemiology of metastases in neuroendocrine tumors. Int J Cancer. 2016;139(12):2679–86.
8. Alexandraki KI, Kaltsas GA, Grozinsky-Glasberg S, Chatzellis E, Grossman AB. Appendiceal neuroendocrine neoplasms: diagnosis and management. Endocr Relat Cancer. 2016;23(1):R7–41.
9. Ford MM. Neuroendocrine tumors of the colon and rectum. Dis Colon Rectum. 2017;60(10):1018–20.
10. Mandair D, Caplin ME. Colonic and rectal NET's. Best Pract Res Clin Gastroenterol. 2014;26(6):775–89.

11. Dasari A, Shen C, Halperin D, Zhao B, Zhou S, Xu Y. Trends in the incidence, prevalence, and survical outcomes in patients with neuroendocrine tumors in the United States. JAMA Oncol. 2017;3:1335–42.
12. Bertani E, Ravizza D, Milione M, Massironi S, Grana CM, Zerini D, Fazio N. Neuroendocrine neoplasms of rectum: a management update. Cancer Treat Rev. 2018;66:45–55.
13. Shah R, Nalamati SPM. Neuroendocrine tumors of the colon and rectum. Semin Colon Rectal Surg. 2015;26(2):60–3.
14. Shim KN, Yang SK, Myung SJ, et al. Atypical endoscopic features of rectal carcinoid. Endoscopy. 2004;36(4):313–6.
15. Bednarczuk T, Bolanowski M, Zemczak A, et al. Neuroendocrine neoplasms of the small intestine and appendix-management guidelines (recommended by the Polish Network of Neuroendocrine Tumours). Endokrynol Pol. 2017;68(2):223–36.
16. Toumpanakis C, Fazio N, Janson ET. al. Unmet Needs in Appendiceal Neuroendocrine Neoplasms. Neuroendocrinology. 2019;108(1):37–44.
17. Pape UF, Niederle B, Costa F, et al. ENETS consensus guidelines for neuroendocrine neoplasms of the appendix (excluding goblet cell carcinomas). Neuroendocrinology. 2016;103(2):144–52.
18. Nagtegaal ID, Odze RD, Klimstra D, Paradis V, Rugge M, Schirmacher P, Washington KM, Carneiro F. Cree IA; WHO classification of Tumours Editorial Board. The 2019 WHO classification of tumours of the digestive system. Histopathology. 2020;76(2):182–8.
19. Anthony LB, Strosberg JR, Klimstra DS, Maples WJ, O'Dorisio TM, Warner RRP, Wiseman GA, Benson 3rd AI, Pommier RF, North American Neuroendocrine Tumor Society (NANETS). The NANETS consensus guidelines for the diagnosis and management of gastrointestinal Neuroendocrine Tumors (Nets): well-differentiated nets of the distal colon and rectum. Pancreas. 2010;39(6):767–74.
20. Caplin M, Sundin A, Nillson O, Paum RP, Klose KJ, Kelestimur F, Plöckinger U, Papotti M, Salazar R, Pascher A, all other Bacerlona Consensus Conference participants. ENETS consensus guidelines for the management of patients with digestive neuroendocrine neoplasms: colorectal neuroendocrine neoplasms. Neuroendocrinology. 2012;95:88–97.
21. de Mestier L, Lorenzo D, Fine C, et al. Endoscopic, transanal, laparoscopic, and transabdominal managements of rectal neuroendocrine tumors. Best Pract Res Clin Endocrinol Metab. 2019;33(5):101293.
22. Basuroy R, Haji A, Ramage JK, Quaglia A, Srirajaskanthan R. Review article: the investigation and management of rectal neuroendocrine tumours. Aliment Pharmacol Ther. 2016;44(4):332–45.
23. Kimura N, Sasano N. Prostate-specific acid phosphatase in carcinoid tumors. Virchows Arch A Pathol Anat Histopathol. 1986;410:247–51.
24. Gade AK, Olariu E, Douthit NT. Carcinoid syndrome: a review. Cureus. 2020;12(3):e7186.
25. Clement D, Ramage J, Srirajaskanthan R. Update of pathophysiology, treatment, and complications of carcinoid syndrome. J Oncol. 2020;21:8341426.
26. Kunz PL, Reidy-Lagunes D, Anthony LB, et al. Consensus guidelines for the management and treatment of neuroendocrine tumors. Pancreas. 2013;42(4):557–77.
27. Howe JR, Cardona K, Fraker DL, et al. The surgical management of small bowel neuroendocrine tumors: consensus guidelines of the North American Neuroendocrine Tumor Society. Pancreas. 2017;46(6): 715–31.
28. Liu EH, Solorzado CC, Katznelson L, Vinik AI, Wong R, Randolph G. AACE/ACE disease state clinical review: diagnosis and management of midgut carcinoids. Endocr Pract. 2015;21(5):534–45.
29. Doherty G. Surgical treatment of neuroendocrine tumors (including carcinoid). Curr Opin Endocrinol Diabetes Obes. 2013;20(1):32–6.

30. Norlén O, Hessman O, Stålberg P, Akerström G, Hellman P. Prophylactic cholecystectomy in midgut carcinoid patients. World J Surg. 2010;34(6):1361–7.
31. Sinnamon AJ, Neuwirth MG, Vining CC, et al. Prophylactic cholecystectomy at time of surgery for small bowel neuroendocrine tumor does not increase postoperative morbidity. Ann Surg Oncol. 2018;25(1):239–45.
32. Starzynska T, Londzin-Olesik M. Baldys-Waligórska et al. Colorectal neuroendocrine neoplasms – management guidelines (recommended by the Polish Network of Neuroendocrine Tumours). Endokrynol Pol. 2017;68(2):250–60.
33. Hrabe J. Neuroendocrine tumors of the appendix, colon and rectum. Surg Oncol Clin N Am. 2020;29(2):267–79.
34. Chablaney S, Zator ZA, Kumta NA. Diagnosis and management of rectal neuroendocrine tumors. Clin Endosc. 2017;50(6):530–6.
35. Naraev BG, Halland M, Halperin DM, et al. Management of diarrhea in patients with carcinoid syndrome. Pancreas. 2019;48(8):961–72.
36. Gangi A, Howe JR. The landmark series: neuroendocrine tumor liver metastases. Ann Surg Oncol. 2020; https://doi.org/10.1245/s10434-020-08787-x.
37. Loughrey PB, Zhang D, Heaney AP. New treatments of the carcinoid syndrome. Endocrinol Metab Clin N Am. 2018;47(3):557–76.
38. Frilling A, Clift AK. Therapeutic strategies for neuroendocrine liver metastases. Cancer. 2015;121(8):1172–86.
39. Alexander ES, Soulen MC. Liver metastases from noncolorectal malignancies (neuroendocrine tumor, sarcoma, melanoma, breast). Cancer J. 2016;22(6):381–6.
40. McStay MK, Maudgil D, Williams M, et al. Large-volume liver metastases from neuroendocrine tumors: hepatic intraarterial ^{90}Y-DOTA-lanreotide as effective palliative therapy. Radiology. 2005;237:718–26.
41. King J, Quinn R, Glenn DM, et al. Radioembolization with selective internal radiation microspheres for neuroendocrine liver metastases. Cancer. 2008;113:921–9.
42. Boudreaux KP, Klimstra DS, Hassan MM, et al. The NANETS consensus guidelines for the diagnosis and management of neuroendocrine tumors. Pancreas. 2010;39:753–66.
43. Alexandraki KI, Griniatsos J, Bramis KI, et al. Clinical value of right hemicolectomy for appendiceal carcinoids using pathologic criteria. J Endocrinol Investig. 2011;34:255–9.
44. Mullen JT, Savarese DMF. Carcinoid tumors of the appendix: a population-based study. J Surg Oncol. 2011;104:41–44.
45. Mitchell BG, Mandava N. Hemicolectomy. In: StatPearls(Internet). Treasure Island: StatPearls Publishing; 2020.
46. Davenport E, Courtney ED, Benson-Cooper S, Bissett IP. Appendiceal neuroendocrine neoplasms in the era of laparoscopic appendicectomy. ANZ J Surg. 2014;84(5):337–40.
47. Byrne RM, Pommier RF. Small bowel and colorectal carcinoids. Clin Colon Rectal Surg. 2018;31(5):301–8.
48. Kinoshita R, Kanehira E, Omura K, et al. Transanal endoscopic microsurgery in the treatment of rectal carcinoid tumor. Surg Endosc. 2007;2186:970–4.
49. Chen WJ, Wu N, Zhou JL, et al. Full-thickness excision using transanal endoscopic microsurgery for treatment of rectal neuroendocrine tumors. World J Gastroenterol. 2015;21(30):9142–9.
50. de Mestier L, Brixi H, Gincul R, Ponchon T, Cardiot G. Updating the management of patients with rectal neuroendocrine tumors. Endoscopy. 2013;45(12):1039–46.
51. Rajput A, Bullard-Dunn K. Surgical management of rectal cancer. Semin Oncol. 2007;34(3):241–9.

52. Pavel M, Baudin E, Couvelard A, et al. ENETS consensus guidelines for the management of patient with liver and other distant metastases from neuroendocrine neoplasms of foregut, midgut, hindgut, and unknown primary. Neuron. 2012;95(2):157–76.
53. Frilling A, Modlin IM, Kidd M, et al. Recommendations for management of patients with neuroendocrine liver metastases. Lancet Oncol. 2014;15(1):e8–21.
54. Elias D, Lasser P, Ducreux M, et al. Liver resection (and associated extra-hepatic resections) for metastatic well-differentiated endocrine tumors: a 15-year single center prospective study. Surgery. 2003;133:375–82.
55. Glazer ES, Tseng JF, Al-Refaie W, et al. Long-term survival after surgical management of neuroendocrine hepatic metastases. HPB (Oxford). 2010;12:427–33.
56. Mazzaferro V, Pulvirenti A, Coppa J. Neuroendocrine tumors metastatic to the liver: how to select patients for liver transplantation? J Hepatol. 2007;47:460–6.
57. Sinno SAJ, Jurdi NMH. Goblet cell tumors of the appendix. A review. Ann Diagn Pathol. 2019;43:151401.
58. Tang LH, Shia J, Soslow RA, et al. Pathologic classification and clinical behavior of the spectrum of goblet cell carcinoid tumors of the appendix. Am J Surg Pathol. 2018;32(10):1429–43.
59. Modlin IM, Lye KD, Kidd M. A 5-decade analysis of 13,715 carcinoid tumor. Cancer. 2003;97(4):934–59.
60. Jann H, Roll S, Couvelard A, et al. Neuroendocrine tumor of midgut and hindgut origin: tumor-node-metastasis classification determines clinical outcome. Cancer. 2011;117:3332–41.
61. Lawrence B, Gustafsson BI, Chan A, et al. The epidemiology of gastroenteropancreatic neuroendocrine tumors. Endocrinol Metab Clin N Am. 2011;40(1):1–18.

Surgical Procedure Steps and Key Points: Whipple Procedure, Enucleations, and Management of Complications

Sami Shoucair and Christopher Wolfgang

Contents

A. L. Shifrin et al. (eds.), *Endocrine Surgery Comprehensive Board Exam Guide*,
https://doi.org/10.1007/978-3-030-84737-1_31

Questions

1. A 61-year-old woman is found on MRI to have a 1.3-cm mass, with characteristics of a neuroendocrine tumor in the tail of the pancreas. Which of the following best describes the association of her symptoms with a given type of pancreatic neuroendocrine tumor?
   A. Insulinoma – diabetes, necrolytic migratory erythema
   B. Glucagonoma – hypoglycemia
   C. Somatostatinoma – neuroglycopenic symptoms
   D. Gastrinoma – acid hypersecretion, diarrhea, gastric and duodenal ulcers
2. A 48-year-old man, who is 3 weeks status-post Whipple operation for a 3-cm gastrinoma, now presents with vague abdominal pain and nausea but otherwise able to tolerate PO intake. He reports he feels extremely bloated after each meal and avoids eating for the rest of the day. He denies any fever or chills. A bedside ultrasound performed in the office showed a distended stomach with some surrounding fluid. Surgical drain was removed on postoperative day 4.

   What is the next best step in management?
   A. Insertion of CT-guided percutaneous drain
   B. Order CT scan of the abdomen and pelvis
   C. Surgical revision of gastro-jejunostomy
   D. Course of oral antibiotics and proton pump inhibitor
   E. Recommend small meals and follow-up in 2 weeks
3. Which of the following symptoms or signs is characteristic of the clinical syndrome associated with glucagon-producing islet cell tumors?
   A. Hypoglycemia
   B. Seizures
   C. Hypokalemia
   D. Watery diarrhea
   E. Migratory skin rash
4. A 45-year-old female patient with a previous history of subtotal parathyroidectomy for hyperparathyroidism presents to the emergency department for abdominal pain, nausea, and intermittent diarrhea. A CT scan of the abdomen and pelvis reveals a 2.5-cm mass in the head of the pancreas.

   Which of the following functional neuroendocrine pancreatic tumors is the most likely diagnosis?
   A. Gastrinoma
   B. Insulinoma
   C. Glucagonoma
   D. VIPomas (vasoactive intestinal peptide–secreting tumors)

5. A 50-year-old otherwise healthy woman presents to the ER with complaints of intermittent, voluminous (sometimes 2–3 liters/day), watery, odorless diarrhea for the past several weeks. Vital signs are within normal limits. A CT scan of the abdomen with oral and intravenous contrast was done which shows a 2-cm hyperdense mass in the tail of the pancreas. On blood tests, which of the following is most likely decreased in this patient?
   A. Calcium
   B. Sodium
   C. VIP
   D. Glucose
   E. Potassium
6. A 65-year-old healthy man is diagnosed with a nonfunctioning neuroendocrine tumor in the tail of her pancreas. On CT scan, tumor size is 1 cm, and not close to the main pancreatic duct. There is no evidence of metastatic or locally advanced disease by CT or octreotide scan. EUS-guided FNA of the lesion shows high-grade features and an elevated Ki67. What is the next step in management?
   A. Pancreaticoduodenectomy
   B. Enucleation
   C. Spleen-sparing distal pancreatectomy
   D. Spleen-sparing total pancreatectomy
   E. Distal pancreatectomy with splenectomy
7. Which of the following procedures is associated with an increased likelihood of delayed gastric emptying postoperatively?
   A. Open pancreaticoduodenectomy of a 2-cm gastrinoma
   B. Robotic pancreaticoduodenectomy of a 2.5-cm pancreatic adenocarcinoma
   C. Pylorus preserving pancreaticoduodenectomy of a 4-cm insulinoma
   D. Enucleation of a 3-cm insulinoma of the head of the pancreas
8. A 52-year-old healthy female presents to the office with complaints of nausea, oral ulcers, and 25 lb. weight loss in the past 3 months. She also reports a history of recurrent rash appearing at different locations over her trunk and lower extremities. CT scan of the abdomen and pelvis shows a 1-cm mass in the head of the pancreas with surrounding enlarged lymph nodes. Metastatic workup is negative.

   Which of the following procedures would be the most appropriate step in management?

   A. Neoadjuvant octreotide treatment
   B. Laparoscopic enucleation with drain placement
   C. Open enucleation with drain placement
   D. Pylorus preserving pancreaticoduodenectomy (PPPP)
   E. Classical pancreaticoduodenectomy (PD)
9. During a Whipple procedure, takedown of the ligament of Treitz should be done carefully to avoid injury to:
   A. Left renal vein
   B. Superior mesenteric vein (SMV)
   C. Inferior mesenteric vein (IMV)
   D. First jejunal branch of the SMV
   E. Right gastric artery arising from the gastroduodenal artery (GDA)
10. Which of the following is true regarding imaging modalities used in the diagnostic workup of pancreatic neuroendocrine tumors?
   A. Octreotide scan has a higher sensitivity than 68Ga-DOTA TATE PET/CT scan.
   B. The sensitivity of a Multi-Detector Computed Tomography (MDCT) does not exceed 82% for the detection of PNETs.
   C. There is no role for Magnetic Resonance Imaging (MRI) in the staging of PNETs.
   D. Octreotide scan has a high accuracy in the diagnosis of functional PNETs especially insulinomas.

31.1 Introduction

Pancreatic neoplasms can be broadly classified into exocrine and endocrine neoplasms. The most common neoplasms include the notoriously aggressive pancreatic ductal adenocarcinoma (pancreatic cancer) and cystic neoplasms of the pancreas accounting for 95% of all pancreatic tumors. The remaining 5% consist of pancreatic neuroendocrine tumors (PNETs) [1]. PNET exhibit a spectrum of biological behaviors ranging from indolent and not requiring resection to aggressive undifferentiated tumors. The majority of PNETs are well differentiated, and although can metastasize and cause cancer-specific mortality, are relatively indolent in comparison to pancreatic cancer. PNET further can be classified along the lines of functional and non-functional. The indications for surgical resection of PNETs are complex and beyond the scope of this chapter. Oncologic resection of PNET of the tail and body of the pancreas is removed through a distal pancreatectomy, and those of the head and neck of the pancreas are resected via a pancreaticoduodenectomy (PD; Whipple Operation) [2]. Finally, certain PNETs can be safely enucleated. This is particularly the case for insulinomas and is controversial in other instances. The scope of this chapter will focus on the technical aspects of PD and enucleation.

31.2 Clinical Presentation

Clinical presentation largely depends on whether a PNET is functional or non-functional; this is defined by the association with a clinically recognizable syndrome. With the widespread use of high-resolution imaging, non-functional tumors have recently become more common than functional tumors. Non-functional PNETs do not present with symptoms due to elevation in hormone levels, and the majority is either detected incidentally on imaging or secondary to a mass effect particularly when localized to the head of the pancreas.

Functional PNETs can be associated with a variety of tumor syndromes with specific pancreatic endocrine hormone elevations subsequently leading to a more or less typical presentation.

- Insulinomas are the most common, 90% benign, and arise from β cells of the pancreatic islets of Langerhans. They are typically associated with a diagnostic triad on presentation (Whipple's triad): hypoglycemic symptoms, drop in serum glucose of >50%, and resolution of symptoms with glucose intake/administration.
- Gastrinomas are largely sporadic (75%) with 25% associated with Multiple Neuroendocrine Neoplasia type 1 (MEN-1) and more commonly localized to the head and neck of the pancreas. Patients typically present with epigastric pain, peptic ulcers, GERD, and diarrhea. The pathophysiology is due to gastric acid hypersecretion; thus diarrhea usually improves with insertion of a nasogastric tube. Glucagonomas are malignant in 75% of cases and arise from α cells in body and tail of pancreas. They are characterized by necrolytic migratory erythema, diabetes (insulin resistance), anemia, and weight loss.
- VIPomas (Vasoactive Intestinal Peptide secreting) also known as Verner-Morrison Syndrome are usually malignant with 50% having metastatic disease at the time of presentation. VIP stimulates insulin and inhibits gastrin causing profuse watery diarrhea, hypokalemia, and achlorhydria (WDHA).
- Glucagonomas are characterized by a constellation of common symptoms that are typical of glucagonoma syndrome. New onset diabetes, anemia, stomatitis, and weight loss are commonly seen. A characteristic skin rash, necrolytic migratory erythema, is pathognomonic of glucagonoma and attributed to hypoaminoacidemia. It exhibits cyclic appearance and migrates to different locations with no particular disposition or pattern.
- Somatostatinomas are mostly localized in the pancreatic head and are usually malignant. Symptoms typically include steatorrhea, hyperglycemia, vomiting, and gallstones.

31.3 Pre-operative Evaluation: Diagnostic Imaging and Staging

High volume centers have been demonstrated to offer a superior outcome to patients undergoing complex surgery [3]. Pancreatic resections require a multidisciplinary approach in the pre-operative setting for staging, neoadjuvant therapy, as well as support specialties such as interventional radiology, advanced gastro-enterology, radiation oncology, and others. A multitude of studies showed that pancreatic resections performed in high volume centers had decreased hospital stay, decreased re-admission rates, and superior survival rates compared to low volume centers [4].

1. *Multi-detector Computed Tomography (MDCT)*

Primarily, Multi-Detector Computed Tomography (MDCT) of the abdomen and pelvis has revolutionized the initial evaluation of patients with suspected pancreatic pathology. This imaging modality involves obtaining images with thin sections (<3 mm or less) and no interval gaps. High concentration intravenous contrast (>300 mgI/L) at an injection rate of 3–5 ml/sec is recommended (so-called pancreas protocol CT) [5]. The acquired phases should include a pancreatic parenchymal phase obtained at 40–50 sec and portal venous phase at 65–70 sec after initiation of contrast injection. PNETs are typically hyperdense on the arterial phase and become iso-dense on the later washout phase of imaging. Unfortunately, the accuracy of CT in detecting PNETs remains at 68–82% sensitivity and depends on the size of tumor.

2. *Endoscopic Ultrasonography (EUS) and EUS-Guided Fine Needle Aspiration (FNA)*

Endoscopic ultrasonography (EUS) utilizes ultrasound technology to obtain high-resolution images by passing an endoscope with a high-frequency transducer at its tip. The high sensitivity of EUS in detecting pancreatic lesions compared to other imaging modalities has been repeatedly confirmed [6]. A meta-analysis evaluating the role of EUS in patients with a suspected pancreatic tumor not identifiable on CT scan determined a sensitivity of 85% and a positive predictive value of 77% [7]. In fact, EUS is particularly valuable in detecting pancreatic tumors ≤20 mm in size [7]. According to the NCCN guidelines, the use of EUS as a routine tool is not recommended and should be offered in cases where there is high suspicion of a pancreatic malignancy not detectable on Multi-Detector or Pancreas Protocol CT scan.

Obtaining a tissue biopsy for pathological confirmation of malignancy is not routinely required prior to surgical resection. If necessary, EUS-guided fine needle aspiration (FNA) or biopsy offers a better diagnostic yield and lower risk of peritoneal seeding compared to CT-guided percutaneous approach [8]. The overall complication rate of EUS-FNA is 0.82%, including complications such as pain (0.38%), bleeding (0.10%), and pancreatitis (0.4%) [8].

3. *Endoscopic Retrograde Cholangiopancreatography (ERCP) and Pre-operative Biliary Drainage*

Pre-operative biliary drainage is a safe and feasible modality to relieve biliary obstruction at the time of presentation. The impact of preoperative biliary drainage through ERCP and common bile duct (CBD) stenting on clinical and survival outcomes has received particular attention in the past several years. Some studies have shown worse survival in patients undergoing preoperative stenting compared to patients who proceeded immediately to surgery. However, a recently published analysis of a cohort of patients from a high-volume center showed no impact of pre-operative biliary stenting and drainage on overall survival and disease-free survival [9].

An interesting study investigated the predictors of stent dysfunction and worsened surgical outcomes in patients undergoing endoscopic biliary stenting prior to pancreaticoduodenectomy. A longer duration from initial stent placement to surgery as well as a stent diameter of 7 Fr or above was associated with a higher risk of complications [10].

4. *Octreotide Scan and Ga-DOTA TATE PET/CT Scan*

An octreotide scan is also called a somatostatin receptor (SSR) scintigraphy scan utilizing somatostatin receptors and octreotide (a somatostatin analogue) to detect and localize neuroendocrine tumors. It has a reported sensitivity of 75–100% in the detection of PNETs [11]. The paucity of somatostatin receptors in non-functional PNETs and insulinomas constitutes a limitation in the application of octreotide scans for all PNETs. The introduction of Gallium-68 (Ga-68) as a radiopharmacological tracer has allowed the application of 68 Ga-DOTA TATE PET/CT scan on somatostatin receptors as a more sensitive tool for the detection of PNETs. Recent studies have demonstrated high accuracy of 68Ga-DOTA TATE for imaging neuroendocrine tumors with a sensitivity of up to 93% [12]. Based on tracer uptake and imaging characteristics, PNETs can also be classified into benign, indeterminate, and malignant categories.

5. *Diagnostic Laparoscopy*

Diagnostic laparoscopy has been advocated as a staging tool to identify occult distant metastases for pancreatic cancer that are not detectable on imaging which occurs in about 20–50% of patients. The role is less clear in PNET, but similar principles apply. With the advent of imaging accuracy, the role of staging laparoscopy for pancreatic cancer has decreased and remains controversial. Some studies have advocated the mandatory use of laparoscopy to avoid missing radiologically negative metastases. Patients with elevated Ca19-9 level at diagnosis were more than twice as likely to have occult metastases detected at the time of surgical resection [13]. Other studies evaluated the impact of staging laparoscopy on prognosis compared to proceeding with exploratory laparotomy at the time of surgery in patients undergoing neoadjuvant therapy. Although staging laparoscopy was able to identify 35% with metastasis and thus prevented unnecessary laparotomies, there was no significant difference in rate of complications or overall survival [14]. Finally, a recently published meta-analysis evaluating the role of staging laparoscopy in both resectable and borderline resectable cases again only showed benefit in reduction of non-therapeutic laparotomy rate [15].

6. *Tumor Markers*

Serum markers can aid in the diagnosis and monitoring of treatment response in neuroendocrine tumor. In non-functional PNETs, baseline serum levels of chromogranin A and pancreatic polypeptide (PP) can be useful prior to surgical resection [16]. Neuron-specific enolase (NSE) can be present in ~50% of PNETs and would raise suspicion to pulmonary metastases [17]. The use of other hormone levels secreted by functional PNETs is generally helpful in diagnosis such as insulin-to-glucose ratio for insulinomas, gastrin and secretin levels of gastrinomas, and elevated VIP levels for VIPomas. However, the role of these hormones as tumor markers for the monitoring treatment response and recurrence is limited.

31.4 Consideration for Method of Surgical Treatment

Surgical therapy for PNETs aims at controlling symptoms of hormone excess, safe resection of maximal tumor mass particularly in malignant cases with preservation of sufficient pancreatic parenchyma. A detailed discussion on indication for resection is beyond the scope of this chapter. The trend toward the non-operative management of asymptomatic well-differentiated PNETs less than 2 cm has added to the complexity of decision-making. In the absence of metastatic disease, surgical resection is the mainstay of therapy in PNETs with the extent of resection depending on the location of the tumor. All patients with localized PNETs should be resected. Small benign tumors, peripheral in location and <2 cm in size that are not close to the main pancreatic duct can be removed by enucleation [18]. Resection of larger >2 cm or malignant appearing PNETs should include total removal of tumor with negative margins and regional lymph nodes.

A formal pancreatic resection should be considered if there is evidence of invasion, lymphadenopathy, or if the tumor is in close proximity to the pancreatic duct or major vessels. Contraindications to surgical resection include recent pancreatitis, uncontrolled coagulopathy, high surgical risk due to medical comorbidities, or widely metastatic disease [19].

31.5 Surgical Technique

The surgical technique of a Whipple procedure has evolved over the years; routine basic steps dictated by most common anatomical variants are relayed in this chapter with focus on critical steps in surgical technique. Despite the complex nature of the Whipple surgery, improvements in surgical technique have decreased perioperative mortality rates to ~3%; however, postoperative morbidity and complications remains a challenge [20].

1. *Open Pancreaticoduodenectomy (Whipple)*

   A midline upper abdominal incision is performed followed by a thorough inspection of all peritoneal surfaces and major abdominal organs to confirm absence of extra-pancreatic metastatic disease. The basic steps of a Whipple procedure involve:

   (i) Isolation of the infra-pancreatic SMV

   The lesser sac is entered separating the greater omentum of the transverse colon and posterior gastric wall attachments from the anterior surface of the pancreas. The junction of the middle colic vein and SMV is exposed by incising the peritoneal attachments at the inferior border of the pancreas.

   (ii) *Cattell-Braasch maneuver for exposure of duodenum*

   The visceral peritoneum of the small bowel mesentery is incised to the Ligament of Treitz allowing cephalad retraction of the colon and small bowel to expose third and fourth portions of the duodenum.

   (iii) *Mobilization of duodenum and pancreatic head through a Kocher maneuver*

   The third portion of the duodenum serving as a starting point, all fibrofatty tissue anterior to the inferior vena cava are elevated along with the pancreatic head and duodenum. The Kocher maneuver is continued to the lateral edge of the aorta exposing the left renal vein. A complete Kocher maneuver is necessary for proper dissection of the pancreatic head from the SMA.

   (iv) *Portal dissection, cholecystectomy, and common hepatic duct (CHD) transection*

   The common hepatic artery proximal and distal to the right gastric and GDA is exposed by removing the lymph node anterior to it using sharp dissection. The right gastric artery and GDA are ligated which allows mobilization of the common hepatic artery off the underlying PV. Prior to transection of the GDA, a test clamp should be performed to ensure that the proper hepatic artery is receiving flow from the common hepatic artery and not retrograde through the GDA. In cases of calcific stenosis of the celiac trunk or median accurate ligament syndrome in which substantial flow to the proper hepatic artery is from the GDA, ligation of the GDA can cause liver ischemia. Cholecystectomy is performed, and the CHD is transected at its junction with the cystic duct. It is important to palpate for pulsation of a replaced or an accessory right hepatic artery arising from the proximal SMA coursing posterolateral to the PV. Biliary fluid cultures may be sent, and any biliary stents removed. PV is further exposed with caution to prevent traction injury and avulsion of the superior pancreaticoduodenal vein which is a constant venous tributary of the PV.

(v) *Transection of stomach and takedown of ligament of Treitz (LOT)*

The stomach is transected with a linear gastrointestinal stapler completing a standard antrectomy. Pylorus preservation can be performed if the tumor is small, does not involve the first and second portion of the duodenum, and no pyloric lymph nodes appearing grossly positive. The loose attachments of the LOT are taken down with attention not to injure the inferior mesenteric vein (IMV). The jejunum is then transected ~20–30 cm distal to the LOT. The mesenteric dissection is carried on proximally to the third and fourth portions of the duodenum to the level of the aorta allowing reflection of the de-vascularized segment beneath the mesenteric vessels to the right upper quadrant.

(vi) *Pancreatic transection and dissection off the SMV-PV confluence and SMA*

Traction sutures are placed on the superior and inferior borders of the pancreas. The pancreas is then transected with electrocautery at the level of PV or where no gross tumor involvement is evident. Proper mobilization of the SMV involves identification of the jejunal branch of the SMV (also often referred to as the first jejunal branch). This branch originates from the right posterolateral aspect of the SMV (at the level of the uncinate process), travels posterior to the SMA, and enters the medial (proximal) aspect of the jejunal mesentery. Once the uncinate process is separated from the distal SMV, medial retraction of the SMV-PV confluence allows one to expose the SMA. The specimen is then separated from the lateral wall of the SMA by dividing the uncinate process which is dissected to its origin at the aorta.

(vii) *Anastomotic reconstruction of the gastrointestinal tract, bile duct, and pancreatic duct*

To enable adequate tension-free anastomosis, the pancreas is mobilized from the retroperitoneum and splenic vein. The transected jejunum is brought in a retro-colic fashion through an incision in the transverse mesocolon to the left of the middle colic vessels. A two-layer end-to-side, duct-to-mucosa pancreato-jejunostomy is performed. A posterior row if interrupted 3-0 seromuscular monofilament sutures is performed first. A full-thickness enterotomy is made, and the anastomosis between the pancreatic duct and small bowel mucosa is done using full-thickness bite of the jejunum and a generous bite of the pancreatic duct. Typically, a 5-0 absorbable monofilament suture is used for this layer. The anastomosis is completed with placement of an anterior row of 3-0 seromuscular monofilament sutures.

A single-layer biliary anastomosis is performed using interrupted 4-0 or 5-0 absorbable monofilament sutures depending on the size and thickness of the common hepatic duct. After that, an ante-colic, end-to-side gastrojejunostomy is constructed in two layers. A posterior row of silk sutures is followed by a full-thickness inner layer of running monofilament sutures; the anterior row of silk sutures completes the anastomosis.

2. Pylorus Preserving Pancreaticoduodenectomy (PPPD)

PPPD is thought to preserve the physiologic function of the antrum and pylorus allowing for fewer nutritional complications, post-operative weight loss, and reduced incidence of bile reflux gastritis. Others argue that this would come at the expense of increased post-operative delayed gastric emptying (DGE) [21]. A propensity-score matched analysis evaluating the risk of DGE showed increased risk in PPPD (38%) compared to 19.2% in classical PD [22]. PPPD involves the same steps of a classical PD except in the approach to the antrum, pylorus, and duodenum. The proximal division is done distal to the pylorus preserving blood supply and vagal innervation to the antrum and pylorus. Careful dissection of the portal structures should avoid inadvertent injury to the nerves of Laterjet leading to increased risk of postoperative gastroparesis. A duodenojejunostomy is subsequently performed in an end-to-side fashion.

Drain placement following PD has been evolving in clinical practice with controversy on the number of drains and duration of placement. Placement of at least 1 drain serves to evacuate pancreatic fluid, blood, or chyle from the surgical bed and help identify early anastomotic leaks. An analysis of over 5000 pancreatectomy patients from >100 institutions in the USA showed that 87% of cases underwent drain placement particularly for ducts <3 mm and soft glands [23]. A recent analysis of NSQIP data showed that routine drain placement following PD decreases post-operative complications including organ space surgical infections with prolonged length of drainage leading to worse outcomes [24].

3. Minimally Invasive Approach: Laparoscopic and Robotic Whipple

A growing body of evidence has emerged in evaluating the feasibility and potential benefit of minimally invasive approaches for pancreaticoduodenectomy using laparoscopic and robotic technologies. With the complexity of the Whipple procedure, it is crucial to highlight the technical challenge and long learning curve associated with the safe performance of minimally invasive pancreaticoduodenectomies which limited its uniform acceptance across institutions [25].

1. *Laparoscopic Pancreaticoduodenectomy (LPD)*

According to international expert consensus on laparoscopic PD (LPD), patient selection plays an important role. Selected patients should have no history of previous upper abdominal surgery and have lower body mass index (BMI $\leq$ 25.0 kg/m^2). It is also recommended to select patients with a pancreatic duct diameter $\geq$3 mm and a bile duct diameter $\geq$10 mm tumors around the ampulla without vascular invasion, as well as benign pancreatic tumors without vascular compression [26]. A systematic review and meta-analysis of randomized controlled trials assessed the value of laparoscopic PD compared to open PD. Laparoscopic PD was associated with a longer operative time and lower intra-operative blood loss with no significant advantage in reducing 90-day mortality, serious post-operative complications, length of stay, bile leak, pancreatic fistulas, reoperation, readmission, or oncologic outcomes [20].

2. *Robotic Pancreaticoduodenectomy (RPD)*

Another minimally invasive platform that is becoming increasingly popular is the robotic approach. The superior robotic technology provides features that could prove to be crucial for successful minimally invasive PD. Optical magnification, 3-D depth perception, augmented instrument articulation, and overall greater precision with suture targeting allow for a shorter learning curve when compared to laparoscopic PD [27]. However, debate over the perioperative benefit of robotic

PD continues to be a topic in current literature. Several retrospective studies have shown that RPD had significantly higher lymph node (LN) yield with no added operative time or blood loss [28]. There was no difference in the rate of bile leaks, infections, hemorrhage, urinary retention, or ileus. Patient undergoing robotic PD had significantly shorter length of stay of 7.5 days compared to 9 days in those undergoing open surgery; however, there were no differences in 30- or 90-day readmissions or 90-day mortality. Although there was a trend toward improved median overall survival in and longer time to recurrence, randomized controlled trials are still underway, and the need for higher level of evidence is still present [28].

4. Enucleation for Neuroendocrine Tumors

Although enucleation has no role in the treatment of pancreatic adenocarcinoma, it remains a hallmark in the management of pancreatic neuroendocrine tumors (PNETs). Enucleation is usually indicated when there is no evidence of advanced disease or neurovascular invasion which is less common in neuroendocrine tumors. It can be performed in an open or laparoscopic approach. Intraoperative ultrasound serves as a valuable imaging modality in identification of small PNETs as well as evaluation of liver metastases.

Tumors of the surface of the pancreas not involving the main pancreatic duct are amenable to enucleation. Imaging involvement of the main pancreatic duct is typically a contraindication to enucleation, and a formal resection must be considered. In terms of the technical aspect of enucleation, once the tumor is identified on the surface of the pancreas, dissection commences along the capsule of the tumor by dividing the pancreatic parenchyma using an energy device. The harmonic scalpel works well for this purpose. Once the tumor is resected, the base of the cavity is inspected for hemostasis and the absence of injury to the main pancreatic duct. A drain is then placed.

31.6 Post-operative Care and Complications

1. *Enhanced Recovery After Surgery*

Enhanced Recovery after Surgery (ERAS) is a multimodal protocol aimed at enhancing perioperative care and thus postoperative outcomes. This includes pre-operative counseling, nutrition optimization with immune-nutrition supplements, adequate thrombophylaxis, and infection prevention measures in the intra-operative and post-operative period [29]. Although the evidence is still controversial, the application of ERAS protocols for Whipple surgeries has the potential to decrease length of stay and morbidity from post-operative complications [30].

A recently published meta-analysis focusing on randomized and non-randomized trials showed that ERAS significantly reduced length of stay after Whipple surgery with decreased rates of incisional surgical site infections, intra-abdominal infections, delayed gastric emptying, and 30-day re-admission rates [31]. Other high evidence publications have replicated the same evidence although the peri-operative protocol had no influence on the rate of post-operative pancreatic fistula [32].
2. *Infectious Complications*

The overall rate of SSI after pancreatic resection was 10.4% with higher incidence in pancreaticoduodenectomies compared to distal pancreatectomy (32% and 23%, respectively) [33]. A recently published meta-regression identified pancreas-specific SSI risk factors, namely, pre-operative biliary drainage, chemotherapy, radiotherapy, and higher risk of intra-abdominal SSI in patients with post-operative pancreatic fistulas (POPF) (47.7%) [34].
3. *Delayed Gastric Emptying (DGE)*

Delayed Gastric Emptying is a common complication after PD with an incidence ranging from 16–40% according to different reports [22]. The International Study Group of Pancreatic Surgery (ISGPS) described a definition of DGE based on a proposed grading system based on NGT requirement, inability to tolerate PO intake, or use of prokinetics. This enabled a more uniform assessment and accurate evaluation of the incidence and predictors of DGE. A national multicenter study of the American College of Surgeons National Surgical Quality Improvement Program (ACS-NSQIP) database identified an incidence of 16.6% of patients undergoing PD [21]. Perioperative factors including advanced age, increased BMI, ASA class of 3 or more, pylorus preservation, and prolonged operative time were associated with increased risk of DGE [21].
4. *Post-operative Pancreatic Fistulas (POPF)*

The occurrence of post-operative pancreatic fistulas (POPF) remains one of the most challenging complications following Whipple surgery and the most common with an incidence of >10% [35]. The International Study Group on Pancreatic Fistula (ISGPF), most recently revised in 2016, classified POPF into biochemical and clinically significant fistula over a range of 3 grades (A, B, and C) [36]. A grade A fistula or a biochemical fistula is defined as fluid output on or after postoperative day 3 with amylase levels three times higher than upper limit of normal serum level. Grade A fistula is not associated with clinically significant morbidity, and most patients continue on their normal post-operative pathway. A grade B fistula is defined by clinical symptoms including infection without organ failure, requiring endoscopic or radiologic intervention for management of fistula, or requirement of surgical drain for more than

3 weeks. If organ failure develops or clinical management deviates from normal clinical pathway requiring re-operation, the fistula is defined as Grade C.

Several studies have identified factors that increase the risk of post-operative pancreatic fistulas after Whipple surgery. Some of these factors are patient-related such as male gender, increased BMI, and small pancreatic duct (≤3 mm), while others are related to surgical technique such as reconstruction method (pancreaticogastrostomy (PG) versus pancreatojejunostomy (PJ)), and anastomotic technique [35].

The comparison of surgical reconstruction method with PG or PJ has shown variable results in a multitude of well-designed RCTs and meta-analyses. Some have shown no difference in the occurrence of grade B or C POPFs except in patients with small pancreatic duct diameter having lower rates of POPF with PG [37]. Other multicenter RCTs have shown no effect of pancreatic duct diameter in depicting the use of PG or PJ [38]. Each reconstruction method offers its own advantages, and the superiority of one over the other in reducing POPF rate is not evident.

Throughout the years, several anastomotic techniques have been reported in the reconstruction of the pancreatic duct drainage. The most secure well-established feature is a "duct-to-mucosa" anastomosis allowing drainage of pancreatic fluid into the intestinal lumen. Blumgart proposed an original method using four to six trans-pancreatic jejunal seromuscular U-shaped sutures to approximate the pancreas and the jejunum which was later modified to include only 1–3 sutures. Some initial evidence showed a dramatic reduction in the rate of POPF (down to 2–6%) with the use of Blumgart's method compared to the conventional interrupted sutures [39]. However, this was not replicated and confirmed in other studies which failed to prove superiority of the Blumgart method.

Further efforts have been applied to design fistula mitigation strategies using internal or external trans-anastomotic stents in PJ reconstruction. The results from several high evidence meta-analyses showed varying results of benefit between stent and no stent placement [35]. Regarding externalized stents, a Fistula risk score for the prediction of clinically relevant fistula after pancreatoduodenectomy was designed based on high risk factors which included gland texture, pathology, pancreatic duct diameter, and intraoperative blood loss [40]. This risk assessment tool assigns a score out of a 10-point scale to identify high-risk situations that would benefit from an externalized stent. Soft gland texture, pathology other than adenocarcinoma, decreased pancreatic duct diameter, and increased intraoperative blood loss were assigned a higher score signifying increased risk. The use of externalized stents continues to be institution-based with multicenter studies showing significant reduction in POPF rate and related hospital stay and complications when applied in a risk-stratified approach [40]. Other surgical modifications such as omental wrapping and the use of topical fibrin glue around the pancreatic anastomosis have been described, but no evidence on significant benefit in reducing POPF rate [39].

31.7 Summary

In conclusion, neuroendocrine tumors of the pancreas have variable presentations with clinical course ranging from indolent to more aggressive depending on pathological type. Surgical resection with curative intent remains the mainstay of treatment in the absence of extra-pancreatic disease through open or minimally invasive approaches for PD as well as enucleation when feasible. Surgical debulking in certain cases can offer a survival advantage which is a feature of neuroendocrine tumors. Advances in surgical technique and increasing evidence on post-operative care protocols continue to evolve offering patients improved morbidity and better overall outcomes.

Answers

1. Correct answer is **D**.

   Somatostatinomas are rare neuroendocrine tumors that secrete somatostatin which inhibits pancreatic enzymes, causing malabsorption, steatorrhea, cholelithiasis from reduced gallbladder emptying, and diabetes. Insulinomas secrete insulin, causing neuroglycopenic symptoms (sweating, shakiness, tachycardia, sensation of hunger), low glucose level during symptoms, and improvement of symptoms with glucose administration, also known as Whipple's triad.

   VIPomas arise from D2 cells of the pancreatic islets and release vasoactive intestinal peptide (VIP) which causes a syndrome of watery diarrhea, hypokalemia, and achlorhydria (WDHA). Gastrinomas release high amounts of gastrin which causes acid hypersecretion and peptic ulcer diathesis (known as Zollinger-Ellison syndrome). Glucagonomas are associated with necrolytic migrating erythema (dermatitis), diabetes, deep venous thrombosis, and depression (the four-D's).

2. Correct answer is **E**.

   The patient in this clinical scenario is most likely presenting with symptoms and signs of Delayed Gastric Emptying (DGE). There are no signs of any infectious processes going on, and no antibiotics are indicated at this time. Although pancreatic leaks and fluid collections can present similarly, some fluid is not un-expected and does not warrant intervention in the setting of low clinical suspicion. At 3 weeks post-operatively, with symptoms being not too severe, no further workup is required, and an attempt of watchful waiting and follow-up in 2 weeks would be sufficient.

3. Correct answer is **E**.

   Glucagonomas are characterized by a constellation of common symptoms that are typical of glucagonoma syndrome. New onset diabetes, anemia, stomatitis, and weight loss are commonly seen. A characteristic skin rash, necrolytic migratory erythema, is pathognomonic of glucagonoma and attributed to hypoaminoacidemia. It exhibits cyclic appearance and migrates to different locations with no particular disposition or pattern. Hypoglycemia and seizures are more likely seen in insulinomas. Watery diarrhea and hypokalemia are characteristic of VIPoma.

4. Correct answer is **A**.

   This patient has a clinical diagnosis of multiple endocrine neoplasia type 1 (MEN1). In patients with MEN1, the most common functional neuroendocrine tumors are gastrinomas (54%), insulinomas (18%), glucagonomas (3%), and VIPomas (vasoactive intestinal peptide–secreting tumors, 3%).

5. Correct answer is **E**.

   This question describes a VIPoma (Verner-Morrison syndrome) with watery diarrhea, hypokalemia, and achlorhydria. It is a rare pancreatic endocrine tumor originating from non-beta islet cells of the pancreas and produces vasoactive intestinal peptide. The massive amounts of VIP in turn cause profound and chronic watery diarrhea and resultant dehydration, hypokalemia, achlorhydria, acidosis, hypercalcemia, and hyperglycemia.

6. Correct answer is **E**.

   Parenchyma-sparing operations are generally safe and effective for the management of small (< 3 cm), nonfunctional pancreatic NETs without overt malignant features; however, even small pancreatic NETs may have lymph node disease, and so traditional resection (pancreatic head resection, pancreatic tail resection) is typically necessary for these lesions instead of enucleation. If the lesion is thought to be benign, splenic preservation may be attempted. When malignancy is suspected, distal pancreatectomy with splenectomy and peripancreatic lymphadenectomy should be performed.

7. Correct answer is **C**.

   Delayed Gastric Emptying is a common complication post pancreaticoduodenectomy. Pylorus preserving pancreaticoduodenectomy (PPPD) is argued to increase the risk of DGE post-operatively. Although it involves the same steps of a classical PD except in the approach to the antrum, pylorus, and duodenum, the proximal division is done distal to the pylorus potentially compromising vagal innervation to the antrum and pylorus during dissection. The pathology and size of the tumor are not known to be risk factors for increased incidence of DGE.

8. Correct answer is **E**.

   Glucagonomas are more likely to be malignant. Even though a size of 1 cm is in favor of performing an enucleation, the presence of enlarged lymph nodes constitutes an increased risk and necessitates complete resection for removal of tumor bulk and surrounding lymph nodes. Classical Pancreaticoduodenectomy would be the best choice for management. Octreotide can assist in symptom control and management in cases with overt symptoms due to increased glucagon.

9. Correct answer is **C**.

   The inferior mesenteric vein courses cephalad and terminates draining into the splenic vein with variations draining into the confluence of the SMV and splenic vein. The IMV residing in the para-duodenal fold can be encountered during takedown of the LOT with risk of traction or thermal injury if not identified and preserved. The first jejunal branch arises from the posterolateral aspect of the SMV and is at risk of injury during dissection of SMV-PV confluence.

10. Correct answer is **B**.

    Octreotide scan has a limited accuracy in the diagnosis of insulinomas and non-functional PNETs due to the low number of somatostatin receptors. It has a lower sensitivity (87%) compared to 93% for 68Ga-DOTA TATE PET/CT scan in the detection of PNETs. MRIs can be useful for characterization and staging of smaller PNETs and those not identified on MDCT which has a limited sensitivity that does not exceed 82%.

References

1. Bray F, Ferlay J, Soerjomataram I, Siegel RL, Torre LA, Jemal A. Global cancer statistics 2018: GLOBOCAN estimates of incidence and mortality worldwide for 36 cancers in 185 countries. CA Cancer J Clin. 2018;68(6):394–424. https://doi.org/10.3322/caac.21492.
2. Nagtegaal ID, Odze RD, Klimstra D, et al. The 2019 WHO classification of tumours of the digestive system. Histopathology. 2020;76(2):182–8. https://doi.org/10.1111/his.13975.
3. Torphy RJ, Friedman C, Halpern A, et al. Comparing short-term and oncologic outcomes of minimally invasive versus open pancreaticoduodenectomy across low and high volume centers. Ann Surg. 2019;270(6):1147–55. https://doi.org/10.1097/SLA.0000000000002810.
4. Lidsky ME, Sun Z, Nussbaum DP, Adam MA, Speicher PJ, Blazer DG. Going the extra mile. Ann Surg. 2017;266(2):333–8. https://doi.org/10.1097/SLA.0000000000001924.
5. Cui SJ, Tang TY, Zou XW, Su QM, Feng L, Gong XY. Role of imaging biomarkers for prognostic prediction in patients with pancreatic ductal

adenocarcinoma. Clin Radiol. 2020;75(6):478.e1–478.e11. https://doi.org/10.1016/j.crad.2019.12.023.

6. Kitano M, Yoshida T, Itonaga M, Tamura T, Hatamaru K, Yamashita Y. Impact of endoscopic ultrasonography on diagnosis of pancreatic cancer. J Gastroenterol. 2019;54(1):19–32. https://doi.org/10.1007/s00535-018-1519-2.
7. Krishna SG, Rao BB, Ugbarugba E, et al. Diagnostic performance of endoscopic ultrasound for detection of pancreatic malignancy following an indeterminate multidetector CT scan: a systemic review and meta-analysis. Surg Endosc. 2017;31(11):4558–67. https://doi.org/10.1007/s00464-017-5516-y.
8. Wang KX, Ben QW, Jin ZD, et al. Assessment of morbidity and mortality associated with EUS-guided FNA: a systematic review. Gastrointest Endosc. 2011;73(2):283–90. https://doi.org/10.1016/j.gie.2010.10.045.
9. Shen Z, Zhang J, Chen H, et al. Does pre-operative biliary drainage influence Long-term survival in patients with obstructive jaundice with resectable pancreatic head cancer? Front Oncol. 2020;10(September):1–9. https://doi.org/10.3389/fonc.2020.575316.
10. Furukawa K, Onda S, Hamura R, et al. Predictive factors and surgical outcomes of stent dysfunction after preoperative endoscopic biliary stenting in patients who underwent pancreaticoduodenectomy. J Laparoendosc Adv Surg Tech. 2020;30(3):256–9. https://doi.org/10.1089/lap.2019.0666.
11. Manyak K, Kasi A. Octreotide Scan. StatPearls Publishing; 2020.
12. Bauckneht M, Albano D, Annunziata S, et al. Somatostatin receptor PET/CT imaging for the detection and staging of pancreatic NET: a systematic review and meta-analysis. Diagnostics. 2020;10(8):80–97. https://doi.org/10.3390/diagnostics10080598.
13. Takadate T, Morikawa T, Ishida M, et al. Staging laparoscopy is mandatory for the treatment of pancreatic cancer to avoid missing radiologically negative metastases. Surg Today. 2020;0123456789 https://doi.org/10.1007/s00595-020-02121-4.
14. Yamamura K, Yamashita YI, Yamao T, et al. Efficacy of staging laparoscopy for pancreatic cancer. Anticancer Res. 2020;40(2):1023–7. https://doi.org/10.21873/anticanres.14037.
15. Ta R, O'Connor DB, Sulistijo A, Chung B, Conlon KC. The role of staging laparoscopy in resectable and borderline resectable pancreatic cancer: a systematic review and meta-analysis. Dig Surg. 2019;36(3):251–60. https://doi.org/10.1159/000488372.
16. Cheng Y, Sun Z, Bai C, et al. Serum chromogranin A levels for the diagnosis and follow-up of well-differentiated non-functioning neuroendocrine tumors. Tumor Biol. 2016;37(3):2863–9. https://doi.org/10.1007/s13277-015-4114-7.
17. Zhang C, Huang Y, Long J, et al. Serum chromogranin a for the diagnosis of gastroenteropancreatic neuroendocrine neoplasms and its association with tumour expression. Oncol Lett. 2019;17(2):1497–504. https://doi.org/10.3892/ol.2018.9795.
18. Cameron JL, Cameron AM. Current surgical therapy. 13th ed. Elsevier Inc.; 2020.
19. Heidsma CM, Tsilimigras DI, van Dieren S, et al. Indications and outcomes of enucleation versus formal pancreatectomy for pancreatic neuroendocrine tumors. HPB. 2020; https://doi.org/10.1016/j.hpb.2020.06.015.
20. Nickel F, Haney CM, Kowalewski KF, et al. Laparoscopic versus open pancreaticoduodenectomy: a systematic review and meta-analysis of randomized controlled trials. Ann Surg. 2020;271(1):54–66. https://doi.org/10.1097/SLA.0000000000003309.
21. Snyder RA, Ewing JA, Parikh AA. Delayed gastric emptying after pancreaticoduodenectomy: a study of the national surgical quality improvement program: delayed gastric emptying after pancreaticoduo-

denectomy. Pancreatology. 2020;20(2):205–10. https://doi.org/10.1016/j.pan.2019.12.003.
22. Cai X, Zhang M, Liang C, Xu Y, Yu W. Delayed gastric emptying after Pancreaticoduodenectomy: a propensity score-matched analysis and clinical nomogram study. BMC Surg. 2020;20(1):1–9. https://doi.org/10.1186/s12893-020-00809-5.
23. El Khoury R, Kabir C, Maker VK, Banulescu M, Wasserman M, Maker AV. Do drains contribute to pancreatic fistulae? Analysis of over 5000 pancreatectomy patients. J Gastrointest Surg. 2018;22(6):1007–15. https://doi.org/10.1007/s11605-018-3702-4.
24. Addison P, Nauka PC, Fatakhova K, Amodu L, Kohn N, Rodriguez Rilo HL. Impact of drain placement and duration on outcomes after pancreaticoduodenectomy: a National Surgical Quality Improvement Program Analysis. J Surg Res. 2019;243:100–7. https://doi.org/10.1016/j.jss.2019.04.071.
25. Triantafyllidis I, Gayet B, Fuks D. Tips and tricks for a safe laparoscopic pancreatoduodenectomy. Wideochirurgia I Inne Tech Maloinwazyjne. 2020;15(3):383–90. https://doi.org/10.5114/wiitm.2020.97977.
26. Qin R, Kendrick ML, Wolfgang CL, et al. International expert consensus on laparoscopic pancreaticoduodenectomy*. Hepatobil Surg Nutr. 2020;9(4):464–483. https://doi.org/10.21037/hbsn-20-446.
27. Baimas-George M, Watson M, Murphy KJ, et al. Robotic pancreaticoduodenectomy may offer improved oncologic outcomes over open surgery: a propensity-matched single-institution study. Surg Endosc. 2020;34(8):3644–9. https://doi.org/10.1007/s00464-020-07564-x.
28. Kamarajah SK, Gujjuri R, Bundred JR, Hilal MA, White SA. Long-term survival after minimally invasive resection versus open pancreaticoduodenectomy for periampullary cancers: a systematic review, meta-analysis and meta-regression. HPB. 2020; https://doi.org/10.1016/j.hpb.2020.09.023.
29. Miyauchi Y, Furukawa K, Suzuki D, et al. Additional effect of perioperative, compared with preoperative, immunonutrition after pancreaticoduodenectomy: a randomized, controlled trial. Int J Surg. 2019;61(November 2018):69–75. https://doi.org/10.1016/j.ijsu.2018.11.028.
30. Lawrence SA, McIntyre CA, Pulvirenti A, et al. Perioperative bundle to reduce surgical site infection after pancreaticoduodenectomy: a prospective cohort study. J Am Coll Surg. 2019;228(4):595–601. https://doi.org/10.1016/j.jamcollsurg.2018.12.018.
31. Wang XY, Cai JP, Huang CS, Huang XT, Yin XY. Impact of enhanced recovery after surgery protocol on pancreaticoduodenectomy: a meta-analysis of non-randomized and randomized controlled trials. HPB. 2020;22(10):1373–83. https://doi.org/10.1016/j.hpb.2020.07.001.
32. Sun YM, Wang Y, Mao YX, Wang W. The safety and feasibility of enhanced recovery after surgery in patients undergoing pancreaticoduodenectomy: an updated meta-analysis. Biomed Res Int. 2020;2020 https://doi.org/10.1155/2020/7401276.
33. Brown JA, Zenati MS, Simmons RL, et al. Long-term surgical complications after pancreatoduodenectomy: incidence, outcomes, and risk factors. J Gastrointest Surg. 2020;24(7):1581–9. https://doi.org/10.1007/s11605-020-04641-3.
34. Mentor K, Ratnayake B, Akter N, et al. Meta-analysis and meta-regression of risk factors for surgical site infections in hepatic and pancreatic resection. World J Surg. 2020;44(12):4221–30. https://doi.org/10.1007/s00268-020-05741-6.
35. Ecker BL, McMillan MT, Asbun HJ, et al. Characterization and optimal management of high-risk pancreatic anastomoses during pancreatoduodenectomy. Ann Surg. 2018;267(4):608–16. https://doi.org/10.1097/SLA.0000000000002327.
36. Bassi C, Marchegiani G, Dervenis C, et al. The 2016 update of the International Study Group (ISGPS) definition and grading of post-

operative pancreatic fistula: 11 years after. Surgery (United States). 2017;161(3):584–91. https://doi.org/10.1016/j.surg.2016.11.014.
37. Topal B, Fieuws S, Aerts R, Weerts J, Feryn T. Pancreaticojejunostomy versus pancreaticogastrostomy reconstruction after pancreaticoduodenectomy for pancreatic or periampullary tumours: a multicentre randomised trial. Lancet Oncol. 2013;14:655.
38. Grendar J, Ouellet JF, Sutherland FR, Bathe OF, Ball CG, Dixon E. In search of the best reconstructive technique after pancreaticoduodenectomy: Pancreaticojejunostomy versus pancreaticogastrostomy. Can J Surg. 2015;58(3):154–9. https://doi.org/10.1503/cjs.010014.
39. Kawaida H, Kono H, Hosomura N, et al. Surgical techniques and postoperative management to prevent postoperative pancreatic fistula after pancreatic surgery. World J Gastroenterol. 2019;25(28):3722–37. https://doi.org/10.3748/wjg.v25.i28.3722.
40. McMillan MT, Ecker BL, Behrman SW, et al. Externalized stents for pancreatoduodenectomy provide value only in high-risk scenarios. J Gastrointest Surg. 2016;20(12):2052–62. https://doi.org/10.1007/s11605-016-3289-6.

Familial Endocrine Syndromes

Contents

Familial Non-medullary Thyroid Carcinoma Syndrome (FNMTC) and Familial Syndromes Associated with Thyroid Cancer

Samira Mercedes Sadowski

Contents

A. L. Shifrin et al. (eds.), *Endocrine Surgery Comprehensive Board Exam Guide*,
https://doi.org/10.1007/978-3-030-84737-1_32

Case Presentation

A 22-year-old female was referred to the Clinic of Gastroenterology for an expert colonoscopy and a decision regarding a subsequent proctocolectomy since polyps were seen during the colonoscopy in the regional hospital. The patient was symptom-free. On admission, her general physical examination was normal. All routine laboratory tests were within a normal range. The patient's personal history was unremarkable; however, her father died from metastatic colorectal cancer at the age of 45. Her mother was healthy. The patient has two siblings, an older sister and a younger brother. The patient's older sister has anemia and underwent a proctocolectomy after FAP was diagnosed at the age of 20. In our patient, the repeat colonoscopy revealed a total of seven polyps that were endoscopically resected. The largest polyp was eight millimeters in diameter. Histology revealed tubular adenomas with low-grade dysplasia and no high-grade dysplasia in any of the polyps. Screening for gastric and proximal small bowel tumors was performed using esophagogastroduodenoscopy, and polyps were not detected.

Questions

1. What is the most likely diagnosis for this young patient and what confirms her diagnosis?
   (a) Peutz-Jeghers syndrome. The presence of a mutation in the serine/threonine-protein kinase 11 gene confirms this diagnosis.
   (b) Familial adenomatous polyposis. The presence of a germline mutation in the adenomatous polyposis coli (*APC*) gene confirms this diagnosis.
   (c) Familial adenomatous polyposis. The presence of a mutation in the *WRN* gene confirms this diagnosis.
   (d) PTEN hamartoma tumor syndrome. The presence of a mutation in the *PTEN* gene confirms this diagnosis.
2. What is clinically pathognomonic for Familial Adenomatous Polyposis (FAP) and what risk is there?
   (a) Primary pigmented micronodular adrenal hyperplasia. There is a risk of Cushing's syndrome.
   (b) Café-au-lait macules, fibrous dysplasia, and loss of vision and/or hearing. There is a risk of endocrinopathies.
   (c) Macrocephaly and intestinal hamartomatous polyps. There is a risk of mental retardation.
   (d) Hundreds of polyps in the intestinal tract. There is a risk of colorectal cancer.
3. What is the likely pattern of inheritance in this clinical case/FAP?
   (a) Autosomal dominant mode
   (b) Mitochondrial inheritance
   (c) X-linked dominant mode
   (d) Autosomal recessive mode

4. What are the clinical features of Gardner's syndrome?
   (a) Osteomas, dental abnormalities, epidermal cysts, desmoids tumors, congenital hypertrophy of the retinal pigment epithelium, and hepatoblastoma
   (b) Premature aging, short stature, age-related disorders, diabetes, peripheral vascular disease, and malignancy
   (c) Gastric and duodenal polyps, and colon and rectal adenomas
   (d) Multiple hamartomas, acral keratosis, and oral papillomatous papules
5. What is the appropriate workup for thyroid nodules in this case?
   (a) Thyroid function labs only
   (b) Physical neck exam only
   (c) Physical neck exam, thyroid function labs, and thyroid ultrasound
   (d) Thyroid function labs and iodine scan
6. When should thyroid screening be performed in patients diagnosed with FAP?
   (a) At age 18
   (b) Only if palpation reveals a thyroid nodule on physical exam
   (c) Never
   (d) Annually if a thyroid nodule is present, every 2 years if there are no nodules, as soon as there is a diagnosis of FAP, and best performed at time of gastrointestinal screen

   Follow-up in clinical case: Proctocolectomy was not indicated in this case, and annual endoscopic surveillance was recommended, which is currently ongoing. Further complementary workup revealed a 1.5-cm thyroid nodule on the left.
7. To inform the patient, what is the rate of TC in patients with FAP and what is the predominant TC histology?
   (a) TC rate of more than 30%. Follicular variant TC histology.
   (b) TC rate below 1%. Anaplastic TC histology.
   (c) TC rate between 2% and 12%. Cribriform-morular variant of papillary TC histology.
   (d) Very rare. Follicular-variant TC histology.
8. What are the clinical features of Carney complex?
   (a) Bilateral sensorineural deafness, thyroid multinodular goiter, and hypothyroidism
   (b) Multiple hamartomas, acral keratosis, and oral papillomatous papules
   (c) Pituitary adenomas; primary pigmented micronodular adrenal hyperplasia, Cushing's syndrome; myxomas of heart, skin, and soft tissue; and thyroid and testicular tumors
   (d) Café-au-lait spots, *neurofibromas, optic glioma, learning disabilities,* and short stature

9. What are the criteria to establish the diagnosis of non-syndromic FNMTC and what is the probability of this being FNMTC?
   (a) Non-syndromic FNMTC is defined when a patient has a positive family history of thyroid cancer. The probability of this being FNMTC is 5%.
   (b) Non-syndromic FNMTC is defined when two or more first-degree relatives are affected, in the absence of other predisposing causes of TC. The probability of this being FNMTC is 31–38%.
   (c) Non-syndromic FNMTC is defined when a patient has a positive history of radiation exposure. The probability of this being FNMTC is 45%.
   (d) Non-syndromic FNMTC is defined when a thyroid tumor is positive for a *BRAF* mutation. The probability of this being FNMTC is 25%.
10. Though the topic is still debated by many investigators, and further studies are needed, what do many large familial studies show regarding aggressiveness in FNMTC versus sporadic NMTC?
   (a) FNMTC was associated with thyroid hyperfunction (hyperthyroidism).
   (b) FNMTC was associated with increased multinodular goiter.
   (c) FNMTC was associated with multiple thyroid tumors.
   (d) FNMTC was associated with a younger age at diagnosis and a higher rate of multifocal and bilateral tumors, extrathyroidal invasion, lymph node metastasis, and recurrence.

32.1 Introduction

Thyroid cancer (TC) accounts for only about 1% of all epithelial malignancies but represents 95% of all endocrine malignancies. The incidence of TC in the United States and Europe increased from 4.56 per 100,000 person-years in 1974–1977 to 14.42 per 100,000 person-years in 2010–2013 and has become the most commonly diagnosed endocrine malignancy in the world [1–3].

TCs arising from parafollicular cells are referred to as medullary TC, whereas those arising from follicular cells are more common (making up 95% of TCs) and are referred to as non-medullary thyroid cancer (NMTC), with papillary thyroid cancer (PTC) comprising more than 85% of these cases. Most NMTCs are sporadic; however, approximately 3–9% of NMTCs are familial [4–6]. Familial non-medullary thyroid cancer (FNMTC) can occur as a minor component of familial cancer syndromes (familial adenomatous polyposis, Gardner's syndrome, Cowden syndrome, Werner syndrome, Carney complex, and others discussed in this chapter) or as non-syndromic familial disease [7, 8]. Most of the susceptibility genes for syndromic FNMTC are known. However, to date, the susceptibility gene(s) for non-syndromic FNMTC are not known. Furthermore, non-syndromic FNMTC is more common than syndromic FNMTC [5].

This chapter will summarize emerging data regarding classifications and definitions of FNMTC, criteria for screening and surveillance in patients with FNMTC, evaluation of the extent of disease, candidate susceptibility genes, and pattern of inheritance in FNMTC. The aim is to provide guidance for managing patients with FNMTC.

32.2 Definition, Screening, and Clinical Management of FNMTC

32.2.1 Syndromic FNMTC

Several inherited syndromes have shown an association with an increased risk of NMTC (syndromic FNMTC). These syndromes include familial adenomatous polyposis (FAP), Cowden syndrome, Carney complex, Werner syndrome, Pendred syndrome, Ataxia-telangiectasia, Bannayan-Riley-Ruvalcaba syndrome, PTEN hamartoma tumor syndrome, Peutz-Jeghers syndrome, DICER1 syndrome, McCune-Albright syndrome, and papillary renal neoplasia (◘ Table 32.1). The susceptibility genes responsible for these syndromes have been identified, and patients with pathogenic germline mutations in these genes or who fulfill clinical criteria for these syndromes have an increased likelihood of developing NMTC and other malignancies.

In general, screening for TC in at-risk individuals with germline mutations or clinical diagnosis of syndromic FNMTC is recommended in all cases (◘ Table 32.1). The optimal age for screening with a thyroid ultrasound (US) and frequency of surveillance in these cases, however, is not clearly established. Individuals could be screened for thyroid nodules/cancer at 18 years of age or the youngest age of NMTC diagnosis in the family, whichever is the youngest. Annual thyroid US in most cases seems reasonable, and specific cases are mentioned in ◘ Table 32.1. The evaluation and workup for TC in patients found to have a thyroid nodule should follow established guidelines, similar to patients with sporadic thyroid nodules [9]. The benefit of this screening and surveillance strategy for TC in patients with syndromic FNMTC is unknown.

Table 32.1 Incidence, Screening, and Clinical Features of Familial and Syndromic NMTC

Syndrome	Susceptibility gene(s)	Inheri-tance	Incidence of TC	Type of TC (Pathology)	Thyroid screening recommendations[a]	Clinical features
Familial adenomatous polyposis	*APC*	AD	2–12%	PTC	Start at time of gastrointestinal screen. If baseline normal, screen every 2 years	Intestinal: gastric and duodenal polyps and >100 colon and rectal adenomas (colorectal cancer) Extraintestinal (Gardner's syndrome): osteomas, dental abnormalities, epidermal cysts, desmoids tumors, CHRPE, hepatoblastoma, medulloblastoma brain tumors (Turcot syndrome)
Cowden's syndrome	*PTEN*	AD	10%	FTC, PTC	Start as soon as DX made, independent of age	Multiple hamartomas, acral keratosis, oral papillomatous papules Benign and malignant disease of the breast, endometrium, colon, and brain
Carney complex	*PRKAR1*	AD	4%; 60% for nodules	FTC, PTC	Routine and long-term screening	Myxomas of heart, skin, and soft tissue, external auditory canal, breast; pituitary adenomas; primary pigmented micronodular adrenal hyperplasia, Cushing's syndrome; schwannomas; testicular tumors; and thyroid disease
Werner syndrome	*WRN*	AR	18%	PTC, FTC, ATC	Routine and long-term screening	Premature aging; short stature; and age-related disorders such as osteoporosis, cataracts, diabetes, peripheral vascular disease, and malignancy: melanoma, soft-tissue sarcoma, or osteosarcoma
Pendred syndrome	*SLC26A4, FOXI1, KCNJ10*	AR	1%	PTC, FTC, ATC	Screening for hypothyroidism	Bilateral sensorineural deafness, thyroid multinodular goiter, and hypothyroidism
Ataxia-telangiectasia	*ATM*	AR	Rare	PTC	Routine and long-term screening	Cerebral ataxia; apraxia of eye movements; oculocutaneous telangiectasia; immunodeficiency; and radiosensitivity
Bannayan-Riley-Ruvalcaba	*PTEN*	NA	Rare	PTC, FTC	NA	Macrocephaly; intestinal hamartomatous polyps; multiple lipomas; developmental delay and mental retardation; and thyroid adenoma and thyroiditis

PTEN hamartoma tumor	*PTEN, SDH, PIK3CA, C160RF72, PTPN2, SEC23B, KLLN*	NA	Age-dependent; see text	DTC, FTC, PTC	Early routine and long-term screening	Cowden's syndrome; Bannayan-Riley-Ruvalcaba syndrome; Proteus syndrome
Peutz-Jeghers syndrome	*STK11*	AD	Rare	PTC, FTC, DTC	NA	Hamartomatous polyps in the gastrointestinal tract; malignancies, such as pancreas, breast, uterus, ovaries, testes and thyroid
DICER1 syndrome	*DICER1*	AD	Age-dependent; see text	DTC, FTC, FVPTC	Start as soon as DX made, early routine and long-term screening	Familial pleuropulmonary blastoma; cystic nephroma, renal sarcoma and Wilms tumor; ovarian Sertoli-Leydig cell tumors; and brain tumors
McCune-Albright syndrome	*GNAS*	Not inherited	Rare	Case reports of PTC	Screening for hyperthyroidism	Café-au-lait macules; fibrous dysplasia; loss of vision and/or hearing; and endocrinopathies: precocious puberty, testicular lesions, benign thyroid lesions +/− hyperthyroidism, and neonatal hypercortisolism
Papillary Renal Neoplasia[b]	Unknown; loci 1q21	Unknown	Rare	Kindred study: PTC and benign nodules	NA	Familial tumor syndrome characterized by a predominance of NMTC associated with renal papillary tumors

[a]Thyroid screening consists of yearly physical examination and thyroid ultrasound. Thyroid function testing should be obtained as clinically indicated and routinely in patients with Pendred and McCune-Albright syndromes

[b]Non-Syndromic, familial NMTC

AD autosomal dominant, *AR* autosomal recessive, *PTC* papillary thyroid cancer, *FTC* follicular thyroid cancer, *FVPTC* follicular variant PTC, *ATC* anaplastic thyroid cancer, *DTC* differentiated thyroid cancer, *DX* diagnosis, *CHRPE* congenital hypertrophy of the retinal pigment epithelium, *GNAS* guanine nucleotide-binding protein (G protein), alpha-stimulating activity polypeptide, *PRKAR1-a* protein kinase A regulatory subunit type 1-alpha, *APC* adenomatous polyposis coli, *NA* not available, *NMTC* non-medullary thyroid cancer, *PTEN* phosphatase and tensin, *PDS* Pendred syndrome, *WRN* Werner

32.2.1.1 Familial Adenomatous Polyposis

FAP is an inherited syndrome characterized by the development of hundreds to thousands of adenomatous polyps in the colon with nearly a 100% lifetime risk of developing colorectal cancer if left untreated. It occurs approximately 1 per 10,000 births. FAP is caused by a germline mutation in the adenomatous polyposis coli (*APC*) gene, which is inherited in an autosomal dominant manner [10, 11]. Because colorectal polyps are not always symptomatic, the first manifestation of FAP or clue to its diagnosis can be colorectal cancer or an extraintestinal manifestation, such as TC. Patients may have extraintestinal manifestations that include osteomas, dental abnormalities, epidermal cysts, desmoids tumors, congenital hypertrophy of the retinal pigment epithelium, hepatoblastoma, medulloblastoma, and TC [12]. Gardner's syndrome is the variant that is characterized by extracolonic disease, and Turcot syndrome includes patients with FAP who have medulloblastoma brain tumors.

Patients with FAP are at risk for developing PTC. Two prospective studies detailing results from thyroid screening programs have revealed higher TC rates, ranging from 2.6% to 11.8% [13, 14]. A recent meta-analysis of 12 studies ($n = 9821$) revealed a 2.6% pooled prevalence of TC in FAP (95% confidence interval (CI) 1.3–4.8), a 48.8% pooled prevalence in benign thyroid nodules (95% CI 33.8–64.0), and a 6.9% pooled prevalence in endocrine thyroid disorders (95% CI 4.5–10.3) [15]. TC diagnosis preceded the diagnosis of FAP in 34% of the patients, and the mean age at diagnosis of FAP and TC was 29 and 31 years, respectively. Ninety-five percent of patients were female, and the most common pathology was a papillary subtype (PTC in 83.3%) (◘ Table 32.1) [15, 16]. The unique pathology is a cribriform-morular variant of PTC, which accounts for less than 1 in 500 cases of PTC. Investigators have identified differences in the location of *APC* germline mutations in FAP patients with and without PTC [17]. Another recent study performing whole-genome sequencing on paired thyroid tumor and normal DNA from 12 FAP patients who developed PTC found that all 12 patients harbored germline mutations in *APC*; seven patients also had somatic mutations in *APC*, and seven patients harbored somatic mutations in *KMT2D*, which encodes a lysine methyltransferase. Most notably, only two of the tumors harbored the somatic *BRAF* V600E mutation, which is the most common driver mutation found in sporadic PTCs. Six of the tumors displayed a cribriform-morular variant of PTC histology and had somatic mutations in *APC* [18].

No optimal screening protocol has yet been established for FAP patients, and, due to the low incidence of FAP-associated PTC, routine screening of all patients has not been recommended. Based on benign nodules in young patients with FAP, some authors suggest initiation of screening at age 16 [13]. Additional research found that TC detected by US screening in FAP patients was smaller and associated with fewer surgical complications, recurrences, and cancer-related deaths. Thus, prospective thyroid screening in this population is important, especially as the survival rate from colonic manifestations improves. A recent prospective study in 264 patients with FAP participating in a US screening program with an average of three follow-up USs over a mean 4.8 years found the development of TC to be low, and no FAP patient with a normal baseline US developed TC during observation. The authors conclude that an annual US in patients with a normal baseline US may not be needed, and extending the screening interval to 2 years could be reasonable until nodules are detected [19]. The recommendation is to perform routine thyroid US screening at the time of gastrointestinal surveillance [13]. Once NMTC is detected, the American Thyroid Association's (ATA) standard management guidelines should be followed [9].

32.2.1.2 Cowden Syndrome

Cowden syndrome is an intestinal polyposis syndrome characterized by the development of hamartomatous polyps and is inherited in an autosomal dominant manner. It is caused by inactivating mutations in the phosphatase and tensin homolog (*PTEN*) gene, a tumor suppressor [20]. In addition to the hamartomas, patients are at an increased risk of developing both benign and malignant breast, uterine, and thyroid tumors. Nearly all patients will have mucocutaneous lesions such as acral keratosis, oral mucosal papillomatous papules, and trichilemmoma (benign neoplasms derived from the outer root sheath epithelium of hair follicles). The International Cowden Consortium outlined the operational criteria for diagnosis in 1995 [11, 21]. Genotype–phenotype correlations for *PTEN* have been investigated; however, so far, no associations have been made that can reliably guide surveillance or predict cancer [22].

The thyroid disease in Cowden syndrome consists of multinodular goiter or multiple follicular adenomas in more than 50% of patients, with follicular cancer (FTC) occurring in up to 10% of patients [22, 23]. Patients have also presented with PTC. The high incidence of thyroid pathology in patients with Cowden syndrome warrants routine thyroid screening with US and a low threshold for recommending thyroidectomy, particularly in patients with indeterminate fine-needle aspiration biopsies or suspicious characteristics on US [22]. Given the association of *PTEN* mutation with both benign and malignant transformation and nodules found in patients as young as 12 years old, thyroid screening should begin at the time of Cowden syndrome diagnosis, regardless of age [21, 22]. The significant risk and hereditary basis of TC in these patients might justify total thyroidectomy when surgery is indicated.

32.2.1.3 Carney Complex

Carney complex was first characterized by J. A. Carney in 1985 with symptoms including "myxomas, spotty pigmentation, and endocrine overactivity." Patients may also have pituitary adenomas, primary pigmented micronodular adrenal hyperplasia with Cushing's syndrome, schwannomas, testicular tumors, and thyroid disease. Most cases of this autosomal dominant condition are associated with a mutation in the protein kinase A regulatory subunit type 1-alpha (*PRKAR1-a*) gene, a tumor suppressor gene [24].

A review of 53 patients with Carney complex in 12 families found clinically significant thyroid disease in 11% of cases [24]. TC was found in two patients (4%), including one FTC and one PTC. Thyroid screening USs in 11 asymptomatic patients confirmed thyroid nodules in 60% of adults and 67% of children. The presence of thyroid nodules is very common, and routine US may lead to early identification of TC. A follow-up review in 26 patients with Carney complex and thyroid abnormalities in 2018 [25] showed pathologic thyroid findings that included benign lesions (follicular hyperplasia, nodular hyperplasia, and follicular adenoma) in 16 patients and carcinomas (follicular or papillary) in 10 patients. FTC had multifocal and bilateral features as well as lymph node metastases, and tumors harbored aggressive outcomes when greater than three centimeters in diameter. Thus, detection and treatment of thyroid neoplasms in these patients requires long-term follow-up.

32.2.1.4 Werner Syndrome

Werner syndrome is a rare premature aging syndrome that typically begins in the third decade. It is an autosomal recessive disease caused by mutations in the *WRN* gene on chromosome 8p11–p12 and has an incidence of 1 in 1,000,000, with as many as 83 known *WRN* mutations [26]. The encoded protein is important in DNA repair and replication. The diagnosis is often made clinically, and molecular analysis is focused on the inability to detect the normal protein of *WRN*. The clinical presentation includes an elderly appearance with thin skin, wrinkles, alopecia, and muscle atrophy. Patients are of short stature and may have age-related disorders such as osteoporosis, cataracts, diabetes, peripheral vascular disease, or malignancy. The mutations of the *WRN* gene are furthermore associated with epithelial-derived malignancies such as melanoma, soft-tissue sarcoma, osteosarcomas, and well-differentiated thyroid cancer (DTC).

Patients present at a younger age and have an approximately threefold increased risk for developing FTC and six times the risk for developing anaplastic thyroid cancer (ATC). The overall incidence of TC in Japanese patients with Werner syndrome is 18% [27]. A recent systematic review in 189 patients harboring 248 neoplasms found the most frequent neoplasms in two thirds of cases to be thyroid neoplasms, malignant melanoma, meningioma, soft-tissue sarcomas, leukemia and pre-leukemic conditions of the bone marrow, and primary bone neoplasms. The highest cancer risk was in patients residing in Japan, ranging from a 53.5-fold increased risk for melanoma of the skin (95% CI: 24.5, 101.6) to an 8.9-fold increased risk for thyroid neoplasms (95% CI: 4.9, 15.0) [28]. The high prevalence of TC in Werner syndrome supports routine thyroid screening in these patients.

32.2.1.5 Pendred Syndrome

Pendred syndrome is an autosomal recessive disorder defined by the combination of sensorineural deafness/hearing impairment, goiter, and an abnormal organification of iodide with or without hypothyroidism. The hallmark of the syndrome is the impaired hearing, which is associated with inner-ear malformations [29]. It is the result of mutations in the *SLC26A4* (*PDS*) gene, which encodes the protein pendrin, an anion transporter at the apical membrane of thyroid cells [30].

The impaired transportation of iodine into the thyroid follicular lumen may lead to impairments in the organification of iodide and subsequent thyroid goiter with possible hypothyroidism [31]. In 16 patients with Pendred syndrome from six different families, thyroid goiter was present in 11 patients, and four had clinical hypothyroidism, all with negative thyroid autoantibodies [30]. Metastatic FTC and a Hürthle cell adenoma were documented in two of three family members with hypothyroidism. The association with TC may be related to long-standing untreated hypothyroidism and chronic stimulation by the thyroid-stimulating hormone, and is thought to contribute to the progression of FTC to ATC [32]. Therefore, the relatively small risk of TC should be reduced with close surveillance to identify and treat hypothyroidism at its onset.

32.2.1.6 Ataxia-Telangiectasia

Ataxia-telangiectasia is a rare, autosomal recessive disorder characterized by progressive cerebellar ataxia, neurodegeneration, radiosensitivity, cell-cycle checkpoint defects, genome instability, and a predisposition to cancer. Defects of the ataxia-telangiectasia mutated (*ATM*) gene play a central role in response to DNA double-strand breaks from radiation, causing DNA damage [33]. Thus, it is possible that inherited functional polymorphisms in *ATM* could influence inherited radiosensitivity, leading to increased predisposition to DTC.

Cases have been reported in syndromic patients, with detection of PTC (follicular variant) within multinodular goiter at the age of 12 [34].

32.2.1.7 Bannayan-Ruvalcaba-Riley Syndrome

Bannayan-Ruvalcaba-Riley syndrome is another *PTEN* hamartoma tumor syndrome [35], which is characterized by neonatal-onset macrocephaly, mental retardation, Hashimoto's thyroiditis, lipomatosis, hemangiomas, hamartomatous polyps, and pigmented macules of the glans penis. These patients have thyroid adenomas and lymphocytic thyroiditis. Somatic *PTEN* mutation has been described in various benign and malignant tumor types. Somatic deletions have been described in follicular adenomas of the thyroid and PTC [36].

32.2.1.8 PTEN Hamartoma Tumor Syndrome

PTEN hamartoma tumor syndrome encompasses several clinical syndromes with germline mutations in the *PTEN* tumor suppressor gene, including Cowden syndrome, which is characterized by an increased risk of cancers in 40% of cases [23]. This inactivating germline *PTEN* mutation leads to subsequent activation of PI3K-AKT-mTOR signaling, predisposing patients to developing TC [37]. A genotype–phenotype analysis in 146 patients with this syndrome found benign thyroid lesions in 71% of patients and malignant thyroid lesions in 17% of patients [23]. The patients with malignant thyroid lesions were diagnosed at a median age of 31 years (range 16–57 years old), with some presenting as precancerous lesions (microPTC (<1 cm) and minimally invasive FTC). In the 22 cases of TC, 13 (59%) were PTC, and 6 (27.5%) were FTC. Based on the findings, the authors recommend annual thyroid US and total thyroidectomy in cases of multiple nodules or multinodular goiter according to ATA guidelines and beginning at 10 years of age, the earliest age of onset [38]. Another study found an almost ninefold (95% CI, 3.08–25.0) risk of pediatric-onset TC in *PTEN* mutation-positive individuals [39].

32.2.1.9 Peutz-Jeghers Syndrome

Peutz-Jeghers syndrome is an autosomal dominant hereditary polyposis syndrome in which a germline mutation of serine/threonine-protein kinase 11 (*STK11*), a tumor suppressor gene, is identified. Clinical features include hamartomatous polyps, mucocutaneous pigmentation, and an increased predisposition to developing malignancies, especially gastrointestinal, but also gynecological, testicular, and thyroid cancers [40]. Case reports have found varied forms of TC, PTC (tall cell variant), and FTC [41, 42]. Some researchers/clinicians recommend surveillance from childhood or beginning at the time of diagnosis.

32.2.1.10 DICER1 Syndrome

DICER1 syndrome is a novel autosomal dominant disorder that increases the risk of benign and malignant tumors, such as pleuropulmonary blastoma and Sertoli-Leydig cell tumors, and has a high prevalence of multinodular thyroid goiter. The mutation in the *DICER1* gene is associated with dysregulated gene expression of five micro RNAs (Let-7, miR-99b, miR-133, miR-345, and miR-194). Multinodular goiter and DTC have been reported in patients with *DICER1* germline mutations (16- to 24-fold increased risk of TC), and chemotherapy treatment may be a risk factor for TC in patients with this syndrome [43, 44].

A recent study in 15 pediatric patients with FTC, including four with DICER1 syndrome (three patients were less than 10 years of age), found multinodular goiter at an early stage in its development with screening; therefore, continuous screening for tumor development is recommended [45]. To date, there are no prospective studies on the efficacy or timing of thyroid screening USs. Guidelines from an inaugural International DICER1 Symposium [46] recommend a thyroid US at approximately 8 years of age in children with DICER1-associated conditions and then every 2–3 years. A baseline thyroid US should be performed at the time of diagnosis for individuals receiving chemotherapy and repeated annually for 5 years after exposure. There is no indication for prophylactic thyroidectomy in patients with DICER1-associated conditions.

32.2.1.11 McCune-Albright Syndrome

McCune-Albright syndrome is a non-inherited disease that is the result of an early embryonic postzygotic somatic-activating pathogenic variant in *GNAS* (encoding the cAMP pathway-associated guanine nucleotide-binding-protein, $G_s\alpha$). It is characterized by café-au-lait skin macules, fibrous dysplasia of the craniofacial and axial skeleton leading to progressive scoliosis, facial deformities, loss of vision and/or hearing, and endocrinopathies including precocious puberty, testicular lesions, thyroid lesions with or without hyperthyroidism, growth hormone excess, and neonatal hypercortisolism [47]. Hyperthyroidism is present in 10–30% of cases, and malignant transformation has rarely been reported in case reports for PTC and clear cells [48]. Thyroid abnormalities have been diagnosed at a very young age; early screening is advised for thyroid function and thyroid disease (cystic/nodules) on USs maintained at regular intervals.

Methimazole is effective for medical management of hyperthyroidism, but because the condition is mostly persistent in this particular situation, definitive treatment such as early total thyroidectomy is preferred [49, 50].

32.2.1.12 Papillary Renal Neoplasia (Non-syndromic FNMTC)

This familial syndrome presents with the usual classical variant of PTC and benign thyroid nodules and is associated with renal papillary neoplasia. A linkage study suggests a significant association caused by a mutant susceptibility gene (designated *fPTC/PRN*), which is mapped to the chromosomal region 1q21 (▣ Table 32.1) [51].

32.2.2 Non-syndromic FNMTC

Population studies have shown that the risk of TC increases ninefold in patients with a first-degree relative with TC [52, 53]. Traditionally, non-syndromic FNMTC is diagnosed when two or more first-degree relatives are affected [54]; this in the absence of other predisposing causes of TC. When three or more first-degree relatives are affected, the probability that the patient's cancer is FNMTC is greater than 95%, compared to 31–38% when only two first-degree relatives are affected [52]. However, given the increased incidence of TC in the general population [2], some have suggested that patients with only two first-degree relatives with NMTC might represent sporadic disease (a chance occurrence) and not an inherited predisposition [52]. Furthermore, since the susceptibility gene(s) for non-syndromic FNMTC have not yet been identified, it is difficult to reliably know whether there actually is an inherited predisposition in the situation of only two first-degree relatives affected with TC.

Several studies have evaluated the risk of TC based on the number of family members affected with NMTC. As mentioned above, because no genetic testing can be performed to assess at-risk family members and the susceptibility genes for non-syndromic FNMTC are unknown to date, clinical screening (thyroid US and physical examination) has been used to determine an inherited predisposition. A prospective screening study by Klubo-Gwiezdzinska et al. [55], which used thyroid US and physical examination in at-risk family members with at least two first-degree relatives affected and evaluated thyroid nodule/cancer following American Thyroid Association guidelines (workup based on US features and tumor size), found 4.6% of at-risk family members in families with two affected first-degree relatives had TC diagnosed on screening, while 22.7% of at-risk family members in families with three or more affected first-degree relatives had a TC diagnosis. The authors found that patients with three or more first-degree relatives had a high rate of TC detected. Additionally, all cases diagnosed by screening had smaller primary tumor size, had a lower rate of central neck lymph node metastases, needed less extensive initial surgical intervention, and had a lower rate of radioiodine therapy compared to patients who presented with clinical disease. The youngest age of TC detection in this study was 18 years old [55]. Rios et al. [56] conducted a screening study in patients with FNMTC and found that 44% of at-risk family members had benign thyroid tumors, and 11.5% had a biopsy suggestive of cancer. The rate of TC was 5.5% in the study group and 1.3% in the control group, but the authors did not analyze whether the first-degree relatives were affected.

The goal of screening and surveillance for inherited or highly prevalent cancers in the general population is to identify and treat cancer early for those who are at risk, assuming this will result in reductions in cancer morbidity and mortality. Screening and surveillance for non-syndromic FNMTC is complicated because the susceptibility gene(s) are unknown, which necessitates screening all first-degree relatives who may be at risk with thyroid USs [57, 58].

The above studies show that screening at-risk family members resulted in earlier detection of low-risk FNMTC and was associated with a less aggressive initial treatment. Screening with thyroid USs should be considered in patients with three or more family members affected by FNMTC [55, 58]. Thus, to exclude sporadic disease—and thereby avoid over-diagnosing clinically insignificant TC that exists in the general population—non-syndromic FNMTC should be defined with the presence of three or more first-degree relatives. However, recent American Thyroid Association guidelines do not recommend screening and surveillance in non-syndromic FNMTC, citing a lack of evidence to date [9].

To summarize, these findings suggest that a reasonable approach is to screen for FNMTC with annual USs in patients age 18 years or older (or the youngest age of a TC diagnosis within the family) who are first-degree relatives with three affected family members. However, to date, it is unknown if earlier detection of less-advanced disease via this proposed screening and surveillance approach for FNMTC would result in a lower rate of TC recurrence and TC-related death or in overdiagnosis and overtreatment.

32.3 Prognosis and Aggressiveness in FNMTC Compared to Sporadic Disease

It is still debated and controversial whether non-syndromic FNMTC is more aggressive than sporadic NMTC, with multiple studies suggesting it is more aggressive and others finding similar outcomes (extent of disease and risk of recurrence and/or death) to sporadic NMTC [59–67].

A meta-analysis of 12 studies with a total of 12,741 participants compared the extent of disease and outcomes in non-syndromic FNMTC versus sporadic NMTC and found that FNMTC was associated with a younger age at diagnosis and higher rate of multifocal and bilateral tumors, extrathyroidal invasion, lymph node metastasis, and recurrence rate [60]. In a recent prospective cohort study comparing 78 patients with FNMTC to 53,571 NMTC patients [59], the investigators found that FNMTC cases presented at a younger age, with a greater rate of T1 disease, lymph node metastasis, and PTC compared to the cancer registry cohort of NMTC patients (US SEER NCI Database). Based on these findings, the investigators suggested that patients with non-syndromic FNMTC should be considered for aggressive initial treatment (prophylactic central neck lymph node dissection) [59]. Similar findings were shown in a retrospective study of 74 families with FNMTC [65], and the authors recommend periodic screening for early detection in FNMTC.

On the other hand, some studies found similar outcomes when comparing FNMTC to sporadic cases. For example, a retrospective controlled study in which 67 patients with FNMTC and 375 controls with sporadic disease were followed for a period of approximately 10 years showed similar long-term disease-free survival rates among FNMTC patients and controls with sporadic disease [66]. Additionally, long-term outcome in families with three or more affected relatives was similar to families with only two affected relatives. And in another smaller retrospective study [67], comparable outcomes were found, despite higher incidence of lymph node metastasis in FNMTC patients.

Some of the discrepancies found in studies evaluating whether non-syndromic FNMTC is more aggressive than sporadic NMTC are due to study design shortcomings, such as variable inclusion criteria/definitions for FNMTC, data based on retrospective studies, and small sample size. Furthermore, most of the patients studied had their disease status diagnosed clinically, instead of screened by thyroid US to provide an accurate (earlier) assessment of affected disease status and extent of disease. Thus, further large prospective studies are needed to fully assess the outcome in patients with FNMTC.

32.4 Susceptibility Genes in Non-syndromic FNMTC

Recently, multiple rare germline variants thought to contribute to FNMTC have been investigated by performing linkage analyses and whole-genome or whole-exome sequencing studies within families with FNMTC. The most recent or important findings from these studies will be discussed here. However, most of these results have not been able to be repeated or validated by other investigators and/or have not been found to account for a large number of FNMTC cases.

A study performing whole-exome sequencing in a family with six affected members found a germline variant in the serine/arginine repetitive matrix 2 gene (*SRRM2*). The heterozygous variant S346F affects downstream splicing of unknown targets and is co-segregated with PTC in this family, but the mutation was not found in 138 affected individuals with PTC [68].

A germline variant A339V in the thyroid transcription factor-1 (*TITF-1/NKX2.1*) was found in four patients with PTC. This germline mutation was dominantly inherited in two families, with some family members bearing the mutation affected with multinodular goiter, associated with either PTC or colon cancer. However, the mutation encoding the A339V substitution was not found among the 349 healthy control subjects nor among the 284 PTC patients who had no history of multinodular goiter [69]. Another study did not find the A339V mutation in 63 patients with PTC belonging to 38 families with NMTC [70].

A *HABP2* germline variant, G534E, was reported in seven affected members of a family with NMTC; functional studies show that HABP2 had a tumor-suppressive effect, with the G534E variant resulting in loss of function [71], but many follow-up studies found that this variant was not present in cases with FNMTC, and it did not segregate with all the affected members in families with non-syndromic FNMTC [72–75].

Recently, investigators have studied known susceptibility genes for other cancers and identified germline variants present in affected members with non-syndromic FNMTC, such as variants in *CHEK2* and *ATM* [76]. *CHEK2* encodes a checkpoint kinase that regulates cell cycle progression and DNA repair and *ATM* produces a protein responsible for cell growth control. These findings have not been validated in follow-up studies.

In 34 families with two or more affected members with FNMTC, Ye et al. [77] found gene mutations in *MAP2K5*: G961A and T110C in 3.85% and 2.59% of FNMTC families, respectively (using whole-exome and target gene sequencing). However, this was not confirmed in a recent follow-up study in Italian families with FNMTC [78]. Another whole-genome sequencing study in 23 affected individuals from five families with FNMTC found genes enriched in tumorigenic signaling pathways, such as MAPK/ERK and PI3K/AKT, implicating a central role of these signaling pathways in familial NMTC [79]. Recent analysis in three affected individuals, including two first-degree relatives and three healthy members of a family with FNMTC, found 28 pivotal genes with rare non-synonymous mutations; seven of these genes were novel candidate FNMTC pathogenic genes (*ANO7*, *CAV2*, *KANK1*, *PIK3CB*, *PKD1L1*, *PTPRF*, and *RHBDD2*), and among them, three genes (*PIK3CB*, *CAV2*, and *KANK1*) are reportedly involved in tumorigenesis through the PI3K/AKT signaling pathway [80].

To summarize, no clear susceptibility gene has been identified for FNMTC to date. As described above, many variants of candidate susceptibility genes appear to be present only in a few/single patients, and are most often not present within all family members affected by NMTC and subsequently not validated across multiple studies (from different populations). Again, some limitations are due to poorly defined inclusion criteria across these studies and the inclusion of families with only two affected members with TC, which reduces the chances of it being a truly familial disease. Additionally, unstudied alternative mechanisms, such as epigenetic mechanisms, might be involved in FNMTC and warrant further investigations. Overall, this supports the need for additional larger well-designed studies to validate the abovementioned genes, elucidate inheritance contributing to FNMTC, and determine the best screening tools and methods of clinical management.

Answers to the Questions

1. (b); 2. (d); 3. (a); 4. (a); 5. (c); 6. (d); 7. (c); 8. (c); 9. (b); 10. (d).

Conflict of interest The author declares no conflict of interest.

References

1. Schlumberger M. [Papillary and follicular thyroid carcinoma]. Ann Endocrinol (Paris). 2007;68(2–3):120–8.
2. Vaccarella S, Franceschi S, Bray F, Wild CP, Plummer M, Dal ML. Worldwide thyroid-cancer epidemic? The increasing impact of overdiagnosis. N Engl J Med. 2016;375(7):614–7.
3. Lim H, Devesa SS, Sosa JA, Check D, Kitahara CM. Trends in thyroid cancer incidence and mortality in the United States, 1974–2013. JAMA. 2017;317(13):1338–48.
4. Moses W, Weng J, Kebebew E. Prevalence, clinicopathologic features, and somatic genetic mutation profile in familial versus sporadic non-medullary thyroid cancer. Thyroid. 2011;21(4):367–71.
5. Vriens MR, Suh I, Moses W, Kebebew E. Clinical features and genetic predisposition to hereditary nonmedullary thyroid cancer. Thyroid. 2009;19(12):1343–9.
6. Lamartina L, Grani G, Durante C, Filetti S, Cooper DS. Screening for differentiated thyroid cancer in selected populations. Lancet Diabetes Endocrinol. 2020;8(1):81–8.
7. Kebebew E. Hereditary non-medullary thyroid cancer. World J Surg. 2008;32(5):678–82.
8. Ammar SA, Alobuia WM, Kebebew E. An update on familial nonmedullary thyroid cancer. Endocrine. 2020;68(3):502–7.
9. Haugen BR, Alexander EK, Bible KC, Doherty GM, Mandel SJ, Nikiforov YE, et al. 2015 American Thyroid Association Management Guidelines for Adult Patients with Thyroid Nodules and Differentiated Thyroid Cancer: The American Thyroid Association Guidelines Task Force on Thyroid Nodules and Differentiated Thyroid Cancer. Thyroid. 2016;26(1):1–133.
10. Richards ML. Familial syndromes associated with thyroid cancer in the era of personalized medicine. Thyroid. 2010;20(7):707–13.
11. Metzger R, Milas M. Inherited cancer syndromes and the thyroid: an update. Curr Opin Oncol. 2014;26(1):51–61.

12. Dinarvand P, Davaro EP, Doan JV, Ising ME, Evans NR, Phillips NJ, et al. Familial adenomatous polyposis syndrome: an update and review of extraintestinal manifestations. Arch Pathol Lab Med. 2019;143(11):1382–98.
13. Jarrar AM, Milas M, Mitchell J, Laguardia L, O'Malley M, Berber E, et al. Screening for thyroid cancer in patients with familial adenomatous polyposis. Ann Surg. 2011;253(3):515–21.
14. Herraiz M, Barbesino G, Faquin W, Chan-Smutko G, Patel D, Shannon KM, et al. Prevalence of thyroid cancer in familial adenomatous polyposis syndrome and the role of screening ultrasound examinations. Clin Gastroenterol Hepatol. 2007;5(3):367–73.
15. Chenbhanich JA-O, Atsawarungruangkit A, Korpaisarn S, Phupitakphol T, Osataphan S, Phowthongkum P. Prevalence of thyroid diseases in familial adenomatous polyposis: a systematic review and meta-analysis. Familial Cancer. 2019;18(1):53–62.
16. Perrier ND, van Heerden J, Goellner JR, Williams ED, Gharib H, Marchesa P, et al. Thyroid cancer in patients with familial adenomatous polyposis. World J Surg. 1998;22(7):738–42.
17. Cetta F, Montalto G, Gori M, Curia MC, Cama A, Olschwang S. Germline mutations of the APC gene in patients with familial adenomatous polyposis-associated thyroid carcinoma: results from a European cooperative study. J Clin Endocrinol Metab. 2000;85(1):286–92.
18. Nicolson NG, Man J, Carling T. Advances in understanding the molecular underpinnings of adrenocortical tumors. Curr Opin Oncol. 2017;
19. Monachese MA-OX, Mankaney G, Lopez R, O'Malley M, Laguardia L, Kalady MF, et al. Outcome of thyroid ultrasound screening in FAP patients with a normal baseline exam. Familial Cancer. 2019;18(1):75–82.
20. Liaw D, Marsh D, Li J, Dahia PL, Wang SI, Zheng Z, et al. Germline mutations of the PTEN gene in Cowden disease, an inherited breast and thyroid cancer syndrome. Nat Genet. 1997;16(1):64–7.
21. Milas M, Mester J, Metzger R, Shin J, Mitchell J, Berber E, et al. Should patients with Cowden syndrome undergo prophylactic thyroidectomy? Surgery. 2012;152(6):1201–10.
22. Tan MH, Jl M, Ngeow J, Rybicki LA, Orloff MS, Eng C. Lifetime cancer risks in individuals with germline PTEN mutations. Clin Cancer Res. 2012;18(2):400–7.
23. Bubien V, Bonnet F, Brouste V, Hoppe S, Barouk-Simonet E, David A, et al. High cumulative risks of cancer in patients with PTEN hamartoma tumour syndrome. J Med Genet. 2013;50(4):255–63.
24. Stratakis CA, Courcoutsakis NA, Abati A, Filie A, Doppman JL, Carney JA, et al. Thyroid gland abnormalities in patients with the syndrome of spotty skin pigmentation, myxomas, endocrine overactivity, and schwannomas (Carney complex). J Clin Endocrinol Metab. 1997;82(7):2037–43.
25. Carney JA, Lyssikatos C, Seethala RR, Lakatos P, Perez-Atayde A, Lahner H, et al. The spectrum of thyroid gland pathology in carney complex: the importance of follicular carcinoma. Am J Surg Pathol. 2018;42(5):587–94.
26. Yokote K, Chanprasert S, Lee L, Eirich K, Takemoto M, Watanabe A, et al. WRN mutation update: mutation spectrum, patient registries, and translational prospects. Hum Mutat. 2017;38(1):7–15.
27. Ishikawa Y, Sugano H, Matsumoto T, Furuichi Y, Miller RW, Goto M. Unusual features of thyroid carcinomas in Japanese patients with Werner syndrome and possible genotype-phenotype relations to cell type and race. Cancer. 1999;85(6):1345–52.
28. Lauper JM, Krause A, Vaughan TL, Monnat RJ Jr. Spectrum and risk of neoplasia in Werner syndrome: a systematic review. PLoS One. 2013;8(4):e59709.

29. Wémeau JL, Kopp P. Pendred syndrome. Best Pract Res Clin Endocrinol Metab. 2017;31(2):213–24.
30. Snabboon T, Plengpanich W, Saengpanich S, Sirisalipoch S, Keelawat S, Sunthornyothin S, et al. Two common and three novel PDS mutations in Thai patients with Pendred syndrome. J Endocrinol Investig. 2007;30(11):907–13.
31. Yoshida A, Taniguchi S, Hisatome I, Royaux IE, Green ED, Kohn LD, et al. Pendrin is an iodide-specific apical porter responsible for iodide efflux from thyroid cells. J Clin Endocrinol Metab. 2002;87(7):3356–61.
32. Camargo R, Limbert E, Gillam M, Henriques MM, Fernandes C, Catarino AL, et al. Aggressive metastatic follicular thyroid carcinoma with anaplastic transformation arising from a long-standing goiter in a patient with Pendred's syndrome. Thyroid. 2001;11(10):981–8.
33. Lavin MF, Shiloh Y. The genetic defect in ataxia-telangiectasia. Annu Rev Immunol. 1997;17:177–202.
34. Ulusoy E, Edeer-Karaca N, Özen S, Ertan Y, Gökşen D, Aksu G, et al. An unusual manifestation: papillary thyroid carcinoma in a patient with ataxia-telengiectasia. Turk J Pediatr. 2016;58(4):442–5.
35. Marsh DJ, Kum JB, Lunetta KL, Bennett MJ, Gorlin RJ, Ahmed SF, et al. PTEN mutation spectrum and genotype-phenotype correlations in Bannayan-Riley-Ruvalcaba syndrome suggest a single entity with Cowden syndrome. Hum Mol Genet. 1999;8(8):1461–72.
36. Eng C. The role of PTEN, a phosphatase gene, in inherited and sporadic nonmedullary thyroid tumors. Recent Prog Horm Res. 1999;54:441–52.
37. Sloot YJE, Rabold K, Netea MG, Smit JWA, Hoogerbrugge N, Netea-Maier RT. Effect of PTEN inactivating germline mutations on innate immune cell function and thyroid cancer-induced macrophages in patients with PTEN hamartoma tumor syndrome. Oncogene. 2019;38(19):3743–55.
38. Tosur M, Brandt ML, Athanassaki ID, Rednam SP. Considerations for total thyroidectomy in an adolescent with PTEN mutation. Ther Adv Endocrinol Metab. 2018;9(9):299–301.
39. Ngeow J, Mester J, Rybicki LA, Ni Y, Milas M, Eng C. Incidence and clinical characteristics of thyroid cancer in prospective series of individuals with Cowden and Cowden-like syndrome characterized by germline PTEN, SDH, or KLLN alterations. J Clin Endocrinol Metab. 2011;96(12):E2063–71.
40. Daniell J, Plazzer JP, Perera A, Macrae F. An exploration of genotype-phenotype link between Peutz-Jeghers syndrome and STK11: a review. Familial Cancer. 2018;17(3):421–7.
41. Wei S, LiVolsi VA, Brose MS, Montone KT, Morrissette JJ, Baloch ZW. STK11 mutation identified in thyroid carcinoma. Endocr Pathol. 2016;27(1):65–9.
42. Jelsig AM, Qvist N, Sunde L, Brusgaard K, Hansen T, Wikman FP, et al. Disease pattern in Danish patients with Peutz-Jeghers syndrome. Int J Color Dis. 2016;31(5):997–1004.
43. Rutter MM, Jha P, Schultz KA, Sheil A, Harris AK, Bauer AJ, et al. DICER1 mutations and differentiated thyroid carcinoma: evidence of a direct association. J Clin Endocrinol Metab. 2016;101(1):1–5.
44. de Kock L, Sabbaghian N, Soglio DB, Guillerman RP, Park BK, Chami R, et al. Exploring the association between DICER1 mutations and differentiated thyroid carcinoma. J Clin Endocrinol Metab. 2014;99(6):E1072–7.
45. Lee YA, Im SW, Jung KC, Chung EJ, Shin CH, Kim JI, et al. Predominant DICER1 pathogenic variants in pediatric follicular thyroid carcinomas. Thyroid. 2020;30(8):1120–31. https://doi.org/10.1089/thy.2019.0233.
46. Schultz KAP, Williams GM, Kamihara J, Stewart DR, Harris AK, Bauer AJ, et al. DICER1 and associated conditions: identification of

at-risk individuals and recommended surveillance strategies. Clin Cancer Res. 2018;24(10):2251–61.
47. Boyce AM, Florenzano P, de Castro LF, Collins MT. Fibrous Dysplasia/ McCune-Albright Syndrome. GeneReviews(®). 2015.
48. Collins MT, Sarlis NJ, Merino MJ, Monroe J, Crawford SE, Krakoff JA, et al. Thyroid carcinoma in the McCune-Albright syndrome: contributory role of activating Gs alpha mutations. J Clin Endocrinol Metab. 2003;88(9):4413–7.
49. Tessaris D, Corrias A, Matarazzo P, De Sanctis L, Wasniewska M, Messina MF, et al. Thyroid abnormalities in children and adolescents with McCune-Albright syndrome. Horm Res Paediatr. 2012;78(3):151–7.
50. Merchant N, Viau-Colindres JM, Hicks KA, Balazs AE, Wesson DE, Lopez ME, et al. McCune-Albright syndrome with unremitting hyperthyroidism at early age: management perspective for early thyroidectomy. Glob Pediatr Health. 2019;(6):2333794X19875153.
51. Malchoff CD, Sarfarazi M, Tendler B, Forouhar F, Whalen G, Joshi V, et al. Papillary thyroid carcinoma associated with papillary renal neoplasia: genetic linkage analysis of a distinct heritable tumor syndrome. J Clin Endocrinol Metab. 2000;85(5):1758–64.
52. Charkes ND. On the prevalence of familial nonmedullary thyroid cancer in multiply affected kindreds. Thyroid. 2006;16(2):181–6.
53. Hemminki K, Eng C, Chen B. Familial risks for nonmedullary thyroid cancer. J Clin Endocrinol Metab. 2005;90(10):5747–53.
54. Malchoff CD, Malchoff DM. Familial nonmedullary thyroid carcinoma. Cancer Control. 2006;13(2):106–10.
55. Klubo-Gwiezdzinska J, Yang L, Merkel R, Patel D, Nilubol N, Merino MJ, et al. Results of screening in familial non-medullary thyroid cancer. Thyroid. 2017;27(8):1017–24.
56. Ríos A, Rodríguez JM, Navas D, Cepero A, Torregrosa NM, Balsalobre MD, et al. Family screening in familial papillary carcinoma: the early detection of thyroid disease. Ann Surg Oncol. 2016;23(8):2564–70.
57. Rosario PW, Mineiro Filho AF, Prates BS, Silva LC, Lacerda RX, Calsolari MR. Ultrasonographic screening for thyroid cancer in siblings of patients with apparently sporadic papillary carcinoma. Thyroid. 2012;22(8):805–8.
58. Sadowski SM, He M, Gesuwan K, Gulati N, Celi F, Merino MJ, et al. Prospective screening in familial nonmedullary thyroid cancer. Surgery. 2013;154(6):1194–8.
59. El Lakis M, Giannakou A, Nockel PJ, Wiseman D, Gara SK, Patel D, et al. Do patients with familial nonmedullary thyroid cancer present with more aggressive disease? Implications for initial surgical treatment. Surgery. 2019;165(1):50–7.
60. Wang X, Cheng W, Li J, Su A, Wei T, Liu F, et al. Endocrine tumours: familial nonmedullary thyroid carcinoma is a more aggressive disease: a systematic review and meta-analysis. Eur J Endocrinol. 2015;172(6):R253–62.
61. Park YJ, Ahn HY, Choi HS, Kim KW, Park Do J, Cho BY. The long-term outcomes of the second generation of familial nonmedullary thyroid carcinoma are more aggressive than sporadic cases. Thyroid. 2012;22(4):356–62.
62. Uchino S, Noguchi S, Kawamoto H, Yamashita H, Watanabe S, Shuto S. Familial nonmedullary thyroid carcinoma characterized by multifocality and a high recurrence rate in a large study population. World J Surg. 2002;26(8):897–902.
63. Lee YM, Yoon JH, Yi O, Sung TY, Chung KW, Kim WB, et al. Familial history of non-medullary thyroid cancer is an independent prognostic factor for tumor recurrence in younger patients with conventional papillary thyroid carcinoma. J Surg Oncol. 2014;109(2):168–73.
64. Mazeh H, Benavidez J, Poehls JL, Youngwirth L, Chen H, Sippel RS. In patients with thyroid cancer of follicular cell origin, a family history of

nonmedullary thyroid cancer in one first-degree relative is associated with more aggressive disease. Thyroid. 2012;22(1):3–8.
65. Tavarelli M, Russo M, Terranova R, Scollo C, Spadaro A, Sapuppo G, et al. Familial non-medullary thyroid cancer represents an independent risk factor for increased cancer aggressiveness: a retrospective analysis of 74 families. Front Endocrinol (Lausanne). 2015;6(117)
66. Robenshtok E, Tzvetov G, Grozinsky-Glasberg S, Shraga-Slutzky I, Weinstein R, Lazar L, et al. Clinical characteristics and outcome of familial nonmedullary thyroid cancer: a retrospective controlled study. Thyroid. 2011;21(1):43–8.
67. Pitoia F, Cross G, Salvai ME, Abelleira E, Niepomniszcze H. Patients with familial non-medullary thyroid cancer have an outcome similar to that of patients with sporadic papillary thyroid tumors. Arq Bras Endocrinol Metabol. 2011;55(3):219–23.
68. Tomsic J, He H, Akagi K, Liyanarachchi S, Pan Q, Bertani B, et al. A germline mutation in SRRM2, a splicing factor gene, is implicated in papillary thyroid carcinoma predisposition. Sci Rep. 2015;5(10566)
69. Ngan ES, Lang BH, Liu T, Shum CK, So MT, Lau DK, et al. A germline mutation (A339V) in thyroid transcription factor-1 (TITF-1/NKX2.1) in patients with multinodular goiter and papillary thyroid carcinoma. J Natl Cancer Inst. 2009;101(3):162–75.
70. Cantara S, Capuano S, Formichi C, Pisu M, Capezzone M, Pacini F. Lack of germline A339V mutation in thyroid transcription factor-1 (TITF-1/NKX2.1) gene in familial papillary thyroid cancer. Thyroid Res. 2010;3(1):4.
71. Gara SK, Jia L, Merino MJ, Agarwal SK, Zhang L, Cam M, Patel D, et al. Germline HABP2 mutation causing familial nonmedullary thyroid cancer. N Engl J Med. 2015;373:448–55.
72. Cantara S, Marzocchi C, Castagna MG, Pacini F. HABP2 G534E variation in familial non-medullary thyroid cancer: an Italian series. J Endocrinol Investig. 2017;40(5):557–60.
73. Zhang T, Xing M. HABP2 G534E mutation in familial nonmedullary thyroid cancer. J Natl Cancer Inst. 2016;108(6):djv415.
74. Kowalik A, Gąsior-Perczak D, Gromek M, Siołek M, Walczyk A, Pałyga I, et al. The p.G534E variant of HABP2 is not associated with sporadic papillary thyroid carcinoma in a Polish population. Oncotarget. 2017;8(35):58304–8.
75. Sahasrabudhe R, Stultz J, Williamson J, Lott P, Estrada A, Bohorquez M, et al. The HABP2 G534E variant is an unlikely cause of familial non-medullary thyroid cancer. J Clin Endocrinol Metab. 2016;10(3):1098–103.
76. Wang Y, Liyanarachchi S, Miller KE, Nieminen TT, Comiskey DF Jr, Li W, et al. Identification of rare variants predisposing to thyroid cancer. Thyroid. 2019;29(7):946–55.
77. Ye F, Gao H, Xiao L, Zuo Z, Liu Y, Zhao Q, et al. Whole exome and target sequencing identifies MAP2K5 as novel susceptibility gene for familial non-medullary thyroid carcinoma. Int J Cancer. 2019;144(6):1321–30.
78. Cirello V, Colombo C, Persani L, Fugazzola L. Absence of the MAP2K5 germline variants c.G961A and c.T1100C in a wide series of familial nonmedullary thyroid carcinoma Italian families. Int J Cancer. 2019;145(2):600.
79. Srivastava A, Kumar A, Giangiobbe S, Bonora E, Hemminki K, Försti A, et al. Whole genome sequencing of familial non-medullary thyroid cancer identifies germline alterations in MAPK/ERK and PI3K/AKT signaling pathways. Biomolecules. 2019;9(10):605. https://doi.org/10.3390/biom9100605.
80. Zhu J, Wu K, Lin Z, Bai S, Wu J, Li P, et al. Identification of susceptibility gene mutations associated with the pathogenesis of familial nonmedullary thyroid cancer. Mol Genet Genomic Med. 2019;7(12):e1015.

Familial Primary Hyperparathyroidism

Leyre Lorente-Poch and Joaquin Gómez-Ramírez

Contents

A. L. Shifrin et al. (eds.), *Endocrine Surgery Comprehensive Board Exam Guide*,
https://doi.org/10.1007/978-3-030-84737-1_33

Case Presentation

Patient is a 43-year-old male who is referred to our clinic after an unsuccessful parathyroidectomy in another center. He had undergone a selective approach parathyroidectomy removing the right inferior gland (weight 800 mg) before. His blood test showed a persistent PHPT with elevated PTH of 125 pg/mL (12.5 pmol/L) and a serum calcium of 11.2 mg/dL (2.85 mmol/L) which were similar to preoperative levels. He has no past medical history. His father underwent a distal pancreatectomy for a benign tumor, and his brother is also under study for hypercalcemia.

Questions

1. *Which of the following would make you suspect the presence of a familial PHPT in the patient of the case presentation?*
   1. Presence of hypercalcemia in a blood test performed when he was 35 years old
   2. The patient being symptomatic
   3. Previous unsuccessful parathyroidectomy
   4. Presence of a prolactinoma
   5. Positive family history of glioblastoma
      - (a) Only (3) and (4) and (5) are correct.
      - (b) Only (2) and (4) and (5) are correct.
      - (c) Only (1) and (3) and (4) are correct.
      - (d) Only (3) and (5) are correct.
      - (e) All are correct.
2. *Which of the following further steps would you take in this patient?*
   1. Treat him with biphosphates.
   2. Check his urine calcium levels.
   3. Request adrenal MRI.
   4. Suggest assessing calcium and PHT levels in his relatives.
   5. Consider bilateral neck exploration.
      - (a) Only (3) and (4) and (5) are correct.
      - (b) Only (2) and (4) and (5) are correct.
      - (c) Only (1) and (3) and (4) are correct.
      - (d) Only (3) and (5) are correct.
      - (e) All are correct.
3. *The patient is positive for MEN 1, which of the following would you include in the preoperative workout?*
   1. Laryngoscopy.
   2. Redo sestamibi scan.
   3. Request intraoperative PTH monitoring.
   4. Request more comprehensive blood tests.
   5. Inform the patient about the risk of further recurrence.
      - (a) Only (3) and (4) and (5) are correct.
      - (b) Only (2) and (4) and (5) are correct.
      - (c) Only (1) and (3) and (4) are correct.
      - (d) Only (3) and (5) are correct.
      - (e) All are correct.

4. *Which of the following would you choose to do in this patient in case the sestamibi and ultrasound scans are concordant?*
    1. Focused parathyroidectomy
    2. Bilateral exploration
    3. Subtotal parathyroidectomy leaving the most normal looking parathyroid gland
    4. Subtotal parathyroidectomy leaving ½ of the most normal-looking parathyroid
    5. Bilateral thymectomy
        (a) Only (3) and (4) and (5) are correct.
        (b) Only (2) and (4) and (5) are correct.
        (c) Only (1) and (3) and (4) are correct.
        (d) Only (3) and (5) are correct.
        (e) All are correct.
5. *Which statements regarding MEN 1 are correct?*
    1. It has an autosomal dominant pattern.
    2. It was first described in 1990.
    3. Non-endocrine manifestations include angiofibromas, leiomyomas, and breast cancer.
    4. First degree family members have a risk of 50% of carrying the disease gene.
    5. The most commonly recommended initial operation is the minimally invasive targeted single gland resection.
        (a) Only (1) and (4) and (5) are correct.
        (b) Only (2) and (4) and (5) are correct.
        (c) Only (1) and (3) and (4) are correct.
        (d) Only (2) and (3) and (4) are correct.
        (e) All are correct.
6. *What are recommendations for surgical management of patients with PHPT-MEN 1?*
    1. When there is unilateral disease dominance by localization studies, the option of a "unilateral neck clearance" exists.
    2. The option of the minimally invasive targeted single-gland resection in patients with clear preoperative localization studies is probably the most adequate.
    3. The most commonly recommended initial operation for MEN 1 patients with PHPT is bilateral neck exploration with the aim of a subtotal parathyroidectomy.
    4. Total parathyroidectomy has clear advantages over subtotal approach.
    5. Standard preoperative localization studies are mandatory in the case of reoperation for persistent or recurrent PHPT.
        (a) Only (1) and (3) and (5) are correct.
        (b) Only (2) and (4) and (5) are correct.
        (c) Only (1) and (3) and (4) are correct.
        (d) Only (2) and (3) and (5) are correct.
        (e) All are correct.

7. *Which statements regarding MEN 2A are correct?*
   1. The "classical" findings in MEN 2A consist of medullary thyroid carcinoma (MTC) in 95%, pheochromocytoma 50–60%, and PHPT in 50–60%.
   2. PHPT is usually the first manifestation of MEN 2A.
   3. Parathyroid multiglandular involvement is less frequent, and the volume of the affected glands tends to be smaller as compared to MEN 1.
   4. Systematic resection of normal glands in patients with medullary thyroid cancer and normal PTH and calcium levels is recommended.
   5. MEN 2A is also known as Sipple syndrome.
      (a) Only (1) and (5) are correct.
      (b) Only (2) and (4) and (5) are correct.
      (c) Only (1) and (3) and (4) are correct.
      (d) Only (3) and (5) are correct.
      (e) All are correct.
8. *What are the main features of MEN 4?*
   1. It is caused by germline mutations of the *CDKN1B* gene.
   2. It has a female predominance.
   3. MEN 4 has been found and described in MEN 1-like patients in the absence of a *MEN1* mutation.
   4. It is characterized by the occurrence of parathyroid and anterior pituitary tumors in possible association with tumors of the adrenals, kidneys, and reproductive organs.
   5. Indications for parathyroid surgery are similar as for MEN 1.
      (a) Only (1) and (5) are correct.
      (b) Only (2) and (4) and (5) are correct.
      (c) Only (1) and (3) and (4) are correct.
      (d) Only (3) and (5) are correct.
      (e) All are correct.
9. *Which statements regarding HPT-JT syndrome are correct?*
   1. PHPT is rarely the first manifestation.
   2. It is generally due to a multiglandular disease.
   3. Parathyroid carcinoma is frequent (15–20%).
   4. HPT-JT is linked to germline inactivating mutations in the tumor suppressor gene *CDC73*.
   5. In the case of preoperative imaging techniques localizing a single gland, selective parathyroidectomy should be recommended.
      (a) Only (3) and (4) and (5) are correct.
      (b) Only (2) and (4) and (5) are correct.
      (c) Only (1) and (3) and (4) are correct.
      (d) Only (3) and (5) are correct.
      (e) All are correct.

10. *Which of the following would you find in a patient affected with FHH?*
    1. Highly elevated PTH
    2. Hypophosphatemia
    3. Hypocalciuria <100 mg/dL
    4. Mild hypercalcemia
    5. Slightly elevated PTH
        (a) Only (3) and (4) and (5) are correct.
        (b) Only (2) and (4) and (5) are correct.
        (c) Only (1) and (3) and (4) are correct.
        (d) Only (3) and (5) are correct.
        (e) All are correct.

33.1 Introduction

Primary hyperparathyroidism (PHPT) is one of the most common endocrinological disorders and is typically characterized by elevated serum calcium and excessive and unregulated secretion of the parathyroid hormone (PTH). The classical pathological pictures of PHPT mainly consist of an sporadic solitary benign parathyroid adenoma (80–85%), followed by multiglandular hyperplasia (10–15%), double adenoma (2%), and parathyroid carcinoma (less than 1%) [1, 2]. Approximately 90% of PHPT cases are estimated to be sporadic, whereas one tenth of PHPT occurs in a genetic and hereditary setting with a mutation in one of the, so far, identified 11 genes (*MEN1, RET, CDKN1A, CDKN1B, CDKN2B, CDKN2C, CASR, CDC73, GNA11, AP2S1*, and *PTH*) [3]. Familial PHPT may be present as part of a hereditary syndrome, together with other endocrine or non-endocrine tumors, namely, Multiple Endocrine Neoplasia Syndrome type 1 (MEN 1), type 2A (MEN 2A), type 4 (MEN 4), and Hereditary Hyperparathyroidism-Jaw Tumor Syndrome (HPT-JT). Less frequently, it may represent the only endocrine abnormality recurring in the affected members of kindreds with Familial Hypercalcemia Hypocalciuric (FHH) forms, Neonatal Severe HPT (NSHPT), and Familial Isolated HPT (FIHPT). Familial PHPT has an earlier onset than the sporadic variants and is mainly transmitted by an autosomal dominant pattern, although penetrance and expressivity are quite variable. Distinction between sporadic and familial cases of PHPT is not always easy, and family history may be absent because affected parents may have died before symptoms developed, the pedigree has not been evaluated carefully, or the patients turn out to be the index case [4]. Identification of hereditary disease is of vital importance for both, patient and affected relatives, who may be offered tailored management according to the presence of the associated mutations. Complete medical history should be performed to rule out familial PHPT (Table 33.1).

Table 33.1 Clinical history features suggesting familial PHTP

Young age of onset (<40 years old)		
Multiglandular involvement		
Persistent or recurrent PHPT		
Positive family history of PHPT		
Syndrome-related endocrinopathies (personal or family history):		
	Endocrine tumors	*Non-endocrine tumors*
MEN 1	PHPT Pituitary adenoma Enteropancreatic tumor Gastric NET Adrenocortical tumor Rarely: Pheochromocytoma Thymic NET Bronchopulmonary NET	Angiofibroma Meningioma Lipoma Breast cancer Rarely: Spinal ependymoma Soft tissue tumors
MEN 2A	Medullary thyroid cancer Pheochromocytoma PHPT	
MEN 4	PHPT Pituitary adenoma Neuroendocrine tumors Rarely: Adrenal tumor Papillary thyroid carcinoma Gonadal tumor	Lipoma Renal tumor
HPT-JT	Parathyroid carcinoma Atypical adenoma	Ossifying jaw fibroma Uterine tumors Kidney tumors

PHPT primary hyperparathyroidism, *NET* neuroendocrine tumor

33

Familial PTHP should be managed differently from sporadic PHPT [5]. Multiglandular involvement is more frequently found than in sporadic cases since all parathyroid tissue is genetically predisposed to be affected. Either synchronous multiglandular involvement may be present at onset or occur metachronously after a widely variable interval. Therefore, intraoperative findings may vary from symmetric or asymmetric hyperplasia to an apparent single-gland adenoma. Accordingly, prevalence of persistent and recurrent disease is higher than in sporadic cases, especially when a hereditary condition is not preoperatively suspected. Surgical strategy should aim achieving normocalcemia for as long as possible, avoiding hypoparathyroidism, and facilitating potential subsequent operation for recurrence [6].

The optimal surgical management generally starts with a bilateral neck exploration. Surgical technique ranges from total parathyroidectomy with autotransplantation and thymectomy to a limited parathyroidectomy according to the variant of familial PHPT, with exception for FHH, in which surgery is contraindicated. Lifelong follow-up is critical.

33.2 Preoperative Localization Studies

Standard preoperative localization studies with nuclear scintigraphy and ultrasound are not routinely recommended by experts since in the context of familial PHTP a bilateral exploration is usually advisable in the majority of forms. Ultrasound and Tc99m-sestamibi had sensitivities of 100 and 85% for localizing an enlarged parathyroid gland. They have been found to be infrequently contributory in first-time surgery in MEN 1 changing strategy in less than 20% of cases. However they may be of benefit identifying ectopic (20–38%) [7] or supernumerary parathyroid tissue. In the case of persistent or recurrent PHPT, however, imagine positive test are mandatory prior to reoperation [8].

33.3 Role of Intraoperative PTH Measurement in Familial HPT

Intraoperative PTH measurements may prove useful in parathyroid surgery for familial PHPT, and some authors have suggested it should be used to confirm the removal of all the functional parathyroid tissue [9]. High PPV for postoperative normocalcemia, for example, in MEN 1 patients has been found [7]. However, some other reports showed a substantially lower reliability with a high rate of false-positive values in the context of hyperplasia or multiglandular disease probably due to the presence of suppressed pathological glands.

To reduce the risk of false-positive results in MEN 1 patients, it has been suggested that more strict criteria should be applied, such as evaluation at 20 minutes and 70% reduction in PTH prior to accepting adequate excision of parathyroid tissue [10].

Intraoperative PTH is generally recommended for reoperative surgery.

33.4 Cryopreservation

Cryopreservation of parathyroid tissue is not widely performed as a routine practice for first surgery for familial PHPT and is not mandatory [11]. It is selectively recommended in cases of reoperation of MEN 1 [12] and MEN 2A patients. The viability of the parathyroid tissue is diminished after 2 years; thus, storage may be not a cost-effective strategy [13].

33.5 The Syndromes

33.5.1 MEN 1

It is the most frequent form of familial PHPT. PHPT is present in ~95% of MEN 1 cases, being usually the first manifestation of the syndrome.

MEN 1 is a rare disease with an estimated prevalence of 2–3 per 100,000 in unselected persons. It has an autosomal dominant pattern of inheritance which was first described by Wermer in 1954 [14]. In 1997, the gene (*MEN1*) causing MEN 1 was identified. The *MEN1* gene is localized on chromosome 11q13 and consists of 10 exons, it encodes for Menin, a tumor suppressor gene (◘ Table 33.2).

33.5.1.1 Clinical Presentation

The most common and first endocrine manifestation of MEN 1 is parathyroid tumors, resulting in primary hyperparathyroidism (75–95%) followed by pancreatic islets and anterior pituitary gland tumors. Parathyroid involvement may be asymmetrical multiglandular hyperplasia or multiple metachronic adenomas.

Pituitary tumors occur from 15% to 55% of which prolactinoma is the most common. Multiple non-secreting or secreting (gastrinomas, insulinomas) gastroenteropancreatic tumors occur in more than 50% of cases. Less frequently, thymic and lung neuroendocrine tumors may be present. Non-endocrine manifestations of MEN 1 include angiofibromas, collagenomas, lipomas, leiomyomas, and meningiomas; more recently, breast cancer has been described as an associated disease [15] (◘ Table 33.1).

33.5.1.2 Natural History

Typically, PHPT is the first clinical presentation in patients with MEN 1, and the age at diagnosis ranges from 20 to 25 years. Its prevalence is similar in both sexes with a penetrance of PHPT near to 100% by the age of 50 years [16].

When an *MEN1* mutation is confirmed, first-degree family members and offspring have a risk of 50% of carrying the disease gene. Second- and third-degree relatives have a risk of 25% and 12.5%, respectively [5].

33.5.1.3 Diagnosis

MEN 1 may be clinically diagnosed in an individual on the basis of the occurrence of two or more MEN 1-associated endocrine tumors [16]. Additionally it can be diagnosed in a

Table 33.2 Main genetic and clinical features of different forms of familial primary hyperparathyroidism

B	OMIN	Chromosome	Gene/Protein	Germline mutation	Age at onset	Parathyroid involvement	Surgical strategy
MEN 1	131,100	11q13	*MEN1*/Menin	Inactivating	20–25	MGD (asymmetric hyperplasia/ multiple adenomas)	SPTX or TPTX with autologous reimplantation + transcervical thymectomy
MEN 2A	171,400	10q11.21	*RET*/RET	Activating	>30	Single adenoma MGD (hyperplasia/adenoma(s))	Selective resection during thyroidectomy SPTX or TPTX with autologous reimplantation + transcervical thymectomy
MEN 4	610,755	12p13.1	*CDKN1B*/P27KIP1	Inactivating	>35	MGD (hyperplasia/ adenoma(s)	SPTX or TPTX with autologous reimplantation + transcervical thymectomy or limited approach in selected cases
HPT-JT	145,001	1q31.2	*CDC73*/Parafibromin	Inactivating	>30	Single (atypical adenoma) MGD (atypical adenomas) Parathyroid carcinoma	Focused parathyroidectomy SPTX or TPTX En block resection plus hemithyroidectomy
FIHPT	145,000	11q13 1q31.2 3q21.1	*MEN1, CDC73, CASR, CDKN1B, GCM2*	Inactivating	Not reported	Single/MGD (hyperplasia/adenoma(s))	Surgery tailored to the intraoperative findings
FHH				Inactivating	At birth	MGD (mild hyperplasia)	No surgery
Type 1	145,980	3q21.1	*CASR*/calcium-sensing receptor				
Type 2	145,981	19p13.3	*GNA11*/calcium-sensing receptor				
Type 3	600,740	19q13.2–q13.3	*AP2S1*/calcium-sensing receptor				
NSHPT	239,200	3q21.1	*CASR*/calcium-sensing receptor	Inactivating	At birth	MGD (Severe hyperplasia)	Emergency TPTX
ADMH	601,199	3q13.3–q21.1	*CASR*/calcium-sensing receptor	Inactivating	45	MGD >Single (Mild hyperplasia/adenoma(s))	Surgery tailored to the intraoperative findings

MGD multiglandular disease, *SPTX* subtotal parathyroidectomy, *TPTX* total parathyroidectomy

patient with an MEN 1-associated tumor and a first degree relative with MEN 1 and in an asymptomatic *MEN1* mutant gene carrier [17]. *MEN1* gene testing may be considered when PHPT occurs before the age of 40 years.

33.5.1.4 Indications for Surgery and Surgical Details

The indications for referral to surgery should be similar to the sporadic form, but the optimal timing for surgery and the number of parathyroid glands to resect remains controversial.

Standard preoperative localization studies with nuclear scintigraphy and ultrasound not officially recommended because they are infrequently contributory in first-time surgery (17%). However, they may be of benefit identifying ectopic (20–38%) [7] or supernumerary parathyroid glands. In the case of persistent or recurrent PHPT, however, imagine positive test is mandatory prior to reoperation [8].

Intraoperative PTH assay is recommended in reoperative surgery while its benefit is unproven in first-time surgery [5].

The surgical management requires a strategy that acknowledges that all of the parathyroid glands are, or will be, abnormal, and that the patient is better treated by having a smaller amount of abnormal parathyroid tissue and further risk of long-term recurrence, than by having none at all and subsequent life-long permanent hypoparathyroidism. Parathyroid involvement is multiglandular asymmetric in size and should be regarded as independent clonal adenomas [16].

The gold standard [5, 6] is a bilateral neck exploration identifying all four glands, and the most accepted first surgery for MEN 1 patients is a subtotal parathyroidectomy (STPX) removing 3 + 1/2 glands and leaving half of the most normal-appearing gland. Specially in children affected with MEN 1-HPTP, this is the approach selected by experts [18]. Marking the remnant with a non-absorbable thread is desirable since the recurrence occurs locally in more than 50% of patients with recurrent PHPT [19]. Since parathyroid tissue has been found in the thymus in 15% of patients with MEN 1, a bilateral cervical thymectomy is recommended.

The second most performed and more radical operation is a total parathyroidectomy (TPTX) with autotransplantion to the brachiocephalic muscle in the forearm. It involves lower risk of persistent and recurrent PHPT at the expense of higher rate of permanent hypoparathyroidism. A reported advantage of this technique would be that reoperation for recurrence in the autograft may be easier than resecting a regrowth remnant in the neck. However, it is not considered the most appropriate approach by the current guidelines.

Lairmore et al. published a randomized, prospective trial comparing subtotal and total parathyroidectomy with autotransplantation. The study showed comparable outcomes for

MEN 1 patients treated by both techniques, but subtotal parathyroidectomy may have advantages because it involves only one surgical incision and avoids an inevitable period of transient postoperative hypoparathyroidism [20].

Another less aggressive option is a "unilateral neck clearance" when there is unilateral disease dominance of localization studies. Both glands from the ipsilateral neck as well as the cervical thymic horn are resected. If a reoperation is required, it will be limited to the contralateral "virgin" neck. Although this approach remains controversial, it might be a good option in selected patients, providing them with a period of parathyroid normal function, especially important in young patients.

The option of the minimally invasive targeted single-gland resection in patients with clear preoperative localization studies is probably the least adequate, due to the high failure rate and some authors consider it contraindicated [21].

33.5.1.5 Outcomes/Prognosis

The reported incidence of recurrent or persistent hyperparathyroidism is 16–54%, and the incidence of hypoparathyroidism is between 10% and 25% [22]. Thorough review of the literature of parathyroidectomy in MEN 1 was crystalized in an European Consensus report of the European Society of Endocrine Surgeons [5] and showed a median recurrence rate of 32% (4–92%) and rate of 31.5% (3–100%) of permanent hypoparathyroidism.

The reported risk of persistence/recurrence according to the type of operation has been more than 50% after less than SPTX, 17% after SPTX, and 19% after TPTX. The risk of hypoparathyroidism has been reported to be 7–24% after less than SPTX, 16–39% after SPTX, and 66–75% after TPTX [23, 24].

A Dutch MEN 1 study showed that patients with nonsense or frameshift mutations in exons 2, 9, and 10 had a significantly lower risk of recurrence than patients with other mutations [23], whereas mutations in exon 3 may be linked to a higher risk of recurrence [24]. Thus, it has been suggested that genotyping may be useful in the future to guide the extent of initial parathyroidectomy [5].

33.5.2 MEN 2A

Unlike MEN 1, PHPT is not the dominant part of the disease, and MEN 2-related HPTP is considered an infrequent syndromic variant of hereditary PHPT.

MEN 2A is rare autosomal dominant inherited tumor syndrome due to germline activating mutations of the *RET* proto-oncogene. MEN 2A is also known as Sipple syndrome. In patients with MEN 2A, most mutations (>70%) are found in codon 634 (exon 11), which actually is more frequently associated with PHTP (30%) [11]. On the other hand, HPTP is uncommon in patients with mutations of codons 609, 611, 618, 620, 790, 791, and 804, rarely present in patients with mutations of codons 630, 649, 768, 790, 804, and 891 [5]. Whereas there is a genotype-phenotype correlation in terms of prevalence, it has no influence on the severity or gland involvement. In MEN 2B, PHPT has not been ever reported.

33.5.2.1 Clinical Presentation

The "classical" tumors combination of MEN 2A is represented by medullary thyroid carcinoma (MTC) in 95%, pheochromocytoma in 50%, and PHPT in 20–30%. PHPT is rarely the first manifestation (less than 8%). MEN 2A-PHTP is moderate, often asymptomatic, especially at a younger age, with only about 15–25% of patients developing clinical signs of disease [4]. The typical symptoms are rarely seen in patients with MEN 2A. MEN 2-related PHPT is not as predictable as in MEN 1, parathyroid multiglandular involvement is less frequent, and the volume of the affected glands tends to be smaller.

33.5.2.2 Natural History

The age of onset is later than in MEN 1, ranging from 35 to 40 years old, and it is 2 times more frequent in female patients. PHTP is typically identified during the preoperatory assessment for medullary carcinoma or pheochromocytoma.

33.5.2.3 Diagnosis

Diagnosis is confirmed by a *RET* mutation analysis in all patients who present with medullary thyroid carcinoma and/or pheochromocytoma. If positive, PHPT should be ruled out.

Screening also should be done if there is familial history of MEN 2 related tumors or any sign suggesting a non-sporadic PHTP (◘ Table 33.1).

If *RET* screening is positive in patient, timing of screening of the kindred for PHPT differs according to the mutation. If mutation is at codon 634, PTH and serum calcium should be checked annually by the age of 11 years, whereas if mutation occurs at other codons such as 609, 611, 618, 620, 790, and 791, screening of PHPT should be done every 2–3 years by the age of 16 years [11, 25].

33.5.2.4 Indications for Surgery and Surgical Details

Prior to surgery due to MTC, the possible coexistence of hyperparathyroidism should be assessed. Surgery is the treatment of choice for MEN 2-related PHPT. The indications for surgery are similar to the symptomatic sporadic form. Usual scenario is an asymptomatic patient who undergoes neck surgery for medullary thyroid carcinoma, in which resection of enlarged parathyroid glands found at the time of thyroidectomy is recommended to avoid reoperation for persistent or recurrent PHPT. Prophylactic parathyroidectomy of normal glands in patients with thyroid medullary carcinoma and still normal calcium and PTH levels is not indicated [26].

Usually, a conservative approach performing selective resection of only grossly enlarged parathyroid glands is recommended by the majority of authors and guidelines [5, 11], although subtotal parathyroidectomy or total parathyroidectomy plus autotransplantation may also be chosen when all four glands are enlarged. Decision-making should be balanced between putting patient at risk of easy manageable mild recurrent PHPT and tedious permanent hypoparathyroidism.

Unlike MEN1, there are no formal recommendations regarding the need for thymectomy in MEN 2A patients, so routine thymectomy is debatable and may only be advisable in selected cases.

33.5.2.5 Outcomes/Prognosis

The reported cure rate for patients with MEN 2A-associated PHPT after an appropriate surgery is high ranging from 77% to 100%, and permanent hypoparathyroidism is reflected to be 20%. Unlike MEN 1, similar success rates are reported, regardless the extent of resection. If present, recurrence is mild and expected beyond 5 years of follow-up [5].

33.5.3 MEN 4

MEN 4 has been found and described in MEN 1-like patients in the absence of a MEN 1 mutation. It is an extremely rare disease. It is caused by germline mutations of the *CDKN1B* gene, codifying for p27 kip1, an inhibitor of cyclin-dependent kinases, involved in the negative control of cell cycle progression [27] (◘ Table 33.2).

33.5.3.1 Clinical Presentation

MEN 4 is characterized by the occurrence of parathyroid and anterior pituitary tumors in possible association with tumors of the adrenals, kidneys, and reproductive organs [17] (◘ Table 33.1).

33.5.3.2 Natural History

MEN 4 shows a female predominance and affects approximately 80% of the reported cases to date. In contrast to MEN 1-PHPT, the MEN 4-PHPT occurs at a later age (mean age 25 years and 56 years, respectively) [28]. PHPT has a high penetrance (>80%) and is often the first endocrinopathy at onset.

33.5.3.3 Diagnosis

Patients with a MEN 1-like phenotype that are *MEN1*-mutation negative should undergo an accurate clinical evaluation for possible MEN 4 manifestations, and genetic analysis for *CDKN1B* mutations should be carried out to confirm the diagnosis.

33.5.3.4 Indications for Surgery and Surgical Details

No definitive conclusion can be drawn from the current literature concerning the optimal surgical management, because of the small number of patients reported. Indications for parathyroid surgery and surgical strategy should probably overlap the ones for MEN 1 [9] but limited approaches may be justified in selected cases.

33.5.4 Hereditary Hyperparathyroidism-Jaw Tumor Syndrome (HPT-JT)

HPT-JT syndrome is a rare autosomal dominant syndrome with incomplete penetrance and variable expression. HPT-JT is linked to germline inactivating mutations in the tumor suppressor gene CDC73 (formerly HRPT2), which encodes for parafibromin.

33.5.4.1 Clinical Presentation

It is characterized by parathyroid tumors (>95%), ossifying fibromas of mandible and/or maxilla (30%), uterine tumors (<50% of female patients), and less frequently, a variety of renal lesions [29, 30].

PHPT related symptoms are usually mild with exception of severe hypercalcemic syndrome in the context of parathyroid carcinoma.

33.5.4.2 Natural History

PHPT is the main manifestation of HPT-JT and affects about 95–100% of carriers at an early adulthood (>third decade). Single-gland involvement at onset occurs in around 80% of patients, often with pathological features of atypical adenoma (cystic aspect, fibrosis, mitosis). Predisposition to neoplastic progression due to germline *CDC73* mutation and a second genetic or epigenetic hit has been postulated as the mechanism for the frequently reported higher rate of single-gland parathyroid involvement in HPT-JT which differs from other variants of hereditary PHPT. Multiglandular disease is unfrequently present at the time of first surgery (20%), and metachronous second adenomas leading to recurrence may be present decades after in around 25% [31]. Parathyroid carcinoma (PC) is relatively frequent in HPT-JT (15–20% of the cases).

33.5.4.3 Diagnosis

Genetic analysis should be assessed in PHPT with cystic, atypical, and/or malignant parathyroid histology, in children diagnosed with ossifying fibroma(s) of the maxilla or mandible, PHPT with the absence of nuclear parafibromin staining in parathyroid tumor, and PHPT with young onset [5].

Parathyroid carcinoma may be preoperatively suspected biochemically by higher serum calcium levels and PTH levels, and larger tumor size or surrounding tissue invasion in imagine tests.

33.5.4.4 Surgery and Surgical Details

The optimal surgical approach has not yet been established and remains controversial, varying between bilateral or selective approach, and extensive or limited parathyroidectomy.

As in previous familial syndromes, the surgical strategy should be aimed to achieve the longest possible recurrence-free period without permanent hypoparathyroidism, minimizing surgical morbidity and facilitating possible future surgery for recurrent disease.

A focused approach with selective parathyroidectomy has been proposed for concordant single- gland localization at preoperative localizing techniques as in sporadic PHPT [5, 27], whereas bilateral neck exploration with subtotal parathyroidectomy might be preferred in cases of negative or discordant pre-operative localization.

When parathyroid carcinoma suspected, "en-bloc" resection including ipsilateral thyroid lobe and central compartment neck dissection, the remaining normal parathyroid and thymus is recommended in order to prevent capsular spillage and local seeding [31].

33.5.4.5 Outcomes/Prognosis

Because of the risk of recurrent and/or new disease, regular lifelong serum testing for biochemical evidence of PHPT is recommended.

According to the largest monocentric series including 20 HPT-JT operated patients, overall persistence/recurrence rate is around 30%. The outcome is significantly worse in parathyroid carcinoma compared to benign involvement (overall cure rate 33.3% vs 100%) [31].

33.6 Non-syndromic PHPT

33.6.1 Familial Isolated Hyperparathyroidism (FIHPT)

FIHPT is characterized by familial clusters typically with early onset of PHPT in the absence of other endocrine syndromic manifestations. It is an exclusion condition (can be postulated as the cause of PHPT only when the other possible genetic variants have been excluded). Its real prevalence remains unknown since it has been difficult to study due to small kindreds and mildly symptomatic cases.

FIHPT is an apparently autosomal dominant condition. Mutations of the *MEN1, CASR, CDKN1B,* or *CDC73* genes have to be excluded since families with germline mutations in these genes but isolated presence of PHPT have been described. It has been recently found that 17% of FIHPT patients have germline activating mutation of the *GCM2* gene encoding for a transcription factor [32].

33.6.1.1 Clinical Presentation and Natural History

Familial clusters of PHPT (usually FIHP kindreds contain a median of only two cases of primary hyperparathyroidism), presence of a history of recurrent PHPT, or multiple gland disease at surgery can suggest FIHPT. It is thought to represent either a stand-alone non-syndromic entity or an incomplete expression of one of the genetic syndromes that include PHPT within their profile such us MEN 1 and HPT-JT.

Patients with FIHP and a *GCM2* germline mutation present as adults with mild hypercalcemia and multiple parathyroid tumors.

33.6.1.2 Diagnosis

After a thorough clinical review excluding features typical of MEN 1 syndrome and HPT-JT syndrome, recommended gene mutational testing can then be performed after appropriate counselling to confirm or exclude the incomplete expression of a syndromic form of hereditary. PHPT gene testing should include the genes *MEN 1, CASR,* and *CDC73.*

33.6.1.3 Surgery and Surgical Details

The rarity of this condition is such that no truly evidence-based surgical strategy can be provided and the disease is best treated empirically [33] At surgery, FIHPT may be either caused by a single adenoma, or multiple gland disease, often with asymmetry. However, while forms of image-guided focused surgery are an option, visualization of all four parathyroid glands is the approach most likely to provide the most long-term cure [5].

33.6.2 Familial Hypocalciuric Hypercalcemia (FHH)

Its prevalence among PHPT patients is about 2%, and since no treatment is required, it is of great importance to rule it out before an unnecessary surgery is planned. FHH is an autosomal dominant inherited condition with 100% of penetrance. The inactivating mutation affects the calcium-sensing receptor

(CASR) causing an insensibility to hypercalcemia, resetting the normal range for serum calcium, so hypercalcemia is perceived as normal.

33.6.2.1 Clinical Presentation and Natural History

FHH is usually asymptomatic. In some cases mild symptoms such as fatigue, weakness, excessive thirst, and poor concentration have been described as well as relapsing pancreatitis, chondrocalcinosis, and premature vascular calcification [34]. Unlike other PHPT, patients with this affection will not develop end organ damage at the renal or bone level (bone mineral density may even be improved) and vitamin D are not altered [35, 36].

So far three genetic types of FHH have been described. The more frequent type (65% of cases) is FHH type 1, characterized by mild hypercalcemia with inappropriately elevated PTH. In this type, newborn from carriers are at a higher risk of developing neonatal severe primary hyperparathyroidism, which can be life-threatening. FHH type 2 (35% of cases) is typically characterized by very marked hypocalciuria, and the distinctive characteristic in FHH type 3 is the presence of mild hypophosphatemia (◘ Table 33.3).

33.6.2.2 Diagnosis

Mild hypercalcemia with inappropriately normal or slightly elevated PTH are detected in the blood test associated with inappropriate low urinary calcium excretion (<100 mg/dL 24 hours). Another distinctive characteristic from normal PHPT is that hypophosphatemia usually is not present (with exception of type III mutation).

Confirmatory test is classically done by assessing urinary calcium/creatinine clearance ratio [5, 37]:

$$\text{CaE} = \frac{\text{24h urine calcium}(\text{mmol})}{\text{24h urine creatinine}(\mu\text{mol})} \times \frac{\text{24h serum creatinine}(\mu\text{mol})}{\text{24h serum calcium}(\text{mmol})} < 100$$

$$\text{CaE} = \frac{\text{24h urine calcium}(\text{mmol}/\text{L})}{\text{24h serum calcium}(\text{mmol}/\text{L})} \times \frac{\text{24h serum creatinine}(\mu\text{mol}/\text{L})/1000}{\text{24h urine creatinine}(\text{mmol}/\text{L})} < 0.01$$

However, the largest series to date evaluating the validity of CCCR in 1000 patients with surgically confirmed PHPT showed that utility of this screening for FHH was limited, as 63% of non-FHH hyperparathyroid patients had low values [38].

When strongly suspicious, genetic mutation testing should be done, more to prevent a potential iatrogenic harm to the individual patient that treatment, since there is no need for it. But in the case of pregnancy it is mandatory to confirm the mutation because of the risk of severe neonatal hypocalcemia due to inhibition of endogenous secretion of PTH secondary to mother's hypercalcemia [5].

Table 33.3 Tips and Tricks

MEN 1	Most frequent form of familial PHPT "3 p": parathyroid, pituitary, and pancreatic tumors Asymmetric multiglandular parathyroid involvement Gold standard: bilateral neck exploration and STPX+ bilateral thymectomy Recurrence expected
MEN2A	PHPT infrequent Typically detected during medullary thyroid carcinoma or pheochromocytoma workout Genotype-phenotype correlation Parathyroid multiglandular involvement less frequent and less predictable Selective resection at the time of thyroidectomy High cure rates
MEN 4	MEN 1-like syndrome in the absence of *MEN1* mutation Later onset (fifth decade) Surgical strategy similar to MEN 1 (scarce literature)
HPT-JT	PHPT frequent Associated jaw, uterine, and renal tumors Single gland involvement more frequent (atypical parathyroid adenoma) High prevalence of parathyroid carcinoma Same surgical strategy as sporadic PHPT If parathyroid carcinoma suspected: "unilateral complete parathyroid clearance" High rate of recurrence
FIHPT	Exclusion condition: non-syndromic familial PHPT without other genetic mutations Variated parathyroid involvement: asymmetric multiglandular disease or single adenoma Bilateral neck exploration and surgery tailored to the intraoperative findings
FHH	Life-long mild hypercalcemia with inappropriately normal or slightly elevated PTH Hypocalciuria <100 mg/dL 24 hours Hypophosphatemia not present (with exception of type III) Usually asymptomatic, no bone or renal damage No treatment, only appropriate diagnostic Surgery contraindicated
NSHPT	Rare form of FHH (kindred of FHH carriers) Early onset (within few days of birth–6 months) Potentially life-threatening if not immediately treated Severe hypercalcemia and massive multiglandular hyperplasia Emergency TPTX
ADMH	Reported in a Swedish family FHH-like but hypercalciuria, hyperphosphaturia, hypermagnesemia, and nephrolithiasis More frequently mild multiglandular hyperplasia Surgery tailored to the intraoperative findings

PHPT primary hyperparathyroidism, *SPTX* subtotal parathyroidectomy, *TPTX* total parathyroidectomy

33

33.6.2.3 Treatment

In FHH there is no need for treatment and surgery is contraindicated. There is no response to diuretics or bisphosphonates.

If unfortunate surgery is performed, intraoperative findings usually are normal or mildly hyperplastic parathyroid glands but also hyperplasia has been described [5].

33.6.2.4 Outcomes/Prognosis

There is no known impact on patient life expectancy.

33.6.3 Neonatal Severe Hyperparathyroidism (NSHPT)

NSHPT is a rare, extreme form of FHH with approximately 100 reported cases. Classically, it was considered that heterozygous and homozygous inactivating mutations of the *CASR* gene were responsible for the occurrence of FHH and NSHPT, respectively. Recent findings, however, have shown that genetic bases of these rare diseases are actually more complex than expected. To date, more than 25 *CASR* mutations have been described involving a wide spectrum of 9 genotype/phenotype pairings [39].

33.6.3.1 Clinical Presentation and Natural History

In homozygous NSHPT, disease typically presents within a few days of birth or within 6 months of age and can be potentially life-threatening if not immediately diagnosed and opportunely treated with a reported mortality of 50%. Biochemically, severe hypercalcemia associated with very elevated serum levels of PTH and a low fractional excretion of urinary calcium are detected.

Early symptoms such as lethargy, hypotonia, failure to thrive, poor feeding and marked dehydration, constipation, vomiting, nephrocalcinosis, polyuria, and weight loss during the first weeks of life due to severe hypercalcemia are common. As serum PTH concentrations are intensively increased, bone disease is severe; thus young NSHPT patients may develop severe diffuse osteopenia, often complicated by multiple fragility fractures with the consequent ribcage instability and deformity that may lead to severe respiratory distress [39].

On the other hand, NHPT patients harboring heterozygous *CASR* mutations may present a milder variant of the neonatal form shortly after birth, usually during the first weeks of life. Actually, an homozygous inactivating *CASR* variant per se is not an obligatory cause of NSHPT as some variants have been presenting with hypercalcemia at later than 6 months of age and well into adulthood (mean onset age of 23 years) [41].

33.6.3.2 Diagnosis

Calcium above 4.5 mmol/L (18 mg/dL) among NSHPT is frequent and unique only to most homozygotes, so this cutoff proves a *CASR* homozygote and promotes optimal parathyroidectomy [41].

Once the emergency situation has been resolved if the genetic abnormality is not already diagnosed, then a genetic counselling review with testing of *CASR, AP2S1*, and *GNA11* is recommended. Moreover, in cases of both parents carrying CASR mutations and/or presenting clinical signs of FHH, prenatal mutational analysis or genetic testing at birth is recommended, although to date, age of initiation and type and frequency of screening have not been defined [9].

33.6.3.3 Medical Treatment, Surgery and Surgical Details

NSHPT is associated with life-threatening hypercalcemia that requires urgent treatment with intravenous saline and bisphosphonates on a pediatric high dependency unit in preparation for an urgent life-preserving total parathyroidectomy. More recently, it has been shown that cinacalcet can be used as another temporizing measure either alone or with a bisphosphonate [42]. Typically, massive hyperplastic parathyroid glands are identified and total parathyroidectomy should be performed.

33.6.3.4 Outcomes/Prognosis

If untreated, NSHPT is often lethal or otherwise catastrophic during infancy. However, once adequate treatment and surgery has been done, there is a promising long-term survival. Unfortunately, neuromotor retardation in the context of microcephaly and/or long-term and intense hypercalcemia may persist after otherwise successful therapy [41].

33.6.4 Autosomal Dominant Moderate Hyperparathyroidism (ADMH)

This non-syndromic variant of hereditary PHPT was first reported 20 years ago in a large kindred of 20 individuals of a Swedish family [43]. The disease is caused by a unique inactivating point mutation located in exon seven of the *CASR* gene affecting the intracytoplasmic tail domain of CaSR with inactivation of the receptor. The atypical disorder demonstrated autosomal dominant inheritance, and an early age at onset similar to FHH.

The monoclonal parathyroid lesions of this family may develop secondary to deletion of novel parathyroid tumor suppressor genes on chromosome arms 7q and 12q. Hypothetically, the germline mutation in the *CASR* gene of the affected family members may promote parathyroid cell proliferation and susceptibility to additional potential specific genetic hits [44].

An overlap with FIHPT is possible given the very similar phenotypes. It has been suggested it could be a subtype of FHH, but his disorder presents with hypercalciuria instead of hypocalciuria, hypermagnesemia, patients may develop nephrolithiasis and it can be reversed by radical parathyroid resection.

33.6.4.1 Clinical Presentation and Natural History

Combination of moderate hypercalcemia, inappropriately high serum PTH levels, elevated urinary calcium excretion, relative hypermagnesemia and hyperphosphaturia, and history of renal stones has been described. Hypercalciuria may be secondary mainly to the hypercalcemia per se, but also mild inactivation of the CaR in renal cells has been postulated as an additional mechanism.

33.6.4.2 Diagnosis

Confirmed by genetic testing.

33.6.4.3 Surgery and Surgical Details

So far parathyroidectomy in 12 out of 22 patients has been reported [45].

Nearly 80% showed mild enlargement with diffuse hyperplasia, and only in 2 of them an apparently single adenoma was found. The majority of them underwent a subtotal parathyroidectomy leaving parathyroid remnants of 10–20 mg.

33.6.4.4 Outcome

Success was achieved in 88% of the patients. Postoperative persistence of hypercalcemia, albeit ameliorated, occurred in the three members who had limited parathyroidectomy of two enlarged parathyroid glands who seemed to require subsequent subtotal parathyroidectomy. Recurrent hypercalcemia was not been observed during an average follow-up of 5.1 years [33].

There is no information regarding the follow-up in the nonsurgical patients.

Answers to the Questions

1. (c); 2. (b); 3. (e); 4. (b); 5. (c); 6. (a); 7. (d); 8. (e); 9. (a); 10. (a)

References

1. Insogna KL. Primary hyperparathyroidism. N Engl J Med. 2018;379(11):1050–9.
2. Bilezikian JP, Bandeira L, Khan A, Cusano NE. Hyperparathyroidism. Lancet. 2018;391(10116):168–78.
3. Bilezikian JP, Brandi ML, Eastell R, Silverberg SJ, Udelsman R, Marcocci C, et al. Guidelines for the management of asymptomatic primary hyperparathyroidism: summary statement from the fourth international workshop. J Clin Endocrinol Metab. 2014;99(10):3561–9.
4. Alberto F. Genetics of parathyroids disorders: overview. Best Pract Res Clin Endocrin Metab. 2018;32(6):781–90.
5. Iacobone M, Carnaille B, Palazzo FF, Vriens M. Hereditary hyperparathyroidism—a consensus report of the European Society of Endocrine Surgeons (ESES). Langenbeck's Arch Surg. 2015;400(8):867–86.
6. Wilhelm SM, Wang TS, Ruan DT, Lee JA, Asa SL, Duh QY, et al. The American association of endocrine surgeons guidelines for definitive management of primary hyperparathyroidism. JAMA Surg. 2016;151(10):959–68.

7. Nilubol N, Weinstein L, Simonds WF, Jensen RT, Phan GQ, Hughes MS, et al. Preoperative localizing studies for initial parathyroidectomy in MEN1 syndrome: is there any benefit? World J Surg. 2012;36(6):1368–74.
8. Mihai R, Barczynski M, Iacobone M, Sitges-Serra A. Surgical strategy for sporadic primary hyperparathyroidism an evidence-based approach to surgical strategy, patient selection, surgical access, and reoperations. Langenbeck's Arch Surg. 2009;394(5):785–98.
9. Tonelli F, Marcucci T, Giudici F, Falchetti A, Brandi ML. Surgical approach in hereditary hyperparathyroidism. Endocr J. 2009;56(7):827–41.
10. Thompson GB, Grant CS, et al. Reoperative parathyroid surgery in the era of ses- tamibi scanning and intraoperative parathyroid hormone monitoring. Arch Surg. 1999;134:699–705.
11. Wells SA, Asa SL, Dralle H, Elisei R, Evans DB, Gagel RF, et al. Revised american thyroid association guidelines for the management of medullary thyroid carcinoma. Thyroid. 2015;25(6):567–610.
12. Keutgen XM, Nilubol N, Agarwal S, Welch J, Cochran C, Marx SJ, et al. Reoperative surgery in patients with multiple endocrine neoplasia type 1 associated primary hyperparathyroidism. Ann Surg Oncol. 2016;23:701–7.
13. Samuel S, Guerrero MA. The evidence for and against parathyroid cryopreservation: should we continue to promote parathyroid cryopreservation? In: Angelos P, Grogan RH, editors. Difficult decisions in endocrine surgery. Springer; 2018. p. 273–81.
14. Wermer P. Genetic aspects of adenomatosis of endocrine glands. Am J Med. 1954;16(3):363–71.
15. Dreijerink KMA, Goudet P, Burgess JR, Valk GD. Breast-cancer predisposition in multiple endocrine neoplasia type 1. New Engl J Med. 2014;371(6):583–4.
16. Thakker RV, Newey PJ, Walls GV, Bilezikian J, Dralle H, Ebeling PR, et al. Clinical practice guidelines for multiple endocrine neoplasia type 1 (MEN1). J Clin Endocrinol Metab. 2012;97(9):2990–3011.
17. Thakker RV. Multiple endocrine neoplasia type 1 (MEN1) and type 4 (MEN4). Mol Cell Endocrinol. 2014;386(1–2):2–15.
18. Nobecourt PF, Zagzag J, Asare EA, Perrier ND. Intraoperative decision-making and technical aspects of parathyroidectomy in young patients with MEN1 related hyperparathyroidism. Front Endocrinol. 2018;618(9):1–9.
19. Salmeron MDB, Gonzalez JMR, Fornos JS, Goday A, Perez NMT, Zambudio AR, et al. Causes and treatment of recurrent hyperparathyroidism after subtotal parathyroidectomy in the presence of multiple endocrine neoplasia 1. World J Surg. 2010;34(6):1325–31.
20. Lairmore TC, Govednik CM, Quinn CE, Sigmond BR, Lee CY, Jupiter DC. A randomized, prospective trial of operative treatments for hyperparathyroidism in patients with multiple endocrine neoplasia type 1. Surg. 2014;156(6):1326–35.
21. Nilubol N, Weinstein LS, Simonds WF, Jensen RT, Marx SJ, Kebebew E. Limited parathyroidectomy in multiple endocrine neoplasia type 1-associated primary hyperparathyroidism: a setup for failure. Ann Surg Oncol. 2016;23(2):416–23.
22. Doherty GM. Multiple endocrine neoplasia type 1. J Surg Oncol. 2005;89(3):143–50.
23. Pieterman CRC, Van Hulsteijn LT, Den Heijer M, Van Der Luijt RB, Bonenkamp JJ, Hermus ARMM, et al. Primary hyperparathyroidism in MEN1 patients: a cohort study with longterm follow-up on preferred surgical procedure and the relation with genotype. Ann Surg. 2012;255(6):1171–8.
24. Fyrsten E, Norlén O, Hessman O, Stålberg P, Hellman P. Long-term surveillance of treated hyperparathyroidism for multiple endocrine neo-

plasia type 1: recurrence or hypoparathyroidism? World J Surg. 2016;40(3):615–21.
25. Brandi ML, Gagel RF, Angeli A, Bilezikian JP, Beck-Peccoz P, Bordi C, et al. Consensus: guidelines for diagnosis and therapy of MEN type 1 and type 2. J Clin Endocrinol Metab. 2001;86(12):5658–71.
26. Guerin C, Romanet P, Taieb D, Brue T, Lacroix A, Sebag F, et al. Looking beyond the thyroid: advances in the understanding of pheochromocytoma and hyperparathyroidism phenotypes in MEN2 and of non-MEN2 familial forms. Vol. 25. Endocr Relat Cancer. 2018;25(2):T15–28.
27. Cetani F, Saponaro F, Borsari S, Marcocci C. Familial and hereditary forms of primary hyperparathyroidism. In: Brandi ML, editor. Parathyroid disorders. Focusing on unmet needs. Front Horm Res. Basel: Karger. 2019. p. 40–51.
28. Cristina EV, Alberto F. Management of familial hyperparathyroidism syndromes: MEN1, MEN2, MEN4, HPT-Jaw tumour, Familial isolated hyperparathyroidism, FHH, and neonatal severe hyperparathyroidism. Best Pract Res Clin Endocrinol Metabol. 2018;32(6):861–75.
29. Mehta A, Patel D, Rosenberg A, Boufraqech M, Ellis RJ, Nilubol N, et al. Hyperparathyroidism-jaw tumor syndrome: results of operative management. Surg. 2014;156(6):1315–25.
30. Carpten JD, Robbins CM, Villablanca A, Forsberg L, Presciuttini S, Bailey-Wilson J, et al. HRPT2, encoding parafibromin, is mutated in hyperparathyroidism-jaw tumor syndrome. Nat Genet. 2002;32(4):676–80.
31. Iacobone M, Camozzi V, Mian C, Pennelli G, Pagetta C, Casal Ide E, et al. Long-term outcomes of parathyroidectomy in hyperparathyroidism-jaw tumor syndrome: analysis of five families with CDC73 mutations. World J Surg. 2020;44(2):508–16.
32. Marx SJ. New concepts about familial isolated hyperparathyroidism. J Clin Endocrinol Metab. 2019;104(9):4058–66.
33. Carling T, Udelsman R. Parathyroid surgery in familial hyperparathyroid disorders. J Intern Med. 2005;257(1):27–37.
34. Egbuna OIBE. Hypercalcaemic and hypocalcaemic conditions due to calcium-sensing receptor mutations. Best Pr Res Clin Rheumatol. 2008;22:129–48.
35. Christensen SE, Nissen PHVP, et al. Plasma 25- hydroxyvitmain D, 1,25-dihydroxyvitmain D, and PTH in familial hypocalciuric hypercalcaemia (FHH) and primary hyperparathyroidism (PHPT). Eur J Endocrinol. 2008;159(6):719–27.
36. Isaksen T, Nielsen CSCS, et al. Forearm bone mineral density in familial hypocalciuric hypercalcemia and primary hyperparathyroidism: a comparative study. Calcif Tissue Int. 2011;89:285–94.
37. Konya J, Aye M, Rj E, Atkin SL. Assessment of hyperparathyroidism. In: Watkinson JC, Scott-Coombes DM, editors. Tips and tricks in endocrine surgery. Springer; 2014. p. 235–43.
38. Moore EC, Berber E, Jin J, Krishnamurthy V, Shin JSA. Calcium creatinine clearance ratio is not helpful in differentiating primary hyperparathyroidism from familial herpercalcemic hypocalciuria: a study of 1000 patients. Endocr Pract. 2018;24(11):988–94.
39. Vannucci L, Brandi ML. Familial hypocalciuric hypercalcemia and neonatal severe hyperparathyroidism. Front Horm Res. 2018;51:52–62.
40. Hannan FM, Babinsky VNTR. Disorders of the calcium-sensing receptor and partner pro- teins: insights into the molecular basis of calcium ho- meostasis. J Mol Endocrinol. 2016;57:R127–42.
41. Marx SJ, Sinaii N. Neonatal severe hyperparathyroidism: novel insights from calcium, PTH, and the CASR gene. J Clin Endocrinol Metab. 2020;105(4):1061–78.
42. Wilhelm-Bals A, Parvex P, Magdelaine CGE. Successful use of bisphosphonate and calcimimetic in neonatal severe primary hyperparathyroidism. Pediatrics. 2012;129:e812–6.

43. Carling T, Szabo E, Bai M, Ridefelt P, Westin G, Gustavsson P, et al. Familial hypercalcemia and hypercalciuria caused by a novel mutation in the cytoplasmic tail of the calcium receptor. J Clin Endocrinol Metab. 2000;85(5):2042–7.
44. Szabo E, Carling T, Hessman O, Rastad J. Loss of heterozygosity in parathyroid glands of familial hypercalcemia with hypercalciuria and point mutation in calcium receptor. J Clin Endocrinol Metab. 2002;87(8):3961–5.
45. Szabo E, Hellman P, Lundgren E, Carling T, Rastad J. Parathyroidectomy in familial hypercalcemia with clinical characteristics of primary hyperparathyroidism and familial hypocalciuric hypercalcemia. Surgery. 2002;131(3):257–63.

Familial Hypocalciuric Hypercalcemia (FHH)

Serkan Teksöz

Contents

A. L. Shifrin et al. (eds.), *Endocrine Surgery Comprehensive Board Exam Guide*,
https://doi.org/10.1007/978-3-030-84737-1_34

Case Presentation

A 40-year-old male presented to the clinic with worsening of constipation over the last year. Abdominal screening and colonoscopy revealed no obvious pathology. On laboratory evaluation, serum calcium level was measured as 11.1 mg/dl (2.78 mmol/l) (normal range: 8.8–10.2 mg/dl; 2.2–2.55 mmol/l), parathyroid hormone (PTH) was 76 pq/ml (10–60 pq/ml), 1,25(OH2) vitamin D was 42 ng/ml (8.8–46.3 ng/ml), albumin was 4.1 mg/dl (3.5–5 mg/dl), and creatinine was 0.9 mg/dl (0.8–1.1 mg/dl).

Questions

1. Which of the following test(s) should be performed next?
   1. A 24-hour urine calcium and creatinine with calculation of the fractional excretion of calcium
   2. Parathyroid sestamibi scan
   3. Referral for parathyroid surgery
   4. Order renal ultrasound and dual-energy X-ray absorptiometry scan
      - (a) Only (1) and (2) and (3) are correct.
      - (b) Only (1) and (2) are correct.
      - (c) Only (1) is correct.
      - (d) Only (1) and (3) and (4) are correct.
      - (e) All are correct.
2. Primary hyperparathyroidism and familial hypocalciuric hypercalcemia are both causes of hypercalcemia. Which of the following(s) can differentiate between these two diseases?
   1. Parathyroid hormone (PTH) level above 100 pg/ml suggests primary hyperparathyroidism.
   2. The absence of family history of hypercalcemia suggests primary hyperparathyroidism.
   3. A calcium/creatinine ratio below 0.01 supports the diagnosis of familial hypocalciuric hypercalcemia.
   4. A calcium/creatinine ratio below 0.01 supports the diagnosis of primary hyperparathyroidism.
      - (a) Only (2) and (3) are correct.
      - (b) Only (2) and (4) are correct.
      - (c) Only (1) is correct.
      - (d) Only (2) is correct.
      - (e) Only (3) is correct.
3. Which statement(s) regarding FHH is (are) correct?
   1. The etiology of FHH is the defect in the parathyroid hormone receptor.
   2. Treatment is not often necessary.
   3. There is an autosomal recessive pattern.
   4. Symptoms usually manifest in the sixth or seventh decade of life.

(a) All are correct.
(b) Only (1) and (2) and (3) are correct.
(c) Only (1) and (3) are correct.
(d) Only (1) is correct.
(e) Only (2) is correct.

4. Which statement(s) regarding FHH is (are) correct?
   1. Urine calcium excretion is generally low.
   2. There is an autosomal dominant pattern.
   3. Vitamin D metabolism is normal with normal seasonal variation, although 1,25- dihydroxy vitamin D is increased compared with normal controls.
   4. Bone mineral density (BMD) and Z-scores are often normal.
      (a) Only (1) and (3) are correct.
      (b) Only (1) and (4) are correct.
      (c) Only (1) is correct.
      (d) Only (1) and (2) and (3) are correct.
      (e) All are correct.
5. Which diagnostic criterion (criteria) regarding FHH is (are) correct?
   1. Recurrent hypercalcemia is seen after parathyroidectomy.
   2. Most persons with FHH are asymptomatic.
   3. Serum phosphate levels are often reduced.
   4. Serum magnesium levels are often reduced.
      (a) Only (1) and (2) are correct.
      (b) Only (1) and (2) and (3) are correct.
      (c) Only (1) and (4) are correct.
      (d) Only (2) is correct.
      (e) All are correct.
6. Which statement(s) regarding FHH is (are) correct?
   1. Genetic testing for CaSR mutations can be helpful when biochemical data are indeterminate.
   2. Intact PTH levels are typically high in 80% of patients with FHH.
   3. Low calcium intake, the presence of vitamin D deficiency, or hypocalciuric drugs (lithium or thiazide diuretics) can also lower renal calcium excretion.
   4. There is an autosomal recessive pattern.
      (a) Only (1) is correct.
      (b) Only (3) is correct.
      (c) Only (1) and (3) are correct.
      (d) Only (2) and (4) are correct.
      (e) All are correct.
7. Which statement(s) regarding FHH is (are) correct?
   1. Calcium-sensing receptor mutational analysis is the best test for diagnosing FHH.
   2. Morbidity is generally high in FHH.
   3. Calcimimetics can be considered in patients with symptomatic FHH.

4. Surgery is the best treatment.
   (a) Only (1) is correct.
   (b) Only (1) and (2) and (3) are correct.
   (c) Only (4) is correct.
   (d) Only (1) and (3) are correct.
   (e) All are correct.

8. Which statement(s) regarding FHH is(are) correct?
   1. Postoperative serum calcium level is normalized.
   2. Creatinine clearance is decreased.
   3. Serum magnesium level is decreased.
   4. The prognosis in FHH is good.
      (a) Only (1) and (2) and (3) are correct.
      (b) Only (1) and (2) are correct.
      (c) Only (2) is correct.
      (d) Only (4) is correct.
      (e) All are correct.
9. The following clinical features can be seen in patients with FHH:
   1. Chondrocalcinosis
   2. Kidney stones
   3. Hypertension
   4. Band keratopathy
   5. Acute pancreatitis
      (a) All are correct.
      (b) Only (2) and (4) are correct.
      (c) Only (1) and (5) are correct.
      (d) Only (1) and (2) and (4) are correct.
      (e) Only (1) and (2) and (5) are correct.
10. Hypercalcemia with high parathyroid hormone (PTH) level is associated with which of the following:
   1. Lithium intake
   2. Familial hypocalciuric hypercalcemia
   3. Milk alkali syndrome
   4. Metastatic parathyroid carcinoma
   5. Sarcoidosis
      (a) All are correct.
      (b) Only (1) and (2) are correct.
      (c) Only (1) and (2) and (3) are correct.
      (d) Only (1) and (2) and (4) are correct.
      (e) Only (2) is correct.

34

34.1 Introduction

Hypercalcemia, a metabolic abnormality often found on routine blood screening, is usually asymptomatic for a prolonged period. Although hypercalcemia has many causes, primary hyperparathyroidism and malignancy are the most common factors in etiology. Small but an important minority of patients has familial hypocalciuric hypercalcemia (FHH) [1].

FHH is a rare autosomal dominant condition. It most often occurs as a result of mutations in the calcium-sensing receptor gene (CaSR) causing decreased receptor activity. Patients can have mild hypercalcemia, hypocalciuria, hypermagnesemia, and hypophosphatemia. Parathyroid hormone level (PTH) is normal or mildly elevated [2]. The true prevalence of FHH is not known but has been estimated to be in the range of 1/78,000, compared to the prevalence of PHPT of 1/1000. The true prevalence is likely to be higher due to its subclinical nature in many cases [3]. Establishing the correct diagnosis is important because surgery is ineffective and usually not required in FHH [4].

34.2 Molecular Genetics

FHH is usually a benign condition in patients who have the heterozygous mutation. In most of the cases, FHH results from loss-of-function mutations in the CaSR on the long arm of chromosome 3 (FHH1; over 85%). Besides chromosome 3, mutation on chromosome 19 was observed: a mutation in the G-protein subunit alpha 11 (GNA11) gene (19p) causes FHH2, and a mutation in the adaptor-related protein complex 2 (AP2S1) gene (19q13.3) is responsible for FHH3 [5–9].

The wide variations of specific mutations in the *CaSR*-gene are easily accessible online [10]. Nevertheless, it has to be taken into account that due to locus heterogeneity and large gene rearrangements, false-negative results may occur even in molecular genetic analysis [11].

Besides genome mutations (FHH1–3), some patients presenting with FHH phenotype show no genetic alterations but have autoantibodies against the CaSR. This needs to be considered in case of negative genetic testing [12, 13].

34.3 Clinical Presentation

In the earlier analyses of index cases and their kindreds in 1985, those who had FHH (genotype unknown at the time) presented with mild hypercalcemia; more symptoms of muscle weakness, fatigue, arthralgias, and increased thirst compared to their normocalcemic relatives were reported [14]. Relapsing pancreatitis may be slightly increased in patients with FHH, but it is not clear that there is a causative association [15]. FHH may also be associated with an increased incidence of chondrocalcinosis and premature vascular calcification [16].

Whereas patients with FHH1 and FHH2 often show high normal PTH values and slightly increased magnesium levels, patients with FFH3 are characterized by elevated PTH, decreased phosphate, and sometimes osteomalacia [9].

Some patients with FHH1 suffer from pancreatitis and chondrocalcinosis or may have concurrent PHPT. Parathyroid adenomas have rarely been described in FHH [17], and parathyroid gland enlargement has been found in some cases of FHH, but the enlargement is not as significant as in primary hyperparathyroidism [3, 18, 19].

However, several authors report patients with both PHPT and FHH. In the reported patients, enlarged parathyroid glands (histologically defined as adenoma) have been removed, followed by a decrease of the serum calcium level, but, nevertheless, it did not lead to a calcium normalization in all patients. At the moment, there is no evidence for genetic factors causing FHH and PHPT in one patient. However, the authors postulate that the CaSR mutation with altered calcium homeostasis may trigger and/or enhance the development of PHPT [17, 20–22].

In FHH, the patients generally have bone mineral density (BMD) and Z-scores comparable to normal controls, with only marginal changes in bone markers and maintained balance between bone resorption and bone formation [23, 24].

34.4 Natural History

The family history is important and should be explored in all cases of hypercalcemia. Relatives with hypercalcemia and relatives who have undergone unsuccessful parathyroid surgery should be identified [23].

Possible symptoms are fatigue, weakness, constipation, polyuria, polydypsia, renal insufficiency, or headache. Other symptoms include chondrocalcinosis or mental problems [2].

Most people with FHH are asymptomatic, and sometimes they are not diagnosed or have such a varied spectrum of clinical presentations that it is actually more prevalent than reported [3].

34.5 Diagnosis

Standard biochemical evaluation of hypercalcemia should be undertaken with more emphasis on collection and interpretation of 24-h urine calcium and creatinine. A 24-hour urinary calcium excretion (24 h-UCa) is decreased. The Ca/Cr excretion ratio (CCCR) is below 0.01 (indicating FHH) or in the "gray area" between 0.01 and 0.02 (FHH or PHPT); CCCR >0.02 indicates PHPT [11]. Calculating CCCR has a sensitivity of 80% and a sensitivity of 88% and is therefore more reliable than measuring calcium excretion alone or calculating 24-h urine calcium-to-creatinine excretion ratio [11, 25].

CCCR is calculated as follows: (UCa x SCr)/(SCa x UCr), where UCa is the urinary calcium concentration, SCr is the serum creatinine. SCa is the serum calcium concentration, and UCr is the urinary creatinine concentration, all in mg/dl. The Ca/Cr clearance ratio is less than 0.01 in 80% of cases [2]. However, it has been shown that neither CCCR nor 24 h-UCa was able to clearly make a distinction between PHPT and FHH [26]. Serum phosphate level is often reduced, and intact PTH level is typically inappropriately (high-)normal in 80% of patients and mildly elevated in the remaining. A 25(OH) vitamin D level is normal, calcitriol level is normal or elevated, renal function is preserved, and mild hypermagnesemia may be present [3].

Serum biochemical studies may not be helpful in differentiating between FHH and primary hyperparathyroidism. If PTH level is normal and Ca/Cr clearance ratio is greater than 0.01 and less than 0.02, in the absence of a family history of hypercalcemia, the differential diagnosis is difficult. Investigation of asymptomatic hypercalcemia in patients younger than 40 years old should be put in the differential diagnosis of FHH higher on the list. In the absence of a family history, evaluation of serum calcium values in first-degree relatives can be helpful [2, 3].

Vitamin D deficiency, very low calcium intake, mild renal insufficiency, and treatment with thiazide diuretics or lithium should also be ruled out as causes of PTH-dependent hypocalciuric hypercalcemia. If the patient has primary hyperparathyroidism, correction of any of these abnormalities will lead to hypercalciuria [2].

Imaging of parathyroid glands with ultrasound is typically unrevealing. Genetic testing should be considered for cases of suspected FHH given the substantial clinical and biochemical overlap with primary hyperparathyroidism cases, especially if surgery has being considered [3, 27]. In patients with persistent disease after parathyroid surgery, genetic testing for FHH may also be considered.

In conclusion, the assessment of the biochemical values helps to eliminate patients that need molecular genetic evaluation for FHH. However, genetic testing is necessary to make a diagnosis of FFH [26].

34.6 Treatment

The majority cases of FHH do not require any treatment. Hypercalcemia in these patients is mostly asymptomatic and has minimal morbidity. Morbidity is often a result of inappropriate surgical intervention [1, 3].

Hypercalcemia in patients with FHH does not respond to medications such as diuretics or bisphosphonates. Calcimimetic drugs could play a role in treatment of FHH when treatment is needed [1, 28].

Educating and reassuring the patient and affected family members about the benign nature of this condition is very important. This communication avoids unnecessary and expensive monitoring and unnecessary parathyroid exploration in the patient and their relatives [2].

34.7 Indications for Surgery and Surgical Details

FHH is benign condition and therefore is not an indication for surgery [1, 2]. It is therefore important to detect subjects with FHH prior surgery due to incorrectly suspected PHPT. However, some patients may have both FHH and PHPT, respectively (see above).

34.8 Prognosis

The prognosis in most patients with FHH is good to excellent. The main argument for establishing the diagnosis is to avoid unnecessary and futile parathyroidectomy [1–3, 23].

Answers to the Questions

1. (c); 2. (e); 3. (e); 4. (e); 5. (b); 6. (c); 7. (d); 8. (d); 9. (c); 10. (d)

References

1. Varghese J, Rich T, Jimenez C. Benign familial hypocalciuric hypercalcemia. Endocr Pract. 2011;17 Suppl 1:13–7.
2. Afzal M, Kathuria P. Familial Hypocalciuric Hypercalcemia. Treasure Island, FL: StatPearls Publishing; 2021.
3. Lee JY, Shoback DM. Familial hypocalciuric hypercalcemia and related disorders. Best Pract Res Clin Endocrinol Metab. 2018;32(5):609–19.
4. Heath DA. Familial hypocalciuric hypercalcemia. Rev Endocr Metab Disord. Kluwer Academic Publishers;. 2000;1(4):291–6.
5. Lloyd SE, Pannett AA, Dixon PH, Whyte MP, Thakker RV. Localization of familial benign hypercalcemia, Oklahoma variant (FBHOk), to chromosome 19q13. Am J Hum Genet. 1999;64(1):189–95.
6. Nesbit MA, Hannan FM, Graham U, Whyte MP, Morrison PJ, Hunter SJ, et al. Identification of a second kindred with familial hypocalciuric hypercalcemia type 3 (FHH3) narrows localization to a <3.5 megabase pair region on chromosome 19q13.3. J Clin Endocrinol Metab. 2010;95(4):1947–54.
7. Pollak MR, Brown EM, Chou YH, Hebert SC, Marx SJ, Steinmann B, et al. Mutations in the human Ca(2+)-sensing receptor gene cause familial hypocalciuric hypercalcemia and neonatal severe hyperparathyroidism. Cell. 1993;75(7):1297–303.
8. Heath H, Jackson CE, Otterud B, Leppert MF. Genetic linkage analysis in familial benign (hypocalciuric) hypercalcemia: evidence for locus heterogeneity. Am J Hum Genet Elsevier. 1993;53(1):193–200.
9. Nesbit MA, Hannan FM, Howles SA, Reed AAC, Cranston T, Thakker CE, et al. Mutations in AP2S1 cause familial hypocalciuric hypercalcemia type 3. Nat Genet. Nature Publishing Group;. 2013;45(1):93–7.

10. Pidasheva S, D'Souza-Li L, Canaff L, Cole DEC, Hendy GN. CASRdb: calcium-sensing receptor locus-specific database for mutations causing familial (benign) hypocalciuric hypercalcemia, neonatal severe hyperparathyroidism, and autosomal dominant hypocalcemia. Hum Mutat. John Wiley & Sons, Ltd;. 2004;24(2):107–11.
11. Christensen SE, Nissen PH, Vestergaard P, Heickendorff L, Brixen K, Mosekilde L. Discriminative power of three indices of renal calcium excretion for the distinction between familial hypocalciuric hypercalcaemia and primary hyperparathyroidism: a follow-up study on methods. Clin Endocrinol. 2008;69(5):713–20.
12. Kifor O, Moore FD, Delaney M, Garber J, Hendy GN, Butters R, et al. A syndrome of hypocalciuric hypercalcemia caused by autoantibodies directed at the calcium-sensing receptor. J Clin Endocrinol Metabol. 2003;88(1):60–72.
13. Pallais JC, Kifor O, Chen Y-B, Slovik D, Brown EM. Acquired hypocalciuric hypercalcemia due to autoantibodies against the calcium-sensing receptor. N Engl J Med. Massachusetts Medical Society;. 2004;351(4):362–9.
14. Law WM, Heath H. Familial benign hypercalcemia (hypocalciuric hypercalcemia). Clinical and pathogenetic studies in 21 families. Ann Intern Med. American College of Physicians;. 1985;102(4):511–9.
15. Auwerx J, Brunzell J, Bouillon R, Demedts M. Familial hypocalciuric hypercalcaemia–familial benign hypercalcaemia: a review. Postgrad Med J. The Fellowship of Postgraduate Medicine;. 1987;63(744):835–40.
16. Volpe A, Guerriero A, Marchetta A, Caramaschi P, Furlani L. Familial hypocalciuric hypercalcemia revealed by chondrocalcinosis. Joint Bone Spine. 2009;76(6):708–10.
17. Burski K, Torjussen B, Paulsen AQ, Boman H, Bollerslev J. Parathyroid adenoma in a subject with familial hypocalciuric hypercalcemia: coincidence or causality? J Clin Endocrinol Metabol. 2002;87(3):1015–6.
18. Forde HE, Hill AD, Smith D. Parathyroid adenoma in a patient with familial hypocalciuric hypercalcaemia. BMJ Case Rep. BMJ Publishing Group Ltd;. 2014;2014(oct15 1):bcr2014206473–3.
19. Thorgeirsson U, Costa J, Marx SJ. The parathyroid glands in familial hypocalciuric hypercalcemia. Hum Pathol. 1981;12(3):229–37.
20. Frank-Raue K, Leidig-Bruckner G, Haag C, Schulze E, Lorenz A, Schmitz-Winnenthal H, et al. Inactivating calcium-sensing receptor mutations in patients with primary hyperparathyroidism. Clin Endocrinol. 2011;75(1):50–5.
21. Yabuta T, Miyauchi A, Inoue H, Yoshida H, Hirokawa M, Amino N. A patient with primary hyperparathyroidism associated with familial hypocalciuric hypercalcemia induced by a novel germline CaSR gene mutation. Asian J Surg. 2009;32(2):118–22.
22. Brachet C, Boros E, Tenoutasse S, Lissens W, Andry G, Martin P, et al. Association of parathyroid adenoma and familial hypocalciuric hypercalcaemia in a teenager. Eur J Endocrinol. BioScientifica;. 2009;161(1):207–10.
23. Christensen SE, Nissen PH, Vestergaard P, Mosekilde L. Familial hypocalciuric hypercalcaemia: a review. Curr Opin Endocrinol Diabetes Obes. 2011;18(6):359–70.
24. Christensen SE, Nissen PH, Vestergaard P, Heickendorff L, Rejnmark L, Brixen K, et al. Skeletal consequences of familial hypocalciuric hypercalcaemia vs. primary hyperparathyroidism. Clin Endocrinol (Oxf). 2009;71(6):798–807.
25. Shinall MC, Dahir KM, Broome JT. Differentiating familial hypocalciuric hypercalcemia from primary hyperparathyroidism. Endocr Pract. American Association of Clinical Endocrinologists;. 2013;19(4):697–702.
26. Bhangu JS, Selberherr A, Brammen L, Scheuba C, Riss P. Efficacy of calcium excretion and calcium/creatinine clearance ratio in the differen-

tial diagnosis of familial hypocalciuric hypercalcemia and primary hyperparathyroidism. Head Neck. 2019;41(5):1372–8.
27. Law WM, Carney JA, Heath H. Parathyroid glands in familial benign hypercalcemia (familial hypocalciuric hypercalcemia). Am J Med. 1984;76(6):1021–6.
28. Marx SJ. Calcimimetic use in familial hypocalciuric hypercalcemia-a perspective in endocrinology. J Clin Endocrinol Metab. 2017;102(11):3933–6.

Hyperparathyroidism-Jaw Tumor Syndrome

Maurizio Iacobone, Cristina Martínez-Santos, and Francesca Torresan

Contents

A. L. Shifrin et al. (eds.), *Endocrine Surgery Comprehensive Board Exam Guide*,
https://doi.org/10.1007/978-3-030-84737-1_35

Case Presentation

A 35-year-old woman presented at the emergency room due to confusion and vomiting. Past medical history includes gastritis, femur fracture, and two miscarriages. At physical examination, dehydration signs were observed. The serum calcium was 15.4 mg/dl (normal value, 9–10.5 mg/dl) and was admitted into the internal medicine unit; the PTH level was 969 pg/ml (normal value, 15–70 pg/ml); the vitamin D25OH level was normal; the 24-hour urine calcium and calcium clearance-to-creatinine ratio were within normal range. After 24 hours of initial treatment with rehydratation and loop diuretics, calcium level decreased to 13.6 mg/dl. Neck ultrasound and SestaMIBI scintigraphy were performed, concordantly suggesting the presence of a left parathyroid tumor.

❓ Questions

1. In the operating room, a left lateral minimally invasive approach using a 20 mm skin incision was performed, and a 4 cm superior parathyroid gland was found grossly adherent to the thyroid. What surgical procedure is indicated?
   (a) Continuing with minimally invasive surgery and resection of the parathyroid tumor.
   (b) Continuing with minimally invasive surgery and removal of both left parathyroid glands.
   (c) Enlargement of incision to standard cervicotomy and resection of the parathyroid tumor en bloc with the ipsilateral thyroid lobe and the surrounding lymph fatty tissue.
   (d) Closure of the incision and external radiotherapy.
   (e) Closure of the incision and medical treatment with cinacalcet (30 mg every 12 hours).
2. The definitive histology report described a parathyroid carcinoma with extensive local invasion and negative immunohistochemical staining for parafibromin. Another parathyroid was founded with cystic changes. What is the most probable diagnosis?
   (a) Sporadic parathyroid carcinoma.
   (b) Hereditary parathyroid carcinoma in the context of MEN 1.
   (c) Hereditary parathyroid carcinoma in the context of MEN 2.
   (d) Hereditary parathyroid carcinoma in relation to hyperparathyroidism-jaw tumor (HPT-JT) syndrome.
   (e) Familial hypocalciuric hypercalcemia.
3. The diagnosis of HPT-JT syndrome must be confirmed by genetic testing. The gene responsible for HPT-JT is:
   (a) *SDH-B.*
   (b) *CDC73.*

(c) *RET.*
(d) *BRAF.*
(e) *TP53.*

4. What is the prevalence of jaw tumors in HPT-JT?
(a) 30%
(b) 50%
(c) 60%
(d) 70%
(e) 100%

5. Most of the reported jaw tumors in HPT-JT syndrome are:
1. Ossifying fibromas.
2. Radiolucent lesions at panoramic X-ray dental imaging.
3. Malignant.
4. Located in maxilla or mandible.
5. Similar to brown tumors.
(a) Only (1) and (2) and (3) are correct.
(b) Only (1) and (2) and (4) are correct.
(c) Only (1) and (2) and (5) are correct.
(d) Only (2) and (3) and (4) are correct.
(e) All are correct.

6. The most common clinical feature of HPT-JT syndrome after pHPT is:
(a) Jaw tumors.
(b) Renal involvement.
(c) Uterine involvement.
(d) Thyroid carcinoma.
(e) Colon carcinoma.

7. Women with HPT-JT syndrome often have a history of:
1. Miscarriage.
2. Impaired ability to bear children.
3. Hysterectomy due to menorrhagia.
4. Benign tumors.
5. Malignant tumors.
(a) Only (1) and (2) and (3) are correct.
(b) Only (1) and (2) and (4) are correct.
(c) Only (1) and (3) and (4) are correct.
(d) Only (2) and (3) and (4) are correct.
(e) All are correct.

8. What statements regarding renal involvement in HPT-JT syndrome are correct?
1. The kidney is involved in 70% of the patients.
2. Wilms' tumor is usually identified in the fifth decade of life.
3. Cystic kidney disease is the most common manifestation of this syndrome.
4. Papillary renal cell carcinoma is frequent.
5. Surgery usually is not needed.
(a) Only (1) and (2) and (3) are correct.
(b) Only (2) and (3) and (4) are correct.

(c) Only (2) and (3) are correct.
(d) Only (5) is correct.
(e) All are correct.

9. The screening for *CDC73* germline mutations is indicated in:
   1. Familial pHPT.
   2. pHPT with old age onset.
   3. Malignant parathyroid tumors.
   4. pHPT and ossifying jaw tumors.
   5. pHPT and uterine tumors.
      (a) Only (1) and (2) are correct.
      (b) Only (1) and (3) are correct.
      (c) Only (1) and (3) and (4) and (5) are correct.
      (d) Only (5) is correct.
      (e) All are correct.
10. In *CDC73* germline mutation carrier families, the screening for primary hyperparathyroidism should be performed before the age of:
    (a) 4
    (b) 10
    (c) 15
    (d) 20
    (e) 25
11. The initial rate of parathyroid benign single gland involvement in HPT-JT syndrome patients is:
    1. Higher than MEN 1.
    2. Higher than MEN 2.
    3. Lower than MEN 1.
    4. Lower than MEN 2.
    5. Similar to MEN 1 and MEN 2.
       (a) Only (1) is correct.
       (b) Only (1) and (4) are correct.
       (c) Only (3) and (4) are correct.
       (d) Only (2) and (3) are correct.
       (e) Only (5) is correct.
12. The recurrence rate of HPT-JT-related pHPT after surgery is:
    (a) 10%
    (b) 12%
    (c) 15%
    (d) 25%
    (e) 50%
13. The optimal surgical approach to HPT-JT-related pHPT is:
    1. Bilateral exploration with prophylactic total parathyroidectomy.
    2. Bilateral exploration with prophylactic subtotal parathyroidectomy.
    3. Bilateral exploration with selective removal of abnormal gland(s).
    4. Focused exploration with selective parathyroidectomy according to preoperative imaging.

5. If parathyroid carcinoma is suspected wide en bloc resection of the mass with the ipsilateral thyroid lobe, the ipsilateral normal parathyroid, and surrounding lymph fatty tissue.
   (a) Only (1) and (2) and (3) are correct.
   (b) Only (4) is correct.
   (c) Only (4) and (5) are correct.
   (d) Only (3) and (4) and (5) are correct.
   (e) Only (2) and (3) and (4) and (5) are correct.

14. With respect to surgical treatment of tumors associated with HPT-JT, the following is correct:
   1. Complete surgical removal of ossifying fibromas of the jaw is recommended.
   2. For renal tumors, nephron-sparing surgery rather than radical surgery is advocated.
   3. For renal tumors, radical surgery rather than nephron-sparing surgery is advocated.
   4. Renal tumors may be multiple and bilateral, and patients would require multiple surgeries over their lifetime.
   5. Women with menorrhagia may require hysterectomy at early age.
      (a) Only (1) and (2) are correct.
      (b) Only (1) and (2) and (4) are correct.
      (c) Only (1) and (3) and (4) are correct.
      (d) Only (1) and (2) and (4) and (5) are correct.
      (e) Only (1) and (3) and (4) and (5) are correct.

15. Our patient should undergo the following screening:
   1. Biannual serum calcium and PTH and parathyroid ultrasound.
   2. Panoramic X-ray dental imaging at least every 5 years.
   3. Renal ultrasound, RM, or CT scan at least every 5 years.
   4. Colonoscopy at least every 2 years.
   5. Regular gynecologic care including pelvic ultrasound.
      (a) Only (1) and (2) and (3) are correct.
      (b) Only (1) and (2) and (4) are correct.
      (c) Only (1) and (2) and (3) and (5) are correct.
      (d) Only (2) and (3) and (4) are correct.
      (e) All are correct.

35.1 Introduction

Primary hyperparathyroidism (pHPT) is a relatively common disease and in 90% occurs as a sporadic form. During the last few decades, different hereditary syndromes causing pHPT have been described, reaching 10% of cases. Most of these familial cases occur in association with multiple endocrine neoplasia (MEN). Other syndromes like hyperparathyroidism-jaw tumor syndrome (HPT-JT) are very uncommon. The earliest report of some manifestations of the syndrome probably occurred in 1958, when Jackson reported a kindred with autosomal dominant transmission of hypercalcemia with seven pHPT members including four fibro-osseous jaw tumors [1]. Dinnen contributed to a preliminary formulation of the syndrome in 1977 reporting a family with benign and malignant parathyroid tumors and ossifying fibroma of the jaw [2].

In recent years, major advances have been made in the understanding of the molecular pathogenesis of HPT-JT syndrome. Szabo mapped the gene in 1995 to 1q21-q31 [3], and finally Carpten in 2002 identified the gene responsible as *HRPT2* (later named *CDC73*) and its encoded product parafibromin [4].

The present chapter emphasizes clinical characteristics and management of HPT-JT syndrome.

35.2 Etiology

HPT-JT syndrome is linked to germline inactivating mutations in the tumor suppressor gene *CDC73*, which contains 17 exons on chromosome *1q31.2* and encodes for a predominantly nuclear, 531-amino-acid protein named parafibromin [5]. Parafibromin is ubiquitously expressed in many organs, including kidney, liver, stomach, renal cortex tubules, and the pars intermedia of the hypophysis [6]. Parafibromin is associated with other proteins in the polymerase-associated factor (PAF1) and induces the downregulation of cyclin D1 expression and direct interaction with ß-catenin, resulting in the activation of transcription of target genes. Studies of the PAF1 complex in yeast and *Drosophila*, as well as in mammalian cells, have revealed that parafibromin induces histone modification, transcription elongation, and chromatin remodeling [7–9].

About 75% of HPT-JT patients have germline *CDC73* mutations within the coding region, and the majority (>80%) are frameshift or nonsense mutations that determine the functional loss of parafibromin by causing a premature truncation of this protein or a rapid loosing of the translated protein via nonsense-mediated mRNA decay. Therefore, the expression of parafibromin is completely lost in HPT-JT-associated tumor tissues. The remaining 25% of HPT-JT patients may have abnormalities in *CDC73* promoter regions, whole exon or gene deletions, mutations in unidentified genes, or epigenetic modifications [10].

As all tumor suppressor genes, the first mutation is usually inherited by one of the parents or, in very rare cases, developed de novo at embryonic level. A second and novel acquired somatic mutation or a loss of heterozygosity in HPT-JT tumor-related tissues is needed, consistent with Knudson's two-hit hypothesis [4–13].

35.3 Clinical Presentation

HPT-JT is a rare autosomal dominant disorder with incomplete penetrance. It is characterized by the development of parathyroid tumors, ossifying fibromas of the mandible and maxilla, cystic and neoplastic renal abnormalities, and hyperplastic and neoplastic uterine involvement [14, 15].

No genotype-phenotype correlations have been fully established to date [16, 17]. However, it has been suggested that missense mutations are more likely to be associated with the disease without typical associated features (familial isolated pHPT), whereas mutations causing gross parafibromin disruption are more likely associated with the classical HPT-JT phenotype [12].

35.3.1 pHPT

pHPT is the main clinical feature and is found in almost 100% of mutation carriers typically in late adolescence or early adulthood. According to the literature review reported by Torresan and Iacobone in 2019 including 154 HPT-JT kindred and 365 patients affected by pHPT, the earliest age of hypercalcemia is 7 years [18, 19]. The median age of diagnosis of pHPT was 27 years, and the mean age ranged between 32 and 36 years [20–22]. In a report of three large kindred, *CDC73*-related pHPT occurred in 87.5% of cases among patients older than 20 years [19], while penetrance of pHPT in a Dutch population was shown to increase with age (8%, 53%, and 75% at age of 25, 50, and 70, respectively) [22].

A single gland parathyroid involvement had been reported more frequently (86.1%) than in other forms of hereditary pHPT like MEN1. Multiglandular involvement occurs rarely at initial surgery (13.9% of cases), but it may affect other glands at long-term follow-up (over decades) in many patients [21–25].

HPT-JT is associated with a higher prevalence of atypical adenomas and parathyroid carcinoma which can be found in 23% of the cases [4, 6–13, 15, 17, 19–22, 24–90], unlike other forms of hereditary pHPT in which parathyroid tumors are typically benign [4, 11]. Cystic changes of parathyroids were originally described as a common histological feature in HPT-JT (previously called familial cystic parathyroid adenomatosis), but it is actually found in only a quarter of the parathyroid tumors (Fig. 35.1) [25]. The adenomas may be cystic, either with micro- or macrocysts, and similar cystic changes can also be present in normal parathyroid glands in these patients [30]. The diagnosis of parathyroid carcinoma in HPT-JT is based on the standard criteria of extensive local invasion and/or metastasis.

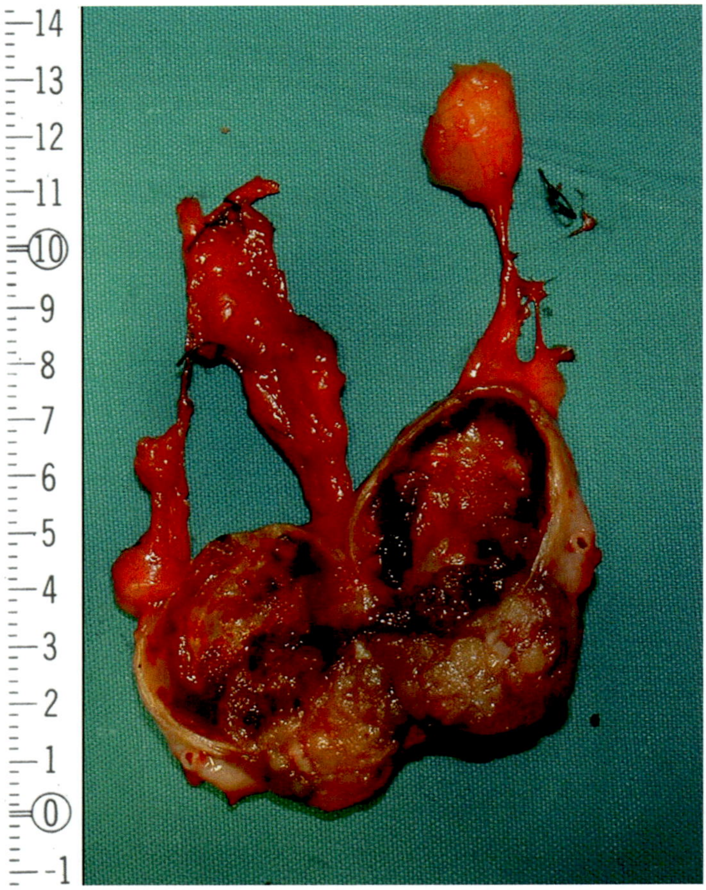

Fig. 35.1 Surgical specimen: parathyroid carcinoma in hyperparathyroidism-jaw tumor syndrome. The parathyroid carcinoma (sectioned) presents cystic and regressive changes. (Reproduced with permission from [91])

pHPT is usually mild or asymptomatic, but, in case of parathyroid carcinoma, severe hypercalcemic crisis may occur [91, 92]. Hence, in the presence of abnormal high serum calcium concentration (>12 mg/dL) and iPTH levels (>3 times the upper limit of normal) and parathyroid lesions larger than 3 cm, parathyroid carcinomas should be suspected. On the other hand, nonfunctioning parathyroid malignancy may very rarely occur in *CDC73*-related disorder [4, 44, 90]. Moreover, parathyroid carcinoma can present as a palpable neck mass associated with hoarseness, difficulty speaking or swallowing, muscle weakness, nausea/vomiting, altered mental status, bone pain, and/or pathologic bone fractures [4, 22, 29, 32, 48].

35.3.2 Jaw Tumors

Despite the nomenclature of the syndrome, jaw tumors may be found only in approximately one third of cases. Jaw tumors in

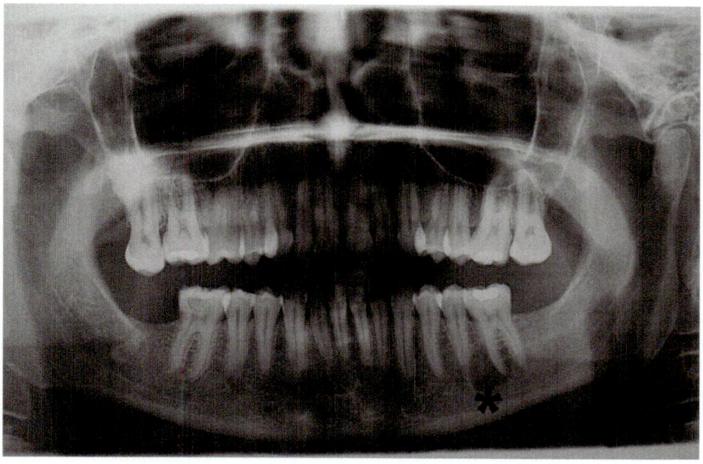

Fig. 35.2 Orthopantomographic X-ray: Ossifying fibroma of the left ramus of the mandible (*) in a young patient with hyperparathyroidism-jaw tumor syndrome. (Reproduced with permission from [91])

HPT-JT are fibro-osseous lesions that typically involve maxilla or mandible often prior to the third decade of life.

Most of the reported jaw tumors in HPT-JT syndrome are ossifying fibromas and benign and generally slow-growing tumors arising from the periodontal ligament in molar or premolar areas [3]. Jaw tumors are usually radiographically radiolucent compared to the mixed radiolucent/radiopaque lesions in the sporadic variants [41]. Sometimes they present with an enlarging visible or palpable mass, but, in other cases, they are only detected on dental X-ray imaging (Figs. 35.2, 35.3, and 35.4). Although benign, ossifying fibroma can disrupt normal dentition, impair breathing, and cause functional and cosmetic symptoms. Ossifying fibroma in HPT-JT syndrome may be bilateral or multifocal and may recur.

The ossifying fibromas are composed of a relatively avascular cellular fibroblast-rich stroma, sometimes with a prominent storiform pattern admixed with bone trabeculae and/or cementum-like spherules. The histology is different from brown tumors of osteitis fibrosa cystica associated with pHPT.

35.3.3 Renal Involvement

The kidney is involved in approximately 20% of patients with HPT-JT. Cystic kidney disease is the most common renal manifestation of this syndrome, but some patients often develop hamartomas and rare renal tumors, such as adult Wilms' tumors and mixed epithelial-stromal tumors (MEST). The Wilms' tumors in HPT-JT have been identified in the fifth decade of life, are usually bilateral, are poorly circumscribed, are smaller than in the classical childhood form, and do not usually metastasize. Moreover, they have also distinctive histo-

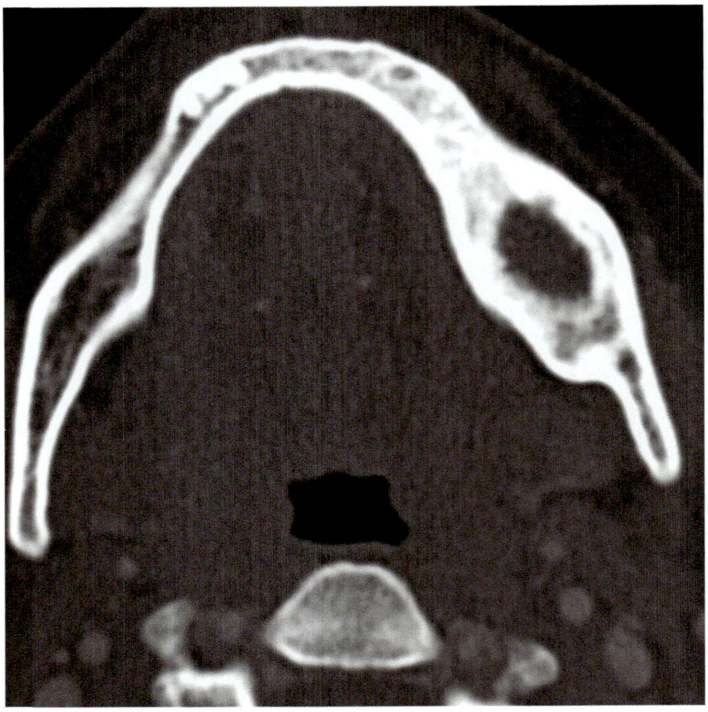

Fig. 35.3 CT scan: Ossifying fibroma of the left ramus of the mandible in a young patient with hyperparathyroidism-jaw tumor syndrome. (Reproduced with permission from [91])

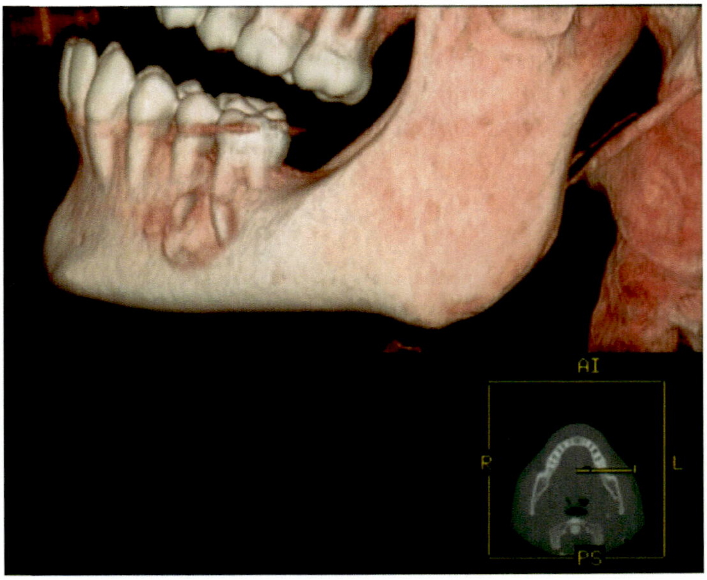

Fig. 35.4 CT scan (reconstruction): Ossifying fibroma of the left ramus of the mandible in a young patient with hyperparathyroidism-jaw tumor syndrome. (Reproduced with permission from [91])

logical features from the childhood form, such as a low number of mitoses, lack of necrosis and hemorrhages, large mesenchymal components, and the presence of cysts [93]. The association between MEST, a predominantly benign tumor characterized by both epithelial and spindle cell stromal components, and HPT-JT syndrome is poorly reported in the literature. Papillary renal cell carcinoma has very rarely been described in HPT-JT [21, 94].

35.3.4 Uterine Involvement

Uterine tumors have been described in association with HPT-JT and are the most common clinical feature after pHPT, affecting more than 50% of HPT-JT female patients in some cohorts [12]. Uterine tumors are frequently accompanied by menorrhagia and often require hysterectomy at an early age (mean 35 years). Affected women often have a history of miscarriage and a significantly impaired ability to bear children when compared with their unaffected female relatives [42].

Histological analysis of the uterine specimens revealed both benign and malignant tumors, such as adenomyosis, adenofibromas, leiomyomas, endometrial hyperplasia, adenosarcomas, or tumors arising from the Müllerian duct system.

35.3.5 Other Features

Thyroid carcinoma, thyrotoxicosis, colon carcinoma, cholangiocarcinoma, chronic lymphatic leukemia, pancreatic adenocarcinoma, and pituitary cyst have also been described, but the association between these tumors and HPT-JT syndrome remains unclear [21, 50, 94].

35.4 Diagnosis

HPT-JT is uncommon, but the exact incidence and prevalence rates are unknown and might be underestimated. In most families, parathyroid tumors are the only lesions at presentation, but when jaw tumors are present in an individual or in a kindred, the diagnosis is strongly suggested [21, 24, 25].

Given the extreme rarity of parathyroid carcinoma in the general population and in other hereditary syndromes associated with hypercalcemia, parathyroid malignancy should be another important clue to the diagnosis of HPT-JT [4]. About 20–30% of patients with apparently sporadic parathyroid carcinomas in fact have germline mutations in *CDC73*, indicating occult HPT-JT syndrome [29, 32].

Parathyroid adenomas and carcinomas and other associated tumors arising in the setting of HPT-JT usually demonstrate negative immunohistochemical staining for parafibromin that is considered a biomarker for *CDC73* or an indirect method to recognize HPT-JT syndrome patients. Nevertheless, *CDC73* immunochemistry should be interpreted with care because some *CDC73* mutations are not associated with loss of *CDC73* expression and therefore normal parafibromin immunohistochemistry does not exclude the diagnosis of HPT-JT [24, 95, 96]. Furthermore, it should be noted that parafibromin is also absent in 60–70% of sporadic parathyroid cancers, 20% of sporadic atypical adenomas, and 1–5% of sporadic parathyroid adenomas.

Finally, the diagnosis of HPT-JT must be confirmed by genetic testing. The screening for *CDC73* germline mutations is indicated in the presence of familial pHPT; pHPT with young age onset (<35 years); multiglandular involvement; cystic, atypical, or malignant parathyroid tumors; or coexistence ossifying jaw fibroma and renal or uterine tumors [12, 29] (▶ Box 35.1).

Box 35.1 Indication for *CDC73* genetic testing

- Personal or family history of HPT-JT.
- Young age onset of primary hyperparathyroidism (<35 years).
- Primary hyperparathyroidism caused by cystic, atypical, or malignant parathyroid involvement.
- Primary hyperparathyroidism due to multiglandular parathyroid involvement.
- Coexistence of primary hyperparathyroidism and ossifying jaw fibroma and renal or uterine tumors.

Following the initial diagnosis, it is necessary to establish the extent of the disease by evaluating standard end organ damage of pHPT, but also the associated jaw tumors and renal and uterine lesions should be systematically searched [26, 28].

Genetic screening for identifying gene carriers should be performed in all family members to start a specific HPT-JT screening program [31]. In *CDC73* mutation carrier families, the screening should be performed also in children before the age of 10, since malignant pHPT has been sometimes described at very early age.

35.5 Treatment

Most patients with a diagnosis of parathyroid adenoma can be cured by surgery, but about 25% of cases may recur [21, 24]. Given the rarity of the disease and the heterogeneity of the phenotype, the optimal surgical approach to *CDC73*-related pHPT has not yet been established and remains controversial, varying between bilateral or targeted neck exploration and extensive or limited parathyroidectomy [12]. In the past, prophylactic total parathyroidectomy has been suggested to minimize the risk of recurrences and parathyroid carcinoma in HPT-JT syndrome and therefore to obtain a definitive cure. However, total parathyroidectomy is clearly not always successful and leads to permanent postsurgical hypoparathyroidism with difficult treatment especially in young patients and increased morbidity. For these reasons, subtotal parathyroidectomy or total parathyroidectomy with autotransplantation has been suggested for HPT-JT-related pHPT as for other variants of hereditary pHPT, even if autotransplantation has been implicated in tumor dissemination in case of malignant involvement [90]. Moreover, in contrast with other variants of hereditary pHPT, a high prevalence of uniglandular involvement at onset has been reported. For that reason, when malignant parathyroid involvement is unlike, targeted approaches (even with minimally invasive procedures with minimal tissue dissection) and selective parathyroid excisions have recently been proposed in the same setting of sporadic pHPT. This strategy is aimed to achieve, whenever possible, the longest possible normocalcemia without permanent hypoparathyroidism, minimizing surgical morbidity and facilitating eventual future surgery for recurrent disease [21]. On the other hand, if parathyroid carcinoma is clinically suspected (large tumor at imaging, palpable neck mass, biochemical and clinical presentation of severe pHPT), wider en bloc resection of the mass with the ipsilateral thyroid lobe (◘ Fig. 35.5), possibly also including the ipsilateral normal parathyroid and the surrounding lymph fatty tissue, should be performed, in order to avoid tumor

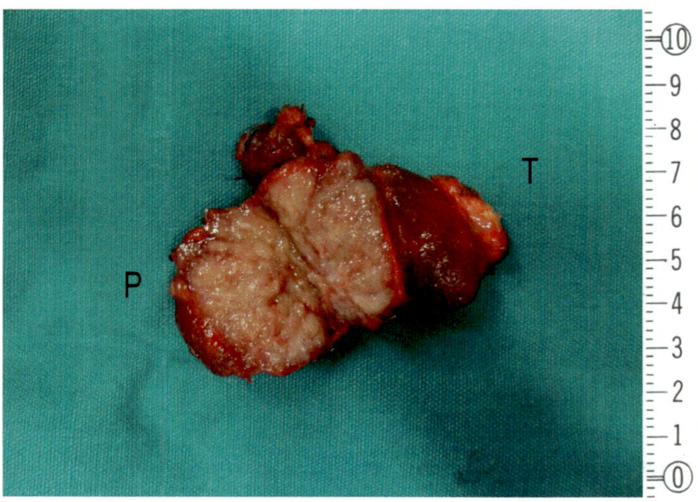

◘ **Fig. 35.5** Surgical specimen: parathyroid carcinoma. The parathyroid carcinoma (P, sectioned) has been removed en bloc with the ipsilateral thyroid lobe (T)

seeding and achieve a "complete unilateral parathyroidectomy" and finally minimize the risk of reoperation in a scarred area [21, 88–91].

However, the strategy remains controversial. In 2008, Sarquis et al. observed, in a series of 11 *CDC73* germline mutated patients from three kindred, a synchronous multiglandular involvement at initial operation in 54.5% of cases, parathyroid malignancy in 9%, and an overall persistence/recurrence rate of 80%; thus, a bilateral exploration with subtotal parathyroidectomy was suggested as the initial approach [25].

In 2014, Mehta et al. suggested a bilateral neck exploration with selective removal only of abnormal gland(s) in HPT-JT syndrome patients, given the high frequency of benign single-gland involvement (69%) and relatively low rate of recurrences (20%) found in their multicentric cohort of 16 individuals from seven HPT-JT families [24].

More recently, Iacobone et al. reported a 95% rate of single gland involvement at initial diagnosis, in a cohort of 20 HPT-JT syndrome patients from five large families. Therefore, in case of concordant results of preoperative functional and anatomical tests suggesting a single gland involvement and in the absence of suspicion of parathyroid malignancy, a focused approach with selective parathyroidectomy was proposed. A subtotal parathyroidectomy was recommended in case of absent or discordant preoperative localization because of the increased risk of multiglandular involvement and recurrent pHPT [88]. However, long-term follow-up is indicated for all patients because of the risk of recurrent disease.

35

Cinacalcet hydrochloride, a calcimimetic that binds to the calcium-sensing receptor, has been approved for the long-term control of hypercalcemia secondary to pHPT in individuals who are unable to undergo parathyroidectomy and for the treatment of parathyroid carcinoma-related hypercalcemia, in case of unresectable or metastatic disease. For severe or symptomatic hypercalcemia, an infusion of bisphosphonates, steroids, or dialysis can be necessary for acute management [18].

In relation to ossifying fibromas of the jaw, a complete surgical removal is the recommended treatment based on the size, location, and symptoms of the lesion. Individuals with a history of jaw tumors should be followed closely because of the possibility of recurrence [97].

With respect to renal involvement, HPT-JT patients may be at risk for multiple and bilateral renal tumors potentially requiring multiple renal surgeries over their lifetime. Sarcomatoid differentiation and metastatic spread is rare. Surgery represents the treatment of choice [98]. Nephron-sparing surgery rather than radical surgery should be preferred, whenever possible, in order to preserve renal function.

Finally, no treatment guidelines for uterine manifestations associated with HPT-JT syndrome have been proposed to date [18]. Given the occurrence of both benign and malignant involvement, individuals with evidence of a uterine tumor should be managed by a gynecologist with a tailor-made treatment. In case of malignancy or in case of severe recurrent menorrhagia, hysterectomy even at an early age (mean 35 years) may be required.

35.6 Surveillance

Even if there are no well-established surveillance guidelines, it has been suggested that *CDC73* mutation carriers should undergo a specific screening [18] including an evaluation of serum calcium and PTH for pHPT screening at least every 6 months, possibly after the age of 5 with periodic parathyroid ultrasound examination; panoramic X-ray dental imaging at least every 5 years; and monitoring for kidney lesions by periodic renal ultrasound examination, magnetic resonance imaging, or computed tomography scan at least every 5 years, starting at age of diagnosis. Moreover, starting at reproductive age, women with a *CDC73*-related disorder should undergo regular gynecologic care, including pelvic ultrasound examination with eventually further imaging studies if clinically indicated (◘ Table 35.1).

◘ **Table 35.1** Clinical features, treatment, and follow-up of HPT-JT

Phenotype	Treatment	Follow-up (frequency)
Primary hyperparathyroidism	Focused parathyroidectomy (in case of preoperatively suspected uniglandular involvement); subtotal or total parathyroidectomy (with/without autotransplantation, in case of suspicion of multiglandular involvement); en bloc resection of the parathyroid tumor with the ipsilateral thyroid lobe, including the ipsilateral normal parathyroid and the surrounding lymph fatty tissue (in case of suspicion of parathyroid carcinoma)	Serum calcium and PTH evaluation, possibly starting after the age of 5 and periodic parathyroid ultrasound examination (every 6 months)
Ossifying jaw fibroma	Radical excision	Panoramic X-ray dental imaging or computed tomography at least every 5 years
Uterine tumors	Uterine polyps excision, hysterectomy	Regular gynecologic care, including pelvic ultrasound examination with eventual further imaging studies if clinically indicated, starting at the reproductive age, at least every 5 years
Renal tumors	Variable	Kidney lesions monitoring by periodic renal ultrasound examination, magnetic resonance imaging, or computed tomography scan at least every 5 years

Answers to the Questions

1. (c); 2. (d); 3. (b); 4. (a); 5. (b); 6. (c); 7. (e); 8. (c); 9. (c); 10. (b); 11. (a); 12. (d); 13. (e); 14. (d); 15. (c).

References

1. Jackson CE. Hereditary hyperparathyroidism associated with recurrent pancreatitis. An Int Med. 1958;49:829–36.
2. Dinnen JS, Greenwood RH, Jones JH, Walker DA, Williams ED. Parathyroid carcinoma in familial hyperparathyroidism. J Clin Path. 1977;30:966–75.
3. Szabó J, Heath B, Hill VM, et al. Heath H. Hereditary hyperparathyroidism-jaw tumor syndrome: the endocrine tumor gene HRPT2 maps to chromosome 1q21-q31. Am J Hum Genet. 1995;56:944–50.
4. Carpten JD, Robbins CM, Villablanca A, et al. HRPT2, encoding parafibromin, is mutated in hyperparathyroidism-jaw tumor syndrome. Nat Genet. 2002;32:676–80.
5. Cascón A, Huarte-Mendicoa CV, Javier Leandro-García L, et al. Detection of the first gross CDC73 germline deletion in an HPT-JT syndrome family. Genes Chrom Cancer. 2011;50:922–9.
6. Porzionato A, Macchi V, Barzon L, Masi G, Iacobone M, Parenti A, et al. Immunohistochemical assessment of parafibromin in mouse and human tissues. J Anat. 2006;209:817–27.
7. Rozenblatt-Rosen O, Hughes CM, Nannepaga SJ, Shanmugam KS, Copeland TD, Guszczynski T, et al. The parafibromin tumor suppressor protein is part of a human Paf1 complex. Mol Cell Biol. 2005;25:612–20.
8. Yart A, Gstaiger M, Wirbelauer C, Pecnik M, Anastasiou D, Hess D, et al. The HRPT2 tumor suppressor gene product parafibromin associates with human PAF1 and RNA polymerase II. Mol Cell Biol. 2005;25:5052–60.
9. Mosimann C, Hausmann G, Basler K. Parafibromin/Hyrax activates Wnt/Wg target gene transcription by direct association with beta-catenin/Armadillo. Cell. 2006;125:327–41.
10. Newey PJ, Bowl MR, Cranston T, Thakker RV. Cell division cycle protein 73 homolog (CDC73) mutations in the hyperparathyroidism-jaw tumour syndrome (HPT-JT) and parathyroid tumours. Hum Mutat. 2010;31:295–307.
11. Kelly TG, Shattuck TM, Reyes-Múgica M, et al. Surveillance for early detection of aggressive parathyroid disease: carcinoma and atypical adenoma in familial isolated hyperparathyroidism associated with a germline HRPT2 mutation. J Bone Miner Res. 2006;21:1666–71.
12. Iacobone M, Carnaille B, Palazzo F, Vriens M. Hereditary hyperparathyroidism—a consensus report of the European Society of Endocrine Surgeons (ESES). Langenbeck's Arch Surg. 2015;400:867–86.
13. Walls GV, Stevenson M, Lines KE, et al. Mice deleted for cell division cycle 73 gene develop parathyroid and uterine tumours: model for the hyperparathyroidism-jaw tumour syndrome. Oncogene. 2017;36:4025–36.
14. Carling T, Udelsman. Parathyroid surgery in familial hyperparathyroid disorders. J Intern Med. 2005;257:27–37.
15. Bradley KJ, Hobbs MR, Buley ID, et al. Uterine tumours are a phenotypic manifestation of the hyperparathyroidism-jaw tumour syndrome. J Intern Med. 2005;257:18–26.
16. Cardoso L, Stevenson M, Thakker RV. Molecular genetics of syndromic and non-syndromic forms of parathyroid carcinoma. Hum Mutat. 2017;38(12):1321–648.

17. Korpi-Hyövalti E, Cranston T, Ryhänen E, et al. CDC73 intragenic deletion in familial primary hyperparathyroidism associated with parathyroid carcinoma. J Clin Endocrinol Metab. 2014;99:3044–8.
18. Torresan F, Iacobone M. Clinical features, treatment and surveillance of hyperparathyroidism-jaw tumor syndrome: an up to date and review of the literature. Int J Endocrinol. 2019;1761030
19. Pichardo-Lowden AR, Manni A, Saunders BD, Baker MJ. Familial hyperparathyroidism due to a germline mutation of the CDC73 gene: implications for management and age-appropriate testing of relatives at risk. Endocr Pract. 2011;17:602–9.
20. Bricaire L, Odou MF, Cardot-Bauters C, et al. Frequent large germline HRPT2 deletions in a French National cohort of patients with primary hyperparathyroidism. J Clin Endocrinol Metab. 2013;98(2):E403–8.
21. Iacobone M, Masi G, Barzon L, et al. Hyperparathyroidism jaw tumor syndrome: a report of three large kindred. Langenbeck's Arch Surg. 2009;394:817–25.
22. van der Tuin K, Tops CMJ, Adank MA, et al. CDC73-related disorders: clinical manifestations and case detection in primary hyperparathyroidism. J Clin Endocrinol Metab. 2017;102(12):4534–40.
23. Jackson CE, Norum RA, Boyd SB, et al. Hereditary hyperparathyroidism and multiple ossifying jaw fibromas: a clinically and genetically distinct syndrome. Surgery. 1990;108:1006–12.
24. Mehta A, Patel D, Rosenberg A, et al. Hyperparathyroidism-jaw tumor syndrome: results of operative management. Surgery. 2014;156:1315–25.
25. Sarquis MS, Silveira LG, Pimenta FJ, et al. Familial hyperparathyroidism: surgical outcome after 30 years of follow up in three families with germline HRPT2 mutations. Surgery. 2008;143:630–40.
26. Iacobone M, Barzon L, Porzionato A, et al. Parafibromin expression, single-gland involvement, and limited parathyroidectomy in familial isolated hyperparathyroidism. Surgery. 2007;142(6):984–91.
27. Masi A, Barzon L, Iacobone M, et al. Clinical, genetic, and histopathologic investigation of *CDC73*-related familial hyperparathyroidism. Endocr Relat Cancer. 2008;15:1115–26.
28. Masi G, Iacobone M, Sinigaglia A, et al. Characterization of a new CDC73 missense mutation that impairs Parafibromin expression and nucleolar localization. PLoS One. 2014;9(5):e97994.
29. Cetani F, Pardi E, Borsari SL, et al. Genetic analyses of the HRPT2 gene in primary hyperparathyroidism: germline and somatic mutations in familial and sporadic parathyroid tumors. J Clin Endocrinol Metab. 2004;89:5583–91.
30. Mallette LE, Malini S, Rappaport MP, Kirkland JL. Familial cystic parathyroid adenomatosis. Ann Intern Med. 1987;107:54–60.
31. Hyde SM, Rich TA, Waguespack SG, Perrier ND, Hu MI. CDC73-Related Disorders. GeneReviews® 2019 [Internet]. Pagon RA, Adam MP, Ardinger HH, et al., Eds. University of Washington, Seattle, WA, USA 2019.
32. Shattuck TM, Valimaki S, Obara T, et al. Somatic and germline mutations of the HRPT2 gene in sporadic parathyroid carcinoma. N Engl J Med. 2003;349:1722–9.
33. Howell VM, Haven CJ, Kahnoski K, et al. HRPT2 mutations are associated with malignancy in sporadic parathyroid tumours. J Med Genet. 2003;40:657–63.
34. Simonds WF, Robbins CM, Agarwal SK, et al. Familial isolated hyperparathyroidism is rarely caused by germline mutation in HRPT2, the gene for the hyperparathyroidism-jaw tumor syndrome. J Clin Endocrinol Metab. 2004;89:96–102.
35. Villablanca A, Calender A, Forsberg L, et al. Germline and de novo mutations in the HRPT2 tumour suppressor gene in familial isolated hyperparathyroidism (FIHP). J Med Genet. 2004;41(3):e32.

36. Cavaco BM, Guerra L, Bradley KJ, et al. Hyperparathyroidism-jaw tumor syndrome in Roma families from Portugal is due to a founder mutation of the HRPT2 gene. J Clin Endocrinol Metab. 2004;89:1747–52.
37. Howell VM, Zori RT, Stalker HJ, et al. A molecular diagnosis of hyperparathyroidism-jaw tumor syndrome in an adolescent with recurrent kidney stones. J Pediatr. 2004;145(4):567.
38. Moon SD, Park JH, Kim EM, et al. A Novel IVS2-1G>A mutation causes aberrant splicing of the HRPT2 gene in a family with hyperparathyroidism-jaw tumor syndrome. J Clin Endocrinol Metab. 2005;90:878–83.
39. Gimm O, Lorenz K, Nguyen Thanh P, et al. Das Familiäre Nebenschilddrüsenkarzinom. Indikation zur prophylaktischen Parathyreoidektomie? Chirurg. 2006;77:15–24.
40. Mizusawa N, Uchino S, Iwata T, et al. Genetic analyses in patients with familial isolated hyperparathyroidism and hyperparathyroidism-jaw tumour syndrome. Clin Endocrinol. 2006;65:9–16.
41. Aldred MJ, Talacko AA, Savarirayan R, et al. Dental findings in a family with hyperparathyroidism-jaw tumor syndrome and a novel HRPT2 gene mutation. Oral Surg Oral Med Oral Pathol Oral Radiol Endod. 2006;101:212–8.
42. Bradley KJ, Cavaco BM, Bowl MR, et al. Parafibromin mutations in hereditary hyperparathyroidism syndromes and parathyroid tumours. Clin Endocrinol. 2006;64(3):299–306.
43. Juhlin C, Larsson C, Yakoleva T, et al. Loss of parafibromin expression in a subset of parathyroid adenomas. Endocr Relat Cancer. 2006;13:509–23.
44. Guarnieri V, Scillitani A, Muscarella LA, et al. Diagnosis of parathyroid tumors in familial isolated hyperparathyroidism with HRPT2 mutation: implications for cancer surveillance. J Clin Endocrinol Metab. 2006;91:2827–32.
45. Yamashita Y, Akiyama T, Mizusawa N, et al. A case of hyperparathyroidism-jaw tumour syndrome found in the treatment of an ossifying fibroma in the maxillary bone. Int J Oral Maxillofac Surg. 2007;36:365–9.
46. Cetani F, Pardi E, Ambrogini E, et al. Different somatic alterations of the HRPT2 gene in a patient with recurrent sporadic primary hyperparathyroidism carrying an HRPT2 germline mutation. Endocr Relat Cancer. 2007;14:493–9.
47. Cetani F, Ambrogini E, Viacava P, et al. Should parafibromin staining replace HRTP2 gene analysis as an additional tool for histologic diagnosis of parathyroid carcinoma? Eur J Endocrinol. 2007;156:547–54.
48. Raue F, Haag C, Frank-Raue K. Hyperparathyroidism-jaw tumor syndrome. A hereditary form of primary hyperparathyroidism with parathyroid carcinoma. Dtsch Med Wochenschr. 2007;132:1459–62.
49. Cetani F, Pardi E, Ambrogini E, et al. Hyperparathyroidism 2 gene (HRPT2, CDC73) and parafibromin studies in two patients with primary hyperparathyroidism and uncertain pathological assessment. J Endocrinol Investig. 2008;31:900–4.
50. Guarnieri V, Bisceglia M, Bonfitto N, et al. Familial hyperparathyroidism: surgical outcome after 30 years of follow-up in three families with germline HRPT2 mutations. Surgery. 2008;144:839–40.
51. Howell VM, Gill A, Clarkson A, et al. Accuracy of combined protein gene product 9.5 and parafibromin markers for immunohistochemical diagnosis of parathyroid carcinoma. J Clin Endocrinol Metab. 2009;94:434–41.
52. Silveira LG, Dias EP, Marinho BC, et al. HRPT2-related familial isolated hyperparathyroidism: could molecular studies direct the surgical approach? Arq Bras Endocrinol Metabol. 2008;52:1211–20.
53. Schmidt BP, Bradrick JP, Gabali A. Hyperparathyroidism jaw tumor syndrome: a case report. J Oral Maxillofac Surg. 2009;67(2):423–7.
54. Rekik N, Ben Naceur B, Mnif M, et al. Hyperparathyroidism-jaw tumor syndrome: a case report. Ann Endocrinol. 2010;71(2):121–6.

55. Panicker LM, Zhang JH, Dagur PK, et al. Defective nucleolar localization and dominant interfering properties of a parafibromin L95P missense mutant causing the hyperparathyroidism-jaw tumor syndrome. Endocr Relat Cancer. 2010;17:513–24.
56. Veiguela B, Isidro ML, Jorge S, Ruano B. An uncommon cause of hypercalcemia: synchronous carcinoma of two parathyroids in the context of hyperparathyroidism-jaw tumor syndrome. Endocrinol Nutr. 2010;57(8):391–3.
57. Cavaco BM, Santos R, Felix A, et al. Identification of de novo germline mutations in the HRPT2 gene in two apparently sporadic cases with challenging parathyroid tumor diagnoses. Endocr Pathol. 2011;22:44–52.
58. Frank-Raue K, Leiding-Bruckner G, Lorenz A, et al. Dtsch Med Wochenschr. 2011;136(38):1889–94.
59. Siu WK, Law CY, Lam CW, et al. Novel nonsense CDC73 mutations in Chinese patients with parathyroid tumors. Familial Cancer. 2011;10(4):695–9.
60. Domingues R, Tomaz RA, Martins C, et al. Identification of the first germline HRPT2 whole-gene deletion in a patient with primary hyperparathyroidism. Clin Endocrinol. 2012;76:33–8.
61. Guerrouani A, Rzin A, El Khatib A. Hyperparathyroidism jaw tumour syndrome detected by aggressive generalized osteitis fibrosa cystica. Clin Cases Miner Bone Metab. 2013;10(1):65–7.
62. Kutcher MR, Rigby MH, Bullock M, et al. Hyperparathyroidism-jaw tumor syndrome. Head Neck. 2013;35(6):E175–7.
63. Ghemigian A, Ghemigian M, Popescu I, et al. Familial isolated primary hyperparathyroidism due to HRPT2 mutation. Hormones. 2013;12(3):454–60.
64. Abdulla AG, O'Leary EM, Isorena JP, et al. Recurrent hyperparathyroidism and a novel nonsense mutation in a patient with hyperparathyroidism-jaw tumor syndrome. Endocr Pract. 2013;19(6):e134–7.
65. Pazienza V, La Torre A, Baorda F, et al. Identification and functional characterization of three NoLS (nucleolar localisation signals) mutations of the CDC73 gene. PLoS One. 2013;8(12):e82292.
66. Kong J, Wang O, Nie M, et al. Familial isolated primary hyperparathyroidism/hyperparathyroidism-jaw tumour syndrome caused by germline gross deletion or point mutations of CDC73 gene in Chinese. Clin Endocrinol. 2014;81(2):222–30, 2.
67. Chiofalo MG, Sparaneo A, Chetta M, et al. A novel CDC73 gene mutation in an Italian family with hyperparathyroidism-jaw tumour (HPT-JT) syndrome. Cell Oncol. 2014;37(4):281–8.
68. Sriphrapradang C, Sornmayura P, Chanplakorn N, et al. Fine-needle aspiration cytology of parathyroid carcinoma mimic hürthle cell thyroid neoplasm. Case Rep Endocrinol. 2014;680876
69. Parfitt J, Harris M, Wright JM, Kalamchi S. Tumor suppressor gene mutation in a patient with a history of hyperparathyroidism-jaw tumor syndrome and healed generalized osteitis fibrosa cystica: a case report and genetic pathophysiology review. J Oral Maxillofac Surg. 2015;73(1):194.e1–9.
70. Shibata Y, Yamazaki M, Takei M, et al. Early-onset, severe, and recurrent primary hyperparathyroidism associated with a novel CDC73 mutation. Endocr J. 2015;62(7):627–32.
71. Khadilkar KS, Budyal SR, Kasliwal R, et al. HRPT2- (cdc73) related hereditary hyperparathyroidism: a case series from western India. Endocr Pract. 2015;21(9):1010–6.
72. Marchiori ÉC, Isom BA, Indresano AT. Management of ossifying fibroma in a suspicious case of hyperparathyroid-jaw tumor syndrome. Craniomaxillofac Trauma Reconstr. 2015;8(3):228–33.

73. Bellido V, Larrañaga I, Guimón M, et al. A novel mutation in a patient with hyperparathyroidism-jaw tumour syndrome. Endocr Pathol. 2016;27(2):142–6.
74. Ennazk L, El Mghari G, El Ansari N. Jaw tumor in primary hyperparathyroidism is not always a brown tumor. Clin Cases Miner Bone Metab. 2016;13(1):64–6.
75. Mathews JW, Winchester R, Alsaygh N, et al. Hyperparathyroidism-jaw tumor syndrome: an overlooked cause of severe hypercalcemia. Am J Med Sci. 2016;352(3):302–5.
76. Mele M, Rolighed L, Jespersen M, et al. Recurrence of hyperparathyroid hypercalcemia in a patient with the HRPT-2 mutation and a previous parathyroid carcinoma in hyperparathyroidism-jaw tumor syndrome. Int J Endocrinol Metab. 2016;14(2):e35424.
77. Piciu D, Piciu A, Barbus E, et al. Primary hyperparathyroidism-jaw tumor syndrome: a confusing and forgotten diagnosis. Clujul Med. 2016;89(4):555–8.
78. Guarnieri V, Seaberg RM, Kelly C, et al. Large intragenic deletion of CDC73 (exons 4-10) in a three-generation hyperparathyroidism-jaw tumor (HPT-JT) syndrome family. BMC Med Genet. 2017;18(1):83.
79. Mamedova E, Mokrysheva N, Vasilyev E, et al. Primary hyperparathyroidism in young patients in Russia: high frequency of hyperparathyroidism-jaw tumor syndrome. Endocr Connect. 2017;6(8):557–65.
80. Redwin Dhas MP, Karthiga KS, Tatu JE, Eugenia SJ. Hyperparathyroidism jaw tumor syndrome: a rare condition of incongruous features. Ethiop J Health Sci. 2017;27(3):309–13.
81. Rubinstein JC, Majumdar SK, Laskin W, et al. Hyperparathyroidism-Jaw Tumor Syndrome associated with large-scale 1q31 Deletion. J Endocr Soc. 2017;1(7):926–30.
82. Koikawa K, Okada Y, Mori H, et al. Hyperparathyroidism-jaw tumor syndrome confirmed by preoperative genetic testing. Intern Med. 2018;57(6):841–4.
83. Bachmeier C, Patel C, Kanowski P, Sangla K. Should all patients with hyperparathyroidism be screened for a CDC73 mutation? Endocrinol Diabetes Metab Case Rep. 2018;170164
84. Kapur A, Singh N, Mete O, et al. A young male with parafibromin-deficient parathyroid carcinoma due to a rare germline HRPT2/CDC73 mutation. Endocr Pathol. 2018;29(4):374–9.
85. Ciuffi S, Cianferotti L, Nesi G, et al. Characterization of a novel CDC73 gene mutation in a hyperparathyroidism-jaw tumor patient affected by parathyroid carcinoma in the absence of somatic loss of heterozygosity. Endocr J. 2019;66(4):319–27.
86. Russo M, Borzì G, Ilenia M, et al. Challenges in the treatment of parathyroid carcinoma: a case report. Hormones. 2019;8(3):325–8.
87. Gill AJ, Lim G, Cheung VKY, et al. Parafibromin-deficient (HPT-JT type, CDC73 mutated) parathyroid tumors demonstrate distinctive morphologic features. Am J Surg Pathol. 2019;43(1):35–46.
88. Iacobone M, Camozzi V, Mian C, et al. Long-term outcomes of parathyroidectomy in Hyperparathyroidism-Jaw Tumor syndrome: analysis of 5 families with CDC73 mutations. World J Surg. 2020;44(4):508–16.
89. Iacobone M, Lumachi F, Favia G. Up to date on parathyroid carcinoma: analysis of an experience of 19 cases. J Surg Oncol. 2004;88:223–8.
90. Iacobone M, Ruffolo C, Lumachi F, Favia G. Results of iterative surgery for persistent and recurrent parathyroid carcinoma. Langenbeck's Arch Surg. 2005;390(5):385–90.
91. Iacobone M, Henry JF. Parathyroid cancer. In: Licata AA, Lerma E, editors. Diseases of the parathyroid gland. New York: Springer; 2012.
92. Chen JD, Morrison C, Zhang C, Kahnoski K, Carpten JD, Teh BT. Hyperparathyroidism-jaw tumour syndrome. J Intern Med. 2003;253(6):634–42.

93. Xie WL, Lian JY, Li B, Tian XY, Li Z. Mixed epithelial and stromal tumor of kidney with renal vein extension: an unusual case report and review of literature. Histol Histopathol. 2017;32:361–9.
94. Haven CJ, Wong FK, van Dam EW, et al. A genotypic and histopathological study of a large Dutch kindred with hyperparathyroidism-jaw tumor syndrome. J Clin Endocrinol Metab. 2000;85:1449–54.
95. Gill AJ, Clarkson A, Gimm O, et al. Loss of nuclear expression of parafibromin distinguishes parathyroid carcinomas and hyperparathyroidism-jaw tumor (HPT-JT) syndrome-related adenomas from sporadic parathyroid adenomas and hyperplasia. Am J Surg Pathol. 2006;30:1140–9.
96. Witteven JE, Hamdy NA, Dekkers OM, et al. Downregulation of CASR expression and global loss of parafibromin staining are strong negative determinants of prognosis in parathyroid carcinoma. Mod Pathol. 2011;24:688–97.
97. Teh Y, Hu DY, Wang TT, et al. CDC73 gene mutations in sporadic ossifying fibroma of the jaws. Diagn Pathol. 2016;11(1):91.
98. Vocke CD, Ricketts CJ, Ball MW, et al. CDC73 germline mutation in a family with mixed epithelial and stromal tumors. Urology. 2019;124:91–7.

Multiple Endocrine Neoplasia Type 1

Alexander A. Leung, Paulien van Galen, A. Micheil Innes, Vicky Parkins, and Janice L. Pasieka

Contents

A. L. Shifrin et al. (eds.), *Endocrine Surgery Comprehensive Board Exam Guide*,
https://doi.org/10.1007/978-3-030-84737-1_36

Case

A 48-year-old male with a past medical history of nephrolithiasis dating back 10 years presented to the emergency department with bitemporal hemianopsia and gynecomastia. He was found to have a prolactin-secreting 2.8-cm anterior pituitary mass. He underwent successful transsphenoidal pituitary surgery. Postoperative investigation revealed a normalization of his prolactin level; however, he had an elevated serum calcium of 2.88 mmol/L with a concordant elevated PTH level of 74 pg/mL. A surgeon-directed bedside neck ultrasound (US) revealed multi-gland parathyroid disease. Additional screening for MEN1 revealed no pancreatic or adrenal lesions on cross-sectional imaging. He did, however, have multiple cutaneous lipomas. An appointment at our multidisciplinary endocrine hereditary clinic with our team, which included a geneticist and a genetic councillor, was done with the patient and his wife revealing they had two healthy biological children aged 12 and 14. Consent was obtained for genetic testing of the MEN1 gene of the patient, and recommendations for both timing of and potential screening of the children were made. A successful subtotal parathyroidectomy was performed on the index patient while awaiting genetic testing results. The genetic testing confirmed the clinical suspicion of an MEN1 mutation. The geneticist upon follow-up found multiple cutaneous lipomas on the patient's 14-year-old son. However, the mother refused to have the children tested for MEN1. The family was lost to follow-up for several years, until the now 22-year-old eldest son appeared in the surgeon's office asking for genetic testing. History revealed, like his father, he had suffered from an episode of nephrolithiasis in the last 6 months. Examination reveals multiple cutaneous lipomas, a neck US demonstrates four enlarged parathyroid glands and laboratory investigations confirm PTH-mediated hypercalcaemia. Both the MRI of his pancreas and pituitary were normal as were the biological screening tests for functional tumours. At the follow-up appointment to discuss surgical treatment of his HPT, he reveals that he and his wife are hoping to start a family in the near future.

Review Questions

1. Which of the following are common sets of manifestations of MEN1?
   (a) Gastrinoma, pituitary macroadenoma, primary hyperparathyroidism
   (b) Primary hyperthyroidism, pheochromocytoma, pituitary macroadenoma
   (c) Pituitary macroadenoma, insulinoma, cortisol-secreting adrenal adenoma
   (d) Primary hyperparathyroidism, medullary thyroid cancer, gastrinoma
2. MEN1 should be suspected in which of the following cases of primary hyperparathyroidism?
   (a) Onset of symptoms during the fifth decade of life
   (b) Multi-gland hyperplasia at the time of parathyroidectomy
   (c) Permanent hypocalcaemia after parathyroidectomy
   (d) Presence of limited bone disease

3. Which of the following tumours is associated with the *lowest* malignant potential?
   (a) Nonfunctioning pancreatic neuroendocrine tumour
   (b) Gastrinoma
   (c) Pituitary macroprolactinoma
   (d) Thymic neuroendocrine tumour
4. In which of the following scenarios is genetic testing for MEN1 routinely recommended?
   (a) Family and personal history of hypercalcaemia refractory to surgery
   (b) First-degree relative of a patient with genetically proven MEN1
   (c) Presence of an isolated anterior pituitary tumour in an older person
   (d) Personal history of severe peptic ulcer disease
5. Subtotal 3½ parathyroidectomy in MEN1-related hyperparathyroidism as a surgical approach is often favoured over total parathyroidectomy with autotransplantation. Which of the statements below explains the rationale?
   (a) It is associated with a lower rate of permanent hypoparathyroidism.
   (b) It is associated with a lower rate of persistent hypercalcaemic disease.
   (c) It is associated with a lower rate of hypercalcaemic disease recurrence.
   (d) It is associated with a lower rate of preoperative localization requirement.
6. The most frequent neuroendocrine tumour in the MEN1 pancreas is:
   (a) Gastrinoma
   (b) VIPoma
   (c) Insulinoma
   (d) Nonfunctioning neuroendocrine tumour
7. Ongoing surveillance of small (<2 cm) NF-pNETs is a reasonable strategy. What is the cited evidence for this?
   (a) Only 15% of NF-pNETs will demonstrate growth over time.
   (b) Of these lesions, 60–70% remain stable on long-term follow-up.
   (c) Regional disease is only seen when the lesions are greater than 3 cm.
   (d) Most of the pancreatic tumours will become functional over time.
8. What percent of individuals who have MEN1 are due to de novo mutations in the *MEN1* gene?
   (a) 10%
   (b) 20%
   (c) 30%
   (d) 1–2%

9. Genetic counselling plays an essential part in providing individuals and families with MEN1 with:
   (a) Discussion on the timing of surgical intervention of the condition
   (b) Limiting the genetic testing to first-degree relatives to minimize the burden
   (c) Developing an appreciation for the lack of randomness in genetic risk
   (d) Understanding the purpose and possible outcomes of genetic testing
10. Which of the following is a diagnostic genetic test available prior to gestation?
    (a) Bespoke NIPD
    (b) Targeted mutational analysis
    (c) Amniocentesis
    (d) PGT-M
11. The menin protein is a tumour suppressor. Which of the following is true?
    (a) MEN1 is an autosomal dominant condition with genetic anticipation.
    (b) MEN1 tumours acquire a second mutation in the somatic tumour tissue.
    (c) MEN1 is an autosomal recessive condition, with two mutations in the gene.
    (d) MEN1-related tumour development is common in childhood years.
12. The yield of genetic testing in individuals with MEN1 features and a positive family history is higher than in isolated patients. Which of the following is an explanation for this?
    (a) Sporadic patients have a mosaic mutation thus not detectable in blood.
    (b) Sporadic patients, particularly of younger ages, have an MEN1 phenocopy.
    (c) The variant has not been seen before and cannot detect it on the assay.
    (d) The pathogenicity of the variant is determined by familial linkage typically.
13. Which of the following is a major factor in determining the pathogenicity of a variant in the *MEN1* gene detected by clinical genetic testing?
    (a) The exon of the *MEN1* gene where the variant occurs
    (b) The impact on epigenetic methylation sites of the variant
    (c) The frequency of the variant in the general population
    (d) The predicted impact on transcription of the variant protein

14. The recommended surveillance for MEN1 incorporates both biochemical and anatomic components. The rationale for the dual assessment is related to:
    (a) The progression of tumours from nonfunctioning to functioning in time.
    (b) Anatomic imaging may miss functioning tumours in up to 20% of patients.
    (c) The biochemical testing is less invasive in the paediatric population.
    (d) The threshold for intervention varies depending on tumour function.
15. An 18-year-old patient newly diagnosed with MEN1 presents to the clinic for assessment. What is the most complete list of investigations that should be ordered?
    (a) CT head-neck-chest-abdomen, calcium/PTH, fasting glucose, gastrin, IGF-1
    (b) MRI sella-chest-abdomen, calcium/PTH, fasting glucose, insulin, prolactin
    (c) Ga68-DOTATATE PET, fasting glucose, insulin, gastrin, VIP, glucagon, calcium
    (d) CT chest, EUS pancreas, calcium/PTH, fasting glucose, insulin, prolactin

36.1 Introduction

Multiple endocrine neoplasia type 1 (MEN1) is a hereditary endocrine tumour syndrome inherited in an autosomal dominant fashion. First described in 1903 by Jacob Erdheim in a patient with acromegaly, pancreatic neuroendocrine tumours and parathyroid hyperplasia, it was not characterized as a syndrome until 1953. Underdahl reported eight patients with a clustering of pituitary, pancreatic and parathyroid tumours from the Mayo Clinic [1]. It was Paul Wermer in 1954 who first acknowledged that these cases were likely a hereditary disorder, coining the phrase multiple endocrine adenomatosis otherwise known as Wermer syndrome at the time [2]. In 1997, Chandrasekharappa discovered the MEN1 tumour suppressor gene on chromosome 11q3 that encodes the protein menin [3]. It is estimated that 1:5000 to 1:50,000 live births have MEN1. Diagnosis and treatment of patients with MEN1 requires a lifelong multidisciplinary approach by experts interested in this condition. Despite advances in the diagnosis and treatment of MEN1-associated tumours, the life expectancy of patients with MEN1 remains lower than that in the general population. Clinical practice guidelines call for early genetic testing and lifelong intensive surveillance to help disease disease-specific morbidity and mortality [4].

36.2 Molecular Genetics of MEN1

MEN1 is an autosomal dominant condition, associated with heterozygous pathogenic germline variants in the *MEN1* gene which encodes the protein menin. The *MEN1* gene has 10 exons, and the encoded protein is 610 amino acids and does not show similarity with any other known human protein [3].

Menin is considered a classic tumour suppressor protein. As such, patients with MEN1 typically have a germline pathogenic variant present at birth in all of their cells. In a somatic cell, a second 'hit' in the *MEN1* gene is acquired leading to nonfunctioning menin protein as part of the early stages of tumorigenesis, as predicted by Knudson's classic 'two-hit' hypothesis.

Over 1000 different germline variants in the MEN1 gene have been reported. They can occur anywhere across the gene. It is important to note, however, that only a portion of these are known to be pathogenic (disease causing). Pathogenic variants in *MEN1* may be of all types including (in decreasing order of frequency) frameshift, nonsense, intronic and missense variants followed by in-frame deletions or insertions. Historically where there was a clinical suspicion of MEN1, targeted (sanger) sequencing of the *MEN1* gene, with or without a test for copy number changes (deletions or duplications), was ordered. Increasingly with newer technologies, the test may be requested as part of a larger custom 'next-generation sequencing' panel which may include other known endocrine disorders or cancer predisposing genes or rarely via whole exome sequencing (sequencing of all of the greater than 20,000 genes in the genome). As costs of such technologies decrease, these are expected to be increasingly preferred as part of first-line testing. Regardless of the testing approach applied, as long as there is good coverage of the *MEN1* gene, a pathogenic variant should be detected in greater than 80–90% of individuals with familial MEN1 and greater than 65% of individuals with simplex (or sporadic) MEN1 [5]. Reasons for the lower yield in simplex cases of MEN1, including phenocopies and mosaicism, are discussed later in this chapter.

No matter which testing approach is used, it is important to consider the possible testing outcomes prior to ordering the test. In patients who meet the operational criteria of MEN1, the majority will have a pathogenic or likely pathogenic variant detected. In some patients, the testing will be completely negative. In such cases, it is worth reviewing the differential diagnosis, in the context of the a priori suspicion of MEN1. However, some individuals will have variants of uncertain significance identified. The American College of Medical Genetics has recently published guidelines to annotate variants and attempt to determine their pathogenicity [6]. While an in-depth discussion of this topic is beyond the scope of the chapter, factors that go into determining the pathogenicity of a variant include the following: the frequency of the variant in the general population (with an awareness of different variant populations in different ethnic groups), predicted impact of the nucleotide change on the amino acid, segregation of the variant appropriately within families (do all affected individuals share the variant), functional (laboratory based) testing of the variant (when available) and previous literature studies. Curated databases of known *MEN1* variants (pathogenic and nonpathogenic) exist (▶ https://databases.lovd.nl/shared/genes/MEN1; ▶ https://www.ncbi.nlm.nih.gov/clinvar/?term=MEN1%5Bgene%5D) and are readily available via the Internet. In general, it is important to note that clinical decisions (including offering genetic testing to at-risk family members) should only be made on variants known to be pathogenic or likely pathogenic. Finally, some individuals will be found through testing to have genetic variants known to be benign based on the above criteria. Importantly, in these cases, it is critical not to label these individuals as having MEN1 due to the presence of a known benign variant, even though it is rare. The implications of these variants on genetic counselling will be discussed further below.

36.3 Clinical Presentation and Diagnosis

MEN1 is characterized by the occurrence of multiple specific endocrine tumours in the same individual [4]. The clinical presentation of MEN1 can be highly variable, even among affected family members, as there is a lack of any clear genotype-phenotype correlation [7]. Manifestations are predominantly determined by the involved endocrine gland and the presence of secreted hormone. Although there may be significant heterogeneity in tumour penetrance, the parathyroid glands, pancreas and anterior pituitary gland are the sites most commonly affected by this condition (◘ Table 36.1).

36.3.1 Primary Hyperparathyroidism

Primary hyperparathyroidism (HPT) is the most common feature of MEN1, is present in more than 90% of patients and is usually the earliest manifestation of the syndrome [4]. Though affected patients may be asymptomatic, some report nonspecific symptoms (e.g. fatigue, malaise, abdominal discomfort,

Table 36.1 Endocrine manifestations of multiple endocrine neoplasia type 1

Condition	Estimated prevalence (%)	Risk of malignancy
Endocrine		
Hyperparathyroidism	>90	Rare
Gastroduodenopancreatic NET	30–70	Variable
Gastrinoma	40[a]	High
Insulinoma	10–30[a]	Low
Glucagonoma	<3[a]	High
VIPoma	<1[a]	Uncertain
Nonfunctional	20–55[a]	Variable
Pituitary adenoma	30–40	Rare
Prolactin-secreting	60[a]	Rare
GH-secreting	25[a]	Rare
ACTH-secreting	<5[a]	Rare
Nonfunctional	<5[a]	Rare
Bronchial NET	2	Low
Thymic NET	2	High
Adrenocortical tumour	25	Variable
Pheochromocytoma	<1	Low

Adapted from Thakker et al. [4]
Abbreviations: *ACTH* adrenocorticotropic hormone, *GH* growth hormone, *NET* neuroendocrine tumour, *PTH* parathyroid hormone, *VIP* vasoactive intestinal polypeptide
[a]Percentages represent estimated proportion of cases within each category. These do not necessarily summate to 100% because of the approximations made

dyspepsia, constipation and polyuria). End-organ damage from hypercalcaemia (e.g. renal calculi, nephrocalcinosis, kidney failure and osteoporosis) may occasionally be present. Laboratory evaluation generally reveals mild hypercalcaemia associated with a concomitantly elevated (or inappropriately normal) parathyroid hormone (PTH). Preoperative localization studies, such as ultrasound (US) and 99m-Tc-sestamibi (MIBI), are usually of limited value given that these patients typically have multi-gland disease.

In contrast to most sporadic cases of primary hyperparathyroidism, patients with MEN1 tend to have an earlier age of onset of disease (e.g. before 30 years), suffer more advanced bone disease, experience a higher risk of recurrence after parathyroidectomy and may report a family history of hyperparathyroidism [8]. Furthermore, parathyroid gland hyperplasia is commonly multicentric (affecting multiple glands) and metachronous (enlarging at different times) in patients with MEN1. As such, long-term follow-up is required to monitor for persistence or recurrence of hypercalcaemia following surgery.

36.3.2 Gastroduodenopancreatic Neuroendocrine Tumours

Gastroduodenopancreatic neuroendocrine tumours (GDP-NETs) occur in around 30–80% of people with MEN1 [4]. Although many of these are associated with syndromes of hormonal hypersecretion, some are nonfunctional and clinically silent.

Gastrinomas are among the most frequently encountered neoplasms, representing around 40% of GDP-NETs in MEN1. They most often arise in the duodenum (>80%) and less commonly in the pancreas. Gastrinomas are typically small (<1 cm) and frequently multicentric and carry a high risk of malignancy. These tumours produce gastrin, resulting in increased gastric acid production and recurrent peptic ulcer disease (Zollinger-Ellison syndrome). Symptoms may include abdominal pain, nausea, vomiting and diarrhoea. Primary hyperparathyroidism, which commonly coexists, can exacerbate underlying dyspepsia. Complications from untreated peptic ulcer disease (e.g. bleeding, obstruction and perforation) can be fatal [9]. Diagnosis is informed by laboratory testing which demonstrates hypergastrinaemia (increased fasting serum gastrin) in association with gastric acid hypersecretion (gastric pH <2), ideally measured in the absence of acid suppression therapy. In equivocal cases, a secretin stimulation test may be required to confirm the diagnosis. Less than half of gastrinomas are identified using traditional imaging studies (e.g. computed tomography (CT), magnetic resonance imaging (MRI), US, endoscopic US and somatostatin receptor scintigraphy) because most tumours are small and situated in the duodenum. Where available, positron emission tomography ((PET) with 68Ga DOTA octreotate)-CT, a more sensitive imaging modality, can be considered for preoperative localization.

Insulinomas are the second most common functional GDP-NET in patients with MEN1 (10–30%). These usually present as a benign, solitary lesion in the pancreas that produces insulin. Symptoms usually occur with prolonged fasting or exercise. Neuroglycopenic symptoms (e.g. fatigue, difficulty concentrating, confusion and headache) typically predominate over autonomic symptoms of hypoglycaemia (e.g. tremulousness, palpitations and diaphoresis). Evaluation includes a thorough review of the history and medication list to exclude the use of hypoglycaemic agents. Laboratory testing confirms the presence of elevated insulin, C-peptide and proinsulin levels in the setting of hypoglycaemia. A prolonged 72-hour supervised fast may occasionally be needed to elicit hypoglycaemia in order to confirm the diagnosis. Endoscopic US is preferred for preoperative localization because these tumours are often not visualized with conventional cross-sectional imaging such as CT or MRI. PET-CT (with 68Ga DOTA octreotate) and selective arterial calcium infusion (with venous sampling for insulin) can also aid in localization.

Other functioning tumours are rare, collectively representing less than 5% of all GDP-NETs in MEN1. Glucagonomas, which secrete glucagon, classically produce a syndrome of depression, weight loss, abdominal pain, steatorrhoea, characteristic rash (necrolytic migratory erythema), stomatitis and thrombosis. Patients frequently have associated laboratory abnormalities such as anaemia and glucose intolerance. These tumours are generally large, often located in the tail of the pancreas and associated with a high rate of malignancy. Vasoactive intestinal polypeptide (VIP)-secreting tumours, also known as VIPomas, are rare and associated with a cholera-like syndrome, characterized by copious amounts of watery diarrhoea unresponsive to fasting, hypokalaemia, metabolic acidosis and achlorhydria.

Notably, the majority of GDP-NETs are not associated with any clinical features and considered to be nonfunctioning (20–55%). This category is highly heterogeneous and includes tumours that produce small amounts of hormone that are not clinically apparent (e.g. pancreatic polypeptide). Importantly, the behaviour of nonfunctioning tumours can be highly variable with some being malignant. Therefore, careful long-term monitoring is required.

36.3.3 Pituitary Tumours

Around 30–40% of patients are affected by anterior pituitary tumours. The majority are macroadenomas (>1 cm) with a tendency to be aggressive, but actual malignancy is very rare [10]. The clinical presentation is largely determined by the hormone secreted. Around 60% of pituitary adenomas in individuals with MEN1 produce prolactin. Patients may present with symptoms and signs of hypogonadism (e.g. amenorrhoea in women and decreased libido in men) and galactorrhoea. Diagnosis is based on a markedly elevated serum prolactin. Growth hormone-secreting adenomas are the second most common type of lesions (25%), and these may co-secrete prolactin. Patients may initially be asymptomatic. Untreated over time, patients may develop acromegaly with features of growth hormone excess (e.g. enlargement of hands and feet, thickening of skin, deepening of voice, hyperhidrosis, frontal bossing, separation of teeth and painful arthropathies). Laboratory evaluation reveals an elevated insulin-like growth factor-1, adjusted for age and sex, and an inability to suppress growth hormone following a 75-g oral glucose tolerance test. Adrenocorticotropic hormone (ACTH)-producing adenomas, which are associated with Cushing's disease, are uncommon (<5%). These produce symptoms and signs of cortisol excess (e.g. proximal muscle weakness, thinning skin, bruising, violaceous striae and high blood pressure). Laboratory testing with a 24-hour urinary free cortisol, low-dose dexamethasone suppression test and/or late-night salivary cortisol reveals evidence of hypercortisolism. Remaining lesions are mostly nonfunctioning pituitary adenomas. Patients are generally asymptomatic, but those harbouring large tumours may experience local mass effects (e.g. headaches), visual disturbances from compression of the optic chiasm (e.g. bitemporal hemianopsia) and/or hypopituitarism.

36.3.4 Adrenal Tumours

Adrenal tumours are present in around 25% of patients with MEN1. Most lesions are nonfunctioning adrenocortical adenomas and detected incidentally on imaging [11]. Hormonal hypersecretion accounts for up to 15% of cases, and these are most commonly associated with aldosterone or cortisol excess. Patients with primary aldosteronism largely have nonspecific symptoms but may report a history of resistant hypertension and/or hypokalaemia. The biochemical hallmark of this condition is an elevated aldosterone-to-renin ratio. Cortisol excess, when present, may lead to Cushing's syndrome with similar symptoms and signs as those encountered with an ACTH-producing pituitary adenoma. The diagnostic evaluation is analogous. Importantly, the differential diagnosis for cortisol excess is broad; the possibility of an ACTH-secreting pituitary adenoma (most common; see above), ectopic ACTH production from a carcinoid tumour (least common; see below) or a cortisol-producing adrenal adenoma should be considered. Patients with MEN1 may also have a higher risk of adrenocortical carcinoma compared to individuals with sporadic adrenal lesions in the general population [11]. Pheochromocytoma however is rare, in contrast to other inherited endocrine tumour syndromes including multiple endocrine neoplasia type 2 (MEN2).

36.3.5 Bronchial and Thymic Neuroendocrine Tumours

Bronchial and thymic neuroendocrine tumours are present in less than 5% of cases of MEN1. Though infrequent, these tumours are important to recognize because they are associated with significant morbidity and mortality [12]. Patients with bronchial carcinoids may have respiratory symptoms (e.g. coughing, wheezing and shortness of breath) or present with syndromes of hormonal excess (e.g. Cushing's syndrome from ectopic ACTH production). These lesions are detected on imaging (e.g. X-ray or CT of the chest) or by bronchoscopy. Among patients with MEN1, around 80% of those with bronchial carcinoids are women. In contrast, nearly all (>90%) of thymic carcinoids in MEN1 occur in men, and smoking may be an additional risk factor for these. There is a high rate of malignancy with these tumours, and complications from local mass effect (e.g. superior vena cava syndrome) or invasion of surrounding structures (e.g. recurrent laryngeal nerve paralysis) are possible. While most cases are found on imaging, some are incidentally discovered following prophylactic thymectomy.

36.3.6 Non-endocrine Tumours

MEN1 is associated with a number of dermatological manifestations. Angiofibromas, which tend to be multiple and located on face, are among the most common and specific cutaneous features of MEN1 [12, 13]. Collagenomas and lipomas may also be present. Certain tumours of the central nervous system are described to occur in higher frequency in MEN1 as well, particularly meningiomas [14]. The presence of MEN1 may also increase the risk of developing breast cancer in women [15]. Thyroid tumours, though variably reported in patients with MEN1, are also highly prevalent in the general population, but the actual risk of thyroid disease may not necessarily be greater in this condition [4, 16].

36.3.7 Diagnosis

Diagnosis of MEN1 is important because it is associated with significant morbidity and mortality [9]. The majority of patients succumb to metastatic disease (e.g. malignant pancreatic or thymic neuroendocrine tumours) and complications from hormonal excess (e.g. gastric bleeding from Zollinger-Ellison syndrome). Accordingly, early recognition of this genetic disorder, surveillance for the occurrence of characteristic tumours and timely treatment may potentially help to improve clinical outcomes [4, 17].

A diagnosis of MEN1 can be established clinically (i.e. in a patient with two or more MEN1-associated endocrine tumours), by family history (i.e. in a patient with one MEN1-associated tumour plus a first-degree relative with a clinical diagnosis of MEN1) or genetically (i.e. detection of a germline *MEN1* pathogenic variant) [4]. However, the use of clinical and familial criteria may be confounded by the presence of phenocopies [17, 18]. Genetic testing can help to confidently establish the diagnosis of MEN1 in such cases, as well as for individuals at risk for MEN1 but without apparent clinical or biochemical manifestations of disease [19]. Germline *MEN1* testing should be routinely offered to index patients and their first-degree relatives, including those who are asymptomatic. Genetic testing should also be considered for individuals where there is a high index of suspicion of disease (e.g. family history of multiple endocrine tumours, personal history of multiple endocrine tumours, personal history of primary hyperparathyroidism with multi-gland hyperplasia or recurrence following parathyroidectomy or personal history of Zollinger-Ellison syndrome).

36.4 Surgical Management

36.4.1 Primary Hyperparathyroidism

Primary HPT is commonly the presenting disease process in MEN1. However, unlike sporadic HPT, these patients present at an early age and have multi-gland disease. In the era of focused, more minimally invasive surgery for HPT, it is important to recognize that the perioperative surgical planning for MEN1 patients differs from sporadic disease. The indications for surgery are very similar with the caveat that earlier intervention is often considered to reduce the end-organ effect of unopposed PTH on the bones and the kidney [20, 21]. Early surgical treatment, however, must be balanced with the significant consequences of hypoparathyroidism, particularly in a young population that has yet to achieve their peak bone mass. The goals for surgery in MEN1-related HPT are to safely achieve a eucalcaemic state for as long as possible while facilitating the ease of re-operative surgery, if necessary, in the future.

The extent of surgery in MEN1-related HPT continues to evolve. Classically, most surgeons would perform either a total parathyroidectomy with autotransplantation (TPTx-AT) or a 3½ gland subtotal parathyroidectomy (STPTx) [8, 9, 20–23]. The rates of persistent (<20%) and recurrent (>50%) disease have been shown to be equivalent with these two approaches, with the majority of endocrine surgeons preferring STPTx in this population because of the reduced risk of permanent hypoparathyroidism (11–33% STPTx vs. 66% in TPTx-AT) [20, 22, 24]. With improvements in preoperative parathyroid imaging, a more limited approach has been proposed in selective patients despite the fact that parathyroid disease is most often asymmetrical and multi-glandular in MEN1 [25]. Montenegro et al. proposed a unilateral clearance in patients in whom preoperative imaging demonstrated focal unilateral disease. In their study cohort of 62 patients with both preoperative US and MIBI scans, 23% had concordant unilateral imaging. These patients would be eligible for a unilateral clearance of the parathyroids, leaving the contralateral side untouched and virgin territory for a persistent/recurrent operation in the future. With the utilization of intra-operative PTH (iPTH) to guide the surgeon, theoretically this limited initial procedure has potential to limit the extent of surgery performed [26]. To date, there are limited data to critically appraise this approach, but it worth considering in highly selected patients with MEN1, recognizing the higher rates of persistent disease and the certain need for a second operation [27].

In primary HPT, preoperative imaging such as MIBI or 4D-CT scans is utilized solely for surgical planning. Since a bilateral operation is needed in the majority of MEN1 patients, there is limited role for these modalities. However, head and neck US is an invaluable tool to assess for concomitant thyroid pathology that should be addressed at the time of surgery. It also may help to select patients for a unilateral clearance approach should this prove to be a valuable approach in the future. Bilateral cervical thymectomies are recommended because of the 6–20% chance of supernumerary glands found in the thymus. However, in the case of a STPTx, if the inferior gland remnant is within the thymus, one should consider a unilateral cervical thymectomy to preserve the viability of the remaining remnant [28].

Utilization of iPTH is an adjunct that some surgeons have found to useful in assessing the adequacy of the exploration and/or amount of remand left behind. However, the criteria used in sporadic disease (>50% drop at 10 minutes) is not adequate in this patient population. Nilubol et al. found that a higher cutoff of >75% drop was adequate in the majority of patients with MEN1 but did not exclude the possibility of persistent disease [29].

36.4.2 Gastroduodenopancreatic Neuroendocrine Tumours

The surgical approach to GPD-NETs in MEN1 continues to evolve. The natural history and cause of death in MEN1 has changed over the last few decades with the development of effective acid-reducing drugs and early treatment of HPT. Over 60% of MEN1-related deaths are from malignant GPD-NETs [4, 30]. Surgical resection remains the mainstay of treatment; however, the timing and extent of resection varies depending on the hormonal secretion, the location and size of the tumour. Unlike sporadic NETs of the pancreas, there are several unique features of the MEN1 pancreatic NETs (pNETs) that complicate therapeutic strategies:

- Almost all patients have small nonfunctioning pancreatic NETs (NF-pNETs). These tend to be multiple and evenly distributed throughout the pancreas. Over time, it is estimated that only 13% will become symptomatic [31]. In a recent review of the literature, 60% of NF-pNETs remained stable, 25% developed new tumours on surveillance and 13% demonstrated growth [32].
- Gastrinomas resulting in Zollinger-Ellison syndrome in MEN1 (ZES/MEN), unlike sporadic ZES, are rarely cured with surgery. The gastrinomas are located in the duodenum, rather than the pancreas, and are usually multiple. Lymph node metastases are found in 60% of patients [31].
- Functional non-gastrin secreting pNETs including insulinomas (18%), glucagonomas (4%) and VIPomas (1–5%) are usually found in a background of NF-pNETs, and, as such, localization of the secreting functional tumour should precede resection.
- Unlike sporadic pNETs, MEN1 NF-pNET patients are younger, and pancreatic surgery has been shown to have higher associated rates of acute and long-term complications [33]. Diabetes develops in 15% of individuals, and pancreatic insufficiency is found in up to 20% of MEN1 patients. This has led many centres to consider pancreatic parenchyma preserving procedures or surveillance strategies for NF-pNETs.

The goals of treating GPD-NET MEN1-related tumours are to reduce hormonal secretion and the associated effects of hormonal excess and to prevent the development of metastatic disease while limiting the long-term morbidity from the therapeutic strategy. There are three clinical scenarios to consider: (a) functioning non-gastrin secreting pNETs, (b) NF-pNETs and (c) ZES/MEN.

Functioning non-gastrin pNETs should undergo surgical resection to address the life-threatening endocrinopathy [4]. However, identifying the secreting tumour when other NF-pNETs are seen in the pancreas is paramount in the surgical planning. Utilizing selective venous sampling or more novel techniques, such as PET-labelled glucagon-like peptide-1 (GLP-1) analogues in insulinomas, allows for the regionalization of the secreting tumour. Although some surgeons have advocated for removal of all visible pNETs in this scenario, knowing which tumour is functioning allows for better pancreatic conservation. Glucagonomas and VIPomas tend to develop in the tail of the pancreas, allowing for a distal pancreatectomy and nucleation of residual NF-pNETs if deemed necessary. Unfortunately, these rare tumours tend to present with metastatic disease, and, as such, the oncological principles of their treatment should be similar to that of sporadic metastatic functioning pNETs. Surgical debulking along with the use of systemic therapies has been shown to minimize associated endocrinopathies [4, 20, 31].

Nonfunctioning pNETs are found throughout the pancreas in 80–100% of MEN1 patients. Improved radiographic imaging has led to increased recognition of these lesions. The goal of surgical intervention is to intervene before regional and distant metastatic disease has developed while preserving exocrine and endocrine function of the pancreas. Like sporadic NF-NETs, the role of surgery versus surveillance is evolving. Although most guidelines and centres of excellence favour surgical resection for lesions ≥2–3 cm or significant growth over a short period of time, there is increasing literature to support selective surveillance [4, 20, 28, 32, 34–38]. The risk of lymph node metastases in NF-pNETs >2–3 cm is 40–50%, and hepatic disease is seen in 25–40% of patients with tumours >4 cm. This has led most centres to consider surgical intervention when an index lesion exceeds 2 cm in size. Longitudinal series have demonstrated that the majority (60–70%) of NF-NETs <2 cm in size remain stable with only 13% demonstrating interval growth [32, 35, 38]. The extent of surgical resection is based on the location and numbers of tumours found. Since complete eradication of NF-pNETs in MEN1 is not possible, surgical strategies to preserve pancreatic parenchyma should be employed [20, 34].

There is no consensus on either the indication or the timing of surgery in *ZES/MEN*. Since symptoms of ZES can be well controlled medically, the role of surgery has been contested for decades [31, 39]. Hypercalcaemia is known to stimulate gastrin production from the gastrinoma, and therefore concomitant HPT should be addressed first before considering any surgical intervention in the ZES/MEN patient. The management strategy for ZES/MEN utilized by many centres following parathyroidectomy for HPT includes:

(a) Proton pump inhibitors and surveillance for ZES/MEN1 patients with no or ≤2 cm NF-pNETs and no nodal or duodenal lesions seen.
(b) Surgical exploration with duodenal evaluation, pancreatic resection/enucleation of NF-pNETs and regional lymph node dissection in patients with pancreatic lesions >2 cm and/or interval growth. The pancreatic lesions are not the source of the gastrin but act as surrogate markers for more aggressive disease. It is therefore important that when operating on ZES/MEN, the duodenum be opened and the small gastrinomas excised locally.
(c) In highly selected patients with metastatic liver disease, duodenal excision of the primaries, lymph node dissection and pancreatic resection with surgical debulking of the liver disease [20, 29, 36, 39].

36.5 Genetic Counselling

As an autosomal dominant condition, MEN1 can be passed by and on to men or women. If an individual carries an *MEN1* pathogenic variant/likely pathogenic variant (PV/LPV), each of his/her children has a 50% chance of inheriting the same *MEN1* PV/LPV. The risks of inheriting the condition for the siblings of an affected individual depend on the genetic status of the parents. If a parent is affected, the risk to the siblings is 50%. The risk to other family members depends on the status of the parents. Approximately 10% of patients with MEN1 are de novo the result of a new PV/LPV that occurred in that person, not carried by either parent [4]. A de novo occurrence can be proven when a pathogenic variant is found in an individual that is not detected in either parent. In this instance, germline mosaicism in a parent is theoretically possible, and genetic testing for the pathogenic variant would still be recommended for the siblings when the parents test negative. Other explanations are alternate paternity or maternity (i.e. assisted reproduction) or undisclosed adoption. If parents are not tested for the MEN1 pathogenic variant but appear clinically unaffected, some risk for the siblings of the probands remains considering clinical variability and the possibility of germline mosaicism.

Genetic counselling plays an integral role in care of individuals and families with MEN1. It helps individuals better understand their condition and benefits of screening and early detection. It provides opportunity to understand the purpose of genetic testing, possible outcomes and how genetic test results may affect them and their family members, particularly when a clear pathogenic variant is identified to allow for predictive testing of at-risk family members. Review of the family history is essential as it can help an individual see the variability of the condition and understand who is at risk. It is also an important adjunct to help individuals through the psychological impacts of testing and diagnosis, specifically understanding the randomness of genetic risk and how it can affect self-image, individual and family identity and dynamics. Providing support and guidance for communication of the condition, risks to family members and addressing concerns for life/disability insurance and/or employment discrimination are an essential part of this process.

36

36.5.1 Family Planning

Predictive genetic testing to clarify a child's genetic status and/or prenatal diagnosis is available if the pathogenic variant is known in the family. If a couple would not change their decisions regarding an affected pregnancy, genetic testing could be considered at the age that screening would start appreciating that MEN1 surveillance would not be required if they test negative. It is important to note that discussions regarding availability of prenatal testing options and preimplantation genetics are ideally provided prior to a pregnancy so couples are aware and have time to make informed decisions about what approach, if any, is best suited to their needs. It is also appropriate to ensure young adults either affected or at risk have opportunity to discuss potential risk to offspring and reproductive options.

36.5.2 Prenatal Testing

Traditionally, prenatal testing has been limited to testing by either chorionic villi sampling (CVS) at 11–13 weeks' gestation or amniocentesis around 15 weeks' gestation, both of which are invasive tests with very small risk for miscarriage [40]. Bespoke noninvasive prenatal diagnosis (NIPD) is an emergent option for some autosomal dominant conditions like MEN1 [41–43]. It is currently most straightforward when the condition is paternally inherited [44]. To facilitate bespoke NIPD, a couple would need to start the process prior to becoming pregnant to determine if a successful assay can be designed. If a successful test is developed, it would allow a couple to complete a noninvasive diagnostic prenatal test as early as 8 weeks' gestation. While prenatal testing primarily provides opportunity for early diagnosis and option for continuing or ending a pregnancy, the emergence of NIPD may make this approach a more acceptable option appreciating it can be completed early in pregnancy and is a safer and more affordable option to preimplantation genetic testing.

36.5.3 Preimplantation Genetic Testing

Preimplantation genetic testing for monogenic disorders (PGT-M) is alternate option for some couples, particularly those who may already be in position of requiring in vitro fertilization (IVF) to achieve a pregnancy. While PGT-M can be completed for almost any condition in which the familial PV/LPV is known, like bespoke NIPD, it requires preparation prior to starting IVF to ensure an accurate test can be developed. PGT-M is a combination of direct mutational analysis and linked markers which ideally requires genetic testing and DNA samples of two affected family members from two generations for the purpose of determining phase in linkage. When no second generation is available, PGT-M is still possible for some cases but not all (i.e. large deletion/duplication-type PV/LPVs). PGT-M is not perfect, and as such diagnostic prenatal testing is still recommended for confirmation [45, 46]. Lastly, the process of IVF and PGT-M has significant financial costs and may not ultimately be successful for all couples. What costs, if any for IVF and/or PGT-M, are covered can vary by country. As such, it may not be a feasible option for all couples interested.

Table 36.2 Surveillance guidelines for patients with multiple endocrine neoplasia type 1

Tumour site	Screening start	Anatomic screening (every 1–5 y)	Biochemical screening (annually)
Parathyroid	8 y		Calcium, PTH
Pancreas Gastrinoma Insulinoma Nonfunctioning	*By tumour* 20 y 5–10 y 10 y	CT, MRI or EUS for all	*By tumour* Gastrin/gastric pH FBG, insulin PPP(+/−), CgA Glucagon, VIP
Pituitary	5–10 y	MRI sella	Prolactin, IGF-1
Adrenal	10 y	CT, MRI	Only if lesion >1 cm
Carcinoid bronchial, thymic, gastric (type 2)	15 y	CT, MRI + ZES-EUS	?CgA With ZES

Adapted from Thakker et al. [4], Kamilaris and Stratakis [28], and Burgess [49]

Abbreviations: *CT* computed tomography, *MRI* magnetic resonance imaging, *EUS* endoscopic ultrasound, *FBG* fasting blood glucose, *PPP* pancreatic polypeptide, *CgA* chromogranin A

36.6 Surveillance

Given the variety of potential tumours arising from an *MEN1* pathogenetic variant, a rational surveillance strategy needs to take all these into account (Table 36.2). For the purpose of this section, it is assumed the need for surveillance is defined by the presence of a PV/LPV giving rise to the MEN1 syndrome. The purpose of surveillance is to detect disease at such a stage as to modify the morbidity and mortality associated with MEN1. Epidemiologic data suggest that patients with MEN1 have higher mortality rates at every tumour site than their non-MEN1 matched cohort [4]. The difficulty of surveillance lies in the presence of functioning and nonfunctioning tumours. Typically, functioning tumours are detected by clinical symptoms and biochemical assessment of their hormone secretion, whereas the nonfunctioning tumours are detected exclusively by anatomic imaging. Thus, the complete surveillance requires judicious use of both types of investigations. The clinician has to balance the intensity and risk of screening tests with the risk of delayed management of MEN1 defining tumours. There may also be a difference in the screening algorithm depending on if the goal is primary detection versus recurrence of previously treated disease. Observations from the Tasman longitudinal cohort suggest that surveillance can focus on individuals in young adulthood and beyond, as *MEN1* positivity did not adversely impact survival in patients up to the age of 22 years [47].

36.6.1 Primary Hyperparathyroidism

Primary HPT is the most common and earliest presenting manifestation of MEN1. Fortunately, the screening for this condition can be readily achieved with a fasting calcium and matched PTH level completed on a yearly basis. In certain populations, assessment of 25-hydroxyvitamin D levels is important in order to rule out secondary HPT from endemic deficiency [48]. There is currently no evidence to suggest that early operative intervention on a patient with MEN1 while they are normocalcaemic will change any meaningful clinical outcome [4]. Inquiry for clinical symptoms of hypercalcaemia should be made at each visit, but it is rare for patients receiving appropriate surveillance to develop symptomatic HPT. For patients who have received surgery for primary HPT, it remains important to screen for recurrent disease, at least, annually.

36.6.2 Gastroduodenopancreatic Neuroendocrine Tumours

The next most common presenting tumour is the pNET. Clinical symptoms of functioning pNETs are important to elicit from all patients. There is debate as to the cost-effectiveness of biochemical screening for functioning pNETs in the absence of clinical symptoms. However, a fasting glucose, insulin and gastrin (provided the patient is not taking a proton pump inhibitor) should be ordered on an annual basis. A further detailed hormonal panel of VIP, somatostatin, glucagon and chromogranin A can also be considered [4, 49]. Anatomic imaging is needed to detect nonfunctioning pNETs. The optimal modality depends on local expertise and availability, but both MRI and CT can be considered. The role of newer functional imaging, such as Ga68 DOTATATE, has not been studied in the MEN1 population to determine if it is superior to conventional imaging and whether the risk of higher radiation doses is justified. The extent of disease (i.e. local, loco-regional, metastatic) needs to be determined to optimize both medical and surgical management. Due to the small nature of gastrinomas, the need for EUS or calcium-stimulated hepatic venous gastrin sampling may arise in the presence of ZES. Similarly, insulinomas can be hard to visualize. Intra-arterial calcium-stimulated hepatic venous insulin sampling and Ga68 DOTATATE PET can aid in localization [28].

36.6.3 Pituitary Adenoma

The surveillance of pituitary adenomas/neuroendocrine tumours follows a similar process as that of PNET [4] and is based on both biochemical and anatomic assessment. MRI is the imaging modality of choice. This should be requested at a frequency in keeping with the cadence of disease, typically every 3–5 years. The rate of functioning tumours is around 50%. Again, clinical symptoms are important to identify both functioning tumours and the consequences of large, nonfunctioning tumours. For the latter, the symptoms are broken down into mass effect, such as bitemporal hemianopsia and double vision due to cavernous sinus/cranial nerve involvement. The other group of symptoms is due to pituitary insufficiency. As such, biochemical screening on an annual basis, at minimum, should be followed. In order to screen for functioning adenomas, a prolactin and insulin-like growth factor-1 are helpful. The prevalence of Cushing's disease is of a rarity that yearly assessment of cortisol oversecretion need not be undertaken unless clinically indicated. The screening for pituitary deficiency would include measurement of a morning serum cortisol and free T4; evaluation for sex hormone deficiency is guided by the presence of compatible symptoms.

36.6.4 Adrenal Tumours

Anatomic surveillance with diagnostic imaging largely overlaps with the screening protocol used to detect GDP-NETs, as above [4]. Biochemical evaluation should be performed in the presence of compatible clinical symptoms of adrenal hormone excess or to evaluate the function of any incidental adrenal lesion detected on imaging.

36.6.5 Bronchial and Thymic Carcinoids

The detection of these tumours is dependent on anatomic imaging as there are no reliable biochemical markers. An MRI or CT can be ordered every 1–2 years for screening [4].

Ultimately, all patients with a pathogenic variant in *MEN1* require lifelong screening and management in the context of a multidisciplinary team. The burden of testing is high, but individualized screening strategies based on a risk-adapted paradigm can be considered, as informed by various factors including patient preferences and disease expression within the patient's kindred. Further study is needed to define these parameters more concretely.

36.7 Summary

MEN1 is a challenging disease to diagnose, treat and manage and therefore requires input from a multidisciplinary team. It is a disease that has implications across the entire lifespan and requires long-term follow-up for both the endocrine tumours and the consequences of the disease and its treatment. Local variations will undoubtedly exist in the provision of care, but key collaborations with endocrinology, neurosurgery, endocrine surgery and medical genetics are important.

With the advent of modern genetic testing, the detection of cases has improved. This has enabled an earlier ability to screen affected individuals and detect earlier stages of disease. The associated morbidity and mortality for patients with MEN1 is anticipated to improve commensurately. However, many questions remain for the timing of surgical management. Ongoing research in these areas through the large, established databases or disease registries is expected to refine the quality of clinical care.

Key Points

- The menin protein is a tumour suppressor. Individuals affected with MEN1 are born with a single germline variant in the gene and acquire a second hit in tumour tissues.
- Genetic testing is widely available for individuals suspected to have MEN1 and in appropriately selected patients that test is of high yield, particularly if there is a positive family history.
- It is important to determine the pathogenicity of a variant in the *MEN1* gene prior to altering clinical decision-making. While the clinical test lab plays an important role in variant classification, the clinician should understand the factors that go into such decisions.
- The clinical presentation of MEN1 is highly variable and predominantly determined by the involved endocrine gland and presence of secreted hormone.
- Primary hyperparathyroidism, gastroduodenopancreatic neuroendocrine tumours and anterior pituitary adenomas are the most common endocrine manifestations of MEN1. This condition is frequently associated with cutaneous lesions and tumours of the central nervous system.
- Diagnosis of MEN1 is important because it is associated with significant morbidity and mortality from metastatic disease and complications from uncontrolled hormonal excess.
- Surgical goals in MEN1-related HPT are to safely achieve a eucalcaemic state for a long as possible while facilitating the ease of re-operative surgery in the future.

- A 3½ gland subtotal parathyroidectomy is the preferred approach due to its lower rate of permanate hypoparathyroidism compared to a total parathyroidectomy and autotransplantation.
- The gastrinomas in MEN1 are located in the duodenum, not the pancreas, and are usually multiple.
- Of NF-pNETs, 60% remained stable, 25% will develop new tumours on surveillance and 13% will demonstrate growth.
- Of individuals with MEN1, 10% are de novo the result of a new pathogenic variant not carried by either parent.
- Genetic counselling is an essential component of care by providing individuals with an understanding of their condition, purpose of genetic testing, benefits of screening, early detection and treatment and providing support for communication of risk to family members.
- The surveillance of patients with genetically confirmed MEN1 is lifelong with both biochemical and imaging modalities.
- The appropriateness of the surveillance protocol balances medical burden/risks of testing against the benefit achieved by early detection and intervention.

Answer Key

1. (a); 2. (b); 3. (c); 4. (b); 5. (a); 6. (d); 7. (b); 8. (a); 9. (d); 10. (d); 11. (b); 12. (a); 13. (c); 14. (d); 15. (b)

References

1. Underdahl LO, Woolner LB, Black BM. Multiple endocrine adenomas; report of 8 cases in which the parathyroids, pituitary and pancreatic islets were involved. J Clin Endocrinol Metab. 1953;13(1):20–47.
2. Wermer P. Genetic aspects of adenomatosis of endocrine glands. Am J Med. 1954;16(3):363–71.
3. Chandrasekharappa SC, Guru SC, Manickam P, et al. Positional cloning of the gene for multiple endocrine neoplasia-type 1. Science. 1997;276(5311):404–7.
4. Thakker RV, Newey PJ, Walls GV, et al. Clinical practice guidelines for multiple endocrine neoplasia type 1 (MEN1). J Clin Endocrinol Metab. 2012;97(9):2990–3011.
5. Giusti F, Marini F, Brandi ML. Multiple endocrine neoplasia type 1. In: Adam MP, Ardinger HH, Pagon RA, Wallace SE, LJH B, Stephens K, Amemiya A, editors. GeneReviews® [Internet]. Seattle: University of Washington, Seattle; 1993–2019; 2005. [updated 2017 Dec 14].
6. Richards S, Aziz N, Bale S, et al. Standards and guidelines for the interpretation of sequence variants: a joint consensus recommendation of the American College of Medical Genetics and Genomics and the Association for Molecular Pathology. Genet Med. 2015;17(5):405–24.

7. Flanagan DE, Armitage M, Clein GP, Thakker RV. Prolactinoma presenting in identical twins with multiple endocrine neoplasia type 1. Clin Endocrinol. 1996;45(1):117–20.
8. Eller-Vainicher C, Chiodini I, Battista C, et al. Sporadic and MEN1-related primary hyperparathyroidism: differences in clinical expression and severity. J Bone Miner Res. 2009;24(8):1404–10.
9. Goudet P, Murat A, Binquet C, et al. Risk factors and causes of death in MEN1 disease. A GTE (Groupe d'Etude des Tumeurs Endocrines) cohort study among 758 patients. World J Surg. 2010;34(2):249–55.
10. Verges B, Boureille F, Goudet P, et al. Pituitary disease in MEN type 1 (MEN1): data from the France-Belgium MEN1 multicenter study. J Clin Endocrinol Metab. 2002;87(2):457–65.
11. Gatta-Cherifi B, Chabre O, Murat A, et al. Adrenal involvement in MEN1. Analysis of 715 cases from the Groupe d'Etude des Tumeurs Endocrines database. Eur J Endocrinol. 2012;166(2):269–79.
12. Goudet P, Bonithon-Kopp C, Murat A, et al. Gender-related differences in MEN1 lesion occurrence and diagnosis: a cohort study of 734 cases from the Groupe d'Etude des Tumeurs Endocrines. Eur J Endocrinol. 2011;165(1):97–105.
13. Vidal A, Iglesias MJ, Fernandez B, Fonseca E, Cordido F. Cutaneous lesions associated to multiple endocrine neoplasia syndrome type 1. J Eur Acad Dermatol Venereol. 2008;22(7):835–8.
14. Asgharian B, Chen YJ, Patronas NJ, et al. Meningiomas may be a component tumor of multiple endocrine neoplasia type 1. Clin Cancer Res. 2004;10(3):869–80.
15. van Leeuwaarde RS, Dreijerink KM, Ausems MG, et al. MEN1-dependent breast cancer: indication for early screening? Results from the Dutch MEN1 study group. J Clin Endocrinol Metab. 2017;102(6):2083–90.
16. Lodewijk L, Bongers PJ, Kist JW, et al. Thyroid incidentalomas in patients with multiple endocrine neoplasia type 1. Eur J Endocrinol. 2015;172(4):337–42.
17. de Laat JM, van Leeuwaarde RS, Valk GD. The importance of an early and accurate MEN1 diagnosis. Front Endocrinol (Lausanne). 2018;9:533.
18. Turner JJ, Christie PT, Pearce SH, Turnpenny PD, Thakker RV. Diagnostic challenges due to phenocopies: lessons from multiple endocrine neoplasia type1 (MEN1). Hum Mutat. 2010;31(1):E1089–101.
19. Giusti F, Cianferotti L, Boaretto F, et al. Multiple endocrine neoplasia syndrome type 1: institution, management, and data analysis of a nationwide multicenter patient database. Endocrine. 2017;58(2):349–59.
20. Kiernan CM, Grubbs EG. Surgical management of multiple endocrine neoplasia 1 and multiple endocrine neoplasia 2. Surg Clin North Am. 2019;99(4):693–709.
21. Wilhelm SM, Wang TS, Ruan DT, et al. The American Association of Endocrine Surgeons guidelines for definitive management of primary hyperparathyroidism. JAMA Surg. 2016;151(10):959–68.
22. Nobecourt PF, Zagzag J, Asare EA, et al. Intraoperative decision-making and technical aspects of parathyroidectomy in young patients with MEN1 related hyperparathyroidism. Front Endocrinol (Lausanne). 2018;9:618.
23. Tonelli F, Giudici F, Cavalli T, et al. Surgical approach in patients with hyperparathyroidism in multiple endocrine neoplasia type 1: total versus partial parathyroidectomy. Clinics (Sao Paulo). 2012;67(Suppl 1):155–60.
24. Schreinemakers JM, Pieterman CR, Scholten A, Vriens MR, Valk GD, Rinkes IH. The optimal surgical treatment for primary hyperparathyroidism in MEN1 patients: a systematic review. World J Surg. 2011;35(9):1993–2005.
25. Montenegro FLM, Brescia MDG, Lourenço DM Jr, et al. Could the less-than subtotal parathyroidectomy be an option for treating young patients

with multiple endocrine neoplasia type 1-related hyperparathyroidism? Front Endocrinol (Lausanne). 2019;10:123.
26. Kluijfhout WP, Beninato T, Drake FT, et al. Unilateral clearance for primary hyperparathyroidism in selected patients with multiple endocrine neoplasia type 1. World J Surg. 2016;40(12):2964–9.
27. Nilubol N, Weinstein LS, Simonds WF, et al. Limited parathyroidectomy in multiple endocrine neoplasia type 1-associated primary hyperparathyroidism: a setup for failure. Ann Surg Oncol. 2016;23(2):416–23.
28. Kamilaris CDC, Stratakis CA. Multiple endocrine neoplasia type 1 (MEN1): an update and the significance of early genetic and clinical diagnosis. Front Endocrinol (Lausanne). 2019;10:339.
29. Nilubol N, Weisbrod AB, Weinstein LS, et al. Utility of intraoperative parathyroid hormone monitoring in patients with multiple endocrine neoplasia type 1-associated primary hyperparathyroidism undergoing initial parathyroidectomy. World J Surg. 2013;37(8):1966–72. https://doi.org/10.1007/s00268-013-2054-1.
30. Ito T, Igarashi H, Uehara H, et al. Causes of death and prognostic factors in multiple endocrine neoplasia type 1: a prospective study: comparison of 106 MEN1/Zollinger-Ellison syndrome patients with 1613 literature MEN1 patients with or without pancreatic endocrine tumors. Medicine (Baltimore). 2013;92(3):135–81.
31. Jensen RT, Norton JA. Treatment of pancreatic neuroendocrine tumors in multiple endocrine neoplasia type 1: some clarity but continued controversy. Pancreas. 2017;46(5):589–94.
32. van Treijen MJC, van Beek DJ, van Leeuwaarde RS, et al. Diagnosing nonfunctional pancreatic NETs in MEN1: the evidence base. J Endocr Soc. 2018;2(9):1067–88.
33. Nell S, Borel Rinkes IHM, Verkooijen HM, et al. Early and late complications after surgery for MEN1-related nonfunctioning pancreatic neuroendocrine tumors. Ann Surg. 2018;267(2):352–6.
34. Sadowski SM, Cadiot G, Dansin E, et al. The future: surgical advances in MEN1 therapeutic approaches and management strategies. Endocr Relat Cancer. 2017;24(10):T243–60.
35. Pieterman CRC, de Laat JM, Twisk JWR, et al. Long-term natural course of small nonfunctional pancreatic neuroendocrine tumors in MEN1-results from the Dutch MEN1 Study Group. J Clin Endocrinol Metab. 2017;102(10):3795–805.
36. Falconi M, Eriksson B, Kaltsas G, et al. ENETS consensus guidelines update for the management of patients with functional pancreatic neuroendocrine tumors and non-functional pancreatic neuroendocrine tumors. Neuroendocrinology. 2016;103(2):153–71.
37. Triponez F, Dosseh D, Goudet P, et al. Epidemiology data on 108 MEN 1 patients from the GTE with isolated nonfunctioning tumors of the pancreas. Ann Surg. 2006;243(2):265–72.
38. Triponez F, Sadowski SM, Pattou F, et al. Long-term follow-up of MEN1 patients who do not have initial surgery for small ≤2 cm nonfunctioning pancreatic neuroendocrine tumors, an AFCE and GTE study: association Francophone de Chirurgie Endocrinienne & Groupe d'Etude des Tumeurs Endocrines. Ann Surg. 2018;268(1):158–64.
39. Albers MB, Manoharan J, Bartsch DK. Contemporary surgical management of the Zollinger-Ellison syndrome in multiple endocrine neoplasia type 1. Best Pract Res Clin Endocrinol Metab. 2019;33(5):101318.
40. Tabor A, Alfirevic Z. Update on procedure-related risks for prenatal diagnosis techniques. Fetal Diagn Ther. 2010;27(1):1–7.
41. Fan HC, Gu W, Wang J, et al. Non-invasive prenatal measurement of the fetal genome. Nature. 2012;487(7407):320–4.
42. Lench N, Barrett A, Fielding S, et al. The clinical implementation of non-invasive prenatal diagnosis for single-gene disorders: challenges and progress made. Prenat Diagn. 2013;33(6):555–62.
43. Lewis C, Hill M, Chitty LS. Non-invasive prenatal diagnosis for single gene disorders: experience of patients. Clin Genet. 2014;85(4):336–42.

44. Jenkins LA, Deans ZC, Lewis C, et al. Delivering an accredited non-invasive prenatal diagnosis service for monogenic disorders and recommendations for best practice. Prenat Diagn. 2018;38(1):44–51.
45. Sullivan-Pyke C, Dokras A. Preimplantation genetic screening and pre-implantation genetic diagnosis. Obstet Gynecol Clin N Am. 2018;45(1):113–25.
46. Basille C, Frydman R, El Aly A, et al. Preimplantation genetic diagnosis: state of the art. Eur J Obstet Gynecol Reprod Biol. 2009;145(1):9–13.
47. Herath M, Parameswaran V, Thompson M. Paediatric and young adult manifestations and outcomes of multiple endocrine neoplasia type 1. Clin Endocrinol. 2019;91(5):633–8.
48. Heaney RP. Functional indices of vitamin D status and ramifications of vitamin D deficiency. Am J Clin Nutr. 2004;80(6 Suppl):1706S–9S.
49. Burgess J. How should the patient with multiple endocrine neoplasia type 1 (MEN 1) be followed? Clin Endocrinol. 2010;72(1):13–6.

Multiple Endocrine Neoplasia Type 2 (MEN 2)

Kyriakos Vamvakidis and Kerstin Lorenz

Contents

A. L. Shifrin et al. (eds.), *Endocrine Surgery Comprehensive Board Exam Guide*,
https://doi.org/10.1007/978-3-030-84737-1_37

Case Presentation

The patient is a 27-year-old female who was referred to our hospital because she was found to have a palpable neck mass. The neck ultrasound examination (◘ Figs. 37.1, 37.2, and 37.3) by an experienced radiologist revealed a 2.9-cm nodule in the left thyroid lobe with increased vascularity, irregular margins, and microcalcifications, suspicious for thyroid cancer. The FNA biopsy was performed with cytological diagnosis of a medullary thyroid carcinoma. The basal serum calcitonin level was markedly elevated at 355 pg/ml.

Preoperative physical examination revealed the presence of increased blood pressure that was not known to the patient. The surgeons, after consulting with hospital endocrinologists, suspected pheochromocytoma and proceeded with measurements of 24-hour urine for metanephrines, which were markedly elevated. An abdominal CT scan was also ordered that revealed a 4.2-cm mass within the left adrenal gland with typical features of PCC. The right adrenal gland appeared normal.

Genetic testing confirmed a mutation in the *RET* proto-oncogene at codon 618. The patient was diagnosed with the MEN 2A syndrome. Genetic testing, to look for the *RET* proto-oncogene mutation, was recommended to be performed for all first-degree family members.

The parathormone and calcium levels were within normal ranges, so the diagnosis of PHPT was excluded.

Because of the findings of PCC, the initially scheduled thyroidectomy with bilateral systematic neck dissection was postponed, and a laparoscopic left adrenalectomy was performed first, after the patient had preoperatively received alpha blockade with per os phenoxybenzamine for 2 weeks.

One month after the left adrenalectomy, the patient underwent a total thyroidectomy with bilateral central and lateral neck dissection. Final histology evaluation was consistent with a medullary thyroid carcinoma in the left thyroid lobe with 12/67 lymph nodes (LN) positive for metastatic disease.

The patient was referred to endocrinologists for the follow-up. Three months after the thyroid surgery, the basal CTN was undetectable.

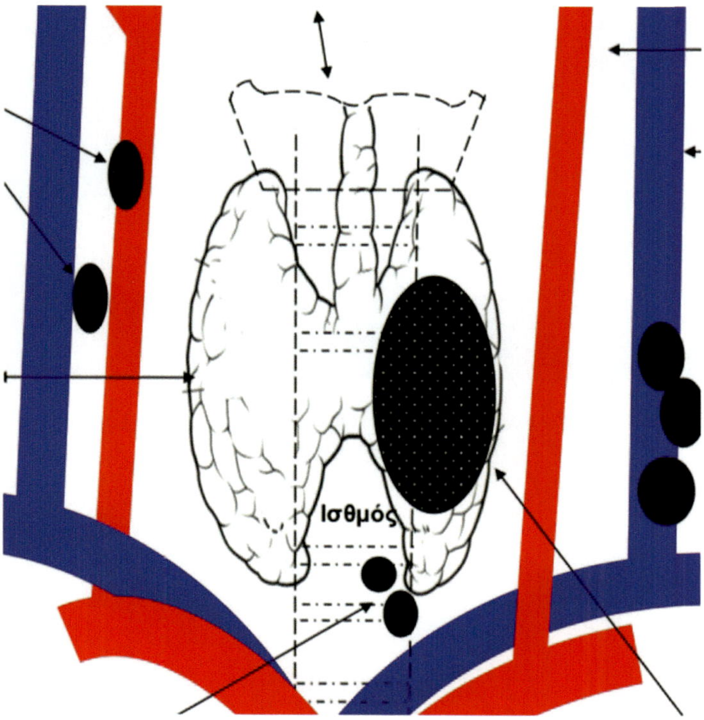

◘ **Fig. 37.1** Neck ultrasound with lymph node mapping arises the suspicion of regional lymph node metastasis

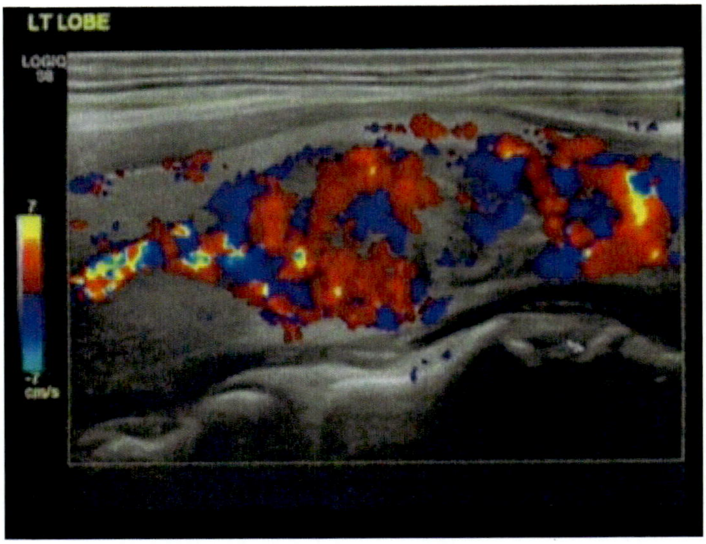

■ **Fig. 37.2** Color Doppler ultrasound of the nodule in the left lobe shows the increased vascularity

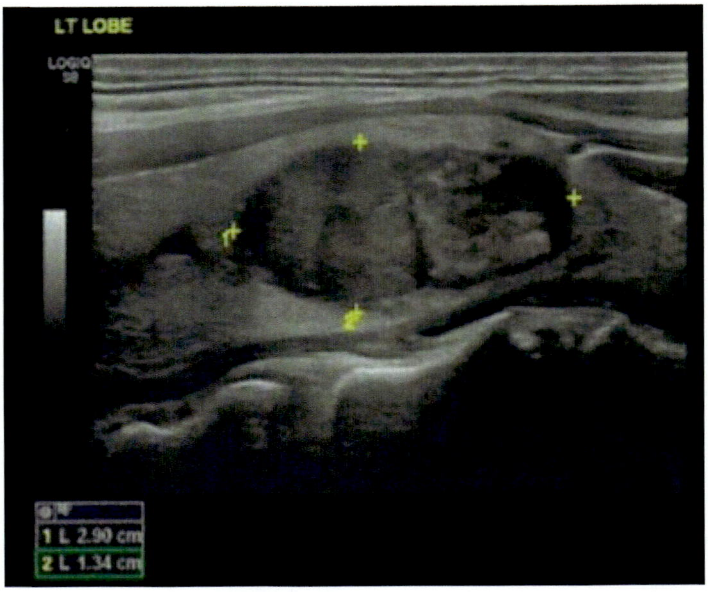

■ **Fig. 37.3** Ultrasound imaging of the medullary thyroid carcinoma with max. diameter of 2.9 cm located in the left thyroid lobe

Questions

1. MEN 2B can be related to the following *RET* mutations:
   1. Codon 620 *RET* mutation
   2. Codon A883F *RET* mutation
   3. Codon M918T *RET* mutation
   4. Codon 634Y *RET* mutation
   5. Codon 620 *RET* mutation
      (a) 1 and 2 are correct.
      (b) 2 and 3 are correct.
      (c) All are correct.
      (d) None are correct.
      (e) Only 3 is correct.
2. The most common *RET* mutation(s) in MEN 2A patients with cutaneous lichen amyloidosis is (are):
   1. Codon 620 *RET* mutation
   2. Codon 634 *RET* mutation
   3. Codon 620 and codon 634 *RET* mutation equally
   4. Codon A883F *RET* mutation
   5. Codon 618 *RET* mutation
      (a) 1 is correct.
      (b) 2 is correct.
      (c) 3 is correct.
      (d) 4 is correct.
      (e) None are correct.
3. The high-risk category *RET* mutations include:
   1. Codon M918T
   2. Codon 634
   3. Codon A883F
   4. Codon 620
   5. Codon 804
      (a) 1 and 2 are correct.
      (b) 2 and 3 are correct.
      (c) Only 3 is correct.
      (d) Only 1 is correct.
      (e) 4 and 5 is correct.
4. The FMTC can include the following manifestations:
   1. PCC
   2. MTC
   3. pHPT
   4. MTC and pHPT
   5. MTC and PCC
      (a) Only 2 is correct.
      (b) 3 and 5 are correct.
      (c) 1 and 2 are correct.
      (d) 2 and 3 are correct.
      (e) 1 and 3 are correct.

5. The usually delayed diagnosis of MEN 2B is due to:
   1. The difficulty of testing of codon M918T
   2. The lack of premonitory symptoms
   3. The absence of specific body characteristics
   4. The fact that most of the carriers have de novo mutations making screening impossible in these cases
   5. The early onset during the first months of the life
      (a) 1 and 2 is correct.
      (b) 5 is correct.
      (c) 4 and 5 are correct.
      (d) 2 and 3 are correct.
      (e) 1, 2, and 3 are correct.
6. In case that PCC is diagnosed synchronously with MTC, what are the next steps:
   1. PCC must be removed first, then surgery for the MTC.
   2. A-blockers for about 2 weeks is recommended.
   3. First the thyroidectomy and then the adrenalectomy.
   4. The possibility of the copresence of pHPT should be examined.
   5. Ideally, both operations at the same time.
      (a) 5 is correct.
      (b) 1 is correct.
      (c) 1, 2, and 4 are correct.
      (d) 3 is correct.
      (e) 1 and 4 are correct.
7. Prophylactic thyroidectomy for MEN 2B patients:
   1. Must be performed between 3 and 5 years old
   2. Must be performed when the calcitonin levels are >40 pg/ml
   3. Must be performed in the first months of life
   4. Is not sure that it must be performed in all patients
   5. Must be performed if a suspicious nodule occurs
      (a) 2 is correct.
      (b) 3 is correct.
      (c) 2 and 5 are correct.
      (d) 4 is correct.
      (e) 1 is correct.
8. The biomarkers for the evaluation of MTC are:
   1. Calcitonin
   2. Precalcitonin
   3. CEA
   4. Thyroglobulin
   5. Parathormone
      (a) 1, 2, and 3 are correct.
      (b) 3, 4, and 5 are correct.
      (c) All are correct.
      (d) 1 and 3 are correct.
      (e) 1 and 2 are correct.

9. Which statements for the MEN 2A with Hirschsprung's disease are correct?
   1. The most common *RET* mutations are related to codons 618 and 620.
   2. The most common *RET* mutations are related to codons 634 and 609.
   3. It is due to a "Janus" mutation that induces a loss-of-function and a gain-of-function activity simultaneously.
   4. Affects usually the entire colon.
   5. Affects usually the distal part of the colon.
      (a) 1 and 4 are correct.
      (b) 1 and 5 are correct.
      (c) 2 and 3 are correct.
      (d) 2 and 5 are correct.
      (e) 1, 3, and 5 are correct.
10. What's the premonitory symptoms of MEN 2B?
   1. Inability to cry tears
   2. Constipation
   3. Weak suckling causing feeding problems
   4. Diplopia
   5. Exophthalmos
      (a) 1 and 2 are correct.
      (b) 1, 2, and 5 are correct.
      (c) 2, 3, and 5 are correct.
      (d) 1, 2, and 3 are correct.
      (e) 2, 3, and 4 are correct.
11. Which statements regarding the extent of the surgery in young MEN 2 patients are correct?
   1. It depends on the basal calcitonin levels.
   2. It depends on the presence of suspected lymph nodes.
   3. Younger patients have increased rate of hypoparathyroidism, so unnecessary neck dissection must be avoided.
   4. The risk for permanent hypoparathyroidism increases by extensive surgery.
   5. The risk of permanent recurrent laryngeal nerve damage decreases by extensive surgery.
      (a) All is correct.
      (b) 1, 2, 3, and 4 are correct.
      (c) 1, 2, 4, and 5 are correct.
      (d) 1 and 2 are correct.
      (e) 1, 2, and 4 are correct.
12. Which statements for the PCC in MEN 2 patients are correct?
   1. Is very often malignant.
   2. Usually follows chronically the MTC.
   3. Occurs in about 50% of MEN 2 patients.
   4. It is rarely lethal.

5. It is never bilateral.
   (a) 1, 2, and 3 are correct.
   (b) 2, 3, and 4 are correct.
   (c) 2 and 3 are correct.
   (d) 1, 2, and 4 are correct.
   (e) 3, 4, and 5 are correct.

13. Which statements for the prognostication of MEN 2 are correct?
    1. It depends on the underlying mutation.
    2. It is related to the course of MTC.
    3. The initial operation is very important.
    4. It depends on the preoperative calcitonin levels.
    5. It depends on the doubling time of calcitonin postoperatively.
       (a) 2, 4, and 5 are correct.
       (b) All are correct.
       (c) 1, 2, and 4 are correct.
       (d) 1, 2, 4, and 5 are correct.
       (e) 1, 3, and 5 are correct.
14. Which statements for the pHPT in MEN 2 patients are correct?
    1. pHPT never occurs in patients with codon M918T *RET* mutation.
    2. pHPT is less common than PCC in MEN 2A patients.
    3. pHPT rarely preexists MTC.
    4. pHPT is always the most delayed manifestation of FMTC.
    5. pHPT initially begins as hyperplasia, but it can evolve into adenomas.
       (a) 1, 2, 3, and 5 are correct.
       (b) 2, 3, and 4 are correct.
       (c) 2, 4, and 5 are correct.
       (d) 1, 2, and 3 are correct.
       (e) All are correct.
15. Which statements for ectopic ACTH secretion by MTCs are correct?
    1. It is a very rare condition of about 0.6% of MTCs.
    2. Its prognosis is very good.
    3. Bilateral adrenalectomy could be a therapeutic choice.
    4. Ketoconazole can be the medical therapy.
    5. It occurs only in the hereditary forms of MTC.
       (a) 1, 2, 3, and 5 are correct.
       (b) 2, 3, and 4 are correct.
       (c) 1, 3, and 4 are correct.
       (d) 1, 3, and 5 are correct.
       (e) All are correct.
16. Which statements regarding FMTC are correct?
    1. The underlying *RET* mutations are mainly noncysteine mutations.
    2. The onset of the MTC is later compared to the other subtypes of MEN 2A.
    3. pHPT is not associated with FMTC.

4. The diagnosis of FMTC is problematic because it is sharing the same manifestations with classical MEN 2A syndrome.
5. The mutation in the codon A883F is strongly related to FMTC.
   (a) 1, 2, 3, and 4 are correct.
   (b) 2, 3, 4, and 5 are correct.
   (c) 1, 3, and 4 are correct.
   (d) 1, 3, and 5 are correct.
   (e) 2, 4, and 5 are correct.

17. Which criteria for the diagnosis of FMTC have been used?
   1. More than ten carriers in the family, over 50 years old, and negative family history for PCC and pHPT.
   2. More than five members in the family with MTC and at least one with PCC.
   3. Family with at least four members with MTC and no signs for PCC or pHPT.
   4. Delayed MTC due to non-cysteine *RET* mutations in codons which are associated with very low risk for the other manifestations.
   5. Each patient belongs to the subgroup of FMTC, if he has any *RET* mutation without signs of PCC or pHPT.
      (a) 1, 2, and 5 are correct.
      (b) 1, 3, and 4 are correct.
      (c) 1, 3, 4, and 5 are correct.
      (d) All are correct.
      (e) 1, 3, and 5 are correct.

18. Which statements about lymphadenectomy in MTC patients are correct?
   1. The systematic compartment-oriented neck dissection has better outcomes when compared with the selective lymphadenectomy.
   2. The lymphadenectomy is associated with increased risk for temporary and permanent hypoparathyroidism.
   3. If the basal calcitonin levels are above 500 pg/ml, a lateral neck dissection is indicated.
   4. The minor therapeutic operation for MTC is total thyroidectomy with at least central neck dissection.
   5. Lymphadenectomy is associated with decreased risk for temporary and permanent recurrent laryngeal nerve damage.
      (a) 1, 3, and 5 are correct.
      (b) 1, 2, 3, and 5 are correct.
      (c) 2, 3, and 4 are correct.
      (d) 1, 3, and 5 are correct.
      (e) 1, 2, 3, and 4 are correct.

37.1 Introduction

The syndrome of multiple endocrine neoplasia type 2 (MEN 2) is an autosomal dominant hereditary syndrome characterized by the synchronous or heterochronous development of malignant or benign tumors of different endocrine organs such as medullary thyroid cancer, pheochromocytoma, hyperplasia, or adenomas of the parathyroid glands and is often associated with other clinical manifestations.

MEN 2 is divided into two main subtypes: the MEN 2A and MEN 2B. The MEN 2A in this classification concerns 95% of cases, while the MEN 2B syndrome is rare and occurs in only 1 in every 20 patients with MEN 2. Although the two subtypes, MEN 2A and 2B, share many similarities, they have important differences regarding epidemiological, clinical, and genetical characteristics.

While in MEN 2A patients there are no specific external recognizable signs, MEN 2B patients have age-related external signs with progressive development. For example, the typical neuromas on the language tip can be missing or minimally developed in infants, while they are fully developed in young adults.

The MEN 2A syndrome can appear in four variants: the classical form of MEN 2A, MEN 2A combined with lichen amyloidosis, MEN 2A with Hirschsprung's disease (HD), and the familial form of medullary thyroid carcinoma (FMTC) without PCC and PHPT.

The MEN 2B syndrome is characterized by very early onset of MTC, practically during the infancy, the marfanoid habitus, raised bumps on the lips and tongue, and an increased aggressiveness of the MTC combined with the absence of PHPT from the clinical manifestations of the disease [1].

The subtypes and variants of MEN 2 are summarized in ◘ Table 37.1, and the clinical manifestations of MEN 2A and MEN 2B are summarized in ◘ Tables 37.2 and 37.3, respectively, while the main differences between MEN 2A and MEN 2B are summarized in ◘ Table 37.4.

◘ **Table 37.1** Subtypes and variants of MEN 2

MEN2 **MEN 2A (95%)**	**MEN 2B (5%)**
1. Classical MEN 2A	
2. MEN 2A with lichen amyloidosis	
3. MEN 2A with HD	
4. FMTC	

Table 37.2 Clinical manifestations of MEN 2A syndrome

MEN 2A	Organ	Manifestation
	Thyroid gland	C-cell hyperplasia
		Medullary thyroid cancer
	Parathyroid	Hyperplasia
		Adenoma
	Adrenals	Pheochromocytoma
	Skin	Cutaneous lichen amyloidosis
	Colon	Absence of enteric innervation

Table 37.3 Clinical manifestations of MEN 2B syndrome

MEN 2B	Organ	Manifestation
	Thyroid gland	Medullary thyroid cancer
	Parathyroid	None
	Adrenals	Pheochromocytoma
	Colon	Enteric neuromas – constipation
	Eye	Thickened corneal nerves – inability to cry
	Lips, tongue	Neuromas – raised bumps
	Whole body	Marfanoid habitus

Table 37.4 Main differences between MEN 2A and MEN 2B

	MEN 2	
	MEN 2A	MEN 2B
Proportion	95%	5%
MTC onset	Often during the first 5 years	During the first months
MTC aggressiveness	Less aggressive than MEN 2B-MTC	Regarded as the most aggressive form
PHPT	The third most common manifestation	Absent
Marfanoid habitus	Absent	Present in the vast majority of patients

37.1.1 RET Proto-Oncogene

The *RET* proto-oncogene possesses a central role in the origin not only in the hereditary MEN 2 syndromes but also in the sporadic forms of MTC.

Initially reported and named in 1985 (Takahashi and colleagues) [2], *RET* (*re*arranged during *t*ransfection) is expressed in thyroid C-cells that originate most possibly, as new data suggests, from the anterior endoderm and not from the neural crest as was previously believed. *RET* is also expressed in adrenal medullary cells, neural cells, cells originated from the branchial arches (parathyroid cells), and the urogenital system. *RET* is located in the pericentromeric part of chromosome10q11.2 with a width of 21 exons.

37.1.2 Medullary Thyroid Cancer

MTC is the central manifestation of MEN 2 syndromes for two reasons: firstly, because it affects almost 100% of all MEN 2 patients and, secondly, because its aggressiveness determines the prognosis of the patient. MTC arises from the parafollicular cells or C-cells of the thyroid and represents about 3% of all types of thyroid carcinomas.

The origin of C-cells was traditionally believed to be of the neural crest, but new data contest this theory that was first proposed by A.G. E Pearce in Hammersmith over 50 years ago [3]. Nilsson et al., in a recent study revising the origin of C-cells, suggested that the anterior endoderm is the source of differentiated C-cells [4, 5].

Sporadic MTC occurs usually as a single nodule, while hereditary MTC often is multifocal involving both thyroid lobes.

The pathogenesis of MTC, either hereditary (25% of cases) or sporadic (75% of cases), is related to the activation of *RET* proto-oncogene. Germline activating point mutations or other alterations are encountered in approximately 98% of hereditary cases, and somatic mutations are encountered in approximately 45–50% of sporadic cases.

Patients diagnosed with MTC should have genetic screening performed for activating *RET* proto-oncogene mutations in order to distinguish between hereditary and sporadic disease [6]:

1. The presence of a *RET* mutation is an indication to search for a coexisting tumor associated with MTC in the index patient.
2. All first-degree relatives of *RET*-positive patients should be tested for the same specific mutation that was identified in the proband. Those that were tested positive should be evaluated for MEN 2-related tumors and advised to proceed with further specific management that would result in early diagnosis and treatment.

3. All first-degree negative relatives can be relieved of further investigation and psychological burden.
4. With a *RET* mutation identified in about 5–10% of patients diagnosed initially with sporadic MTC, one can assume that a number of cases were either misclassified or that a de novo *RET* mutation was identified.

37.1.3 Medullary Thyroid Carcinoma and Biomarkers

A relatively specific biomarker for MTC is calcitonin (CTN). CTN is a 32-amino-acid monomeric peptide and is specifically secreted by C-cells of the thyroid gland. CTN originates from pre-procalcitonin and procalcitonin (PCTN) after proteolytic splitting.

Calcitonin level can be elevated in numerous other conditions than MTC or C-cell hyperplasia such as thyroiditis, elevated calcium levels, renal insufficiency, pregnancy, and lactation. Furthermore, in rare circumstances, some other malignant diseases that are derived by other than thyroid organs could overproduce CTN (i.e., lung, breast, pancreas, leukemia) [7, 8].

In general, CTN level >100 pg/ml is diagnostic for MTC in both genders [9]. The differences in the secretion of calcitonin due to the different C-cell mass between women and men led to the use of gender-specific thresholds, which are more precise for the accurate diagnosis of occult MTC when compared to unisex thresholds.

A study by Machens et al. reported a 100% specificity and 100% positive predictive value for the diagnosis of MTC in women when basal calcitonin levels are more than 50 pg/ml [10].

In cases when basal CTN level is mildly elevated within the "gray zone," the calcitonin stimulation test (CST) with pentagastrin or calcium gluconate can been used to establish the biochemical diagnosis of MTC. A study by Niederle et al. reports equal diagnostic power in both tests if gender-specific cutoff values are used [11].

In case of MTC, the levels of CTN should be increased manifold from the baseline. The above tests (CST with pentagastrin and CST with calcium gluconate) have significant differences in the increase of calcitonin levels, so their results are not comparable. Lorenz et al. reported that CST with calcium gluconate yields significantly higher calcitonin levels compared to CST with pentagastrin, so that the generalization of pentagastrin-CST to calcium-CST thresholds is precluded [8]. CTN could be within a normal range in rare cases of an advanced dedifferentiation of the MTC that is associated with worse prognosis and shorter survival [12].

During the last years, the use of PCTN is proposed as a promising alternative for the evaluation of MTC because both PCTN and CTN have a similar diagnostic value. The biphasic half-life, the isoforms, and the different fragments of CTN led to the suggestion for the use of PCTN that is devoid from the above problems [13, 14]. On the other hand, the lack of a threshold for MTC, its increase by inflammatory processes, and the fact that it is not widely available are significant limitations of PCTN. Thus, at present, the use of CTN remains the primary biomarker for the diagnosis and follow-up of MTC patients [15].

Serum carcinoembryonic antigen (CEA) is another parameter related to MTC. CEA is not a specific biomarker for MTC mainly because it can be secreted by other benign conditions and especially by non-thyroid malignancies. Therefore, the diagnosis of MTC cannot be made based on CEA. With regard to MTC, CEA is usually elevated in either advanced disease or in the rare cases of low differentiation disease that makes it useful during the follow-up. Progression of MTC combined with elevation of CEA without increase of CTN levels or even with decrease of CTN is a sign of dedifferentiation and/or poor differentiation of the tumor with bad prognosis. Thus, CEA can be used as a sensitive marker to distinguish more aggressive biological behavior in MTC patients [16]. High preoperative levels of CEA are associated with a decreased chance of biochemical cure. CEA values >500 ng/ml are related to increased mortality [17].

37.1.4 MTC and Ectopic ACTH Secretion

MTC has a rare association with the ectopic secretion of ACTH that can result in a Cushing's syndrome [18]. Barbosa et al. report that about 0.6% of the patients with MTC (either sporadic or hereditary) can have Cushing's syndrome due to ectopic production by the MTC.

The management of the patients included surgery for the MTC, bilateral adrenalectomy, ketoconazole, and somatostatin analogs.

The prognosis of the disease, as seen in the aforementioned study, was poor; half of the patients died due to the MTC, while the other half died of complications of Cushing's syndrome [19].

During the last years, the use of vandetanib is reported by many authors as an efficient therapy for the long-term control of Cushing's syndrome in MTC [20–22].

37.2 Clinical Presentation

37.2.1 MEN 2A

37.2.1.1 Classical Type of MEN 2A

The typical clinical manifestation of an MEN 2A patient almost always includes a medullary thyroid cancer, a pheochromocytoma in about 40–50% (usually with coexisting diffuse nodular adrenal medullary hyperplasia), and less frequently PHPT due to hyperplasia or adenomas of the parathyroid glands.

The multiple gland disease is more frequent in MEN 2A patients compared to the sporadic cases, while parathyroid cancer in association with MEN 2A mutation has not been described so far. The PHPT manifestations in these patients mainly appear after the age of 30 years.

The mutations found in patients with MEN 2A are mainly located on exon 10 (codons 609, 611, 618, and 620) or on exon 11 (codons 630 and 634) with codon 634 being the most prevalent underlying RET mutation at a rate of 85%.

37.2.1.2 MEN 2A with CLA

MEN 2A can be combined with cutaneous lichen amyloidosis (CLA). These patients suffer from stress-exacerbated pruritus located predominantly in the scapula regions. CLA affects the dermatomes C8-D3 and results in a scaly rash that could lead to the early diagnosis of the MEN 2A syndrome.

37.2.1.3 MEN 2A with HD

Another subtype of MEN 2A is the association with HD. This association can be explained by common mutations in the *RET* proto-oncogene. These mutations occur on exon 10 and are of special scientific interest because they simultaneously induce a loss-of-function and a gain-of-function activity. They are called "Janus" mutations, a name that is derived from the Roman mythological god who had two faces looking in opposite directions. HD is a congenital pathologic situation characterized by the absence of enteric innervation, which in the majority of patients affects only the distal part of the colon (80%); nevertheless, it can be present in multiple segments or even in the entire colon.

In a systematic review which studied the association of HD and MEN 2A by D. Coyle et al., it was found that the most common mutations were related to codons 620 and 618, on exon 10. Those patients with the aforementioned mutations had higher risk for long-segment disease or even total colonic aganglionosis [23].

37.2.1.4 FMTC

In the FMTC variant, the presence of the MTC is the only clinical feature and thus not associated with parathyroid or adrenal pathology. Recent data associate FMTC with non-cysteine *RET* mutations, while the MEN 2A is developed due to cysteine RET mutations [24].

37.2.2 MEN 2B

The onset of the disease in patients with the MEN 2B syndrome is very early, compared to the manifestation of the disease in patients with the MEN 2A syndrome, and usually occurs in the first year of life. All patients develop MTC, while 50% of them develop pheochromocytoma. MTC and pheochromocytoma are more aggressive in patients with the MEN 2B syndrome compared to the patients with the MEN 2A syndrome, while PHPT is absent.

The patients appear thin and tall, having the characteristic marfanoid habitus with long upper and lower extremities combined by increased joint flexibility.

The mucosal neuromas create a further morphological characteristic which are raised bumps on the lips and tongue (◘ Fig. 37.4), while the intestinal neuromas can affect the intestinal motility and cause frequent constipation. Severe constipation can be an early clinical sign during infancy in MEN 2B patients [25].

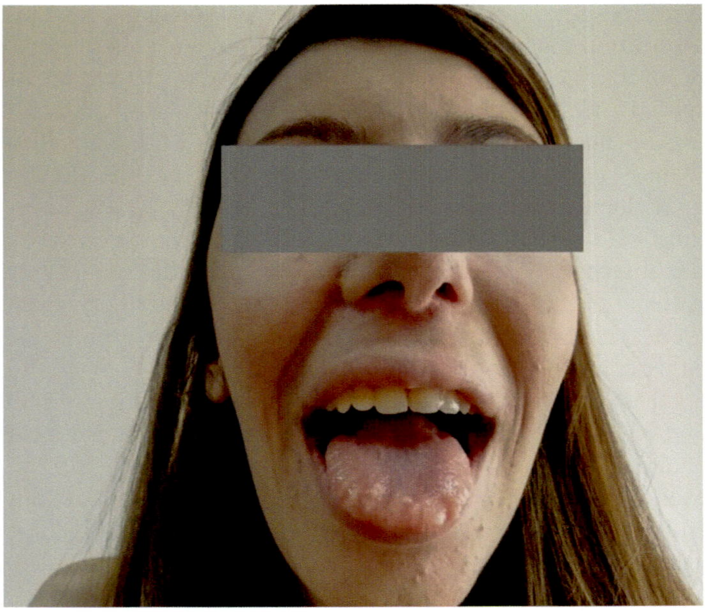

◘ **Fig. 37.4** Characteristic mucosal neuromas on the lips and tongue in a MEN 2B-patient. (Courtesy of Dr. A. Saltiki)

A very interesting premonitory symptom of MEN 2B was described in detail by Brauckhoff et al., as an infant inability to shed tears. The mechanism proposed by the authors is the decreased activity of the thickened corneal nerves which affect eye surface sensitivity. Along with the inability of an infant to cry and development of constipation, the authors also reported the presence of feeding problems due to weak suckling function. The inability to cry may be the first clinical sign of MEN 2B syndrome [26].

Megacolon is a common clinical manifestation among MEN 2B patients. A retrospective data analysis by D. Gibbons et al. in Mayo Clinic reports, along with the megacolon, described serious problems with esophageal motility (achalasia and Zenker's diverticulum) which is most likely the result of neuromuscular incoordination [27].

37.3 Natural History

37.3.1 Classical MEN 2A Syndrome

The classical MEN 2A syndrome initially develops as C-cell hyperplasia which progresses to MTC. The time that MTC will occur varies and depends on the specific underlying mutation. In general, the MTC in hereditary cases, when compared to the sporadic cases, is associated with multiple and bilateral lesions in younger ages [28].

The second timely manifestation of the classical MEN 2A syndrome is the PCC which is present in about 40–50% of patients. The risk of malignancy for the PCC in MEN 2 is extremely low. The definitive diagnosis of malignancy can be made only in the presence of metastases in other organs, i.e., by the presence of chromaffin cells in organs which do not physiologically possess these types of cells. Although the development of PCC usually appears 5–10 years after the diagnosis of MTC (metachronously), it may be diagnosed synchronously. In some cases, PCC can occur before MTC. Two studies which analyzed the data from 212 and 563 MEN 2 patients reported the diagnosis of PCC prior to MTC at 17% and 15%, respectively [29, 30].

The last and least frequent manifestation of the MEN 2A syndrome is PHPT that usually develops initially as a parathyroid cell hyperplasia that can evolve into an adenoma. The coexistence of hyperplasia and adenoma is not rare. The presence of PHPT in MEN 2A is generally mild or even asymptomatic and may syn- or metachronously involve more than one PG. The frequency of PHPT in MEN 2A patients was estimated at 20–30%. Some recent studies with large a series of patients, though, report that the prevalence of PHPT in MEN

2A is significantly less (between 4% and 8%). A possible explanation for this is that with the increase of genetic testing in recent years, more cases of MEN 2A were diagnosed, which probably belong to the subgroup of FMTC, which is also characterized by the absence of PHPT [31]. The latter is clearly supported by the study by Romei et al. This study, after analyzing the data of *RET* genetic screening in a large population of 1556 patients, revealed that 68 out of the 1007 apparently sporadic cases (6.7%) were hereditary. These cases, totaling nearly 90%, were classified as FMTC cases (61/68) [24].

PHPT which precedes MTC and PCC is extremely rare. A recent international retrospective multicenter study by LV Larsen et al. showed that of the 1085 MEN 2A cases only 0.9% (10/1085) had PHPT as the first clinical manifestation of the syndrome [32].

37.3.2 MEN 2A with CLA

In these patients, the first symptom is usually an intense pruritus with onset occurring during infancy. Sunlight exposure has beneficial effects, while stress has the opposite effect of aggravating it. Over time, hyperpigmented lesions are developed, probably as a result of intense scratching. Light microscopy can reveal orthokeratotic hyperkeratosis and concretions of amorphous material in the superficial dermis, while when placed under ultraviolet light, the deposit of amyloid in the dermis can be confirmed by the presence of thioflavin T-positive staining. The underlying mutation is related to codon 634 of the RET, which is associated with the early onset of MTC usually within the first 5 years, while the process of CLA begins in infancy.

The fact that CLA precedes the occurrence of MTC can be a premonitory symptom that can lead to early diagnosis and effective treatment of MTC [33].

37.3.3 MEN 2A and HD

HD is a rare condition characterized by the absence of autonomic ganglion cells within the colonic parasympathetic plexus that can cause enteric obstruction and megacolon. The disease, when coexisting with the MEN 2A syndrome, is related to mutations in the codons 609, 618, and 620 (most frequent) on exon 10 of the *RET* proto-oncogene. Symptoms have an early onset in childhood and include abdominal pain, reduced weight, constipation, vomiting, and diarrhea. The evolution of the disease makes colonic surgery unavoidable [34].

37.3.4 MEN 2B

MEN 2B is the most aggressive type of MEN 2 syndromes which in the vast majority of cases originates from a mutation in codon 918 of the RET. The onset of the disease is usually in the first months of life, so that any precursory symptom of the syndrome is of great importance for early diagnosis and effective treatment.

The latter becomes even more important because most affected patients show a de novo germline *RET* mutation combined with a negative family history for MEN, making early diagnosis through previous family genetic testing not applicable for many patients.

A review by Gfroerer et al. analyzing the data of 55 MEN 2B patients regarding gastrointestinal problems reveals that although more than half of the patients had the first obstructive signs during early infancy, the median age of diagnosis was 13 years.

Of the patients, 73% suffered constipation, which was, by far, the most common gastrointestinal symptom, while 29% of patients were found to have colonic dilatation. Diarrhea, vomiting, abdominal pain, and weight loss are included in the enteric discomforts [35]. Therefore, it is suggested that MEN 2B syndrome be included in the working diagnosis of constipation in newborns.

37.4 Diagnosis

The diagnosis of MEN 2 syndrome can be made as follows:

- By the identification of a germline RET mutation after genetic screening in asymptomatic first-degree relatives of RET-positive patients
- By the identification of a germline RET mutation:
  (a) In apparently sporadic cases of MTC
  (b) Rarely in apparently sporadic cases of PCC or PHPT

Although the most important step, before the identification of germline mutation by genetic screening, for the diagnosis of MEN 2 in patients without family history of MEN 2, is the diagnosis of MTC, in rare cases, when either PCC or PHPT preexists MTC, the initial step for the diagnosis can be the appearance of PCC or PHPT, respectively.

The preoperative diagnosis of MTC may be confirmed in two ways: (1) basal CTN levels (>100 pg/ml) and (2) the cytology by fine needle aspiration (FNA) of the suspected nodule. In a study by Bugalho et al., it was shown that CTN levels had higher sensitivity (98%) when compared to the cytology results (63%) [36]. Furthermore, CTN levels can inform the surgeon about the extent of the disease and arising biochemical suspicion for either lymph node (LN) or even distant metastases [37].

MEN 2A syndrome can be diagnosed [38]:

- By identifying a *RET* mutation associated with MEN 2A in a patient with one or two clinical features of the disease (MTC, PCC, PHPT)
- By identifying the clinical features of the disease at least in one first-degree relative of a patient with one or two clinical features of MEN 2A
- Clinically, if two of the manifestations of the disease are present, in cases of negative genetic testing

Where a germline RET mutation is present with no clinical features of MEN 2A, the affected individuals are at risk of developing the MEN 2A syndrome and require suitable medical attention.

To categorize a patient with FMTC instead of the classical variant of MEN 2A, the following criteria have been proposed:

- More than ten carriers in the family, multiple carriers or affected members over 50 years old, and a negative family history for pheochromocytoma and PHPT [39]
- Families with at least four members with MTC without any sign for PCC or PHPT [40]
- Kindreds with late-onset MTC due to non-cysteine RET mutations on exons 13–15, which are associated with very low risk for the other manifestations of MEN 2A [41]

The classification of MEN 2A patients in the group of FMTC instead of the classical form of MEN 2A is problematic because the manifestation of FMTC is included in MEN 2A syndrome. In a family which includes members only with MTC and is initially classified as FMTC, if years later a family member develops PCC or PHPT, the whole family should be reclassified as MEN 2A [1].

MEN 2B can be diagnosed [38]:

- By identifying a *RET* mutation associated with MEN 2B in a patient with one or two clinical features of the disease (MTC, PCC, marfanoid habitus)
- By identifying the clinical features of the disease at least in one first-degree relative of a patient with one or two clinical features of MEN 2B
- Clinically, if a majority of the clinical features of the disease are present in cases of negative genetic testing

Every patient with MTC, even those without any family history, should be investigated for the presence of a germline *RET* mutation to exclude the possibility of the hereditary forms. In a study by R. Elisei et al., about 7% of those patients who seemingly suffered from sporadic MTC were proven to carry a germline *RET* mutation that reclassified them as hereditary cases of MTC. Most carriers only had MTC after a follow-up of mean 8.1 years, except for one patient who developed a PCC 6 years after the initial diagnosis of MTC. This reclassification has led to the genetic testing of their relatives, of which 35.5% were gene carriers [42].

37.5 Treatment

The treatment of MEN 2 patients is dependent on the manifestations of the disease and the variety of their clinical symptoms.

Priority must be given to the surgical therapy of MTC, which is the most aggressive component of the syndrome. Before dealing with the MTC, the coexistence of a PCC must be excluded. If a unilateral PCC is concomitantly present, it is necessary to treat it first, preferably with a laparoscopic or retroperitoneoscopic subtotal adrenalectomy. The reason for the priority to be dealing with the PCC first is that a possible pronounced hypertensive crisis during the thyroid operation could put the patient at mortal risk. Regarding PCC surgery, an adrenal tissue-sparing procedure is suggested in order to avoid adrenal insufficiency, especially in cases of bilateral PCC (◘ Fig. 37.5). In the rare cases of malignant PCC, an open adrenalectomy could be the best approach, if there are doubts that the laparoscopic procedure can achieve an adequate oncological result. Prior to adrenalectomy, the blocking of the PCC with a-blockers for a period of up to 2 weeks is recommended. After the exclusion or the effective treatment of the PCC, the patient has to be operated on for the MTC.

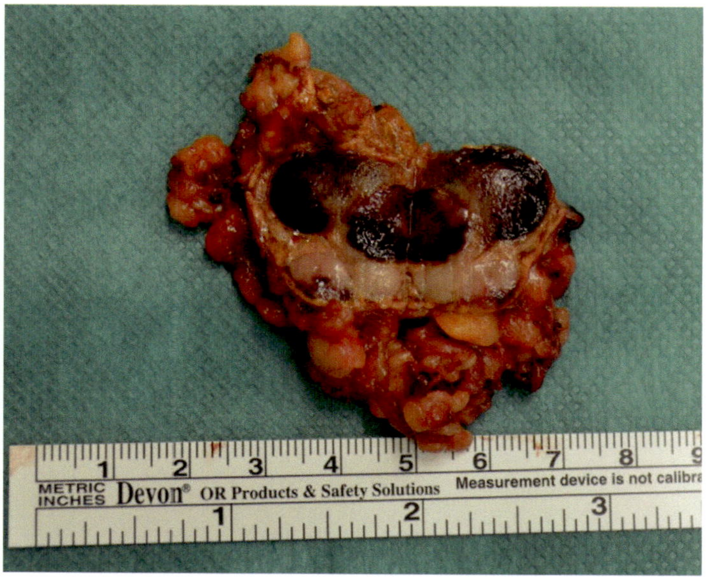

◘ **Fig. 37.5** Subtotal adrenal resection in MEN 2A patient with bilateral PCC

37.5.1 Risk Categories for Hereditary MTC

Before proceeding to the treatment of MTC in MEN 2 patients, it is important to assess the effect of the underlying *RET* mutation on the biological behavior of MTC.

According to many studies that have been conducted over recent years, it is clear that the aggressiveness and prognosis of MTC in MEN 2 patients depends on the underlying mutation in the *RET* proto-oncogene.

The new revised ATA guidelines for the management of MTC suggest three risk categories regarding the biological behavior of MTC, which are based on the early onset and the metastatic potential: the highest risk (HST) category that includes M918T mutation in MEN 2B patients, the high-risk (H) category that includes codon 634 of exon 11 mutations, and the moderate-risk (MOD) category that includes the remaining RET mutations [37].

Regarding the A883F mutation, a rare (<5%) *RET* mutation in MEN 2B patients, a recent international collaborative study by Mathiesen et al., investigating the risk profile of this rare mutation in 13 carriers, suggested that it has to be included in the ATA high-risk category [43].

MEN 2 is a rare syndrome, and the A883F mutation is expected to appear in less than 1 in every 400 MEN 2 patients (1/400). Concerning the rarity of this A883F mutation, it is concluded that the data provided by the aforementioned study are important and practically determine the risk profile of this mutation.

Thus, the risk categories for hereditary MTC are summarized as follows [44] (◘ Table 37.5):

- Highest risk: M918T (MEN 2B patients)
- High risk: codon 634 mutations and A883F mutation
- Moderate risk: all other remaining RET mutations

◘ **Table 37.5** Risk classification for MTC in MEN 2 patients

Risk categories for hereditary MTC	
Risk category	**RET mutation**
Highest risk	918T (responsible for MEN 2B in 95%)
High risk	Codon 634 mutations, A883F
Moderate risk	All remaining mutations

Table 37.6 The possibility of ipsilateral lateral LN infiltration based on the number of infiltrated central LN

Number of infiltrated LN in central cervical compartment	Possibility of LN metastasis in the ipsilateral lateral compartment (%)
0	10
1–3	77
>4	98

Based on the publication by Machens et al. [45]

37.5.2 Extent of the Initial Surgery for MTC

The decision regarding the extent of the initial operation depends on many parameters such as basal calcitonin and CEA levels and preoperative mapping of cervical LN and on the underlying mutation. Total thyroidectomy with central neck dissection is considered by the revised ATA guidelines for the management of MTC (Recommendation 24) as the least extensive surgical procedure [37].

Machens et al. report that the possibility of LN metastasis in the lateral compartment is related to the number of infiltrated LN in the central compartment. The possibility for ipsilateral lateral LN metastases was 10%, 77%, and 98% in cases of 0, 1–3, and more than 4 infiltrated LN in the central compartment, respectively (Table 37.6), while the possibility for contralateral LN metastases is 38% and 77% in cases of 1–9 and 10 or more infiltrated LN in the central compartment, respectively [45].

Another study by Bae et al. reported 100% ipsilateral lateral LN metastases if there are metastases in the contralateral central cervical compartment, while 96% of the patients with ipsilateral lateral LN metastases had LN metastases in the ipsilateral central compartment [46].

In cases where the removal of the regional LN is indicated, a selective lymphadenectomy must be avoided. Dralle et al. revealed the superiority of the compartment-oriented microdissection, i.e., a systematic lymphadenectomy, which includes LN and adipose and connective tissue of the entire cervical compartment. Those patients who underwent systematic lymphadenectomy needed fewer reoperations and had better results regarding their survival compared to patients who underwent a selective approach [47].

Reoperations can be considered during the follow-up if there is evidence of persistent/recurrent disease with elevated CTN levels.

A study which analyzes data of those patients who underwent reoperation for persistent MTC reported that the possibility of biochemical cure was 44% if the basal CTN levels were <1000 pg/ml and if no infiltrated LN were removed during the initial operation. If the CTN levels were <1000 and one to five infiltrated LN were removed during the first operation, biochemical cure was only 18%. If the CTN levels were >1000 pg/ml, the biochemical cure rate was disappointingly low at 1% [48].

Systematic staging in MTC patients is indicated if the preoperative basal calcitonin levels are above 500 pg/ml or if there is evidence of distant metastasis or extensive disease in the neck. The systematic staging should include CT or MRI for the liver, CT of thorax for the assessment of lungs and mediastinal LN metastases, and bone scintigraphy [37].

MRI should be preferable for the staging of hereditary MTC in MEN 2 children and young adult patients due to the absence of ionizing radiation [49].

Regarding the treatment of PHPT in MEN 2 patients, which is present in a minority of these patients and occurs usually as the last manifestation of the syndrome, it is practically the same as in sporadic cases of PHPT. Nevertheless, hereditary PHPT is characterized by an earlier onset compared to sporadic forms and in about 50% of the patients affects multiple glands even if the glands are not simultaneously affected. Thus, in the beginning, the PHPT in MEN 2 patients can be masked as a single-gland disease and may affect the remaining parathyroid glands years later. The multiglandular disease in MEN 2 patients is characterized either by diffuse hyperplasia or by the coexistence of hyperplasia and adenomas. The parathyroidectomy (PTx) can be either selective or, in cases of four-gland disease, subtotal or total with autologous reimplantation [50].

PTx can be performed simultaneously with the thyroidectomy in cases of concomitant presence with MTC or can be performed years later after the thyroidectomy. The situation that PHPT precedes MTC is improbable. Due to the asynchronous and asymmetric character of PHPT in MEN 2 patients, recurrences are not rare. Reoperation for persistent/recurrent disease is not always curable [31]. Recurrent or persisted PHPT could be treated alternatively using calcimimetics which has shown to have good results [51, 52].

37.5.3 Systematic Treatment

The systematic treatment of MTC in MEN 2 patients, as in the patients of sporadic form, is indicated by unresectable locally advanced disease or in the presence of distant metastasis. The systematic treatment is based mainly on tyrosine kinase inhibitors (TKIs). Vandetanib and cabozantinib have been approved for systematic therapy in patients with recurrent/metastatic disease. The adverse effects may include skin reactions, diarrhea, hypertension, nausea and vomiting, fatigue, and headaches [53, 54].

An important issue regarding systematic therapy is the proper timing for beginning this therapy in an attempt to control the disease and maintain an acceptable quality of life for the patient. The therapy should begin while the disease is progressing and causing symptoms to the patient. In patients who are not eligible for surgery, the use of TKIs like vandetanib and cabozantinib can be effective and can result in a protraction of the progression-free survival of the patient. In particular, MEN 2B patients with codon M918T RET mutation showed excellent response to TKI treatment [55]. In a report of a phase I/II trial by Fox et al., the use of vandetanib in MEN 2B children resulted in an objective partial response rate of 47%, while the therapy was very well tolerated [56].

Milner et al. reported a very encouraging case of a child with MEN 2B-MTC with encasement of the carotid artery and distant metastases to the lungs at the time of diagnosis. After therapy with vandetanib, the tumor decreased by 68%, making the operation feasible. The patient was in a stable condition for 6 years [57].

Clinical research is ongoing with the purpose of explaining the mechanisms for the progression of MTC in order to find suitable therapy to intercept it.

37.6 Surgical Considerations in MEN2 Patients

The indication for surgery regarding the thyroid gland is given by the diagnosis of MEN syndrome. In cases where the patient is diagnosed after the appearance of the MTC, the patient should undergo the appropriate therapeutic surgery with central and/or lateral neck dissection (as described in the previous part of this chapter), from the moment that the coexistence of a PCC has been ruled out.

In cases in which the diagnosis has been made by genetic testing in asymptomatic patients, then the appropriate treatment is the prophylactic thyroidectomy. There are two issues concerning the prophylactic thyroidectomy:

- The proper time (age) for the prophylactic thyroidectomy.
- Is a prophylactic neck dissection necessary?

37.6.1 Complications Related to Surgery for MTC

The thyroidectomy has two main possible, specific complications. The first is the damage of the inferior laryngeal nerve, and the second is the postoperative hypocalcemia, both of which can be either temporary or permanent. The damage of the external branch of the superior laryngeal nerve is often not considered a major complication because of its subtle and frequently overlooked symptomatology but is a disastrous complication in voice professionals [58]. After the initial debate regarding the possibility of increased complication rates following thyroidectomy combined with central neck dissection, today, we accept that the rate of temporary and permanent inferior laryngeal nerve damage remains the same, while the rate of temporary and permanent hypocalcemia is increased [59].

Regarding the remaining non-endocrine-specific complications like hematoma, postoperative bleeding (POB), and surgical site infection (SSI), they are rare and often related to predisposing factors. Hematomas and POB are related to antithrombotic drugs, hypertension, old age, reoperations, and extent of surgery [60].

Thyroidectomy is considered a clean operation, and SSI, following neck surgery, is generally very low (<1%), while the antibiotic prophylaxis is not routinely recommended [61, 62].

37.6.2 What About Parathyroid Transplantation During Thyroidectomy in MEN 2 Patients?

The revised ATA guidelines suggest that if the parathyroid glands are not viable, or are accidentally removed during the operation, then slivers of them should be transplanted orthotopic in the sternocleidomastoid muscle only in patients without or with a limited possibility of developing PHPT in the future. Thus, all patients with MEN 2B and FMTC, as well as patients with MEN 2A with an underlying *RET* mutation associated with a very low possibility of PHPT, are candidates for orthotropic transplantation. Patients with mutation of codons 609, 611, 618, 620, and 791 are unlikely to develop PHPT, while carriers of mutation in codons 630, 649, 768, 790, 804, and 891 are even more unlikely to develop it [31, 50]. For the remaining MEN 2A patients with higher rates of the development of PHPT, especially for those with the mutation of codon 634, the best option is the heterotopic transplantation [37].

37.6.3 Excluding Pheochromocytoma Before Neck Surgery

As half of all MEN 2 patients have PCC as a second manifestation, it is of great importance to rule out its presence before proceeding with the thyroidectomy with or without neck dissection.

The reason for this is that an unexpected pronounced hypertensive crisis, as a result of an excessive catecholamine secretion by the tumor, could put the patient's life at risk during the thyroidectomy.

About 30–50% of MTC in MEN 2 patients are diagnosed simultaneously with a PCC. In a study from Japan by T. Imai et al. with 493 MEN 2 patients, 212 of them had PCC, and for 49% of them (102/212) the diagnosis of MTC and PCC was made simultaneously [29]. In another study by F. Castinetti et al., 563 out of 1210 MEN 2 patients had PCC, and the diagnosis was made simultaneously with MTC in 169 out of 563, i.e., 30% [30].

Thus, before proceeding to the surgical treatment of MTC, excluding PCC is a mandatory step. Biochemically fractional plasma or urine metanephrines and normetanephrines can confirm the diagnosis [63].

A PCC can possess the following characteristics: cystic, necrotic, fibrous, and hemorrhagic. Despite this variety in appearance and the imaging diversity of PCC, the CT or MRI can usually confirm the diagnosis.

The unenhanced density is usually >10 Hounsfield units (with a washout less than 50%).

In those rare cases where malignant PCC is suspected in a MEN 2 patient, functional imaging studies, like MIBG scintigraphy, have to be applied so that multifocal disease can be assessed.

A possible diagnosis of PCC will change the priority of the surgical treatment of MTC. Once the patient has been prepared with the oral administration of a-blockers (for about 2 weeks), an adrenalectomy should first take place.

An endoscopic approach is the gold standard procedure (laparoscopic or retroperitoneoscopic) with the exception of very large tumors or invasive PCC. Adrenal sparing surgery, when feasible, must always be taken into consideration, especially when bilateral PCC is diagnosed synchronously or is metachronously expected [63, 64].

The preparation for the removal of the PCC is well described by Lenders et al. in the endocrine society clinical practice guidelines for PCC and paraganglioma. The authors suggest adrenergic receptor blockers as the first choice combined with a high-sodium diet and fluid intake. The duration of the treatment should be 1–2 weeks preoperatively in order to normalize blood pressure and heart rate [64].

37.6.4 Prophylactic Thyroidectomy

The purpose of prophylactic thyroidectomy is either the elimination of the risk for MTC or the cure at a very early stage that ensures a favorable prognosis for the patient. The strategy that should be followed by the physicians depends on the subjacent mutation, the calcitonin levels, and the preoperative imaging for the detection of infiltrated LN. The proper time and the extent of surgery are the main issues that must be addressed.

In patients with MEN 2B and the highest risk mutation M918T in *RET*, there is no doubt that the prophylactic thyroidectomy must be performed during infancy, in the first year of life. In these patients, not only does MTC exist within the first year, but it can have already metastasized to LN or even to distant organs [65]. Brauckhoff et al., in a retrospective study of MEN 2B patients, reported that surgical intervention could be curative if it is performed before the age of 4 years. In that study, 41 out of 44 MEN 2B patients had de novo M918T *RET* mutations, and only three had inherited mutations. The high percentage of de novo *RET* mutations in MEN 2B makes the familial screening improbable and worsens the prognosis of the disease due to delayed diagnosis [66, 67].

In patients belonging to the high-risk category of MEN 2A (codon 634 mutations and possibly with recent data the A883F mutation), prophylactic thyroidectomy should be performed during the first 5 years of life in asymptomatic patients, unless increased calcitonin levels or clinical evidence of disease is manifested during the annual examination, which is recommended to begin at the age of 3 years.

The revised ATA guidelines for the high-risk category suggest a central neck dissection if calcitonin levels are >40 pg/ml or if there is imaging evidence of LN metastasis [37]. A recent study of 50 patients who underwent prophylactic thyroidectomy due to codon 634Y mutation suggested an age <5 years for the surgical intervention [68].

Regarding patients in the moderate-risk category, the operation must be performed ideally at the time before the onset of the MTC. Considering that the annual examination in these patients is recommended to start at the age of 5, the time of surgery is usually after this age. The decision about the time and the extent of the operation is based mainly on the calcitonin levels and on the preoperative imaging [37].

The concept of the prophylactic operation for MEN 2A patients shows an extended age spectrum, because the time of the increase of CTN levels varies even among patients with mutation in the same codon. The risk-benefit judgment must include the hormonal substitution need and the operation specific risks such as the hypoparathyroidism and the RLN damage.

Choosing the suitable age gains greater importance because there are data that support that the endocrine-specific complications of the thyroidectomy are increased in the pediatric population when compared to adults.

Furthermore, data showed that the younger the patient, the more frequent the complications. In a cross-sectional analysis of data by Sosa et al., out of the 1199 patients who were younger than 17 years and underwent thyroidectomy/parathyroidectomy, the complication rates were 22%, 15%, and 11% for the ages 0–6, 7–12, and 13–17, respectively [69].

Therefore, the prophylactic thyroidectomy especially in children and young adults has to be performed by experienced endocrine surgeons.

In a series of 21 asymptomatic children diagnosed with MEN 2 syndrome, the histology after prophylactic thyroidectomy revealed nine microcarcinomas (9/21). All children with high-risk *RET* mutations in this series had a medullary microcarcinoma [70].

Taking into consideration the genetic disposition for multifocal lesions of MTC as well as C-cell hyperplasia, total thyroidectomy is the indicated surgical procedure.

Regarding the necessity of LN dissection simultaneously with the prophylactic thyroidectomy in MEN 2 patients, Machens et al., after analyzing the data from 308 *RET* mutation carriers, suggest the avoidance of LN dissection in patients with calcitonin levels within the normal range and without clinical evidence of LN metastasis [71].

It is important that the surgery take place during a "window of opportunity" in which either MTC is not yet developed or is isolated in the thyroid gland and no LN metastasis is yet evident. This way, total thyroidectomy alone suffices to eliminate the disease without the need for neck dissection that could increase the complication rates [72].

37.7 Prognosis and Follow-Up

Prognosis of the MEN 2 patients is associated mainly with the aggressiveness of MTC. A study of four families with 116 MEN 2A carriers showed that before the annual screening of family members began (1975), most deaths were related to the PCC and not to MTC. According to this study, prior to annual screening, 29 out of 36 deaths occurred due to PCC, while only seven happened because of MTC. After the annual screening of the family members became standard practice, the main cause of death was MTC [73].

In a recent international multicentric study, where the data of 563 MEN 2 patients with PCC were analyzed, the mortality rate was found to be less than 1% (5/563), mainly due to hypertensive crisis. Mortality, because of diffuse metastases from a malignant PCC in this study, was encountered in only one patient in this series [30].

In another study by Thosani et al., after retrospective data analysis of MEN 2 patients, the possible association of the presence of PCC with more aggressive behavior of MTC was investigated. The authors studied patients with codon 634 mutation, which is the most common mutation related to PCC in MEN 2, and compared the MTC aggressiveness in cases with and without PCC, concluding that there were no differences either in overall survival or in the stage of MTC at the time of diagnosis [74].

Taking into consideration that:

- PCC in MEN 2 is rarely malignant (less than 5%) and more rarely fatal
- PCC concerns only half of the MEN 2 patients and usually follows the diagnosis of MTC chronically, so that physicians are well prepared for its effective treatment,

we can conclude that the PCC has no significant impact on the mortality in MEN 2 patients and that the prognosis of MEN 2 mainly depends on the course of the MTC.

In general, the prognosis of the hereditary MTC (with the exception of MEN 2B) is better when compared to sporadic cases. A study by Saltiki et al. reported a more favorable prognosis in hereditary MTC when compared with sporadic MTC, with a probability of 10-year stable disease of 86.4% versus 65%, respectively [75].

After the initial surgery, the most important prognostic factors of MTC are the calcitonin and CEA levels and the evidence or absence of structural disease. Lindsey et al. calculated the risk stratification evaluating a "response to initial therapy" staging system proposed by M. Tuttle and I. Ganly [76], which is based on the abovementioned parameters. Three categories were proposed depending on the results after the initial therapy: (i) "excellent," if there is no evidence of structural disease and calcitonin and CEA levels are undetectable and normal respectively; (ii) "biochemical incomplete," if there is no evidence of disease but calcitonin and CEA levels are detectable and abnormal, respectively; and (iii) "structural incomplete," if structural disease is present regardless of calcitonin and CEA levels. After the follow-up of 287 patients with MTC, the authors report that the possibility of MTC-related death was 3%, 11%, and 56% in categories (i), (ii), and (iii), respectively [77].

Filimon et al. suggested a novel prognostic factor that could be useful for the prognostication of MTC. This is the Calcitonin Secretory Index (CSI) that is calculated by the division of preoperative basal CTN (pg/ml) to the maximum diameter of the tumor (mm) [78].

Preoperative calcitonin levels make up an important prognostic indicator for the remission of the MTC postoperatively. Machens et al., after analyzing 177 node-positive MTC patients, reported a zero possibility of biochemical remission postoperatively if the preoperative basal CTN was above 3000 pg/ml [79]. In contrast, preoperative CTN levels <500 pg/ml are associated with a 100% possibility of clinical remission postoperatively [78].

37.7.1 The Importance of the Initial Operation

It is very important for a favorable prognosis that an adequate first operation regarding the surgical treatment of MTC is achieved. Verbeek et al. published data supporting that a primary operation in referred centers according to the ATA guidelines was associated not only with fewer reoperations for the control of locoregional disease but also with increased biochemical cure rates [80].

37.7.2 What About the Impact of HD in the Prognosis of MEN 2A Patients?

Although mutations involving codons on exon 10 are classified as of moderate risk, one has to take into consideration that these mutations, especially those in codons 620 and 618, are associated with the appearance of HD and the high risk of the long segmental type of the disease or even with the total colonic aganglionosis that increase the risk of colon perforation, which is a life-threatening situation and can affect the prognosis of MEN 2A syndrome. The HD-associated enterocolitis, which affects many children, is presented by diarrhea, abdominal distention, and fever and if left untreated may lead to a potentially fatal outcome [81].

37.7.3 Follow-Up

The follow-up of MEN 2 patients regarding the MTC is mainly based on the biochemical profile: Calcitonin and CEA levels are the most important values, not only for the prognostication, but also for the early detection of the recurrent disease.

The earliest time for the normalization of basal CTN after successful surgery is not well established. In a recent study, where the data of 395 primary operations for MTC were analyzed, basal CTN was normalized in a mean of 4.7, 5.2, 7.0, and 57.1 days in patients with 0, 1–5, 6–10, and more than 10 positive LN, respectively [82].

Apart from the basal levels of calcitonin and CEA, it seems that the doubling time (DT) of calcitonin (to a higher degree) and CEA (to a lower degree) has a significant role in making decisions regarding possible reoperation or medical therapy [83]. A clinical study of MTC patients by Giraudet et al. supported that DT of CTN and CEA greater than about 2 years is related to a stable disease without progression, while DT of CTN and CEA less than 2 years is associated with progressive disease [84]. In general, calcitonin DT seems to be a better prognostic factor compared to the initial staging of MTC patients [85].

If basal CTN levels are below 150 pg/ml, then the disease is expected to be isolated in the neck. A basal CTN measurement, along with a clinical examination and neck US, is adequate; there is no need for further imaging studies. For basal CTN levels above 150 pg/ml, a detailed imaging with thorax CT, liver MRI, and bone scintigraphy should be undertaken in order to exclude distant metastasis.

In rare cases of advanced MTC but normal or inappropriate low serum levels of calcitonin, the possibility of a dedifferentiated MTC with poor prognosis must be suspected [37].

Answers to Questions

1. (b); 2. (b); 3. (b); 4. (a); 5. (c); 6. (c); 7. (b); 8. (a); 9. (e); 10. (d); 11. (b); 12. (b); 13. (b); 14. (a); 15. (c); 16. (a); 17. (b); 18. (e)

References

1. Frank-Raue K, Raue F. Hereditary medullary thyroid cancer genotype-phenotype correlation. Recent Results Cancer Res. 2015;204:139–56. Available from: http://www.ncbi.nlm.nih.gov/pubmed/26494387.
2. Takahashi M, Ritz J, Cooper GM. Activation of a novel human transforming gene, ret, by DNA rearrangement. Cell. 1985;42(2):581–8.
3. Pearse AGE, Polak JM. Cytochemical evidence for the neural crest origin of mammalian ultimobranchial C cells. Histochemie. 1971;27(2): 96–102.
4. Johansson E, Andersson L, Örnros J, Carlsson T, Ingeson-Carlsson C, Liang S, et al. Revising the embryonic origin of thyroid C cells in mice and humans. Development. 2015;142(20):3519–28.
5. Nilsson M, Williams D. On the origin of cells and derivation of thyroid cancer: C cell story revisited. Eur Thyroid J. 2016;5(2):79–93.
6. Elisei R, Bottici V, Cappagli V, Ramone T, Tacito A, Ciampi R, et al. Clinical utility of genetic diagnosis for sporadic and hereditary medullary thyroid carcinoma. Utilité clinique de diagnostic génétique dans le cancer médullothyroïdien héréditaire et sporadique. Ann Endocrinol. 2019;80:187–90.
7. Soh SB, Aw TC. Laboratory testing in thyroid conditions – pitfalls and clinical utility. Ann Lab Med. 2018;39(1):3–14.
8. Lorenz K, Elwerr M, MacHens A, Abuazab M, Holzhausen HJ, Dralle H. Hypercalcitoninemia in thyroid conditions other than medullary thyroid carcinoma: a comparative analysis of calcium and pentagastrin stimulation of serum calcitonin. Langenbeck's Arch Surg. 2013;398(3):403–9.
9. Costante G, Meringolo D, Durante C, Bianchi D, Nocera M, Tumino S, et al. Predictive value of serum calcitonin levels for preoperative diagnosis of medullary thyroid carcinoma in a cohort of 5817 consecutive patients with thyroid nodules. J Clin Endocrinol Metab. 2007;92(2): 450–5.
10. Machens A, Hoffmann F, Sekulla C, Dralle H. Importance of gender-specific calcitonin thresholds in screening for occult sporadic medullary thyroid cancer. Endocr Relat Cancer. 2009;16(4):1291–8.
11. Niederle MB, Scheuba C, Gessl A, Li S, Koperek O, Bieglmayer C, et al. Calcium-stimulated calcitonin – the "new standard" in the diagnosis of thyroid C-cell disease-clinically relevant gender-specific cut-off levels for an "old test". Biochem Med. 2018;28(3):2020.
12. Dora JM, Da Silva Canalli MHB, Capp C, Puñales MK, Vieira JGH, Maia AL. Normal perioperative serum calcitonin levels in patients with advanced medullary thyroid carcinoma: case report and review of the literature. Thyroid. 2008;18(8):895–9.
13. Machens A, Lorenz K, Dralle H. Utility of serum procalcitonin for screening and risk stratification of medullary thyroid cancer. J Clin Endocrinol Metab. 2014;99(8):2986–94.
14. Trimboli P, Seregni E, Treglia G, Alevizaki M, Giovanella L. Procalcitonin for detecting medullary thyroid carcinoma: a systematic review. Endocr Relat Cancer. 2015;22(3):R157–64.

15. Karagiannis AKA, Girio-Gragkoulakis C, Nakouti T. Procalcitonin: a new biomarker for medullary thyroid cancer? A systematic review. Anticancer Res. 2016;36(8):3803–10.
16. Mendelsohn G, Wells SA, Baylin SB. Relationship of tissue carcinoembryonic antigen and calcitonin to tumor virulence in medullary thyroid carcinoma. An immunohistochemical study in early, localized, and virulent disseminated stages of disease. Cancer. 1984;54(4):657–62.
17. Turkdogan S, Forest VI, Hier MP, Tamilia M, Florea A, Payne RJ. Carcinoembryonic antigen levels correlated with advanced disease in medullary thyroid cancer. J Otolaryngol Head Neck Surg. 2018;47(1):1–7.
18. Wijewardene AA, Glastras SJ, Learoyd DL, Robinson BG, Tsang VHM. ACTH-secreting medullary thyroid cancer: a case series. Endocrinol Diabetes Metab Case Rep. 2017;2017:16-0110.
19. Barbosa SLS, Rodien P, Leboulleux S, Niccoli-Sire P, Kraimps JL, Caron P, et al. Ectopic adrenocorticotropic hormone-syndrome in medullary carcinoma of the thyroid: a retrospective analysis and review of the literature. Thyroid. 2005;15(6):618–23.
20. Paepegaey AC, Cochand-Priollet B, Louiset E, Sarfati PO, Alifano M, Burnichon N, et al. Long-term control of hypercortisolism by vandetanib in a case of medullary thyroid carcinoma with a somatic RET mutation. Thyroid. 2017;27(4):587–90.
21. Baudry C, Paepegaey AC, Groussin L. Reversal of Cushing's syndrome by vandetanib in medullary thyroid carcinoma. N Engl J Med. 2013;369(6):584–6.
22. Nella AA, Lodish MB, Fox E, Balis FM, Quezado MM, Whitcomb PO, et al. Vandetanib successfully controls medullary thyroid cancer-related Cushing's syndrome in an adolescent patient. J Clin Endocrinol Metab. 2014;99(9):3055–9.
23. Coyle D, Friedmacher F, Puri P. The association between Hirschsprung's disease and multiple endocrine neoplasia type 2a: a systematic review. Pediatr Surg Int. 2014;30(8):751–6.
24. Romei C, Tacito A, Molinaro E, Agate L, Bottici V, Viola D, et al. Twenty years of lesson learning: how does the RET genetic screening test impact the clinical management of medullary thyroid cancer? Clin Endocrinol. 2015;82(6):892–9.
25. Zhang L, Guo Y, Ye L, Lu W, Dong Z, Wang W, et al. Severe constipation as the first clinical manifestation in multiple endocrine neoplasia type 2B: a case report and literature review. BMC Pediatr. 2020; 20(1):1–6.
26. Brauckhoff M, Machens A, Hess S, Lorenz K, Gimm O, Brauckhoff K, et al. Premonitory symptoms preceding metastatic medullary thyroid cancer in MEN 2B: an exploratory analysis. Surgery. 2008;144(6): 1044–51.
27. Gibbons D, Camilleri M, Nelson AD, Eckert D. Characteristics of chronic megacolon among patients diagnosed with multiple endocrine neoplasia type 2B. United European Gastroenterol J. 2016;4(3):449–54.
28. Machens A. Early malignant progression of hereditary medullary thyroid cancer [1]. N Engl J Med. 2004;350(9):943.
29. Imai T, Uchino S, Okamoto T, Suzuki S, Kosugi S, Kikumori T, et al. High penetrance of pheochromocytoma in multiple endocrine neoplasia 2 caused by germ line RET codon 634 mutation in Japanese patients. Eur J Endocrinol. 2013;168(5):683–7.
30. Castinetti F, Qi XP, Walz MK, Maia AL, Sansó G, Peczkowska M, et al. Outcomes of adrenal-sparing surgery or total adrenalectomy in phaeochromocytoma associated with multiple endocrine neoplasia type 2: an international retrospective population-based study. Lancet Oncol. 2014;15(6):643–55.

31. Alevizaki M, Saltiki K. Primary hyperparathyroidism in MEN2 syndromes. Recent Results Cancer Res. 2015;204:179–86.
32. Larsen LV, Mirebeau-Prunier D, Imai T, Alvarez-Escola C, Hasse-Lazar K, Censi S, et al. Primary hyperparathyroidism as first manifestation in multiple endocrine neoplasia type 2A: an international multicenter study. Endocr Connect. 2020;9(6):489–97.
33. Verga U, Fugazzola L, Cambiaghi S, Pritelli C, Alessi E, Cortelazzi D, et al. Frequent association between MEN 2A and cutaneous lichen amyloidosis. Clin Endocrinol. 2003;59(2):156–61.
34. Cohen MS, Phay JE, Albinson C, DeBenedetti MK, Skinner MA, Lairmore TC, et al. Gastrointestinal manifestations of multiple endocrine neoplasia type 2. Ann Surg. 2002;235(5):648–55.
35. Gfroerer S, Theilen TM, Fiegel H, Harter PN, Mittelbronn M, Rolle U. Identification of intestinal ganglioneuromatosis leads to early diagnosis of MEN2B: role of rectal biopsy. J Pediatr Surg. 2017;52(7):1161–5.
36. Bugalho MJM, Santos JR, Sobrinho L. Preoperative diagnosis of medullary thyroid carcinoma: fine needle aspiration cytology as compared with serum calcitonin measurement. J Surg Oncol. 2005;91(1):56–60.
37. Wells SA, Asa SL, Dralle H, Elisei R, Evans DB, Gagel RF, et al. Revised American Thyroid Association guidelines for the management of medullary thyroid carcinoma. Thyroid. 2015;25(6):567–610.
38. Kloos RT, Eng C, Evans DB, Francis GL, Gagel RF, Gharib H, et al. Medullary thyroid cancer: management guidelines of the American Thyroid Association. Thyroid. 2009;19(6):565–612.
39. Brandi ML, Gagel RF, Angeli A, Bilezikian JP, Beck-Peccoz P, Bordi C, et al. Consensus: guidelines for diagnosis and therapy of MEN type 1 and type 2. J Clin Endocrinol Metab. 2001;86(12):5658–71.
40. Eng C, Clayton D, Schuffenecker I, Lenoir G, Cote G, Gagel RF, et al. The relationship between specific ret proto-oncogene mutations and disease phenotype in multiple endocrine neoplasia type 2: international RET mutation consortium analysis. J Am Med Assoc. 1996;276(19): 1575–9.
41. Wells SA, Pacini F, Robinson BG, Santoro M. Multiple endocrine neoplasia type 2 and familial medullary thyroid carcinoma: an update. J Clin Endocrinol Metab. 2013;98(8):3149–64.
42. Elisei R, Romei C, Cosci B, Agate L, Bottici V, Molinaro E, et al. Brief report: RET genetic screening in patients with medullary thyroid cancer and their relatives: experience with 807 individuals at one center. J Clin Endocrinol Metab. 2007;92(12):4725–9.
43. Mathiesen JS, Habra MA, Bassett JHD, Choudhury SM, Balasubramanian SP, Howlett TA, et al. Risk profile of the RET A883F germline mutation: an international collaborative study. J Clin Endocrinol Metab. 2017;102(6):2069–74.
44. Raue F, Frank-Raue K. Update on multiple endocrine neoplasia type 2: focus on medullary thyroid carcinoma. J Endocr Soc. 2018;2(8):933–43.
45. Machens A, Hauptmann S, Dralle H. Prediction of lateral lymph node metastases in medullary thyroid cancer. Br J Surg. 2008;95(5):586–91.
46. Bae SY, Jung SP, Choe JH, Kim JS, Kim JH. Prediction of lateral neck lymph node metastasis according to preoperative calcitonin level and tumor size for medullary thyroid carcinoma. Kaohsiung J Med Sci. 2019;35(12):772–7.
47. Dralle H, Damm I, Scheumann GF, Kotzerke J, Kupsch E, Geerlings H, et al. Compartment-oriented microdissection of regional lymph nodes in medullary thyroid carcinoma. Surg Today. 1994;24(2):112–21. Available from: http://www.ncbi.nlm.nih.gov/pubmed/8054788.
48. MaChens A, Dralle H. Benefit-risk balance of reoperation for persistent medullary thyroid cancer. Ann Surg. 2013;257(4):751–7.

49. Kushchayev SV, Kushchayeva YS, Tella SH, Glushko T, Pacak K, Teytelboym OM. Medullary thyroid carcinoma: an update on imaging. J Thyroid Res. 2019;2019:1893047.
50. Iacobone M, Carnaille B, Palazzo FF, Vriens M. Hereditary hyperparathyroidism—a consensus report of the European Society of Endocrine Surgeons (ESES). Langenbeck's Arch Surg. 2015;400(8):867–86.
51. Silva BC, Cusano NE, Bilezikian JP. Primary hyperparathyroidism. Best Pract Res Clin Endocrinol Metab. 2018;32(5):593–607.
52. Marcocci C, Chanson P, Shoback D, Bilezikian J, Fernandez-Cruz L, Orgiazzi J, et al. Cinacalcet reduces serum calcium concentrations in patients with intractable primary hyperparathyroidism. J Clin Endocrinol Metab. 2009;94(8):2766–72.
53. Tsang VHM, Robinson BG, Learoyd DL. The safety of vandetanib for the treatment of thyroid cancer. Expert Opin Drug Saf. 2016;15(8): 1107–13.
54. Milling RV, Grimm D, Krüger M, Grosse J, Kopp S, Bauer J, et al. Pazopanib, cabozantinib, and vandetanib in the treatment of progressive medullary thyroid cancer with a special focus on the adverse effects on hypertension. Int J Mol Sci. 2018;19(10):19103258.
55. Pappa T, Alevizaki M. Management of hereditary medullary thyroid carcinoma. Endocrine. 2016;53(1):7–17.
56. Fox E, Widemann BC, Chuk MK, Marcus L, Aikin A, Whitcomb PO, et al. Vandetanib in children and adolescents with multiple endocrine neoplasia type 2b associated medullary thyroid carcinoma. Clin Cancer Res. 2013;19(15):4239–48.
57. Milner TD, Ronghe M, Shaikh MG, MacGregor FB, Reed N. Vandetanib tumor shrinkage in metastatic medullary thyroid cancer allowing surgical resection of the primary site: a case report. J Pediatr Hematol Oncol. 2019;41(5):e329–32.
58. Wang K, Cai H, Kong D, Cui Q, Zhang D, Wu G. The identification, preservation and classification of the external branch of the superior laryngeal nerve in thyroidectomy. World J Surg. 2017;41(10):2521–9.
59. Giordano D, Valcavi R, Thompson GB, Pedroni C, Renna L, Gradoni P, et al. Complications of central neck dissection in patients with papillary thyroid carcinoma: results of a study on 1087 patients and review of the literature. Thyroid. 2012;22(9):911–7.
60. Fan C, Zhou X, Su G, Zhou Y, Su J, Luo M, et al. Risk factors for neck hematoma requiring surgical re-intervention after thyroidectomy: a systematic review and meta-analysis. BMC Surg. 2019;19(1):1–12.
61. Vamvakidis K, Rellos K, Tsourma M, Christoforides C, Anastasiou E, Zorbas K, et al. Antibiotic prophylaxis for clean neck surgery. Ann R Coll Surg Engl. 2017;99(5):410–2. Available from: http://www.ncbi.nlm.nih.gov/pubmed/28462662.
62. Bures C, Klatte T, Gilhofer M, Behnke M, Breier AC, Neuhold N, et al. A prospective study on surgical-site infections in thyroid operation. Surgery (United States). 2014;155(4):675–81.
63. Amodru V, Taieb D, Guerin C, Romanet P, Paladino N, Brue T, et al. Correction to: MEN2-related pheochromocytoma: current state of knowledge, specific characteristics in MEN2B, and perspectives. Endocrine. 2020;69(3):695. https://doi.org/10.1007/s12020-020-02332-2.
64. Lenders JWM, Duh QY, Eisenhofer G, Gimenez-Roqueplo AP, Grebe SKG, Murad MH, et al. Pheochromocytoma and paraganglioma: an endocrine society clinical practice guideline. J Clin Endocrinol Metab. 2014;99(6):1915–42.
65. Waguespack SG, Rich TA, Perrier ND, Jimenez C, Cote GJ. Management of medullary thyroid carcinoma and MEN2 syndromes in childhood. Nat Rev Endocrinol. 2011;7(10):596–607.

66. Brauckhoff M, Machens A, Lorenz K, Bjøro T, Varhaug JE, Dralle H. Surgical curability of medullary thyroid cancer in multiple endocrine neoplasia 2b: a changing perspective. Ann Surg. 2014;259(4):800–6.
67. Elisei R, Matrone A, Valerio L, Molinaro E, Agate L, Bottici V, et al. Fifty years after the first description, MEN 2B syndrome diagnosis is still late: descriptions of two recent cases. J Clin Endocrinol Metab. 2019;104(7):2520–6.
68. Febrero B, Rodríguez JM, Ríos A, Segura P, Pérez-Sánchez B, Torregrosa N, et al. Prophylactic thyroidectomy in multiple endocrine neoplasia 2 (MEN2) patients with the C634Y mutation: a long-term follow-up in a large single-center cohort. Eur J Surg Oncol. 2019;45(4):625–30.
69. Sosa JA, Tuggle CT, Wang TS, Thomas DC, Boudourakis L, Rivkees S, et al. Clinical and economic outcomes of thyroid and parathyroid surgery in children. J Clin Endocrinol Metab. 2008;93(8):3058–65.
70. Bussières V, Roy S, Deladoey J, Rousseau É, St-Vil D, Piché N. Prophylactic thyroidectomies in MEN2 syndrome: management and outcomes. J Pediatr Surg. 2018;53(2):283–5. Available from: https://pubmed.ncbi.nlm.nih.gov/29336779/.
71. MacHens A, Lorenz K, Dralle H. Individualization of lymph node dissection in RET (rearranged during transfection) carriers at risk for medullary thyroid cancer: value of pretherapeutic calcitonin levels. Ann Surg. 2009;250(2):305–10.
72. Machens A, Dralle H. Advances in risk-oriented surgery for multiple endocrine neoplasia type 2. Endocr Relat Cancer. 2018;25(2):T41–52.
73. Lips C, Landsvater RM, Hoppener J, Hoppener JWM, Geerdink RA, Blijham G, et al. Clinical screening as compared with DNA analysis in families with multiple endocrine neoplasia type 2A. N Engl J Med. 1994;331(13):828–35.
74. Thosani S, Ayala-Ramirez M, Palmer L, Hu MI, Rich T, Gagel RF, et al. The characterization of pheochromocytoma and its impact on overall survival in multiple endocrine neoplasia type 2. J Clin Endocrinol Metab. 2013;98(11):1813–9.
75. Saltiki K, Simeakis G, Anagnostou E, Zapanti E, Anastasiou E, Alevizaki M. Different outcomes in sporadic versus familial medullary thyroid cancer. Head Neck. 2019;41(1):154–61.
76. Tuttle RM, Ganly I. Risk stratification in medullary thyroid cancer: moving beyond static anatomic staging. Oral Oncol. 2013;49(7):695–701.
77. Lindsey SC, Ganly I, Palmer F, Tuttle RM. Response to initial therapy predicts clinical outcomes in medullary thyroid cancer. Thyroid. 2015;25(2):242–9.
78. Filimon S, Payne RJ, Black MJ, Hier MP, Mlynarek AM, Forest VI, et al. Calcitonin secretory index and unsuspected nodal disease in medullary thyroid carcinoma. Endocr Pract. 2018;24(5):460–7.
79. Machens A, Schneyer U, Holzhausen HJ, Dralle H. Prospects of remission in medullary thyroid carcinoma according to basal calcitonin level. J Clin Endocrinol Metab. 2005;90(4):2029–34.
80. Verbeek HHG, Meijer JAA, Zandee WT, Kramp KH, Sluiter WJ, Smit JW, et al. Fewer cancer reoperations for medullary thyroid cancer after initial surgery according to ATA guidelines. Ann Surg Oncol. 2015;22(4):1207–13.
81. Haricharan RN, Georgeson KE. Hirschsprung disease. Semin Pediatr Surg. 2008;17(4):266–75.
82. Machens A, Lorenz K, Dralle H. Time to calcitonin normalization after surgery for node-negative and node-positive medullary thyroid cancer. Br J Surg. 2019;106(4):412–8.
83. Viola D, Elisei R. Management of medullary thyroid cancer. Endocrinol Metab Clin N Am. 2019;48(1):285–301.

84. Giraudet AL, Al Ghulzan A, Aupérin A, Leboulleux S, Chehboun A, Troalen F, et al. Progression of medullary thyroid carcinoma: assessment with calcitonin and carcinoembryonic antigen doubling times. Eur J Endocrinol. 2008;158(2):239–46.
85. Barbet J, Campion L, Kraeber-Bodéré F, Chatal JF. Prognostic impact of serum calcitonin and carcinoembryonic antigen doubling-times in patients with medullary thyroid carcinoma. J Clin Endocrinol Metab. 2005;90(11):6077–84.

Multiple Endocrine Neoplasia Type 4 (MEN 4)

Oliver Gimm and Natalia S. Pellegata

Contents

A. L. Shifrin et al. (eds.), *Endocrine Surgery Comprehensive Board Exam Guide*,
https://doi.org/10.1007/978-3-030-84737-1_38

Case

A 41-year-old woman having serum calcium 11.65 mg/dl (8.4–10.2 mg/dl) and parathyroid hormone (PTH) 189 pg/ml (10–65 pg/ml) was diagnosed with primary hyperparathyroidism (pHPT). She then underwent inferior left and right parathyroidectomy. The two superior parathyroid glands were identified, biopsied, and found to be histologically normal. The histological examination of both inferior parathyroid glands showed an oxyphil chief cell adenoma.

Serum calcium levels normalized after surgery, and no further biochemical testing was performed until the age of 48 years when a relapse of pHPT was diagnosed (serum calcium 11.3 mg/dl and PTH 201 pg/ml). At the age of 50 years, the patient underwent clinical and biochemical evaluation which confirmed the diagnosis of relapsing pHPT, and she underwent a second surgery. The superior right parathyroid gland was removed, and the histological examination showed a 20-mm oxyphil chief cell adenoma.

At follow-up, gastro-entero-pancreatic NETs were found, which were initially treated with proton pump inhibitors and somatostatin analogs and then successfully by surgery.

At 54 years of age, the patient had a follow-up evaluation, which identified a relapse of pHPT. Total serum calcium and PTH were 10.6 mg/dl and 138 pg/ml, respectively. A 99 m-Tc-sestamibi scan showed an uptake in the left paratracheal region.

Further investigation showed that the anterior pituitary function was normal, and a pituitary MRI showed only slight enlargement of the left side of the gland, in the absence of focal lesions. Surveillance was advised.

One year later, the patient underwent surgery, and the left superior parathyroid gland was removed.

Genetic Analyses

The search for mutations in the *MEN1* gene in the entire coding region and splice sites gave negative results.

Thus, the *CDKN1B* gene was sequenced, and a novel germline heterozygous deletion was found in exon 1 of the *CDKN1B* gene, c.374_375delCT (the +1-position corresponding to the A of the ATG translation initiation codon in the reference sequence).

The two-nucleotide deletion caused a frameshift and ultimately led to a stop codon (TGA) at codon 125 (S125X) and to a truncated P27 variant consisting of only 124 amino acids. The P27_S125X protein lacks the C-terminal domain, which contains the NLS required to enter the nucleus where the protein binds to cyclin-CDK complexes.

The somatic DNA from the patient's tumoral parathyroid tissue did not show loss of the wild-type allele, as assessed by sequencing.

Questions (the Correct Answers Can Be Found at the End of the Chapter)

1. What statements are correct?
    1. MEN 4 in humans is clinically more similar to MEN 1 than to MEN 2.
    2. MEN 4 in humans is clinically more similar to MEN 2 than to MEN 1.
    3. The genetic cause for MEN 4 is known.
    4. The genetic cause for MEN 4 is not known.
        - (a) Only statements 1 and 3 are correct.
        - (b) Only statements 1 and 4 are correct.
        - (c) Only statements 2 and 3 are correct.
        - (d) Only statements 2 and 4 are correct.

2. What statements are correct?
   1. Patients with MEN 4 are clinically easily identified.
   2. Patients with MEN 4 are clinically more difficult to be identified as compared to patients with MEN 1 and MEN 2.
   3. When diagnosed patients with MEN 4 are typically older than patients with MEN 1.
   4. When diagnosed patients with MEN 4 are typically younger than patients with MEN 1.
      (a) Only statements 1 and 3 are correct.
      (b) Only statements 1 and 4 are correct.
      (c) Only statements 2 and 3 are correct.
      (d) Only statements 2 and 4 are correct.
3. What statements are correct?
   1. Germline *CDKN1B* mutations have been shown to be associated with MEN 4.
   2. Germline *CDKN1B* mutations have been shown to be associated with apparently sporadic endocrine tumors.
   3. Germline *CDKN1B* mutations have been shown to be associated with non-endocrine tumors.
   4. Germline *CDKN1B* polymorphisms have been shown to be associated with various types of tumors.
      (a) Only statements 1, 2, and 3 are correct.
      (b) Only statements 1, 2, and 4 are correct.
      (c) Only statements 1, 3, and 4 are correct.
      (d) Statements 1, 2, 3, and 4 are all correct.
4. What statements are correct?
   1. Primary hyperparathyroidism is the most common phenotype in MEN 4.
   2. Primary hyperparathyroidism in MEN 4 is as often multiglandular as in MEN 1.
   3. Patients with MEN 4-associated primary hyperparathyroidism are older than patients with MEN 1-associated primary hyperparathyroidism.
   4. Germline mutations in *CDKN1B* have been found in patients with apparently sporadic parathyroid adenoma.
      (a) Only statements 1, 2, and 4 are correct.
      (b) Only statements 1, 3, and 4 are correct.
      (c) Only statements 2, 3, and 4 are correct.
      (d) Statements 1, 2, 3, and 4 are all correct.
5. What statements are correct?
   1. Pituitary adenomas are the most common phenotype in MEN 4.
   2. Pituitary adenomas in MEN 4 can be functioning and nonfunctioning.
   3. A polymorphism in *CDKN1B* has been shown to be associated with the development of pituitary adenomas.

4. Germline mutations in *CDKN1B* have been found in patients with apparently sporadic pituitary adenoma.
    (a) Only statements 1, 2, and 4 are correct.
    (b) Only statements 1, 3, and 4 are correct.
    (c) Only statements 2, 3, and 4 are correct.
    (d) Statements 1, 2, 3, and 4 are all correct.

6. What statements are correct?
    1. MEN 4 appears to be less common than MEN 1.
    2. MEN 4 appears to be more common than MEN 2.
    3. MEN 4 has been more often reported in women than men.
    4. MEN 4 has been more often reported in men than women.
        (a) Only statements 1 and 2 are correct.
        (b) Only statements 1 and 3 are correct.
        (c) Only statements 2 and 3 are correct.
        (d) Only statements 2 and 4 are correct.
7. What statements concerning genetic counseling with regard to MEN 4 are correct?
    1. Offsprings of a patient with MEN 4 each have a risk of 50% inheriting the mutated gene.
    2. More than 10% of patients with typical clinical signs for MEN 1 but without a germline *MEN 1* mutation can be expected to have MEN 4.
    3. More than 10% of patients with an apparently sporadic parathyroid adenoma can be expected to have MEN 4.
    4. More than 10% of patients with an apparently sporadic pituitary adenoma can be expected to have MEN 4.
        (a) Only statement 1 is correct.
        (b) Only statements 1 and 2 are correct.
        (c) Only statements 2 and 3 are correct.
        (d) Only statements 2 and 4 are correct.
8. What statements regarding surgery of primary hyperparathyroidism in a patient with MEN 4 are correct?

    1. Either subtotal parathyroidectomy or total parathyroidectomy with autotransplantation is recommended in all cases.
    2. Bilateral exploration with removal of only enlarged parathyroid glands may be a justified approach.
    3. In cases where an enlarged parathyroid gland is localized preoperatively, a limited surgical approach preferably including intraoperative PTH measurement may also be reasonable.

4. Current data strongly indicates that unilateral approaches should be avoided.
   (a) Only statements 1 and 2 are correct.
   (b) Only statements 1 and 4 are correct.
   (c) Only statements 2 and 3 are correct.
   (d) Only statements 2 and 4 are correct.

38.1 Introduction

A variety of multiple endocrine neoplasia (MEN) syndromes are known. Multiple endocrine neoplasia type 1 (MEN 1) is associated with an increased risk of developing primary hyperparathyroidism (pHPT), adenomas of the anterior pituitary gland, and neuroendocrine neoplasms (NENs) in the foregut (most common in the pancreas and duodenum, rarely in the stomach). Less common are lipomas, angiofibromas, thyroid adenomas, adrenocortical adenomas, angiomyolipomas, and spinal cord ependymomas. Incomplete expression has been observed, and some families develop pHPT only (familial isolated hyperparathyroidism). Nevertheless, by the age of 50 years, the penetrance is around 95%. The *MEN1* gene was identified in 1997 [1].

Multiple endocrine neoplasia type 2 (MEN 2) is subdivided into MEN 2A and MEN 2B. MEN 2A is associated with an increased risk of developing medullary thyroid carcinoma (MTC), pheochromocytoma, and pHPT. Cutaneous lichen amyloidosis, a skin disorder associated with pruritus, has also been occasionally described. The clinical penetrance of MEN 2A is estimated to be higher than 60% by the age of 70 years. Under screening conditions, the manifestation has been reported to be higher than 90% by the age of 30 years. Similar to MEN 1, the expression in MEN 2A can be incomplete, and some families develop MTC only (familial MTC = FMTC). Like MEN 2A, MEN 2B is also associated with an increased risk of developing MTC and pheochromocytoma. However, pHPT is not part of MEN 2B. In contrast, mucosal neuromas, thickened corneal nerves, and a marfanoid habitus are associated with MEN 2B. The *RET* gene responsible for MEN 2A, MEN 2B, and FMTC was identified in 1993 [2, 3].

Initially, MEN 2B was named MEN 3 since the phenotype of these patients differed from those having MEN 2A. However, when it was shown that mutations in the same gene, namely, the *RET* gene, also are responsible for MEN 2B [4], the name MEN 3 was abandoned.

In 2006, yet another multiple endocrine neoplasia syndrome was reported in both rats and humans which was caused by mutations of the *Cdkn1b* gene or its human homolog *CDKN1B*, respectively [5]. In rats, this syndrome was named MENX, whereas in patients it was named MEN 4 [6].

38.2 The MENX Syndrome

MENX-affected rats are homozygous for an underlying inactivating *Cdkn1b* mutation which codes for a very unstable p27KIP1 mutant protein [5]. MENX rats develop medullary thyroid tumors, pheochromocytoma, and pituitary adenomas with complete penetrance and with a clear progression over time [7]. Thus, MENX rats have a phenotype that shares features with both MEN 1 and MEN 2 [5, 7].

38.3 Molecular Genetics of MEN 4

MEN 4 is caused by heterozygous germline mutations in the *CDKN1B* gene, indicating an autosomal dominant inheritance. *CDKN1B* encodes the cyclin-dependent kinase (CDK) inhibitor P27KIP1. A summary of the germline p27KIP1 mutations so far identified in patients is illustrated in ◘ Fig. 38.1. In the nucleus, P27KIP1 binds to and inhibits cyclin/CDK complexes and is the main regulator of quiescence in adult cells. P27KIP1

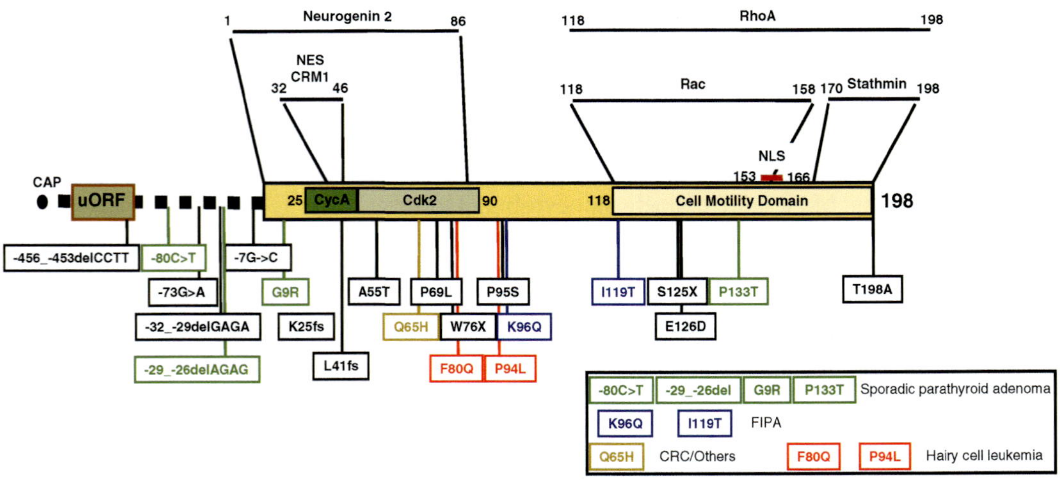

◘ **Fig. 38.1** Schematic representation of the 5′ region of the human *CDKN1B* gene and of the p27KIP1 protein. The main domains of the protein, their location along the protein sequence, and the interaction partners are reported. The germline/somatic mutations identified in patients with endocrine and non-endocrine tumors are also illustrated. *ORF* open reading frame, *NES* nuclear export signal, *CycA* cyclin A, *NLS* nuclear localization signal, *FIPA* familial isolated pituitary adenoma, *CRC* colorectal cancer

inhibits cell cycle progression at the G1-to-S phase transition by preventing CDK2 from phosphorylating the tumor suppressor Rb, event required to move cells into the S phase [8]. Some of the *CDKN1B* mutations identified in MEN 4 patients were characterized in vitro and were found to be mostly inactivating [9]. Indeed, they were associated with reduced or absent expression of P27KIP1 or with a cytoplasmic mislocalization of the mutant protein in both pathological and non-pathological tissues. Interestingly, although *CDKN1B* is rarely mutated in human malignancies, it is frequently under-expressed and/or mislocalized [10]. The precise molecular mechanisms linking reduced or absent P27KIP1 expression to the formation of endocrine tumors, however, are still only partially understood.

38.4 Clinical Presentation of MEN 4

In contrast to rats with MENX, MEN4 patients show a variety of features like pituitary adenomas causing acromegaly and pHPT, which are typical for MEN 1 but not MEN 2. Pheochromocytomas have not yet been reported in humans with germline mutations in *CDKN1B* [11]. Further, patients with germline mutations in *CDKN1B* may develop tumors not associated with any type of multiple endocrine neoplasia like testicular cancer [5].

Of note, the phenotype of MEN 4 is still ill-defined mainly because of the limited number of patients identified to date. Initially, all patients reported as having both an inactivating mutation in *CDKN1B* and a clinical MEN 4 phenotype were women [12]. Thus, it was hypothesized that either sexual hormones or genetic imprinting might be responsible for the disease. Later, male patients were also reported [13]; however, more than 75% of the patients identified so far are women.

38.4.1 Primary Hyperparathyroidism

As in MEN1, pHPT is the most common phenotype in MEN 4. In a large Danish family, all available mutation carriers had hypercalcemia due to pHPT (▪ Table 38.1) [13]. In contrast to individuals affected by the MEN 1 syndrome, in about 50% of MEN4 patients presenting with pHPT, only one gland has been reported to be affected [12].

38.4.2 Pituitary Adenomas

Adenomas of the anterior pituitary are the second most common manifestation of the MEN4 syndrome [12]. In the aforementioned large Danish family, about 30% of all available

Table 38.1 Phenotypes of patients belonging to a large Danish family with multiple endocrine neoplasia type 4

Female	? years: pHPT
Female	? years: pHPT
	? years: neuroendocrine neoplasm (pancreas)
Female	? years: pHPT
	? years: pituitary microadenoma (nonfunctioning)
Female	? years: pHPT
	? years: goiter
Male	? years: pHPT
	? years: pituitary microadenoma (nonfunctioning)
Female	? years: pHPT
Male	? years: pHPT
	? years: pituitary adenoma (nonfunctioning)
Female	? years: pHPT
Female	36 years: pHPT
	37 years: pituitary microadenoma (ACTH-producing)
Male	? years: pHPT
Female	? years: pHPT
Female	? years: pHPT
Male	? years: pHPT

Modified from [13]
All patients harbor the mutation c.121_122delTT that leads to a frameshift mutation at codon 41 which creates a premature stop codon at codon 83
pHPT primary hyperparathyroidism

38

mutation carriers had a pituitary adenoma [13]. Both functioning (GH-, ACTH-, prolactin-, somatotropin-secreting) and nonfunctioning pituitary adenomas have been reported. The polymorphism rs2066827 (V109G) in P27KIP1 has been shown to be associated with pituitary adenomas, particularly those that are ACTH-secreting [14].

38.4.3 Neuroendocrine Neoplasms

NENs are also seen in MEN 4 but are less common in comparison with MEN 1. In the aforementioned large Danish family, less than 10% of all available mutation carriers developed such a tumor [13]. NENs in MEN4 patients can be either functioning (gastrin-secreting) or nonfunctioning and develop in the foregut (lungs, stomach, duodenum, and pancreas). As such, their location resembles that of the MEN 1 syndrome. Of interest, the advent of next-generation sequencing technologies has enabled to identify somatic mutations of *CDKN1B* in 8% of patients with small bowel neuroendocrine tumors [15] which is not part of MEN 1.

38.4.4 Other Endocrine Tumors Associated with Mutation of p27KIP1

A variant in the noncoding part of the *CDKN1B* gene has been associated with various types of thyroid cancers and in particular with follicular variant of papillary thyroid cancer [16].

38.4.5 Non-endocrine Tumors and Other Conditions Associated with Mutation of p27KIP1

Of interest, a variety of non-multiple endocrine neoplasia-related tumors including lipomas and meningiomas have also been found in patients with germline *CDKN1B* mutations. Interestingly, in a three-generation family, presenting with colorectal carcinoma and other cancers, a germline *CDKN1B* variant was found to segregate with the tumor phenotype [17]. Further, polymorphisms in the *CDKN1B* gene have been shown to be associated with an increased risk of developing prostate cancer (c.-79C > T) [18] but a decreased risk of ovarian cancer (rs2066827, V109G) [19]. Using a next-generation sequencing panel, somatic mutations of *CDKN1B* have been detected in 16% of patients with hairy cell leukemia [20].

38.5 Diagnosis

The typical clinical presentation of MEN 4 is still not well defined given that the clinical spectrum varies widely and that the number of patients so far identified is low. There seems to be a clinical overlap in particular with MEN 1. The definitive diagnosis is made by identifying a pathogenic germline mutation in the *CDKN1B* gene.

38.6 Genetic Counseling

Like MEN 1, MEN 4 is a hereditary endocrine tumor syndrome inherited in an autosomal dominant fashion. As for other syndromes inherited in this fashion, genetic screening is considered useful to identify mutation carriers who then can be monitored for the clinical manifestations of associated diseases. In addition, individuals tested negative can forego unnecessary surveillance.

Missense, nonsense, and frameshift mutations as well as a mutation in the upstream open reading frame of the *CDKN1B* gene have been described [12]. There is no indication to date that there is a genotype-phenotype correlation for MEN 4. Also, the precise phenotypic features of MEN 4 are still not completely defined. This makes the clinical identification of patients having MEN 4 very difficult.

Of interest, about 10% of patients with clinically typical signs of MEN 1 do not harbor a germline mutation or a large genomic alteration in *MEN1* [9]. Therefore, the newly identified susceptibility gene (i.e., *CDKN1B*) that appeared to be associated with a syndrome very similar to MEN 1 could account for these remaining cases and therefore was of great interest. In some studies, inactivating mutations in *CDKN1B* have been found in about 2% of patients with an MEN 1 phenotype not harboring *MEN1* mutations [12, 21, 22], whereas others found slightly higher frequencies [23, 24].

Interestingly, in one study analyzing patients with pHPT due to apparently sporadic parathyroid adenomas, 2 out of 86 patients (2.3%) harbored a germline mutation in *CDKN1B* [25], which is similar to the frequency (2.0%) reported by another study of 147 patients with such sporadic tumors [26].

Of note, germline mutations in *CDKN1B* have even been found in familial isolated pituitary adenoma (FIPA) [27] but appear to affect less than 3% of the patients. In addition, a lack of clear segregation with FIPA patients has been observed [27]. Hence, routine analysis of *CDKN1B* in patients with FIPA is not recommended. Overall, *CDKN1B* germline mutations have been considered to be rare in these patients.

Of interest, most of the clinical manifestations in female patients arose around the age of menopause or even later [12]. Thus, in contrast to patients with MEN 1, those with MEN 4 are rather diagnosed at an older age, but exceptions exist (Table 38.2) [9].

Due to the rarity of the syndrome, guidelines regarding the screening for MEN 4 are currently lacking. It has been recommended that patients that clinically classify as MEN 1 but carry no germline mutations in the *MEN1* gene should undergo mutation analysis of *CDKN1B* [9].

38.7 Surgical Management

Surgical resection is the standard of care for many neuroendocrine tumors. Since the number of patients diagnosed with germline *CDKN1B* mutations is still very low, recommenda-

Table 38.2 Genotypes and phenotypes published in multiple endocrine neoplasia type 4

Gender	Mutation (consequence)	"MEN"-related phenotype	References
Female	c.227G>A	30 years: pituitary adenoma (GH-secreting)	[5]
	(nonsense W76X)	46 years: pHPT	
Female	c.59_77dup19	45 years: neuroendocrine carcinoma (neck)	[21]
	(frameshift; protein 69 amino acids shorter than wild type, complete different amino acid sequence after codon 25)	46 years: pituitary adenoma (ACTH-secreting)	
		47 years: pHPT (one gland)	
Female	ATG-7G>C in the 5′-UTR	61 years: pHPT (one gland)	[22]
	(?)	63 years: bilateral adrenal tumor (nonfunctioning)	
Female	c.283C>T	50 years: pHPT (two glands)	[22]
	(missense P95S)	50 years: ZES (tumors in the duodenum and pancreas)	
Female	c.595T>C	50 years: pHPT (three glands)	[22]
	(STOP>199Q; protein 60 amino acids longer than wild type)		
Female	c.206C>G	67 years: neuroendocrine neoplasm (lungs)	[23]
	(missense P69L)	67 years: pHPT (one gland)	
		79 years: pituitary microadenoma (nonfunctioning)	
Male	c.25G>A	68 years: pHPT	[25]
	(missense G9R)		
Male	c.397C>A	53 years: pHPT (one gland)	[25, 29]
	(missense P133T)	56 years: pHPT (one gland = second gland)	
Female	c.-32_-29delGAGA	69 years: neuroendocrine neoplasm (stomach)	[30]
	(GAGA deletion which is predicted to modify the "stem and loop" structure in 5′-UTR responsible for ribosome recruitment)	74 years: pHPT	
Female	c.163G>A	42 years: ZES (tumor location?)	[31]
	(missense A55T)	51 years: pHPT	
Female	c.286A>C	? years: pituitary adenoma (prolactin-secreting)	[27]
	(missense K96Q)		
Female	c.356T>C	? years: pituitary adenoma (somatotropin-secreting)	[27]
	(missense I119T)		

(continued)

Table 38.2 (continued)

Gender	Mutation (consequence)	"MEN"-related phenotype	References
Female	c.-456_-453del CCTT	62 years: pituitary adenoma (GH-secreting)	[24]
	(CCTT deletion in 5′-UTR)	62 years: neuroendocrine neoplasm (pancreas, nonfunctioning)	
Female	c.371_372delCT	41 years: pHPT (two glands)	[12]
	(frameshift mutation at codon 125; creates a premature stop codon at codon 145)	50 years: neuroendocrine neoplasm (pancreas, gastrin-secreting)	
		50 years: pHPT (one gland = third gland)	
		51 years: neuroendocrine neoplasm (duodenum, nonfunctioning?)	
		55 years: pituitary microadenoma? (nonfunctioning)	
		55 years: pHPT (one gland = forth gland)	
Female	c.378G>C	15 years: pHPT	[32]
	(missense E126D)		
Female	c.-29_-26delAGAG	5 years: pituitary adenoma (GH-secreting)	[33]
	(AGAG deletion which is predicted to modify the "stem and loop" structure in 5′-UTR responsible for ribosome recruitment)		
Male	c.-80C>T	38 years: pHPT	[26]
	(?)		
Female	c.397C>A	49 years: pHPT	[26]
	(missense P133T)		
Female	c.-29_-26delAGAG	61 years: pHPT	[26]
	(AGAG deletion which is predicted to modify the "stem and loop" structure in 5′-UTR responsible for ribosome recruitment)		

Modified from [9, 12]
MEN multiple endocrine neoplasia, *pHPT* primary hyperparathyroidism, *ZES* Zollinger-Ellison syndrome

tions on the clinical management of diseases associated with MEN 4 have to be given cautiously.

With regard to pHPT, it can be stated that multiglandular involvement has been reported. However, it seems that many patients do not develop multiglandular disease. Therefore, bilateral exploration with removal of only enlarged parathyroid glands seems to be a justified approach [9, 28]. However, in those cases where an enlarged parathyroid gland is localized preoperatively, a limited surgical approach including the use of intraoperative PTH measurement may also be reasonable since many patients only seem to develop uniglandular disease.

With regard to pituitary adenomas, they appear to be smaller and less aggressive as compared to MEN 1 [9]. Whether this means that the surgical treatment of these adenomas is associated with a higher rate of cure and lower rate of side effects remains to be seen.

Relatively few cases of NENs have been reported in MEN 4. As in MEN 1, they have been found in the foregut. Due to the very limited number of patients, no specific recommendations can be given with regard to the surgical treatment of these tumors. Based on the overall relatively low incidence of NENs in MEN 4 as compared to MEN 1, it could be speculated that the overall "recurrence" rate also will turn out to be lower as compared to MEN 1, but this remains to be confirmed. In order to be able to give recommendations on the surgical extent, the behavior and aggressiveness of MEN 4-associated NENs also needs to be characterized better.

38.8 Surveillance and Follow-Up

A variety of tumors associated with germline variants of *CDKN1B,* together with their overall rarity and the lack of any known genotype-phenotype correlation, make it challenging to formulate specific recommendations regarding the screening of these patients.

As of today, surveillance for the development of any of the abovementioned tumors in patients with MEN 4 has been recommended to be performed on a case-by-case basis and following existing guidelines for other MEN syndromes [9]. The same applies to the follow-up of such patients.

38.9 Summary

MEN 4 appears to be a multiple endocrine neoplasia syndrome that shows clinical overlap with MEN 1. Studies have shown that even in patients with a typical MEN 1 phenotype but no germline mutation in *MEN1*, germline mutations in *CDKN1B* are only found in about 2–3% of cases. Interestingly, about the same frequency of germline mutations in *CDKN1B* have been found in patients only having apparently sporadic parathyroid or pituitary adenomas. If the latter frequencies prove to be correct, the overall number of patients with germline mutations in *CDKN1B* should be much higher than currently assumed. Future research should focus on the natural course of the various tumors/diseases associated with MEN 4 and on whether any genotype-phenotype correlation exists. This will help to provide better recommendations also with regard to the surgical treatment.

Answers to the Questions

1. (a); 2. (c); 3. (d); 4. (b); 5. (c); 6. (b); 7. (a); 8. (c)

References

1. Chandrasekharappa SC, Guru SC, Manickam P, et al. Positional cloning of the gene for multiple endocrine neoplasia-type 1. Science. 1997;276:404–7.
2. Mulligan LM, Kwok JB, Healey CS, et al. Germ-line mutations of the RET proto-oncogene in multiple endocrine neoplasia type 2A. Nature. 1993;363:458–60.
3. Donis-Keller H, Dou S, Chi D, et al. Mutations in the RET proto-oncogene are associated with MEN 2A and FMTC. Hum Mol Genet. 1993;2:851–6.
4. Carlson KM, Dou S, Chi D, et al. Single missense mutation in the tyrosine kinase catalytic domain of the RET protooncogene is associated with multiple endocrine neoplasia type 2B. Proc Natl Acad Sci U S A. 1994;91:1579–83.
5. Pellegata NS, Quintanilla-Martinez L, Siggelkow H, et al. Germ-line mutations in p27Kip1 cause a multiple endocrine neoplasia syndrome in rats and humans. Proc Natl Acad Sci U S A. 2006;103:15558–63.
6. Georgitsi M. MEN-4 and other multiple endocrine neoplasias due to cyclin-dependent kinase inhibitors (p27(Kip1) and p18(INK4C)) mutations. Best Pract Res Clin Endocrinol Metab. 2010;24:425–37.
7. Pellegata NS. MENX and MEN4. Clinics (Sao Paulo). 2012;67(Suppl 1):13–8.
8. Lee M, Pellegata NS. Multiple endocrine neoplasia syndromes associated with mutation of p27. J Endocrinol Investig. 2013;36:781–7.
9. Alrezk R, Hannah-Shmouni F, Stratakis CA. MEN4 and CDKN1B mutations: the latest of the MEN syndromes. Endocr Relat Cancer. 2017;24:T195–208.
10. Chu IM, Hengst L, Slingerland JM. The Cdk inhibitor p27 in human cancer: prognostic potential and relevance to anticancer therapy. Nat Rev Cancer. 2008;8:253–67.
11. Molatore S, Kugler A, Irmler M, et al. Characterization of neuroendocrine tumors in heterozygous mutant MENX rats: a novel model of invasive medullary thyroid carcinoma. Endocr Relat Cancer. 2018;25:145–62.
12. Tonelli F, Giudici F, Giusti F, et al. A heterozygous frameshift mutation in exon 1 of CDKN1B gene in a patient affected by MEN4 syndrome. Eur J Endocrinol. 2014;171:K7–K17.

13. Frederiksen A, Rossing M, Hermann P, et al. Clinical features of multiple endocrine neoplasia type 4: novel pathogenic variant and review of published cases. J Clin Endocrinol Metab. 2019;104:3637–46.
14. Sekiya T, Bronstein MD, Benfini K, et al. p27 variant and corticotropinoma susceptibility: a genetic and in vitro study. Endocr Relat Cancer. 2014;21:395–404.
15. Francis JM, Kiezun A, Ramos AH, et al. Somatic mutation of CDKN1B in small intestine neuroendocrine tumors. Nat Genet. 2013;45:1483–6.
16. Landa I, Montero-Conde C, Malanga D, et al. Allelic variant at −79 (C>T) in CDKN1B (p27Kip1) confers an increased risk of thyroid cancer and alters mRNA levels. Endocr Relat Cancer. 2010;17:317–28.
17. Esteban-Jurado C, Vila-Casadesus M, Garre P, et al. Whole-exome sequencing identifies rare pathogenic variants in new predisposition genes for familial colorectal cancer. Genet Med. 2015;17:131–42.
18. Chang BL, Zheng SL, Isaacs SD, et al. A polymorphism in the CDKN1B gene is associated with increased risk of hereditary prostate cancer. Cancer Res. 2004;64:1997–9.
19. Lu Y, Gao K, Zhang M, et al. Genetic association between CDKN1B rs2066827 polymorphism and susceptibility to cancer. Medicine (Baltimore). 2015;94:e1217.
20. Dietrich S, Hullein J, Lee SC, et al. Recurrent CDKN1B (p27) mutations in hairy cell leukemia. Blood. 2015;126:1005–8.
21. Georgitsi M, Raitila A, Karhu A, et al. Germline CDKN1B/p27Kip1 mutation in multiple endocrine neoplasia. J Clin Endocrinol Metab. 2007;92:3321–5.
22. Agarwal SK, Ozawa A, Mateo CM, et al. The MEN1 gene and pituitary tumours. Horm Res. 2009;71(Suppl 2):131–8.
23. Molatore S, Marinoni I, Lee M, et al. A novel germline CDKN1B mutation causing multiple endocrine tumors: clinical, genetic and functional characterization. Hum Mutat. 2010;31:E1825–35.
24. Occhi G, Regazzo D, Trivellin G, et al. A novel mutation in the upstream open reading frame of the CDKN1B gene causes a MEN4 phenotype. PLoS Genet. 2013;9:e1003350.
25. Costa-Guda J, Marinoni I, Molatore S, et al. Somatic mutation and germline sequence abnormalities in CDKN1B, encoding p27Kip1, in sporadic parathyroid adenomas. J Clin Endocrinol Metab. 2011;96:E701–6.
26. Borsari S, Pardi E, Pellegata NS, et al. Loss of p27 expression is associated with MEN1 gene mutations in sporadic parathyroid adenomas. Endocrine. 2017;55:386–97.
27. Tichomirowa MA, Lee M, Barlier A, et al. Cyclin-dependent kinase inhibitor 1B (CDKN1B) gene variants in AIP mutation-negative familial isolated pituitary adenoma kindreds. Endocr Relat Cancer. 2012;19:233–41.
28. Marini F, Cianferotti L, Giusti F, et al. Molecular genetics in primary hyperparathyroidism: the role of genetic tests in differential diagnosis, disease prevention strategy, and therapeutic planning. A 2017 update. Clin Cases Miner Bone Metab. 2017;14:60–70.
29. Bugalho MJ, Domingues R. Uncommon association of cerebral meningioma, parathyroid adenoma and papillary thyroid carcinoma in a patient harbouring a rare germline variant in the CDKN1B gene. BMJ Case Rep. 2016;2016:bcr2015213934.
30. Malanga D, De Gisi S, Riccardi M, et al. Functional characterization of a rare germline mutation in the gene encoding the cyclin-dependent kinase inhibitor p27Kip1 (CDKN1B) in a Spanish patient with multiple endocrine neoplasia-like phenotype. Eur J Endocrinol. 2012;166:551–60.

31. Belar O, De La Hoz C, Perez-Nanclares G, et al. Novel mutations in MEN1, CDKN1B and AIP genes in patients with multiple endocrine neoplasia type 1 syndrome in Spain. Clin Endocrinol. 2012;76:719–24.
32. Elston MS, Meyer-Rochow GY, Dray M, et al. Early onset primary hyperparathyroidism associated with a novel germline mutation in CDKN1B. Case Rep Endocrinol. 2015;2015:510985.
33. Sambugaro S, Di Ruvo M, Ambrosio MR, et al. Early onset acromegaly associated with a novel deletion in CDKN1B 5′UTR region. Endocrine. 2015;49:58–64.

Non-MEN Familial Endocrine Syndromes: Von Recklinghausen Disease, Von Hippel-Lindau Syndrome, Pheochromocytoma/Paraganglioma

Orhan Agcaoglu and Özer Makay

Contents

A. L. Shifrin et al. (eds.), *Endocrine Surgery Comprehensive Board Exam Guide*,
https://doi.org/10.1007/978-3-030-84737-1_39

Case Presentation

A 27-year-old woman presented with intermittent abdominal pain over the last 2 years. The pain was localized to right lumbar region with no specific exacerbating or relieving factors. On questioning, she reported that the family physician had diagnosed hypertensive episodes, accompanied by intermittent attacks of severe flushing, perspiration, and ectopic heartbeat 3 years ago and that she is currently requiring more than three antihypertensive drugs for optimal control. Detailed physical examination revealed a blood pressure of 160/90 mmHg, heart rate between 100 and 110/min, multiple soft to firm nodular swellings over the entire body including the face, multiple brown macules, and generalized freckling of the skin. On ophthalmic examination, yellow-brown pigmentation on the iris was seen, and abdominal examination was unremarkable. Family history revealed similar nodular lesions in her mother and sister with no major illness in them or other family members. Ultrasonography of the abdomen revealed a mass lesion in the right adrenal gland, and CT scan showed a 4.6 × 3.8 cm mass arising from right adrenal gland. Her laboratory findings revealed that 24-h urinary metanephrines and normetanephrines were elevated. Investigations for neck pathologies including thyroid and parathyroid diseases were negative.

Questions

1. What is the most likely diagnosis?
   (a) Von Hippel-Lindau syndrome
   (b) Neurofibromatosis type 1
   (c) Addison's disease
   (d) Kallmann's syndrome
2. All of the following regions of the adrenal cortex and medulla with its producing hormones are given correctly *except*:
   (a) Zona glomerulosa – mineralocorticoids
   (b) Zona fasciculate – glucocorticoids
   (c) Zona reticularis – aldosterone
   (d) Medulla – epinephrine and norepinephrine
3. Neural crest cells migrate to the adrenal glands to form which region?
   (a) Zona glomerulosa
   (b) Zona fasciculate
   (c) Zona reticularis
   (d) Medulla
4. Which is the secretory cell found in the adrenal medulla?
   (a) Chromaffin cells
   (b) Neuroglial cells
   (c) Follicle cells
   (d) Oxyphil cells

5. Pheochromocytoma can secrete excess amounts of all of the following *except*:
   (a) Cortisol
   (b) Dopamine
   (c) Norepinephrine
   (d) Epinephrine
6. Which of the following imaging technique is important whether the malignant form of the tumor can be treated with lutetium?
   (a) Computed tomography (CT) scan
   (b) Magnetic resonance imaging (MRI) scan
   (c) Metaiodobenzylguanidine (MIBG) scan
   (d) Ga-DOTATATE PET/CT
7. The preoperative preparation of a patient with pheochromocytoma should include all of the following *except*:
   (a) An alpha-adrenergic blocker such as phentolamine
   (b) A beta-adrenergic blocker such as propranolol
   (c) Intravenous hydration to avoid volume depletion
   (d) Systemic steroids to adrenal insufficiency
8. Which familial endocrine syndrome and the related gene is given correctly?
   (a) Von Hippel-Lindau syndrome – PTEN
   (b) Neurofibromatosis type – neurofibromin gene
   (c) Von Recklinghausen disease – SDHx genes
   (d) Hereditary paraganglioma – VHL tumor suppressor gene

? Open-Ended Oral Exam Questions

1. Please define hereditary endocrine syndromes affecting the adrenal glands.
2. Please define the affected organs and characteristic lesions in patient with von Hippel-Lindau syndrome.
3. Please define the short-term and long-term stress response for adrenal hormones.
4. What are the three regions of the adrenal cortex and what hormones do they produce?

39.1 Hereditary Pheochromocytoma and Paraganglioma

39.1.1 Introduction

Rare neuroendocrine tumors, pheochromocytomas and paragangliomas, also known as extra-adrenal pheochromocytomas, originate from neural crest cells of the autonomic nervous system. In a significant proportion of hereditary pheochromocytomas, the gene mainly responsible for the origin of these tumors relates to genetic control of succinate dehydrogenase (SDH) [1, 2].

In relation to the autonomic nervous system, it has been reported that the organ of Zuckerkandl and the adrenal medulla are related to the sympathetic paraganglia, while the carotid bodies are related to the parasympathetic paraganglia. The WHO defined pheochromocytoma in 2004 as "tumors derived from neural crest origin chromaffin cells which arise in the adrenal medulla." While tumors from neural crest cells that arise from the adrenal medulla are called pheochromocytomas, those that arise extra-adrenally are referred to as paragangliomas [3].

Pheochromocytomas display a relatively less malignant (10%) pattern when compared to paragangliomas. Paragangliomas are found mostly in the abdomen, in which case they have proven to be 15–35% more malignant when compared to the other regions in which they can be found. The paragangliomas can also be found in the head and neck region, where they tend to be painless masses which are vertically fixed but laterally mobile, a characteristic termed Fontaine's sign [4].

39.1.2 Epidemiology and Genetics

Historically, pheochromocytoma was referred to as the 10% tumor because it was regarded as 10% malignant, 10% familial, 10% extra-adrenal, and 10% bilateral. Currently, however, both paragangliomas and pheochromocytomas are actually considered to be 30% hereditary [5]. Pheochromocytomas are considered rare tumors as the incidence of these tumors is 2–9.1 per million among adults per year [6]. Men and women are equally at risk of developing these tumors, but paragangliomas and pheochromocytomas tend not to be present in the pediatric populations [6]. However, when these syndromes do occur in pediatric patients, they are usually hereditary and multifocal in nature.

There is variety among the familial genetic syndromes related to paragangliomas and pheochromocytomas [7]. Such an example is the result of a mutation on chromosome 3 at a tumor suppressor gene that causes the autosomal dominant VHL syndrome, which has an estimated prevalence of 1/35,000.

The syndrome can affect the eyes, brain, pancreas, ears, adrenal glands (causing pheochromocytomas in 20–80% of VHL patients), and prostate. Another example is the *SDHx* gene mutations which were found to be related to familial paragangliomas [8]. A chronic hypoxic signal is produced in the mitochondrial II complex due to these mutations which causes cellular proliferation [9]. There is an association between the familial paragangliomas of the abdomen or thorax that are likely to be malignant with the *SDHB* gene and those of the head and neck which are less likely to be malignant with *SDHD* subunits, which are both located on chromosome 1. Both of the subunits have a weak association with pheochromocytoma [8]. However, paragangliomas of the head and neck region are diagnosed later in life than pheochromocytomas. This is in part due to the catecholamine-associated symptoms in pheochromocytomas [10]. The hereditary tendency of *SDHx* genes is autosomal dominant. It should be noted that the *SDHD* gene, if transmitted maternally, exhibits a carrier state without affecting the phenotype [11]. Paragangliomas and pheochromocytomas can be associated also with tuberous sclerosis, ataxia-telangiectasia, Sturge-Weber, and Carney complex [12].

39.1.3 Clinical Presentation

Pheochromocytoma and paraganglioma patients usually suffer from hypertension that can be episodic, new onset, and refractory or persistent despite standard pharmacological agents. In addition to hypertension, patients can exhibit signs and symptoms such as palpitations, headaches, and diaphoresis. Some other manifestations of these patients include tremor, anxiety, pallor, tachycardia, flushing, visual disturbances, orthostatic hypotension, fever, heat intolerance, abdominal pain, vomiting, constipation, hematuria (due to a bladder paraganglioma), polyuria, hyperglycemia, polydipsia, and hypercalcemia [13]. On the other hand, because pheochromocytomas tend to have cystic degeneration, even if the tumor reaches extreme sizes, some patients can be asymptomatic. While these lesions are generally benign, pheochromocytomas may be malignant from 5% to 10%, and paragangliomas may be malignant from 15% to 35% [14]. Malignant tumors that produce catecholamines are present clinically with symptoms identical to those of their benign counterparts. Upon metastasis, the tumors spread mostly to the regional lymph nodes, liver, bone, and lung [15].

39.1.4 Diagnosis and Indications for Surgery

The workup of suspected pheochromocytoma or paraganglioma includes initial biochemical screening. Diagnosis is imperative, as lack of identification of these syndromes may lead to stroke or even sudden death. Recognition of the excessive production of catecholamines is the first part of the informed evaluation. Comorbidities, such as severe congestive heart failure, acute MI, acute alcohol withdrawal, acute clonidine withdrawal, emotional or physical stress, subarachnoid hemorrhage, or cerebral tumors causing comatose state, and interfering substances, in particular levodopa, amphetamines, pseudoephedrine, dietary caffeic acid, acetaminophen, reserpine, prochlorperazine, ethanol, labetalol, methylglucamine of contrast media with iodine, and mostly tricyclic antidepressants and phenoxybenzamine, are all important factors that have to be taken into account. If the blood and urine analyses indicate different results, then the clonidine suppression test is used to make a distinction between essential hypertension and pheochromocytoma. Essential hypertension is indicated if there is more than 50% suppression, and no suppression suggests that the patient has pheochromocytoma.

Regarding the catecholamines produced, while pheochromocytomas secrete epinephrine, paragangliomas secrete norepinephrine. Moreover, it should be noted that norepinephrine is produced in excess in VHL-associated tumors, whereas both epinephrine and norepinephrine are produced in MEN 2-associated tumors. Dopamine is secreted in malignancy due to alterations in catecholamine synthesis. Since pheochromocytomas and paragangliomas are neuroendocrine tumors, serum chromogranin A can be used as a biomarker for identification [16]. It is important to keep in mind that measurement of serum chromogranin A may result in false positives in many instances including renal insufficiency patients.

39.1.5 Preoperative Management and Radiological Studies

Paragangliomas and pheochromocytomas are evaluated radiologically via CT, MRI, and MIBG scintigraphy [17]. Although CT is initially the preferred modality, its specificity is relatively poor, at 50% [17]. CT scans are recommended before and after the injection of IV contrast medium for evaluation of pheochromocytomas. If CT imaging excludes the presence of paragangliomas intra-abdominally, the head and neck region of the patient should also be examined for the possible presence of tumors at the carotid bodies and the mediastinum.

In cases which patients are ineligible for CT scans (e.g., pregnancy, allergy, pediatrics), MRI should be preferred instead. Due to increased vascularity around the paragangliomas and pheochromocytomas, T2-weighted images show increased signal intensity. Signal intensity on T2 can be diminished if the tumor is large enough to be associated with hemorrhaging or necrosis. MRI has a higher specificity (50–100%) and higher sensitivity (90–100%) when compared to CT. If biochemical testing suggests the presence of pheochromocytoma in a patient, but a CT scan contradicts the results, then MRI can be used for additional investigation [12].

Surgical intervention to remove pheochromocytoma and paraganglioma in a patient is the preferred treatment route among several other options. Because the tumors are highly vascular, upon diagnosis of pheochromocytoma or paraganglioma, patients should never have a FNAB that may potentially cause hemorrhage, hypertensive crisis, or even death. In general, α-blockade is recommended to be administered at least 2 weeks preoperatively, in particular phenoxybenzamine. If the patient has tachycardia, β-blockade ought to be added to the ongoing treatment. Preoperative treatment must continue up to the morning of the operation. Blood pressure alterations are anticipated during the operation. Therefore, the patient must be monitored hemodynamically and have an optimal IV access for serious changes. Norepinephrine may need to be added to the postoperative treatment for routine monitoring and maintenance of blood pressure.

Genetic counseling should be offered to those with a positive or suspected family history of pheochromocytoma or paragangliomas. If a patient is 50 years old or younger with a positive family history, possible *VHL, SDHB, SDHD*, and *RET* mutations must be tested.

39.1.6 Surgical Techniques

The gold standard surgical intervention for pheochromocytoma patients is minimally invasive (either laparoscopic or retroperitoneoscopic) adrenalectomy, along with cortical-sparing adrenalectomy which is especially important for cases with hereditary disease and a high risk for bilateral pheochromocytoma [18]. Even though data for robotic adrenalectomy is scarce, the technique is widely accepted among surgeons [19]. Several studies conducted in order to compare laparoscopic and robotic surgeries failed to show a statistically significant difference in perioperative outcomes [19]. Surgical technique should be chosen based on patient demographics, tumor features, and most importantly the surgeon's experience [19]. Intraoperatively, in order to evaluate real-time hemodynamic volatility, invasive blood pressure monitoring must be done. Esmolol or sodium nitroprusside (short-acting vasodilators) are best for optimal hypertension control [18].

Many elements factor into the decision of radical or conservative adrenalectomy in pheochromocytoma patients. Due to the risk of recurrence or residual disease, unilateral total adrenalectomy is preferred in patients with sporadic occurrence. However, in young patients with hereditary pheochromocytomas due to germline mutations, the tumors can present bilaterally, which can call for the removal of both of the adrenal glands [20]. However, resection of both adrenal glands can lead to unwanted complications since the patients will be dependent on long-term supplementation of glucocorticoid, affecting patient quality of life [21]. Patients can avoid these complications by opting to "cortex-sparing" surgery, benefitting from the remaining adrenal cortex, as deemed appropriate [22]. It should also be considered that those patients that present with hereditary pheochromocytomas tend to have benign tumors. Even when the adrenal medulla is left in situ, postoperative ipsilateral recurrence rates of 3–7% have been reported after a median interval 8–10 years [23, 24]. Therefore, all aspects of the extent of surgery should be considered carefully to improve clinical outcome and quality of life of the patients.

For familial paragangliomas, surgical resection – if possible – remains the only choice of curative treatment. However, due to the multifocal nature of paragangliomas, the morbidity of the operation may necessitate alternative treatments to the surgical intervention (e.g., radiotherapy, active surveillance) [25]. Without proper treatment compliance, patients with an *SDHB* germline mutation that have had a unilateral adrenalectomy carry the risk of going through an adrenal crisis. Usually, adrenal-sparing surgery would not be considered for those patients with *SDHB* mutations due to the advanced nature of the disease, and total adrenalectomy would be favored in these patients to avoid preventable metastasis. But, in situations in which patients are disregarding their condition and run the risk of adrenal crisis, the risk of metastasis may be overlooked in relation to the risk of adrenal crisis, and cortex-sparing adrenalectomy may be advantageous [24].

39.1.7 Postoperative Follow-Up and Prognosis

Due to the possibility of recurrence of paragangliomas and pheochromocytomas, patients –especially those with a hereditary history – ought to be followed up throughout their entire life. As the rate of recurrence for both pheochromocytomas and paragangliomas is hard to foretell, authors have investigated factors that correlate with the recurrence. Due to their more difficult resection, right-sided tumors have a higher risk of recurrence than their left counterparts. The prognosis for such patients is inconsistent; half have more than a 20-year life expectancy, whereas the other half suffer recurrence and disease progression within the first 1–3 years after the diagnosis. The probability of new event occurrence is higher in younger patients and also in those with hereditary and larger tumors than the sporadic and smaller tumors in elder patients [15].

39.2 Von Hippel-Lindau Syndrome

39.2.1 Introduction

Hippel-Lindau (VHL) is relatively rare (1 in 35,000 incidence ratio) autosomal dominant syndrome, caused by mutations in the *VHL* tumor suppressor gene located on chromosome 3p25-26. The mutation causes vascular endothelial growth factor (VEGF) upregulation. VHL is related to tumors in several organs such as the adrenal glands, kidneys, eyes, inner ears, CNS, pancreas, and epididymis [26]. The specific tumors related to VHL include pheochromocytoma, renal cell carcinoma (RCC), hemangioblastoma of the CNS, endolymphatic sac tumors, retinal angiomas, pancreatic cysts, and neuroendocrine tumors [26]. If a patient has a missense mutation, then this patient is classified as VHL type 2 and usually also has pheochromocytoma. If other mutations are present, the patient is classified as VHL type 1 [27].

39.2.2 Epidemiology and Genetics

One in 36,000 are born with VHL syndrome, which by the age of 65 has a 90% penetrance [28]. Historically, the median age of survival was less than 50 before CT alongside other imaging techniques, and screening methods for the affected individuals were developed. RCC or CNS hemangioblastoma was the cause of death in those individuals. With the development of the aforementioned diagnostic modalities, survival rates increased.

39.2.3 Clinical Presentation

VHL affects several organs such as the adrenal glands, eyes, pancreas, CNS, inner ears, and epididymis [26]. Even asymptomatic patients can be diagnosed by utilizing routine genetic tests and imaging techniques. Clinical diagnosis of pheochromocytoma is confirmed by a positive family history of VHL as well as positive test results indicating a diagnosis for pheochromocytoma, CNS hemangioblastoma, or renal manifestations. If the patient is diagnosed de novo, then she must meet the criteria of having a visceral tumor with one CNS manifestation or two or more CNS hemangioblastomas.

Clinical presentations of the affected organs aforementioned differ from each other. Therefore, they have been depicted in different groups below and will be further characterized: visceral lesions, CNS lesions, retina, and inner ear [29].

39.2.3.1 Visceral Lesions

Comorbidity of pheochromocytomas in VHL patients is 20% with a mean age of 30 years. Lesions can be bilateral as well as extra-adrenal paragangliomas.

Patients with VHL are more likely to develop both solid lesions of the kidneys and renal cystic disease – up to 25–45% – which can be multifocal and bilateral with the mean age of 39 years. Due to the possibility of malignancy of RCC, it is one of the most significant causes of death. If left untreated, 13–42% of the patients will have tumors that metastasize [27].

From 17% up to 56% of VHL patients with the comorbidity of pancreatic lesions will develop cystic lesions – serous cystadenomas – that can be single or multiple. Even if the lesions lack malignancy potential, they may occupy both the endocrine and exocrine portions of the pancreas, leading to insufficiency and obstruction of the intestine and bile duct. Always nonfunctional but potentially malignant, pancreatic neuroendocrine tumors (PNETs) can be seen in 12–17% of VHL patients. Even if PNETs become malignant, they are not a common cause of death [10].

39.2.3.2 CNS Lesions

Almost 80% of VHL patients, with a mean age of 33 years, suffer from hemangioblastomas which makes it the most common tumor in patients with VHL. They never cause malignancy, but depending on their size or location, hemangioblastomas can cause swelling and result in symptoms that correlate with their specific location along the craniospinal axis.

39.2.3.3 Retina

Up to 60% of the VHL patients – with a relatively early mean of age of 25 years – have retinal hemangioblastomas which can be both multifocal and bilateral. Even if the lesion is benign, it may cause vision loss [29].

39.2.3.4 Inner Ear

A less common manifestation of VHL patients is endolymphatic sac tumors that may lead to equilibrium disorders and hearing loss [29].

39.2.4 Diagnosis and Indications for Surgery

In order to determine gene rearrangements and deletions, complete gene sequencing methods are used to detect the germline mutations of VHL [26].

If a patient with VHL has a PNET, the tumor is always nonfunctional. This leads to a failure of detection of the tumor in biochemical screening tests. Plasma and 24-h urinary metanephrine levels should be controlled before any intervention is carried out due to the possibility of overlooking a case of pheochromocytoma and risking a hypertensive crisis.

39.2.5 Preoperative Management and Radiological Studies

The gold standard for screening and follow-up of visceral lesions related to this disease is contrast-enhanced abdominal CT. This modality is preferred also due to its feasibility and accessibility. MRI can be used alternatively to the CT in the case of an allergy or similar constraints.

Biochemical analysis and radiological modalities are used together to identify adrenal masses. CT is used if the catecholamine levels are elevated. If the CT result is negative, then the nuclear MIBG scan is used to identify any extra-adrenal paragangliomas.

Preoperative management of the patients is complicated due to the involvement of multiple lesions in multiple organs. Thus, a team with individuals of multidisciplinary backgrounds such as neurosurgeons, endocrine surgeons, ophthalmologists, and urologists is needed to manage these syndromes.

39.2.6 Surgical Techniques

Surgical techniques employed for treatment depend on the clinical presentation of the VHL disease. When weighing options for extent of surgery in von Hippel-Lindau disease, in vitro studies have shown that genetic changes tend to be missense mutations rather than deletions or other kinds of mutations that would lead to a nonfunctional pVHL in pheochromocytomas [30, 31], though this does not necessarily mean that the possibility of recurrence can be excluded. Yet, it should be noted that these VHL-related chromaffin tumors have a relatively low malignancy rate as 1–5% [24, 32], making subtotal adrenalectomy a plausible alternative to the radical route, and has been executed successfully in both adults and children with VHL [33]. The clinical presentation of pheochromocytoma and paraganglioma is further discussed, and treatment options are considered in the previous chapter as either minimally invasive or robotic adrenalectomy.

The main treatment options for retinal hemangioblastomas are cryotherapy and laser photocoagulation. If retinal detachment occurs from traction and exudation, vitreoretinal surgery can be performed. Anti-VEGF therapy in the intravitreal compartment should be considered if the optic nerve is at risk due to its proximity with the hemangioblastoma [34].

Treatment of endolymphatic sac tumors calls for the surgical resection of the tumor as the gold standard. The resection may relieve hearing-related symptoms [34]. For RCC lesions less than 3 cm in diameter, surgical resection is advised. Total nephrectomy has been replaced by partial nephrectomy (nephron sparing). Also, radiofrequency ablation is an alternative technique used in addition to surgery in order to enhance results [34].

39.2.7 Postoperative Follow-Up and Prognosis

Gaps of 6–12 months are arranged between the CT imaging along with history taking and physical examinations in patients with renal lesions. Improvement of the quality of life of VHL patients is evident, thanks to the development of imaging modalities, cumulative clinical knowledge of such patients, and novel genetic techniques. Such improvements also contribute to better prognosis in these patients.

39.3 Neurofibromatosis Type 1 (Von Recklinghausen Disease)

39.3.1 Introduction

The autosomal disorder neurofibromatosis type 1 (NF-1) arises due to mutations at c17q11 in the *NF1* tumor suppressor gene which is a very large gene with several mutations identified. No correlation between phenotype and genotype has been found. Café au lait spots and benign cutaneous neurofibromas are the characteristic features. Some NF patients (less than 4%) tend to develop pheochromocytoma that is 10% bilateral and 10% malignant. Of the disease, 96% is intra-adrenal and may show a mixed pathology, such as ganglioneuroma and neuroblastoma. In NF-1, duodenal periampullary somatostatinomas with psammomatous calcification are almost pathognomonic. Rarely there may be associated HPT and MTC endocrine tumors [35].

39.3.2 Epidemiology and Genetics

Mutations on chromosome 17 at the tumor suppressor gene cause an autosomal dominant NF1 disease with a prevalence rate of 1/3000 people. Two percent of the NF1 patients have paragangliomas and pheochromocytomas, whereas 20–80% of VHL patients have paragangliomas and pheochromocytomas [8]. A greater prevalence is estimated if there is a comorbidity with hypertension or duodenal carcinoids [35].

39.3.3 Clinical Presentation

The patients may be found to have café au lait macules, bone lesions, optic glioma, several types of neurofibromas, Lisch nodules, freckles in areas of opposing skin such as the axilla or inguinal area, pheochromocytoma, and paraganglioma.

Café au lait macules are well-defined and regular macules with hyperpigmentation in their typical forms. If they are atypical, they exhibit an irregular border and a heterogenic pigmentation [36]. The aforementioned osseous lesions can be listed as osteoporosis, osteopenia, scoliosis, pseudoarthrosis, and sphenoid wing dysplasia. As scoliosis patients have a 21–49% likelihood of having comorbidity with the NF-1 disease, the pediatric routine clinical examination must be executed carefully. The evaluation must take into consideration the potential of a patient having NF-1 symptoms [36]. The NF-1-associated pheochromocytomas and paragangliomas are diagnosed at similar ages compared to the sporadic counterparts [37]. The NF-1-associated pheochromocytomas and paragangliomas tend to be active biochemically, MIBG-positive, and unilateral [37].

39.3.4 Diagnosis and Indications for Surgery

The diagnostic criteria of NF-1 according to the National Institutes of Health (NIH) are met if two or more of these symptoms are seen [36]:

1. Six or more café au lait macules that are larger than 15 mm in diameter in postpubertal patients and macules larger than 5 mm in diameter in prepubertal patients
2. A distinguishable osseous lesion
3. Optic glioma
4. Two or more of any type of neurofibromas or one plexiform neurofibroma
5. Two or more Lisch nodules
6. Axillary or inguinal freckles
7. Positive first-degree family history

39.3.5 Preoperative Management and Radiological Studies

The main aim of preoperative management is to identify potentially treatable symptoms and complications. The types of neurofibromas can differ from spinal nerve root, nodular or diffuse plexiform, dermal, or neurofibromatous neuropathy. The management of dental neurofibromatosis mostly involves surgical intervention. Alternatively, laser ablation, emollients, electrodessication, psychological support, or camouflage makeup may be used.

More than half of NF-1 patients also have internal tumors which can be evaluated by the volumetric whole-body MRI modality to observe their tumor growth and burden characteristics.

Recent studies conducted in mice models showed that imatinib, mTOR inhibitors, and selective MEK inhibitor therapies resulted in tumor size reduction [38].

Due to the possible peri-/postoperative complications of the cardiovascular system such as cardiovascular crisis, screening with plasma or urine free fractionated metanephrine levels should be done before any surgical intervention [37].

39.3.6 Surgical Techniques

NF-1 patients are monitored via active surveillance without the application of any medical or surgical treatments. Yet, some particular cases need such treatment [39]. Radiotherapy provides only a local and symptomatic treatment of NF-1 and does not contribute to the overall survival of the patients according to retrospective studies. Due to the increased risk of secondary malignancy in plexiform neurofibroma, radiotherapy should be avoided specifically in this situation. Thus, surgical intervention along with medical treatments can be used, when necessary [39].

Surgical intervention is comprised of surgical resection, laser treatment, and orthopedic surgery. Surgical resection can be favored in cutaneous and plexiform neurofibromas. Yet, recurrence is common in such resections. Approximately 10–25% of pheochromocytoma patients have NF1-related bilateral adrenal disease [40, 41]. Low occurrence of pheochromocytoma in NF1 patients makes it less suitable for subtotal adrenalectomy, yet when these adrenal neoplasms do develop, they tend to do so bilaterally. These could be regarded as pheochromocytoma-prone NF1 mutations, though further evaluations are needed to characterize this association. Although subtotal adrenalectomy may not be favored for an adrenal tumor on one side, the malignancy rates of adrenal neoplasms range between 1% and 7% [40, 42], and cortex-sparing surgery may be performed on the opposite gland if the tumor is bilateral. Malignant peripheral nerve sheath tumor is the main indication for surgical resection in NF-1 patients [39]. Moreover, if the freckles and café au lait macules affect the quality of life of a patient, laser removal can be considered. Orthopedic surgeries can be carried out in order to correct osseous lesions [39].

39.3.7 Postoperative Follow-Up and Prognosis

NF-1 patients have the highest Clavien-Dindo graded complication rates for pheochromocytoma or paraganglioma as compared to those arising in MEN 2 and VHL, and among these three hereditary types of pheochromocytomas and paragangliomas, NF-1 patients also have the most intraoperative hemodynamic volatility [43].

Answers

1. (b); 2. (c); 3. (d); 4. (a); 5. (a); 6. (d); 7. (d); 8. (b)

Answers to Open-Ended Oral Exam Questions

1. MEN 2A, MEN 2B, MEN 4, von Hippel-Lindau syndrome, Neurofibromatosis type I, hereditary pheochromocytoma/paraganglioma
2. VHL affects several organs such as the adrenal glands, eyes, pancreas, CNS, inner ears, and epididymis. Clinical presentations of the affected organs have been depicted in different groups as follows and will be further characterized: visceral lesions, CNS lesions, retina, and inner ear.
3. The short-term stress response involves the hormones epinephrine and norepinephrine, which work to increase the oxygen supply to organs important for extreme muscular action such as the brain, lungs, and muscles. In the long-term stress response, the hormone cortisol is involved in catabolism of glycogen stores, proteins, and triglycerides, glucose and ketone synthesis, and downregulation of the immune system.
4. The regions from the most outer layer are the zona glomerulosa, the zona fasciculate, and the zona reticularis which produces aldosterone and glucocorticoids such as cortisol and androgens, respectively.

References

1. Nazar E, Khatami F, Saffar H, Tavangar SM. The emerging role of succinate dehydrogenase genes (SDHx) in tumorigenesis. Int J Hematol Oncol Stem Cell Res. 2019;13(2):72–82.
2. Albattal S, Alswailem M, Moria Y, Al-Hindi H, Dasouki M, Abouelhoda M, et al. Mutational profile and genotype/phenotype correlation of non-familial pheochromocytoma and paraganglioma. Oncotarget. 2019;10(57):5919–31.
3. Fishbein L. Pheochromocytoma and paraganglioma: genetics, diagnosis, and treatment. Hematol Oncol Clin North Am. 2016;30(1):135–50.
4. Shepherd JJ. The natural history of multiple endocrine neoplasia type 1. Highly uncommon or highly unrecognized? Arch Surg. 1991;126(8):935–52.
5. Farrugia FA, Martikos G, Tzanetis P, Charalampopoulos A, Misiakos E, Zavras N, et al. Pheochromocytoma, diagnosis and treatment: review of the literature. Endocr Regul. 2017;51(3):168–81.
6. Farrugia FA, Charalampopoulos A. Pheochromocytoma. Endocr Regul. 2019;53(3):191–212.

7. Tassone F. Pheochromocytoma and paraganglioma. N Engl J Med. 2019;381(19):1882–3.
8. Turchini J, Cheung VKY, Tischler AS, De Krijger RR, Gill AJ. Pathology and genetics of phaeochromocytoma and paraganglioma. Histopathology. 2018;72(1):97–105.
9. Aldera AP, Govender D. Gene of the month: SDH. J Clin Pathol. 2018;71(2):95–7.
10. Muth A, Crona J, Gimm O, Elmgren A, Filipsson K, Stenmark Askmalm M, et al. Genetic testing and surveillance guidelines in hereditary pheochromocytoma and paraganglioma. J Intern Med. 2019;285(2):187–204.
11. Baysal BE. Mitochondrial complex II and genomic imprinting in inheritance of paraganglioma tumors. Biochim Biophys Acta. 2013;1827(5):573–7.
12. Ikram A, Rehman A. Paraganglioma. Treasure Island: StatPearls; 2020.
13. Pacak K, Tella SH. Pheochromocytoma and Paraganglioma. In: Feingold KR, Anawalt B, Boyce A, Chrousos G, de Herder WW, Dungan K, et al., editors. Endotext. South Dartmouth: MDText.com, Inc.; 2000.
14. Bourdeau I, El Ghorayeb N, Gagnon N, Lacroix A. MANAGEMENT OF ENDOCRINE DISEASE: differential diagnosis, investigation and therapy of bilateral adrenal incidentalomas. Eur J Endocrinol. 2018;179(2):R57–67.
15. Plouin PF, Amar L, Dekkers OM, Fassnacht M, Gimenez-Roqueplo AP, Lenders JW, et al. European Society of Endocrinology Clinical Practice Guideline for long-term follow-up of patients operated on for a phaeochromocytoma or a paraganglioma. Eur J Endocrinol. 2016;174(5):G1–G10.
16. Morita SY, Dackiw APB, Zeiger MA. McGraw-Hill manual endocrine surgery. The McGraw-Hill Companies, Inc; 2010.
17. Itani M, Mhlanga J. Imaging of Pheochromocytoma and Paraganglioma. In: Mariani-Costantini R, editor. Paraganglioma: a multidisciplinary approach. Brisbane: Codon Publications; 2019.
18. Shank J, Prescott JD, Mathur A. Surgical approach to endocrine hypertension in patients with adrenal disorders. Endocrinol Metab Clin N Am. 2019;48(4):875–85.
19. Agcaoglu O, Aliyev S, Karabulut K, Mitchell J, Siperstein A, Berber E. Robotic versus laparoscopic resection of large adrenal tumors. Ann Surg Oncol. 2012;19(7):2288–94.
20. Welander J, Soderkvist P, Gimm O. Genetics and clinical characteristics of hereditary pheochromocytomas and paragangliomas. Endocr Relat Cancer. 2011;18(6):R253–76.
21. Oksnes M, Ross R, Lovas K. Optimal glucocorticoid replacement in adrenal insufficiency. Best Pract Res Clin Endocrinol Metab. 2015;29(1):3–15.
22. Janetschek G, Finkenstedt G, Gasser R, Waibel UG, Peschel R, Bartsch G, et al. Laparoscopic surgery for pheochromocytoma: adrenalectomy, partial resection, excision of paragangliomas. J Urol. 1998;160(2):330–4.
23. Castinetti F, Qi XP, Walz MK, Maia AL, Sanso G, Peczkowska M, et al. Outcomes of adrenal-sparing surgery or total adrenalectomy in phaeochromocytoma associated with multiple endocrine neoplasia type 2: an international retrospective population-based study. Lancet Oncol. 2014;15(6):648–55.
24. Rossitti HM, Soderkvist P, Gimm O. Extent of surgery for phaeochromocytomas in the genomic era. Br J Surg. 2018;105(2):e84–98.
25. Iacobone M, Belluzzi A, Torresan F. Surgical approaches and results of treatment for hereditary paragangliomas. Best Pract Res Clin Endocrinol Metab. 2019;33(5):101298.

26. Li SR, Nicholson KJ, McCoy KL, Carty SE, Yip L. Clinical and biochemical features of pheochromocytoma characteristic of Von Hippel-Lindau syndrome. World J Surg. 2020;44(2):570–7.
27. Crespigio J, Berbel LCL, Dias MA, Berbel RF, Pereira SS, Pignatelli D, et al. Von Hippel-Lindau disease: a single gene, several hereditary tumors. J Endocrinol Investig. 2018;41(1):21–31.
28. Binderup MLM. von Hippel-Lindau disease: diagnosis and factors influencing disease outcome. Dan Med J. 2018;65(3):B5461.
29. van der Horst-Schrivers ANA, Sluiter WJ, Kruizinga RC, van Leeuwaarde RS, Giles R, Olderode-Berends MJW, et al. The incidence of consecutive manifestations in Von Hippel-Lindau disease. Familial Cancer. 2019;18(3):369–76.
30. Ong KR, Woodward ER, Killick P, Lim C, Macdonald F, Maher ER. Genotype-phenotype correlations in von Hippel-Lindau disease. Hum Mutat. 2007;28(2):143–9.
31. Peng S, Shepard MJ, Wang J, Li T, Ning X, Cai L, et al. Genotype-phenotype correlations in Chinese von Hippel-Lindau disease patients. Oncotarget. 2017;8(24):38456–65.
32. Pamporaki C, Hamplova B, Peitzsch M, Prejbisz A, Beuschlein F, Timmers H, et al. Characteristics of Pediatric vs adult pheochromocytomas and paragangliomas. J Clin Endocrinol Metab. 2017;102(4):1122–32.
33. Volkin D, Yerram N, Ahmed F, Lankford D, Baccala A, Gupta GN, et al. Partial adrenalectomy minimizes the need for long-term hormone replacement in pediatric patients with pheochromocytoma and von Hippel-Lindau syndrome. J Pediatr Surg. 2012;47(11):2077–82.
34. Chittiboina P, Lonser RR. Von Hippel-Lindau disease. Handb Clin Neurol. 2015;132:139–56.
35. Adil A, Singh AK. Neurofibromatosis type 1. Treasure Island: StatPearls; 2020.
36. Ly KI, Blakeley JO. The diagnosis and management of neurofibromatosis type 1. Med Clin North Am. 2019;103(6):1035–54.
37. Petr EJ, Else T. Pheochromocytoma and paraganglioma in neurofibromatosis type 1: frequent surgeries and cardiovascular crises indicate the need for screening. Clin Diabetes Endocrinol. 2018;4(1):15.
38. Gutmann DH, Ferner RE, Listernick RH, Korf BR, Wolters PL, Johnson KJ. Neurofibromatosis type 1. Nat Rev Dis Primers. 2017;3:17004.
39. Sabatini C, Milani D, Menni F, Tadini G, Esposito S. Treatment of neurofibromatosis type 1. Curr Treat Options Neurol. 2015;17(6):355.
40. Gruber LM, Erickson D, Babovic-Vuksanovic D, Thompson GB, Young WF Jr, Bancos I. Pheochromocytoma and paraganglioma in patients with neurofibromatosis type 1. Clin Endocrinol. 2017;86(1):141–9.
41. Bausch B, Borozdin W, Mautner VF, Hoffmann MM, Boehm D, Robledo M, et al. Germline NF1 mutational spectra and loss-of-heterozygosity analyses in patients with pheochromocytoma and neurofibromatosis type 1. J Clin Endocrinol Metab. 2007;92(7):2784–92.
42. Moramarco J, El Ghorayeb N, Dumas N, Nolet S, Boulanger L, Burnichon N, et al. Pheochromocytomas are diagnosed incidentally and at older age in neurofibromatosis type 1. Clin Endocrinol. 2017;86(3):332–9.
43. Butz JJ, Yan Q, McKenzie TJ, Weingarten TN, Cavalcante AN, Bancos I, et al. Perioperative outcomes of syndromic paraganglioma and pheochromocytoma resection in patients with von Hippel-Lindau disease, multiple endocrine neoplasia type 2, or neurofibromatosis type 1. Surgery. 2017;162(6):1259–69.

Endocrine Emergencies

Contents

Thyroid Storm

Pietro Princi and Ioannis Koutelidakis

Contents

A. L. Shifrin et al. (eds.), *Endocrine Surgery Comprehensive Board Exam Guide*,
https://doi.org/10.1007/978-3-030-84737-1_40

Case Presentation

A 38-year-old woman had been referred to the general practitioner because she was irritable with fever, upper abdominal pain, tachycardia, and previously unrecognized thyroid disease, before being referred to our hospital for emergency access.

At the emergency department, the patient is admitted to red room for the rapidly worsening clinical condition, because of highly elevated fever (>39 °C). The electrocardiogram (ECG) shows atrial fibrillation with over 140 beats per minute. Elevated values of serum liver function and creatinine are noted, but the myocardial enzymes are in the normal range.

The white blood cell (WBC) count is mildly elevated. Hydration and diuretics are started at the emergency department. Cardiologist evaluation and intensive care admission are necessary after 12 h for ulterior worsening condition. Serum T4 and T3 free fraction showed elevated value, and TSH are suppressed. Thyrostatic treatment with propylthiouracil and propranolol is administered.

After 48 h from admission in ICU, the vital signs are stabilized, the fever disappeared, and the patient is discharged from ICU after 4 days, but the consciousness of patient is not completely recovered. After 9 days, T3 and T4 become normal even if TSH is suppressed. Then an urgent neck exploration is planned with total thyroidectomy performed with prior administration for 5 days of Lugol's solution (ten drops three times per day).

The patient is discharged in a euthyroid condition and fully conscious state 18 days after admission with normal renal function and serum calcium. Calcium and vitamin D supplementation is necessary for 2 weeks.

Questions

1. Concerning the definition of thyroid storm:
   1. It is a life-threatening medical emergency that results from an extreme hyperthyroidism with possible multiorgan dysfunction.
   2. It is a really rare condition, but it could be extremely dangerous and fatal if not treated in time.
   3. It is related to hypothyroidism.
   4. It was first described by Lahey in 1926.
      - (a) Only 1, 2, and 4 are correct.
      - (b) Only 3 is correct.
      - (c) Only 1, 2, and 3 are correct.
      - (d) All answers are correct.
2. Regarding the clinical presentation of thyroid storm:
   1. Fever is the most uncommon symptoms.
   2. The main symptoms are related to the thyrotoxicosis crisis with all the aspects included.
   3. The finding of thyroid disease is evident in all cases.
   4. Atrial fibrillation has never been registered.
      - (a) Only 1, 2, and 4 are correct.
      - (b) Only 2 is correct.
      - (c) Only 2 and 4 are correct.
      - (d) Only 4 is correct.
3. Among symptoms related to thyroid storm:
   1. Psychological signs could be developed with tremor and severe agitation.
   2. They can progress to severe psychosis, stupor, and coma.

3. Epilepticus status and stroke are very common.
4. Confusion and delirium may be present.
   (a) All answers are correct.
   (b) Only 1, 2, and 3 are correct.
   (c) Only 1, 2, and 4 are correct.
   (d) Only 4 is correct.

4. Regarding gastrointestinal symptoms:
   1. Abdominal pain, vomiting, and nausea may be present.
   2. It could suggest an abdominal surgical emergency.
   3. Liver dysfunction is frequently reported.
   4. Jaundice has been registered.
      (a) Only 1, 3, and 4 are correct.
      (b) Only 2 and 3 are correct.
      (c) Only 1 is correct.
      (d) All are correct.
5. Regarding the etiology of thyroid storm:
   1. Thyroid surgery is considered the most common cause.
   2. Autonomous interruption of drug administration exposes the patients to a higher risk during surgery.
   3. Use of radioiodine increased the risk of thyroid storm.
   4. Better preoperative preparation increases its incidence.
      (a) Only 1 and 2 are correct.
      (b) Only 1, 2, and 3 are correct.
      (c) Only 2, 3, and 4 are correct.
      (d) Only 1 is correct.
6. Among all precipitating factors of thyroid storm:
   1. Infection is considered the most common.
   2. Delivery is reported as a factor in case of unrecognized thyrotoxicosis.
   3. Major trauma is not reported as precipitating factor.
   4. They are not clearly identified in 25–43% of the patients.
      (a) Only 4 is correct.
      (b) All are correct.
      (c) Only 1, 2, and 4 are correct.
      (d) Only 2 and 4 are correct.
7. Concerning the diagnosis of thyroid storm:
   1. Early diagnosis is fundamental to reduce the incidence of a fatal outcome.
   2. It is based on clinical features.
   3. Burch and Wartofsky introduced a specific scoring system in 1993.
   4. More than 45 points in Burch and Wartofsky score system indicate the diagnosis of thyroid storm.
      (a) Only 1 and 3 are correct.
      (b) Only 2 and 4 are correct.
      (c) All are correct.
      (d) Only 1, 3, and 4 are correct.

8. With regard to the diagnosis of thyroid storm according to the Japanese Thyroid Association, it can be stated:
   1. The diagnosis is based on the association of thyrotoxicosis with other symptoms (central nervous system symptoms, fever, tachycardia, hearth failure, and gastrointestinal/hepatic symptoms)
   2. The suspected patient does not need to have an underlying diagnosis of thyrotoxicosis.
   3. The diagnosis of TS2 thyroid storm could be related to, at least, five features.
   4. The Japanese Thyroid Association scoring system is more sensitive and more specific than the Burch and Wartofsky scoring system.
      (a) All are correct.
      (b) Only 2 and 3 are correct.
      (c) Only 4 is correct.
      (d) Only 1 is correct.
9. The treatment option of thyroid storm is:
   1. An urgent operation
   2. Mainly based on drugs
   3. Immediate use of glucocorticoids
   4. Only beta-blockers are useful
      (a) Only 1 is correct.
      (b) Only 2 is correct.
      (c) Only 3 is correct.
      (d) Only 4 is correct.
10. The initial treatment for patients with clinical features of thyroid storm or severe thyrotoxicosis who do not fully meet the criteria for thyroid storm is:
    1. A beta-blocker (propranolol) and either propylthiouracil (PTU) or methimazole
    2. Glucocorticoids and beta-blockers
    3. Propylthiouracil only
    4. Methimazole only
       (a) Only 1 is correct.
       (b) Only 2 is correct.
       (c) Only 3 is correct.
       (d) Only 4 is correct.
11. In patients with thyroid storm or severe thyrotoxicosis:
    1. Glucocorticoids and iodine solutions are mandatory.
    2. Only glucocorticoids must be administrated the first hours.
    3. It is better to use iodine 1 h after the first dose of thionamide.
    4. Iodine blocks the release of T4 and T3 from the gland within hours.
       (a) Only 1 and 2 are correct.
       (b) Only 1 is correct.
       (c) Only 3 is correct.
       (d) Only 3 and 4 are correct.

12. In patients with airway problems and thyroid storm:
    1. Cardio-selective beta-blockers such as metoprolol or atenolol could be considered but with care.
    2. ICU treatment is mandatory.
    3. Only propranolol is effective.
    4. In patients with severe asthma who cannot take beta-blockers, rate control can be achieved with calcium-channel blockers such as diltiazem.
        (a) Only 1 and 2 are correct.
        (b) Only 2 and 3 are correct.
        (c) Only 1 and 4 are correct.
        (d) Only 4 is correct.
13. The best operation for patients with thyroid storm:
    1. Is total thyroidectomy
    2. Is subtotal thyroidectomy
    3. Depends on the pathology of the thyroid
    4. Must be postponed for 3 months
        (a) Only 1 and 4 are correct.
        (b) Only 1 is correct.
        (c) Only 2 is correct.
        (d) Only 3 and 4 are correct.
14. The operation is urgent:
    1. In every condition when thyroid storm is present
    2. If the patient is unable to take antithyroid drugs
    3. If the patient has no comorbidities
    4. If the patient is under the age of 40
        (a) Only 1 and 2 and 3 are correct.
        (b) Only 1 and 4 are correct.
        (c) Only 1 and 3 are correct.
        (d) Only 2 is correct.
15. Concerning the prognosis of thyroid storm:
    1. Recent reviews reported the mortality of treated thyroid storm to be less than 10%.
    2. It depends on early recognition and treatment.
    3. It still has a poor prognosis and high mortality.
    4. Multiorgan failure develops very often in thyroid storm.
        (a) Only 3 and 4 are correct.
        (b) Only 1 and 2 are correct.
        (c) Only 1 correct.
        (d) Only 2 is correct.

40.1 Introduction

Thyroid storm is a life-threatening medical emergency that results from an extreme hyperthyroidism with possible multiorgan dysfunction [1–6]. Even if this is a rare condition, it could be extremely dangerous and fatal if not treated in time.

It was first described by Lahey in 1926 as the "crisis of exophthalmic goiter" related to the patients who presented exacerbation of symptoms for Basedow-Graves' disease [7].

Today, this condition rarely occurs after thyroid operations. Nevertheless, it is important for surgeons to understand its clinical manifestations, pathophysiology, and the effective treatment.

Furthermore, thyroid storm could be precipitated by trauma, infections, or other causes, and patients with untreated or inadequately treated preexisting hyperthyroidism may require urgent operations [8, 9].

The contemporary involvement of cardiovascular system as well as the thermoregulatory, gastrointestinal, hepatic, and central nervous system is included in the actual definition as reported by Burch and Wartofsky [3] who develop a specific scoring system for diagnosis.

Actually, the diagnosis of this clinical condition is difficult for physicians even if different teams around the world tried to define clear diagnostic criteria to improve the treatment of thyroid storm and to decrease its mortality with early aggressive therapy and ICU (intensive care unit) support, when necessary.

Thyroid storm accounts for between 1% and 2% of all hospital admissions for thyrotoxicosis, but some reports estimate the incidence may be as high as 10% [3].

The decrease of incidence in the last years may be due to more frequent screening for thyroid blood test with subsequent early diagnosis of hyperthyroidism and prevention of thyroid storm with administration of medical therapy.

40.2 Clinical Presentation

Thyroid storm must be early recognized for prompt definition of medical therapy because it could be burdened by a mortality ranged from 8% to 25% in hospitalized populations according to the most recent reports [4, 9, 10].

The clinical presentation is mainly the thyrotoxicosis crisis with all the aspects included.

Fever is one of the most common symptoms, with temperature occasionally exceeding 40 °C, and is usually considered a leading factor in differentiating thyroid storm from non-storm thyrotoxicosis [9]. It must be treated because, if not, it could lead to the death of patients within 48 h. Patients with thyroid storm present warm skin and often flushing, with profuse diaphoresis. The finding of thyroid disease with diffuse goiter as well as exophthalmos may not be evident. It is possible to register tachycardia higher than 150 beats/min and atrial fibrillation as well as tachypnea, acute pulmonary edema, and ventricular dysfunction or heart failure [11–17]. Psychic signs and symptoms could be developed with tremor and severe agitation, emotional liability, confusion, and delirium that may progress to severe psychosis, stupor, and coma and rarely epilepticus status and stroke [18, 19].

Other symptoms could affect the gastrointestinal system like abdominal pain, vomiting, nausea, and diarrhea that should suggest an abdominal surgical emergency, and hepatomegaly, liver dysfunction, and jaundice sometimes indicate a hepatocellular dysfunction [20–24].

Leukocytosis occasionally is present especially with coexisting infections or trauma [25–27].

Diabetic ketoacidosis is rare in concomitancy of thyroid storm but could be dangerous for patients [28]. Then efforts should be made to maximize patient compliance to antithyroid and antidiabetic agents in treating such patients [4].

40.3 Natural History

Thyroid surgery has been considered the most common cause of thyroid storm, even if in the last years it has become rare because of a better preoperative therapeutic preparation of patients with administration of antithyroid and beta-blocker drugs. Furthermore, the increased use of radioiodine, especially in older patients, has decreased the incidence of this disorder. Among this subgroup of patients, there are some with incompletely treated hyperthyroidism or autonomous interruption of drug intake that expose them to an increased risk of thyroid storm during surgery [4].

A wide list of condition is reported in ► Box 40.1, like nonthyroidal surgery, major trauma, infection, imaging studies with iodinated contrast, and delivery in patients with unrecognized thyrotoxicosis [4, 29–32]. In all the cases, these conditions have the main role as precipitating factor of thyroid storm.

The basis of thyroid storm is essentially related to the pathophysiology of thyroid hormones.

The complete passages that lead from a simple toxicosis to a severe and multiorgan acute crisis are not well and completely known even if a major insult is required [32].

All the primary causes of hyperthyroidism can follow into acute crisis of thyroid storm even if the most common etiology is a history of Graves' disease [22, 33, 34]. Plummer disease and multinodular toxic goiter were reported as well as amiodarone-associated thyrotoxicosis or autoimmune thyroiditis.

Actually, infection is the most common cause of thyroid storm in the inpatient setting even if from 25% to 43% of the patients present without a clearly identifiable precipitating factor [3, 26, 30].

The mechanism underlying the pathogenesis of thyroid storm is not completely known. A dramatic increase in serum free T4 level is commonly observed and may precipitate the onset of thyroid storm. Additional factors such as poor nutrition and complicating medical, surgical, and emotional effects on thyroid hormone binding are other important contributors as well as increased catecholamines [35].

The development of heart failure and cardiomyopathy in case of thyroid storm is reported in 20 cases even if the mortality rate is nearly 25%. Recognizing this condition is imperative in preventing left ventricular dysfunction and cardiogenic shock and for early treatment with specific medical therapy.

Thyroid storm combined with thyroid cancer, primary hyperparathyroidism, or hypercalcemic crisis is reported [36–38]. Elevated serum calcium level could increase the action of T4 through the second messenger way with subsequent set off the crisis.

Box 40.1: Factors Precipitating the Thyroid Storm

Thyroid surgery/surgical storm
Non-thyroidal surgery
Trauma and sepsis
Infections (pneumonia)
Vigorous manipulation of the thyroid gland
Thyroiditis
Parturition burn
Myocardial infarct and pulmonary embolism
Cerebrovascular incidents
Medications such as anesthetics, salicylates, pseudoephedrine, and amiodarone
Interferon treatment
Radioactive iodine treatment
Exposure to iodinated contrast
Withdrawal of antithyroid treatment
Diabetic ketoacidosis
Hypoglycemia acute ingestion of high doses of thyroid hormone
Metastatic thyroid cancer
Struma ovarii
Molar pregnancy
H1N1 infection
Emotional stress
Intense exercise
Extreme hyperparathyroidism

40.4 Diagnosis

The successful management of thyroid storm is based on early diagnosis and therapy that must be started as soon as possible because a delay may increase the risk of a fatal outcome.

Serum concentration of triiodothyronine (T3), thyroxine (T4), and free T4 is usually nondiagnostic, because these tests are similar in patients with storm and non-storm thyrotoxicosis.

The real challenge of this clinical condition is the diagnosis.

Characteristic features such as Bayley's symptom complex of insomnia, anorexia, vomiting, diarrhea, marked sweating, and great emotional instability are reliable in predicting impending storm [39]. A temperature greater than 38 ° C, marked tachycardia, accentuated symptoms and signs of thyrotoxicosis, and central nervous system (CNS), cardiovascular, or gastrointestinal system dysfunction indicate storm [9, 10].

In 1993, Burch and Wartofsky [2] introduced a specific scoring system for the diagnosis of thyroid storm:

- Temperature: 5 points per 1 °F above 99 F (no more than 30 points)
- Central nervous system dysfunction: 10 points for mild (agitation), 20 points for moderate (delirium, psychosis, or extreme lethargy), and 30 points for severe (seizure or coma)
- Tachycardia: 5 points for 99–109, 10 points for 110–119, 15 points for 120–129, 20 points for 130–139, and 25 points for frequency greater than 140
- Presence of atrial fibrillation:10 points
- Heart failure: 5 points for mild (pedal edema), 10 points for moderate (bi-basilar rales), 15 points for severe (pulmonary edema)
- Gastrointestinal dysfunction: 10 points for moderate (diarrhea, nausea/vomiting, or abdominal pain) and 20 for severe (unexplained jaundice)
- Presence of precipitating factor: 10 points

A score of 25 to 44 using the scale of "Burch and Wartofsky" is suggestive of impending storm, and a score of 45 or higher is highly suggestive of storm. A score less than 25 points does not suggest a thyroid storm status. One should be aware that patients rarely have thyroid storm and apathetic thyrotoxicosis, coma, cerebral infarction, status epilepticus, rhabdomyolysis, and acute renal failure.

Another score system based on similar clinical findings has been defined in 2012 by the Japanese Thyroid Association [3, 30]. Thyrotoxicosis (elevated FT3 and/or FT4) is fundamental, but other different symptoms are required:

- Central nervous system symptoms (restlessness, delirium, psychosis/mental aberration, lethargy/somnolence, coma)
- Fever (38 C/100.4 F or greater)
- Tachycardia (130/min or higher)
- Hearth failure (pulmonary edema, rales, cardiogenic shock, or NYHA class IV)
- GI/hepatic manifestation (nausea, vomiting, diarrhea, total bilirubin 3 mg/dl or more)

The diagnosis has been made for thyroid storm (TS1): thyrotoxicosis (elevated FT3 and/or FT4) combined with:

- At least one central nervous system manifestation and one or more other symptoms (fever, tachycardia, cardiologic disease, gastrointestinal/hepatic) *or* a combination of at least three symptoms among GI/hepatic, hearth failure or tachycardia, and fever

  Thyroid storm (TS2) could be suspected with:
- Thyrotoxicosis (elevated FT3 and/or FT4)

- A combination of at least two features among tachycardia, hearth failure, gastrointestinal or liver dysfunction, and fever *or* a patient with thyroid disease and presence of goiter and exophthalmos who meets criteria for TS1 but TF hormones are not available

These scoring systems are guidelines albeit the actual diagnosis is based on clinical judgment. According to the Burch and Wartofsky scoring system, a score of 45 or more is more sensitive but less specific than JTA scoring systems TS1 or TS2 to detect thyroid storm cases. A chest X-ray may be done to assess heart failure. Head CT scan may help exclude a neurological cause in some patients. An ECG is often done to monitor arrhythmias.

Differential diagnosis could be made with sepsis, infection, psychosis, cocaine abuse, pheochromocytoma, neuroleptic malignant syndrome, and hyperthermia.

40.5 Treatment

The treatment options of thyroid storm are mainly based on drugs [1, 3, 4]. The therapeutic options for thyroid storm are varying from those used for uncomplicated hyperthyroidism, with additional drugs often used such as glucocorticoids and an iodine solution. Also support of the patient in an ICU is essential sometimes since the mortality rate of thyroid storm is 2.5–7% [5, 9, 11, 14]. The principles of treatment are based on clinical experience and case studies since there are no prospective studies. They are mostly used to patients with severe hyperthyroidism who do not fully suffer from thyroid storm. The therapeutic drugs are numerous, each of which has a different mechanism of action:

- A beta-blocker for the symptoms and signs provoked by increased adrenergic tone.
- A thionamide to block new hormone synthesis.
- An iodine solution for blocking the release of thyroid hormone.
- An iodinated radiocontrast agent (if available) to stop the peripheral conversion of T4 to T3.
- Glucocorticoids to reduce T4 to T3 conversion, activate vasomotor stability, reduce the autoimmune process in Graves' disease, and treat an associated relative adrenal insufficiency.
- Bile acid sequestrants may also benefit in severe cases the decrease of enterohepatic recycling of thyroid hormones [31–33, 39].

For patients with clinical features of thyroid storm or severe thyrotoxicosis who do not fully meet the criteria for thyroid storm, we begin treatment with a beta-blocker (propranolol) and either propylthiouracil (PTU) or methimazole. PTU is better than methimazole because of PTU's effect to decrease T4 to T3 conversion. One hour after the first dose of thionamide is taken, we administer iodine (saturated solution of potassium iodide [SSKI] or Lugol's solution) [40].

For patients with symptoms of thyroid storm, we also administer glucocorticoids (hydrocortisone). Cholestyramine may also be beneficial in severe cases to reduce enterohepatic recycling of thyroid hormones. Many patients require high amounts of fluid, but others may require diuresis because of congestive heart failure. Infection has to be identified and treated, and hyperpyrexia should be immediately corrected mainly with acetaminophen.

In patients with thyroid storm or severe thyrotoxicosis, it is mandatory immediate treatment with a beta-blocker. Japanese guidelines recommend esmolol over propranolol due to increased mortality in patients with congestive heart failure treated with propranolol [3, 40, 41]. If thyroid storm is accompanied by reactive airway disease, cardio-selective beta-blockers such as metoprolol or atenolol could be considered but with care. In patients with severe asthma who cannot take beta-blockers, rate control can be achieved with calcium-channel blockers such as diltiazem [41].

Thionamides inhibit thyroid hormone synthesis in 1–2 h after administration. But they have no effect on the release of hormones from the thyroid gland. For patients with thyroid storm or severe thyrotoxicosis, we begin immediate treatment with either PTU or methimazole [41, 42]:

- PTU is suggested for the acute treatment of life-threatening thyroid storm in an ICU setting.
- Methimazole is better for severe, but not life-threatening, hyperthyroidism due to longer duration of action and, after weeks of treatment, leads to more rapid normalization of serum T3 compared with PTU and also is less hepatotoxic.

The dose of thionamide given to patients with thyroid storm should be higher than that required to fully block thyroid hormone synthesis [43, 44].

Iopanoic acid and other iodinated radiocontrast agents used for oral cholecystography have been used to treat hyperthyroidism but with little data published for their use in thyroid storm. They are strong inhibitors of T4 to T3 conversion, and release of iodine in pharmacologic quantities from these agents has the important benefit of blocking thyroid hormone release [45, 46]. They have been useful in treating severe hyperthyroidism and preparing hyperthyroid patients for urgent surgery. Due to their iodinization, they should be given 1 h after the thionamide in order to prevent the iodine from being used as substrate for new hormone synthesis [47].

Iodine-containing solutions have mostly been used for the treatment of thyroid storm since iodine blocks the release of T4 and T3 from the gland within hours. In patients with thyroid storm or severe thyrotoxicosis, it is better to use iodine 1 h after the first dose of thionamide. Oral doses are potassium iodide-iodine (Lugol's) solution, or SSKI [48, 49].

Glucocorticoids also reduce the T4 to T3 conversion. In addition, they may have a direct effect on the underlying autoimmune process if the reason of thyroid storm is Graves' disease and treat potentially associated limited adrenal reserve. Glucocorticoids should not be used in patients with severe, but not life-threatening, hyperthyroidism [42, 50].

Thyroid hormones are metabolized in the liver and conjugated with glucuronide and sulfate, and their products are excreted in the bile. Free thyroid hormones are released and reabsorbed in the intestine. Bile acid sequestrants such as cholestyramine have been found to reduce thyroid hormone levels in thyrotoxic patients by interfering with enterohepatic circulation and recycling of thyroid hormone. They are useful adjunctive therapy in patients with thyroid storm but mostly in patients who are intolerant of thionamides [44, 51, 52].

Other therapies such plasmapheresis has been tried when traditional therapy has not been successful [12, 39, 53–56]. Plasmapheresis removes cytokines, antibodies, and thyroid hormones from plasma. Lithium also is used to block the release of thyroid hormone. However, it may provoke renal and neurologic toxicity [57–60].

In patients with Graves' disease, radioactive iodine or thyroidectomy as definitive therapy is important to prevent a recurrence of thyroid storm. Radioiodine therapy could be suggested as first choice for definitive therapy of hyperthyroidism in the absence of orbitopathy due to its lower cost and lower complication rate compared with surgery.

In summary, the treatment of thyroid storm is based on the reduction of thyroid hormone production and secretion. Further, the therapy must be directed against systemic disturbances, amelioration of the peripheral actions of thyroid hormones, and treatment of any precipitating or underlying illness (► Box 40.2).

After the thyroid storm has been treated, permanent treatment of the hyperthyroidism should be administered. The initial therapy should be slowly diminished after the acute hospitalization, and the patient should be closely followed as an outpatient before definitive therapy. Many of the patients will receive iodine therapy as part of their acute treatment strategy. During this interval period, it is important to continue thionamides and check thyroid function to assess stabilization. If surgery is planned, preparation and control of hyperthyroidism should be accomplished prior to operation. Finally, continuation of therapy with thionamide agents is an alternative in those patients.

Box 40.2: Treatment of Thyroid Storm

1. *Reduction of thyroid hormone synthesis and secretion*

   Inhibition of T4 and T3 synthesis: propylthiouracil and methimazole

   Inhibition of T4 and T3 secretion: potassium iodide, Lugol's solution, radiographic contrast agents, iopanoic, acid, lithium, thyroidectomy
2. *Therapy directed against systemic disorders*

   Treatment of fever: acetaminophen

   Correction of volume and nutrition: iv fluids and electrolytes, glucose, vitamins

   Supportive therapy: oxygen, vasopressor drugs

   Treatment of congestive heart failure: diuretics, digoxin
3. *Amelioration of the peripheral actions of thyroid hormones*

   Inhibition of extrathyroidal conversion of T4 to T3: propylthiouracil, radiographic contrast agents, glucocorticoids, propranolol

   Removal of T4 and T3 from serum: cholestyramine, plasmapheresis, hemodialysis, hemoperfusion
4. *Treatment of any precipitating or underlying illness*

40.6 Indications for Surgery and Surgical Details

The indications for surgery are the same with those who have to be operated on due to hyperthyroidism. The operation indicated is total thyroidectomy. Before surgery though, thyroid storm must be treated and the patient should be euthyroid. The main indication for urgent operation is if the patient is unable to take antithyroid drugs and all the drugs mentioned above. Also another category of urgent operation is those patients who clinically deteriorate or do not improve within 24–48 h despite intensive medical treatment, develop side effects from the treatment, or need immediate treatment of their hyperthyroidism due to severe underlying cardiac or pulmonary comorbidities. Surgery is mandatory for patients with hyperthyroidism due to a very large or obstructive goiter [9, 41, 61].

Some patients are unable to continue thionamides due to side effects such as agranulocytosis or hepatotoxicity or because of allergy. In those patients who need urgent treatment of hyperthyroidism, thyroidectomy is the treatment of choice. Also, there is a category of patients who are in coma due to hyperthyroidism and cannot be treated with drugs, and plasmapheresis might be a treatment of choice. In case reports, when therapy with drugs mentioned above has not been successful, plasmapheresis has been used to prepare patients with thyroid storm for thyroid surgery. Iodinated contrast agents have also been used to prepare patients for urgent surgery, but they are no longer available in many countries. In those patients, total thyroidectomy might be a useful addition in the definitive treatment of thyroid storm [5, 39, 55].

If an operation is mandatory, treatment is recommended to be continued for up to 5–7 days. Surgery should not be delayed for more than 8–10 days. The reason is a phenomenon called escape from the Wolff-Chaikoff effect. High doses of exogenous iodine inhibit the organification of iodine in the thyroid gland (the Wolff-Chaikoff effect). This effect is mostly transient. The iodide transport system is able to adapt to higher concentrations of iodine, allowing thyroid hormone synthesis, with potential exacerbation of thyrotoxicosis [41, 62].

40.7 Outcomes and Prognosis

The outcomes of thyroid storm depend mainly on the immediate delivery of the appropriate treatments described previously. Initial case series described mortality rates as high as 37.5%, but more recent reviews report the mortality of treated thyroid storm to be at 10.7%. This can be due to the advances made in treatment options and in earlier recognition of this endocrine emergency. In a Japanese survey with cases of thyroid storm, multiorgan failure and congestive heart failure were the main causes of death [41].

Even when mortality is avoided, significant morbidity, such as brain injury, diffuse atrophy of the muscles, cerebrovascular disease, renal function impairment, and even psychosis, can lead to long-term complications.

Answers to the Questions

1. (a); 2. (b); 3. (c); 4. (d); 5. (a); 6. (c); 7. (c); 8. (d); 9. (b); 10. (a); 11. (d); 12. (c); 13. (b); 14. (d); 15. (b)

References

1. Ross DS, Burch HB, Cooper DS, Greenlee MC, Laurberg P, Maia AL, Rivkees SA, Samuels M, Sosa JA, Stan MN, Walter MA. 2016 American Thyroid Association guidelines for diagnosis and management of hyperthyroidism and other causes of thyrotoxicosis. Thyroid. 2016;26(10):1343–421.
2. Burch HB, Wartofsky L. Life-threatening thyrotoxicosis. Thyroid storm. Endocrinol Metab Clin North Am. 1993;22(2):263–77.
3. Akamizu T, Satoh T, Isozaki O, Suzuki A, Wakino S, Iburi T, Tsuboi K, Monden T, Kouki T, Otani H, Teramukai S, Uehara R, Nakamura Y, Nagai M, Mori M, Japan Thyroid Association. Diagnostic criteria, clinical features, and incidence of thyroid storm based on nationwide surveys. Thyroid. 2012;22(7):661–79.
4. Angell TE, Lechner MG, Nguyen CT, Salvato VL, Nicoloff JT, LoPresti JS. Clinical features and hospital outcomes in thyroid storm: a retrospective cohort study. J Clin Endocrinol Metab. 2015;100(2):451–9.
5. Sarlis NJ, Gourgiotis L. Thyroid emergencies. Rev Endocr Metab Disord. 2003;4(2):129–36.
6. Nayak B, Burman K. Thyrotoxicosis and thyroid storm. Endocrinol Metab Clin N Am. 2006;35(4):663–86.
7. Lahey FH. Apathetic thyroidism. Ann Surg. 1931;93(5):1026–30.
8. Tietgens ST, Leinung MC. Thyroid storm. Med Clin North Am. 1995;79(1):169–84.

9. Chiha M, Samarasinghe S, Kabaker AS. Thyroid storm: an updated review. J Intensive Care Med. 2015;30(3):131–40.
10. Pokhrel B, Aiman W, Bhusal K. Thyroid storm. In: StatPearls. Treasure Island: StatPearls Publishing; 2020.
11. Jacobi J. Management of endocrine emergencies in the ICU. J Pharm Pract. 2019;32(3):314–26.
12. Ba JH, Wu BQ, Wang YH, Shi YF. Therapeutic plasma exchange and continuous renal replacement therapy for severe hyperthyroidism and multi-organ failure: a case report. World J Clin Cases. 2019;7(4):500–7.
13. Neiva J, Fernandes G, Carvalho D, Ferreira B, Duarte R, Araújo R. Thyroid storm and myxoedema: two reversible causes of acute heart failure. Acute Med. 2018;17(4):229–31.
14. Ringel MD. Management of hypothyroidism and hyperthyroidism in the intensive care unit. Crit Care Clin. 2001;17(1):59–74.
15. Klein I, Danzi S. Thyroid disease and the heart. Circulation. 2007;116(15):1725–35.
16. Klein I, Ojamaa K. Thyroid hormone and the cardiovascular system. N Engl J Med. 2001;344(7):501–9.
17. Eliades M, El-Maouche D, Choudhary C, Zinsmeister B, Burman KD. Takotsubo cardiomyopathy associated with thyrotoxicosis: a case report and review of the literature. Thyroid. 2014;24(2):383–9.
18. Lee TG, Ha CK, Lim BH. Thyroid storm presenting as status epilepticus and stroke. Postgrad Med J. 1997;73(855):61.
19. Ishii M. Endocrine emergencies with neurologic manifestations. Continuum (Minneap Minn). 2017;23(3, Neurology of Systemic Disease):778–801.
20. Choudhary AM, Roberts I. Thyroid storm presenting with liver failure. J Clin Gastroenterol. 1999;29(4):318–21.
21. Dillmann WH. Thyroid storm. Curr Ther Endocrinol Metab. 1997;6: 81–5.
22. Lee CH, Lin HD. Thyroid emergencies: thyroid storm and myxedema coma. In: Clark OH, Duh QY, Kebebew E, editors. Textbook of endocrine surgery. 2nd ed. Philadelphia: Elsevier Saunders; 2005. p. 216–9.
23. Wartofsky L. Thyrotoxic storm. In: Braverman L, Utiger R, editors. Werner and Ingbar's the thyroid. 8th ed. Philadelphia: Lippincott Williams and Wilkins; 2000. p. 679–84.
24. Harwood-Nuss AL, Martel TJ. An unusual cause of abdominal pain in a young woman. Ann Emerg Med. 1991;20(5):574–82.
25. Vora NM, Fedok F, Stack BC Jr. Report of a rare case of trauma induced thyroid storm. Ear Nose Throat J. 2002;81(8):570–2, 4.
26. Migneco A, Ojetti V, Testa A, De Lorenzo A, Gentiloni SN. Management of thyrotoxic crisis. Eur Rev Med Pharmacol Sci. 2005;9(1):69–74.
27. Yanai H, Hakoshima M, Katsuyama H. Clinical, biochemical, hematological, endocrinological and immunological differences between Graves' disease patients with and without thyroid storm. J Clin Med Res. 2019;11(6):452–7.
28. Rathish D, Karalliyadda S. Concurrent presentation of thyroid storm and diabetic ketoacidosis: a systematic review of previously reported cases. BMC Endocr Disord. 2019;19(1):49.
29. Goodier CG. Endocrine emergencies in obstetrics. Clin Obstet Gynecol. 2019;62(2):339–46.
30. Akamizu T. Thyroid storm: a Japanese perspective. Thyroid. 2018;28(1):32–40.
31. Swinburne JL, Kreisman SH. A rare case of subacute thyroiditis causing thyroid storm. Thyroid. 2007;17(1):73–6.
32. Brooks MH, Waldstein SS. Free thyroxine concentrations in thyroid storm. Ann Intern Med. 1980;93(5):694–7.
33. Feldt-Rasmussen U, Emerson CH. Further thoughts on the diagnosis and diagnostic criteria for thyroid storm. Thyroid. 2012;22(11):1094–5.
34. Stathatos N, Wartofsky L. Thyrotoxic storm. J Intensive Care Med. 2002;17(1):1–7.

35. Bilezikian JP, Loeb JN. The influence of hyperthyroidism and hypothyroidism on alpha- and beta-adrenergic receptor systems and adrenergic responsiveness. Endocr Rev. 1983;4(4):378–88.
36. Naito Y, Sone T, Kataoka K, Sawada M, Yamazaki K. Thyroid storm due to functioning metastatic thyroid carcinoma in a burn patient. Anesthesiology. 1997;87(2):433–5.
37. Yokomoto M, Minamoto M, Utsunomiya D, Umakoshi H, Fukuoka T, Kondo S. Hypercalcemic crisis due to primary hyperparathyroidism occurring concomitantly with Graves' disease. Intern Med. 2015;54(7):813–8.
38. Chen K, Xie Y, Zhao L, Mo Z. Hyperthyroidism-associated hypercalcemic crisis: a case report and review of the literature. Medicine (Baltimore). 2017;96(4):e6017.
39. Wyble AJ, Moore SC, Yates SG. Weathering the storm: a case of thyroid storm refractory to conventional treatment benefiting from therapeutic plasma exchange. J Clin Apher. 2018;33(6):678–81.
40. Brunette DD, Rothong C. Emergency department management of thyrotoxic crisis with esmolol. Am J Emerg Med. 1991;9:232.
41. Isozaki O, Satoh T, Wakino S, Suzuki A, Iburi T, Tsuboi K, Kanamoto N, Otani H, Furukawa Y, Teramukai S, Akamizu T. Treatment and management of thyroid storm: analysis of the nationwide surveys: the taskforce committee of the Japan Thyroid Association and Japan Endocrine Society for the establishment of diagnostic criteria and nationwide surveys for thyroid storm. Clin Endocrinol. 2016;84(6):912.
42. Andrade Luz I, Pereira T, Catorze N. Thyroid storm: a case of haemodynamic failure promptly reversed by aggressive medical therapy with antithyroid agents and steroid pulse. BMJ Case Rep. 2018;14:11(1).
43. Carroll R, Matfin G. Endocrine and metabolic emergencies: thyroid storm. Ther Adv Endocrinol Metab. 2010;1(3):139–45.
44. Solomon BL, Wartofsky L, Burman KD. Adjunctive cholestyramine therapy for thyrotoxicosis. Clin Endocrinol. 1993;38:39.
45. Langley RW, Burch HB. Perioperative management of the thyrotoxic patient. Endocrinol Metab Clin N Am. 2003;32(2):519–34. https://doi.org/10.1016/s0889-8529(03)00010-0. PMID: 12800544.
46. Pandey CK, Raza M, Dhiraaj S, Agarwal A, Singh PK. Rapid preparation of severe uncontrolled thyrotoxicosis due to Graves' disease with Iopanoic acid--a case report. Can J Anaesth. 2004;51(1):38–40.
47. Deng Y, Zheng W, Zhu J. Successful treatment of thyroid crisis accompanied by hypoglycemia, lactic acidosis, and multiple organ failure. Am J Emerg Med. 2012;30(9):2094 e2095–6.
48. Davies TF, Larsen PR. Thyrotoxicosis. In: Kronenberg H, Melmed S, Polonsky K, Larsen PR, editors. Williams textbook of endocrinology. 11th ed. Philadelphia: Saunders Elsevier; 2007. p. 333–75.
49. Piantanida E. Preoperative management in patients with Graves' disease. Gland Surg. 2017;6(5):476–81. https://doi.org/10.21037/gs.2017.05.09.
50. Cooper DS. Anti-thyroid drugs. N Engl J Med. 2005;352(9):905–17.
51. Suwansaksri N, Preechasuk L, Kunavisarut T. Nonthionamide drugs for the treatment of hyperthyroidism: from present to future. Int J Endocrinol. 2018;2018:5794054.
52. Fumarola A, Di Fiore A, Dainelli M, Grani G, Calvanese A. Medical treatment of hyperthyroidism: state of the art. Exp Clin Endocrinol Diabetes. 2010;118(10):678–84.
53. Ngo SY, Chew HC. When the storm passes unnoticed—a case series of thyroid storm. Resuscitation. 2007;73(3):485–90.
54. Carhill A, Gutierrez A, Lakhia R, Nalini R. Surviving the storm: two cases of thyroid storm successfully treated with plasmapheresis. BMJ Case Rep. 2012;2012:006696.
55. Simsir IY, Ozdemir M, Duman S, Erdogan M, Donmez A, Ozgen AG. Therapeutic plasmapheresis in thyrotoxic patients. Endocrine. 2018;62(1):144–8.

56. Miller A, Silver KD. Thyroid storm with multiorgan failure treated with plasmapheresis. Case Rep Endocrinol. 2019;2019:2475843.
57. Szczepiorkowski ZM, Bandarenko N, Kim HC, et al. Guidelines on the use of therapeutic apheresis in clinical practice: evidence-based approach from the Apheresis Applications Committee of the American Society for Apheresis. J Clin Apher. 2007;22(3):106–75.
58. Ezer A, Caliskan K, Parlakgumus A, Belli S, Kozanoglu I, Yildirim S. Preoperative therapeutic plasma exchange in patients with thyrotoxicosis. J Clin Apher. 2009;24(3):111–4.
59. Ashkar FS, Katims RB, Smoak WM 3rd, Gilson AJ. Thyroid storm treatment with blood exchange and plasmapheresis. JAMA. 1970;214(7):1275–9. Muller C, Perrin P, Faller B, Richter S, Chantrel F. Role of plasma exchange in the thyroid storm. Ther Apher Dial. 2011;15(6):522–31.
60. Chen JH, Yeh JH, Lai HW, Liao CS. Therapeutic plasma exchange in patients with hyperlipidemic pancreatitis. World J Gastroenterol. 2004;10(15):2272–4.
61. Scholz GH, Hagemann E, Arkenau C, et al. Is there a place for thyroidectomy in older patients with thyrotoxic storm and cardiorespiratory failure? Thyroid. 2003;13(10):933–40.
62. Woeber KA. Iodine and thyroid disease. Med Clin North Am. 1991;75(1):169–78.

Hypercalcemic Crisis

Denise Carneiro-Pla, Roswitha Koeberle-Wuehrer, and Carmen C. Solórzano

Contents

A. L. Shifrin et al. (eds.), *Endocrine Surgery Comprehensive Board Exam Guide*,
https://doi.org/10.1007/978-3-030-84737-1_41

Case

A 53-year-old female presented to the emergency room with severe nausea and vomiting, along with mental status changes. She reported weakness and trouble swallowing over the last few months, and in the last few days, she suffered from polyuria and nocturia. The patient reports a history of gastrointestinal infection for the past 3 days. Although she denied hypercalcemia, previous laboratory tests showed calcium levels ranging from 10.5 to 10.8 mg/dL (2.62–2.69 mmol/L) over 4 years. No other significant medical history was reported. Laboratory tests revealed corrected total serum calcium of 19.6 mg/dL (4.9 mmol/L) and a creatinine of 2.4 mg/dL (NR 0.6–1.1 mg/dL). The patient was also anuric. The PTH level was 971 pg/mL (102 pmol/L). After aggressive hydration with intravenous fluids, her calcium decreased to 12 mg/dL (2.9 mmol/L). Other causes of hypercalcemia, such as sarcoidosis, calcium intake, malignancy, multiple myeloma, and hyperthyroidism, were ruled out. Despite aggressive hydration, corrected calcium levels ranged from 10.9 to 11.5 mg/dL (2.72–2.87 mmol/L). The endocrine surgical team was consulted. Neck ultrasound (◘ Fig. 41.1a, b) was performed, and a large right hypoechoic lesion was found posterior to the thyroid lobe with possible infiltration into the thyroid lobe. CT scan of the neck is shown in ◘ Fig. 41.2. The preoperative laryngoscopy diagnosed the symmetric movement of the vocal cords. While medical management with IV fluids, loop diuretics, bisphosphonate, and calcimimetics was maintained, the surgical team planned parathyroidectomy during the index hospitalization.

Intraoperatively, the parathyroid gland was large, and tissue planes with the thyroid were obscured. The lesion also extended behind the right recurrent laryngeal nerve, between the esophagus and trachea, and reached the left lobe of the thyroid. Because of the above findings, parathyroid cancer was suspected even though on palpation, the consistency of the parathyroid lesion was soft. The right thyroid lobe was resected en bloc with the right superior parathyroid gland with care not to violate the parathyroid capsule. There was no lymphadenopathy (◘ Figs. 41.3 and 41.4).

Intraoperative PTH was monitored with a pre-incision level of 1103 pg/mL (116 pmol/L). The 10-minute PTH sample was collected after the en bloc resection, and it had dropped significantly to 164 pg/mL (17 pmol/L). This adequate PTH drop from a very high initial level suggested that the remaining glands were not overproducing PTH and the procedure was terminated. PTH at wound closure assured further reduction in PTH to 83 pg/mL (8.8 pmol/L). On postoperative day 1, calcium level was 10.3 mg/dL with PTH of 20 pg/mL (2.1 pmol/L), and calcium levels continued to drop to within normal limits over the next day. Oral calcium supplementation was started on postoperative day 2 to prevent severe hypocalcemia. Vitamin D was low preoperatively and was aggressively replaced with ergocalciferol 50,000 IU once a week for 6 weeks. The calcium level was within the normal range at 9.2 mg/dL with PTH of 52 pg/mL (5.5 pmol/L) 1 month postoperatively as well as creatinine 1.1 mg/dL. Final pathology revealed a giant parathyroid adenoma with cystic changes without signs of malignancy (5.5 cm) and normal right thyroid lobe.

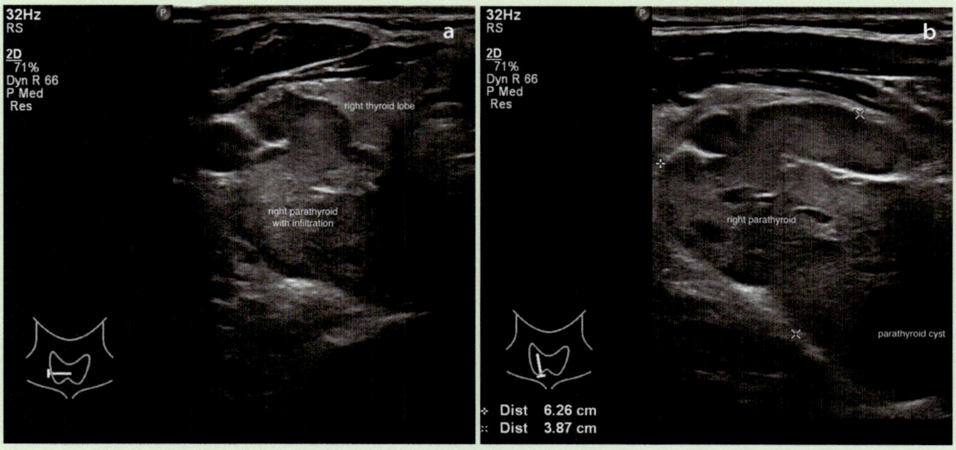

Fig. 41.1 Traverse and longitudinal ultrasound views of the neck demonstrating the right thyroid gland and a large right parathyroid extending posteriorly and inferiorly in the neck with signs of infiltration into the thyroid. (Courtesy of T. Lutz institute of radiology KSBL)

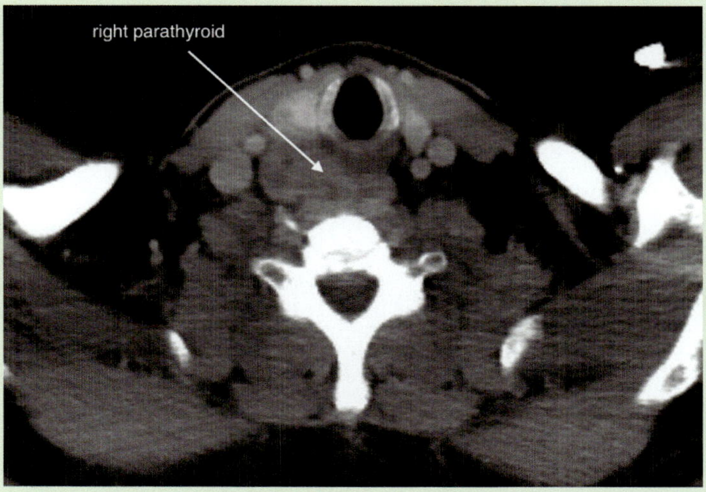

Fig. 41.2 Computed tomography scan axial views showing the extension of the parathyroid between trachea and esophagus which was not evident on the ultrasound. (Courtesy of T. Lutz Institute of Radiology KSBL)

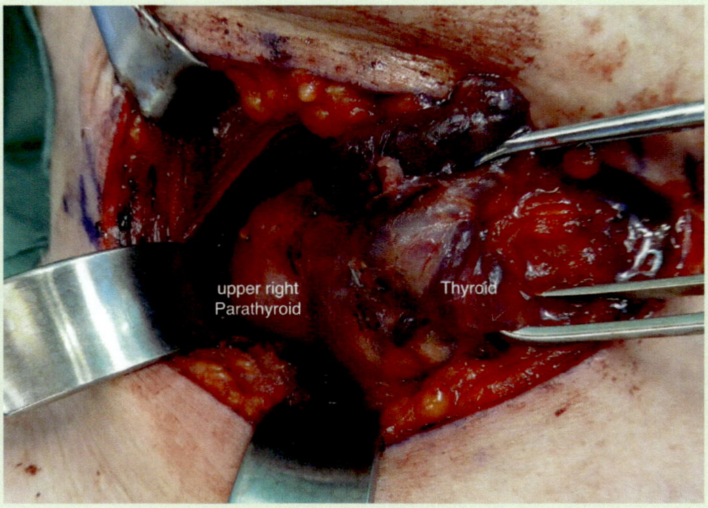

Fig. 41.3 Surgical field showing the right thyroid lobe and a large posteriorly located parathyroid gland intimately related to the thyroid

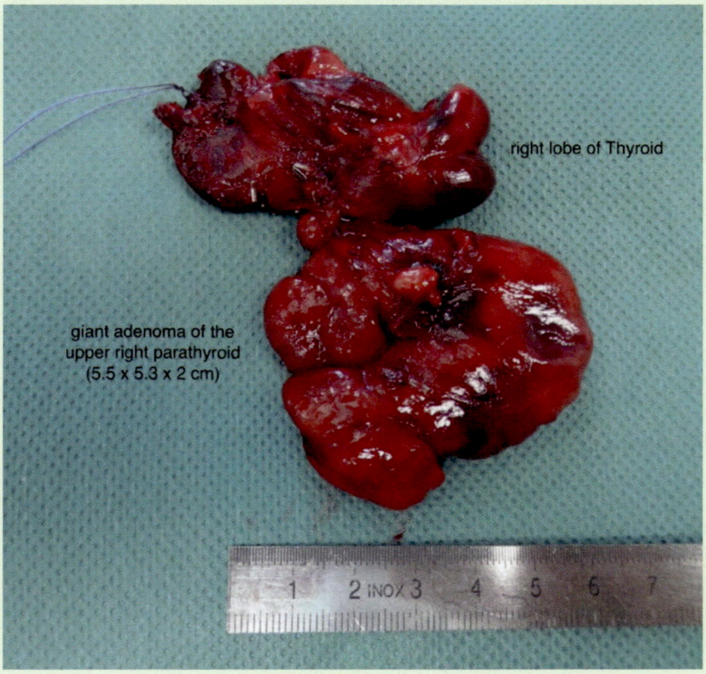

Fig. 41.4 Surgical specimen including right thyroid lobe and right superior parathyroid gland

Questions

1. In patients with hypercalcemic crisis (HC) caused by hyperparathyroidism, the *most common* parathyroid pathology observed is:
   1. Multiple gland disease
   2. Parathyroid adenoma
   3. Parathyroid carcinoma
   4. Parathyroid cyst
   5. Atypical parathyroid adenoma
      - (a) 1 and 3
      - (b) 1, 3, and 5
      - (c) 1, 2, 3, and 4
      - (d) 2
      - (e) All are correct.
2. The possible causes of HC include:
   1. Osteitis fibrosa cystica
   2. Lytic bone metastases
   3. Paraneoplastic tumor production of PTHrp
   4. Primary hyperparathyroidism
   5. Severe osteoporosis with fragility fractures
      - (a) 1 and 2
      - (b) 1, 2, and 3
      - (c) 2, 3, and 4
      - (d) 1, 2, 3, and 4
      - (e) All are correct.
3. A 25-year-old pregnant patient presents with dehydration, nausea, vomiting, fatigue, and a calcium level of 18 mg/dL (4.49 mmol/L) with a PTH level of 560 pg/mL (59.3 pmol/L). The *initial* management should include?
   1. Immediate CT scan with IV contrast to look for the location of the parathyroid
   2. Immediate and liberal use of bisphosphonates to decrease calcium levels
   3. Immediate and liberal use of cinacalcet to reduce calcium level
   4. Immediate i.v. hydration with normal saline or lactated ringers to decrease calcium levels
   5. Loop diuretics to induce calciuria once the patient is hydrated
      - (a) 1 and 2
      - (b) 4 and 5
      - (c) 1, 4, and 5
      - (d) 1, 2, and 3
      - (e) All are correct.

4. During a parathyroidectomy, for a patient originally admitted with HC, a large 4-cm firm parathyroid attached to the thyroid lobe without a plane and no enlarged lymph nodes was noted. A preoperative sestamibi scan and ultrasound showed a right lower cervical parathyroid. Which is the appropriate management of this patient?
   1. Obtain an intraoperative ultrasound to evaluate the thyroid.
   2. Examine the ipsilateral central neck for any involvement of other organs or structures.
   3. Excise the parathyroid and right thyroid lobe en bloc and also remove the central lymph nodes prophylactically.
   4. Excise the parathyroid and the right lobe of the thyroid en bloc.
   5. Carefully excise the parathyroid and the central lymph nodes without violating the capsule.
      (a) 1, 2, and 3
      (b) 2 and 3
      (c) Only 5
      (d) 2 and 4
      (e) 1, 2, and 4
5. Which localization studies have the highest accuracy and are most appropriate in a patient with HC and anuria?
   1. Surgeon-performed cervical US
   2. Four-dimensional CT scan with IV contrast
   3. MRI of the neck
   4. Sestamibi scan
   5. Sestamibi with SPECT/CT
      (a) 1, 3, 4, and 5
      (b) 1 and 5
      (c) 1, 3, and 4
      (d) 1, 2, and 3
      (e) All are correct.
6. A 55-year-old male presenting with HC has preoperative calcium of 13 mg/dL (3.24 mmol/L) and PTH of 670 pg/mL (71 pmol/L) and creatinine 1.8 mg/dL just before his parathyroid operation. On postoperative day 1, total serum calcium is 10.5 mg/dL (2.62 mmol/L) with a PTH level of 30 pg/mL (3.1 pmol/L). This biochemical presentation is likely due to:
   1. Persistent hyperparathyroidism
   2. Vitamin D deficiency
   3. Slow decrease of postoperative calcium levels in a successfully treated patient
   4. Sarcoidosis
   5. Renal insufficiency
      (a) Only 3
      (b) 1 and 2
      (c) 2 and 3
      (d) 1, 2, and 4
      (e) All are correct.

7. A 52-year-old female was admitted with total serum calcium 15 mg/dL (3.74 mmol/L) and was found to have a PTH of 35 mg/dL (3.7 pmol/L). The surgical team was consulted for the possible diagnosis of primary hyperparathyroidism. The sestamibi scan is shown in the figure below. What is the likely diagnosis(es) of this patient?

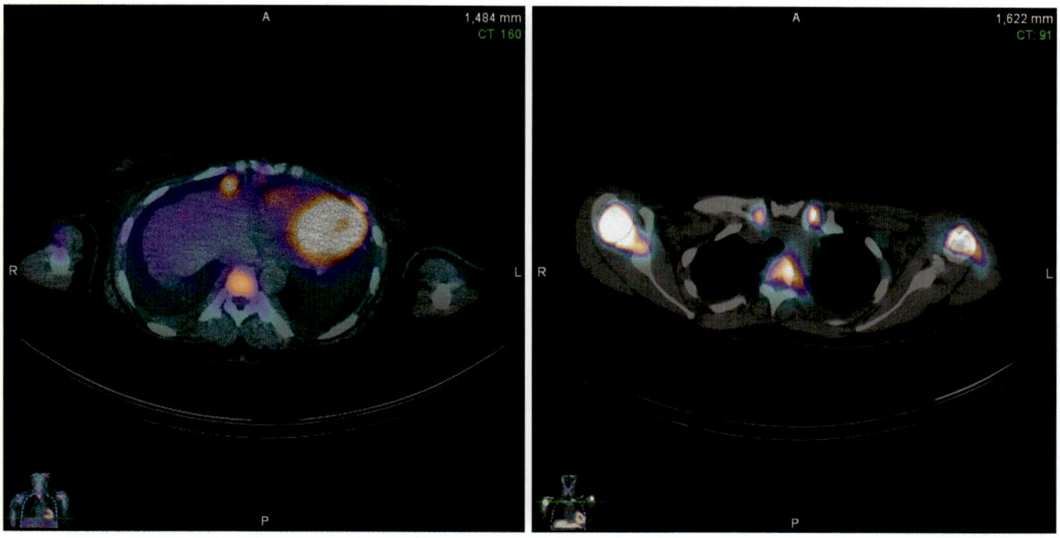

1. Sarcoidosis
2. Multiple myeloma
3. Primary hyperparathyroidism with inappropriate secretion of PTH
4. Parathyroid cancer with metastasis
5. Breast cancer with bone metastasis
   (a) Only 3
   (b) 1 and 3
   (c) 2 and 3
   (d) 3 and 4
   (e) Only 2

8. A 48-year-old male with a history of HC presents with PTH levels of 90 pg/mL (9.5 pmol/L) (NR 17–72 pg/mL or 1.8–7.6 pmol/L) 7 days after parathyroidectomy. Total serum calcium levels are 8.7 mg/dL (2.17 mmol/L) (NR 8.7–10.2 mg/dL or 2.17–2.54 mmol/L), and vitamin D level is 24 ng/mL (NR 30–80 ng/mL). This PTH elevation is likely due to:
1. Persistent hyperparathyroidism
2. Parathyroid cancer
3. Vitamin D deficiency
4. Hungry bone syndrome
5. Multiple myeloma
   (a) 1 and 2
   (b) 1 and 3

   (c) 3 and 4
   (d) 5 and 3
   (e) Only 2
9. A 75-year-old woman presents with HC symptoms. Which of her medications could have triggered severely elevated calcium levels?
   1. Calcium antagonist
   2. Thiazide diuretic
   3. Thyroid hormone replacement
   4. Vitamin D supplement
   5. Lithium
      (a) Only 3
      (b) 1 and 3
      (c) 2 and 3
      (d) 2, 4, and 5
      (e) All of the above
10. A 72-year-old woman was admitted with progressive weakness, obstipation, and nausea over the last few months. She suffers from schizoaffective disorder and osteoporosis treated with bisphosphonates and calcium supplementation. A month later, her calcium level was 18 mg/dL (4.49 mmol/L), and she developed rapid renal function decline. Further laboratory work revealed leukocytosis, elevated CRP, and PTH level of 25 pg/mL (2.6 pmol/L). She had no lymphadenopathy or pulmonary lesions. Physical exam showed tenderness to percussion over both kidneys. This patient shortly after required hemodialysis for renal failure, and a kidney biopsy was performed. What is a possible diagnosis?
    1. Nephritis
    2. Nephrolithiasis
    3. Sarcoidosis
    4. Hyperparathyroidism
    5. Hypercalcemic crisis due to malignancy
       (a) Only 3
       (b) 1 and 2
       (c) 2 and 4
       (d) 1, 2, and 4
       (e) All of the above

41.1 Introduction

41

Hypercalcemic crisis (HC) is a rare but potentially life-threatening medical emergency induced by calcium intoxication. It impacts numerous organ systems and requires acute hospitalization. An agreed definition does not exist, but HC is usually considered with calcium levels exceeding 14 mg/dL (>3.5 mmol/L) and acute symptoms of calcium intoxication, which can be reversed by correcting the hypercalcemia [1, 2].

A variety of clinical conditions can cause compensated hypercalcemia, but mainly primary hyperparathyroidism (PHPT) and advanced malignancy can decompensate from a chronic disease to HC [3]. Neurological, gastrointestinal, renal, and cardiovascular symptoms may develop first subtly but lead to subsequent rapid deterioration. When HC is recognized, immediate medical treatment has to follow irrelevant of the cause. After the patient is medically stabilized, in the case of HC due to PHPT, parathyroidectomy in expert hands treats the underlying disorder with low morbidity and mortality. Modern intensive care of these critically ill patients and preoperative medical management are essential to avoid mortality, which is reduced to <4.5% for HC due to PHPT. Underlying pathologies are parathyroid adenomas and carcinomas in >85% and 4% of cases, respectively. Following localization studies such as ultrasound, SPECT Tc-99 m sestamibi scan (MIBI), 18F-fluorocholine-PET-CT, and/or four-dimensional computed tomography (4D CT), surgery can be planned [4]. According to the suspected underlying parathyroid pathology, surgery can be performed as minimally invasive parathyroidectomy, bilateral exploration, or with en bloc resections of the ipsilateral thyroid lobe when parathyroid carcinoma is suspected intraoperatively. When appropriate, minimally invasive focused parathyroidectomy has proven successful with excellent short- and long-term outcomes [5]. Early diagnosis and prompt, effective treatment improve prognosis [6].

41.2 Clinical Presentation

The onset of symptoms of HC is variable. There is no clear correlation between serum calcium level and hypercalcemic symptoms. Most patients are symptomatic at calcium levels of >14 g/dL (>3.5 mmol/L) but may be asymptomatic at levels as high as 20 mg/dL (5 mmol/L), while others might have crisis symptoms at levels of <14 mg/dL (>3.5 mmol/L) [7]. A variety of clinical conditions can cause HC, which will be discussed below.

Symptoms of crisis are dehydration, often leading to impairment in the neurocognitive, renal, gastrointestinal, and cardiovascular systems. Simultaneous symptoms are more suggestive of HC, but clinical findings can be subtle, particularly if isolated symptoms are present. Therefore, clinicians should have a high index of suspicion [8]. Fortunately, calcium levels are now part of automated routine laboratory tests assisting in the early diagnosis of HC.

Neurologic symptoms present in the mild stages of hypercalcemia as anxiety, depression, lack of concentration/initiative, headache, insomnia, and fatigue. Severe hypercalcemia is hallmarked by altered mental status, psychosis, confusion, lethargy, somnolence, and coma. Hypercalcemia-induced delirium has been described with sudden alterations of mental status, accompanied by auditory hallucinations, paranoia, and persecutory delusions [8]. High calcium levels can be a catalyst for neuronal demise. Excitotoxicity and alteration of key neurotransmitters lead to altered mental status and psychotic presentations [9, 10]. This neuropsychiatric manifestation is easily missed particularly in the elderly population due to overlapping symptoms with aging and dementia [10].

Musculoskeletal complaints and fatigue were the most common symptoms in one of the largest retrospective reports of parathyroidectomy for the treatment of HC [5].

Renal symptoms comprise polyuria, nocturia, and polydipsia referred to as *diabetes hypercalcemicus*. Hypercalcemia has a diuretic effect, and it is accompanied by potassium loss leading to hypokalemia [8]. Chronic renal manifestations are kidney stones and nephrocalcinosis. When hypercalcemia reaches a critical level of >16 mg/dL (4 mmol/L), polyuria may develop into oliguria and finally into anuria, especially in the case of exsiccosis [7]. When hypercalcemia goes untreated, renal deficiency can be lethal.

Intestinal symptoms are anorexia, malaise, constipation, nausea, vomiting, and abdominal pain. High levels of calcium can increase gastric acid production causing peptic ulcers and increase pancreatic enzymes resulting in pancreatitis, which is a severe complication.

Cardiac symptoms are shortened QT interval and tachycardia and seldom ventricular tachycardia. High calcium and PTH levels have arrhythmogenic potential through calcium inflow into myocardial cells [11]. Chronic hyperparathyroidism induces hypertension, which is not clearly understood.

Bone disease with changes in bone mineral density (BMD) such as osteopenia and osteoporosis, especially in the distal radius, is adverse effect of PHPT and develops over time with compensated serum calcium levels. Osteitis fibrosa cystica with cystic bone lesions, brown tumors, and subperiosteal resorption of the phalange is the chronic change of severe PHPT. These changes sustain HC development but are not the dynamic, rapid changes typical for HC. Bone pain deriving from these changes is a symptom of HC.

Visceral calcinosis is described in case reports when deleterious calcium precipitation leads to calcium deposits in the alveolar epithelium of the lung or renal tubules. This causes a lethal rapid onset of multiorgan failure [12, 13].

Non-uremic calciphylaxis is a condition with high mortality (80%) where a calcific uremic arteriolopathy causes thrombosis, mural, and extravascular calcification leading to ischemia and necrosis of skin and soft tissue. This disorder is also reported with PHPT and other hypercalcemic states, not necessarily with HC [14]. Patients with PHPT and calciphylaxis who had a parathyroidectomy had a more favorable outcome, especially when performed before skin lesions progress [15].

Physical exam can show a palpable cervical mass either due to a large adenoma or in the presence of parathyroid carcinoma.

41.3 HC Due to PHPT in Pregnancy

PHPT is rare during pregnancy with an incidence in women of childbearing age of 8/100.000 per year [16, 17]. During pregnancy, physiological changes in intestinal calcium reabsorption occur to meet the fetal need and maintain the mother's calcium stores. Maternal PTH decreases during the first trimester of pregnancy, and active vitamin D increases intestinal absorption. The ionized calcium level remains unaltered during the hypoalbuminemia state. The placenta produces PTH-related peptide (PTHrP) and 1-alpha-hydrolase enzyme to enhance calcium absorption.

The symptoms of HPT and hypercalcemia during pregnancy can easily be mistaken for symptoms of normal first-trimester gestation. Symptoms of HC may present as *hyperemesis gravidarum* or preeclampsia [18]. Pregnant patients in HC suffer from anorexia, protracted vomiting, depression, muscle weakness, constipation, nephrolithiasis, hypertension, confusion, pancreatitis, and lastly coma. Serum calcium levels should be checked if a pregnant patient is presenting with these symptoms. HC in pregnancy can also arise from other causes such as thyrotoxicosis, granulomatous diseases, milk- or calcium-alkali syndrome, vitamin A or D intoxication, use of thiazide diuretics, and lithium as well as humoral hypercalcemia from PTHrP produced by benign leiomyomas [19].

During pregnancy, severe hypercalcemia causes intrauterine growth retardation, sometimes even miscarriage. Polyhydramnios can develop from fetal polyuria due to fetal hypercalcemia. Therefore, calcium measurement should be part of the investigation in otherwise unexplained polyhydramnios [20].

The second phase of HC risk is the postpartum period. During pregnancy, the placenta actively shifts maternal calcium to the fetus, which is protective for the mother against the development of HC. After childbirth, this mechanism is missing, and the mother is at increased risk for HC. In contrast, the neonate is unable to mobilize calcium from the bones because of the suppression of the fetus' parathyroid glands by the maternal hypercalcemia. This results in newborn hypocalcemia and tetany. In untreated mothers with PHPT, fetal complications have been reported to be as high as 80%. Even in conservatively treated mothers, the neonatal complication rate has been reported to be as high as 53%, of which 23–31% are neonatal stillbirths and deaths [16, 21]. PHPT should be screened for in pregnancy, and treatment and/or surgery should be indicated in the approved timeframe of the second trimester. Treatment during the first trimester should be hydration, diuresis, and electrolyte replacement along with close follow-up. Calcitonin may be used for treatment in pregnancy because there is no passage through the placenta. Bisphosphonates should be avoided because of their impact on fetal bone development. If the patient remains acutely ill and calcium cannot be reduced sufficiently (to <12 mg/dL or <3 mmol/L), parathyroidectomy is urgently indicated and should be carried out in a multidisciplinary fashion and by experienced endocrine surgeons [21]. Emergency parathyroidectomy during the third trimester is of high risk and should only be considered after risk/benefits have been thoroughly discussed. Calcimimetics lack safety data and have a delayed onset of action. This medication might have the potential for use in the third trimester to bridge for postpartum surgery, but further investigation is needed.

41.4 HC in Young Patients

Adolescent patients appear to present with more severe forms of primary HPT [22–24]. Young patients are often symptomatic and with a more severe presentation, higher serum calcium levels, and lower PTH levels than adults. As reported by Pashtan et al., young patients present with HC (4%) more often than adults with PHPT (1%) [25]. The most frequent symptom triad is fatigue, weakness, and depression. Renal stones were found in 52% of the adolescent patients, as well as abdominal and bone pain, which are symptoms that should trigger a workup for hyperparathyroidism. A single gland disease cause is found in the same proportion in children as in adults (about 85%), but the size of the parathyroid gland in children may be smaller, leading to a lower sensitivity of MIBI scans. Furthermore, only 1 of 21 patients in this series had a genetic syndrome as the underlying cause of HPT [25]. In the absence of positive family history and other endocrinopathies, single adenomas are more likely to be the cause of PHPT in adolescents. Nonetheless, endocrine surgeons should continue to be aware of possible genetic causes of PHPT in young patients presenting with hypercalcemia.

41.5 Natural History

The reported incidence of HC in PHPT derives mainly from case reports and retrospective analysis of databases. It appears to have decreased to 1.6–6% due to the availability of auto-analyzers that measure calcium and PTH, allowing earlier surgical intervention. Diagnosis and treatment of PHPT occur in much earlier stages of the disease, and fewer patients present with the classic symptoms of HC. Several milestones in the treatment of PHPT have improved the early diagnosis and treatment of this disease (▶ Box 41.1).

Lack of access to medical care and/or health insurance influences the incidence of HC in PHPT patients. In a series from India, HC occurs in 21% of the patients presenting with pancreatitis. PHPT patients are younger with skeletal muscular and renal symptoms. In China, women seem to suffer from more advanced PHPT than in the United States. Published series of underinsured patients in the United States demonstrated that these patients presented with higher mean serum calcium and were more likely to be diagnosed with HC [26]. In countries with modern medical services, about 1.6–6% of patients with PHPT develop HC [17, 27]. Mortality has decreased to 1–4.5% in contemporary studies, in contrast to reaching almost 100% in historical reports when timely diagnosis and therapy were not available [5, 28].

Box 41.1: Important Milestones in the Management of Hypercalcemia Due to Hyperparathyroidism in the Last Century

1925 Ability to measure serum calcium

1925 Parathyroid hormone discovery

1925 First parathyroidectomy performed by Mandl in Europe

1934 Multiglandular primary hyperplasia described by Albright

1939 First description of hyperparathyroid crisis due to parathyroid adenoma by Hanes

1959 Automated serum calcium analysis by the "Robot Chemist" by Baruch

1963 Radioimmunoassay for measurement of parathyroid hormone fragments

1973 Ability to measure the intact form of parathyroid hormone

1980 Sestamibi scan use for parathyroid localization

1988 First parathyroidectomy with intraoperative parathyroid hormone monitoring by Nussbaum

1990s First commercially available intraoperative rapid PTH assay

2004 Surgeon-performed US for parathyroid localization

41.6 Histopathological Characteristics in HC

As mentioned before, the most common underlying pathology causing PHPT-induced HC is a parathyroid adenoma, which is usually larger and heavier. Carcinoma is present in a higher percentage than in non-HC crisis patients (4% vs. 1%). Multiglandular disease (MGD) is found in 5% of patients presenting with HC [17]. Gucek refers to the enlarged glands as giant adenomas in 87.5% of the HC cases, with some of them measuring 10 cm in diameter. In one report, parathyromatosis accounted for 4% of all patients with HC [27]. Starker et al. described the pathologic findings in adenomas causing HC as showing microcystic chief cell pattern and significant intraglandular fibrosis with streaking throughout the gland rather than overwhelming it, as is typically seen in carcinoma [29]. In the literature, parathyroid adenomas with cystic changes are often mentioned as the underlying pathologic cause of many patients with PHPT-induced HC. Acute cystic degeneration, because of rapid growth, partial necrosis, or infarction of a parathyroid adenoma, may lead to a sudden release of large amounts of hormone from the damaged epithelium [30, 31]. Of the parathyroid cysts, 10% are located in the mediastinum, usually originating from the inferior parathyroid glands probably descended through weight and intrathoracic pressure, especially in elderly patients [32–34]. MIBI scans are often falsely negative in parathyroid cysts due to the sparse parenchyma at the periphery of the cyst and the rapid washout of the tracer [35]. Spontaneous hemorrhage of parathyroid glands can cause HC as described in a report of Chodack 1965 [36].

Most crucial for the performance of an adequate oncologic resection is the awareness that the underlying cause of HC could be parathyroid cancer. Quinn et al. analyzed their series of "aggressive parathyroid tumors" dividing them as atypical adenomas and parathyroid carcinomas. Carcinomas were found to account for more HC presentations. The PTH and calcium levels were higher than in non-carcinomas. Intraoperatively atypical adenomas showed a capsule, were easier to dissect, and had a soft texture when compared to the firm densely scarred parathyroid carcinomas with obliteration of normal tissue planes [37]. The invasive carcinomas oblige for en bloc resection of the thyroid lobe, as described in the parathyroid cancer chapter.

Postoperative hypocalcemia was more common in carcinomas as well. Besides the obvious features of capsular/vascular invasion or invasion of surrounding tissues with necrosis, parathyroid carcinomas and atypical adenomas showed no difference in cellular atypia or the pattern of Ki-67 and parafibromin staining. These differences are important for the follow-up of such patients. Being aware of the pathologic and imaging features allows the surgeon to choose the best operative strategy and to adapt the intraoperative technique.

41.7 Assessment of the Risk of Developing HC

Lowell et al. studied whether HC could be predicted in patients with PHPT. They showed that patients with serum calcium levels >13.2 mg /dL (>3.3 mmol/L) and a history of kidney stones were more likely to develop dehydration and at greater risk of developing HC. Patient's comorbidities also play a role in the development of HC due to the difficulty in those patients to compensate for the elevated calcium. A Charlson Comorbidity Index score > 4 as well as a PTH >394 pg/mL (42 pmol/L) indicated a higher risk of developing HC. If these thresholds were reached, 91% of the patients had HC. The urgency of parathyroidectomy could be determined according to these risk stratifications [38].

41.8 Diagnosis of HC

PHPT and humoral hypercalcemia from malignancies make up for 90% of HC. Diagnosis of HC due to parathyroid disease is similar to the diagnosis of PHPT except calcium levels should be >14 mg/dL (>3.5 mmol/L) along with signs and symptoms of acute calcium intoxication. These patients rarely have PTH levels within normal limits as their parathyroid glands are usually quite large and not suppressible. When HC occurs with PTH levels within normal limits, other causes of hypercalcemia should be investigated.

HC, due to PHPT, often presents with gastrointestinal symptoms and anorexia with possible hypoalbuminemia. Therefore, it is important to measure ionized calcium levels or correct the total serum calcium to albumin levels (corrected calcium (mg/dL) = measured total Ca (mg/dL) + 0.8 (4.0 − measured serum albumin [g/dL]), where 4.0 represents the average albumin level).

Although the presence of HC raises suspicion of parathyroid cancer, the great majority of these patients simply have a long history of hypercalcemia and untreated PHPT [17, 39, 40].

41.9 Differential Diagnosis of HC (▶ Box 41.2)

Malignancy is the cause of hypercalcemia in up to 30% of cases. Bone metastases cause high serum calcium by osteolysis. Hypercalcemia caused by malignancy also develops through the paraneoplastic production of PTHrP, which acts as a PTH analog, or the secretion of calcitriol and hypercalcemic cytokines (IL-1, IL-3-6, TNF-a, RANKL). Malignancies associated with humoral hypercalcemia mediated by PTHrP are lymphoma, chronic myeloid leukemia, and lung, renal, bladder, breast, ovarian, prostate, and colorectal carcinomas.

Malignancies with osteolytic metastasis are breast cancer, multiple myeloma, lymphoma, and leukemia. Multiple myeloma is especially associated with extensive tumor-induced, osteoclast-mediated bone destruction. Potentially life-threatening severe hypercalcemia is the most common metabolic complication of multiple myeloma and occurs in as many as one-third of such patients [41].

Vitamin D intoxication can result from overuse of prescription or over-the-counter vitamin D-containing supplements. 1,25(OH)2D promotes increased absorption of calcium from the intestine and mobilization of calcium from the bone leading to hypercalcemia [42].

In *chronic granulomatous disorders* such as sarcoidosis and tuberculosis, 1-alpha hydroxylase converts 25-OH vitamin D to 1,25 OH vitamin D or calcitriol, which mediates the increased intestinal calcium resorption causing hypercalcemia. HC caused by granulomatosis due to silicone injections has been reported. In elderly patients with granulomatous disorders, a combination of factors such as the use of thiazide medications, vitamin D supplements and/or calcium intake, and immobilization could precipitate HC [43].

Medications like lithium used in the treatment of bipolar disorder trigger hypercalcemia through the PTH pathway in 15–60% of treated patients. The prevalence of hypercalcemia correlates with the cumulative time lithium was used [44]. The use of thiazide diuretics can also precipitate HC due to PHPT and should be avoided in patients with significant hypercalcemia [45].

Endocrinopathies such as hyperthyroidism lead to bone resorption and hypercalcemia. In thyrotoxicosis, the symptoms of hyperthyroidism may be masked by HC, and it is very important for the clinician to be aware that the cause of hypercalcemia is the hyperthyroid state, which requires treatment and monitoring [17]. Conversely, hypercortisolism may mask HC. Glucocorticoids have a calcium-lowering effect; therefore, when cortisol levels decrease acutely, following adrenalectomy for Cushing's, or in the setting of Addison's disease, the abrupt decrease in cortisol can lead to hypercalcemia.

Immobilization reduces the inflow of calcium into skeletal tissue, and calcium is released into the circulation. When the patient's homeostatic capacity is already under distress because of predisposing diseases, hypercalcemia can develop [8]. This is of potential concern in patients with high bone turnover, like children or in patients with Paget's disease [28].

Milk-alkali syndrome, better described today as *calcium-alkali syndrome*, is one of the leading causes of hospitalization for hypercalcemia because of the routine intake of calcium and vitamin D supplements by the general population. The demographics of patients at risk for hypercalcemia have changed toward postmenopausal or pregnant women, solid organ transplant recipients, bulimic, and dialysis patients. Elderly patients with a reduced calcium buffer capacity in their bone mass and who are ingesting other medication (thiazide diuretics, inhibitors of the renin-angiotensin system, nonsteroidal anti-inflammatory drugs, and over-the-counter dyspepsia remedies) are susceptible for hypercalcemia with renal and cardiovascular morbidity [46]. A mildly elevated or normal PTH in the face of severe hypercalcemia should prompt consideration of additional underlying processes, as listed above.

Box 41.2: Differential Diagnosis of HC

Malignancy including multiple myeloma
- Hyperparathyroidism
- Medications such as thiazide diuretics and lithium
- Sarcoidosis
- Vitamin D intoxication
- Milk-alkali or calcium-alkali syndrome
- Hyperthyroidism
- Tuberculosis
- Immobilization
- Rhabdomyolysis and acute renal failure
- Addisonian crisis

41.10 Medical Management of HC Due to PHPT

The main goal of medical management is to bring calcium levels below 14 mg/dL (3.5 mmol/L) and as close as possible to the normal range while waiting for definitive treatment with parathyroidectomy. Initially, aggressive hydration and diuresis are implemented to lower calcium levels as soon as possible. Intravenous fluid boluses of normal saline 0.9% (NS) or lactate ringer (LR) can be used until adequate urinary output (UO) is achieved as severe hyperparathyroidism causes dehydration. When adequate hydration is achieved, loop diuretics can be used to decrease calcium levels while preventing fluid overload. Loop diuretics block calcium reabsorption in the ascending limb of the loop of Henle, inducing calciuresis, and can be administered a few times during the day depending on calcium levels and degree of response with this therapy. Following boluses, high volume maintenance rates (150–200 mL/h) should be given to lower calcium as close to the normal range as possible while the surgical team is consulted. Intravenous fluid needs should be individualized based on underlying cardiac and other comorbidities. Bisphosphonates are indicated for HC; however, its effect peaks in 2 days and lasts for 6 days, which is longer than desired if patients are expeditiously surgically treated. Calcitonin lowers calcium levels by reducing osteoclastic bone resorption and stimulating calciuresis, and it can be used for HC; however, short-term changes in calcium levels are not significant. Emergent low-calcium hemodialysis has been described for HC treatment; however, it is rarely needed for hypercalcemia due to PHPT [47]. As per the authors' clinical observations, cinacalcet is quite effective in lowering calcium levels when used along with hydration and diuresis. Although no large studies are describing the use of calcimimetics for patients with HC, it is successful in controlling hypercalcemia in patients with PHPT without HC [48]. Cinacalcet can be started at 30 mg once a day and increased up to 90–120 mg daily. It is important to remember that cinacalcet can cause nausea making this drug at times not well tolerated. Also, cinacalcet is not as widely available to patients in the ambulatory setting due to its cost as insurance companies often do not cover this medication for PHPT.

As soon as the diagnosis of PHPT is confirmed, the surgical team should be consulted since the only definitive treatment for this condition is parathyroidectomy. Better operative outcomes have been demonstrated when parathyroidectomy is performed during the first 72 h from the admission with a reported mortality of <14% [5, 17]. Mortality of HC has been reported to be 60–93% in historical studies, but it approaches <4.5% in contemporary studies [17]. The authors recommend parathyroidectomy, preferably during the same admission. When a reliable patient can be discharged from the hospital, the surgeon can perform the parathyroidectomy in an elective fashion, particularly if the crisis has been controlled, and the patient can be monitored closely.

41.11 Surgical Management

Since most patients with HC behave similarly to patients with PHPT without HC, the majority have a single parathyroid adenoma, making targeted parathyroidectomy the operative approach of choice [39].

As in PHPT, preparation for operative intervention starts with localization. The authors recommend ultrasonography (US) not only to localize the parathyroid gland(s) but also to evaluate the thyroid gland for any pathology [49].

Surgeon-performed US (SUS) can be the only localization study needed in these patients, as it is for PHPT without HC [50]. When performed in radiology, the sensitivity of US in localizing the parathyroid gland(s) is lower when compared to SUS [51–53]. As these patients are usually admitted, the surgeon can utilize US systems that are widely available in the hospital and often used for venous catheter placement. Probes for small parts/vascular (8–13 MHz range) can easily be deployed for this purpose. If the US is not conclusive or the surgeon/endocrinologist is not comfortable with the cervical US results, other modalities can be used alone or in combination, such as planar or SPECT MIBI or 4D CT scans [54, 55]. The latter requires intravenous contrast and should be avoided in patients with severe renal dysfunction, which is commonly found in patients with HC. The choice of imaging modality or a combination of methods should be driven by local expertise and available technology.

Once preoperative localization is obtained, and it localizes a parathyroid, these patients are great candidates for targeted or minimally invasive parathyroidectomy guided by intraoperative PTH monitoring (IPM). Bilateral neck exploration with visualization and excision of abnormal glands is the gold standard approach when IPM is not available and localization is not conclusive or when preferred by the experienced operating surgeon.

IPM is essential to achieve a successfully focused parathyroidectomy. Still, depending on the intraoperative criteria used to predict operative success, conversion to full bilateral exploration might be higher for these patients, particularly if the intraoperative criteria used to predict operative success require the PTH to fall into the normal range after resection of the parathyroid. Patients with HC often have very high PTH levels, which intraoperatively might not be returned to normal range in 10 minutes after gland excision. Protocols accepting a higher percent of PTH drop (i.e., reduction of 65–70% from baseline) to predict operative success might increase the possibility of a successfully targeted parathyroidectomy [56].

It has been described that ectopic and larger parathyroid glands more often cause HC [17]. When parathyroid carcinoma is suspected intraoperatively due to invasion of tissue planes and the thyroid gland, ipsilateral thyroid lobectomy should be performed at the initial procedure. En bloc resection of the affected parathyroid, ipsilateral thyroid lobe, and any tissue invaded by the parathyroid should be performed. If suspicious/positive lymph nodes are present as visualized by the surgeon, a therapeutic central neck dissection is also indicated. The comprehensive surgical management of parathyroid cancer will be discussed elsewhere.

41.12 Outcome for Parathyroidectomy for HC

HC occurs in 2.8–6.7% of patients with PHPT, and surgical outcomes for this condition are similar to parathyroidectomy for PHPT without HC, as long as the hypercalcemia is medically treated, and the procedure is performed expeditiously [5, 17, 28, 29, 39, 40]. The success rate of parathyroidectomy in these patients has been reported to be 96%, with the majority of operative failures being due to parathyroid cancer. When left untreated, the mortality of HC can be as high as 93% [17, 29].

Following parathyroidectomy for HC, hypocalcemia due to hungry bone syndrome tends to be severe, at times delayed, and should be treated aggressively with oral calcium and vitamin D replacement [57]. If oral calcium replacement is not sufficient, intravenous calcium gluconate infusions should be deployed to prevent severe hypocalcemic symptoms.

Patients with HC due to PHPT should be followed postoperatively with calcium and PTH levels 6 months after the initial operation and then yearly thereafter. After a successful procedure, patients with HC will have normal calcium levels, but their PTH level may be variably elevated.

The cause of this normocalcemic PTH elevation is multifactorial. A common cause of postoperative PTH elevation is vitamin D deficiency, and this should be treated aggressively. Parathyroid carcinoma is associated with higher operative failure rates as well as recurrence; therefore, such patients should be followed carefully.

For an optimal outcome, a multidisciplinary team consisting of endocrinologists, surgeons, pathologists, and radiologists should be involved in the management of HC patients due to PHPT. Adequate medical management and preoperative planning leading to an expeditious parathyroidectomy in expert hands are crucial for the successful management of these critically ill patients.

Answers to the Questions

1. (d); 2. (c); 3. (b); 4. (d); 5. (b); 6. (a); 7. (e); 8. (c); 9. (d); 10. (a)

References

1. Edelson GW, Kleerekoper M. Hypercalcemic crisis. Med Clin North Am. 1995;79(1):79–92.
2. Kebebew E, Clark OH. Parathyroid adenoma, hyperplasia, and carcinoma: localization, technical details of primary neck exploration, and treatment of hypercalcemic crisis. Surg Oncol Clin N Am. 1998;7(4):721–48.
3. Burkhardt E, Kistler HJ. Hypercalcemia in hospitalized patients. Diagnostic and prognostic aspects. Schweiz Med Wochenschr. 1981;111(51):2017–23.
4. Quak E, Blanchard D, Houdu B, Le Roux Y, Ciappuccini R, Lireux B, et al. F18-choline PET/CT guided surgery in primary hyperparathyroidism when ultrasound and MIBI SPECT/CT are negative or inconclusive: the APACH1 study. Eur J Nucl Med Mol Imaging. 2018;45(4):658–66.
5. Lew JI, Solorzano CC, Irvin GL 3rd. Long-term results of parathyroidectomy for hypercalcemic crisis. Arch Surg. 2006;141(7):696–9; discussion 700
6. Keeling CA, Abrahamson MJ, Harloe DG. Fatal hyperparathyroid crisis. Postgrad Med J. 1987;63(736):111–2.

7. Frame B, Jackson GM, Kleerekoper M, Rao DS, DeLorenzo AJ, Garcia M. Acute severe hypercalcemia in a la Munchausen. Am J Med. 1981;70(2):316–9.
8. Ziegler R. Hypercalcemic crisis. J Am Soc Nephrol. 2001;12(Suppl 17):S3–9.
9. Nagy L, Mangini P, Schroen C, Aziz R, Tobia A. Prolonged hypercalcemia-induced psychosis. Case Rep Psychiatry. 2020;2020:6954036.
10. Parks KA, Parks CG, Onwuameze OE, Shrestha S. Psychiatric complications of primary hyperparathyroidism and mild hypercalcemia. Am J Psychiatry. 2017;174(7):620–2.
11. Guimaraes T, Nobre Menezes M, Cruz D, do Vale S, Bordalo A, Veiga A, et al. Hypercalcemic crisis and primary hyperparathyroidism: cause of an unusual electrical storm. Rev Port Cardiol. 2017;36(12):959 e1–5.
12. Pallauf A, Schopohl J, Makeschin M, Kirchner T, Reincke M. Lethal generalized calcinosis and hypercalcemic crisis in primary hyperparathyroidism. J Clin Endocrinol Metab. 2015;100(1):17–8.
13. Sun HM, Chen F, Yin HL, Xu XY, Liu HB, Zhao BL. Rapid development of metastatic pulmonary calcifications in primary hyperparathyroidism: a case report and literature review. Diagn Pathol. 2017;12(1):38.
14. Nigwekar SU, Wolf M, Sterns RH, Hix JK. Calciphylaxis from nonuremic causes: a systematic review. Clin J Am Soc Nephrol. 2008;3(4):1139–43.
15. Bishop J, Brown E, Podesta A, Troy C, Dong XE. Surgical management of calciphylaxis associated with primary hyperparathyroidism: a case report and review of the literature. Int J Endocrinol. 2010;2010:823210.
16. Carella MJ, Gossain VV. Hyperparathyroidism and pregnancy: case report and review. J Gen Intern Med. 1992;7(4):448–53.
17. Phitayakorn R, McHenry CR. Hyperparathyroid crisis: use of bisphosphonates as a bridge to parathyroidectomy. J Am Coll Surg. 2008;206(6):1106–15.
18. Yilmaz BA, Altay M, Degertekin CK, Cimen AR, Iyidir OT, Biri A, et al. Hyperparathyroid crisis presenting with hyperemesis gravidarum. Arch Gynecol Obstet. 2014;290(4):811–4.
19. Rahil A, Khan FY. Humoral hypercalcemic crisis in a pregnant woman with uterine leiomyoma. J Emerg Trauma Shock. 2012;5(1):87–9.
20. Shani H, Sivan E, Cassif E, Simchen MJ. Maternal hypercalcemia as a possible cause of unexplained fetal polyhydramnion: a case series. Am J Obstet Gynecol. 2008;199(4):410 e1–5.
21. Schnatz PF, Curry SL. Primary hyperparathyroidism in pregnancy: evidence-based management. Obstet Gynecol Surv. 2002;57(6):365–76.
22. Cronin CS, Reeve TS, Robinson B, Clifton-Bligh P, Guinea A, Delbridge L. Primary hyperparathyroidism in childhood and adolescence. J Paediatr Child Health. 1996;32(5):397–9.
23. Wang W, Kong J, Nie M, Jiang Y, Li M, Xia W, et al. Primary hyperparathyroidism in Chinese children and adolescents: a single-centre experience at Peking Union Medical College Hospital. Clin Endocrinol. 2017;87(6):865–73.
24. Lou I, Schneider DF, Sippel RS, Chen H, Elfenbein DM. The changing pattern of diagnosing primary hyperparathyroidism in young patients. Am J Surg. 2017;213(1):146–50.
25. Pashtan I, Grogan RH, Kaplan SP, Devon K, Angelos P, Liu D, et al. Primary hyperparathyroidism in adolescents: the same but different. Pediatr Surg Int. 2013;29(3):275–9.
26. Jabiev AA, Lew JI, Garb JL, Sanchez YM, Solorzano CC. Primary hyperparathyroidism in the underinsured: a study of 493 patients. Surgery. 2012;151(3):471–6.

27. Gucek Haciyanli S, Acar N, Gur EO, Celik SC, Karaisli S, Dilek ON, et al. Severe hypercalcaemia of primary hyperparathyroidism: could giant adenoma be the real culprit rather than carcinoma? Ann R Coll Surg Engl. 2020;102(5):363–8.
28. Ahmad S, Kuraganti G, Steenkamp D. Hypercalcemic crisis: a clinical review. Am J Med. 2015;128(3):239–45.
29. Starker LF, Bjorklund P, Theoharis C, Long WD 3rd, Carling T, Udelsman R. Clinical and histopathological characteristics of hyperparathyroidism-induced hypercalcemic crisis. World J Surg. 2011;35(2):331–5.
30. Marienhagen K, Due J, Hanssen TA, Svartberg J. Surviving extreme hypercalcaemia--a case report and review of the literature. J Intern Med. 2005;258(1):86–9.
31. El-Housseini Y, Hubner M, Boubaker A, Bruegger J, Matter M, Bonny O. Unusual presentations of functional parathyroid cysts: a case series and review of the literature. J Med Case Rep. 2017;11(1):333.
32. Gurbuz AT, Peetz ME. Giant mediastinal parathyroid cyst: an unusual cause of hypercalcemic crisis--case report and review of the literature. Surgery. 1996;120(5):795–800.
33. Alghamdi KB, AlReefi MA. Delayed diagnosis of a hyper functioning parathyroid cyst. A case report and genetic analysis. Acta Endocrinol (Buchar). 2016;12(2):215–8.
34. Wirowski D, Wicke C, Bohner H, Lammers BJ, Pohl P, Schwarz K, et al. Presentation of 6 cases with parathyroid cysts and discussion of the literature. Exp Clin Endocrinol Diabetes. 2008;116(8):501–6.
35. Benard F, Lefebvre B, Beuvon F, Langlois MF, Bisson G. Rapid washout of technetium-99m-MIBI from a large parathyroid adenoma. J Nucl Med. 1995;36(2):241–3.
36. Chodack P, Attie JN, Groder MG. Hypercalcemic crisis coincidental with hemorrhage in parathyroid adenoma. Arch Intern Med. 1965;116:416–23.
37. Quinn CE, Healy J, Lebastchi AH, Brown TC, Stein JE, Prasad ML, et al. Modern experience with aggressive parathyroid tumors in a high-volume New England referral center. J Am Coll Surg. 2015;220(6):1054–62.
38. Lowell AJ, Bushman NM, Wang X, Ma Y, Pitt SC, Sippel RS, et al. Assessing the risk of hypercalcemic crisis in patients with primary hyperparathyroidism. J Surg Res. 2017;217:252–7.
39. Beck W, Lew JI, Solorzano CC. Hypercalcemic crisis in the era of targeted parathyroidectomy. J Surg Res. 2011;171(2):404–8.
40. Cannon J, Lew JI, Solorzano CC. Parathyroidectomy for hypercalcemic crisis: 40 years' experience and long-term outcomes. Surgery. 2010;148(4):807–12; discussion 12–3
41. Oyajobi BO. Multiple myeloma/hypercalcemia. Arthritis Res Ther. 2007;9(Suppl 1):S4.
42. Genzen JR. Hypercalcemic crisis due to vitamin D toxicity. Lab Med. 2014;45(2):147–50.
43. Chan JY, Kanthaya M. Hypercalcaemic crisis in an elderly patient with pulmonary tuberculosis. Oxf Med Case Reports. 2015;2015(11):354–7.
44. Twigt BA, Houweling BM, Vriens MR, Regeer EJ, Kupka RW, Rinkes IH, et al. Hypercalcemia in patients with bipolar disorder treated with lithium: a cross-sectional study. Int J Bipolar Disord. 2013;1:18.
45. Riss P, Kammer M, Selberherr A, Bichler C, Kaderli R, Scheuba C, et al. The influence of thiazide intake on calcium and parathyroid hormone levels in patients with primary hyperparathyroidism. Clin Endocrinol. 2016;85(2):196–201.
46. Patel AM, Adeseun GA, Goldfarb S. Calcium-alkali syndrome in the modern era. Nutrients. 2013;5(12):4880–93.
47. Trabulus S, Oruc M, Ozgun E, Altiparmak MR, Seyahi N. The use of low-calcium hemodialysis in the treatment of hypercalcemic crisis. Nephron. 2018;139(4):319–31.

48. Shoback DM. Bilezikian JP, Turner SA, McCary LC, Guo MD, Peacock M. The calcimimetic cinacalcet normalizes serum calcium in subjects with primary hyperparathyroidism. J Clin Endocrinol Metab. 2003;88(12):5644–9.
49. Wilhelm SM, Wang TS, Ruan DT, Lee JA, Asa SL, Duh QY, et al. The American Association of Endocrine Surgeons Guidelines for definitive management of primary hyperparathyroidism. JAMA Surg. 2016;151(10):959–68.
50. Deutmeyer C, Weingarten M, Doyle M, Carneiro-Pla D. Case series of targeted parathyroidectomy with surgeon-performed ultrasonography as the only preoperative imaging study. Surgery. 2011;150(6):1153–60.
51. Michaud L, Balogova S, Burgess A, Ohnona J, Huchet V, Kerrou K, et al. A pilot comparison of 18F-fluorocholine PET/CT, ultrasonography and 123I/99mTc-sestaMIBI dual-phase dual-isotope scintigraphy in the preoperative localization of hyperfunctioning parathyroid glands in primary or secondary hyperparathyroidism: influence of thyroid anomalies. Medicine (Baltimore). 2015;94(41):e1701.
52. Mohammadi A, Moloudi F, Ghasemi-rad M. The role of colour Doppler ultrasonography in the preoperative localization of parathyroid adenomas. Endocr J. 2012;59(5):375–82.
53. Akinci B, Demir T, Yener S, Comlekci A, Binicier O, Ozdogan O, et al. Beneficial effect of endocrinologist-performed ultrasonography on preoperative parathyroid adenoma localization. Endocr Pract. 2009;15(1):17–23.
54. Solorzano CC, Lee TM, Ramirez MC, Carneiro DM, Irvin GL. Surgeon-performed ultrasound improves localization of abnormal parathyroid glands. Am Surg. 2005;71(7):557–62; discussion 62–3
55. De Gregorio L, Lubitz CC, Hodin RA, Gaz RD, Parangi S, Phitayakorn R, et al. The truth about double adenomas: incidence, localization, and intraoperative parathyroid hormone. J Am Coll Surg. 2016;222(6): 1044–52.
56. Singh DN, Gupta SK, Chand G, Mishra A, Agarwal G, Verma AK, et al. Intra-operative parathyroid hormone kinetics and influencing factors with high baseline PTH: a prospective study. Clin Endocrinol. 2013;78(6):935–41.
57. Ariyan CE, Sosa JA. Assessment and management of patients with abnormal calcium. Crit Care Med. 2004;32(4 Suppl):S146–54.

Endocrine Hypertensive Emergencies

Caitlin Egan, Jacques Greenberg, and Thomas J. Fahey III

Contents

Caitlin Egan and Jacques Greenberg contributed equally to the preparation of this chapter.

A. L. Shifrin et al. (eds.), *Endocrine Surgery Comprehensive Board Exam Guide*,
https://doi.org/10.1007/978-3-030-84737-1_42

Case Presentation

Patient is a 55-year-old male presenting with intermittent headaches, palpitations, and sweating. He often notes these symptoms after exercise. He has no other complaints. Past medical history was unremarkable. He recalls an issue with sedation during his screening colonoscopy where his blood pressure was very high. He has no family history of cancer or endocrine tumors. He is on baby aspirin for "heart health." He has no previous abdominal imaging or surgeries. On physical exam, vital signs are within normal range; no other abnormalities are detected. Basic chemistries were within normal limits. Plasma fractionated metanephrines were significantly elevated.

Questions

1. What are criteria to establish the diagnosis of pheochromocytoma?
   (a) Elevated 24-h urine metanephrines and catecholamines
   (b) Elevated plasma fractionated metanephrines
   (c) MRI or CT scan with adrenal mass
   (d) (a) or (b) and (c)
   (e) (a) and (c)
2. What medications need to be started prior to surgical resection of pheochromocytoma?
   (a) Alpha-blockade for at least 7 days
   (b) Beta-blockade if tachycardic
   (c) (b) and then (a)
   (d) (a) and (b)
   (e) (a) and then (b)
3. Which of the following are causes of primary hyperaldosteronism?
   (a) Aldosterone-secreting adenoma
   (b) Adrenocortical carcinoma
   (c) Adrenal hyperplasia
   (d) (a) and (b)
   (e) (a) and (c)
   (f) All of the above
4. What are common lab findings in primary hyperaldosteronism?
   (a) Hypokalemia
   (b) Normokalemia
   (c) Alkalosis
   (d) Hypernatremia
   (e) (a), (c), (d)
   (f) (b), (c), (d)
   (g) All of the above

5. Which endocrine disorder is the most common cause of secondary hypertension?
   (a) Pheochromocytoma
   (b) Primary hyperaldosteronism
   (c) Cushing's syndrome
   (d) Thyroid storm
6. A 63-year-old woman presents with new-onset adiposity confined to her neck and trunk, intermittent low back aches, and fatigability, with new-onset systolic hypertension with SBP 172 mmHg. She was hitherto healthy but does carry a 15-pack-year smoking history. Her last colonoscopy was 3 years ago without diagnostic abnormality. She is ultimately diagnosed with Cushing's syndrome based on a two late-night salivary cortisol levels. Which of the following represents the most likely cause of the patient's Cushing's syndrome?
   (a) Functioning adrenal adenoma
   (b) Adrenal carcinoma
   (c) Colonic neuroendocrine tumor
   (d) Pancreatic neuroendocrine tumor
7. Which of the following is true with respect to diagnostic considerations in Cushing's disease or syndrome?
   (a) Obese patients have a preponderance to hypertension independent of circulating cortisol levels and therefore cannot be diagnosed with Cushing's syndrome based on a late-night salivary cortisol test.
   (b) While the most accurate method of diagnosing Cushing's disease involves measuring a central-to-peripheral ACTH gradient, patients may be spared this procedure if an MRI identifies a tumor exceeding 6 mm in size.
   (c) Octreotide scintigraphy has a >85% sensitivity in identifying occult ACTH-secreting tumors that are unable to be identified by CT or MRI.
   (d) Radiocholesterol scintigraphy remains the most commonly employed imaging modality in diagnosing a functional adrenal adenoma in the United States.
8. Which of the following is true with respect to the development of hypertension in Cushing's disease or syndrome?
   (a) Transsphenoidal resection of an ACTH-pituitary tumor achieves long-term resolution of hypertension in all patients with Cushing's disease and causes normalization of blood pressure with respect to sex and age-matched cohorts.
   (b) Hepatic synthesis of angiotensinogen typically increases in patients with Cushing's syndrome, while renin levels are either downregulated or remain normal.
   (c) Hypertension secondary to Cushing's syndrome is typically resistant treatment with an ACEi or ARBs.
   (d) Catecholamine receptor density is dramatically decreased in patients with Cushing's syndrome.

9. Which of the following features of thyroid-related hypertension is true?
   (a) The primary driver of hypertension in hypothyroidism is an increase in diastolic blood pressure due to an increase in systemic vascular resistance.
   (b) Esmolol is the preferred beta-blocker used during thyroid storm as it blocks the peripheral conversion of T4 to T3.
   (c) Hyperthyroidism is typically associated with systolic hypertension and a widened pulse pressure.
   (d) Diagnosis of thyroid storm mandates the presence of T4 twice the upper limit of normal and at least one of the following: sustained SBP > 150 mmHg, hyperpyrexia >39°, altered mental status, or cardiac dysfunction.

10. Which of the following is false with respect to the contribution of cortisol to hypertension in Cushing's disease and syndrome?
   (a) Mineralocorticoid receptors within the cell nucleus typically bind aldosterone with higher affinity than cortisol.
   (b) Functional mineralocorticoid excess is typically prevented by the presence of 11 beta-hydroxysteroid dehydrogenase type 2, which converts excess cortisol to cortisone.
   (c) Mifepristone, a selective glucocorticoid receptor blocker, lowers blood pressure to a greater extent than either spironolactone or eplerenone in patients with Cushing's syndrome.
   (d) An enhanced pressor response is often observed in patients with Cushing's disease.

42.1 Introduction

The American Heart Association (AHA) defines high blood pressure as sustained systolic or diastolic blood pressure greater than or equal to 130 or 80 mmHg, respectively. A hypertensive crisis is defined by the AHA as blood pressure of 180/120 mmHg or greater [1]. Hypertensive crisis with signs of end organ damage—including vision changes, chest pain, stroke symptoms, and shortness of breath—is defined as a hypertensive emergency.

Hypertensive emergencies require initial blood pressure control and potentially further treatment depending on the cause of the hypertension. Endocrine sources of high blood pressure, including pheochromocytomas and thyrotoxicosis, are considered secondary hypertension and can result in hypertensive emergencies. A thorough history and physical exam can often differentiate secondary hypertension from essential hypertension. Secondary endocrine sources of hypertension often have abrupt onset, no family history, no age criterion, and increased severity [2]. Moreover, hypertension can be the presenting sign for 15 different endocrine disorders [3]. Endocrine hypertensive emergencies, once diagnosed, can be cured or prevented with surgery or medication or a combination of the two. Endocrine disorders associated with hypertension and hypertensive emergencies include pheochromocytomas and paragangliomas, primary hyperaldosteronism, Cushing's disease and syndrome, and disorders of the thyroid.

42.2 Pheochromocytoma

Pheochromocytomas are tumors of neuroectodermal origin, arising from the chromaffin cells of the adrenal medulla, that produce catecholamines. If the tumor is extra-adrenal, it is a considered a paraganglioma and may or may not produce functional catecholamines [4]. The elevated level of catecholamines secreted by pheochromocytomas and functional paragangliomas increases blood pressure and causes other signs and symptoms seen with pheochromocytomas [5]. Pheochromocytomas are a rare cause of hypertension, causing less than 1% of cases [2]. They can be sporadic or hereditary and have been associated with neurofibromatosis type 1 (NF1), multiple endocrine neoplasia type 2 (MEN2) types A and B, von Hippel-Lindau (VHL) syndrome, and mutations in succinate dehydrogenase gene family, among others [6, 7].

42.2.1 Diagnosis

The classic triad presentation for pheochromocytoma includes headache, sweating, and palpitations. Weight loss and anxiety can also be seen. Blood pressure patterns vary in patients with pheochromocytomas and include sustained hypertension, hypertension with crisis level blood pressure spikes, or normotension with blood pressure spikes. Of patients with pheochromocytomas, 50% have been noted to have orthostatic hypotension [8].

Suspicion of an underlying pheochromocytoma is probably the most important step in making a diagnosis of a "pheo." Patients with paroxysmal signs and symptoms suggestive of pheochromocytoma—including volatile hypertension new in onset or discovered during surgery or anesthesia, genetic predisposition, and incidental adrenal nodule—should be evaluated for the presence of a pheo [7]. Biochemical evidence of excessive catecholamine production is the next step in confirming a diagnosis of pheochromocytoma. Plasma metanephrines should be the first test, followed by 24-h urinary metanephrines if the plasma metanephrines are indeterminate [9, 10]. Once blood or urine tests confirm excess catecholamines, magnetic resonance (MR), computerized tomography (CT), or 123-I-metaiodobenzyeguanidine (MIBG) imaging of the abdomen and pelvis is performed to localize the tumor [7, 11, 12].

42.2.2 Treatment

Today, surgical resection of pheochromocytoma is considered safe and usually curative [13]. Laparoscopic surgical resection of metabolically active pheochromocytomas or paragangliomas is the treatment of choice if the patient can tolerate surgery [14]. Open adrenalectomy for pheochromocytoma in a retrospective study was associated with increased vasopressor needs, longer length of stay, and increased complications compared to minimally invasive adrenalectomy [15]. Preoperative optimization including volume expansion and hypertension control with alpha-adrenergic blockade or the calcium channel blocker nicardipine is of great importance to prevent catecholamine-induced complications during surgery, with the goal of systolic blood pressure of 130 mmHg or lower [14, 16]. While the gold standard for preoperative preparation was phenoxybenzamine for many years, its limited availability and excessive cost have caused a search for alternatives. Nicardipine has been an excellent preoperative blocking agent and has as an advantage of a greater simplicity in dosing as compared to phenoxybenzamine [17]. For tachycardia, beta-blockade can be initiated after alpha-blockade to avoid precipitating a hypertensive crisis from an unopposed alpha-adrenergic response [16]. The current guidelines from the Society of Surgical Oncology (SSO) Endocrine and Head and Neck Disease Site Working Group recommend at least 7 days of pharmacological treatment preoperatively [16]. During laparoscopic resection, the abdominal cavity should be surveyed for metastatic disease. While many authors advocate for ligation of the adrenal vein as an early step in the procedure, this is sometimes impractical and furthermore can lead to venous congestion of the gland and the potential for a higher likelihood of capsular disruption and seeding of the tumor [14] (◘ Fig. 42.1). We routinely choose to ligate the adrenal vein only after the arterial supply has been taken.

42.3 Primary Hyperaldosteronism

Primary hyperaldosteronism (PA) may be the underlying cause of hypertension in up to 10% of patients and is due to increased aldosterone secretion [2, 3]. It is the most common cause of secondary hypertension but less likely to be the cause of a

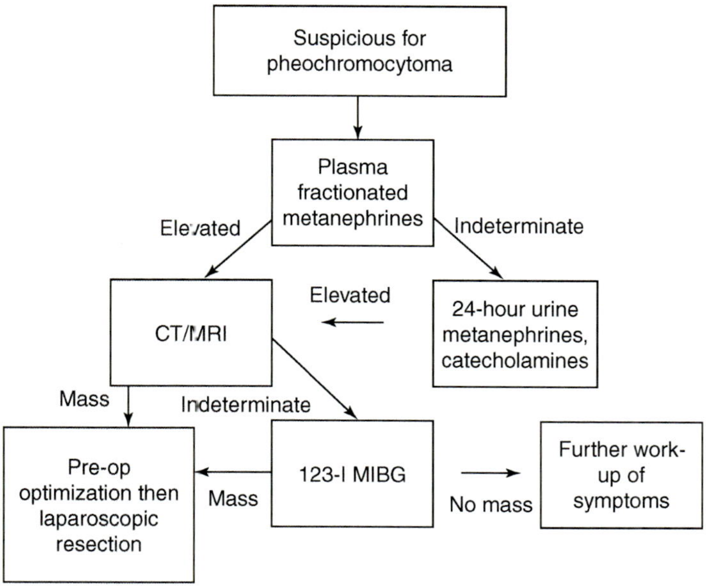

Fig. 42.1 Workup for pheochromocytoma

hypertensive crisis than a pheochromocytoma [18–20]. Elevated aldosterone levels cause increased sodium reabsorption with loss of potassium and hydrogen ions in the nephrons leading to hypertension, hypokalemia, and alkalosis and have been occasionally associated with hypertensive emergencies [21]. PA can be caused by unilateral aldosterone-producing adenoma (APA) or bilateral adrenal hyperplasia [22]. Aldosterone-producing adrenal cortical carcinoma is a rare cause of PA [23].

42.3.1 Diagnosis

PA classically presents with hypertension with hypokalemia but more often presents as normokalemic hypertension or resistant hypertension [20]. Resistant hypertension is defined as hypertension while taking three classes of properly dosed antihypertensives including a diuretic [24]. Patients with resistant hypertension or hypertension with hypokalemia should be screened for PA by calculating the aldosterone/renin ratio (ARR) [24]. The ARR is the ratio of the patient's plasma aldosterone concentration to the plasma renin activity and is elevated in patients with primary hyperaldosteronism [25]. In one prospective study using a cutoff of 32 ng/ng for the ARR, the sensitivity was 100% for patients for APA [26].

Confirmatory testing for PA can be done with oral or intravenous (IV) sodium load and measurement of aldosterone in the urine [24, 27]. Other confirmatory tests include the fludrocortisone suppression and captopril challenge tests [24]. However, confirmatory testing is not usually required for making a diagnosis of primary hyperaldosteronism. Once a diagnosis of primary hyperaldosteronism is made, the subtype must be identified to guide treatment, as APA is typically treated by surgical resection, while bilateral hyperplasia is currently treated medically [28, 29]. Further workup includes CT imaging of the adrenal glands to assess for nodules and micronodular changes and possible adrenal vein sampling (AVS) to localize [24, 30]. CT localization alone has been found by some to be reliable for adenomas greater than 1 cm in young patients, while there is benefit to AVS when equivocal CT scan findings are present [31]. We recommend AVS in most patients, unless they are 35 years old or younger with an obvious unilateral adenoma greater than 1 cm.

For unilateral APA based on imaging and AVS, laparoscopic adrenalectomy is recommended and can cure primary hyperaldosteronism [24]. Laparoscopic transabdominal and retroperitoneal approaches are comparable for surgical resection and guided by surgeon preference and patient surgical history [32]. For bilateral adenomas, bilateral hyperplasia, or if a patient cannot tolerate surgery, treatment is medical with aldosterone antagonists—spironolactone or eplerenone—and continued antihypertensive medications [24] (Fig. 42.2).

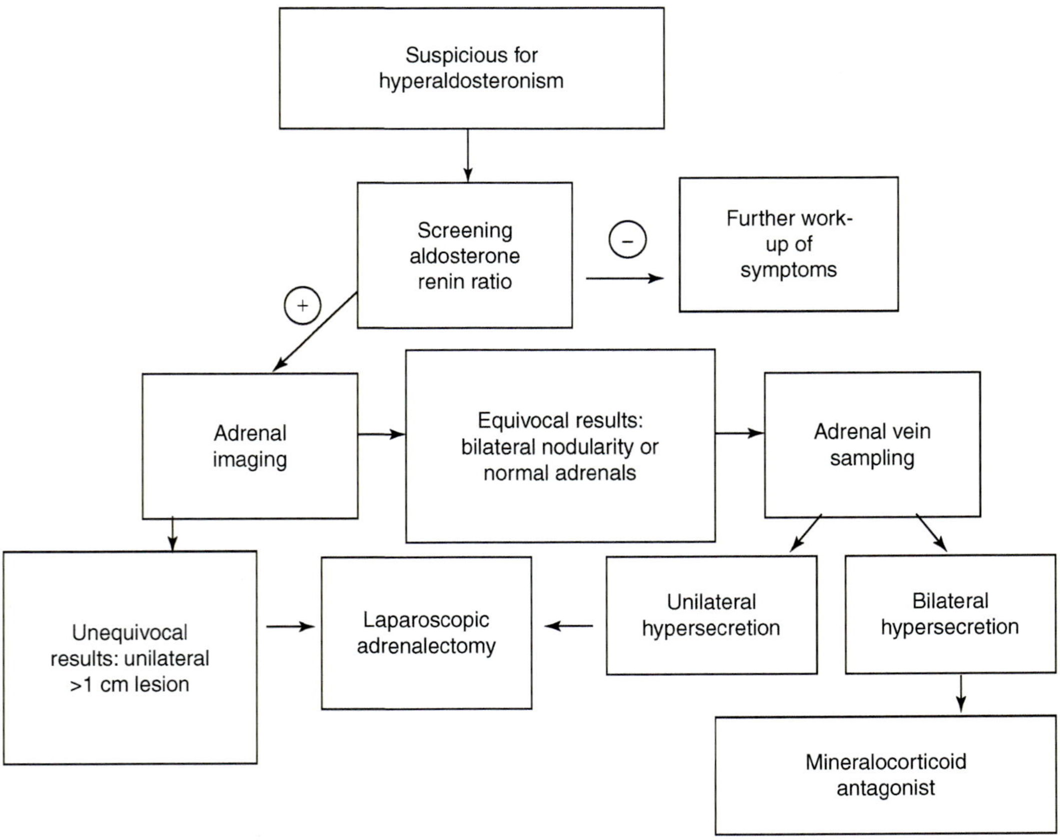

Fig. 42.2 Workup for primary hyperaldosteronism

42.4 Cushing's Disease and Syndrome

In 1932, Harvey Cushing, then at the Brigham Hospital in Boston, reported on 12 patients with the following characteristic features: "(a) a rapidly acquired, peculiarly disposed and usually painful *adiposity*…confined to face, neck and trunk, the extremities being spared; (b) a tendency to become round-shouldered (kyphotic)…; (c) a sexual dystrophy shown by early amenorrhea in the females and ultimate functional impotence in males; (d) An alteration in normal hirsuties shown by a tendency to hypertrichosis of face and trunk…; (e) a dusky or plethoric appearance of the skin with purplish lineae atrophicae; (f) Vascular hypertension…it varied from… 230/170 to …178/100; (g) a tendency to erythraemia…; (h) Variable backaches, abdominal pains, fatigability and ultimate extreme weakness" [33]. He ascribed many of these changes arising secondary to a "basophil adenoma" of the pituitary gland, and the clinical picture embodied by the aforementioned phenotypes rapidly became known as "Cushing's syndrome." By the 1940s, it had become clear that the syndromic characteristics ultimately arose secondary to excess circulating cortisol. Today, the majority of Cushing's syndrome arises due to exogenous sources of cortisol via the pharmacological administration of synthetic glucocorticoids (iatrogenic Cushing's syndrome). Cushing's syndrome arising from endogenous hypercortisolism is much rarer and is generally divided into corticotropin (ACTH)-dependent or corticotropin-independent hypercortisolism. While a detailed description will be reviewed elsewhere in this textbook, a focused overview will be provided here as it pertains to the profound hypertension occasionally observed in these patients, sometimes to the point of representing hypertensive emergencies.

ACTH-dependent Cushing's syndrome arises secondary to excessive stimulation of the adrenal cortex. The two sources of this excessive ACTH are (1) an ACTH-secreting pituitary adenoma (as initially described by Cushing, thus begetting the term Cushing's disease) or (2) an ectopic source of ACTH, typically from a neuroendocrine tumor—usually small-cell lung cancer, thymic malignancy, pancreatic endocrine tumors, or more rarely carcinoid tumors, medullary thyroid cancers, or pheochromocytomas [34–36].

ACTH-independent Cushing's syndrome arises from adrenal adenoma or carcinoma [36] or far more rarely from primary bilateral macronodular hyperplasia (BMAH) or primary pigmented nodular adrenocortical hyperplasia. While BMAH was initially thought to arise sporadically [37–40], several familial variants have been identified [41–47].

The overall incidence of Cushing's syndrome is very low, and thus its contribution to true hypertensive emergency is rare. In one Danish study analyzing all patients with Cushing's disease and syndrome over an 11-year period, the incidence of Cushing's disease was 1.2–1.7 per million per year. Cushing's syndrome arises from adrenal adenoma (0.6 per million per year) or carcinoma (0.2 per million per year), with neuroendocrine tumors of the lung, thymus, colon, and appendix having an incidence of 0.1 per million per year [36].

As described by Cushing, hypertension is one of the key characteristics of the clinical picture, and it has maintained its syndromic prevalence at a rate of 25–93% [48–69]. Typically, both systolic and diastolic blood pressures are increased to a similar extent in patients with Cushing's syndrome [69, 70]. While hypertension is a common feature of Cushing's syndrome, only rarely does it drive elevations in blood pressure to acutely dangerous levels [71]. In a review of 14 studies identifying 842 patients with Cushing's disease and Cushing's syndrome due to an adrenal adenoma or due to ectopic ACTH production, mean SBP was only elevated to slightly above 140 mmHg [70]. This does stand in contrast to those patients described by Dr. Cushing himself, whose peak systolic blood pressures were noted to be as high as 230 mmHg—a true endocrine emergency.

42.4.1 Diagnosis

A patient presenting in true hypertensive emergency warrants a prompt and aggressive approach to obtaining a diagnosis with respect to the driving disease pathology. The diagnostic workup for Cushing's syndrome is principally based on the 2008 Endocrine Society guidelines [72]. Initial screening can proceed with one of the following tests: late-night salivary cortisol (two measurements), 24-h urinary free cortisol excretion (two measurements), or the overnight dexamethasone suppression test (classically 1 mg given at 11 PM). A number of conditions may lead to physiologic hypercortisolism which may resemble Cushing's syndrome and must be noted in the workup of the pathology. These include pregnancy, obesity, and physiologic stress states such as depression, illness, hospitalization, poorly controlled diabetes mellitus, alcoholism, and sleep apnea [73–76]. Of these, some have a preponderance toward hypertension independent of a patient's cortisol status—obesity and sleep apnea, for example.

Historically, a high-dose dexamethasone suppression test has been performed to determine whether Cushing's syndrome is ACTH-dependent (pituitary) or ACTH-independent (ectopic). Theoretically, the pituitary gland maintains responsiveness to the glucocorticoid negative feedback loop, and cortisol levels should be suppressed following high-dose dexamethasone administration [77]. In contrast, nonpituitary tumors excreting ACTH, such as a small-cell lung cancer, lack the negative feedback loop and will lack cortisol suppression following a high-dose dexamethasone suppression test. More recently, the CRH test has been used to better evaluate the etiology of a patient's hypercortisolism [78, 79]. Dehydroepiandrosterone sulfate (DHEA(S)), which is ACTH-dependent and the most common steroid in the body, has been shown to be highly correlated with circulating cortisol levels. Due to its long half-life, some authors have proposed that DHEA(S) best reflects ambient ACTH levels over a long period and may also serve to identify patients with subclinical Cushing's and adrenal incidentalomas [80–82]. Indeed, utilization of an age-adjusted DHEA(S) ratio has recently been proposed as a screening test for subclinical Cushing's following identification of adrenal incidentalomas and is being added to the armamentarium of tests in the workup of hypercortisolism [83].

The suspected pathological process driving a patient's Cushing's disease or syndrome helps guide further imaging or diagnostic abnormalities. In patients suspected of having Cushing's disease due to a pituitary tumor, the most direct way to measure ACTH hypersecretion is to measure a central-to-peripheral ACTH gradient via petrosal sinus sampling [84–86]. However, prior to performing this invasive procedure, MRI with and without gadolinium contrast should be obtained to exclude a tumor >6 mm in size as tumors of this magnitude obviate the need for petrosal sinus sampling. MRI is only able to localize 50% of tumors, with a positive predictive value of 86% but with an associated false-positive rate exceeding 18% [87–89].

Ectopic ACTH-secreting tumors may be found anywhere throughout the body, but focused imaging in the chest is likely the highest yield given the preponderance of small-cell lung cancer as a cause of the disease. CT and MRI appear to have largely similar sensitivities in identifying tumors [90]. Octreotide scintigraphy can detect occult tumors secreting ACTH with a sensitivity of 30–53% [90–93].

Imaging for primary adrenal disease usually starts with thin-section CT. MRI may be obtained when the unenhanced CT attenuation values are >10 Hounsfield units as this may provide extra information regarding the malignant potential of the neoplasm [94]. Radiocholesterol scintigraphy may also provide additional information, though this test is now largely unavailable [95]. When bilateral adrenal masses are identified and suspicion of Cushing's syndrome or subclinical Cushing's syndrome exists, adrenal venous sampling can be performed [96].

Not unexpectedly, few of these diagnostic modalities will provide the physician with an immediate answer regarding any level of contribution of Cushing's syndrome to a patient's hypertension, nor is a definitive diagnosis necessary to initiate treatment. As such, the aforementioned can be pursued in an appropriately timed fashion in conjunction with appropriate treatment.

42.4.2 Treatment

Hypertension is an independent predictor of mortality in patients with Cushing's disease [53, 54, 97]. The definitive therapeutic intervention of Cushing's syndrome -related hypertension involves surgical removal of the suspected neoplasm. When a pituitary tumor is the cause of a patient's Cushing's disease, transsphenoidal resection provides long-term cure in greater than 70% of cases, but there appear to be higher rates of hypertension 5 years after cortisol normalization in these patients when compared to sex and age-matched cohorts [51, 55, 59, 61, 98, 99]. In children with Cushing's syndrome, 93.5% had preoperative systolic hypertension, with a decrease to only 5.5% at 12-month follow-up [100] after surgical resection of the cortisol-secreting neoplasm. In cases of Cushing's syndrome due to an occult ACTH-secreting tumor, bilateral adrenalectomy can resolve hypertension in nearly two-thirds of patients [101].

A variety of mechanisms have been implicated in the development of hypertension in Cushing's syndrome. Principal among these are the renin-angiotensin system, mineralocorticoid activity, the sympathetic nervous system, and the vasoregulatory system [70]. The most extensively studied mechanism contributing to hypertension in Cushing's syndrome is the renin-angiotensin system. Hepatic synthesis of angiotensinogen increases [71], whereas renin may be either downregulated (as expected) [102] or more commonly normal [71]. Angiotensin II itself has also been reported to be normal [103], but the total number of angiotensin II receptors is increased, and an enhanced response to angiotensin II infusion is noted [104]. An acute decrease in blood pressure has been noted in patients with Cushing's syndrome following the oral administration of an angiotensin I-converting enzyme inhibitor (ACEi) [71, 105], which has become the first choice class of drugs along with angiotensin receptor blockers (ARBs) in patients with Cushing's syndrome [70].

While the renin-angiotensin system represents the primary mechanistic pathway involved in hypertension seen in Cushing's syndrome, the mineralocorticoid system is also extensively involved. The mineralocorticoid receptor is expressed on the cell nucleus and binds both aldosterone and cortisol with equal affinity [106]. 11beta-hydroxysteroid dehydrogenase type 2 (11beta-HSD2) typically protects against a functional mineralocorticoid excess by converting cortisol to cortisone [107]. However, in the setting of pathologically elevated cortisol in patients with Cushing's syndrome, 11beta-HSD2 becomes overwhelmed, and an effective hyperaldosteronism is observed with respect to the development of hypokalemia [108]. Paradoxically and somewhat counterintuitively, this hypertension appears sodium-independent, as chronically elevated cortisol has been associated with both normal circulating levels and excretion of sodium [102, 109]. Perhaps this is best explained by the existence of another isoform of 11beta-HSD, the type 1 (11beta-HSD1) which reconverts cortisone into cortisol [107]. Indeed, there is suggestion that this reactivated cortisol itself is at least partially responsible for the hypertension observed in patients with Cushing's syndrome, as mifepristone, a selective glucocorticoid receptor blocker, lowers blood pressure more than spironolactone or eplerenone in these patients [110, 111].

Catecholaminergic receptor density is typically preserved in patients with Cushing's syndrome [103], and a hyperacute sympathetic response is controversially implicated in the development of hypertension in Cushing's syndrome. For example, an enhanced pressor response to norepinephrine (alpha 1, alpha 2, and beta 1 agonism) has been noted in patients with pituitary Cushing's disease, but this was not reproduced when individuals with Cushing's syndrome were treated with the selective alpha-1 agonist phenylephrine [112, 113].

A number of vasoregulatory substances have also been variably implicated in hypertension in the setting of Cushing's syndrome. Endothelin-1 (ET-1), erythropoietin (EPO), nitric oxide synthase (NOS), prostaglandins, prostacyclins, and compounds of the kallikrein-kinin system have all been reported to be deranged [71, 114–118].

There are numerous targets in the medical therapy of hypertension in Cushing's syndrome, although none necessarily in the emergent setting. An algorithm has been proposed by the "Altogether to Beat Cushing's" (ABC) [70]. ACEi or ARBs serve as first-line medications, with a goal of achieving normotension (◘ Fig. 42.3). Further management is dependent on the presence or absence of hypokalemia. If hypokalemia is present, spironolactone or eplerenone may be added. If addition of either of these fails to properly control a patient's blood pressure, then addition of an alpha-blocker, nitric oxide donor, or calcium channel blocker can be considered. If blood pressure yet remains uncontrolled, then careful use of diuretics or beta-blockers should be added. Targeted therapy addressing the source of hypercortisolism should also be pursued. Modulation of pituitary and ectopic ACTH release can be achieved with somatostatin analogs and dopamine agonists. Drugs that inhibit steroidogenesis such as ketoconazole and metyrapone as well as those blocking the glucocorticoid receptor (mifepristone) also play a role [119–121]. Pasireotide, a somatostatin analog, and cabergoline, a dopamine agonist, have both demonstrated significant improvement in hypertension in patients with Cushing's disease [122, 123]. Synergistic effects have been demonstrated with the addition of ketoconazole [124]. While there are clearly a number of treatment modalities addressing Cushing's associated hypertension, the need for directed and immediate control of any hypertensive emergency takes precedence.

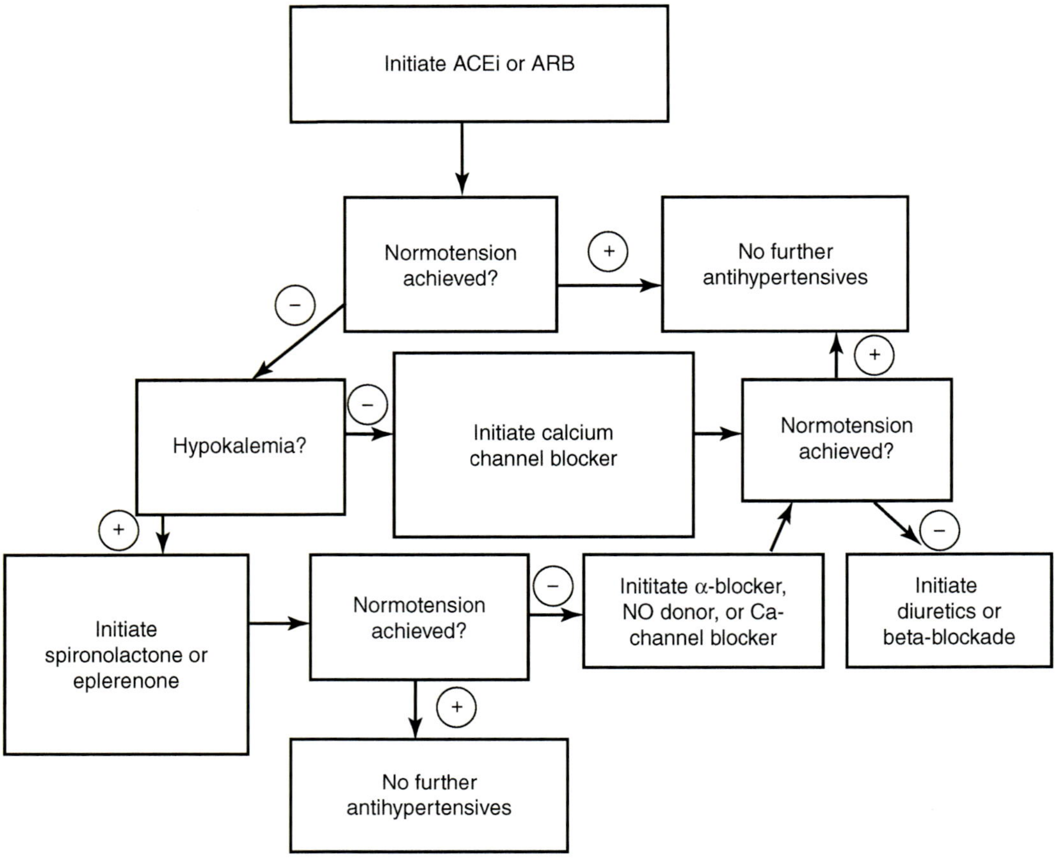

Fig. 42.3 Management of hypertension in Cushing's syndrome. While the management of hypercortisolemia is pursued, antihypertensive medications can be added in a targeted manner to control elevations in blood pressure. ACEi/ARB should be initiated first, followed by spironolactone or eplerenone if hypokalemia is present or calcium channel blockers if hypokalemia is absent. Following the addition of spironolactone or eplerenone, if blood pressure remains poorly controlled in patients with hypokalemia, then an alpha-blocker, nitric oxide donor, or calcium channel blocker can be added. Diuretics and beta-blockers are instituted as last line

42.5 Thyroid Disease

Diseases of the thyroid can often lead to disturbances in a patient's blood pressure, though these disturbances are rarely profound enough to lead to a hypertensive emergency. Nevertheless, both hypothyroidism and hyperthyroidism have been noted to lead to mild hypertension, and some cases of hypertensive emergencies have been reported [125].

Hypothyroidism primarily increases mean arterial pressure by increasing the diastolic blood pressure [126]. The catecholaminergic system has been implicated as the cause of hypertension in hypothyroidism. Higher levels of norepinephrine have been reported in hypothyroid patients when compared to normal controls [127, 128]. Furthermore, an increase in alpha-receptor responsiveness with an associated decrease in beta-adrenergic receptors has also been reported [129, 130], as has inappropriate secretion of antidiuretic hormone [130]. With that said, there are reports of patients presenting with profound hypothyroidism with systolic blood pressure >220 mmHg and diastolic blood pressure >140 mmHg [125].

Hyperthyroidism is generally associated with systolic hypertension with a widened pulse pressure. This arises secondary to the physiologic changes associated with elevated thyroid hormones—including an increase in cardiac output by 50–300% via a decrease in systemic vascular resistance (thus accounting for the decrease in diastolic blood pressure), an increase in heart rate, an increase in left ventricular output, and an increase in circulating blood volume [131, 132]. However, the presentation of hypertensive emergency is rare, and in one study assessing the effects of treatment on patients with hyperthyroidism, the average pre-intervention systolic blood pressure was 132 +/− 2 mmHg, with no records of systolic blood pressure exceeding 150 mmHg [133]. These findings have been replicated in other studies of hypertension in hyperthyroidism [134].

Thyroid storm typically manifests as an exaggeration of hyperthyroid symptoms, and profound hypertension has historically been reported as a feature of this emergent disease pathology [135, 136]. However, as our understanding of emergent thyrotoxicosis has evolved, we've come to recognize a transient diastolic hypertension prior to the development of a supervening cardiogenic shock [135] rather than any overt hypertensive emergency.

42.5.1 Diagnosis

The diagnosis of hypothyroidism, hyperthyroidism, and thyroid storm will primarily be reviewed elsewhere within this book. Briefly, however, the diagnosis of thyroid storm will be reviewed here as it is the only thyroid emergency with respect to hypertension. Diagnosis is primarily clinical and based on the presence of severe, life-threatening symptoms including hyperpyrexia (generally greater than 39 °C), cardiac dysfunction, and altered mental status with biochemical evidence of hyperthyroidism. A number of scoring systems exist to aid in the diagnosis, including that proposed by Burch and Wartofsky in 1993 [137]. Thyroid function tests should also be ordered and assessed, although there exist no diagnostic criteria for the degree of hyperthyroidism during thyroid storm. The underlying etiology of the thyrotoxicosis should also be determined—often, Grave's disease or a toxic adenoma or multinodular goiter is implicated, as have checkpoint inhibitors utilized in cancer treatments [138]. A physiologic stress usually precedes the development of storm such as surgery, trauma, infection, or parturition [139–142]. Diagnoses of the underlying driver for the storm are essential as it helps guide management of the disease.

42.5.2 Treatment

The treatment of hypertension associated with thyroid storm focuses on the management of the storm rather than the hypertension itself. A beta-blocker, either propranolol or esmolol, may be used to blunt the sympathetic response related to excessive thyroid hormone [143]. Propranolol has the added benefit of inhibiting the conversion of T4 to T3. Antithyroid therapy is initiated to inhibit the production of new hormone—propylthiouracil is preferred over methimazole due to its peripheral inhibition of T4 to T3 conversion [143–145]. Glucocorticoids have also been employed, as has plasmapheresis/plasma exchange [146, 147]. Emergency thyroidectomy has also been employed, although it is imperative to note that these interventions are undertaken for the cardiovascular collapse that follows the progression of thyroid storm rather than the any features of the initial hypertension [148]. As the natural progression of thyroid storm continues, any hypertension will rapidly be replaced with profound hypotension as cardiovascular collapse develops.

Answers to the Questions

1. (d); 2. (e); 3. (f); 4. (g); 5. (b); 6. (a); 7. (b); 8. (b); 9. (c); 10. (a)

References

1. Whelton PK, Carey RM, Aronow WS, Casey DE, Collins KJ, Himmelfarb CD, et al. 2017 ACC/AHA/AAPA/ABC/ACPM/AGS/APhA/ASH/ASPC/NMA/PCNA guideline for the prevention, detection, evaluation, and management of high blood pressure in adults: a report of the American College of Cardiology/American Heart Association Task Force on Clinical Practice Guidelines. Hypertension. 2018;71(6):e13–e115.
2. Sica DA. Endocrine causes of secondary hypertension. J Clin Hypertens (Greenwich). 2008;10(7):534–40.
3. Young WF Jr, Calhoun DA, Lenders JWM, Stowasser M, Textor SC. Screening for endocrine hypertension: an endocrine society scientific statement. Endocr Rev. 2017;38(2):103–22.
4. Erickson D, Kudva YC, Ebersold MJ, Thompson GB, Grant CS, van Heerden JA, et al. Benign paragangliomas: clinical presentation and treatment outcomes in 236 patients. J Clin Endocrinol Metab. 2001;86(11):5210–6.
5. Izzo L, Sympathoadrenal Activity J. Catecholamines, and the pathogenesis of vasculopathic hypertensive target-organ damage. Am J Hypertens. 1989;2(12_Pt_2):305S–12S.
6. Bryant J, Farmer J, Kessler LJ, Townsend RR, Nathanson KL. Pheochromocytoma: the expanding genetic differential diagnosis. J Natl Cancer Ints. 2003;95(16):1196–204.
7. Lenders JW, Eisenhofer G, Mannelli M, Pacak K. Phaeochromocytoma. Lancet. 2005;366(9486):665–75.
8. Streeten DH, Anderson GH Jr. Mechanisms of orthostatic hypotension and tachycardia in patients with pheochromocytoma. Am J Hypertens. 1996;9(8):760–9.

9. Lenders JW, Pacak K, Walther MM, Linehan WM, Mannelli M, Friberg P, et al. Biochemical diagnosis of pheochromocytoma: which test is best? JAMA. 2002;287(11):1427–34.
10. Christensen TT, Frystyk J, Poulsen PL. Comparison of plasma metanephrines measured by a commercial immunoassay and urinary catecholamines in the diagnosis of pheochromocytoma. Scand J Clin Lab Invest. 2011;71(8):695–700.
11. Ilias I, Pacak K. Current approaches and recommended algorithm for the diagnostic localization of pheochromocytoma. J Clin Endocrinol Metab. 2004;89(2):479–91.
12. Shapiro B, Copp JE, Sisson JC, Eyre PL, Wallis J, Beierwaltes WH. Iodine-131 metaiodobenzylguanidine for the locating of suspected pheochromocytoma: experience in 400 cases. J Nucl Med. 1985;26(6):576–85.
13. Kinney MA, Warner ME, vanHeerden JA, Horlocker TT, Young WF Jr, Schroeder DR, et al. Perianesthetic risks and outcomes of pheochromocytoma and paraganglioma resection. Anesth Analg. 2000;91(5):1118–23.
14. Kercher KW, Novitsky YW, Park A, Matthews BD, Litwin DE, Heniford BT. Laparoscopic curative resection of pheochromocytomas. Ann Surg. 2005;241(6):919–26; discussion 26–8
15. Kiernan CM, Du L, Chen X, Broome JT, Shi C, Peters MF, et al. Predictors of hemodynamic instability during surgery for pheochromocytoma. Ann Surg Oncol. 2014;21(12):3865–71.
16. Patel D, Phay JE, Yen TWF, Dickson PV, Wang TS, Garcia R, et al. Update on pheochromocytoma and paraganglioma from the SSO endocrine and head and neck disease site working group, part 2 of 2: perioperative management and outcomes of pheochromocytoma and paraganglioma. Ann Surg Oncol. 2020;27(5):1338–47.
17. Brunaud L, Boutami M, Nguyen-Thi PL, Finnerty B, Germain A, Weryha G, et al. Both preoperative alpha and calcium channel blockade impact intraoperative hemodynamic stability similarly in the management of pheochromocytoma. Surgery. 2014;156(6):1410–7; discussion7–8
18. Stowasser M, Gordon RD, Gunasekera TG, Cowley DC, Ward G, Archibald C, et al. High rate of detection of primary aldosteronism, including surgically treatable forms, after 'non-selective' screening of hypertensive patients. J Hypertens. 2003;21(11):2149–57.
19. Fardella CE, Mosso L, Gómez-Sánchez C, Cortés P, Soto J, Gómez L, et al. Primary Hyperaldosteronism in essential hypertensives: prevalence, biochemical profile, and molecular biology*. J Clin Endocrinol Metabol. 2000;85(5):1863–7.
20. Rossi GP, Bernini G, Caliumi C, Desideri G, Fabris B, Ferri C, et al. A prospective study of the prevalence of primary aldosteronism in 1,125 hypertensive patients. J Am Coll Cardiol. 2006;48(11):2293–300.
21. Labinson PT, White WB, Tendler BE, Mansoor GA. Primary hyperaldosteronism associated with hypertensive emergencies. Am J Hypertens. 2006;19(6):623–7.
22. Al Fehaily M, Duh QY. Clinical manifestation of aldosteronoma. Surg Clin North Am. 2004;84(3):887–905.
23. Griffin AC, Kelz R, LiVolsi VA. Aldosterone-secreting adrenal cortical carcinoma. A case report and review of the literature. Endocr Pathol. 2014;25(3):344–9.
24. Funder JW, Carey RM, Mantero F, Murad MH, Reincke M, Shibata H, et al. The management of primary aldosteronism: case detection, diagnosis, and treatment: an Endocrine Society Clinical Practice Guideline. J Clin Endocrinol Metab. 2016;101(5):1889–916.
25. Nishizaka MK, Pratt-Ubunama M, Zaman MA, Cofield S, Calhoun DA. Validity of plasma aldosterone-to-renin activity ratio in African

American and white subjects with resistant hypertension. Am J Hypertens. 2005;18(6):805–12.
26. Ducher M, Mounier-Véhier C, Baguet JP, Tartière JM, Sosner P, Régnier-Le Coz S, et al. Aldosterone-to-renin ratio for diagnosing aldosterone-producing adenoma: a multicentre study. Arch Cardiovasc Dis. 2012;105(12):623–30.
27. Holland OB, Brown H, Kuhnert L, Fairchild C, Risk M, Gomez-Sanchez CE. Further evaluation of saline infusion for the diagnosis of primary aldosteronism. Hypertension. 1984;6(5):717–23.
28. Aronova A, Gordon BL, Finnerty BM, Zarnegar R, Fahey TJ 3rd. Aldosteronoma resolution score predicts long-term resolution of hypertension. Surgery. 2014;156(6):1387–92; discussion 92–3
29. Wachtel H, Cerullo I, Bartlett EK, Kelz RR, Cohen DL, Karakousis GC, et al. Long-term blood pressure control in patients undergoing adrenalectomy for primary hyperaldosteronism. Surgery. 2014;156(6):1394–402; discussion402–3
30. Kempers MJ, Lenders JW, van Outheusden L, van der Wilt GJ, Schultze Kool LJ, Hermus AR, et al. Systematic review: diagnostic procedures to differentiate unilateral from bilateral adrenal abnormality in primary aldosteronism. Ann Intern Med. 2009;151(5):329–37.
31. Zarnegar R, Bloom AI, Lee J, Kerlan RK Jr, Wilson MW, Laberge JM, et al. Is adrenal venous sampling necessary in all patients with hyperaldosteronism before adrenalectomy? J Vasc Interv Radiol. 2008;19(1):66–71.
32. Lombardi CP, Raffaelli M, De Crea C, Sollazzi L, Perilli V, Cazzato MT, et al. Endoscopic adrenalectomy: is there an optimal operative approach? Results of a single-center case-control study. Surgery. 2008;144(6):1008–14; discussion 14–5
33. Cushing H. Basophilic activation of neurohypophysis and its bearing on certain diseases characterized by hypertension. P Soc Exp Biol Med. 1933;30(9):1424–5.
34. Orth DN. The Cushing syndrome: quest for the holy grail. Ann Intern Med. 1994;121(5):377–8.
35. DN O. Ectopic hormone production. In: BJ FP, Broadus AE, Frohman LA, editors. Endocrinology and metabolism. 2nd ed. New York: McGraw-Hill; 1987.
36. Lindholm J, Juul S, Jorgensen JO, Astrup J, Bjerre P, Feldt-Rasmussen U, et al. Incidence and late prognosis of cushing's syndrome: a population-based study. J Clin Endocrinol Metab. 2001;86(1):117–23.
37. Malchoff CD, Rosa J, DeBold CR, Kozol RA, Ramsby GR, Page DL, et al. Adrenocorticotropin-independent bilateral macronodular adrenal hyperplasia: an unusual cause of Cushing's syndrome. J Clin Endocrinol Metab. 1989;68(4):855–60.
38. Swain JM, Grant CS, Schlinkert RT, Thompson GB, vanHeerden JA, Lloyd RV, et al. Corticotropin-independent macronodular adrenal hyperplasia: a clinicopathologic correlation. Arch Surg. 1998;133(5):541–5; discussion 5–6
39. Cheitlin RA, Westphal M, Cabrera CM, Fujii DK, Snyder J, Fitzgerald PA. Cushing's syndrome due to bilateral adrenal macronodular hyperplasia with undetectable ACTH: cell culture of adenoma cells on extracellular matrix. Horm Res. 1988;29(4):162–7.
40. Kirschner MA, Powell RD Jr, Lipsett MB. Cushing's syndrome: nodular cortical hyperplasia of adrenal glands with clinical and pathological features suggesting adrenocortical tumor. J Clin Endocrinol Metab. 1964;24:947–55.
41. Findlay JC, Sheeler LR, Engeland WC, Aron DC. Familial adrenocorticotropin-independent Cushing's syndrome with bilateral macronodular adrenal hyperplasia. J Clin Endocrinol Metab. 1993;76(1):189–91.

42. Lee S, Hwang R, Lee J, Rhee Y, Kim DJ, Chung UI, et al. Ectopic expression of vasopressin V1b and V2 receptors in the adrenal glands of familial ACTH-independent macronodular adrenal hyperplasia. Clin Endocrinol. 2005;63(6):625–30.
43. Minami S, Sugihara H, Sato J, Tatsukuchi A, Sugisaki Y, Sasano H, et al. ACTH independent Cushing's syndrome occurring in siblings. Clin Endocrinol. 1996;44(4):483–8.
44. Miyamura N, Taguchi T, Murata Y, Taketa K, Iwashita S, Matsumoto K, et al. Inherited adrenocorticotropin-independent macronodular adrenal hyperplasia with abnormal cortisol secretion by vasopressin and catecholamines: detection of the aberrant hormone receptors on adrenal gland. Endocrine. 2002;19(3):319–26.
45. Nies C, Bartsch DK, Ehlenz K, Wild A, Langer P, Fleischhacker S, et al. Familial ACTH-independent Cushing's syndrome with bilateral macronodular adrenal hyperplasia clinically affecting only female family members. Exp Clin Endocrinol Diabetes. 2002;110(6):277–83.
46. Vezzosi D, Cartier D, Regnier C, Otal P, Bennet A, Parmentier F, et al. Familial adrenocorticotropin-independent macronodular adrenal hyperplasia with aberrant serotonin and vasopressin adrenal receptors. Eur J Endocrinol. 2007;156(1):21–31.
47. Watson TD, Patel SJ, Nardi PM. Case 121: familial adrenocorticotropin-independent macronodular adrenal hyperplasia causing Cushing syndrome. Radiology. 2007;244(3):923–6.
48. Albiger N, Testa RM, Almoto B, Ferrari M, Bilora F, Petrobelli F, et al. Patients with Cushing's syndrome have increased intimal media thickness at different vascular levels: comparison with a population matched for similar cardiovascular risk factors. Horm Metab Res. 2006;38(6):405–10.
49. Bolland MJ, Holdaway IM, Berkeley JE, Lim S, Dransfield WJ, Conaglen JV, et al. Mortality and morbidity in Cushing's syndrome in New Zealand. Clin Endocrinol. 2011;75(4):436–42.
50. Clayton RN, Jones PW, Reulen RC, Stewart PM, Hassan-Smith ZK, Ntali G, et al. Mortality in patients with Cushing's disease more than 10 years after remission: a multicentre, multinational, retrospective cohort study. Lancet Diabetes Endocrinol. 2016;4(7):569–76.
51. Colao A, Pivonello R, Spiezia S, Faggiano A, Ferone D, Filippella M, et al. Persistence of increased cardiovascular risk in patients with Cushing's disease after five years of successful cure. J Clin Endocrinol Metab. 1999;84(8):2664–72.
52. Dekkers OM, Biermasz NR, Pereira AM, Roelfsema F, van Aken MO, Voormolen JH, et al. Mortality in patients treated for Cushing's disease is increased, compared with patients treated for nonfunctioning pituitary macroadenoma. J Clin Endocrinol Metab. 2007;92(3):976–81.
53. Dekkers OM, Horvath-Puho E, Jorgensen JO, Cannegieter SC, Ehrenstein V, Vandenbroucke JP, et al. Multisystem morbidity and mortality in Cushing's syndrome: a cohort study. J Clin Endocrinol Metab. 2013;98(6):2277–84.
54. Etxabe J, Vazquez JA. Morbidity and mortality in Cushing's disease: an epidemiological approach. Clin Endocrinol. 1994;40(4):479–84.
55. Faggiano A, Pivonello R, Spiezia S, De Martino MC, Filippella M, Di Somma C, et al. Cardiovascular risk factors and common carotid artery caliber and stiffness in patients with Cushing's disease during active disease and 1 year after disease remission. J Clin Endocrinol Metab. 2003;88(6):2527–33.
56. Giordano C, Guarnotta V, Pivonello R, Amato MC, Simeoli C, Ciresi A, et al. Is diabetes in Cushing's syndrome only a consequence of hypercortisolism? Eur J Endocrinol. 2014;170(2):311–9.

57. Giordano R, Picu A, Marinazzo E, D'Angelo V, Berardelli R, Karamouzis I, et al. Metabolic and cardiovascular outcomes in patients with Cushing's syndrome of different aetiologies during active disease and 1 year after remission. Clin Endocrinol. 2011;75(3):354–60.
58. Gomez RM, Albiger NM, Diaz AG, Moncet D, Pitoia FA, Bruno OD. Effect of hypercortisolism control on high blood pressure in Cushing's syndrome. Medicina (B Aires). 2007;67(5):439–44.
59. Hassan-Smith ZK, Sherlock M, Reulen RC, Arlt W, Ayuk J, Toogood AA, et al. Outcome of Cushing's disease following transsphenoidal surgery in a single center over 20 years. J Clin Endocrinol Metab. 2012;97(4):1194–201.
60. Jyotsna VP, Naseer A, Sreenivas V, Gupta N, Deepak KK. Effect of Cushing's syndrome – endogenous hypercortisolemia on cardiovascular autonomic functions. Auton Neurosci. 2011;160(1–2):99–102.
61. Lambert JK, Goldberg L, Fayngold S, Kostadinov J, Post KD, Geer EB. Predictors of mortality and long-term outcomes in treated Cushing's disease: a study of 346 patients. J Clin Endocrinol Metab. 2013;98(3):1022–30.
62. Mancini T, Kola B, Mantero F, Boscaro M, Arnaldi G. High cardiovascular risk in patients with Cushing's syndrome according to 1999 WHO/ISH guidelines. Clin Endocrinol. 2004;61(6):768–77.
63. Muiesan ML, Lupia M, Salvetti M, Grigoletto C, Sonino N, Boscaro M, et al. Left ventricular structural and functional characteristics in Cushing's syndrome. J Am Coll Cardiol. 2003;41(12):2275–9.
64. Ntali G, Asimakopoulou A, Siamatras T, Komninos J, Vassiliadi D, Tzanela M, et al. Mortality in Cushing's syndrome: systematic analysis of a large series with prolonged follow-up. Eur J Endocrinol. 2013;169(5):715–23.
65. Pereira AM, Delgado V, Romijn JA, Smit JW, Bax JJ, Feelders RA. Cardiac dysfunction is reversed upon successful treatment of Cushing's syndrome. Eur J Endocrinol. 2010;162(2):331–40.
66. Pikkarainen L, Sane T, Reunanen A. The survival and well-being of patients treated for Cushing's syndrome. J Intern Med. 1999;245(5):463–8.
67. Torpy DJ, Mullen N, Ilias I, Nieman LK. Association of hypertension and hypokalemia with Cushing's syndrome caused by ectopic ACTH secretion: a series of 58 cases. Ann N Y Acad Sci. 2002;970:134–44.
68. Valassi E, Santos A, Yaneva M, Toth M, Strasburger CJ, Chanson P, et al. The European Registry on Cushing's syndrome: 2-year experience. Baseline demographic and clinical characteristics. Eur J Endocrinol. 2011;165(3):383–92.
69. Pivonello R, Isidori AM, De Martino MC, Newell-Price J, Biller BM, Colao A. Complications of Cushing's syndrome: state of the art. Lancet Diabetes Endocrinol. 2016;4(7):611–29.
70. Isidori AM, Graziadio C, Paragliola RM, Cozzolino A, Ambrogio AG, Colao A, et al. The hypertension of Cushing's syndrome: controversies in the pathophysiology and focus on cardiovascular complications. J Hypertens. 2015;33(1):44–60.
71. Saruta T, Suzuki H, Handa M, Igarashi Y, Kondo K, Senba S. Multiple factors contribute to the pathogenesis of hypertension in Cushing's syndrome. J Clin Endocrinol Metab. 1986;62(2):275–9.
72. Nieman LK, Biller BM, Findling JW, Newell-Price J, Savage MO, Stewart PM, et al. The diagnosis of Cushing's syndrome: an Endocrine Society Clinical Practice Guideline. J Clin Endocrinol Metab. 2008;93(5):1526–40.
73. Gold PW, Loriaux DL, Roy A, Kling MA, Calabrese JR, Kellner CH, et al. Responses to corticotropin-releasing hormone in the hypercortisolism of depression and Cushing's disease. Pathophysiologic and diagnostic implications. N Engl J Med. 1986;314(21):1329–35.

74. Pfohl B, Sherman B, Schlechte J, Stone R. Pituitary-adrenal axis rhythm disturbances in psychiatric depression. Arch Gen Psychiatry. 1985;42(9):897–903.
75. Pfohl B, Sherman B, Schlechte J, Winokur G. Differences in plasma ACTH and cortisol between depressed patients and normal controls. Biol Psychiatry. 1985;20(10):1055–72.
76. Kirkman S, Nelson DH. Alcohol-induced pseudo-Cushing's disease: a study of prevalence with review of the literature. Metabolism. 1988;37(4):390–4.
77. Liddle GW. Tests of pituitary-adrenal suppressibility in the diagnosis of Cushing's syndrome. J Clin Endocrinol Metab. 1960;20:1539–60.
78. Nieman LK, Oldfield EH, Wesley R, Chrousos GP, Loriaux DL, Cutler GB Jr. A simplified morning ovine corticotropin-releasing hormone stimulation test for the differential diagnosis of adrenocorticotropin-dependent Cushing's syndrome. J Clin Endocrinol Metab. 1993;77(5):1308–12.
79. Ritzel K, Beuschlein F, Berr C, Osswald A, Reisch N, Bidlingmaier M, et al. ACTH after 15 min distinguishes between Cushing's disease and ectopic Cushing's syndrome: a proposal for a short and simple CRH test. Eur J Endocrinol. 2015;173(2):197–204.
80. Akehi Y, Kawate H, Murase K, Nagaishi R, Nomiyama T, Nomura M, et al. Proposed diagnostic criteria for subclinical Cushing's syndrome associated with adrenal incidentaloma. Endocr J. 2013;60(7):903–12.
81. Yener S, Yilmaz H, Demir T, Secil M, Comlekci A. DHEAS for the prediction of subclinical Cushing's syndrome: perplexing or advantageous? Endocrine. 2015;48(2):669–76.
82. Zeiger MA, Thompson GB, Duh QY, Hamrahian AH, Angelos P, Elaraj D, et al. American Association of Clinical Endocrinologists and American Association of Endocrine Surgeons Medical Guidelines for the Management of Adrenal Incidentalomas: executive summary of recommendations. Endocr Pract. 2009;15(5):450–3.
83. Dennedy MC, Annamalai AK, Prankerd-Smith O, Freeman N, Vengopal K, Graggaber J, et al. Low DHEAS: a sensitive and specific test for the detection of subclinical hypercortisolism in adrenal incidentalomas. J Clin Endocrinol Metab. 2017;102(3):786–92.
84. Doppman JL, Oldfield E, Krudy AG, Chrousos GP, Schulte HM, Schaaf M, et al. Petrosal sinus sampling for Cushing syndrome: anatomical and technical considerations. Work in progress. Radiology. 1984;150(1):99–103.
85. Oldfield EH, Chrousos GP, Schulte HM, Schaaf M, McKeever PE, Krudy AG, et al. Preoperative lateralization of ACTH-secreting pituitary microadenomas by bilateral and simultaneous inferior petrosal venous sinus sampling. N Engl J Med. 1985;312(2):100–3.
86. Oldfield EH, Girton ME, Doppman JL. Absence of intercavernous venous mixing: evidence supporting lateralization of pituitary microadenomas by venous sampling. J Clin Endocrinol Metab. 1985;61(4):644–7.
87. Hall WA, Luciano MG, Doppman JL, Patronas NJ, Oldfield EH. Pituitary magnetic resonance imaging in normal human volunteers: occult adenomas in the general population. Ann Intern Med. 1994;120(10):817–20.
88. Ilias I, Torpy DJ, Pacak K, Mullen N, Wesley RA, Nieman LK. Cushing's syndrome due to ectopic corticotropin secretion: twenty years' experience at the national institutes of health. J Clin Endocrinol Metab. 2005;90(8):4955–62.
89. Wind JJ, Lonser RR, Nieman LK, DeVroom HL, Chang R, Oldfield EH. The lateralization accuracy of inferior petrosal sinus sampling in 501 patients with Cushing's disease. J Clin Endocrinol Metab. 2013;98(6):2285–93.

90. Pacak K, Ilias I, Chen CC, Carrasquillo JA, Whatley M, Nieman LK. The role of [(18)F]fluorodeoxyglucose positron emission tomography and [(111)in]-diethylenetriaminepentaacetate-D-Phe-pentetreotide scintigraphy in the localization of ectopic adrenocorticotropin-secreting tumors causing Cushing's syndrome. J Clin Endocrinol Metab. 2004;89(5):2214–21.
91. Reincke M, Allolio B, Arlt W, Korber C. Comment on primary localization of an ectopic ACTH-producing bronchial carcinoid tumor by indium111 pentetreotide scintigraphy. J Clin Endocrinol Metab. 1999;84(9):3399–400; author reply 402–3
92. Tabarin A, Valli N, Chanson P, Bachelot Y, Rohmer V, Bex-Bachellerie V, et al. Usefulness of somatostatin receptor scintigraphy in patients with occult ectopic adrenocorticotropin syndrome. J Clin Endocrinol Metab. 1999;84(4):1193–202.
93. Torpy DJ, Chen CC, Mullen N, Doppman JL, Carrasquillo JA, Chrousos GP, et al. Lack of utility of (111)in-pentetreotide scintigraphy in localizing ectopic ACTH producing tumors: follow-up of 18 patients. J Clin Endocrinol Metab. 1999;84(4):1186–92.
94. Ilias I, Sahdev A, Reznek RH, Grossman AB, Pacak K. The optimal imaging of adrenal tumours: a comparison of different methods. Endocr Relat Cancer. 2007;14(3):587–99.
95. Lumachi F, Zucchetta P, Marzola MC, Bui F, Casarrubea G, Angelini F, et al. Usefulness of CT scan, MRI and radiocholesterol scintigraphy for adrenal imaging in Cushing's syndrome. Nucl Med Commun. 2002;23(5):469–73.
96. Raff H, Carroll T. Cushing's syndrome: from physiological principles to diagnosis and clinical care. J Physiol. 2015;593(3):493–506.
97. Clayton RN, Raskauskiene D, Reulen RC, Jones PW. Mortality and morbidity in Cushing's disease over 50 years in Stoke-on-Trent, UK: audit and meta-analysis of literature. J Clin Endocrinol Metab. 2011;96(3):632–42.
98. Biller BM, Sheppard M. The network for the enhancement of endocrinology and oncology knowledge: a case-based consideration of current practice in Cushing's disease and acromegaly. Best Pract Res Clin Endocrinol Metab. 2009;23(Suppl 1):S1–4.
99. Graversen D, Vestergaard P, Stochholm K, Gravholt CH, Jorgensen JO. Mortality in Cushing's syndrome: a systematic review and meta-analysis. Eur J Intern Med. 2012;23(3):278–82.
100. Magiakou MA, Mastorakos G, Zachman K, Chrousos GP. Blood pressure in children and adolescents with Cushing's syndrome before and after surgical care. J Clin Endocrinol Metab. 1997;82(6):1734–8.
101. Chow JT, Thompson GB, Grant CS, Farley DR, Richards ML, Young WF Jr. Bilateral laparoscopic adrenalectomy for corticotrophin-dependent Cushing's syndrome: a review of the Mayo Clinic experience. Clin Endocrinol. 2008;68(4):513–9.
102. Connell JM, Whitworth JA, Davies DL, Lever AF, Richards AM, Fraser R. Effects of ACTH and cortisol administration on blood pressure, electrolyte metabolism, atrial natriuretic peptide and renal function in normal man. J Hypertens. 1987;5(4):425–33.
103. Ritchie CM, Sheridan B, Fraser R, Hadden DR, Kennedy AL, Riddell J, et al. Studies on the pathogenesis of hypertension in Cushing's disease and acromegaly. Q J Med. 1990;76(280):855–67.
104. Shibata H, Suzuki H, Maruyama T, Saruta T. Gene-expression of angiotensin-II receptor in blood-cells of Cushing's-syndrome. Hypertension. 1995;26(6):1003–10.
105. Yasuda G, Shionoiri H, Umemura S, Takasaki I, Ishii M. Exaggerated blood pressure response to angiotensin II in patients with Cushing's syndrome due to adrenocortical adenoma. Eur J Endocrinol. 1994;131(6):582–8.

106. Fuller PJ, Young MJ. Mechanisms of mineralocorticoid action. Hypertension 2005;46(6):1227–35.
107. Quinkler M, Stewart PM. Hypertension and the cortisol-cortisone shuttle. J Clin Endocrinol Metab. 2003;88(6):2384–92.
108. Isidori AM, Kaltsas GA, Pozza C, Frajese V, Newell-Price J, Reznek RH, et al. The ectopic adrenocorticotropin syndrome: clinical features, diagnosis, management, and long-term follow-up. J Clin Endocrinol Metab. 2006;91(2):371–7.
109. Bailey MA, Mullins JJ, Kenyon CJ. Mineralocorticoid and glucocorticoid receptors stimulate epithelial sodium channel activity in a mouse model of Cushing syndrome. Hypertension. 2009;54(4):890–6.
110. McMahon EG. Recent studies with eplerenone, a novel selective aldosterone receptor antagonist. Curr Opin Pharmacol. 2001;1(2):190–6.
111. Williamson PM, Kelly JJ, Whitworth JA. Dose-response relationships and mineralocorticoid activity in cortisol-induced hypertension in humans. J Hypertens Suppl. 1996;14(5):S37–41.
112. Heaney AP, Hunter SJ, Sheridan B, Brew Atkinson A. Increased pressor response to noradrenaline in pituitary dependent Cushing's syndrome. Clin Endocrinol. 1999;51(3):293–9.
113. McKnight JA, Rooney DP, Whitehead H, Atkinson AB. Blood pressure responses to phenylephrine infusions in subjects with Cushing's syndrome. J Hum Hypertens. 1995;9(10):855–8.
114. Axelrod L. Inhibition of prostacyclin production mediates permissive effect of glucocorticoids on vascular tone. Perturbations of this mechanism contribute to pathogenesis of Cushing's syndrome and Addison's disease. Lancet. 1983;1(8330):904–6.
115. Kelly JJ, Martin A, Whitworth JA. Role of erythropoietin in cortisol-induced hypertension. J Hum Hypertens. 2000;14(3):195–8.
116. Radomski MW, Palmer RM, Moncada S. Glucocorticoids inhibit the expression of an inducible, but not the constitutive, nitric oxide synthase in vascular endothelial cells. Proc Natl Acad Sci U S A. 1990;87(24):10043–7.
117. Ruschitzka F, Quaschning T, Noll G, deGottardi A, Rossier MF, Enseleit F, et al. Endothelin 1 type a receptor antagonism prevents vascular dysfunction and hypertension induced by 11beta-hydroxysteroid dehydrogenase inhibition: role of nitric oxide. Circulation. 2001;103(25):3129–35.
118. Wallerath T, Witte K, Schafer SC, Schwarz PM, Prellwitz W, Wohlfart P, et al. Down-regulation of the expression of endothelial NO synthase is likely to contribute to glucocorticoid-mediated hypertension. Proc Natl Acad Sci U S A. 1999;96(23):13357–62.
119. Nieman LK. Medical therapy of Cushing's disease. Pituitary. 2002;5(2):77–82.
120. Nieman LK. Update in the medical therapy of Cushing's disease. Curr Opin Endocrinol Diabetes Obes. 2013;20(4):330–4.
121. Fleseriu M, Biller BM, Findling JW, Molitch ME, Schteingart DE, Gross C, et al. Mifepristone, a glucocorticoid receptor antagonist, produces clinical and metabolic benefits in patients with Cushing's syndrome. J Clin Endocrinol Metab. 2012;97(6):2039–49.
122. Lacroix A, Bronstein MD, Schopohl J, Delibasi T, Salvatori R, Li Y, et al. Long-acting pasireotide improves clinical signs and quality of life in Cushing's disease: results from a phase III study. J Endocrinol Invest. 2020;43(11):1613–22.
123. Pivonello R, De Martino MC, Cappabianca P, De Leo M, Faggiano A, Lombardi G, et al. The medical treatment of Cushing's disease: effectiveness of chronic treatment with the dopamine agonist cabergoline in patients unsuccessfully treated by surgery. J Clin Endocrinol Metab. 2009;94(1):223–30.

124. Feelders RA, de Bruin C, Pereira AM, Romijn JA, Netea-Maier RT, Hermus AR, et al. Pasireotide alone or with cabergoline and ketoconazole in Cushing's disease. N Engl J Med. 2010;362(19):1846–8.
125. Chiu MH, Sharma NC. A case of hypertensive emergency, primary hypothyroidism and large pericardial effusion with early tamponade. J Cardiol Cases. 2018;18(1):29–32.
126. Ittermann T, Thamm M, Wallaschofski H, Rettig R, Volzke H. Serum thyroid-stimulating hormone levels are associated with blood pressure in children and adolescents. J Clin Endocrinol Metab. 2012;97(3):828–34.
127. Coulombe P, Dussault JH, Letarte J, Simmard SJ. Catecholamines metabolism in thyroid diseases. I. Epinephrine secretion rate in hyperthyroidism and hypothyroidism. J Clin Endocrinol Metab. 1976;42(1):125–31.
128. Coulombe P, Dussault JH, Walker P. Catecholamine metabolism in thyroid disease. II. Norepinephrine secretion rate in hyperthyroidism and hypothyroidism. J Clin Endocrinol Metab. 1977;44(6):1185–9.
129. Bilezikian JP, Loeb JN. The influence of hyperthyroidism and hypothyroidism on alpha- and beta-adrenergic receptor systems and adrenergic responsiveness. Endocr Rev. 1983;4(4):378–88.
130. Fletcher AK, Weetman AP. Hypertension and hypothyroidism. J Hum Hypertens. 1998;12(2):79–82.
131. Klein I, Ojamaa K. Thyroid hormone: targeting the vascular smooth muscle cell. Circ Res. 2001;88(3):260–1.
132. Pappachan JM, Buch HN. Endocrine hypertension: a practical approach. Adv Exp Med Biol. 2017;956:215–37.
133. Marcisz C, Jonderko G, Kucharz E. Changes of arterial pressure in patients with hyperthyroidism during therapy. Med Sci Monit. 2002;8(7):CR502–7.
134. Iglesias P, Acosta M, Sanchez R, Fernandez-Reyes MJ, Mon C, Diez JJ. Ambulatory blood pressure monitoring in patients with hyperthyroidism before and after control of thyroid function. Clin Endocrinol. 2005;63(1):66–72.
135. Ingbar SH. Management of emergencies. IX. Thyrotoxic storm. N Engl J Med. 1966;274(22):1252–4.
136. Mc AJ, Rawson RW, et al. Thyrotoxic crisis; an analysis of the thirty-six cases at the Massachusetts General Hospital during the past twenty-five years. J Am Med Assoc. 1947;134(10):868–74.
137. Burch HB, Wartofsky L. Life-threatening thyrotoxicosis. Thyroid storm. Endocrinol Metab Clin N Am. 1993;22(2):263–77.
138. Ferrari SM, Fallahi P, Galetta F, Citi E, Benvenga S, Antonelli A. Thyroid disorders induced by checkpoint inhibitors. Rev Endocr Metab Disord. 2018;19(4):325–33.
139. Akamizu T. Thyroid storm: a Japanese perspective. Thyroid. 2018;28(1):32–40.
140. Akamizu T, Satoh T, Isozaki O, Suzuki A, Wakino S, Iburi T, et al. Diagnostic criteria, clinical features, and incidence of thyroid storm based on nationwide surveys. Thyroid. 2012;22(7):661–79.
141. Rivas AM, Larumbe E, Thavaraputta S, Juarez E, Adiga A, Lado-Abeal J. Unfavorable socioeconomic factors underlie high rates of hospitalization for complicated thyrotoxicosis in some regions of the United States. Thyroid. 2019;29(1):27–35.
142. Swee du S, Chng CL, Lim A. Clinical characteristics and outcome of thyroid storm: a case series and review of neuropsychiatric derangements in thyrotoxicosis. Endocr Pract. 2015;21(2):182–9.
143. Ross DS, Burch HB, Cooper DS, Greenlee MC, Laurberg P, Maia AL, et al. 2016 American Thyroid Association guidelines for diagnosis and management of hyperthyroidism and other causes of thyrotoxicosis. Thyroid. 2016;26(10):1343–421.
144. Abuid J, Larsen PR. Triiodothyronine and thyroxine in hyperthyroidism. Comparison of the acute changes during therapy with antithyroid agents. J Clin Invest. 1974;54(1):201–8.

145. Cooper DS, Saxe VC, Meskell M, Maloof F, Ridgway EC. Acute effects of propylthiouracil (PTU) on thyroidal iodide organification and peripheral iodothyronine deiodination: correlation with serum PTU levels measured by radioimmunoassay. J Clin Endocrinol Metab. 1982;54(1):101–7.
146. Chopra IJ, Williams DE, Orgiazzi J, Solomon DH. Opposite effects of dexamethasone on serum concentrations of 3,3′,5′-triiodothyronine (reverse T3) and 3,3′5-triiodothyronine (T3). J Clin Endocrinol Metab. 1975;41(5):911–20.
147. Muller C, Perrin P, Faller B, Richter S, Chantrel F. Role of plasma exchange in the thyroid storm. Ther Apher Dial. 2011;15(6):522–31.
148. Scholz GH, Hagemann E, Arkenau C, Engelmann L, Lamesch P, Schreiter D, et al. Is there a place for thyroidectomy in older patients with thyrotoxic storm and cardiorespiratory failure? Thyroid. 2003;13(10):933–40.

Carcinoid Crisis

Alexandra Gangi and James R. Howe

Contents

A. L. Shifrin et al. (eds.), *Endocrine Surgery Comprehensive Board Exam Guide*,
https://doi.org/10.1007/978-3-030-84737-1_43

Questions

1. A 67-year-old female presents to her primary care physician with facial flushing and diarrhea of 2 months duration. CT scan shows a mesenteric mass and liver lesions. Appropriate immediate next steps include:
   1. A 24-h urinary 5-HIAA testing
   2. Serum 5-HIAA testing
   3. Initiation of somatostatin analog therapy
   4. Lower extremity duplex
   5. Surgical intervention and debulking
      (a) 1, 2, and 3 are correct.
      (b) 1, 3, and 4 are correct.
      (c) 1, 2 and 5 are correct.
      (d) 2, 3, and 5 are correct.
      (e) All are correct.
2. When counseling the patient, you inform her that as part of her preoperative workup, you would like to obtain a transthoracic echocardiogram because:
   1. As many as 40% of patients with CS may have carcinoid heart disease.
   2. You would like to evaluate the right-sided heart valves.
   3. You need an echocardiography for standard preoperative evaluation.
   4. Her flushing and diarrhea are related to hormone oversecretion which can also affect the heart.
   5. She is over 65 years of age.
      (a) 1, 2, and 3 are correct.
      (b) 1, 2, and 4 are correct.
      (c) 1 and 2 are correct.
      (d) 1 and 3 are correct.
      (e) All are correct.
3. The patient is evaluated by the surgical team, and her disease is deemed resectable. What are predictors of possible development of carcinoid crisis in this patient?
   1. Flushing which resolved with monthly SSA therapy
   2. Presence of carcinoid heart disease
   3. High elevation of plasma serotonin
   4. Elevated urinary 5-HIAA
   5. Diarrhea at time of presentation
      (a) 1, 3, and 5 are correct.
      (b) 1, 2, and 4 are correct.
      (c) 2 and 4 are correct.
      (d) 1, 3, 4, and 5 are correct.
      (e) All are correct.
4. During the procedure, while resecting left lobar liver metastases, the patient becomes acutely hypotensive and tachycardic. The next step should be:
   1. Clear communication between the procedural team indicating the patient's hemodynamic status
   2. Pause of the procedure until stability is restored
   3. Epinephrine administration

4. Evaluation for bronchospasm
5. Blood transfusion
   (a) 1, 2, and 4 are correct.
   (b) 1, 2, and 5 are correct.
   (c) 1, 3, and 4 are correct.
   (d) 1, 3, and 5 are correct.
   (e) All are correct.

5. The anesthesia team notices that the patient is experiencing severe bronchospasm. It is appropriate to consider medicating the patient with:
   1. Octrectide
   2. β-agonists
   3. Steroids
   4. Alpha blockers
   5. Dobutamine
      (a) 1 only
      (b) 1, 2, and 3 are correct.
      (c) 1, 3, and 4 are correct.
      (d) 3, 4, and 5 are correct.
      (e) All are correct.

6. Current international guidelines suggest that carcinoid crisis can be managed with:
   1. An octreotide drip
   2. Octreotide bolus
   3. Fluid administration
   4. Inotropic support
   5. Steroids
      (a) None of the above
      (b) 1, 2, and 3 are correct.
      (c) 1, 2, 3, and 5 are correct.
      (d) 1, 2, 3, and 4 are correct.
      (e) All are correct.

7. When significant hypotension occurs during surgery for carcinoid tumors despite being on an octreotide infusion, options for management include:
   1. Vasopressin
   2. 500-mcg octreotide bolus
   3. Epinephrine
   4. Dobutamine
   5. Phenylephrine
      (a) 1, 2, and 3
      (b) 1, 2, and 5
      (c) 2, 3, and 4
      (d) 1, 3, 4, and 5
      (e) All are correct.

8. Carcinoid crisis is a life-threatening condition that may manifest with symptoms of:
   1. Profound flushing
   2. Fluctuating blood pressure, most commonly hypotension
   3. Bronchospasm

4. Tachycardia
5. Bradycardia
   (a) 2 and 3 are correct.
   (b) 1, 2, 3, and 5 are correct.
   (c) 1, 2, 4, and 5 are correct.
   (d) 1, 2, 3, and 4 are correct.
   (e) All are correct.

9. A 39-year-old female with known carcinoid syndrome from metastatic small bowel NET presents for embolization of a solitary enlarging liver metastasis. She is otherwise healthy and is being treated with monthly injections of lanreotide and has no symptoms since initiation of therapy. In the interventional radiology suite, as she is sedated and upon administration of propofol, she is noted to develop a brief hypotensive episode and no other abnormalities. This is likely related to:
   1. Metastatic NET with carcinoid crisis
   2. Administration of propofol
   3. Excessive release of histamine
   4. Carcinoid heart disease
   5. Bronchospasm
      (a) 1 and 2
      (b) 1 and 3
      (c) 2 only
      (d) 1 only
      (e) 1 and 4

10. Carcinoid crisis can occur
    1. At the time of tumor biopsy
    2. With surgery
    3. Secondary to anesthesia
    4. At the time of tumor embolization
    5. Spontaneously
       (a) 1, 2, 3, and 4
       (b) 1, 2, and 3
       (c) 1 and 2
       (d) 2 only
       (e) All are correct.

11. A 58-year-old female presents to her primary care physician with a 1-month history of facial and chest flushing, as well as intermittent diarrhea and occasional difficulty breathing. On physical exam, a new-onset systolic ejection murmur is heard and is loudest at the left second intercostal space. Subsequent echocardiography reveals leaflet thickening secondary to fibrous plaque deposition on both the pulmonic and tricuspid valves. Which of the following laboratory abnormalities would most likely be seen in this patient?
    1. Decreased serum chromogranin A
    2. Elevated pro-brain natriuretic peptide
    3. Elevated urinary vanillylmandelic acid

4. Elevated serum potassium
5. Elevated urinary 5-hydroxyindoleacetic acid
   (a) 5 only
   (b) 4 and 5
   (c) 1 only
   (d) 2 and 5
   (e) All are correct.

43.1 Introduction

Carcinoid syndrome (CS) may develop in patients with hormone-producing neuroendocrine tumors (NETs) when systemic hormones levels are elevated. The classical symptoms of CS are flushing, diarrhea with abdominal cramps, bronchospasm and wheezing, and potential for development of right-sided heart failure. NETs can produce multiple hormones of which 5-hydroxytryptamine (serotonin) is the most recognized, as well as histamine, kallikrein, bradykinin, tachykinins, and prostaglandins. The overproduction of serotonin leads to CS symptoms and also stimulates fibrosis, which may result in the development of carcinoid-associated complications such as mesenteric fibrosis and carcinoid heart disease. Management of CS focuses on reducing serotonin levels with somatostatin analogs (SSAs). Additional described symptoms of CS are anxiety, depression, and cognitive impairment, but these are less frequently observed and not always recognized or treated. Carcinoid crisis is a life-threatening complication of CS which can appear spontaneously but is most commonly observed peri-procedurally in the setting of surgery, interventional radiological procedures, and possibly chemotherapy and peptide receptor radiotherapy administration. Carcinoid crisis can result in rapid patient deterioration and must be handled in an emergent fashion to avoid serious complications. This chapter reviews considerations for management of carcinoid crisis.

43.2 Diagnosis and Management of CS

NETs synthesize biogenic amines, which can be secreted into the bloodstream, leading to a number of symptoms. CS is characterized by episodic facial flushing (60–85%), diarrhea (60–80%), abdominal cramping, and, in its more advanced stages, hypotension and intermittent bronchial wheezing [1]. Symptoms are commonly associated with elevations of serum serotonin or urinary 5-hydroxyindoleacetic acid (5-HIAA). Most patients with CS have metastatic disease to the liver, which is where most of these hormones are metabolized. Tumors in the liver release their hormones directly into the systemic circulation, which can also occur in patients with bronchial or ovarian NETs without metastases, leading to symptoms of CS.

The diagnosis of CS can be confirmed by high concentrations of urinary 5-HIAA, a metabolite of serotonin, one of the main mediators of CS. Urinary excretion tests measuring 5-HIAA have a sensitivity of over 90% and specificity of 90% for CS [2]. A 24-h urinary 5-HIAA measurement can be performed preoperatively for both screening of CS and to predict the risk of carcinoid heart disease. Patients must avoid intake of serotonin- and tryptophan-rich foods (various fruits and nuts, avocados, tomatoes, eggplant) and medicines (antihistamines, compazine, monoamine oxidase inhibitors, various antihypertensives) at the time of testing. More recently, plasma 5-HIAA tests have been developed that are more convenient for patients. Studies have shown that plasma concentration are comparable to urinary measurements and therefore plasma measurements can be considered as an alternative, but these findings have not yet been validated as standard of care [3].

Once patients are confirmed to have CS, treatment with SSAs is commonly initiated. Somatostatin (SST) inhibits the secretion of a range of hormones by binding to SST receptors and inhibiting the release of serotonin and other hormones. About 80% of gastrointestinal NETs are thought to express SST receptors, making SSA therapy useful for these patients [4, 5]. Patients with CS are typically treated with monthly intramuscular injections of long-acting release octreotide (Sandostatin LAR) at a dose of 20–30 mg [6]. For patients with refractory symptoms, doses may be adjusted or supplemented with doses of short-acting octreotide. Lanreotide, another long-acting formulation, is also available for monthly injection at doses of 90 or 120 mg [7]. Both octreotide and lanreotide are typically well tolerated, but some patients may complain of abdominal discomfort, nausea, and steatorrhea at the initiation of therapy.

As part of their management, patients with known CS should also be evaluated for carcinoid heart disease. This is a feared complication and is characterized by degeneration of right-sided heart valves secondary to fibrosis [8]. As many as 40% of patients with CS may have carcinoid heart disease. Carcinoid heart disease is diagnosed via transthoracic echocardiography. According to the European Neuroendocrine Tumor Society (ENETS), transthoracic echocardiography should be performed in patients with elevated urinary 5-HIAA levels regardless of the presence of CS. Previous literature has shown that urinary 5-HIAA level ≥ 300 μmol within a 24-h period is a strong predictor for the development and progression of carcinoid heart disease [9, 10]. Elevated level of pro-brain natriuretic peptide are a reliable marker to make a rapid and accurate differentiation between patients with and without carcinoid heart disease. Pro-brain natriuretic peptide is mainly produced and excreted in the atria of the heart in response to increased wall tension, and there is a correlation between the degree of dilatation and levels of natriuretic peptides. Patients with normal levels of pro-brain natriuretic peptide are also reported to have better survival rate compared to those with elevated levels [11]. If carcinoid heart disease is diagnosed, patients are managed appropriately to control symptoms and disease progression. In most scenarios, patients may require valve replacement surgery to treat their right-sided heart failure.

43.3 Carcinoid Crisis

Carcinoid crisis is a potentially fatal form of CS that is typically triggered by anesthesia, operations, or other invasive procedures [12–16]. It is most commonly observed in patients who have metastatic gastroenteropancreatic NETs but, as mentioned previously, can also occur in patients with primary bronchial or ovarian NETs. Patients who develop carcinoid crisis typically have a constellation of symptoms which include severe hemodynamic instability, cardiac arrhythmia, cardiac failure, and refractory bronchoconstriction and can lead to complete circulatory collapse and death. Historically, the two most well-known risk factors for development of carcinoid crisis are the presence of liver metastases and a history of CS [17]. However, carcinoid crisis has been observed during procedures in NET patients without known risk factors; therefore, ample pre-procedural preparation to manage potential symptoms is necessary [9, 18].

43.4 Perioperative Delivery and Management of Octreotide

It has been the practice of most clinicians to give octreotide during procedures to prevent or ameliorate carcinoid crises. The optimal administration of octreotide has not been established, however, and there have been many different approaches described in the literature. Options include preoperative depot administration of long-acting SSAs or immediate subcutaneous injection of short-acting octreotide, intermittent intraoperative boluses of octreotide, or continuous infusions of the drug. The doses reported in various studies have varied widely, and there is no generally agreed upon optimal regimen. The need for prophylaxis is also related to the risk of the procedure prompting the carcinoid crisis, with direct surgical interventions and embolizations being more likely to require intravenous infusions or boluses and lower risk, non-carcinoid-related procedures (dental work, endoscopy, minor surgeries) requiring more expectant management. Patients who are likely to secrete high levels of biogenic amines are at the most risk, which include those with significant CS symptoms, usually accompanied by elevation of 5-HIAA and/or serotonin levels. This is most commonly seen in patients with liver metastases, and the presence of these metastases with or without symptoms may justify prophylaxis.

Even if octreotide is the treatment of choice for carcinoid crisis according to its efficacy in CS, data on its value for the management and prevention of carcinoid crisis are still limited and inconsistent [12, 17, 19–23]. Current data are based on retrospective studies which evaluated patients with various primary tumor sites, stages of disease, octreotide regimens, and differing definitions of carcinoid crisis. In 2001, Kinney et al. published the first and only study demonstrating effective perioperative octreotide prophylaxis. They evaluated 119 patients with metastatic NETs undergoing surgical intervention and considered blood pressure deviations (hypo- or hypertension), bronchospasm, flushing, irregular heart rate, acidosis, and need for pressors for blood pressures <80 mm Hg as complications of carcinoid crisis. Events were noted to occur in 10% of patients (7 of 67) who received no SSA therapy and 17% (1 of 6) who received preoperative SSAs only. In those patients who were treated with intraoperative octreotide (n = 45), no intraoperative complications were noted (p = 0.02), and doses ranged from 30 to 4000 mcg (median 350 mcg). Elevated preoperative 5′-HIAA levels and known carcinoid heart disease were found to be predictive for development of complications and death. Despite these results, the authors felt that their findings were not adequate to assess the effectiveness of intraoperative octreotide therapy in the prevention of carcinoid crisis. Interestingly, the current use of intraoperative octreotide therapy is based on patients treated in this study [12].

Some publications have described low rates of carcinoid crisis (range from 0% to 3.4%) with the systematic use of octreotide, and others a high rate of carcinoid crisis (ranging from 24% to 34%) despite the use of intraoperative octreotide [17, 19, 20, 24, 25]. One of the latter studies evaluated 97 patients who underwent abdominal operations for gastrointestinal NETs between 2007 and 2011 where patients were treated with a preoperative intravenous bolus of 500 mcg of octreotide and 250–500-mcg intravenous boluses were given for blood pressure changes, bronchospasm, flushing, tachycardia, or bradycardia. These issues occurred in 24% of patients, with no consistency in the timing of the event (such as anesthesia induction, incision, or resection). Additionally, events were even noted in patients who had no previous symptoms of CS and were significantly decreased by routine monthly preoperative octreotide LAR administration or an immediate preoperative octreotide bolus dose. Multivariate analysis identified the presence of liver metastases as the strongest predictor of CS-associated events. Among patients receiving prophylactic octreotide, 54% received at least one additional intraoperative dose, and almost half of these patients still had an intraoperative event. Patients with intraoperative events were more likely to experience 30-day morbidity [17].

At another institution, patients were treated with an octreotide drip at 500 mcg/hr. preoperatively and through the perioperative period in 179 cases of surgical cytoreduction for SBNETs [20]. Most patients in the study had CS preoperatively (85%) and were on long-acting SSAs preoperatively. In this cohort, only 6/179 (3.4%) patients were described as having carcinoid crisis events. The authors suggested that a continuous infusion of octreotide was more effective than a preoperative bolus based on these findings.

The group at Oregon changed their prophylactic regimen to a preoperative octreotide bolus of 500 mcg and continuous infusion of 500 mcg/hr. They still reported an intraoperative event rate of 34% in 150 procedures for gastrointestinal NETs [19]. Examination of multiple factors revealed that preoperative CS and hepatic metastases, but not elevated preoperative 5′-HIAA and chromogranin levels, were associated with carcinoid crisis events. Since their earlier study found that postoperative morbidity was higher in patients experiencing intraoperative crisis events [17], they treated intraoperative hypotension (<80 mm Hg systolic) with vasopressors. Using this strategy, they found that carcinoid crisis events were only associated with higher postoperative complications if the low blood pressure lasted for more than 10 min. This study suggested that intraoperative octreotide infusions did not necessarily prevent crises but that treating hypotension expeditiously could improve postoperative outcomes.

The same group then did an elegant prospective study of 46 patients with SBNETs or lung NETs undergoing surgery who had been on long-acting SSAs. All were given a 500-mcg preoperative bolus of octreotide, followed by an intraoperative infusion of 500 mcg/h. All patients had a transesophageal echocardiography (TEE) performed intraoperatively, and a pulmonary artery catheter placed. Blood samples were drawn for hormone collection before the incision, before closing, and when there were intraoperative crisis events, which occurred in 35% of patients. During crisis events, there were no changes seen on TEE, mild decrease in systemic vascular resistance and pulmonary arterial pressure, and no difference in pre-incision and crisis levels of serotonin, histamine, kallikrein, or bradykinin. They concluded that the combination of hypotension without decreased cardiac function or increased peripheral vascular resistance was consistent with distributive shock with vasodilatation and decreased venous return. If this is indeed the case, then octreotide would not be expected to improve the situation, and the proper treatment would be increasing volume and vasopressor agents [26].

As has been suggested from the studies above, it is unclear whether prophylactic octreotide will prevent carcinoid crisis, and the ideal prophylactic octreotide dose and scheme of administration has not been clearly established. The ENETS guideline advises a schedule of octreotide at 50–100 μg/h. intravenously for up to 12 h before and 48 h after surgery [22]. The North American Neuroendocrine Tumor Society (NANETS) guideline advises that routine administration of octreotide does not prevent a carcinoid crisis but suggests that octreotide at 100–500 μg/h. intraoperatively will likely not cause harm [23]. The United Kingdom and Ireland Neuroendocrine Tumor Society (UKINETS) guidelines provide a complicated algorithm with different patient categories and procedure types with doses and duration of octreotide administration [27].

43.5 Use of Octreotide Prophylaxis in Procedures

Given the conflicting data currently available for management of carcinoid crisis at the time of operative intervention, it is important to consider the role of octreotide prophylaxis in NET patients undergoing the various less invasive procedures they may undergo for workup, staging, and treatment. These may include tumor localization, staging, and/or therapy, which may include colonoscopy, upper endoscopy, double balloon enteroscopy, endoscopic ultrasound, biopsy of liver tumors, hepatic arterial embolization, and interventional radiology directed tumor ablation. Patients have been described with carcinoid crisis after a number of these procedures [13, 15, 16, 28–34], and some have recommended prophylactic octreotide, but it is unclear how frequent these events occur and whether they would be prevented by pre-procedure or intra-procedural octreotide. In higher risk procedures like embolization or percutaneous ablation, one might consider an octreotide infusion of 100–500 mcg/h. It is perhaps even more important to recognize that carcinoid crisis events may occur during these procedures and to closely monitor NET patients for hypotension, which can be treated with fluid and vasopressors, such as phenylephrine or vasopressin.

43.6 Recommendations Concerning Anesthesia

There are three phases of anesthesia care: the preoperative period, intraoperative period, and postoperative period. During the preoperative phase or "premedication" phase, the focus of care is on alleviating existing symptoms and preparing for potential intraoperative complications. As such, current recommendations suggest that maintenance medications should be continued, and the patient's anxiety is managed with anxiolytics. During the intraoperative phase, adequate invasive monitoring should be available including consideration for central venous pressure and invasive blood pressure monitoring via an arterial line. These monitoring methods could assist in prompt identification of hemodynamic compromise, allowing for rapid fluid management and vasopressor use in the setting of instability [12]. Additionally, airway pressure monitoring should be available to quickly detect the presence of bronchospasm. Medications that stimulate the sympathetic nervous system or can cause excessive histamine release should be avoided. In patients with carcinoid heart disease, the anesthesiologist must avoid right ventricular overload and strain to prevent right ventricular heart failure and cardiac instability [8].

Hypotension should be treated with sympathomimetics as previously discussed. If hypotension occurs secondary to manipulation of bulky metastases, clear communication with the surgical team is critical. Stopping the procedure until hemodynamic control is restored may be required. Bronchospasm, if severe, may require treatment and management with ß-receptor agonists, and steroids can be considered if necessary. Given all the potential complications that can arise, the anesthesiologist must be adequately prepared to manage all potential scenarios that may ensue with carcinoid crisis [22].

In the postoperative period, in patients being treated with an octreotide infusion intraoperatively, the drug can be stopped or tapered off over the course of the next 24 h. In those receiving only bolus doses, octreotide should be given only on an as needed basis. Management of hypovolemia and pain should be as per standard practices of the surgical team, and the patient should be closely observed for further symptoms or recurrence of carcinoid crisis if there was instability intraoperatively.

43.7 Conclusion

Carcinoid crisis is a life-threatening form of CS that may be triggered by tumor manipulation or by anesthesia. The most common sign is wide blood pressure fluctuations with a predominance of hypotension. When major surgery or interventional procedures are planned in patients with CS, prophylactic administration of SSAs should be considered to prevent a potential carcinoid crisis, even in those patients receiving long-acting formulations of these agents. Despite limited prospective randomized evidence, octreotide should be readily available during surgical procedures. However, despite the use of preoperative prophylactic octreotide and intraoperative bolus doses or continuous infusions of octreotide, intraoperative complications can still occur. As such, the treating team should be adequately prepared to treat the symptoms of carcinoid crisis with vasopressors and fluids as required for hypotension and antihypertensives as needed to avoid severe complications. Given the possibility of profound bronchospasm, tachycardia, and widely fluctuating blood pressure, it is also important to avoid sympathomimetics or histamine-releasing drugs.

Answers to the Questions

1. (a); 2. (b); 3. (e); 4. (a); 5. (b); 6. (e); 7. (b); 8. (d); 9. (c); 10. (e); 11. (d)

References

1. Ito T, Lee L, Jensen RT. Carcinoid-syndrome: recent advances, current status and controversies. Curr Opin Endocrinol Diabetes Obes. 2018;25(1):22–35.
2. Sjöblom SM. Clinical presentation and prognosis of gastrointestinal carcinoid tumours. Scand J Gastroenterol. 1988;23(7):779–87.
3. Allen KR, Degg TJ, Anthoney DA, Fitzroy-Smith D. Monitoring the treatment of carcinoid disease using blood serotonin and plasma 5-hydroxyindoleacetic acid: three case examples. Ann Clin Biochem. 2007;44(Pt 3):300–7.
4. O'Toole D, Ducreux M, Bommelaer G, Wemeau JL, Bouché O, Catus F, et al. Treatment of carcinoid syndrome: a prospective crossover evaluation of lanreotide versus octreotide in terms of efficacy, patient acceptability, and tolerance. Cancer. 2000;88(4):770–6.
5. Fisher GA, Wolin EM, Liyanage N, Pitman Lowenthal S, Mirakhur B, Pommier RF, et al. Patient-reported symptom control of diarrhea and flushing in patients with neuroendocrine tumors treated with lanreotide depot/autogel: results from a randomized, placebo-controlled, double-blind and 32-week open-label study. Oncologist. 2018;23(1):16–24.
6. Rubin J, Ajani J, Schirmer W, Venook AP, Bukowski R, Pommier R, et al. Octreotide acetate long-acting formulation versus open-label subcutaneous octreotide acetate in malignant carcinoid syndrome. J Clin Oncol Off J Am Soc Clin Oncol. 1999;17(2):600–6.
7. Ruszniewski P, Ducreux M, Chayvialle JA, Blumberg J, Cloarec D, Michel H, et al. Treatment of the carcinoid syndrome with the long-acting somatostatin analogue lanreotide: a prospective study in 39 patients. Gut. 1996;39(2):279–83.
8. Davar J, Connolly HM, Caplin ME, Pavel M, Zacks J, Bhattacharyya S, et al. Diagnosing and managing carcinoid heart disease in patients with neuroendocrine tumors: an expert statement. J Am Coll Cardiol. 2017;69(10):1288–304.
9. Niederle B, Pape U-F, Costa F, Gross D, Kelestimur F, Knigge U, et al. ENETS consensus guidelines update for neuroendocrine neoplasms of the Jejunum and Ileum. Neuroendocrinology. 2016;103(2):125–38.
10. Bhattacharyya S, Toumpanakis C, Chilkunda D, Caplin ME, Davar J. Risk factors for the development and progression of carcinoid heart disease. Am J Cardiol. 2011;107(8):1221–6.
11. Zuetenhorst JM, Korse CM, Bonfrer JMG, Bakker RH, Taal BG. Role of natriuretic peptides in the diagnosis and treatment of patients with carcinoid heart disease. Br J Cancer. 2004;90(11):2073–9.
12. Kinney MA, Warner ME, Nagorney DM, Rubin J, Schroeder DR, Maxson PM, et al. Perianaesthetic risks and outcomes of abdominal surgery for metastatic carcinoid tumours. Br J Anaesth. 2001;87(3):447–52.
13. Kharrat HA, Taubin H. Carcinoid crisis induced by external manipulation of liver metastasis. J Clin Gastroenterol. 2003;36(1):87–8.
14. Lewis MA, Jaramillo S, Roberts L, Fleming CJ, Rubin J, Grothey A. Hepatic artery embolization for neuroendocrine tumors: postprocedural management and complications. Oncologist. 2012;17(5):725–31.

15. Majeed F, Porter TR, Tarantolo S, Duhachek-Stapelman A, Xie F, Elhendy A. Carcinoid crisis and reversible right ventricular dysfunction after embolization in untreated carcinoid syndrome. Eur J Echocardiogr J Work Group Echocardiogr Eur Soc Cardiol. 2007;8(5):386–9.
16. Magabe PC, Bloom AL. Sudden death from carcinoid crisis during image-guided biopsy of a lung mass. J Vasc Interv Radiol JVIR. 2014;25(3):484–7.
17. Massimino K, Harrskog O, Pommier S, Pommier R. Octreotide LAR and bolus octreotide are insufficient for preventing intraoperative complications in carcinoid patients. J Surg Oncol. 2013;107(8):842–6.
18. Boudreaux JP, Klimstra DS, Hassan MM, Woltering EA, Jensen RT, Goldsmith SJ, et al. The NANETS consensus guideline for the diagnosis and management of neuroendocrine tumors: well-differentiated neuroendocrine tumors of the Jejunum, Ileum, Appendix, and Cecum. Pancreas. 2010;39(6):753–66.
19. Condron ME, Pommier SJ, Pommier RF. Continuous infusion of octreotide combined with perioperative octreotide bolus does not prevent intraoperative carcinoid crisis. Surgery. 2016;159(1):358–65.
20. Woltering EA, Wright AE, Stevens MA, Wang Y-Z, Boudreaux JP, Mamikunian G, et al. Development of effective prophylaxis against intraoperative carcinoid crisis. J Clin Anesth. 2016;32:189–93.
21. Clement D, Ramage J, Srirajaskanthan R. Update on pathophysiology, treatment, and complications of carcinoid syndrome. J Oncol. 2020;2020:8341426.
22. Kaltsas G, Caplin M, Davies P, Ferone D, Garcia-Carbonero R, Grozinsky-Glasberg S, et al. ENETS consensus guidelines for the standards of care in neuroendocrine tumors: pre- and perioperative therapy in patients with neuroendocrine tumors. Neuroendocrinology. 2017;105(3):245–54.
23. Howe JR, Cardona K, Fraker DL, Kebebew E, Untch BR, Wang Y-Z, et al. The surgical management of small bowel neuroendocrine Tumors: consensus guidelines of the North American Neuroendocrine Tumor Society. Pancreas. 2017;46(6):715–31.
24. Marsh HM, Martin JK, Kvols LK, Gracey DR, Warner MA, Warner ME, et al. Carcinoid crisis during anesthesia: successful treatment with a somatostatin analogue. Anesthesiology. 1987;66(1):89–91.
25. Kvols LK, Martin JK, Marsh HM, Moertel CG. Rapid reversal of carcinoid crisis with a somatostatin analogue. N Engl J Med. 1985;313(19):1229–30.
26. Condron ME, Jameson NE, Limbach KE, Bingham AE, Sera VA, Anderson RB, et al. A prospective study of the pathophysiology of carcinoid crisis. Surgery. 2019;165(1):158–65.
27. Ramage JK, Ahmed A, Ardill J, Bax N, Breen DJ, Caplin ME, et al. Guidelines for the management of gastroenteropancreatic neuroendocrine (including carcinoid) tumours (NETs). Gut. 2012;61(1):6–32.
28. Bissonnette RT, Gibney RG, Berry BR, Buckley AR. Fatal carcinoid crisis after percutaneous fine-needle biopsy of hepatic metastasis: case report and literature review. Radiology. 1990;174(3 Pt 1):751–2.
29. Mehta AC, Rafanan AL, Bulkley R, Walsh M, DeBoer GE. Coronary spasm and cardiac arrest from carcinoid crisis during laser bronchoscopy. Chest. 1999 115(2):598–600.
30. Janssen M, Salm EF, Breburda CS, van Woerkens LJ, de Herder WW, v/d Zwaan C, et al. Carcinoid crisis during transesophageal echocardiography. Intensive Care Med. 2000;26(2):254.
31. Ozgen A, Demirkazik FB, Arat A, Arat AR. Carcinoid crisis provoked by mammographic compression of metastatic carcinoid tumour of the breast. Clin Radiol. 2001;56(3):250–1.
32. Sinha V, Dyer P, Shuvro R-C, Geh JI, Karandikar S. Case of carcinoid crisis following a fine-needle biopsy of hepatic metastasis. Eur J Gastroenterol Hepatol. 2009;21(1):101–3.

33. Morrisroe K, Sim I-W, McLachlan K, Inder WJ. Carcinoid crisis induced by repeated abdominal examination. Intern Med J. 2012;42(3):342–4.
34. Jacobs REA, Bai S, Hindman N, Shah PC. Carcinoid abdominal crisis: a case report. J Surg Oncol. 2014;110(3):348–51.

Miscellaneous

Contents

Ethics in Endocrine Surgery

Megan K. Applewhite and Peter Angelos

Contents

A. L. Shifrin et al. (eds.), *Endocrine Surgery Comprehensive Board Exam Guide*,
https://doi.org/10.1007/978-3-030-84737-1_44

44.1 Introduction

Although there are many different ways of conceptualizing the ethical issues that arise in the practice of endocrine surgery, any such exploration must, in some fashion, consider the four central principles of medical ethics: autonomy, beneficence, nonmaleficence, and justice. In the upcoming paragraphs, we will explore these four principles as a means to understand the central ethical issues in the practice of endocrine surgery.

44.2 Autonomy

44.2.1 Informed Consent

In this section, we will address the ethical aspects of endocrine surgery as they relate to autonomy. Respect for patient autonomy dictates that individuals with capacity are self-determining and entitled to make decisions for themselves without undue pressure or coercion. This is the basis for informed consent. Because it is unusual for patients to need an emergency endocrine surgery operation, surgeons and patients are frequently in the fortunate position of having time in the clinic to discuss the risks, benefits, and alternatives to surgery prior to the operative date. This outpatient setting also makes possible the surgeon's establishing a relationship with the patient prior to the day of surgery. Developing such a relationship is important in that it allows the surgeon to get a sense of the patient's understanding of the goals of surgery and how extent of an operation will impact the patient's life.

The data are varied on how much information is retained from the discussion of risks and benefits of endocrine operations. One study evaluating rate of recall related to the complications and side effects of head and neck surgeries (including thyroidectomy and parathyroidectomy) found the ability to recall information given at the time of surgery evaluated within 2 months was 48% overall [1]. Those patients more likely to remember information were younger and had higher levels of education. Some data show that giving out informational packets that discuss surgery does not enhance retention of risks and benefits [2], while other data suggest the opposite, with the rate of recall of complications increasing significantly with written and verbal information (about 50%) versus verbal information alone (about 30%) [3]. Another approach that has shown promising results is the idea of increasing patient engagement in the informed consent discussion by way of a "question prompt list" given to patients before their visit with the surgeon [4]. Although this approach did not enhance engagement or outcomes, the study did find that surgeons overwhelmingly supported the use of the question prompt list, with the hope that it could encourage patient participation in the clinic conversation and decrease the unilaterality of the consult appointments, which frequently is the case given the amount of information that surgeons must explain to patients regarding the operations. A commentary suggests that such a preoperative question prompt list might facilitate shared decision-making as surgeons would be listening more and talking less, potentially allowing for patient goals and objectives to be better understood [5]. Regardless of the approach to informed consent, the element of trust between the surgeon and patient is essential to a successful relationship.

The risks of endocrine-related complications of thyroid and parathyroid surgery are few and low in incidence for high-volume surgeons [6] but are certainly impactful to the quality of life of patients who suffer them [7]. Vocal fold paralysis has been found to occur about 1% of the time, hypocalcemia between 9% and 12% of the time depending on surgeon volume, and postoperative bleeding 0.1–1.7% and wound infection <1% [8, 9]. Due to the impact of permanent injuries to the recurrent laryngeal nerve or parathyroid glands, an honest disclosure of the effects of these risks is a critical component to informed consent in thyroid and parathyroid operations. Balancing the informed consent discussion to make sure the patient understands the risk of impairments while still being reasonable about the low likelihood of their occurrence can be difficult to master. It is important to prevent the "hanging of crepe" in these discussions. This is a strategy described in the medical literature by Dr. Mark Siegler, wherein a "no-lose" scenario is created by a physician by communicating prognoses in a very grim way, such that if the patient does well, there is a sense of victory and relief, but if the patient does poorly, that was the expected outcome so more acceptable [10]. This concept was initially described to reflect critically ill patients and the likelihood of survival, but it can also be used to include communication of the likelihood of any negative outcome in healthcare. Balancing the communication is critical to establishing a durable trust in the relationship between the surgeon and the patient.

As it is typically thought of, informed consent refers particularly to the act of the operation and the intended benefits and possible complications associated with the immediate perioperative period. However, there is tremendous value in truly informing the patient of not only the short-term but probable long-term life changes that come with any given operation. Not part of the formal "informed consent" discussion, it could be argued that it is part of the process and is perhaps better termed "setting realistic expectations." For many patients, setting realistic expectations in the setting of the risks of surgery may allow them to experience less concern and feel they have more control throughout the perioperative period and even years after surgery. There is a lot to be learned from recent quality of life studies published in the endocrine surgery literature that can help patients understand postoperative life [11–13]. While quality of life studies are not without their flaws, due to sampling and other biases, they can certainly offer valuable insight about what is experienced by patients many years after surgery that can help to set appropriate expectations. As such, it is important for surgeons to have an honest discussion surrounding the indications for and the extent of necessary surgery in light of the operative risks.

The listed risks of surgery do not necessarily reflect the range of preoperative experiences that patients have. For example, with thyroid surgery, while the risk of permanent injury to the recurrent laryngeal nerve is about 1%, a quality of life survey completed by >1000 thyroid cancer survivors showed that about 55% of patients reported that they had some amount of change to their voice postoperatively [7]. If a patient is educated about the incidence of permanent nerve injury as well as the possibility of other subtle voice changes, they are less likely to think they are in the minority (1%) of patients with a permanent nerve injury if they experience a subtle subjective voice change. One can imagine that the quality of life of someone who believes they have suffered a 1% complication is probably worse than someone who knows they are experiencing an outcome that over half of others undergoing the same operation also experience.

Informed consent as trust alone represents the idea that the patient has heard all of the information as it relates to the treatment of their disease and that they trust the surgeon to act in their best interest and protect them from harm.

44.2.2 Operative Volume and the Role of Trainees

Patient perceptions of the operating room are frequently very different from reality. Unless a patient is a medical professional who works in the operating rooms or perioperative care areas, they are unlikely to understand the environment in the operating room, and this relative ignorance can heighten the fear and anxiety of surgery.

A common question asked particularly of junior to mid-career surgeons in the preoperative clinic is: "How many of these have you done?" It is an important question, as evidenced by the multiple studies demonstrating that high-volume thyroid, parathyroid, and adrenal surgeons have better outcomes than low-volume surgeons [8, 14, 15]. Before asking the question, patients frequently apologize, as they do not want to appear as though they are insulting the surgeon; however, this question should be applauded. Patients have the right to fully understand the ability of their surgeon to recognize and manage "routine" intraoperative findings as well as the more complex (and at times unanticipated) anatomy and pathology that can require complex intraoperative decision-making and creative solutions. Having participated in more operations allows a surgeon to feel comfortable with a broad spectrum of situations and maximize the likelihood of a good outcome for the patient. An honest answer and fully engaging in this discussion with the patient allows the surgeon to respect the patient's autonomy and enhances the surgeon-patient relationship.

In academic centers, the role of surgical trainees in the form of residents and medical students is another topic that often makes patients uneasy. The misconceptions of the role of trainees may stem from television shows and mass media wherein they are frequently portrayed as having significantly more responsibility and influence than is reality. Although historically surgical residents were much more autonomous with unlimited work hours and significant leeway with independent operating, the current restrictions intended to protect patients make modern operating rooms a much more controlled environment from the perspective of attending oversight. Patients frequently confirm with the attending, "...but you are the one doing the surgery, right?" and this is such a fascinating question. What does it mean to actually be doing the operation? Is the individual wielding the sharp instrument (blade, scissors, cautery) the one operating, or is the person who is giving the exposure and doing the dissection to develop and deliver the tissue that needs to be divided the person doing the operation? Surgeons and residents would likely uniformly agree that the latter is the surgeon and the former is the assistant, but certainly to the observer it could appear the other way around.

Embracing questions about case volume, operating room relationships, and the role of trainees respects patients' autonomy and is critical to adequate informed consent. For most patients, helping to conceptualize the poorly understood nature of the operating room and the interactions of surgeons and trainees can create a stronger surgeon-patient relationship.

44.3 Beneficence

44.3.1 Surgical Decision-Making

Beneficence is the obligation to act for the benefit of others, in the best interest of the patient. The principle of beneficence is at the center of surgery, as surgeons propose operative plans for therapeutic or diagnostic purposes in an effort to benefit the patient. Although performing surgery also benefits the surgeon, it is critical and expected by patients that recommendations for surgery are appropriately made only based on patient benefit rather than surgeon benefit.

Decisions regarding the extent of surgery both preoperatively and intraoperatively are integral to endocrine surgery. In the preoperative setting, for patients with small unilateral thyroid cancers, performing lobectomy or total thyroidectomy is a common conversation to have between surgeon and patient. Depending on patient preferences, and surgeon recommendations, weighing risks of recurrent laryngeal nerve injury, hypoparathyroidism, and bleeding with the benefits of being able to monitor thyroglobulin levels and preventing the potential need for a second operation are points that should be thoughtfully discussed at the individual patient level. While molecular testing may be appropriate for some, that burden of additional testing is not necessarily prudent for all. Recognizing that the goals and priorities of patients vary, it is not possible to state uniformly optimal operations for every patient. In this context, shared decision-making with regard to extent of surgery for thyroid cancer is essential [16].

Discussing extent of surgery also requires attention to the question of when to decide not to offer surgery at all or when to suggest active surveillance for some endocrinopathies. Preoperative decision-making may at times include offering the option of nonoperative treatment if, based on the patient preferences, surgery does not fulfill their goals of care. For those with asymptomatic hyperparathyroidism, or with an incidentally discovered aldosteronoma with well-controlled blood pressures on minimal medications, or a substernal multinodular goiter without concerning appearance of the nodules radiologically, do patients really need to undergo surgery? The question that needs to be asked is, "Just because we can, does that mean we should?" The same diagnosis might necessitate a clear-cut recommendation for surgery in one patient and a recommendation for active surveillance with another patient for whom medical comorbidities pose a more imminent threat than the diagnosis at hand. At what point is it the responsibility of the surgeon to counsel the patient about nonoperative options and the likelihood of their success? Because surgeons do not typically engage in long-term follow-up with patients who decline surgery, the responsibility for this discussion must also include the endocrinologist or primary care physician who may better equipped to answer their questions and set realistic expectations for long-term nonoperative outcomes.

Decisions surrounding extent of surgery do not stop after preoperative discussions. In endocrine surgery in particular, there are frequently intraoperative decisions that need to be made. The experience and discretion of the surgeon dictate the extent of surgery in many cases, which requires the implicit trust of the patient. For example, when performing a four-gland parathyroid exploration, the surgeon must determine which gland to leave behind and how much of the gland should remain. Recognizing that the complication of permanent hypoparathyroidism may be a worse problem for many than living with the effects of primary hyperparathyroidism, that decision holds a significant amount of responsibility. The ability of the surgeon to look for and identify abnormal central neck lymph nodes in order to perform lymphadenectomy in the presence of a thyroid cancer that will optimize the efficacy of postoperative radioactive iodine is another intraoperative decision that results in significant postoperative effects. These are but two of the many possible examples of decisions that a surgeon must thoughtfully execute for the good of the patient intraoperatively. Respecting patient autonomy and demonstrating beneficence with regard to preoperative and intraoperative decision-making defines the trust of the surgeon-patient relationship.

44.4 Non-maleficence

44.4.1 Complications

Non-maleficence is acting to avoid intentionally creating harm or injury. This is fundamental in the commitment made in the Hippocratic Oath to "do no harm." Complications are unavoidable in the practice of surgery. Regardless of the rigor of their training, their focus in the operating room, and care taken postoperatively, surgery is a "contact sport," and any surgeon who operates will have some adverse outcomes. The definition of "complication" adopted by some in the surgical literature is: "A surgical complication is any undesirable, unintended and direct result of surgery affecting the patient, which would not have occurred had the surgery gone as well as could reasonably be hoped." [17] When a patient asks a surgeon if she/he has ever transected a recurrent laryngeal nerve, avulsed the adrenal vein, or needed to reoperate for an airway threatening bleed, while they may hope for confirmation that this has never happened in their surgeon's experience, more experienced surgeons will reassure them that if anyone operates enough, they will have complications. The key is knowing how to address the complication, both intraoperatively and postoperatively, and abide with the patient consistently throughout their course, seeking consultation with other surgical and medical specialties as needed to lend a clear perspective.

44.4.2 Disclosure

The intent and effort to avoid harm to patients and to act in their best interests is the foundation of trust in the surgeon-patient relationship. As discussed above, complications are unavoidable even when the surgeon genuinely is acting in the best interest of the patient and doing their best to protect them from harm. When it comes to disclosure of these complications, it is out of respect for patient autonomy and the goal of non-maleficence that an honest discussion be carried out with the patient and/or family [18]. A patient is entitled to know if a complication has occurred, both out of respect for their human form and for their knowledge of their own medical and surgical history.

Complications that result in permanent injury are certainly deserving of the time and compassion of a genuine discussion with the patient. Frequently, these are risks that had been discussed preoperatively, but it would be unlikely that a patient would undergo surgery if they knew they were going to suffer an adverse outcome. Suboptimal intraoperative events that do not result in permanent injury are more in the gray area of whether or not disclosure is helpful to the patient. These events may be considered errors but not complications. The question must be asked at what point communicating every unanticipated intraoperative event with a patient becomes harmful to the patient if the patient's outcome is the same, and the small errors were handled safely.

The data are clear that high-volume surgeons are less likely to have complications, thereby supporting the role of fellowships and focused postgraduate training in endocrine surgery. Recognizing that finding a specialty-trained surgeon is not always possible, and that non-specialty trained general surgeons and otolaryngologists perform the majority of thyroidectomies, further reinforces the importance of the commitment academic endocrine surgeons make to training residents in a way that gives them the fundamental skills to perform thyroidectomy safely in the community, should they include thyroid and parathyroid operations in their surgical career.

44.4.3 Innovation in Surgery

Innovation in surgery is adopted by surgeons at varying rates. Without any oversight of surgical techniques, creativity is a critical component of intraoperative decision-making. It remains an important ethical question of how to integrate innovations of technique and technology into the operating room [19]. Given the obstacles encountered in the operating room, it is not always possible to anticipate when innovation will be necessary. Creativity in solving challenges in the operating room is a regular requirement of the job, but appreciating when creativity extends to innovation and research is important so that, when possible, the patient can be brought into the conversation to preserve the patient's autonomy.

How, when, and for whom innovative techniques are employed is deserving of a thoughtful discussion, and the answers to these questions will vary from surgeon to surgeon. The principle of non-maleficence represents the surgeon's obligation to do their best to prevent injury to the patient whenever possible. Some surgeons may view early adoption of innovative techniques as putting patients at unacceptable risk of harm, whereas others view employment of innovation as beneficence, that is, as a way to do the best possible good they can for a patient.

While it can present challenges early on, progressive utilization of novel technologies in endocrine operations is an important part of pushing our capabilities forward and enhancing patient care over time. The early adopters of new techniques and technologies have the obligation to record and report their outcomes in order for quality improvement and patient safety to be optimized for future widespread implementation. As mentioned previously in the discussion surrounding informed consent, the incidence of the complications after endocrine operations (including adrenalectomy) is very low. As such, proving superiority of a novel technology over current standard of care often requires a large sample size, which makes practice changes based on randomized studies difficult. For example, surgeons are increasingly utilizing indocyanine green to determine vascular supply to parathyroid glands following subtotal parathyroidectomy [20] and total thyroidectomy [21]. Since one of the most common postoperative complications of subtotal parathyroidectomy and total thyroidectomy is hypoparathyroidism (albeit very low incidence), having a way to determine if a parathyroid is going to function in situ or if it needs to be autotransplanted could significantly improve the quality of life of some patients. This type of potentially dramatic reduction in surgical risk is one that certainly is deserving of large-scale studies and implementation if the outcomes are favorable.

Robotic surgery and, more recently, transoral endoscopic thyroidectomy are other advances in surgical approaches that have taken on an increasing presence in the practice of some endocrine surgeons [22–24]. Ideally, the utilization of robotic and transoral surgery is preserved for surgeons with adequate training, who genuinely feel the approach will benefit the patient beyond traditional approaches [25]. Whether this be due to decreased pain, improved operative times, cosmetic outcome, or enhanced capabilities to visualize critical structures such that the intervention is safer, utilization of such approaches should ultimately serve to improve patient outcomes. Ethically employing technology and innovative approaches to surgery requires the best judgment of the surgeon for the sake of the individual patient and, when possible, solid peer-reviewed evidence to support its utilization. These should guide the decision-making of the surgeon, rather than business-driven marketing campaigns, which can be misleading and potentially harm patients for whom other approaches are safer and offer more long-term benefit [26].

44.5 Justice

The fourth central principle of medical ethics, justice, dictates the duty of the physician to do his or her best to ensure costs and benefits are fairly distributed. As described by Aristotle [27], justice is a form of fairness, insofar as it is giving to each that which is due. In the context of endocrine surgery, as throughout all healthcare, the central ethical issue in justice is the need to ensure that efforts are undertaken to mitigate the disparities of outcomes for different patient groups whether based on gender, race, or socioeconomic status. As the recent experience with COVID-19 has further emphasized, race continues to play a significant role in access to medical care and in outcomes at least in some countries. Surgeons must not assume that the outcomes of surgical patients are immune to the impact of race and socioeconomic status. Quite the contrary, surgeons must remain ever vigilant to the potential impact that different healthcare policies can have on their patient's outcomes and how the policies mitigate or exacerbate the disparities that are so commonly seen.

44.6 Conclusions

Although the ethical issues in the practice of endocrine surgery are not unique and different from the issues in other surgical specialties, they nevertheless play a significant role in the relationships between surgeons and patients. The four central principles of medical ethics, i.e., autonomy, beneficence, non-maleficence, and justice, all impact the ways that endocrine surgeons should optimally interact with their patients. The ethical dimension of the practice of endocrine surgeon should not be ignored without risking significant erosion in the surgeon-patient relationship that will eventually have a negative impact on both patients and surgeons.

References

1. Hekkenberg RJ, Irish JC, Rotstein LE, Brown DH, Gullane PJ. Informed consent in head and neck surgery: how much do patients actually remember? J Otolaryngol. 1997;26(3):155–9.
2. Alsaffar H, et al. Informed consent: do information pamphlets improve post-operative risk-recall in patients undergoing total thyroidectomy: prospective randomized control study. J Otolaryngol Head Neck Surg. 2016;45:14.

3. Chan Y, Irish JC, Wood SJ, et al. Patient education and informed consent in head and neck surgery. Arch Otolaryngol Head Neck Surg. 2002;128(11):1269–74.
4. Schwarze ML, Buffington A, Tucholka JL, et al. Effectiveness of a question prompt list intervention for older patients considering major surgery: a multisite randomized clinical trial [published online October 30, 2019]. JAMA Surg. 2020;155(1):6–13.
5. Angelos P. Interventions to improve informed consent: perhaps surgeons should speak less and listen more. JAMA Surg. 2020;155(1):13–4.
6. Adam M, et al. Is there a minimum number of thyroidectomies a surgeon should perform to optimize patient outcomes? Ann Surg. 2017;265(2):402–7.
7. Aschebrook-Kilfoy B, et al. Risk factors for decreased quality of life in thyroid cancer survivors: initial findings from the North American Thyroid Cancer Survivorship Study. Thyroid. 2015;25(12):1313–21.
8. Hauch A, Al-Qurayshi Z, Randolph G, et al. Total thyroidectomy is associated with increased risk of complications for low- and high-volume surgeons. Ann Surg Oncol. 2014;21:3844–52.
9. Promberger R, Ott J, Kober F, et al. Risk factors for postoperative bleeding after thyroid surgery. Br J Surg. 2012;99(3):373–9.
10. Siegler M. Pascal's wager and the hanging of crepe. N Engl J Med. 1975;293(17):853–7.
11. Nickel B, Tan T, Cvejic E, et al. Health-related quality of life after diagnosis and treatment of differentiated thyroid cancer and association with type of surgical treatment. JAMA Otolaryngol Head Neck Surg. 2019;145(3):231–8.
12. Ejlsmark-Svensson H, Sikjaer T, Webb SM, Rejnmark L, Rolighed L. Health-related quality of life improves 1 year after parathyroidectomy in primary hyperparathyroidism: a prospective cohort study. Clin Endocrinol. 2019;90(1):184–91.
13. Greenhill C. QOL improves after adrenalectomy. Nat Rev Endocrinol. 2010;6:243.
14. Al-Qurayshi Z, Robins R, Buell J, Kandil E. Surgeon volume impact on outcomes and cost of adrenal surgeries. Eur J Surg Oncol. 2016;42(10):1483–90.
15. Adam MA, Thomas S, Youngwirth L, et al. Is there a minimum number of thyroidectomies a surgeon should perform to optimize patient outcomes? Ann Surg. 2017;265(2):402–7.
16. Wang TS, Sosa JA. Thyroid surgery for differentiated thyroid cancer – recent advances and future directions. Nat Rev Endocrinol. 2018;14(11):670–83.
17. Sokol D, Wilson J. What is a surgical complication? World J Surg. 2008;32:942–4.
18. Adedeji A, et al. Ethics of surgical complications. World J Surg. 2009;33:732–7.
19. Angelos P. The ethics of introducing new surgical technology into clinical practice: the importance of the patient-surgeon relationship. JAMA Surg. 2016;151(5):405–6.
20. Vidal Fortuny J, Belfontali V, Sadowski SM, Karenovics W, Guigard S, F. TriponezParathyroid gland angiography with indocyanine green fluorescence to predict parathyroid function after thyroid surgery. Br J Surg. 2016;1035:537–43.
21. Lang BH, Wong CK, Hung HT, Wong KP, Mak KL, Au KB. Indocyanine green fluorescence angiography for quantitative evaluation of in situ parathyroid gland perfusion and function after total thyroidectomy. Surgery. 2017;161(1):87–95.
22. Berber E, Mitchell J, Milas M, Siperstein A. Robotic posterior retroperitoneal adrenalectomy: operative technique. Arch Surg. 2010;145(8):781–4.

23. Garstka ME, Alameer ES, Awwad SA, Kandil E. Conventional robotic endoscopic thyroidectomy for thyroid cancer. Endocrinol Metab Clin N Am. 2019;48(1):153–63.
24. Jongekkasit I, Jitpratoom P, Sasanakietkul T, Anuwong A. Transoral endoscopic thyroidectomy for thyroid cancer. Endocrinol Metab Clin N Am. 2019;48(1):165–80.
25. AAGL Advancing Minimally Invasive Gynecology Worldwide. Guidelines for privileging for robotic-assisted gynecologic laparoscopy. J Minim Invasive Gynecol. 2014;21(2):157–67.
26. Christian F, Pitt DF, Bond J, et al. Professionalism--connecting the past and the present and a blueprint for the Canadian Association of General Surgeons. Can J Surg. 2008;51(2):88–91.
27. Aristotle in 23 Volumes, Vol. 19, translated by H. Rackham. Cambridge, MA, Harvard University Press; London, William Heinemann Ltd. 1934.

How to Read and Interpret a Scientific Paper

Özer Makay and Kerstin Lorenz

Contents

A. L. Shifrin et al. (eds.), *Endocrine Surgery Comprehensive Board Exam Guide*,
https://doi.org/10.1007/978-3-030-84737-1_45

45.1 Introduction

> The art of knowing is knowing what to ignore. – Jalaleddin Rumi[1]

In the aim to provide optimal patient care, we are appointed to continuously update our medical knowledge. The increasing number of publications, the accelerating new data accessible, and the claim to conform to the standards of evidence-based medicine make it challenging to keep oneself up to date [1]. All the more it is important to select and direct the reading to valuable scientific reports. To invest the necessary time into rewarding reports, some skills of critical appraisal of scientific publications can be refined by applying some basic principles. Next to grasping the medical content of a scientific paper, it is important to interpret and evaluate the data presented; thus, the statics used need to be regarded [2]. However, specifics of statistical analysis will not be addressed in detail in this outline. In the following, the basic principles for evaluation of scientific publications that can be generalized for the fields of experimental, clinical (text and video), and epidemiological medical research are outlined with emphasis on clinical research reports.

45.2 What Scientific Report to Read?

The decision which paper to read is closely linked to the intention behind the reading. In case one keeps up to date by continuous periodical perusal of publications in journals dedicated to the field of one's interest, it is most likely a choice made by a catching title, indication of a novelty, change of established proceedings, and personal interest. For a rough orientation, reading the abstract helps to decide whether to read the full article. Generally, the abstracts mirror the articles' structures (aims, methods, results, conclusions, and keywords) and provide a brief account on the primary objective investigated and the content, so the reader has an idea of what to expect. In case a certain aspect in a given field is to be explored or a quick orientation in a subject is warranted, reading most recent review article(s), ideally by renowned experts in the field, are advisable. For a more in-depth exploration of the chosen topic, the reader can primarily refer to the article's references and from there in the references listed in the cited publications. For fur-

1 Also known as "Mevlana," Rumi was a thirteenth-century poet and Sufi mystic, originally from Greater Khorasan in Greater Iran. Rumi's influence transcends national borders and ethnic divisions. His poems have been widely translated into many of the world's languages and transposed into various formats. Like other mystic and Sufi poets of Persian literature, Rumi's poetry speaks of love which infuses the world. Rumi has been described as the "most popular poet" and the "best selling poet" in the United States (source: ► www.en.wikipedia.org).

ther exploration and search of the most recent update in the topic as in case there are no current reviews available, search of medical databases (PubMed, Cochrane, EBSCOhost, Medscape, Ovid, Embase, etc.) is advised. The given keywords can also be used to search the databases for corresponding publications.

45.3 How to Structure the Reading?

By implication, the reading follows the article's structure. As stated above, the abstract provides a rough orientation of the full article. In case the reader looks for information referring strictly to a certain group of patients, efficient selection of articles will be directed to find inclusion or exclusion criteria firstly in the title and secondly in the methods part of the abstract, and if not found there, consult the methods section in the full article. Whenever the article is valued worthwhile thorough reading by perusal of the abstract, the reader follows the given structure [3, 4]. Most scientific medical publications adhere to this structure:

1. Abstract (see above)
2. Introduction
3. Methods
4. Results
5. Discussion
6. Conclusions
7. References
8. Amendments

2. In the introduction, the reader can expect to be briefed about the objective of the current investigation in the light of previous or ongoing research and basic preconditions that entailed the specific question that is addressed now. The clinical or scientific background presented here is usually backed by the most important and recent accompanying findings and statements from other researchers, and the references are adequately provided.
3. The methods section can be referred to as an indicator for the quality and validity of the study presented. Generally, all procedures and the course of actions as well as the choice of study design are described and argued. Importantly, the study design must be aligned to the aim targeted. Thus, the nature of the study can vary from description to exploration or confirmation. Irrespective of the study type, a precise definition of the endpoint(s) and precise data on the study's details should be described to the degree that a reproduction study according to the information provided can be designed. The methods description correlates with the nature of

the investigation: for laboratory and experimental studies, more details addressing the model used or the execution of the procedural steps are warranted compared to clinical studies. The statistical methods applied should be accurately described and be suitable for the study design and endpoint chosen [2]. According to the nature of the study, some elements are required and indicate the quality of the investigation:

- Experimental/laboratory study: study plan, study protocol, pilot study, study cohort (patient/animal/cell line), control cohort, study location(s), study period, ethics approval, study design, study execution, and accuracy.
- Clinical study: prospective/retrospective, unicentric/bicentric/multicentric, sample size estimation (power calculation), control group (historical, actual, placebo), randomized/non-randomized, and blinded/unblended. Review of the Consolidated Standards of Reporting Trials (CONSORT) diagram typically illustrates the subject recruitment.
- Epidemiological study (intervention, cohort, case control, cross-sectional, ecological): rare diseases/tumors, environmental influences/exposure/agents, single/multiple agents, multiple endpoints, cause/effect and cofactors, standardized conditions/measurement (reliability/validity), scale type, choice of statistical test, description measures (table/graph), mean values, confidence intervals, p-values, and appropriate sample size [5].

4. In the results section, account of all findings is presented ideally without interpretation. The reader should be able to objectively receive the data structured according to the aim of the study and detailed study cohort. Thus, the findings are firstly described followed by all necessary statistical parameters (case number, mean value, confidence interval, variation, statistical significance, effect size), and for clarity, the main findings may be depicted in tables or graphs. It is commonplace that study results with statistical significance will be more likely to be published and recognized; however, this harbors a publication bias as the clinical impact of insignificant results may be important [5]. In some journals, extensive additional data may be presented in a supplement. This data may be positively confirmatory and provide very detailed information for the dedicated reader. Perusal of these supplements is recommended to elucidate the findings and to exclude masking of contradictory data.
5. In the discussion section, the outlined basis initially presented in the introduction is picked up again, and the results of the current study are clearly stated and mir-

rored against previous or actual comparable studies. The reader should be aware if the results presented are plausible and in accord with the methods applied and data provided. Furthermore, it should be made clear if the current data add to the state of knowledge in the field and if the data are reliable enough so that the conclusions will influence or change the presently established practice. Possibly, the current findings need to initiate further investigations before any change on established procedures may be considered or new and unanticipated questions arise. In case the findings of the current study have strong implications to influence the established practice, comparison to other or previous studies should positively correlate in line with the adjustments suggested. Whenever there result contradictory conclusions to current practice or the main corpus of corresponding publications, the discussion section should provide plausible and clear arguments. Any vague or imprecise explanation or missing comment should alert the reader that weaknesses regarding the evidence or the study design may be missed, underreported, or masked.

High standard articles address in the discussion section the limitations identified and clarify whether these will affect the results [3, 4]. Generally, the more open and direct the limitations are detailed, the more sustainable the data presented appear. In critical discussion, possible bias with systematic or random effect will be checked. Selection bias and group discrepancies are particularly detailed. Special attention can be directed to the completeness or lacking of data in the follow-up, e.g., how many patients were lost or dropped out of a study. Good-quality studies describe the reasons for and characteristics of dropouts and estimate the effect of missing data. Furthermore, important factors that can produce errors in clinical studies are confounders. These confounders should ideally be identified and evaluated by the authors, or in lack thereof, the error margin and potential bias should be addressed. Whenever dependent variables are closely associated, the precise impact of a factor may not be discriminated, and this needs to be adjusted for the specific confounder in question. In the discussion section, the prevalent study's findings are to be compared to equivalent investigations. The apparent and important confirmatory as well as differing results are debated by the authors, and the strengths and potential weaknesses of the study introduced are weighed against the prevalent literature.

6. In the conclusions, the authors highlight the most relevant findings of the study presented. Ideally, the potential conclusions are firstly indicated when the results are presented since they must be deduced from the results

and backed by the trial's data. Again, as prepared for in the discussion section, the authors should indicate how the limitations of the study may have affected the results and weigh if the conclusions formulated withstand these arguably. In case the presented study confirms other study's findings, this should be mentioned, as well as authors should explore possible reasons and potential errors in case they arrive at conflicting conclusions. Even studies that state their findings as outlined and do not reach significant results support their credibility and harbor clinical impact.

7. The references section should be complete with regard to the citations used and represent an adequate selection of the important and recent publication in the topic addressed. Sometimes historical references will be essential to include.
8. Bonus information that can help to reflect the credibility of an article can be found in the following:
   - Author's list: are all expected contributors (e.g., all specialties involved in a clinical trial) listed?
   - Institutions: are the authors and institutions by accord likely to be credible?
   - Funding and conflict of interest statement: is any form of funding involved and does this harbor potential conflict of interest to the conduct of the study; is a conflict of interest statement provided and is it plausible with regard to the study?
   - Acknowledgments: some journals restrict the number of authors listed, then contributions by other researchers may be acknowledged in an amendment statement, or the contribution provided is judged to not comply with an authorship.

45.4 What About Evidence and Its Grading in Medicine?

In prevalent clinical questions, especially when contradictory practice patterns and recommendations exist, evidence is desired to choose wisely. In such scenario, one can consult the most recent professional society's guidelines that specify the problem in question or turn to systematic reviews and meta-analyses [6]. With regard to clinical research articles, the lowest level of evidence is represented by case reports and the highest level by data from multicentric randomized studies (RCT). Research articles that present data of a clinical study will usually represent only low grades of evidence and strength of recommendation as its findings will most likely need to be confirmed by others and further studies. Guidelines are ranked by the level of evidence research and the corresponding grading of recommendations they are based on. In meta-analyses, the level of evidence is rarely stated but can be derived from the quality of the primary studies included. Depending on the adequate and comprehensible statistics applied, meta-analyses can also provide improved levels of evidence compared to primary studies. Systematic reviews are based on a specific clinical problem that can be structured by, e.g., the PICO model (P = patient/population/problem, I = intervention, C = comparison/control, O = outcome/effect).

To quickly find and determine the quality of the best available evidence, it is possible to label the existing evidence. The use of best available evidence in making decisions and the use of levels of evidence and grades of recommendations will improve clinical practice. Several evidence rating scales are available. One of these is the GRADE: Grading of Recommendations Assessment, Development and Evaluation Working Group (modified by the EBM Guidelines Editorial Team) (◘ Table 45.1) [7].

Levels of evidence and grades of recommendations according to the SIGN grading system [8–10]:

◘ Table 45.1 Level of evidence in medicine

Code	Quality of evidence	Definition
A	High	Further research is very unlikely to change our confidence in the estimate of effect
		Several high-quality studies with consistent results
		In special cases: one large, high-quality multicenter trial
B	Moderate	Further research is likely to have an important impact on our confidence in the estimate of effect and may change the estimate
		One high-quality study
		Several studies with some limitations
C	Low	Further research is very likely to have an important impact on our confidence in the estimate of effect and is likely to change the estimate
		One or more studies with severe limitations
D	Very Low	Any estimate of effect is very uncertain
		Expert opinion
		No direct research evidence
		One or more studies with very severe limitations

- **Levels of Evidence**

1++ – High-quality meta-analyses, systematic reviews of RCTs, or RCTs with a very low risk of bias

1+ – Well-conducted meta-analyses, systematic reviews, or RCTs with a low risk of bias

1− – Meta-analyses, systematic reviews, or RCTs with a high risk of bias

2++ – High-quality systematic reviews of case control or cohort or studies

High-quality case control or cohort studies with a very low risk of confounding or bias and a high probability that the relationship is causal

2+ – Well-conducted case control or cohort studies with a low risk of confounding or bias and a moderate probability that the relationship is causal

2− – Case control or cohort studies with a high risk of confounding or bias and a significant risk that the relationship is not causal

3 – Non-analytic studies, e.g., case reports, case series

4 – Expert opinion

- **Grades of Recommendations**

A – At least one meta-analysis, systematic review, or RCT rated as 1++ and directly applicable to the target population

A body of evidence consisting principally of studies rated as 1+, directly applicable to the target population, and demonstrating overall consistency of results

B – A body of evidence including studies rated as 2++, directly applicable to the target population, and demonstrating overall consistency of results

Extrapolated evidence from studies rated as 1++ or 1+

C – A body of evidence including studies rated as 2+, directly applicable to the target population, and demonstrating overall consistency of results

Extrapolated evidence from studies rated as 2++

D – Evidence level 3 or 4

Extrapolated evidence from studies rated as 2+

In the following, a choice of questions and aspects is provided to roughly assess research publications like clinical trial data (Table 45.2).

Table 45.2 Quick checkbox on quality and credibility of articles

Question/aspect	Benefit/intention	Check for/caveat	*In favor for* quality/credibility of article	*Against* quality/credibility of article
Study design				
Aim of the study	Primary endpoint clearly defined	Primary/secondary endpoints maintained	Primary/secondary endpoints maintained	Change in endpoints
Question of clinical value/interest/relevance/innovative			+++	
Comparative statements/data	Research environment	Citation correctness/comprehensiveness	Support of statements/data	
Data support conclusions			+++	
Conflict of author statement	Credibility, independence of data	Imprecise/missing statements		
Study methods				
Type of study determined	Confirmatory vs. exploratory vs. descriptive study design	Study type in line with aim	Type of study clearly stated; defined goals are followed	Missing declaration of study type
Study population	Area, period, recruitment, power calculation	Imprecise/missing statements	Adequate number included, power adequate	Cohort too small/dropouts or exits too high
Dropouts/exits	Traceability of study subjects	Imprecise/missing statement, only exits	Coherent numbers and reasons for dropouts/crossovers	Contradictory numbers, no dropout information or only exit
Monitoring	Data completeness/confounders	Missing data/lack of identification of confounders		

(continued)

Table 45.2 (continued)

Question/aspect	Benefit/intention	Check for/caveat	*In favor for* quality/ credibility of article	*Against* quality/ credibility of article
Study statistics				
Multicenter trial	Larger/diverse sample size, rare disease/event	Firm regulation/ adherence protocol Outcome validated/ reproducible	Compromise standardization intervention + outcome	Sites are covariates
Dichotomous outcome measure	Treatment comparison	Clear definition of endpoint		
Continuous outcome measure	More power to detect differences between groups			
Correlation and p-value	Differences distinct	p-value may be very sensitive for weak correlations	95% confidence interval (CI) provided	No 95% confidence interval (CI) provided

45.5 Checkbox Basic Questions on Study Quality and Credibility

- Sample size adequate?
- Recruitment method and study population adequate?
- Difference of samples in population relevant?
- Number of subjects in study arms and number of and reasons for dropouts or crossover.
- Bias in study design? Subject in treatment study arm, blinding (single/double, process successful/unsuccessful?), and comparator.
- Randomized study: intention-to-treat (ITT) analysis provided?
- Study type: what is tested for – superiority, equivalence, non-inferiority? Are the definitions of the treatment arms different at the start? Check sample-size calculation; larger samples are needed for equivalence/non-inferiority. Inappropriate subsequent change of study type?
- Definition of success? How is it measured? Is it validated? Precise and reproducible? Is it clinically relevant?
- Primary outcome: focus kept?
- Surrogate (secondary) outcomes: strong independent association of surrogate and desired outcome? Surrogate and clinical outcome improve concordantly.
- Dichotomous and continuous outcomes, correlations, time-to-event endpoints: are endpoints defined clearly?
- Confidence interval 95% provided?

References

1. Sackett DL, Rosenberg WM, Gray JA, Haynes RB, Scott RW. Evidence base medicine: what is and what isn't. BMJ. 1996;312:71–2.
2. Govani SM, Higgins PD. How to read a clinical trial paper: a lesson in basic trial statistics. Gastroenterol Hepatol. 2012;8:241–8.
3. Du Prel JB, Röhrig B, Blettner M. Critical appraisal of scientific articles. Dtsch Arztebl Int. 2009;106:100–5.
4. Röhrig B, du Prel JB, Blettner M. Study design in medical research. Dtsch Arztebl Int. 2009;106:184–9.
5. Amrhein V, Greenland S, MCShane B. Retire statistical significance. Nature. 2019;567:305–7.
6. Mak A, Cheung MW, Fu EY, Ho RC. Meta-analysis in medicine: an introduction. Int J Rheumat Dis. 2010;13:101–4.
7. Guyatt GH, Oxman AD, Vist GE, Kunz R, Falck-Ytter Y, Alonso-Coello P, et al. GRADE: an emerging consensus on rating quality of evidence and strength of recommendations. BMJ (Clin Res ed). 2008;336(7650):924–6.
8. Harbour R, Miller J. A new system for grading recommendations in evidence based guidelines. BMJ. 2001;323(7308):334–6.
9. The GRADE working group. Grading quality of evidence and strength of recommendations. BMJ. 2004;328:1–8.
10. Siglo BA, Murad MH, Schünemann HJ, Kunz R, Vigersky R, Guyatt GH, Montori VM. A case for clarity, consistency, and helpfulness: state-of-the-art clinical practice guidelines in endocrinology using the Grading of recommendations, Assessment, Development, and Evaluation system. J Clin Endocrinol Metab. 2008;93:666–7.

Training and Board Certification in Endocrine Surgery

Oliver Gimm and *Marco Raffaelli*

Contents

A. L. Shifrin et al. (eds.), *Endocrine Surgery Comprehensive Board Exam Guide*,
https://doi.org/10.1007/978-3-030-84737-1_46

46.1 Introduction

Training and examination in any medical specialty should be strongly intertwined since training without any form of examination must be questioned if the task one has been trained for entails responsibility and/or a degree. It is therefore remarkable that, according to a European survey from 2018, at least four European countries do not have any form of examination at the end of their training program for surgical residents [1].

When it comes to surgical subspecialization, the existing discrepancy between training and examination in many European countries becomes even more obvious. With regard to endocrine surgery, seemingly only about 25% of the European countries do have any form of examination which in general is part of a broader surgical examination [1]. Here is where the European Union of Medical Specialist (UEMS) comes into play. The UEMS has the mandate to organize medical examinations on the European level. It currently consists of 43 specialist sections and boards including the Section of Surgery. The Division of Endocrine Surgery (DES) is one of the divisions within the Section of Surgery. Since 2003, the DES has organized examinations in endocrine surgery (including the thyroid gland, the parathyroid glands, the adrenal glands, and neuroendocrine neoplasms of the gastro-entero-pancreatic tract). Successful candidates get a European Board of Surgery Qualification (EBSQ) certificate. Since 2008, examinations are even organized for the neck part only (i.e., the thyroid gland and the parathyroid glands). This enables even surgeons who specialize in head and neck endocrine surgery including otolaryngologists to take the exam. As of July 2020, a total of 162 surgeons/otolaryngologists have passed the EBSQ exam – 108 have passed the exam in endocrine surgery and 54 in neck endocrine surgery. Successful candidates are considered fellows of the DES and entitled to bear the title Fellow of the European Board of Surgery (either FEBS, endocrine surgery, or FEBS, neck endocrine surgery). A similar exam does not exist in any other country including the United States. However, the UEMS EBSQ exam is open even to non-Europeans, and 13 out of the current 162 fellows are practicing outside the European Union.

Examinations in endocrine surgery have now been carried out for 17 years. However, how does one harmonize training and examination since it is the European national surgical boards that determine the content of their surgical training programs? Here, once again, the UEMS comes into play since the UEMS not only has the mandate to organize examinations on the European levels but it is also setting the standard for training and practice in medical specialties. With regard to surgery, in order to achieve this, the divisions of the Section of Surgery are defining European Training Requirements (ETRs).

Nevertheless, it is still the European national boards that determine the content of their surgical training programs. However, if the European national boards have any interest that their surgeons are considered as qualified as surgeons from any other European country, then those boards should ensure that their national surgical training programs are in accordance with the ETRs.

With regard to endocrine surgery, this task can be more challenging as opposed to other surgical subspecialties, e.g., vascular surgery. Training in endocrine surgery always has been challenging for a variety of reasons. One reason is that the organs involved, namely, the thyroid gland, the parathyroid glands, the adrenal glands, and neuroendocrine neoplasms (NENs) of the gastro-entero-pancreatic (GEP) tract, are taken care of by otolaryngologists, head and neck surgeons, general surgeons, upper and lower gastrointestinal surgeons, surgical oncologists, and urologists. In contrast to many other subspecialties, this makes endocrine surgery a subspecialty that is best viewed as a "community" of subspecialties. The overall ongoing subspecialization within the broad field of surgery also contributes to the difficulty to be able to offer the broad spectrum of surgical procedures encompassing all endocrine organs as defined above. For example, some departments offer surgery of the thyroid gland, while the lymph nodes, in particular, in the lateral compartments are taken care of by otolaryngologists/head and neck surgeons. Also, surgery of NENs of the gastrointestinal tract and pancreas is more and more performed by (upper) gastrointestinal surgeons.

46.2 Training and Volume

Training in surgery starts already during residency. During residency, the surgical trainee is confronted with a variety of different surgical procedures in order to become a surgical specialist. While endocrine surgery is part of the training of most European residency programs, the number of required operations is very low [1]. Therefore, fellowships in endocrine surgery are of great importance. During such a fellowship, fellows in endocrine surgery have to acquire a much more profound knowledge in the various surgical aspects and approaches to diseases of the thyroid gland and the parathyroid and adrenal glands as well as NENs of the GEP tract.

46.2.1 Thyroid Gland Surgery and Neck Dissections

According to the literature, the exposure of both residents and fellows in endocrine surgery to thyroid gland operations has increased dramatically during the recent decades. For US residents in otolaryngology, the numbers for performed thyroidectomies increased from about 16 in 1996 to about 55 in 2015 [2]. With regard to fellows in endocrine surgery, an average number exceeding 100 operations has been reported [3]. Of interest, 60 operations have been considered to be required to achieve competency [4].

Nevertheless, as the aforementioned European survey from 2018 has shown, the current training of residents in general surgery with regard to thyroid surgery varies considerably [1]. The required minimum number of thyroid operations during surgical residency as defined by the European national boards often is not considered sufficient to enable the young specialist to perform this type of operation independently and safely. European national delegates considered only 15 performed operations to be an appropriate number of operations for residents [1]. With regard to fellows in endocrine surgery, 20–30 total thyroidectomies and 20–40 hemithyroidectomies were considered appropriate [1] which is in agreement with the 60 thyroidectomies considered appropriate in the aforementioned study [4]. These numbers are very close to what is demanded by the DES. Currently 50 performed thyroid operations are the minimum requirement.

In comparison to the total number of thyroidectomies, fewer numbers of neck dissections used to be performed by surgical residents. According to one report, less than two neck dissections are performed on average. Luckily, fellows in endocrine surgery use to perform between 6 and 15 neck dissections [3, 4]. In this regard, it is of interest that 12 neck dissections have been considered appropriate to achieve the required competence according to one publication [4] which is very similar to the minimum number ($n = 10$) considered appropriate by the European national delegates [1].

In accordance with this, at least ten central or lateral neck dissections are the recommended minimum number of performed procedures for fellows in (neck) endocrine surgery [1].

46.2.2 Parathyroid Gland Surgery

According to the data of the Residency Review Committee (RRC) of the Accreditation Council for Graduate Medical Education (ACGME), there seems to be an obvious increase of parathyroidectomies performed by graduating general surgery residents from about four in 1986 to more than nine in 2015 [3, 5–10]. Results for otolaryngology-head and neck surgery residency programs showed that the number of performed parathyroidectomies was even higher, about 16 such operations in 2015 [8, 10, 11]. Despite these seemingly low numbers, most American Association of Endocrine Surgeons (AAES) members (almost 80%) responding to a survey reported that a final-year resident from their institution could autonomously perform a parathyroidectomy in a patient with concordant imaging [11]. The AAES reported that endocrine surgery fellows graduated with a median of 80–90 parathyroid procedures [3, 4].

These numbers exceed the estimated numbers ($n = 50$) of performed cases considered appropriate to be competent [3, 4]. The latter are more in accordance with the opinion of the European national delegates. According to them, 25 performed focused procedures and 15 performed bilateral neck explorations are considered appropriate [1]. Currently, the minimum number of performed parathyroidectomies as required by the DES is 15, but another 20 assisted procedures are required as well.

46.3 Adrenal Gland Surgery

Most surgical residents do not perform any adrenalectomy during their training [9], and this number has been low for decades. It is of importance to note that it has been shown that resident participation will lead to a longer operative time but is not associated with significant differences in the outcomes including complications and mortality [12]. Strikingly, one study even showed that operations performed with the participation of either residents or fellows were associated with a lower rate of serious complications as compared to operations without the participation of any trainee (fellows 2.8%, residents 6.0%, no trainee 7.9%). Unfortunately, it is not known whether the cases without any trainee participation were more difficult, and, therefore, conclusions have to be drawn cautiously. In another study, no significant difference was found concerning the rates of wound infections, medical complications, reoperations, or overall morbidity between cases operated by attendings alone or with the involvement of residents/fellows [13].

According to the European national delegates, 20 performed adrenalectomies are considered appropriate for fellows in endocrine surgery [1]. Of note, this number is well over the annual workload of many units performing adrenal surgery. This would be an argument why training in adrenal surgery might have to be centralized to units with an annual workload of over 20 cases. Studies have shown that probably between 30 and 40 laparoscopic operations are required to master the procedure [14, 15]. Interestingly, when applying a stage training, these numbers obviously can be lowered [16]. Others have considered 15 laparoscopic adrenalectomies to be sufficient to achieve competency [4].

It is now recommended that the minimum number of both performed and assisted adrenalectomies for fellows in endocrine surgery is 15 [1].

46.4 Surgery of Gastro-Entero-Pancreatic Neuroendocrine Neoplasms

When it comes to surgery of gastro-entero-pancreatic neuroendocrine neoplasms (GEP-NENs), being able to offer sufficient training to achieve competency is even more challenging. The main reasons are that the relatively low numbers of patients and the fact that surgery on these organs more often may be performed by other surgical subspecialties. When it comes to surgery of the stomach, intestine, and pancreas, the majority of tumors operated on are non-endocrine. This differs surgery of GEP-NENs from surgery of tumors in the aforementioned endocrine organs.

Literature addressing training of surgical residents or fellows with regard to GEP-NENs is almost non-existing. Since the surgical strategy of both primary tumors but even metastases of NENs may differ from the strategy for the more common adenocarcinoma counterparts [17], the absence of almost any literature on training in this regard is remarkable. Nevertheless, there exist some literatures with regard to other procedures on the stomach, intestine, and pancreas. With regard to gastric operations, some investigators reported that resident participation seems to lead to an increase of the incidence of superficial site infection [18, 19] which is most likely due to longer operating times, but it has been considered to be clinically insignificant. With regard to training in intestinal surgery, laparoscopic procedures have been investigated at a larger scale. Concerning laparoscopic colorectal surgery, it was demonstrated that final-year residents can achieve results that do not affect patient safety and short-term outcome adversely [20]. To achieve independency, fellows may have to perform 50 laparoscopic colorectal procedures [21, 22]. Of interest, there is one study from 1996 analyzing the experience of residents with regard to some rare endocrine diseases including endocrine pancreatic surgery [23]. While some residents performed up to ten such procedures, close to 85% of the residents did not perform any such procedure at all. With regard to non-endocrine hepato-pancreatobiliary surgery, less than 50% of the residents were considered competent by the program directors despite that fact that the residents completed about 70% of all operations. This may not be surprising since more than half of all operations were performed during their final years [24]. Obviously, it would be desirable to expose residents sooner to more complex procedures [25]. Nevertheless, in contrast to resident programs, current fellowship programs in the United States seem to be able to offer quite sufficient numbers of operations [26].

According to the European survey in 2018, the national surgical boards require that surgical residents have performed only a few intestinal procedures (mean 5) but close to zero gastric and pancreatic operations [1]. According to the European national delegates, surgical residents should perform at least about 15 operations on the stomach, intestine, and pancreas. Nevertheless, one cannot achieve proficiency with such little experience.

Of note, the numbers for fellows in endocrine surgery were only slightly higher. For gastric, intestinal, and pancreatic procedures, a median minimum of 17 procedures was recommended to be performed by fellows in endocrine surgery according to the European national delegates [1]. It is worth noting that surgery of GEP-NENs is not part of endocrine fellowship program in most European countries.

The current recommendation is that fellows in endocrine surgery perform and assist a minimum number of ten operations on GEP-NENs [1].

46.4.1 Summary

Training has the goal to prepare individuals to achieve competency. Surgical residents only achieve competency in a few surgical procedures, and endocrine operations certainly do not belong to them [4]. Why surgical residents are not exposed more to endocrine procedures is unclear. Yes, it has been shown that involving residents in endocrine surgery procedures is associated with longer operative times, but it has also been shown that it is not associated with clinically significant increased complication rates [13, 27, 28]. Therefore, involvement of residents should be started early and be progressive and standardized based on the surgical procedure and the complexity of the surgical steps [11]. Also, it has been shown that early exposure is a critical factor in fellows' decisions to pursue endocrine surgery [4]. Another aspect that seems to be important is to pay meticulous attention to operative technique and anatomical details already at an early stage in order to ensure that competency is lasting [29]. With this in mind, trainees should be an integral part of the surgical team, and patients should be reassured about their outcomes not being compromised when it comes to endocrine surgical procedures.

Obviously, the operating theater is of particular importance for surgeons in training since it is mainly there where the trainee learns technical skills. Traditionally, training in any field of surgery followed the master-apprentice model of learning [30]. However, comprehensive surgical coaching consisting of performance analysis, debriefing, feedback, and behavior modeling has been shown to be superior as compared to conventional training [31].

Of note, residents who graduated in programs in which at least one faculty member was an endocrine surgeon were significantly more often exposed and trained in endocrine surgical procedures compared with the average general surgery residents [4, 6]. Also, not surprisingly, it has been shown that general surgery specialists who apply for endocrine surgery fellowships during residency were more often exposed and trained in endocrine surgical procedures as compared to their peers [4]. Also, it has been shown that surgical residents may benefit from additional training in their final year [10]. Following surgical residency, an additional 2-year fellowship is now being advocated as an appropriate way to prepare surgeons for their future tasks [32].

Already about 20 years ago, it has been noted that the individual surgeon plays an important prognostic factor in endocrine surgical diseases [26]. Therefore, it is striking that no stringent criteria for fellowship programs in endocrine surgery exist. Implementation and standardization of such fellowship programs should be focused on both at national and international levels. Overall, when having to train younger surgical colleagues, one challenge is to provide sufficient training for different programs (resident versus fellow) since the number of procedures is limited. The results in the literature are not consistent, but according to one study, only a few program directors considered fellow programs having a positive effect on the residence program [33]. Obviously, when the number of cases is high enough, fellows do not negatively affect the training of surgical residents [34].

With an obviously limited number of operations, it is important to know that an increasing number of publications have shown a relationship between hospital/surgeon volume and patient outcomes [35–40]. Nevertheless, the number of procedures performed only represents a rough tool to evaluate someone's proficiency. One solution might be the implementation of techniques like animal models and virtual reality training [1]. However, it is important to underline that operating numbers often are used as an indicator for surgical experience of trainees despite the fact that it also has been demonstrated that there is no evidence in any surgical specialty that thresholds of operative experience are equivalent to a particular level of ability [41].

Competence in a certain surgical subspecialty should be regarded as the combination of detailed basic and clinical knowledge and reasoning and clinical and surgical experience. Consequently, although the demonstration of operative experience would seem to be a reliable criterion for evaluating competence in endocrine surgery practice, probably more efficient methods of achieving and evaluating competence would be necessary.

46.5 Board Certification

In order to ensure that the training has reached the required level of knowledge and skills, standardized examinations should be mandatory. In 2018, a European survey with regard to surgical residents revealed that European countries have established a variety of ways on how to perform their examinations [1]. An oral exam only is mandatory in ten European countries. In other ten European countries, a written exam followed by an oral exam at the end of surgical residency is mandatory. A practical exam (e.g., OSCE) is organized in only 12 out of 16 responding European countries, and a three-stage exam (oral, written, and practical) is mandatory in 6 European countries. Of note, no mandatory exam at the end of the surgical residency exists in four European countries.

With regard to fellows in endocrine surgery, the same European survey [1] revealed that no obligatory exam exists in 12 European countries which equals 75% of those countries where a response was given. An oral exam only is mandatory in one European country, whereas a written exam followed by an oral exam at the end of the fellowship in endocrine surgery is mandatory in three European countries. Of interest, a practical exam (e.g., OSCE) is organized in only one European country, and it is a part of a three-stage exam (written, oral, and practical).

Due to this obvious absence of examinations in endocrine surgery in the European countries, the examination offered by the DES is a very attractive surrogate to get confirmation and proof that one has achieved a certain degree of skills and knowledge in this field. And since the exam is even open for non-Europeans that otherwise may face the same challenge as their European colleagues when it comes to achieving a diploma in endocrine surgery, the EBSQ in endocrine surgery is gaining in popularity even outside the European Union. Nevertheless, it is important knowing that the diploma given by the DES is not in itself a license to practice in any European country. However, some European countries have started to accept some EBSQ diplomas due to the absence of national alternatives.

So how can the DES ensure that the candidates passing the exam have achieved a certain degree of skills and knowledge? Operative performance rating system for evaluating surgery residents has been developed [42]. However, already from the beginning of the EBSQ exam in endocrine surgery, it was felt that surgical skills in itself are very difficult to examine. Here, the training surgeon has a very important role. Many ETRs of the UEMS now have included a concept called Entrustable Professional Activity (EPA). An EPA is a critical part of professional work that can be identified as a unit to be entrusted to a trainee once sufficient competence has been reached. With regard to technical skills, the highest level is the one where the trainee "can be trusted to carry out the procedure, independently, without assistance or need for advice." Obviously, such a complex assessment would be very difficult to make during an examination even with an advanced Objective Structured Clinical Examination (OSCE). Therefore, this assessment is put into the hands of the training surgeon. Preferably, the training surgeon should be board certified herself/himself.

The concept of the EBSQ exam of the DES which is in place since 2003 is mainly to test the clinical knowledge in the form of cases that are presented to the examinee. A total of four examiners scrutinize the knowledge in two "viva voce" sessions with two examiners each. It is aimed for to cover the entire spectrum of endocrine surgery. Where it is of importance, preclinical knowledge is examined as well. In addition, the examinee is given two scientific articles that are discussed in a critical manner. The examinee is expected to identify major flaws. The DES considers this an important part of the examinations. We live in a world with unlimited information easily available to almost everyone. However, a lot of data presented is far from being reliable and correctly interpreted. For a specialist, it is important being able to distinguish the wheat from the chaff. About 10% of all candidates taking the exam fail at each occasion. These failing candidates are discussed by the heads of the DES and the four examiners. The fact that there has not been a single case in 17 years where the decision was not uniform speaks for the current concept of the examination as offered by the DES.

46.6 Conclusion

Surgical trainees with an interest in endocrine surgery are recommended to work in surgical departments with a recognized interest in this specialty in order to ensure that appropriate clinical exposure can be secured. Therefore, fellowships in endocrine surgery should only be available in centers where multidisciplinary approaches to complex endocrine cases can offer the trainees the best chance for learning a comprehensive management of endocrine surgical diseases.

Following the fellowship in endocrine surgery, the trainee should aim to obtain a formal certification of qualification through a national and/or the European examination as provided by the DES.

References

1. Gimm O, Barczynski M, Mihai R, et al. Training in endocrine surgery. Langenbeck's Arch Surg. 2019;404:929–44.
2. Kay S, Miller R, Kraus D, et al. Evolving phenotype of the head and neck surgeon. Laryngoscope. 2019;129(5):1150–4.
3. Sosa JA, Wang TS, Yeo HL, et al. The maturation of a specialty: workforce projections for endocrine surgery. Surgery. 2007;142:876–83.
4. Solorzano CC, Sosa JA, Lechner SC, et al. Endocrine surgery: where are we today? A national survey of young endocrine surgeons. Surgery. 2010;147:536–41.
5. Harness JK, Organ CH Jr, Thompson NW. Operative experience of U.S. general surgery residents in thyroid and parathyroid disease. Surgery. 1995;118:1063–9; discussion 1069–1070
6. Prinz RA. Endocrine surgical training--some ABC measures. Surgery. 1996;120:905–12.
7. Parsa CJ, Organ CH Jr, Barkan H. Changing patterns of resident operative experience from 1990 to 1997. Arch Surg. 2000;135:570–3; discussion 573–575
8. Terris DJ, Chen N, Seybt MW, et al. Emerging trends in the performance of parathyroid surgery. Laryngoscope. 2007;117:1009–12.
9. Le D, Karmali S, Harness JK, et al. An update: the operative experience in adrenal, pancreatic, and other less common endocrine diseases of U.S. general surgery residents. World J Surg. 2008;32:232–6.
10. Zarebczan B, McDonald R, Rajamanickam V, et al. Training our future endocrine surgeons: a look at the endocrine surgery operative experience of U.S. surgical residents. Surgery. 2010;148:1075–80; discussion 1080–1081
11. Phitayakorn R, Kelz RR, Petrusa E, et al. Expert consensus of general surgery residents' proficiency with common endocrine operations. Surgery. 2017;161:280–8.
12. Venkat R, Valdivia PL, Guerrero MA. Resident participation and postoperative outcomes in adrenal surgery. J Surg Res. 2014;190:559–64.
13. Goldfarb M, Gondek S, Hodin R, et al. Resident/fellow assistance in the operating room for endocrine surgery in the era of fellowships. Surgery. 2010;148:1065–71; discussion 1071–1062
14. Goitein D, Mintz Y, Gross D, et al. Laparoscopic adrenalectomy: ascending the learning curve. Surg Endosc. 2004;18:771–3.
15. Guerrieri M, Campagnacci R, De Sanctis A, et al. The learning curve in laparoscopic adrenalectomy. J Endocrinol Investig. 2008;31:531–6.
16. Yang Q, Du J, Zhao ZH, et al. Is laboratory training essential for beginners in learning laparoscopic adrenalectomy? Surg Laparosc Endosc Percutan Tech. 2013;23:184–8.
17. Nagorney DM. Ask the experts: management of hepatic metastases from neuroendocrine cancer. Hepat Oncol. 2014;1:177–80.
18. Doyon L, Moreno-Koehler A, Ricciardi R, et al. Resident participation in laparoscopic Roux-en-Y gastric bypass: a comparison of outcomes from the ACS-NSQIP database. Surg Endosc. 2016;30:3216–24.
19. Krell RW, Birkmeyer NJ, Reames BN, et al. Effects of resident involvement on complication rates after laparoscopic gastric bypass. J Am Coll Surg. 2014;218:253–60.
20. Nijhof HW, Silvis R, Vuylsteke R, et al. Training residents in laparoscopic colorectal surgery: is supervised surgery safe? Surg Endosc. 2017;31:2602–6.
21. Kim JH, Lee IK, Kang WK, et al. Initial experience of a surgical fellow in laparoscopic colorectal cancer surgery under training protocol and supervision: comparison of short-term results for 70 early cases (under supervision) and 73 late cases (without supervision). Surg Endosc. 2013;27:2900–6.

22. Akiyoshi T, Kuroyanagi H, Ueno M, et al. Learning curve for standardized laparoscopic surgery for colorectal cancer under supervision: a single-center experience. Surg Endosc. 2011;25:1409–14.
23. Harness JK, Organ CH Jr, Thompson NW. Operative experience of U.S. general surgery residents with diseases of the adrenal glands, endocrine pancreas, and other less common endocrine organs. World J Surg. 1996;20:885–90; discussion 890–881
24. Sachs TE, Ejaz A, Weiss M, et al. Assessing the experience in complex hepatopancreatobiliary surgery among graduating chief residents: is the operative experience enough? Surgery. 2014;156:385–93.
25. Relles DM, Burkhart RA, Pucci MJ, et al. Does resident experience affect outcomes in complex abdominal surgery? Pancreaticoduodenectomy as an example. J Gastrointest Surg. 2014;18:279–85; discussion 285
26. Pasieka JL. The surgeon as a prognostic factor in endocrine surgical diseases. Surg Oncol Clin N Am. 2000;9:13–20, v-vi.
27. Feeney T, Price LL, Chen L, et al. Resident and fellow participation in thyroid and parathyroid surgery: an ACS-NSQIP clinical outcomes analysis. J Surg Res. 2017;220:346–52.
28. Gurrado A, Bellantone R, Cavallaro G, et al. Can total thyroidectomy be safely performed by residents?: a comparative retrospective multicenter study. Medicine (Baltimore). 2016;95:e3241.
29. Reeve TS, Curtin A, Fingleton L, et al. Can total thyroidectomy be performed as safely by general surgeons in provincial centers as by surgeons in specialized endocrine surgical units? Making the case for surgical training. Arch Surg. 1994;129:834–6.
30. Akhtar KS, Chen A, Standfield NJ, et al. The role of simulation in developing surgical skills. Curr Rev Musculoskelet Med. 2014;7:155–60.
31. Bonrath EM, Dedy NJ, Gordon LE, et al. Comprehensive surgical coaching enhances surgical skill in the operating room: a randomized controlled trial. Ann Surg. 2015;262:205–12.
32. Harness JK, van Heerden JA, Lennquist S, et al. Future of thyroid surgery and training surgeons to meet the expectations of 2000 and beyond. World J Surg. 2000;24:976–82.
33. Smithson L, Delvecchio K, Mittal VK. Accreditation Council for Graduate Medical Education compliance and resident competence in hepatopancreaticobiliary surgery during general surgery residency: a program director review. J Surg Educ. 2015;72:818–22.
34. Hallowell PT, Dahman MI, Stokes JB, et al. Minimally invasive surgery fellowship does not adversely affect general surgery resident case volume: a decade of experience. Am J Surg. 2013;205:307–11; discussion 311
35. Thompson NW. The evolution of endocrine surgery as a subspecialty of general surgery. Fragmentation or enhancement? Arch Surg. 1996;131:465–71.
36. Wang TS. Endocrine surgery. Am J Surg. 2011;202:369–71.
37. Krishnamurthy VD, Jin J, Siperstein A, et al. Mapping endocrine surgery: workforce analysis from the last six decades. Surgery. 2016;159:102–10.
38. Adam MA, Thomas S, Youngwirth L, et al. Is there a minimum number of thyroidectomies a surgeon should perform to optimize patient outcomes? Ann Surg. 2017;265:402–7.
39. Meltzer C, Klau M, Gurushanthaiah D, et al. Surgeon volume in thyroid surgery: surgical efficiency, outcomes, and utilization. Laryngoscope. 2016;126:2630–9.
40. Nouraei SA, Virk JS, Middleton SE, et al. A national analysis of trends, outcomes and volume-outcome relationships in thyroid surgery. Clin Otolaryngol. 2017;42:354–65.
41. De Siqueira JR, Gough MJ. Correlation between experience targets and competence for general surgery certification. Br J Surg. 2016;103:921–7.
42. Larson JL, Williams RG, Ketchum J, et al. Feasibility, reliability and validity of an operative performance rating system for evaluating surgery residents. Surgery. 2005;138:640–7; discussion 647–649

Center Accreditation for Endocrine Surgery

Jesús M. Villar-del-Moral and Thomas J. Musholt

Contents

A. L. Shifrin et al. (eds.), *Endocrine Surgery Comprehensive Board Exam Guide*,
https://doi.org/10.1007/978-3-030-84737-1_47

47.1 Introduction

The main objectives of the health systems, scientific societies, and clinics devoted to endocrine surgery should be the promotion and maintenance of high standards in the clinical practice of this field and the promotion of education and research. In order to achieve this goal, the European Society of Endocrine Surgeons (ESES), in addition to other measures, has proposed to implement an accreditation system for endocrine surgery units in Europe. Similar interest has been shown by the American College of Surgeons or the American Association of Endocrine Surgeons.

Although the effectiveness of accreditation in medicine has not been demonstrated in studies to date, it is generally accepted as one of a suite of measures that can maintain and improve the quality of patient care and surgical outcomes. A general definition of accreditation is outlined in the European Norm ISO 9001:2015, which specifies generic requirements for a quality management system that are applicable to any organization regardless of its type or size or the products and services it provides. The norm is useful for organizations that (a) need to demonstrate their ability to consistently provide products and services that meet customer and applicable statutory and regulatory requirements and (b) aim to enhance customer satisfaction through the effective application of the system, including processes for improvement of the system and the assurance of conformity to customer and applicable statutory and regulatory requirements. It is hoped that accreditation will permit patients and physicians to identify high-quality endocrine surgery centers more easily and that, in their efforts to comply with the requirements for such process, centers for endocrine surgery will improve the quality of care that they deliver.

The design of a common continental accreditation system is a significant challenge, because the overarching goal of ensuring a minimum quality standard based on scientific guidance and clinical experience has to be adapted to different regional and national healthcare structures and clinic resources. In addition, in certain European countries, accreditation of endocrine surgery centers has already been implemented (e.g., Italy and Germany) or is currently being defined (Spain). Other disease-specific (but not surgical specialty-specific) European accreditation systems are the certification of centers for neuroendocrine tumors by the European Neuroendocrine Tumor Society (ENETS) and the recently established European Reference Network that focuses on the treatment of rare diseases and includes a section for endocrinology and endocrine tumors. Therefore, any proposed model should take account of these systems.

47.2 Accreditation Process: Aspects to Be Certified – Hierarchy of Units

The process of quality improvement encompasses aspects of structural quality (e.g., training/education, research activities, continuing professional development, clinic facilities and organization), process quality (diagnostic algorithms, collaborations with other units, adherence to national and international treatment protocols/guidelines), and quality of outcomes (improvement or cure of diseases, patient satisfaction, complications, morbidity, and mortality). Putative quality indicators and standards of endocrine surgery also should include aspects such as volume-outcome relationships.

While not all endocrine surgery units will meet quality standards, certified units will gain national/European recognition. Therefore, the accreditation process has to be robust, defendable, unambiguous, and transparent.

The ESES working group intensively analyzed the European healthcare situation in the field of endocrine surgery, examined details of existing and developing accreditation models in different European countries, and employed surveys to associates in order to evaluate which model would be supported by the majority of ESES members. The results of the surveys and the analysis of existing accreditation systems suggested that a two-level model defining Competence and Reference Centers for neck endocrine surgery and endocrine surgery might be a generally accepted solution.

The level of Competence Center is the most basic to be certified. To obtain it, it is necessary to demonstrate that certain requirements are met, regarding human resources including certified surgeons, material, infrastructure, and processes needed to perform endocrine surgery under safe conditions. Also, it forces the unit to comply with a series of standards regarding its results and to participate in teaching and research activities.

Reference Centers should include high-volume clinics, used to receive patients from other units and manage complex cases, with a superior technology endowment, clear definition of processes, and higher number of certified surgeons. Usually these units are involved in the design of national or supranational guidelines, being on the top of the research and teaching.

While the hierarchy of a two-level model remains a final goal, ESES working group decided to start with the implementation of Competence Centers in order to gather more information about the spectrum of endocrine surgery units and to use this information to improve the accreditation model as an evolving system. The embedding of Reference Centers is planned as the second stage.

47.3 Requirements

47.3.1 Minimum Number of Interventions

47.3.1.1 Thyroid Surgery

The definition for low-volume thyroid surgeons ranges from <10 to <50 and for high-volume thyroid surgeons from >23 to >100 surgeries per year [1–9]. Surgeon volume and, to a lesser degree, hospital volume are inversely related to the prevalence of recurrent laryngeal nerve injury and postoperative hypoparathyroidism. Different correlation analyses between surgeon [6, 8, 10–13] or hospital volume [10, 14–17] and postoperative bleeding have revealed conflicting results.

Surgery for thyroid cancer is a predictor of increased risk of recurrent laryngeal nerve injury and postoperative hypoparathyroidism and therefore should be performed by high-volume surgeons [3, 4, 9, 18]. The survey among ESES members revealed a cutoff value for Competence Centers of 100 annual thyroidectomies for benign disease, 25 for thyroid cancer and 10 systematic cervical lymph node dissections of the lateral lymph node compartment, which is in accordance with the existing literature (◘ Table 47.1) [1].

47.3.1.2 Parathyroid Surgery

In the literature, the definition for low-volume parathyroid surgeons ranges from <4 to <20 and for high-volume parathyroid surgeons from 20 to >100 surgeries per year [2, 16, 19–24]. The

◘ **Table 47.1** Proposed minimum case volume for Competence Centers of neck endocrine and endocrine surgery

Type of intervention	Competence Center
Benign goiter	100
Thyroid malignancy	25
Systematic cervical lymph node dissection of the lateral lymph node compartments	10
Hyperparathyroidism	
pHPT	25
sHPT and hereditary HPT	5
Additional for endocrine surgery	
Adrenal or paraganglioma excision	10
GEP-NET	5

Taken from Musholt TJ et al. [1], with permission
pHPT primary hyperparathyroidism, *sHPT* secondary hyperparathyroidism, *GEP-NET* gastroenteropancreatic neuroendocrine tumors

experience, and therefore the individual surgeon volume, seems to be more relevant than the hospital volume, especially in nonstandard cases (multi-glandular disease, hereditary primary hyperparathyroidism (PHPT), ectopic or unlocalized glands). A volume-outcome association was found with regard to higher cure rates [23–25], less persistent disease [25], fewer reoperations [26], and fewer avoidable reoperations [20, 27].

Surveys among ESES members revealed a common proposal for cutoff value for Competence Centers of 25 operations per annum for primary HPT and 5 for secondary and/or hereditary HPT (bilateral cervical neck exploration), which is in accordance with the existing literature [1].

47.3.1.3 Adrenal or Paraganglioma Surgery

The definition for low-volume adrenal surgeons ranges from <3 to <6 surgeries per year [28–33]. A volume-outcome association was found with regard to lower morbidity and mortality rates, shorter length of hospital stay, and less overall costs.

Higher annual numbers of operations might be required for the treatment of adrenocortical carcinoma. Accordingly, we found a cutoff value of 10 adrenal or paraganglioma operations per annum for Competence Centers in the survey among ESES members [1].

47.3.1.4 Gastroenteropancreatic Neuroendocrine Neoplasms (GEP-NEN)

Due to the low incidence and broad range of different gastroenteropancreatic neuroendocrine tumors, a minimum number of annual GEP-NET operations appear reasonable for an appropriate specialized knowledge in the peri- and intraoperative management. Based on our survey among ESES members, we found a cutoff value of 5 annual GEP-NET resections for Competence Centers [1].

47.3.2 Quality Indicators

In order to assess and compare the quality of endocrine surgery centers, tracer diagnoses have to be selected that are performed in all hospitals with significant volume, include a relatively homogeneous group of patients, and are easy to evaluate during onsite audits. The following quality indicators were suggested by the majority of the respondents in the ESES survey [1].

47.3.2.1 Thyroid Surgery

1. *Early postoperative unilateral recurrent laryngeal nerve (RLN) paresis*

It is defined as vocal cord paresis within the first week after surgery, diagnosed by postoperative laryngoscopy, or documented by intraoperative neural monitoring following the International Standard Guideline Statement (clinical monitoring of voice quality is insufficient) [34, 35]. Early postoperative RLN injury occurs in 0.8% of patients with standard thyroidectomy [36] and 2.5% of patients with high-risk thyroidectomy (reoperation, thyroidectomy due to malignancy, thyrotoxicosis, or retrosternal goiter) [37]. In accordance with the results of our survey, a cutoff value of RLN injury in standard thyroidectomy of <5% per nerves at risk with a dropout rate of <2% was defined for Competence Centers. The rate should be reduced by 50% after a follow-up of 6 months [1].

2. *Postoperative hemorrhage requiring re-intervention*

Post-thyroidectomy hemorrhage occurs in 1.5% of patients [38]. A cutoff value of <2% for postoperative bleeding requiring re-intervention for Competence Centers was therefore proposed [1].

47.3.2.2 Parathyroid Surgery

1. *Rate of normalized parathyroid function following resection of sporadic primary hyperparathyroidism (pHPT)*

It is defined as normalized or decreased PTH level on the first postoperative day [39]. Persistence or recurrence in pHPT occurs in 2.5–5% [40]. Based on a cutoff value of 25 annual operations for pHPT for Competence Centers, we defined a normalization rate of ≥92% [1].

47.3.3 Requirements: Equipment, Staff, and Multidisciplinary Collaboration

The advantage for patients with endocrine pathology of being referred to an accredited unit is the possibility of obtaining a customized and up-to-date treatment for their condition [41]. Endocrine diseases require a multi-professional team that need access to specialist laboratory-based testing and imaging, combined with medical and surgical management [42]. Thyroid surgery should preferably be performed in centers with adequate quality, volume of procedures, structure, and technology standards [41, 42].

Unfortunately, the evidence base for this issue is almost non-existent. So the following recommendations are a synthesis of the German [42] and Italian [43] accreditation systems, as well as the UK NHS requirements for specialized endocrine units [44] and training requirements for endocrine surgery [45].

47.3.3.1 Structure

The accreditation models in Italy and Germany define that endocrine surgery, as a part of General Surgery Department, must have:

- In-patient capacity: within the General Surgery Department
- Outpatient clinic: at least once a week [42, 43]
- Administrative and teaching rooms within the Department
- Operating theater capacity to perform:
  - Competence Centers: ≥50 [43] or ≥165 [42] thyroid surgeries/year
  - Reference Centers: ≥200 [42] or ≥500 [43] thyroid surgeries/year

The figures determined by the accreditation systems consulted [42, 43] provide a very wide range of minimum volumes, which requires a consensus. The proposed figures are in keeping with those derived from ESES members and the determination of high-volume surgeons by an ESES working group. Thus, in Competence Centers for neck surgery, the required annual volume would total 135 thyroidectomies (including cancer, recurrences, and neck dissection) and 30 parathyroidectomies, adding 10 adrenalectomies and 5 neuroendocrine tumors, for accreditation in endocrine surgery (◘ Table 47.1) [1]. The caseload for Reference Centers will depend on the results of the first stage of implementation of the accreditation model (Competence Centers).

47.3.3.2 Staff

The unit must have at least two accredited surgeons, dedicated to endocrine surgery, who meet a number of requirements (specialist training, continued medical education, multidisciplinary links, demonstrable academic/professional skills) [42, 43, 45]. Ideally, they should be members of the scientific societies that promote the accreditation program, in this case the ESES [1].

An accredited surgeon should be present either as lead surgeon or assistant for every operation [43]. Regarding the professional qualification, they must be specialized in general surgery plus a subject-specific EBSQ qualification or have performed at least 250 procedures in endocrine surgery during the last 5 years [43]. In Reference Centers, it is proposed that the number of accredited surgeons increases to a minimum of three [43].

Accredited surgeons require constant training, and, consequently, they must demonstrate their attendance at both courses and related conferences (national or international), adding up to a total of at least 24 h (e.g., 3 days with 8 h per day) [1].

47.3.3.3 Equipment and Diagnostic Procedures

Within the hospital infrastructure, Competence Centers in neck endocrine surgery must have access to ultrasound and intraoperative neural monitoring [1, 43]. Alongside this, the Reference Centers should be able to perform intraoperative determination of PTH [43].

Any Reference Center for endocrine surgery will also have access to intraoperative ultrasound and minimally invasive techniques for adrenal surgery, in addition to the equipment previously mentioned [43].

All accredited centers must have the possibility of performing a pre- or postoperative laryngoscopy [43].

These recommendations are in accordance with the results of the working group surveys which consider as basic technical resources access to intraoperative PTH, frozen section pathology, neural monitoring, and laryngoscopy [1]. In future Reference Centers, the required equipment will be more sophisticated and will include intraoperative ultrasound for open and laparoscopic surgery, expertise available to perform sternotomy, radioiodine or radiopeptide treatment, local ablation (radiofrequency, HIFU, laser), interventional radiology for transarterial chemoembolization or selective internal radiotherapy, and external beam radiation treatment [1].

47.3.3.4 Multidisciplinary Collaboration

Due to the frequent complex clinical situations and necessary diagnostic procedures associated with optimal management and treatment of endocrine diseases, the best practice requires a multidisciplinary team and cooperation between specialists. Collaborating disciplines should be preferably located in the same hospital, but cooperation with selected outside units is also accepted, if formal service-level agreements with another provider exist. The list below summarizes the necessary team to provide a high-quality service [1]:

- Anesthesiology [42, 44]
- Intensive care unit (ICU) [42, 44]
- Cardiology [42, 44]
- Pathology [41–45]: cytology, histology, frozen section, immunohistochemical analysis
- Radiology [41–45]: CT, ultrasound, intraoperative ultrasound, MRI
- Interventional radiology [42]
- Endocrinology [42–45] and/or internal medicine [43]
- Otolaryngology [42–44]
- Speech therapy [42, 44]
- Nuclear medicine [41–45]: scintigraphic diagnosis, investigation, and therapy
- Laboratory testing service [42–44]
- Blood transfusion service with blood and its products [42]
- Thoracic surgery [42–44]

- Vascular or cardiovascular surgery [42–44]
- Oncology [42, 43]
- Radiotherapy [42, 43]
- Clinical genetics [42]
- Endoscopic ultrasound for endocrine surgery centers [42]
- Cryopreservation of oocytes/semen (not mandatory in the same unit)

In the survey, ESES members agreed with this multidisciplinary approach and considered it necessary that malignant endocrine diseases are presented and discussed in interdisciplinary tumor board meetings in both Reference and Competence Centers. Regarding the partner services, the following core services should be present in-house: pathology, otolaryngology, radiology, endocrinology, and ICU. Nuclear medicine, oncology, radiotherapy, psycho-oncology, and quality improvement unit may apply for Reference Centers and will be defined in the future [1].

47.3.4 Training and Research

The scarcity of evidence in the literature regarding appropriate provision of training and research in accreditation means that any proposals are necessarily based upon existing guidelines, expert opinion, an attempt to be inclusive and pragmatic, and what is achievable within the various European healthcare systems.

47.3.4.1 The Trainee and Training Center

Although several countries (e.g., the Netherlands, the United Kingdom, and the United States) are transitioning from a traditional time-based model of training to one that is competency-based [46], much of the literature on training is based upon observation of what residents and fellows achieve during a predetermined time [47]. Therefore, it may not be truly indicative of the number of procedures or duration of training required to gain operative competence. Furthermore, training involves other activities including obtaining of non-technical and professional skills, evidence of research activity, and demonstration of knowledge. While the latter may be examined at EBSQ or DES level, many of the other skills are assumed rather than assessed. At present, the recommended minimum numbers as a main operator required for EBSQ accreditation as a specialist are:

- Fifty thyroidectomies
- Two central neck dissections
- Two lateral neck dissections
- Fifteen parathyroidectomies (including ten bilateral neck explorations)
- Two adrenalectomies
- Two GEP-NEN operations

47

Table 47.2 Proposed minimum caseload for accreditation as a specialist surgeon in neck endocrine and endocrine surgery

Type of intervention	Surgeon
Benign goiter	50
Thyroid malignancy	15
Systematic cervical lymph node dissection of the lateral lymph node compartments	5
Hyperparathyroidism	
pHPT	15
sHPT and hereditary HPT	3
Additional for Endocrine Surgery	
Adrenal or Paraganglioma	5
GEP-NET	3

Taken from Musholt TJ et al. [1], with permission
pHPT primary hyperparathyroidism, *sHPT* secondary hyperparathyroidism, *GEP-NET* gastroenteropancreatic neuroendocrine tumors

Based upon these indicative numbers, there is a minimum caseload to which the trainee must be exposed, and this is likely to only be achievable in high-volume centers. There must also be opportunities for research, presentation to learned societies, and exposure to the broad range of surgical endocrine disease. Along with supervision and feedback from accredited surgical staff (see ▶ Sect. 47.3.3.2), Competence Centers provide a minimum caseload per annum as defined in Table 47.1. In Table 47.2, the proposed minimum caseload for accreditation as a specialist in neck endocrine and endocrine surgery derived from the ESES working group is displayed [1].

The gradient (competence vs. procedure number) of learning curves for procedures in general surgery has been examined in general surgical procedures [47, 48], and it may be that similar work in endocrine surgery will determine the true nature of skill acquisition for future endocrine surgery trainees. Therefore, the minimum indicative numbers required for training may change in light of evolving evidence.

47.3.4.2 Research

Research drives innovation in patient care and is an integral part of surgical training. It is also an important component of continued professional development and a requirement for many European training programs. There was broad agreement among ESES respondents in the survey that both Competence and future Reference Centers should participate in research activity to some degree [1]. Following the panel dis-

cussion, it was proposed that Competence Centers should participate in the following research activities:
- Oral and poster communications to endocrine surgical conferences
- Local research

It is proposed that in future, accredited Reference Centers should participate in the above and the following:
- Minimum of one peer-reviewed publication per annum
- Recruitment of patients to randomized or multicenter trials
- Research of multicentric registries (such as Eurocrine®)
- Hosting of visiting surgeons

47.4 Quality Control and Auditing

Documentation of the quality of surgical procedures performed – especially on the number and seriousness of surgical complications recorded for a given surgeon or surgical clinic – is a demand raised by health insurance companies, patient organizations, and the public and is an obligatory part of certifications of surgical excellence. Due to the needs on patient data protection, such documentation in a database nowadays requires a professional setup for software, hardware, and maintenance – which often exceeds the possibilities of smaller clinics – as well as a positive ethic committee vote on data collection in database or registry. Auditing for the purpose of certifications ensures completeness and plausibility of the documented data. Ideally, such information should be accessible to the respective surgeon or to an auditor in an ad hoc fashion, to enable random picking of patient cases to audit, equivalent to randomly pulling out case files. Furthermore, questions of the auditor on patient groups or clusters of complications, etc. should ideally be answered while being raised during the audit.

Since the European registry Eurocrine fulfils all listed requirements and is easily accessible, ESES certification auditing is based on surgical data documentation within Eurocrine.

47.5 Conclusions

Accreditation of clinics in Europe in the field of endocrine surgery should be implemented as one of several measures that aim to maintain and improve quality standards. Although local healthcare structures differ significantly, ESES members agree on a basic definition of high-quality care in endocrine surgery, necessary requirements, and evaluation procedures. The quality standards and requirements defined for the proposed accreditation model comply with detailed analysis of volume-outcome relations as well as training for endocrine surgery. The requirements for the application and the decision process must be unambiguous and transparent. However, in the process of implementation of the proposed accreditation model, refinements will be necessary depending on results of audits performed in the initial round of accredited clinics. The implementation will therefore start with the accreditation of Competence Centers as a first stage. It is hoped that the criteria for Reference Centers will be agreed and implemented as a second stage.

Compliance with Ethical Standards

Conflict of Interest: The authors declare that they have no conflict of interest.

References

1. Musholt TJ, Bränstrom R, Kaderli RM, Muñoz N, Raffaelli M, Stetchman MJ. Accreditation of endocrine surgery units. Langenbeck's Arch Surg. 2019;404:779–93. https://doi.org/10.1007/s00423-019-01820-y.
2. Sosa JA, Bowman HM, Tielsch JM, Powe NR, Gordon TA, Udelsman R. The importance of surgeon experience for clinical and economic outcomes from thyroidectomy. Ann Surg. 1998;228:320–30.
3. Gourin CG, Tufano RP, Forastiere AA, Koch WM, Pawlik TM, Bristow RE. Volume-based trends in thyroid surgery. Arch Otolaryngol Head Neck Surg. 2010;136:1191–8. https://doi.org/10.1001/archoto.2010.212.
4. Loyo M, Tufano RP, Gourin CG. National trends in thyroid surgery and the effect of volume on short-term outcomes. Laryngoscope. 2013;123:2056–63. https://doi.org/10.1002/lary.23923.
5. Gonzalez-Sanchez C, Franch-Arcas G, Gomez-Alonso A. Morbidity following thyroid surgery: does surgeon volume matter? Langenbeck's Arch Surg. 2013;398:419–22. https://doi.org/10.1007/s00423-012-1027-4.
6. Kandil E, Noureldine SI, Abbas A, Tufano RP. The impact of surgical volume on patient outcomes following thyroid surgery. Surgery. 2013;154:1346–52; discussion 1352–53. https://doi.org/10.1016/j.surg.2013.04.068.
7. Al-Qurayshi Z, Robins R, Hauch A, Randolph GW, Kandil E. Association of surgeon volume with outcomes and cost savings following thyroidectomy: a national forecast. JAMA Otolaryngol Head Neck Surg. 2016;142:32–9. https://doi.org/10.1001/jamaoto.2015.2503.
8. Adam MA, Thomas S, Youngwirth L, Hyslop T, Reed SD, Scheri RP, et al. Is there a minimum number of thyroidectomies a surgeon should perform to optimize patient outcomes? Ann Surg. 2017;265:402–7. https://doi.org/10.1097/sla.0000000000001688.
9. Nouraei SA, Virk JS, Middleton SE, Aylin P, Mace A, Vaz F, et al. A national analysis of trends, outcomes and volume-outcome relationships in thyroid surgery. Clin Otolaryngol. 2017;42:354–65. https://doi.org/10.1111/coa.12730.
10. Thomusch O, Sekulla C, Billmann F, Seifert G, Dralle H, Lorenz K. Risk profile analysis and complications after surgery for autoimmune thyroid disease. Br J Surg. 2018;105:677–85. https://doi.org/10.1002/bjs.10770.
11. Meltzer C, Klau M, Gurushanthaiah D, Tsai J, Meng D, Radler L, Sundang A. Surgeon volume in thyroid surgery: surgical efficiency, out-

comes, and utilization. Laryngoscope. 2016;126:2630–9. https://doi.org/10.1002/lary.26119.
12. Adkisson CD, Howell GM, McCoy KL, Armstrong MJ, Kelley ML, Stang MT, et al. Surgeon volume and adequacy of thyroidectomy for differentiated thyroid cancer. Surgery. 2014;156:1453–9.; discussion 1460. https://doi.org/10.1016/j.surg.2014.08.024.
13. Promberger R, Ott J, Kober F, Koppitsch C, Seemann R, Freissmuth M, Hermann M. Risk factors for postoperative bleeding after thyroid surgery. Br J Surg. 2012;99:373–9. https://doi.org/10.1002/bjs.7824.
14. Maneck M, Dotzenrath C, Dralle H, Fahlenbrach C, Paschke R, Steinmuller T, et al. Complications after thyroid gland operations in Germany: a routine data analysis of 66,902 AOK patients. Chirurg. 2017;88:50–7 https://doi.org/10.1007/s00104-016-0267-1.
15. Weiss A, Lee KC, Brumund KT, Chang DC, Bouvet M. Risk factors for hematoma after thyroidectomy: results from the nationwide inpatient sample. Surgery. 2014;156:399–404. https://doi.org/10.1016/j.surg.2014.03.015.
16. Dehal A, Abbas A, Al-Tememi M, Hussain F, Johna S. Impact of surgeon volume on incidence of neck hematoma after thyroid and parathyroid surgery: ten years' analysis of nationwide in-patient sample database. Am Surg. 2014;80:948–52.
17. Hauch A, Al-Qurayshi Z, Randolph G, Kandil E. Total thyroidectomy is associated with increased risk of complications for low- and high-volume surgeons. An Surg Oncol. 2014;21:3844–52. https://doi.org/10.1245/s10434-014-3846-8.
18. Dralle H, Sekulla C, Haerting J, Timmermann W, Neumann HJ, Kruse E, et al. Risk factors of paralysis and functional outcome after recurrent laryngeal nerve monitoring in thyroid surgery. Surgery. 2004;136:1310–22. https://doi.org/10.1016/j.surg.2004.07.018.
19. Stavrakis AI, Ituarte PH, Ko CY, Yeh MW. Surgeon volume as a predictor of outcomes in inpatient and outpatient endocrine surgery. Surgery. 2007;142:887–99; discussion 897–899. https://doi.org/10.1016/j.surg.2007.09.003.
20. Mitchell J, Milas M, Barbosa G, Sutton J, Berber E, Siperstein A. Avoidable reoperations for thyroid and parathyroid surgery: effect of hospital volume. Surgery. 2008;144:899–906; discussion 906–907. https://doi.org/10.1016/j.surg.2008.07.022.
21. Noureldine SI, Abbas A, Tufano RP, Srivastav S, Slakey DP, Friedlander P, Kandil E. The impact of surgical volume on racial disparity in thyroid and parathyroid surgery. Ann Surg Oncol. 2004;21:2733–9. https://doi.org/10.1245/s10434-014-3610-0.
22. Meltzer C, Klau M, Gurushanthaiah D, Tsai J, Meng D, Radler L, Sundang A. Surgeon volume in parathyroid surgery-surgical efficiency, outcomes, and utilization. JAMA Otolaryngol Head Neck Surg. 2017;143:843–7. https://doi.org/10.1001/jamaoto.2017.0124.
23. Sosa JA, Tuggle CT, Wang TS, Thomas DC, Boudourakis L, Rivkees S, Roman SA. Clinical and economic outcomes of thyroid and parathyroid surgery in children. J Clin Endocrinol Metab. 2008;93:3058–65. https://doi.org/10.1210/jc.2008-0660.
24. Neychev VK, Ghanem M, Blackwood SL, Aragon Han P, Fazeli R, Schneider E, et al. Parathyroid surgery can be safely performed in a community hospital by experienced parathyroid surgeons: a retrospective cohort study. Int J Surg (London, England). 2016;27:72–6. https://doi.org/10.1016/j.ijsu.2015.11.026.
25. Malmaeus J, Granberg PO, Halvorsen J, Akerstrom G, Johansson H. Parathyroid surgery in Scandinavia. Acta Chir Scand. 1988;154:409–13.
26. Abdulla AG, Ituarte PH, Harari A, Wu JX, Yeh MW. Trends in the frequency and quality of parathyroid surgery: analysis of 17,082 cases over 10 years. Ann Surg. 2015;261:746–50. https://doi.org/10.1097/sla.0000000000000812.

27. Chen H, Wang TS, Yen TW, Doffek K, Krzywda E, Schaefer S. Operative failures after parathyroidectomy for hyperparathyroidism: the influence of surgical volume. Ann Surg. 2010;252:691–5. https://doi.org/10.1097/SLA.0b013e3181f698df.
28. Park HS, Roman SA, Sosa JA. Outcomes from 3144 adrenalectomies in the United States: which matters more, surgeon volume or specialty? Arch Surg. 2009;144:1060–7. https://doi.org/10.1001/archsurg.2009.191.
29. Lindeman B, Hashimoto DA, Bababekov YJ, Stapleton SM, Chang DC, Hodin RA, Phitayakorn R. Fifteen years of adrenalectomies: impact of specialty training and operative volume. Surgery. 2018;163:150–6. https://doi.org/10.1016/j.surg.2017.05.024.
30. Anderson KL Jr, Thomas SM, Adam MA, Pontius LN, Stang MT, Scheri RP, et al. Each procedure matters: threshold for surgeon volume to minimize complications and decrease cost associated with adrenalectomy. Surgery. 2018;163:157–64. https://doi.org/10.1016/j.surg.2017.04.028.
31. Palazzo F, Dickinson A, Phillips B, Sahdev A, Bliss R, Rasheed A, et al. Adrenal surgery in England: better outcomes in high-volume practices. Clin Endocrinol. 2016;85:17–20. https://doi.org/10.1111/cen.13021.
32. Al-Qurayshi Z, Robins R, Buell J, Kandil E. Surgeon volume impact on outcomes and cost of adrenal surgeries. Eur J Surg Oncol. 2016;42:1483–90. https://doi.org/10.1016/j.ejso.2016.06.392.
33. Kazaure HS, Roman SA, Sosa JA. Adrenalectomy in older Americans has increased morbidity and mortality: an analysis of 6,416 patients. Ann Surg Oncol. 2011;18:2714–21. https://doi.org/10.1245/s10434-011-1757-5.
34. Schneider R, Randolph GW, Dionigi G, Wu CW, Barczynski M, Chiang FY, et al. International neural monitoring study group guideline 2018 part I: staging bilateral thyroid surgery with monitoring loss of signal. Laryngoscope. 2018;128(Suppl 3):s1–s17. https://doi.org/10.1002/lary.27359.
35. Wu CW, Dionigi G, Barczynski M, Chiang FY, Dralle H, Schneider R. International neuromonitoring study group guidelines 2018: part II: optimal recurrent laryngeal nerve management for invasive thyroid cancer-incorporation of surgical, laryngeal, and neural electrophysiologic data. Laryngoscope. 2018;128(Suppl 3):s18–27. https://doi.org/10.1002/lary.27360.
36. Yang S, Zhou L, Lu Z, Ma B, Ji Q, Wang Y. Systematic review with meta-analysis of intraoperative neuromonitoring during thyroidectomy. Int J Surg. 2017;39:104–13. https://doi.org/10.1016/j.ijsu.2017.01.086.
37. Wong KP, Mak KL, Wong CK, Lang BH. Systematic review and meta-analysis on intra-operative neuro-monitoring in high-risk thyroidectomy. Int J Surg. 2017;38:21–30. https://doi.org/10.1016/j.ijsu.2016.12.039.
38. Liu J, Sun W, Dong W, Wang Z, Zhang P, Zhang T, Zhang H. Risk factors for post-thyroidectomy haemorrhage: a meta-analysis. Eur J Endocrinol. 2017;176:591–602. https://doi.org/10.1530/eje-16-0757.
39. Kaderli RM, Riss P, Geroldinger A, Selberherr A, Scheuba C, Niederle B. Primary hyperparathyroidism: dynamic postoperative metabolic changes. Clin Endocrinol. 2018;88:129–38. https://doi.org/10.1111/cen.13476.
40. Guerin C, Paladino NC, Lowery A, Castinetti F, Taieb D, Sebag F. Persistent and recurrent hyperparathyroidism. Updat Surg. 2017;69:161–9. https://doi.org/10.1007/s13304-017-0447-7.
41. Suffat LP, Mondini G, Demaria F, Perino P, Bertotti L, Rosato L. A proposal for thyroid surgery: criteria to identify the references of endocrine surgery. Updat Surg. 2017;69:431–4. https://doi.org/10.1007/s13304-017-0487-z.
42. Deutsche Gesellschaft für Allgemein- und Viszeralchirurgie. Das Zertifizierungssystem der DGAV (zertO 5.1). 2016. www.dgav.de/filead-

min/media/texte_pdf/zertifizierung/zerto/Zertifizierungsordnung_Kurzform_CAEK.pdf. Accessed April 2019.
43. Società Italiana Unitaria di Endocrinochirurgia. Programma Valutativo di Accreditamento delle UO di Endocrinochirurgia per la patologia della tiroide SIUEC. siuec.it/download/file/Regolamento%20per%20Accreditamento%20UO%20SIUEC.pdf. Accessed April 2019.
44. NHS England. 2013/14 NHS STANDARD CONTRACT FOR SPECIALISED ENDOCRINOLOGY SERVICES (ADULT). 2013. https://www.england.nhs.uk/wp-content/uploads/2013/06/a03-spec-endo-adult.pdf. Accessed April 2019.
45. The British Association of Endocrine Surgeons. Guidelines for the surgical management of endocrine disease and the training requirements for endocrine surgery. 2003. https://www.baets.org.uk/wp-content/uploads/2013/02/BAETS-Guidelines-2003.pdf. Accessed April 2019.
46. De Siqueira JR, Gough MJ. Correlation between experience targets and competence for general surgery certification. Br J Surg. 2016;103:921–7. https://doi.org/10.1002/bjs.10145.
47. Gimm O, Barczynski M, Mihai R, Raffaelli M. Training in endocrine surgery. Langenbeck's Arch Surg. 2019;404:929–44. https://doi.org/10.1007/s00423-019-01828-4.
48. Brown C, Abdelrahman T, Patel N, Thomas C, Pollitt MJ, Lewis WG. Operative learning curve trajectory in a cohort of surgical trainees. Br J Surg. 2017;104:1405–11. https://doi.org/10.1002/bjs.10584.

Index

A

B

C

D

E

F

G

H

I

N

O

P

R

S

T

U

V

W

Z

GPSR Compliance

The European Union's (EU) General Product Safety Regulation (GPSR) is a set of rules that requires consumer products to be safe and our obligations to ensure this.

If you have any concerns about our products, you can contact us on ProductSafety@springernature.com

In case Publisher is established outside the EU, the EU authorized representative is:

Springer Nature Customer Service Center GmbH
Europaplatz 3
69115 Heidelberg, Germany

Batch number: 10508680

Printed by Printforce, the Netherlands